HISTOPATHOLOGY OF PRECLINICAL TOXICITY STUDIES:

INTERPRETATION AND RELEVANCE IN DRUG SAFETY EVALUATION

Histopathology of Preclinical Toxicity Studies:

Interpretation and Relevance in Drug Safety Evaluation

P. Greaves M.B., Ch.B., F.R.C. Path.

ICI Pharmaceuticals, Alderley Park
Macclesfield, Cheshire, England

1990

Elsevier

Amsterdam · New York · Oxford

ISBN 0-444-81311-X

This book is printed on acid-free paper.

Published by:
Elsevier Science Publishers B.V.
(Biomedical Division)
P.O. Box 211
1000 AE Amsterdam
The Netherlands

Sole distributors for the USA and Canada:
Elsevier Science Publishing Company, Inc.
655 Avenue of the Americas
New York,
NY 10010
USA

Library of Congress Cataloging-in-Publication Data

Greaves, P. (Peter)
    Histopathology of preclinical toxicity studies : interpretation
  and relevance in drug safety evaluation / P. Greaves.
        p.   cm.
    Includes bibliographical references and index.
    ISBN 0-444-81311-X (alk. paper)
    1. Drugs--Toxicology. 2. Toxicity testing. 3. Laboratory
  animals--Histopathology.   I. Title.
    [DNLM: 1. Animals, Laboratory. 2. Drug Screening. 3. Histology.
  4. Pathology.   QV 771 G787h]
  RA1238.G74   1990
  615.9--dc20
  DNLM/DLC
  for Library of Congress   90-14138
                                                                    CIP

Printed in the Netherlands

Contents

Preface

Histopathological assessment of tissue sections is an important component of many preclinical studies which are conducted to support the safety and clinical development of novel therapeutic agents for use in the treatment of human diseases. The pathologist is not only required to distinguish spontaneous laboratory animal pathology from drug-induced pathological lesions but also to indicate the likely pathogenesis of any treatment-induced effects. It is also important to discriminate between drug-induced tissue alterations which are the consequence of direct adverse effects on vital cellular mechanisms from those which are the result of an exaggerated or unexpected pharmacological effect at excessive doses or due to an exacerbation of spontaneous disease unique to a particular laboratory animal species. Each of these processes may have quite different significance for the human safety of a novel drug.

This remains a major challenge for pathologists despite the improvements in data handling and animal husbandry with its consequent reduction in confounding intercurrent laboratory animal disease. As noted by Zbinden (1988), concepts of drug safety evaluation based on high dose toxicity tests have not kept pace with the rapid developments in biomedical sciences. The drug discovery process, aided by modern biotechnology, is now capable of generating highly potent, pharmacologically active agents which are capable of disturbing body homeostasis in novel ways when administered at high doses. This in turn, can give rise to quite unusual constellations of tissue pathology, particularly at doses which produce inanition and non-specific stress. It has been demonstrated that stress may not only produce lesions in lymphoid tissue, gastrointestinal tract, endocrine organs, and gonads (Selye, 1936), but may also amplify other quite unrelated pathological processes (Tapp and Natelson, 1988). It is, therefore, of greatest importance that pathological changes are evaluated in the light of drug dispositon data where tissue changes can be related to concentrations of drug and metabolites achieved in the target organs (Smith, 1988; Zbinden, 1988).

Questions of terminology, grading, quantitation and peer review are also of increasing importance in the assessment of pathological lesions in preclinical safety evaluation. The pathologist must remain acutely aware that although several different terms for a lesion may be accurate from a purely diagnostic point of view, each may not convey the same sense of importance to the non-specialist reader. Degree or severity of pathological changes have to be clearly defined because terms such as "minimal", "moderate" or "marked" can be misleading if used inappropriately or without clarification.

The complexity and the number of histopathological findings in individual studies indicate the need for particular lucidity in the descriptions and conclusions in pathology reporting. Balanced, objective reports are also vital in view of the complexities of the medicolegal aspects of product liability (Price, 1987).

Unfortunately, it is not unusual to find pathological changes in toxicity studies for which no satisfactory descriptions exist in the available literature. Although more toxicity data is being published than previously, this is frequently scattered in a variety of sources and not always accompanied by detailed descriptions of histopathological changes. Drug-related pathology occurring in man is frequently reported in more detail. However, histopathological examination is usually undertaken only in cases of severe drug-induced disease in patients, following idiosyncratic reactions with no equivalent in laboratory animals, or complicated by underlying disease processes.

In the light of these difficulties, this text is aimed towards bringing together into one volume a description of histopathological changes which relate to toxicity testing of therapeutic agents in the usual test species: rat, mouse, dog and non-human primate. An attempt has been made to discuss lesions which have a particular relevance to drug safety evaluation. Where possible, descriptions of drug-induced changes in conventional toxicity studies have been provided. Unfortunately much data which relate to the toxic effects of drugs in laboratory animals remains unpublished, so reference has been made to other animal models and chemical compounds where it has appeared appropriate. Comparative anatomy, physiology and human pathology is also discussed in some detail in order to provide a basis for understanding pathogenesis and relevance of drug-induced pathological findings in animals for man.

Over the last decade there has been an explosion in the application of new techniques in experimental and human diagnostic pathology, notably immunocytochemistry but also enzyme cytochemistry, autoradiography, electron microscopy, quantitative methodology and most recently, in-situ hybridization. These techniques are finding a wider application in toxicological pathology in view of the additional demands being made on pathologists for the elucidation of unusual tissue and organ responses to drugs. These techniques are, therefore, also discussed.

As always, any work of this type reflects the limitations of the reviewer. Although no one author can hope to provide a fully comprehensive catalogue of spontaneous and drug-induced pathology of laboratory animals, it is hoped that this volume will provide the reader with a useful starting point for the analysis of drug-induced findings in toxicity studies. The format of the book follows that used in a previous monograph (Creaves and Faccini, 1984).

REFERENCES

GREAVES, P. and FACCINI, J.M. (1984): *Rat Histopathology. A Glossary for use in Toxicity and Carcinogenicity Studies.* Elsevier, Amsterdam.

PRICE, J.M. (1987): The liabilities and consequences of medical device development. *J. Biomed Mater. Res.,* 21, 35–58.

SELYE, H. (1934): A syndrome produced by diverse nocuous agents. *Nature,* 138, 32.

SMITH, R.L. (1988): The role of metabolism and disposition studies in the safety assessment of pharmaceuticals. *Xenobiotica,* 18, suppl 1, 89–96

TAPP, U.N. and NATELSON, B.H. (1988): Consequences of stress: a multiplicative function of health status. *FASEB J.,* 2, 2268–2271.

ZBINDEN, G. (1988): Biopharmaceutical studies, a key to better toxicology. *Xenobiotica,* 18, Suppl 1, 9–14.

Acknowledgements

This book has been written in several different laboratories in both Europe and North America and has consequently benefited from the help and courtesy of many friends and colleagues too numerous to mention by name. However, I owe much to Dr Felix de la Iglesia, Vice President, Pathology and Experimental Toxicology, Parke-Davis, Ann Arbor, Michigan, USA, for his encouragement and his particularly forward-looking policy with respect to the publication of toxicology studies. Special thanks are necessary to all the friends and colleagues at the Parke-Davis Research Institute, Sheridan Park, Mississauga, Ontario, Canada where most of this book was drafted and especially Denise Zucchiati who prepared many drafts of the manuscript. Likewise, thanks are due to Dr Nick Read for illustrations and to other colleagues at Wellcome Laboratories, Beckenham, England for fruitful discussions on numerous aspects of drug safety evaluation. In addition, I must thank Anne Flynn and staff in the Secretarial Service and Technical Documentation Unit in the Safety of Medicines Department, ICI Pharmaceuticals, Mereside, Cheshire, England for latterly completing the word processing and John Clinton of the Information Systems Department for placing the manuscript into appropriate magnetic form.

For many of the illustrations I am also grateful for the help provided by Derrick Mills as well as Sue Margetson of the Photographic Department, ICI Pharmaceuticals for most of the line diagrams.

Finally, I must thank my wife Dr Anne Greaves who has endured the writing of this book for many months and has graciously read and helped in the corrections of the final draft.

I. Integumentary System

SKIN AND SUBCUTANEOUS TISSUE

Skin lesions are among some of the most common adverse reactions to drugs in clinical practice. Morbilliform rashes, urticaria and generalized puritis which are believed to be generally allergic responses to systemically administered drugs, occur in 2–3% of hospitalized patients (Bigby et al., 1986). However, some skin reactions such as toxic epidermal necrolysis or Lyell's syndrome can be very severe and even life-threatening if treatment is not discontinued (Furness et al., 1986). Phototoxic and photoallergic reactions also occur as a result of systemically administered therapeutic agents (Bleehan, 1981; Maurer, 1987). Drugs applied topically can be irritant, or likewise produce immune-mediated reactions such as allergic contact dermatitis and photoallergic changes.

Despite tremendous advances in our knowledge of the role of skin in the modulation of cutaneous immune responses, it may not be possible to predict the occurrence of cutaneous immune reactions in man, based on animal models. Such reactions may still only become evident in large scale clinical trials or in general clinical practice following marketing of novel agents.

Different components of the skin may form the target for cutaneous toxicity. Compounds with a high affinity for melanin have been associated with skin changes in man and therefore new drugs which bind to melanin or inhibit enzymes associated with melanin biosynthesis should be assessed carefully in animal models for toxicity in melanin-containing organs. Cutaneous blood vessels or sebaceous glands can also be the targets of drug treatment (Schaefer, 1986).

Despite the undoubted usefulness of histopathological examination of the skin in the assessment of drug induced cutaneous lesions in man, particularly when used with modern immunocytochemical techniques (Furness et al., 1986), histopathological study is less widely applied in animal models used in the preclinical assessment of skin toxicity. Nevertheless, histopathology is a useful adjunct in the study of skin changes in laboratory animals.

It should also be kept in mind that the skin may exhibit alterations which are the result of systemic pathological processes. For instance, damage to blood

1

vessels or failure of blood coagulation can lead to purpura and bleeding. Pituitary and thyroid disorders, changes in endocrine pancreas and derangement of calcium balance are also associated with cutaneous manifestations (Feingold and Elias, 1987).

The epidermis as part of the immune system

Over the past decade it has become apparent that the skin functions in a unique way as an immunological organ. Keratinocytes, Langerhans cells, epidermotropic T-lymphocytes and peripheral lymph nodes have been collectively regarded as forming an integrated system of skin-associated lymphoid tissues (SALT) which mediates cutaneous immunosurveillance (Streilein, 1985) (see Haemopoietic and Lymphatic Systems, Chapter III).

Langerhans cells are a small population of highly dendritic bone marrow-derived cells present in the suprabasal zone of epidermis which represent the most peripheral outpost of the immune system, important for the induction of contact hypersensitivity and in graft rejection (Shimada and Katz 1988). The surface of Langerhans cells possess molecules characteristic of cells involved in antigen presentation: class II major histocompatability complex (MHC) antigens, Fc receptors for immunoglobulin and a receptor for the third component of complement (Streilein, 1985).

Langerhans cells are difficult to visualize in tissue sections by ordinary light microscopy techniques, but can be located in man and laboratory animals by cytochemical, immunocytochemical and ultrastructural techniques. Membrane-bound adenosine triphosphatase (ATPase) has been shown to be a reliable cytochemical marker for Langerhans cells in humans, non-human primates, mice and guinea pigs (Wolff and Stingl, 1983; Halliday et al., 1986). They also demonstrate β-glucuronidase activity (Mackenzie and Bickenback, 1985).

Since Langerhans cells express Ia antigens, monoclonal antibodies directed against Ia antigens can be used to stain Langerhans cells by immunocytochemical methods in man, non-human primates, dogs and rodents (Stingl et al., 1978; Tamaki et al., 1979). Murine monoclonal antibodies to Ia antigens on interdigitating reticulum cells, follicular dendritic cells and Langerhans cells in both humans and rhesus monkeys have also been shown to cross-react with similar canine cells expressing Ia antigens (Iwaki et al., 1983; Moore, 1968a,b). They also stain with other monoclonal antibodies to antigens on mouse macrophages and lymphoid cells such as Mac-1 and Mac-3. (Haines et al., 1983; Flotte et al., 1973; Shimada and Katz, 1988). The immunocytochemical staining patterns of cells possessing dendritic morphology include Langerhans cells, as well as interdigitating cells in lymph nodes, follicular dendritic cells and thymic mesenchymal cells in both man and rodent have been reviewed by Flotte and colleagues, (1983) (see Haemopoietic and Lymphatic Systems, Chapter III).

In formalin-fixed paraffin embedded sections, immunocytochemical demonstration of S-100 protein can also locate Langerhans cells. S-100 protein is an acidic calcium-binding protein initially detected in the brain of several mammalian species and called S-100 because of its solubility in 100% ammonium sulphate. In the skin, it is located specifically in Langerhans cells and melanocytes. Immunocytochemical detection of S-100 is therefore used in the diagnosis of melanoma or detection of Langerhans cells in several species (Cocchia et al., 1981; Kahn et al., 1983a, b; Sandusky et al., 1985).

Ultrastructural study reveals that in addition to possessing abundant mitochondria, well developed endoplasmic reticulum, Golgi apparatus and lysosomes, there are characteristic plate-like cytoplasmic organelles termed Langerhans or Birbeck granules in man and rodents (Birbeck et al., 1961).

In most species these techniques show Langerhans cells as dendritic cells in the suprabasal position in the epidermis and skin appendages as well as in some stratified squamous mucosa such as that lining the oral cavity. There are, however, species and regional differences in the density of Langerhans cells in the skin. For instance, in the mouse, Langerhans cells are far less numerous in the epidermis of the tail than on the abdomen and such differences may relate to immunological properties of different sites (Bergstresser et al., 1980). Epidermal Langerhans cell density has also been shown to decrease with advancing age in aging female BALB/C mice, although this was not associated with any marked decrease in allergic contact sensitivity to trinitrochlorobenzene (Choi and Sauder, 1987).

Whereas it has been shown that ultraviolet light alone can reduce Langerhans cell functions in vitro and in vivo, it is of note here that ultraviolet B irradiation combined with oral methoxypsoralen therapy has been shown to decrease the density of Langerhans cells expressing Ia antigen and ATPase (Breathnach and Katz, 1986). Similarly, topical and systemicaly administered corticosteroids cause dose-related decreases in similar Langerhans cell markers in rodents and in man (Berman et al., 1983).

Other epidermal cells of possible importance in immunity are the dendritic Thy-1 antigen-bearing bone marrow derived cells, distinct from Langerhans cells in mouse epidermis (Bergstresser et al., 1983; Tschachler et al., 1983) but possessing a cell-surface phenotype of very early T-lineage cells (Kuziel et al., 1987).

Keratinocytes also synthesize and secrete thymic hormone-like substances, interferon-α, prostaglandins, granulocyte-monocyte colony stimulating factor and an interleukin-1 like molecule called epidermal-derived thymocyte activating factor (Shimada and Katz, 1988) Although Ia antigens are not normally expressed by keratinocytes, they may be expressed in lymphocyte-mediated skin diseases in man or be induced by γ-interferon (Morhenn et al., 1985).

Non-neoplastic changes

Spontaneous inflammation and necrosis

Inflammation of the skin and subcutaneous tissues may occur following loss of integrity of the epidermal barrier as a result of the abrasions and minor everyday

3

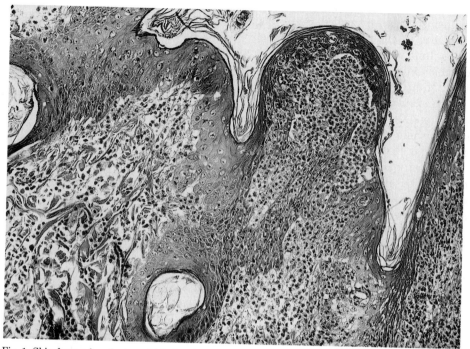

Fig. 1. Skin from a beagle dog which developed non-specific inflammatory and ulcerative skin lesions at minor, intercurrent trauma sites during the course of a conventional high-dose toxicity study. There is intense acute inflammation associated with both degenerative and reactive changes in the epidermis. (HE, ×350.)

traumas occurring naturally among laboratory animals. The nature and distribution of these lesions usually allows the toxicologist to make a clear distinction between intercurrent lesions and drug induced changes, although compounds which affect the proliferative or regenerative capacity of the germinal epithelium or the inflammatory response may be capable of accentuating the appearance of ulcers and erosions at trauma sites (Fig. 1). Excessive blood sampling or intravenous injection into the tails of rodents may also induce inflammation and marked scarring (Weichbrod et al., 1987).

Spontaneous localized infections or infestations of the skin and soft tissues also give rise to inflammatory changes. It also must not be forgotten that some systemic bacterial and viral diseases cause inflammation and necrosis of the skin and subcutaneous tissues in toxicity studies. It has recently been shown that sequential infections with two unrelated viruses, neither of which alone produce soft tissue damage can produce subcutaneous fat necrosis in the rat (Yang et al., 1985).

Mouse pox or infectious ectromelia is a well-known skin infection of mice which can develop in laboratory animal colonies. It is characterised histologically by a variable infiltration of the dermis by lymphocytes and macrophages and thickening of the overlying epidermis as a result of cell swelling or hyperplasia. Keratinocytes in the superficial epidermis and in hair follicles contain large eosinophilic cytoplasmic inclusions (Marshall bodies or type A inclusions) surrounded by clear halos, features similar to those seen in the skin of humans or other animals infected with pox viruses (Allen and Lock, 1989).

Viral skin infections have also been reported in primates in toxicity studies. This is well illustrated by the development of subcutaneous nodules in rhesus monkeys in a toxicity study as a result of spontaneous development of Yaba disease, due to a poxvirus which is characterized by nodular proliferation of histiocytic cells (Spencer, 1985). In this condition, subcutaneous nodules are composed of polymorphic cells with granular cytoplasm and single or occasionally multiple eosinophilic or basophilic cytoplasmic inclusions of variable shape containing virus particles.

An outbreak of poxvirus infection has also been reported in laboratory marmosets (Callithrix jacchus) (Gough et al., 1982). In this outbreak, papular skin lesions developed over the entire body of affected animals. Lesions were characterised by acanthosis of the epithelial cells associated with full-thickness epidermal necrosis and ulceration. Eosinophilic, granular intracytoplasmic inclusion bodies showing ultrastructural evidence of brick-shaped virus particles, typical of poxviruses were described (Gough et al., 1982).

Spontaneous inflammatory or thrombotic conditions of the vasculature can also involve surrounding soft tissues either as a result of ischaemia or direct spread of the inflammatory process in the blood vessel wall to the adjacent tissues (see Cardiovascular System, Chapter VI).

Inflammation induced by topically administered substances

The assessment of topical irritancy or sensitizing potential of agents to be applied to the human skin is important, although skin irritancy reactions in man are much more common than the better studied allergic contact skin reactions (Lazar, 1977). Although histopathological examination of the skin is not performed routinely in the preclinical assessment of irritancy or sensitizing potential of therapeutic agents, it can be helpful in the characterisation of the nature of localized effects on the skin or underlying soft tissues. Phototoxicity and photosensitisation are other forms of drug-induced skin inflammation.

Influence of species differences on effects of topically administered substances

The principle barrier function of the skin resides in the stratum corneum and there are considerable species and regional differences in the thickness of this layer. Man, like the pig, possesses a thicker stratum corneum than the rabbit, guinea pig or mouse. The practice of shaving the skin of test species may also influence absorption because this can affect the natural protective capacity of animal skin which is partly provided by dense hair cover. A study of the in-vivo percutaneous absorption of xenobiotics in Fischer 344 rats showed that age-related differences in penetration also occur although no consistent age-related pattern was observed (Shah et al., 1987). On the basis of in-vivo studies with various labelled chemicals, Bartek et al., (1972) showed that permeability of animal skin could be ranked in decreasing order of permeability: rabbit, rat, pig and man with the skin of the miniature pig skin possessing the closest permeability characteristics to that of human skin.

More recently, a careful comparative study of the percutaneous absorption of C14 radiolabelled benzoic acid, benzoic acid sodium salt, caffeine and acetylsalicyclic acid on the backs of hairless Sprague-Dawley rats and several anatomic sites in man, showed a similar rank order in the absorption of the molecules between man and rat. Although the ratios of absorption between rat and the different sites in man were different, they remained constant (Rougier et al., 1967). These results suggested that by careful control of the conditions of application such as area, dose, vehicle and contact time, it may be possible to predict the absorption of a compound in humans. However, it must be remembered that only normal intact skin remains relatively impermeable and loss of integrity of the epidermal barrier as a result of trauma or disease processes profoundly affect the absorption of foreign substances.

In general, skin penetration of test substances is a reflection of the properties of the inert stratum corneum and differences in the physicochemical characteristics of the test substances such as lipid/water partition coefficient and permeability constraints.

Another morphological difference which may influence absorption includes the much more profuse dermal vasculature in man compared with laboratory animals (Hood, 1977).

In addition to the passive barrier of the stratum corneum, there may also be significant biotransformation of topically applied substances by the viable epidermis and this activity may also show considerable species variation (Kao et al., 1985). Furthermore, there may be increased exposure of the underlying connective tissue, skeletal muscle and joints to high concentrations of therapeutic substances administered topically (Rabinowitz et al., 1982). This factor has been exploited for therapy of soft tissues, but may need to be considered in dermal toxicity studies.

(a) Skin irritancy

The predictive potential of the various animal models proposed for the assessment of irritancy potential of therapeutic agents remains uncertain and controversial. Draize-type testing (Draize et al., 1944) using the rabbit and incorporating various techniques such as hair shaving, abraiding and use of occlusive patches remains widely used. The albino guinea pig is also used and is believed by some authorities to react to skin irritants in a way more similar to humans than the rabbit (National Academy of Sciences, 1977). A model using the mouse ear has also been proposed as being particularly useful for mechanistic studies and better for more accurate quantitation (Patrick et al., 1985).

Various interspecies comparisons of the skin irritancy potential of certain chemicals have shown that neither the rabbit and guinea pig skin models are entirely reliable as predictive models for man and that there may be a degree of over- or under-prediction, depending on the type or potency of the irritant substances (Brown, 1971; Philips et al., 1972; Nixon et al., 1975; Griffith and Buehler, 1977). In general terms, most animal models are capable of predicting compounds which will cause severe irritation, but uncertainties remain in the prediction of mild or moderate irritancy potential (Steinberg, 1984).

Recent mechanistic studies of skin irritation induced in mice by chemical agents of different types have shown that the time course in development of inflammation is not solely due to differences in rates of penetration but also a result of differences in the nature of the induced inflammatory process (Patrick et al., 1985, 1987). Not all chemicals produce skin irritation through a common pathway and histopathological examination may serve to show differences in the various components of the inflammatory process. It may be possible using carefully timed histopathological examination, in combination with other techniques, to distinguish different vascular and cellular responses in the early phases of chemically induced skin irritation (Patrick et al., 1985).

It should be noted that some compounds such as pyrethroid insecticides which are employed as topical therapeutic agents for the treatment of skin infestations, produce an irritant response in human skin without morphological changes. This is probably the result of a pharmacological effect on cutaneous sensory nerve terminals. Such reactions are not detected in classical animal skin irritation tests (McKillop et al., 1987).

Histological changes in skin irritancy studies Histological examination of the skin affected by irritant substances may show a variable constellation of changes. Erosion or ulceration of the epidermis accompanied by acute inflammation or granulation tissue occurs in severe reactions, but may also be seen focally in controls where skin abrasion techniques have been employed as part of the study (Fig. 2). Usually in most mild or moderate reactions, the epidermis remains intact but reactive changes occur. These include hyperkeratosis with increased prominence of the granular cell layer and acanthosis (Figs. 3 and 4). Increased numbers of mitoses may be evident in the basal cell layer. An inflammatory infiltrate, principally lymphoid in type is usually present in the dermis. Oedema fluid, increased numbers of polymorphonuclear cells, fibroblasts and increased prominence of the dermal vasculature is also seen. In view of experimental variables and tissue sampling factors, a simple semiquantitative analysis of each of these components of the skin reaction is usually sufficient for histological assessment of primary skin irritancy. This form of histopathological assessment using a simple scoring scheme for each feature separately is a useful semiquantitative adjunct to visual assessment (Ingram and Grasso, 1975).

(b) Contact dermatitis

Allergic contact dermatitis following exposure to low molecular weight chemicals is distinct from typical primary irritant dermatitis because its development is based on immunological mechanisms which require an initial sensitizing exposure to the precipitating agent. The reaction is mediated by T-lymphocytes and requires penetration of allergen, complexing of the allergen with skin protein to form a relevant antigen and involvement of Langerhans or other antigen presenting cells. The presented antigen reacts with specifically sensitized T cells with production of lymphokines and recruitment of further effector cells to produce an inflammatory response. Contact dermatitis is typically characterized by a delayed response (24–96 hours) to a patch test with a non-irritating concentration of the agent (Andersen, 1987).

Preclinical testing for contact allergens has generally employed outbred guinea pigs but mouse sensitization assays are also sometimes used (Andersen, 1987). High concentrations of test substance are repeatedly applied to the skin or other technical manoevers are used to enhance the penetration of allergen. The guinea pig maximization test employs complete Freund's adjuvant in order to potenti-

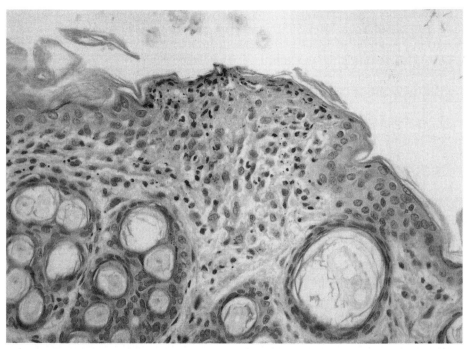

Fig. 2. Rabbit skin subjected only to the simple abrasion technique used in topical irritancy studies. There is a focal abraded area showing loss of epidermal cells, infiltration by inflammatory cells and mild hyperplasia of adjacent epidermis. (HE, ×400.)

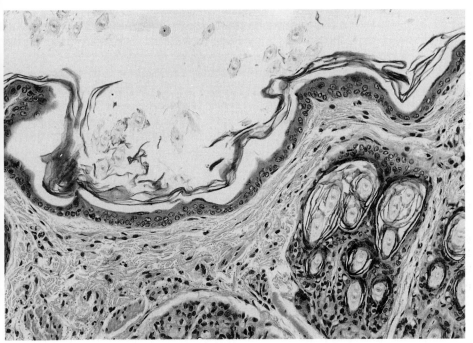

Fig. 3. Skin from the back of an untreated albino rabbit showing normal keratinization, the usual epidermal thickness of two or three cell layers and a scanty scattering of chronic inflammatory cells in the dermis. For comparison with Figure 4. (HE, ×250.)

ate the reaction and detect weak contact allergens. (Magnusson and Kligman, 1977)

Results from these protocols are not always predictive for contact allergenicity in man, particularly for weak sensitizing chemicals which are also primary irritants. As the end-result of an immune-mediated inflammatory skin reaction is non-specific inflammation, histopathological examination using routine techniques is not considered particularly useful in making the distinction between primary irritant and contact dermatitis. However, immunohistochemical techniques using markers for Langerhans cells and subpopulations of T-cells, may prove useful in the more precise characterization of immune mediated skin reactions in the various animal models, as they have proved to be in the histopathological evaluation of inflammatory skin conditions and contact dermatitis in man (Wood et al., 1986).

Immunocytochemical study has shown that in the human skin, contact dermatitis is characterized by an infiltrate of mature helper T cells with an admixture of Langerhans cells (McMillan et al., 1985). The demonstration of Ia antigen expression in the skin of guinea pigs has been recently used in the study of the mechanisms in delayed hypersensitivity reactions (Sobel and Colvin, 1986).

9

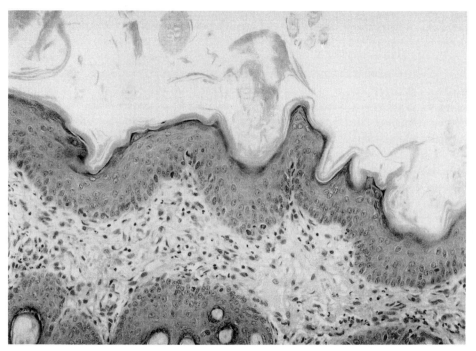

Fig. 4. Rabbit skin from the same site as in Figure 3, but following the repeated application of a mildly irritant substance. There is moderate hyperplasia of the epidermis which is several cell layers thick, increased prominence of the granular cell layer and a slight increase in the number of dermal mononuclear cells. (HE, ×250.)

Langerhans cells have been shown to alter their ultrastructural characteristics following topical application of sensitizing or irritant substances. Irritants such as croton oil, sodium lauryl sulphate and benzalkonium chloride produce cytoplasmic vacuolization and degeneration of Langerhans cells when applied to the skin of BALB/c mice whereas application of contact sensitizers 2,4-dinitrofluorobenzene and picryl chloride produce activation of Langerhans cells characterized by increased numbers of Birbeck granules and coated vesicles. (Kolde and Knop, 1987).

(c) Cutaneous phototoxicity

A variety of drugs may cause phototoxic or photoallergic reactions when they are applied to the skin or reach it via the blood stream. A number of in vivo and in vitro tests have been devised for preclinical testing of photoallergic potential, although there are no standardized methods and the experimental variables are quite diverse (Maurer, 1987). The guinea pig and hairless mouse models have been quite widely used, each employing visual assessment of the irradiated skin or measurement of the test skin thickness with vernier skin fold calipers (Lowe, 1986) rather than histopathological examination.

Histologically, changes of acute phototoxic damage is that of a non-specific inflammatory response.

Injection site inflammation

Inflammatory changes may be produced in the subcutaneous tissues by substances intended for parenteral administration to man. Although skin necrosis from extravasation of intravenous material into soft tissues is an uncommon complication of therapy in man, it can occur particularly in children following infusion of electrolyte solutions containing potassium and calcium salts, 10% dextrose solutions, vasopressors, radiological dyes, methylene blue and chemotherapeutic agents (Dufresne, 1987).

Although a number of special animal models are used for the assessment of local irritant effects, careful histopathological examination at and around the administration sites used in the routine parenteral toxicity studies can be as effective for the assessment of the local irritant effects of potential therapeutic agents intended for parenteral use. Both the intensity and the nature of the local inflammatory response can be assessed, and regional effects such as those occurring in the more proximal vasculature or in lymphoid tissue can also be observed. The actual distribution in lymph nodes of some oily vehicles can also be evaluated by histological examination (Svendsen and Aaes-Jorgensen, 1979).

Inflammation induced by implanted biomaterials

Histological assessment of the tissue response to plastics and other polymeric materials implanted in the soft tissues in rodents or rabbits is an important part of the safety assessment for substances destined for medical applications, particularly for those uses for which there will be direct contact with human tissues (Darby, 1987). These materials are implanted for varying lengths of time into the soft tissues of rabbits or rats using appropriate control materials and the tissue reaction assessed in a semiquantitative way by standard histological techniques. One of the most popular tests for irritancy of a biomaterial is intramuscular implantation in rabbits or rats (see Musculoskeletal System, Chapter IV). The subcutaneous implantation site is also used in these species, although intraperitoneal implantation may not give such a reliable prediction of tissue reactivity in man (Autian, 1972).

Various methods of histopathological evaluation have been employed, but most employ a semiquantitative assessment of the various components of the tissue response. The amount of necrosis, the character and intensity of inflammation especially whether polymorphonuclear or lymphocytic, the presence of plasma cells, macrophages and giant cells and the degree of vascularity and fibrosis are assessed in a semiquantitative manner to arrive at a final score for tissue reactivity (Autian, 1972). It is important to assess the tissue response at several time points in order to avoid false positive and false negative results (Darby, 1987). A negative control such as silicone and a positive control substance such as polyvinyl chloride (PVC) are also helpful (Henderson et al., 1987).

Cytochemical assessment of enzyme activity may also be useful in the assessment of tissue response to implanted materials. For example, the more toxic substances cause the greatest inhibition of succinic and lactate dehydrogenase activity in surrounding muscle cells and the largest increase in lysosomal enzyme activity (eg. acid phosphatase) in surrounding giant cells and macrophages (Salthouse and Willigan, 1972). Electron microscopic examination may also be helpful in the visualization of changes in cells immediately adjacent to implants.

Inflammation and ulceration induced by systemic drug administration

A striking *loss of nails (onychoptosis)* associated with desquamation, erosion or ulceration of the foot pads has been reported in beagle dogs treated with therapeutic agents possessing a radiomimetic-like effect on squamous mucosa.

The antibiotic bleomycin, isolated from streptomyces verticillus, possesses anti-neoplastic activity against squamous cell neoplasms probably as a result of interference with mitosis and inhibition of DNA synthesis (Suzuki et al., 1969). This agent, well known for its pulmonary toxicity (see Respiratory Tract, Chapter V), produces foot pad ulceration when administered to beagle dogs. Epithelial lesions commence as alopecia and dermatitis of the tail tip and foot pad desquamation. This is followed by ulceration, loss of nails, decubital ulcers and stomatitis (Thompson et al., 1972). The lesions occur on average after about 40 days of treatment but may occur after about one week or following periods as long as 13 weeks after initiation of treatment.

In the toxicity studies with bleomycin reported by Ito and colleagues, (1980) onset of skin lesions was earlier and more severe at high doses than at lower dose levels. The severity of the lesions is also influenced by the degree of physical trauma on the feet and tail tip. Thompson et al., (1972) observed that the foot pad ulceration was much less severe if dogs were housed on solid plastic floors rather than wire grid floors. The tail tip lesions also appear to result from trauma associated with tail wagging in the confined space of wire grid cages.

Similar nail loss and foot pad erosions have been also reported in beagle dogs following administration of high doses of synthetic nucleoside analogues with antiviral activity, BW134U and acyclovir (Tucker et al., 1983; Szczeck and Tucker, 1985). These lesions also occurred between a few days to four or five weeks following initiation of treatment.

Histologically, these foot pad lesions were characterized by a defect in maturation of the basal cell layer of the squamous epithelium of the foot pads and claw beds and by loss of polarity of the basal cells. The basal cells contained large hypochromatic nuclei and ballooned cell cytoplasm. The keratin layer became disrupted with development of erosions, ulcers and nail loss accompanied by active chronic inflammation

Although the pathogenesis of these lesions is not certain, it has been postulated that these therapeutic agents primarily affect squamous cell maturation, as a result of a direct interaction with cellular components such as DNA or keratin proteins (Thompson et al., 1972). When such changes coexist with the weight bearing and trauma, which normally occur on the paws, erosion, ulceration and nail loss results (Szczech and Tucker, 1985).

The relevance of such lesions in the safety assessment of these compounds for use in man is unclear but it is important to assess tissue exposure levels occurring in the affected animals relative to those likely to be achieved in man. In this respect, it is of interest to note that extremely high concentrations of acyclovir achieved locally at injection site in man have produced vesicular skin eruptions (Sylvester et al., 1986; Arndt, 1988). Under normal clinical circumstances, it appears that insufficiently high local concentration are achieved to produce skin damage.

Bleomycin is however associated with skin toxicity in man in the usual therapeutic dosage range. Changes include hyperpigmentation, induration and nodule formation on the skin of the hands characterized histologically by epidermal acanthosis and focal cellular atypia followed by gangrene (Cohen et al., 1973). However, bleomycin attains high concentrations in both skin and lung in clinical practice and this may explain its unique organ toxicity.

The dermis, connective and parenchymal tissues of rats were also shown to develop an infiltration of lymphocytes and eosinophils following intravenous or intraperitoneal injection of high doses of purified human recombinant interleukin-2 (Anderson and Hayes, 1989). The eosinophilic infiltration induced in interleukin-2 treated rats is believed to be secondary to an eosinophilic cytokine produced by interleukin-2 stimulated lymphocytes (see Respiratory Tract, Chapter V).

Unrelieved vasoconstriction produced by systemic administration of high doses of ergot derivatives can give rise to the necrosis of the tails of rats, the margins of the external ears in dogs and rabbits as well as produce ischaemic changes in the peripheral parts of the limbs in man (Griffith et al., 1978). Superficial epithelial necrosis of dependent ear margins is also reported in dogs treated for prolonged periods with the ergot compound, bromocriptine (Richardson et al., 1984).

Skin: changes in pigmentation, hyperpigmentation, hypopigmentation

Increased pigmentation of the human skin results from treatment with a number of systemically administered drugs. Some agents such as corticotrophin, oral contraceptive agents, oestrogens, hydantoin derivatives and cytotoxic drugs appear to stimulate increased melanogenesis either by a direct effect on melanocytes or mediated by the pituitary peptide hormones (Krebs, 1987).

Typically, corticotrophin and MSH produce a diffuse pigmentation accentuated in light exposed areas but also involving the oral mucosa, whereas oestrogen-induced pigmentation affects primarily the sex hormone-dependent skin over the mammary glands, genitalia and linea alba (Krebs, 1987).

Other substances such as chloroquine, chlorpromazine, β-carotene, gold salts and minocycline are believed to produce skin pigmentation through the local development of drug-pigment complexes, without increasing melanin deposition.

For instance, patients treated for long periods with phenothiazines may develop skin pigmentation in sun-exposed areas as a result of lipofuscin-like pigments accumulating in the upper dermis (Dencker et al., 1969). Not only does minocycline produce pigmentation of the thyroid gland in patients but also rarely a blue-black discolouration of the skin in patients receiving long-term therapy (McGrae and Zelickson, 1980; Sato et al., 1981). This appears to be the result of an accumulation of iron-containing, electron-dense cytoplasmic granules in macrophages and monocytes of the upper dermis, somewhat similar to the pigment granules reported in the thyroid gland of patients treated with minocycline (see Thyroid Gland, Chapter XII).

Chemical compounds are also reported to cause discolouration of the skin and hair when administered to dogs and rodents in toxicity studies, although correlation between these effects in animals and those in man appears poor. An example is the orange discolouration of the fur of albino Sprague-Dawley rats treated with high doses of β-carotene (Heywood et al., 1985).

Increased melanin deposition was reported in the hormonal-responsive skin of dogs treated with the doperminergic and prolactin inhibiting agent, bromocriptine (Richardson et al., 1984). Brown discolouration of the perianal fur and steel blue coloration of the hairless skin of uncertain significance was reported in albino Wistar rats but not Swiss mice treated for up to two years with β-blocker, levobunolol (Rothwell et al., 1989).

A number of therapeutic agents such as fluphenazine, chloroquine, or corticosteroids may rarely produce hypopigmentation of the skin or hair in human subjects particularly when high local tissue drug concentrations are achieved (McCormack et al., 1984; Dupré et al., 1985; Krebs, 1987). Hypopigmentation can result from a reduction in the number of melanocytes, decreased synthesis of melananosomes or their incomplete melanization. Postulated mechanisms include cytotoxicity, interaction with enzymes involved in melanin synthesis and oxidation of melanin.

A striking example of a skin colour loss in dogs and rats is that produced by an investigational inhibitor of platelet aggregation PD-89454, (2-[2(-3azabicyclo (3.2.2)non-3-yl)ethyl]-5,6-dimethoxy-1,2-benzisothiazol-3(2H)-one). Treatment of Long-Evans rats for four weeks produced loss of pigment in the cranial pigmented hair. Hypopigmentary changes were also observed in the skin of the nose, around the mouth and eyes as well as the oral mucous membrane in beagle dogs after treatment for four weeks (Gracon et al., 1982; Walsh and Gough, 1989). The skin of pigmented C578B/Crl mice was however unaffected by treatment.

Histological examination of the affected skin in rats revealed a reduction or loss of pigment in the hair follicle and hair matrix (skin being pigment-free in

14

this strain) and loss or lessening of pigment in the basal layer of the skin in dogs. The decrease in pigment was confirmed with Masson-Fontana stain and in both species, the DOPA (dihydroxyphenylalanine) reaction was reduced in affected zones. Electron microscopy of the affected skin in dogs showed that melanocytes contained fewer, smaller and incompletely pigmentated melanosomes (Walsh and Gough, 1989).

The exact mechanism was not clear but the dimethoxy substitution of the phenyl ring of this compound suggested that it may have inhibited tyrosinase, an enzyme associated with melanin biosynthesis (Gracon et al., 1982).

Another example is provided by the greying of the dark hair reported in Long-Evans rats treated with the antihypertensive agent medroxalol hydrochloride, for two years (Sells and Gibson, 1987). It was postulated that this change related to the binding of medroxalol to melanin because autoradiographic study showed uptake of labelled medroxalol by melanin-containing tissues.

The selective cytotoxicity of some phenolic compounds to melanocytes in pigmented laboratory rodents has been proposed as a rational basis for their application in melanoma chemotheraphy (Ito and Jimbow, 1987; Ito et al., 1987). The subcutaneous administration of 4-S-cysteaminylphenol to C57BL/6J mice produced localized depigmentation of hair associated with histological evidence of swelling, lysis and necrosis of melanocytes in black hair follicles whereas no degenerative changes were noted in hair follicles of A/J albino mice when administered the same agent (Ito and Jimbow, 1987). It was postulated that this agent mediated its melanocyte toxicity by interference with melanin synthesis.

Solar elastosis

Solar elastosis, found in sun-damaged skin and associated with solar keratosis and squamous carcinoma in man, is sometimes observed in sun exposed skin in animals (Knowles and Hargis, 1986). It can also be induced in the skin of rats and mice by chronic exposure to artificial ultraviolet light (Nakamura and Johnson, 1968; Bergeretal., 1980). Histologically, it is characterized by accumulation of thickened basophilic staining elastic fibres in the upper dermis of treated animals.

Atrophy

In man, atrophy of the skin is a well-known side-effect of prolonged corticosteroid therapy either following systemic administration or topical application (Snedden, 1976; Thomas and Black, 1985; Lavker et al., 1986). Similar alterations have been shown to occur in rodents or pigs following systemic administration of ACTH or corticosteroids as well as topical application of corticosteroids (Baker et al., 1948; Kirby and Munro, 1976; Winter and Burton, 1976; Winter and Wilson, 1976).

These changes appear primarily related to the potency of the corticosteroid and duration of administration. However, changes can occur within days in man

15

and factors such as body site and age influence the degree of atrophy and its reversibility (Kirby and Monro, 1976; Thomas and Black, 1985).

Studies of normal human skin following topical application of a potent corticosteroid (clobetasol-13-propionate) have shown that epidermal atrophy, accompanied by compaction of the papillary dermis, is clearly evident after treatment for three weeks (Lavker et al., 1986). After six weeks, the atrophy was shown to be more marked but the changes also involved the deeper reticular dermis.

Cortiocosteroid-induced thinning of the epidermis in man is typically characterized by loss of the granular layer, flattening of the epidermal-dermal border, the presence of pyknotic nuclei in the basal layers and tendency for clusters of epidermal cells to appear above the normal plane of the granular layer (Winter and Burton, 1976) Reductions in the number of Fc-rosetting, C3b-rosetting and Ia antigen-bearing Langerhans cells have been shown to occur in a dose-related fashion, to some extent dependent on the specific corticosteroid employed (Berman et al., 1983).

The dermis shows loss of collagen and glycosaminoglycans. Fibroblasts become smaller, more ovoid with reduction in cytoplasmic mass and the mast cell population diminishes in number (Lavker et al., 1986).

Similar histological alterations occur in the skin of animals following topical administration of corticosteroids. Studies in the domestic pig given topical corticosteroids for seven weeks also showed loss of the granular layer, flattening of the epidermal-border although the dermis was less affected in this model than in man (Winter and Wilson, 1976).

Our understanding of the mechanisms involved in steroid-induced skin atrophy is incomplete but corticosteroids have been shown to be capable of lowering epidermal cell mitotic rate, lowering dermal collagen content, decreasing mean diameter of collagen fibrils and decreasing fibroblast cell growth as well as collagen biosynthesis (Thomas and Black, 1985).

Alopecia

Hair loss in laboratory animals may occur in association with skin lesions induced by systemic administration or local application of drugs or chemicals, as a result of viral or bacterial infection affecting the skin, or in association with infestation with ectoparasites.

Hair loss also results from grooming activity particularly in certain strains of mice when housed together. A recent study in mice has shown that this type of alopecia is limited to grooming regions, most frequently the head but also shoulders, back and pelvic regions and that this fur chewing is preceded by whisker trimming (Militzer and Wecker, 1986). These behavioral patterns appear to be partly genetically determined in mice for they are highly strain dependent. Nevertheless, whisker trimming and fur chewing may be potentiated in rodents by administration of therapeutic agents, particularly those with activity on the central nervous system.

Behavioral-associated alopecia is characterized histologically by hair loss, hyperkeratosis and acanthosis of the epidermis, keratotic plugs in the hair follicles with a mild inflammatory reaction and foreign body type granulomas in the dermis (Thornburg et al., 1973). In pigmented strains, there may be scattered melanin pigmentation in the deep dermis and regenerated hair in black mice may be grey in colour.

Drug-induced hair loss has been observed in toxicity studies with a wide range of agents, particularly anticancer drugs possessing an effect on rapidly proliferating cells or those causing other skin lesions such as bleomycin (Ito et al., 1980). Progressive hair loss has also been observed in female Wistar rats treated with high doses of a progestogen-oestrogen combination (Lumb et al., 1985). Hair loss was initially observed at the base of the tail and over the lumbar region and progressed cranially and ventrally until complete alopecia was observed after 50 weeks of treatment. The alopecia appeared irreversible even following withdrawal of treatment for 30 weeks.

Hair loss or impaired hair growth was also observed in the chronic toxicity studies performed in both rats and dogs with bromocriptine, an ergot analogue which inhibits prolactin secretion (Richardson et al., 1984). It is probable that these effects were the result of prolactin inhibition, although the mechanism is obscure. Hair loss is also reported in man treated with bromocriptine although clear evidence that it is definitely caused by treatment is lacking (Richardson et al., 1984).

Increased hair growth

It has been recently reported that cyclosporin A stimulates hair growth in nude mice, possibly by inducing a temporary keratinization of hair in the abnormally keratinizing hair follicles in this strain (Sawada et al., 1987).

Mineralization

Although mineralization is particularly liable to occur in organs such as the kidney, stomach mucosa, large arteries and myocardium, mineral deposits are sometimes observed in the subcutaneous and soft tissues. In rats, this can occur spontaneously under circumstances which favour mineralization in other organs such as a high dietary calcium:phosphate ratio and treatment with substances such as dihydrotachysterol which mobilize calcium stores (Von Gialamas et al., 1985).

Histologically, this form of mineralization is characterized by fine or course grains of calcium in the dermis and subcutaneous tissue which may be associated with foreign body giant cells and an infiltration of histiocytes, lymphocytes, fibroblasts and fibrosis. When the deposits become massive, ulceration of the skin occurs. Zones most affected in rats are trauma sites such as those around shoulders and legs and in mammary soft tissues in breeding females (Von Gialamas et al., 1985).

17

Changes in sebaceous glands

A number of different drugs and hormones are capable of modulating sebaceous gland activity and morphology, and this may become evident in toxicity studies by alterations to the normal silky appearance of the pelage of laboratory animals.

Study of the modulating effects of drugs and hormones on sebaceous gland activity has been conducted in some detail using the hamster flank organ or pilosebaceous units located on the ventral aspect of the hamster pinna (Plewig and Luderschmidt, 1977; Gomez, 1985).

Following castration, the large sebaceous glands of the flank organ show atrophy characterized initially by degeneration of sebaceous cells leaving a rim of intact cells at the edge of the gland. Six weeks after castration the glands resemble small sebaceous glands found in normal hamster skin (Gomez, 1985). Administration of antiandrogens also leads to similar alterations in the flank organ or in the large sebaceous units of the hamster pinna.

Sebaceous glands decrease in size and labelling index in a dose related manner in hamsters treated with spironolactone (Luderschmidt et al., 1982). Conversely administration of testosterone to immature castrated female or even intact male hamsters has been shown to increase the size and pigmentation of the flank organ (Gomez, 1985).

Retinoids also cause atrophy of the hamster flank organ and their activity in the gland appears to correlate with their therapeutic effects on acne in man (Gomez, 1985).

Hyperplasia

Hyperplasia of the epidermis is observed in the skin of laboratory animals as a response to a variety of insults including spontaneous or induced inflammatory processes, application of irritant or toxic substances, repeated abrasion of the superficial stratum corneum and prolonged exposure to ultraviolet light.

As an endocrine-responsive tissue, skin thickening also occurs as a response to growth hormone and somatotrophins. In acromegaly in man, much of the thickening is a result of dermal connective tissue proliferation accompanied by increase in coarse body hair and size and function of sebaceous and sweat glands (Feingold and Elias, 1987).

Hyperplasia also occurs as a response to the application of carcinogens and may be manifest during the course of neoplastic progression (see below).

The precise histological changes are to a certain extent dictated by the inciting stimulus, but include varying degrees of hyperkeratosis, parakeratosis, prominance of the granular cell layer, increase in the thickness of the squamous cell layer which when marked may be characterized by acanthosis and papillomatosis.

It is important to recognise the presence of atypical cellular features such as nuclear and cellular pleomorphism, excessive or disordered mitotic activity,

18

abnormal keratinization or dyskeratosis and loss of the normal maturation pattern. In both man and laboratory animals loss of normal maturation is associated with neoplastic progression. It has been recently suggested that a morphometric approach is particularly helpful in distinguishing various types of nuclear alterations in skin hyperplasia induced in mice by irritant and carcinogenic substances (Kosma et al., 1986). Furthermore, Ingram and Grasso (1987) have suggested that morphometric analysis of nuclear enlargement in the epidermis of mice treated with non-carcinogenic and carcinogenic oils for short periods might be useful in discriminating carcinogens from non-carcinogens.

Neoplasms of epidermal origin

Skin cancer can develop following the local application or systemic administration of drugs and other chemicals to both man and experimental animals. Cutaneous application of powerful carcinogens such as 7,12-dimethylbenz(a)-anthracene (DMBA) followed by promotors, typically 12-0-tetradecanoyl phorbol,13-acetate (TPA), have been used to study the initiation and promotion sequence in the skin of mice for many years. A similar sequence has been observed in the skin of rabbits, rats and hamsters (Stenbäck, 1980; Schweizer et al., 1982; Goerttler et al., 1984; Parkinson, 1985) and squamous carcinomas also occur in the skin of man exposed to polycyclic hydrocarbons for long periods.

Stenbäck (1980), using DMBA followed by promotion with croton oil, has demonstrated the existance of considerable species and strain differences in sensitivity to the development of skin neoplasia. Squamous neoplasms developed readily in Swiss, strain A, Balb/c and C57B1 mice, New Zealand and outbred rabbits, but with difficulty in AKR mice and minipigs.

Cutaneous cancer has also been described in man following the systemic administration of therapeutic agents. Notable among these is the drug, methoxsalen (8-methoxypsoralen), which is used in the treatment of severe psoriasis and cutaneous T-cell lymphoma. This drug is administered orally but is photoactivated by exposure of the diseased skin to ultraviolet light which transforms the inert drug to a transiently excited state in which it is capable of covalently cross linking DNA to achieve a therapeutic effect (Song and Tapley, 1979). Whereas this procedure avoids toxicity to internal organs, low grade cutaneous epithelial neoplasms are associated with this therapy in man (Parrish et al., 1974; Stern et al., 1984; Cox et al., 1987). In view of this experience in human therapy, it is of interest therefore to record that inflammation, hyperplasia and epithelial atypia have been reported in a 13 week toxicity study in which hairless mice were given 8-methoxypsoralen and ultravoilet A radiation in a manner similar to that used in human therapy (Dunnick et al., 1987). This suggests that no major qualitative differences in response exist between man and rodent.

Classification of skin tumours

Neoplasms of epidermal origin can be divided into two main groups for the purpose of safety assessment, 1) tumours of the surface epidermis; and 2) tumours of the epidermal appendages.

A wide variety of different tumour types have been described under these general headings in man, particularly those showing various types of differentiation towards epithelial appendages. Many, but not all of these tumour types have also been described in domestic animals, particularly in dogs (Weiss and Frese, 1974) and indeed neoplasms of the skin are one of the most frequently recognized group of neoplasms in domestic animals (Madewell, 1981). Tumour subtypes showing a variety of epithelial differentiation patterns are observed in aged rodents but they have been generally less well categorized. Therefore, in rodent safety studies where tumours of similar histogenesis are often grouped for statistical analysis, it is prudent to use a fairly simple classification.

Whereas neoplasms induced in the mouse skin by cutaneous application of carcinogens tend to be relatively restricted histological subtypes, a far wider spectrum of skin neoplasms appears to occur when similar substances are applied to the rat and hamster skin (Schweizer et al., 1982; Goerttler et al., 1984).

A major problem in diagnosis is making the distinction between epidermal hyperplasia, benign neoplasia and invasive carcinoma. This may be particularly difficult in skin which is altered by inflammation or is ulcerated for long periods because reactive changes in the epithelium may develop a pseudocarcinomatous appearance. Another important part of the evaluation of such complex lesions is close examination of the skin surrounding any neoplastic change or skin changes in animals from the same treatment groups not actually developing neoplasms. As in many tumour systems, evaluation of the non-neoplastic alterations which precede or are associated with the development of neoplasia can give important clues to pathogenesis.

The nature of associated non-neoplastic changes, the presence or absence of inflammation, and the distribution of neoplasms are important in the safety assessment of skin neoplasms developing in safety studies. Any findings need to be assessed in the context of genetic toxicity, pharmacology, disposition data and the intended clinical indications for the drug.

Squamous papilloma

These neoplasms are superficial papillary or pedunculated neoplasms characterized by irregular infolded squamous epithelium showing marked acanthosis, papillomatosis and hyperkeratosis and with a fibrovascular core. There is no evidence of infiltration or invasion of the underlying connection tissues. These lesions occur sporadically in aged untreated rats (Anver et al., 1982), mice (Ward et al., 1979) and hamsters (Coggin et al., 1985). They also occur in rats, mice and hamsters following local application of powerful carcinogens where they are believed to arise from the glabrous epithelium rather than from the hair follicle

(Ghadially, 1961). Squamous papillomas also occur commonly in the skin of dogs where they are believed to be caused by a virus from the papilloma virus group but one which is different from the one that transmits canine oral papillomatosis. Histologically, these canine papillomas contain clusters of cells in the stratum granulosum characterized by clear cytoplasm and eosinophilic intranuclear inclusions.

Although there are many different papilloma viruses, they appear to possess at least one common antigenic determinant. This allows the immunocytochemical demonstration of papilloma viruses in different species including those of the dog using the same antibodies (Sundberg et al., 1984). However, the immunocytochemical study of Sundberg and his colleagues (1984) failed to demonstrate the presence of papilloma virus in the skin neoplasms of rat and hamster, although a hamster papilloma virus has been detected in skin papillomas in certain hamster colonies (Coggin et al., 1985).

Sebaceous adenoma

These neoplasms are composed of proliferating masses of epithelial cells which show a close morphological resemblance to sebaceous glands. These benign neoplasms remain sharply localized, and do not infiltrate the underlying tissues, although cystic change and squamous metaplasia may be focally present. They are found occasionally in both untreated rats (Anver et al., 1982) and can be induced in the hamster by topical administration of carcinogens (Goerttler et al., 1984).

Keratoacanthoma

The study of cutaneous neoplasms induced in rabbits, mice, rats and hamsters by local application of carcinogens has led to the delineation of a group of distinctive squamous neoplasms which are morphologically similar to keratoacanthomas in man and which appear to develop from the hair follicle (Ghadially, 1961). This contrasts with squamous papillomas which develop from the glabrous epithelium. Histologically, these experimental keratoacanthomas are characterized by well defined cup- or bud-shaped proliferations of basal and squamous epithelial cells with a central crater-like mass or cystic formations of excessive, whorled keratin.

In studying the evolution and histogenesis of these tumours, Ghadially (1961) described two main types of keratoacanthomas. The common cup- or bud-shaped variety (type I) develops from the superficial part of the hair follicle and the dome- or berry-shaped type (type II) arises from the deeper parts of the hair follicle or hair germ.

Many of the experimental keratoacanthomas appear to regress and can be considered benign neoplasms. Studies of regression in transplantation experiments have suggested that regression has its origin in the hair follicle and is not an immune-mediated phenomenon (Ramselaar et al., 1980). Similar tumours are sporadically seen in untreated rats, mice and hamsters (Ward et al., 1979; Van Hoosier and Trentin, 1979).

Tumours showing hair follicle differentiation

Neoplasms of the skin may show differentiation towards hair follicles and have been reported as trichoepitheliomas or pilomatrixomas in mice, rats, and hamsters (Anver et al., 1982; Ward et al., 1979; Goerrtler et al., 1984; Maekawa 1989).

Carcinoma

Carcinomas of the skin present a variety of different histological appearances and can be grouped according to the principle cell type, i.e. basal cell carcinoma, squamous cell carcinoma or sebaceous carcinoma. Undoubtedly, some malignant epithelial tumours show differentiation towards hair follicles, although such neoplasms are usually classified as squamous carcinomas. Mixed differentiation patterns also occur, the most notable of these being the so-called sebaceous squamous carcinoma, arising in the rat, usually in the auditory sebaceous (Zymbal's) gland.

Histologically, sebaceous squamous carcinomas are composed of proliferating irregular masses or cords of squamous, sebaceous or basal cells showing variable degrees of mitotic activity and cellular pleomorphism. Squamous carcinoma cells may be particularly pleomorphic and show individual keratinization or spindle cell differentiation resembling mesenchymal cells. Single cells, groups or cords of cells penetrate into the dermis and invade deeper tissues. Eventually, there may be involvement of local lymph nodes and distant organs.

Cutaneous carcinomas are found sporadically in aged treated rats, mice and hamsters in carcinogenicity bioassays. They can also be induced in all three species by the cutaneous application of carcinogens and promoting agents as well as in the skin of rabbits (Stenbäck 1980; Schweizer et al., 1982; Goerttler et al., 1984).

Squamous carcinomas have been reported in fairly young beagle dogs housed under conditions of high solar radiation. These squamous carcinomas develop in sparsely-haired, lightly pigmented ventral body skin, typically associated with *solar keratosis* (Hargis et al., 1977). Solar keratosis is characterized by hyperkeratosis, parakeratosis, acanthosis and collagenous thickening of the upper dermis. Solar elastosis may also be observed (see above).

Neoplasms of the melanogenic system

Pigmented strains of rodent occasionally develop neoplasms of melanogenic cells with advancing age so these neoplasms may be found sporadically in carcinogenicity bioassays performed in these strains (Burek, 1978; Ward et al., 1979; Sher, 1982). Melanomas can also be induced in pigmented rodents such as the hamster and C57BL/6 mice by the cutaneous application of carcinogens (Goerttler et al.,

1984; Berkelhammer and Oxenhandler, 1987). Neoplasms of melanin-producing cells are also widespread among certain domestic animals particularly in heavily pigmented species (Madewell, 1981). In man, benign neoplasms of pigment cells (naevi) are present in most people. The easy access of melanocytic lesions in man and recent advances in tissue culture techniques have shown that tumour development in human epidermal melanocytes embraces all the sequential steps of tumour progress which have been defined in other experimental models (Herlyn et al., 1987). Melanocytic tumours occurring in mice, rats and hamsters have been reviewed in detail (Kanno, 1989, a,b; Zurcher and Roholl, 1989).

Whereas in human diagnostic pathology the term *melanoma* is usually reserved for malignant melanoma, in veterinary pathology, the term melanoma is more widely employed to embrace various forms of benign neoplasms which are usually described as naevi in man (Weiss and Frese, 1974).

Naevi (benign melanoma)

As in man, junctional, compound and intradermal naevi are recognised in animals (Weiss and Frese, 1974). A junctional naevus is one in which clusters or nests of rounded or polygonal melanocytic cells are present at the dermoepidermal junction. In the intradermal naevus, nests or bundles of well-differentiated, rounded melanocytes are located exclusively in the dermis. The so-called compound naevus combines features of both junctional and intradermal types.

Also found are intradermal naevi resembling the so-called *blue naevus* described in man. This naevus is characterized histologically by an ill-defined dermal proliferation of spindle shaped or fibrous dermal melanocytes which are usually laden with melanin pigment. They may be found in pigmented strains of mice (Bogovski, 1979), hamsters and rats.

Malignant melanoma

These neoplasms show broadly similar histological patterns to benign naevi but are composed of atypical or pleomorphic cells which may show marked mitotic activity. They can be composed of cells or epithelioid type which may both spread along the epidermis or into the dermis or be composed of fibrous or spindle cells.

In the hamster both the epithelioid type with junctional activity and the spindle or fibrous cell forms are well-described (Fortner, 1957). Spindle cell forms appear to be more commonly described in pigmented strains of rats and mice.

Burek (1978) described eight malignant melanomas of aged Brown-Norway rats out of a population of 310. Unlike the hooded Long-Evans which possesses pigmented hair, the Brown-Norway rat has heavily pigmented skin and brown hair. Burek (1978) found most of the melanomas on the extremities and they invaded local tissues and spread to local lymph nodes. Ward (1979) found only two malignant melanomas in 5,065 pigmented $B_6C_3F_1$ mice.

23

In C57BL/6 mice treated with 7,12 dimethylbenz(a)anthracene and croton oil, malignant melanomas were of dermal spindle cell type and there appeared to be a progression from benign naevi similar to human blue naevi, through to premalignant cellular blue naevi (Berkelhammer and Oxenhandler, 1987).

Subcutaneous (soft tissue or mesenchymal neoplasms)

Although the histopathological diagnosis of soft tissue neoplasms remains one of the more difficult issues in tumour pathology, such neoplasms are found relatively infrequently in routine rodent carcinogenicity bioassays. The problems that they pose in safety assessment more frequently relate to how a few heterogeneous mesenchymal tumours should or should not be grouped prior to statistical analysis of tumour distribution within treatment groups (see Parker et al., 1984, for example).

Of course exceptions occur and one of the most remarkable of these is the development of mesenchymal sarcomas at sites of repeated injection of quite inocuous therapeutic agents, or at the site of implantation of inert substances. This phenomenon remains unexplained, for it does not fit easily into current concepts of tumour initiation, promotion and progression. Therefore, tumours developing at sites of repeated injections have uncertain relevance in terms of human safety assessment.

Classification

Undoubtedly, the histological types of soft tissue neoplasms show some interspecies variation. However, it is probable that there are fewer differences between the soft tissue tumours occurring in the usual experimental species and man than has commonly been supposed, particularly if their morphological and biological charactertistics are critically compared and appropriate recognition is given to the precise circumstances in which neoplasms occur.

For instance, one of the marked differences between man and rats has been the frequency which fibrosarcomas are reported. In the rat, it has been considered a common sarcoma with a wide spectrum of different histological appearances ranging from monomorphic spindle cell tumours to highly pleomorphic types (Carter, 1973). In man, fibrosarcomas are considered fairly uncommon neoplasms of monomorphic spindle cell arranged in interlacing fascicles or herringbone pattern (Enterline, 1981). In man, the malignant fibrous histiocytoma is now considered the most common soft tissue type of adult life, a tumour barely recognised in experimental pathology until recent years. It is now accepted that many of the sarcomas previously regarded as fibrosarcomas in rats closely resemble malignant fibrous histiocytoma in man (Greaves and Faccini, 1981; Greaves, 1989). Similar observations have been made in other species including mouse (Stewart 1979; Becker et al., 1982), hamster (Fig. 5) and dog (Gleiser et al., 1979).

24

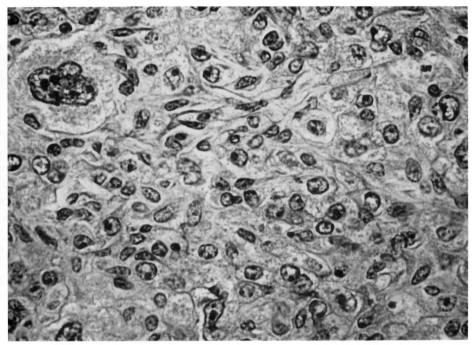

Fig. 5. Malignant histiocytoma found in the soft tissues of a 16-month-old Syrian hamster. It is composed of rounded, macrophage-like cells with abundant eosinophilic cytoplasm with occasional giant cells characterised by large irregular nuclei. (HE, ×750.)

Another example of a similarity between rodent and human tumours which has been often ignored, is the spindle cell pattern found in virally-induced rodent sarcomas. This pattern was recognised as being similar to Kaposi sarcoma found in man twenty years ago (Chesterman et al., 1966). This may be particularly pertinent since the observation that Kaposi sarcoma develops in patients affected by the human T-cell lymphotrophic virus type III (acquired immunodeficiency syndrome, AIDS). Immunosuppression may also play an important part in the development and clinical progression of Kaposi sarcoma. It has been suggested that treatment with corticosteroids or other immunosuppressive drugs may enhance its progression in AIDS patients (Real et al., 1986; Dictor 1987).

Therefore, it appears particularly helpful in the diagnosis of all mesenchymal tumours in safety studies to adopt a common, modern classification, as proposed for man and rat (Enzinger and Weiss, 1983; Greaves and Barsoum, 1990).

Histogenesis

Some of the difficulties in the understanding and diagnosis of mesenchymal neoplasms relates to their diverse histological appearances and the considerable

25

overlap observed in morphological features between neoplasms of different types. This has been accentuated more recently by the demonstration of certain ultrastructural features common to many mesenchymal neoplasms, notably the presence of primitive cells and immunocytochemical demonstration of common antigenic constituents. Such features can only be adequately explained by the concept that sarcomas do not develop from mature cells but from pluripotential primitive mesenchymal cells which fail to differentiate or remain arrested in development along one or more of the many possible pathways of differentiation of these cells (Brookes, 1986; Hajdu, 1986).

Immunocytochemistry

Immunocytochemical techniques have an important role in the diagnosis of human soft tissue tumours and are increasingly being used in the analysis of experimental soft tissue sarcomas (Barsoum et al., 1984; Altmannsberger et al., 1985; Gough et al., 1986). Not only does immunocytochemistry provide a method of cell identification which is independent of the traditional subjective morphological criteria, but provides insights into the histogenesis of soft tissue sarcomas (Brookes, 1986).

It has become increasingly evident in both human and animal tissues that aberrant or unexpected antigen expression can occur, particularly in mesenchymal neoplasms. For appropriate tumour diagnosis, it is essential that immunocytochemistry is applied within the context of other relevant clinical, macroscopic and microscopic information.

Immunocytochemistry can be used to study both cytoplasmic and stromal antigens, some of which are restricted to cells of certain types. For instance, myoglobin, the oxygen binding haem protein, is restricted to striated muscle and its immunocytochemical demonstration is useful in the diagnosis of rhabdomyosarcoma. (Altmannsberger et al., 1985). Lysozyme and to a lesser extent α1-antitrypsin and α1-antichymotrypsin which are found in histiocytes can be helpful in the characterization of rodent histiocytic neoplasms (Barsoum et al., 1984).

Antibodies to intermediate filaments are potentially useful tools in rodent tumour pathology because their tissue specificity outweighs their species divergence, although formalin fixation is not ideal for their optimum immunocytochemical demonstration in tissue sections. However, antibodies to cytokeratins are of value in the differentiation of undifferentiated spindle cell tumours of epithelial origin from mesenchymal neoplasms (Fig. 8). Demonstration of desmin is reliable for identification of neoplasms showing smooth muscle differentiation in rodents, although exceptions to this are reported in cases of human neoplasia (Gough et al., 1986).

Protein S-100, a highly acidic calcium binding protein, initially identified in bovine brain, has also been used as a marker for neuroectodermal tumours (Kahn et al., 1983; Gough et al., 1986). This can be particularly helpful in the differential diagnosis of spindle cell tumours of Schwann cell type from other mesenchymal neoplasms, although under certain circumstances S-100 is expressed by a variety of other tissues in man (Haimoto et al., 1987). In the rat, S-100 protein has been demonstrated immunocytochemically in normal bile ducts, bronchial epithelium and chondrocytes (Gough et al., 1986). It has also been shown that immuno-staining for S-100 protein is more intense in chondrocyte clusters in degenerating cartilage than in individual chondrocytes in normal cartilage (Hamerman et al., 1988; Nakamura et al., 1988).

Although immunocytochemistry using antibodies to factor VIII-related antigens and histochemistry using the lectin, Ulex europeus, have been used for the identification of human endothelial cells, these reagents do not reliably stain rodent endothelium (Alroy et al., 1987; Roussel and Dalion, 1988). However, factor VIII has been demonstrated by immunocytochemistry in canine endothelium following acetone fixation (Schmitt and Schmidt, 1986). Other lectins such as wheat germ lectin stain endothelial cells in rodents (Alroy et al., 1987).

Immunocytochemistry is also useful in the characterization of extracellular matrix produced by mesenchymal neoplasms. An example of this is immunocytochemical demonstration of laminin, the major glycoprotein of basement membrane which may help in the differentiation of mesenchymal tumours such as those of smooth muscle and Schwann cell type which produce basement lamina from fibrosarcomas and other neoplasms which do not.

Fibroma

This term is limited to subcutaneous nodules or masses composed of dense interwoven bands of collagen, interspersed with a sparse scattering of small fibroblast-like cells showing little or no cellular pleomorphism or mitotic activity. These lesions are well localized and usually solid, although focal myxomatous degeneration may be seen.

Fibromas are seen in untreated aged rats where they may be difficult to distinguish from mammary fibroadenomas in which atrophy of glandular elements has occurred (Greaves and Faccini, 1984).

Fibrosarcoma

Providing the group of fibrohistiocytic tumours are recognised, the diagnosis of fibrosarcoma is limited to monomorphic sarcomas composed of spindle cells with oval nuclei and basophilic cytoplasm arranged in interlacing fascicles or interwoven in a herringbone pattern. These neoplasms show variable mitotic activity which can be intense and there is usually a collagenous intercellular matrix. Other features such as giant cells, the storiform pattern of smooth muscle differentiation are typically not seen.

Ultrastructurally, the spindle cells are characterized by cytoplasm which is usually dominated by rough endoplasmic reticulum either as slender profiles or dilated by moderately electron-dense amorphous material. Fibrosarcoma cell cytoplasm characteristically also contains cytoplasmic intermediate filaments (7–10 nm diameter) of the vimentin type (Virtanen et al., 1981; Miettinen et al.,

1982). Thin filaments (4–6 nm diameter) have also been described in rat fibrosarcomas, usually arranged in bundles near the cell membrane, features suggestive of myofibroblast differentiation (Katenkamp and Neupert, 1982).

Thus defined, these fibrosarcomas, both in animals and man behave as locally invasive neoplasms, spreading widely in skeletal muscle with relatively late and infrequent metastatic spread.

Tumours of fibrohistiocytic type

Malignant tumours of this group are considered some of the most commonly occurring soft tissue sarcomas in man, particularly in older age groups (Weiss and Enzinger, 1978; Enjoji et al., 1980). Similar neoplasms have also been well characterized in the rat where they occur spontaneously (Greaves and Faccini, 1981) or can be induced by chemical and inert subcutaneous implants (Konishi et al., 1982; Mii et al., 1982; Greaves et al., 1985; Sakamoto et al., 1986. Similar neoplasms occur in other species including dog, cat, horse (Ford et al., 1975; Gleiser et al., 1975; Renlund and Pritzker, 1984), mouse (Stewart 1979) and hamster (Fig 5).

Histological features are somewhat variable, ranging from a fairly well-ordered storiform or cartwheel pattern of plump spindle cells to patterns composed of highly pleomorphic mixtures of spindle cells, small rounded cells, multinucleated and bizarre giant cells. A mononuclear or polymorphonuclear infiltrate may also be seen and blood vessels may be prominant. Collagen formation is usually marked in spindle cell areas and myxoid change may be seen. Haemorrhage, necrosis and focal accumulation of iron pigment also occurs. Giant cells may present strap-like features suggestive of skeletal muscle differentiation. However, cross-striations are not seen and myoglobin is not detected in the tumour cell cytoplasm by immunocytochemical techniques.

Most of the fibrous histiocytomas in the rat with the histological characteristics described above are malignant neoplasms showing extensive local infiltration into surrounding soft tissues forming metastatic deposits in lymph nodes, lungs and liver relatively late in their development (Greaves and Faccini, 1981; Mii et al., 1982). Smaller, localized fibrous lesions showing a uniform storiform pattern, abundant collagen formation and relatively little mitotic activity are considered benign neoplasms, at least in the rat (Greaves and Faccini, 1981).

Enzyme cytochemical study of these neoplasms both in man and rat have shown the presence of lysosomal enzyme activity such as acid phosphatase, β-glucuronidase, α-naphthyl butyrate or α-naphthyl acetate esterase, characteristic, although, not diagnostic of tissue histiocytes (Greaves et al., 1985; Sakamoto, 1986). Ultrastructural study has shown fine structural features of both fibroblasts and histoiocytes as well as the presence of primitive cells with no differentiated features.

Study of cell lines and fibrous histiocytic neoplasms induced by subcutaneous implantation of inert materials in rodents suggests that these tumours are derived from a primitive local tissue mesenchymal cell rather than a cell of

28

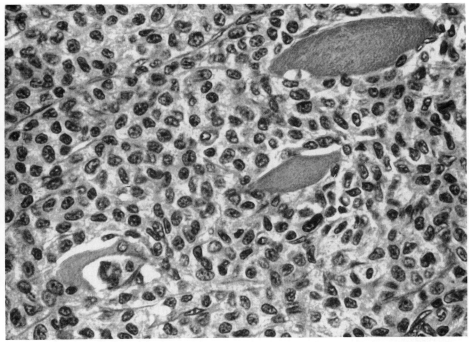

Fig. 6. Malignant histiocytoma infiltrating the soft tissues of a 24-month-old female Sprague-Dawley rat. It is composed almost exclusively of uniform histiocyte-like cells but it infiltrates along skeletal muscle fibres leaving residual islands of atypical muscle cells deep within the neoplasm. (HE, ×350.)

histiocytic lineage (Greaves and Barsoum, 1989; Greaves, 1989). Likewise in man, immunocytochemical investigation using modern immunocytochemical techniques and batteries of antisera to specific cell markers have also tended to suggest that most tumours of so called fibrohistiocytic type are also derived from a primitive extramedullary stem cell (Rohol et al., 1985; Lawson et al., 1987; Fletcher, 1987).

Malignant histiocytoma, histiocytic sarcoma (Fig. 6)

Well described in the rat, the histiocytic sarcoma or malignant histiocytoma possesses certain histological features in common with fibrous histiocytomas, notably their histiocytic appearances and enzymatic characteristics. However, they also present in a diffuse or lymphomatous manner in the rat and as it now appears that unlike fibrous histiocytomas, they are probably of true histiocytic lineage, they are best considered separately. Therefore, these histiocytic tumours in rat and other species are more appropriately discussed with the lymphomas (see Haemopoietic and Lymphatic Systems, Chapter III).

Canine cutaneous histiocytoma

This is one of the few neoplasms not uncommonly observed in toxicity studies using the beagle dog, simply as a result of its prevalence in young dogs. The annual incidence is calculated to be over 100 per 100,000 dogs and 50% of these cases are in dogs under two years of age and commonly found on the head (Taylor et al., 1969). Despite the name histiocytoma, this canine tumour is unlike neoplasms of the same name in man and rodents for it possesses distinctive histological features and it frequently regresses spontaneously. The cause of these neoplasms is unknown.

Light microscope examination of cutaneous histiocytomas in dogs reveals a superficial accumulation of moderately pleomorphic histiocytic-like cells, with oval or indented nuclei, high mitotic activity and plentiful pale eosinophilic, vacuolated or granular cytoplasm. The overlying epidermis may be ulcerated and associated with purulent inflammatory exudate. A characteristic component of this neoplasm is a lymphocytic infiltrate. This may be marked and occur in nodular aggregates, associated with foci of coagulation necrosis of tumour cells (Cockerell and Slausen, 1979). Indeed, Cockerell and Slausen (1979) suggested that these lymphoid aggregates associated with tumour degeneration were evidence of a host-mediated anti-tumour immune response.

The tumour cells show activity for α-naphthyl acetate esterase and possess ultrastructural features consistent with the concept that the tumour cells are of histiocytic/monocytic lineage (Glick et al., 1976). More recently, immunocytochemical study of these lesions for the presence of lysozyme, only 11 out of 32 tumours examined expressed this particular marker in an intense manner, suggesting that some of the tumour cells represent a more primitive phenotype, less able to synthesize lysozyme (Moore, 1986b).

Mast cell tumour

Mast cell tumours are fairly commonly found in certain breeds of dog and similar lesions are occasionally found in other species including laboratory rodents and man (Hottendorf and Nielsen, 1966; Cotchin, 1984; Wilcock et al., 1986; Takashi and Miyakawa, 1987). Histologically, they are usually well-circumscribed lesions in the skin and subcutaneous tissues composed of sheets and cords of cuboidal or rounded cells with eosinophilic and variably granular cytoplasm. Metachromatic cytoplasmic granules are usually clearly evident after staining with toluidine blue, methylene blue or Romanovsky stains. Canine mastocytomas characteristically contain eosinophils and show degeneration and necrosis of associated collagen fibres (Hottendorf and Nielsen, 1966).

They are generally perceived as benign neoplasms although they may show cytological atypia and develop an aggressive behaviour with infiltration of local lymph nodes and spread to the viscera.

Lipoma

Believed to be true neoplasms of fatty tissue, these lesions are soft, lobulated masses of mature fat cells separated by connective tissue septa. Focal fibrosis, fat necrosis and inflammatory cells may be found but myxoid areas, cellular pleomorphism and abundant mitotic activity are not seen because these features are believed to be those of liposarcomas. Lipomas are found at any soft tissue site but in the rat they are most frequently in subcutaneous tissue, within the thoracic cavity or in the mesentery. They are also seen sporadically in both mice and hamsters (Ward et al., 1979; Sher, 1982).

Hibernoma (brown fat tumour)

This neoplasm is characterized histologically by brown fat differentiation. Tumour cells are round, oval or polygonal with dense basophilic nuclei of variable size and pale foamy cytoplasm, which stains with the oil red 0 stain for fat in frozen sections. Electron microscopic study shows numerous mitochondria and small lipid droplets. Usually these neoplasms are well demarcated and show no definite histological evidence of malignancy, although nuclear pleomorphism, marked mitotic activity, local tissue invasion and pulmonary metastases have been reported in rat neoplasms of this type (Coleman, 1980; Stefanski et al., 1987).

They are rare tumours in man and laboratory species. About 80 cases of hibernoma have been reported in man in the world literature (Rigor et al., 1986). In man, they develop in the usual anatomical sites for brown fat, particularly the back, neck, mediastinum and posterior abdominal wall. Clinical observation reveals that they are biologically usually benign neoplasms. A similar anatomical distribution has been reported for hibernomas in the rat (Coleman, 1980; Al Zubaidy and Finn, 1983; Stefanski et al., 1987).

Liposarcoma

Liposarcomas are variable in histological appearances. Although they can show mixed features, they are, by definition, neoplasms which are capable of forming fat. Cells may be rounded or oval with large central or eccentric nuclei and cell cytoplasm is typically vacuolated and stains with oil red 0 or osmium. The stroma is usually well vascularized and a myxoid appearance may also be evident. Spindle cells, undifferentiated cells can also be found and mitotic activity may be intense. In man, they are fairly common neoplasms and various well-defined subgroups have been characterized. In laboratory animals liposarcomas are less well characterized but are found in carcinogenicity bioassays performed in the rat (Port et al., 1979), in the mouse (Ward et al., 1979) and hamster (Van Hoosier and Trentin, 1979).

Rhabdomyosarcoma

Rhabdomyosarcoma remains a difficult diagnosis to make in carcinogencity bioassays in rodents, because a variety of other sarcomas may contain large tumour cells with abundant eosinophilic cytoplasm which superficially resemble rhabdomyoblasts. This difficulty is compounded by the tendancy of many sarcomas to infiltrate along skeletal muscle fibres so that degenerate or altered skeletal muscle cells appear as integral parts of the neoplasms. Indeed, care must be taken in the immunocytochemical demonstration of myoglobin, a muscle-specific constituent. It has been shown that myoglobin can be taken up into the cytoplasm of total unrelated neoplasms when they infiltrate skeletal muscle and this myoglobin may be present in sufficient quantities to stain immuno-cytochemically.

In view of these difficulties, it is clear that an accurate diagnosis of rhabdomyosarcoma can be made only when there is unequivocal evidence of skeletal muscle differentiation in tumour cells. This can be shown by cross striations at light microscopic level, the presence of Z lines at ultrastructural level or immunocytochemical demonstration of myoglobin in parts of the tumour, distinct from any involved non-tumorous skeletal muscle.

Although various types of rhabdomyosarcoma are reported in man, these groups have been less well defined in rodents, although in the rat some of these histological appearances have been described. Rat rhabdomyosarcomas may be composed of bundles of well-differentiated muscle cells with abundant eosinophilic cytoplasm with cross striations (Glaister, 1981). Multinucleated giant cells may be seen and round cell differentiation has also been described in rat rhabdomyosarcomas (Allen et al., 1975; Altmansberger et al., 1985). Rhabdomyosarcomas are also occasionally seen in untreated aged mice and hamsters (Ward et al., 1979; McMartin, 1979).

Leiomyoma

Benign tumours of smooth muscle are occasionally observed in the soft tissues of aged rodents, although they are found more commonly in the female genital organs or other tissue with abundant smooth muscle such as the gastrointestinal tract. In all sites they are characterized histologically by interlacing bundles of uniform spindle cells with typically blunt ended or cigar shaped nuclei and cytoplasm containing longitudinal myofibrils which can be demonstrated by phosphotungstic acid hematoxylin stain. Mitotic activity is low. Indeed, any undue mitotic activity and cellular pleomorphism should be taken as evidence of potential malignancy. These neoplasms show fairly consistent immuno-cytochemical staining for desmin.

Ultrastructural features, although not entirely diagnostic, include a cytoplasm packed with thin filaments with focal densities, some mitochondria, sparse profiles of endoplasmic reticulum and a Golgi apparatus situated adjacent to the nuclear poles, abundant micropinocytic vesicles, and dense plaques at the points of attachment of myofilaments to the cell membrane. A poorly developed basal lamina may be present.

Leiomyosarcoma

This neoplasm is similar to the leiomyoma but mitotic activity and cellular pleomorphism is more marked. As such neoplasms are less well differentiated, the distinction between leiomyosarcomas, fibrosarcomas and Schwann cell neoplasms may be particularly difficult at light microscope level, although immunocytochemical staining for desmin and protein S-100 may be helpful.

They are seen in the soft tissues occasionally in untreated mice (Ward et al., 1979), hamsters (Van Hoosier and Trentin, 1979) and rats (Greaves and Barsoum, 1990).

Haemangioma (angioma, haemangioendothelioma, haemangiopericytoma)

There is little merit in a detailed histological subdivision of benign vascular tumours found in routine rodent bioassays. However, it is important to separate the small non-proliferative lesions composed small blood-filled channels lined by a single layer of flat endothelial cells and found in subcutaneous tissues, liver, spleen and lymph nodes, from other vascular tumours. It is generally believed that these small lesions are usually congenital or developmental malformations rather than true neoplasms. Other vascular tumours consist of closely packed capillary structures with little stroma *(capillary haemangiomas)*, or vascular structures lined by multilayered benign-looking endothelial cells *(haemangioendothelioma)* or proliferating spindle and oval cells outside of, but compressing capillary structures *(haemangiopericytoma)*.

Haemangiosarcoma (angiosarcoma, haemangiosarcoma)

These neoplasms may show a variety of different vascular patterns, similar to those observed in benign neoplasms. In addition, there is evidence of cellular pleomorphism, endothelial cells may be plump and pleomorphic or foci of undifferentiated or spindle cells may be present and these may show marked mitotic activity. These are seen sporadically in mice (Ward et al., 1979), rats (Anver et al., 1982) and hamsters (Van Hoosier and Trentin, 1979).

The classical ultrastructural features used to identify vascular endothelial cells during ultrastructural study of human tissues, the rod shaped microtubular body described by Weibel and Palade (1964), may not be a useful diagnostic feature in rodent tumours. This organelle was not identified in a series of 12 haemangiomas and haemangiosarcomas found in several strains of mice (Murray, 1987).

33

In view of the immense variety of histological appearances of neoplasms of mesenchymal cells, it may not always be possible to place an accurate diagnosis on mesenchymal neoplasms. This is especially true if the pathologist does not have adequately fixed material available for ultrastructural examination or a battery of appropriate antisera for immunocytochemical demonstration of antigens for diagnosis. Thus, it is often more appropriate to place such neoplasms in an undefined category for appropriate grouping with other mesenchymal neoplasms in the final analysis of tumour distribution.

Whereas it may not be necessary to define accurately, cell mesenchymal neoplasms in rodent bioassays, care needs to be taken to separate neoplasms of totally different type such as mammary tumours showing myoepitheliomatous differentiation, spindle cell neoplasms of Schwann cell type, or carcinomas with pseudosarcomatous appearances (Figs. 7 and 8). Neoplasms of this latter type are exemplified by some pancreatic exocrine carcinomas found in man and rat which show appearances of malignant fibrous histiocytomas (see Pancreas, Chapter VIII). In these cases, cytochemical and ultrastructural study reveals evidence of glandular and epithelial differentiation.

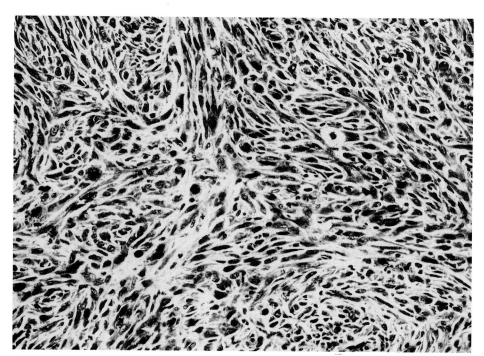

Fig. 7. This is a poorly differentiated squamous carcinoma found on the head of a 24-month-old Wistar rat. In this field there is a distinctly sarcomatous appearance. (HE, ×350.)

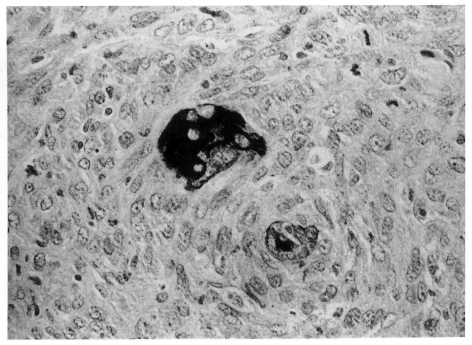

Fig. 8. Another view of the poorly differentiated seen in figure 7. Here, an epithelioid pattern with small groups of cells containing keratin shown by immunocytochemical staining for cytokeratin. (Immunoperoxidase, ×350.)

A particularly difficult differential diagnosis is the distinction of Schwann cell neoplasms from spindle cell tumours of other types. Schwannomas are characterized by the presence prominant pallisading of nuclei, a prominant external lamina, elongated cytoplasmic processes, desmosomal-like intercellular junctions, laminated cytoplasmic inclusions suggestive of myelin sheaths and immune-reactive S-100 protein (Gough et al., 1986). However, some of these features are found in other spindle cell tumours and S-100 protein can be expressed in cells of non-neurogenic type (Egan et al., 1986). See Nervous System, Chapter XIII.

Induced subcutaneous soft tissue sarcomas

In rats and mice, subcutaneous administration of powerful carcinogenic chemicals such as polycyclic hydrocarbons as well as the repeated subcutaneous injection of agents not generally considered carcinogenic, may give rise to sarcomas around the injection sites after varying periods of time. Agents among the latter class include concentrated solutions of glucose and other sugars, sodium chloride, certain water soluble food colourings and surfactants, carboxymethycellulose and macromolecular dextrans (Grasso and Goldberg 1966a,b; Carter, 1970; Hooson et al., 1973).

Some of these materials are pharmaceutical agents such as macromolecular iron dextrans which have been used therapeutically in man by the parenteral route for many years (Carter, 1970). In addition, subcutaneous implantation of inert plastics and other materials of certain dimensions can likewise give rise to sarcomas around implantation sites in rodents, the so called 'Oppenheimer effect' or 'solid state' carcinogenesis. (Oppenheimer et al., 1953; Autian, 1972; Brand et al., 1976).

Whilst the development of sarcomas following injection of polycyclic hydrocarbons and other agents accepted as powerful carcinogens is consistent with current concepts of carcinogenesis, no ready theory is available to explain the development of sarcomas following repeated injection of non-toxic, non-carcinogenic substances or implantation of inert plastics. Thus, as noted by Grasso and Goldberg (1966b) now over 20 years ago, a basic difficulty remains in making the distinction between agents that produce sarcomas by mechanisms which have no relevance for man, from those for which sarcoma development is a reflection of their true carcinogenic potential.

Also unexplained is the development of spindle cell neoplasms on the ear tips of rats treated for long period with ergotamine, at the site of tissue damage produced by this agent (Fitzhugh et al., 1944).

Even though the development of sarcomas at injection sites is not perhaps now generally considered to indicate potential cancer hazard to man for agents administered by other routes (Gross, 1982; Grasso, 1987), the difficulties in interpretation are more usually simply circumvented where possible by the avoidance of the subcutaneous route for long-term toxicity studies. However, the increasing need to assess the safety of agents by parenteral routes to avoid first pass metabolism because of lack of absorption from the gastrointestinal tract and the need to assess new plastic biomaterials may necessitate consideration of these local effects at injection or implantation sites.

Sequential studies of local tissue reactions to repeated subcutaneous injections of non-carcinogenic substances have tended to show a correlation between the nature of the early lesions and the ultimate formation of sarcomas. It appears that if injected substances do not elicit a massive macrophage response, cause little or no damage and are adequately absorbed from the injection site, neoplasia does not result (Grasso and Goldberg, 1966a). By contrast, agents which elicit a response characterized by severe inflammation, tissue damage, a macrophage response, fibroblastic proliferation and fibroplasia tend to be associated with the development of sarcoma (Grasso and Goldberg, 1966a). Early tissue responses observed around implanted inert plastics of dimensions appropriate to produce sarcomas, are also characterized by inflammation, monocytic and macrophage response, fibroblastic proliferation and dense fibrosis (Brand et al., 1979). The importance of the macrophage is of interest as it is now known that macrophages can release the potent mitogen, platelet-derived growth factor (Martinet et al., 1987).

Although no clear relationship between the type of tissue response and chemical structure of the injected or implanted material can be discerned, it has been suggested that the pattern of initial tissue response is related to physical characteristics of the material such as surface activity, lipid solubility and protein binding (Carter, 1970; Grasso, 1987). In the case of subcutaneous implants, size, shape and form appear to be the most critical elements in sarcoma development in these models (Autian, 1972). This latter situation parallels the tumorigenicity of fibrous mineral particles in rodents which appears to be largely dependent on dimensions and durability of fibres rather than their precise chemical structure (Stanton et al., 1981).

In contrast to the tissue responses around inert plastics and the various non-carcinogenic agents, it has been shown that the early tissue response and the latent period before development of sarcomas is quite different with frankly carcinogenic agents. Carcinogens such as N-methyl-N-nitrosourea and N-nitroquinoline-N-oxide appear to *inhibit* connective tissue repair and produce morphologically bizarre fibroblasts as early responses (Hooson et al., 1973). Furthermore, sarcomas develop in rats after a relatively short period of about 20 weeks, in contrast to the 50 weeks or more taken for sarcomas to develop in rats around inert plastic implants and non-carcinogenic chemicals (Hooson et al., 1973).

The established sarcomas which follow injection or implantation of a variety of different agents have usually been classified as fibrosarcomas of variable differentiation or simply as spindle cell or pleomorphic sarcomas. However, fibromas, osteogenic sarcomas, rhabdomyosarcomas, histiocytomas and liposarcomas have all been reported (see reviews by Carter, 1970 and Brand et al., 1976). More recent comparative study of the sarcomas induced by millipore filters in rats, has suggested that most of the spindle cell and pleomorphic neoplasms are similar to the malignant fibrous histiocytomas reported in man and that other tumour phenotypes develop far less frequently (Greaves et al., 1985).

There appears to be generally no clear differences in tumour types induced by different agents, although Roe and Carter (1967) suggested that histopathological characteristics of the established tumours arising in rats at the sites of injection of iron dextran were dose-dependent. It appeared that the more pleomorphic tumours developed after high doses of iron dextran whereas lower doses produced more fibrous and spindle cell subtypes (Roe et al., 1964; Roe and Carter, 1967)

Whilst the relevance of these experimental findings for man remain unclear, sporadic reports of sarcoma development around metallic and non-metallic foreign bodies in both human subjects and domestic animals raises the concern that 'solid state carcinogenesis' or the 'Oppenheimer effect' may have some relevance to the implantation of medical devices and prostheses for long periods. Various histological types of sarcoma including osteosarcoma, fibrosarcoma, malignant fibrous histiocytoma and undifferentiated sarcomas have been reported in man around the site of shrapnal fragments and orthopedic metallic and ceramic prostheses (Ryu et al., 1985; Sunderman, 1989). However, following review of these case reports, paying attention to both the nature of the implants

37

and the experimental data on the carcinogencity of metals in rodent bioassays, Sunderman (1989) suggested that this tumorigenic effect may be related to certain metals in the implanted alloys, notably nickel and cobalt, particularly under circumstances in which corrosion occurs with release of these metallic ions into the surrounding tissues.

REFERENCES

ALLEN, J.R., HSU, I.-C. and CARSTENS, L.A. (1975): Dehydroretronecine-induced rhabdomyosarcomas in rats. *Cancer Res.*, 35, 997–1002.

ALLEN, A.M. and LOCK A. (1989): Mousepox, skin, mouse. In: T.C. Jones, U. Mohr and R.D. Hunt (Eds): *Integument and Mammary glands, Monograph on Pathology of Laboratory Animals*, pp. 158–171. Springer-Verlag, Berlin.

ALROY J., GOYAL V and STUTELSKY E. (1987): Lectin histochemistry of mammalian endothelium. *Histochemistry*, 86, 603–607.

ALTMANNSBERGER, M., WEBER, K., DROSTIE, R. and OSBORN, M. (1985): Desmin is a specific marker for rhabdomyosarcomas of human and rat origin. *Am.J.Pathol.*, 118, 85–95.

AL ZUBAIDY, A.J. and FINN, J.P. (1983): Brown fat tumors (hibernomas) in rats: Histopathological and ultrastructural study. *Lab.Anim.*, 17, 13–17.

ANDERSEN K.E. (1987): Testing for contact allergy in experimental animals. *Pharmacol.Toxicol.*, 61, 1–8

ANDERSON T.D. and HAYES T.J. (1989): Toxicity of human recombinant interleukin-2 in rats. Pathologic changes are characterised by marked lymphocytic and eosinophilic proliferation and multisystem involvement. *Lab.Invest.*, 60, 331–346.

ANVER, M.R., COHEN, B.J., LATTUADA, C.P. and FOSTER, S.J. (1982): Age associated lesions in barrier-raised male Sprague-Dawley rats. A comparison between Hap:(SD) and CrL:COBS-CD(SD) stocks. *Exp. Aging Res.*, 8, 3–24.

ARNDT K.A. (1988): Adverse reactions to acyclovir: Topical, oral and intravenous. *J.Am.Acad.Dermatol.*, 18, 188–190.

AUTIAN, J. (1972): The new field of plastics toxicology: methods and results. *CRC Crit.Rev.Toxicol.*, 2, 1–40.

BAKER, B.L., INGLE, D.J., LI, C.H., and EVANS, H.M. (1948): Growth inhibition of the skin induced by parenteral administration of adrenocorticotropin. *Anat.Rec.*, 102, 313–331

BARTEK, M.J., LABUDDE, J.A. and MAIBACH, H.I. (1972): Skin permeability in vivo: Comparison in rat, rabbit, pig and man. *J.Invest.Dermatol.*, 58, 114–123.

BARSOUM, N.J., HANNA, W., GOUGH, A.W., SMITH, S.G., STURGESS, J.M. and DE LA IGLESIA, F.A. (1984): Histiocytic sarcoma in Wistar rats. A light microscopic, immunohistochemical and ultrastructural study. *Arch.Pathol.Lab.Med.*, 108, 802–807.

BECKER, F.F., NAVARES, D. and MACKAY, B. (1982): Transplantable lines of spontaneous mouse fibrosarcomas. *Vet.Pathol.*, 19, 206–209.

BERGER, H., TSAMBAOS, D. and MAHRLE G. (1980): Experimental elastosis induced by chronic ultraviolet exposure. *Arch. Dermatol.Res.*, 269, 29–49.

BERGSTRESSER, P.R., FLETCHER, C.R. and STREILEIN, J.W. (1980): Surface densities of Langerhans cells in relation to rodent epidermal sites with special immunological properties. *J.Invest.Dermatol.*, 74, 77–80

BERGSTRESSER, P.R., TIGELAAR, R.E., DEES, J.H and STREILEIN, J.W. (1983): Thy-l antigen-bearing dendritic cells populate murine epidermis. *J.Invest.Dermatol.*, 81, 286–288.

BERKELHAMMER, J and OXENHANDLER, R.W. (1987): Evaluation of premalignant and malignant lesions during the induction of mouse melanomas. *Cancer. Res.*, 47, 1251–1254.

BERMAN, B., FRANCE, D.S., MARTINELLI, G.P. and HASS, A. (1983): Modulation of expression of epidermal Langerhans cell properties following in situ exposure to glucocorticosteroids. *J.Invest.Dermatol.*, 80, 168–171.

BIGBY, M., JICK, S., JICK, H. and ARNDT, K. (1986): Drug-induced cutaneous reactions. A report from Boston Collaborative Drug Surveillance Program on 15438 consecutive inpatients, 1975 to 1982. *J.A.M.A.*, 256, 3358–3363.

BIRBECK, M.S., BREATHNACH, A.S. and EVERALL, J.D. (1961): An electron microscopic study of basal melanocytes and high level clear cells (Langerhans cell) in vitiligo. *J.Invest.Dermatol.*, 37, 51–64.

BLEEHEN, S.S. (1981): Light, chemicals and the skin: Contact photodermatitis. *Br.J.Dermatol.*, 105, Suppl.21, 23–27.

BOGOVSKI, P. (1979): Tumours of the skin. In: V.S. Turusov (Ed.), *Pathology of Tumours in Laboratory Animals, Tumours of the Mouse*, pp. 1–41. IARC Scientific Publ. No. 23, Lyon.

BRAND, K.G., JOHNSON, K.H. and BUOEN, L.C. (1976): Foreign body tumorigenesis. *CRC Crit.Rev.Toxicol.*, 4, 353–394.

BREATHNACH, S.M. and KATZ, S.I. (1986): Cell-mediated immunity in cutaneous disease. *Hum.Pathol.*, 17, 161–167.

BROOKES, J.J. (1986): The significance of double phenotypic patterns and markers in human sarcomas. A new model of mesenchymal differentiation. *Am.J.Pathol.*, 125, 113–123.

BROWN, V.K.H. (1971): A comparison of predictive irritation tests with surfactants on human and animal skin. *J.Soc.Cosmet.Chem.*, 22, 411–420.

BUREK, J.D. (1978): Age-associated pathology. In: *Pathology of Aging Rats,* Chap. 4, pp. 29–167. CRC Press, West Palm Beach, FL.

CARTER, R.L. (1970): Induced subcutaneous sarcomata: Their development and critical appraisal. In: F.J.C. Roe (Ed.), *Metabolic Aspects of Food Safety*, Chap. 20, pp. 569–591. Blackwell, Oxford.

CARTER, R.L. (1973): Tumours of the soft tissues. In: V.S. Turusov (Ed.), *Pathology of Tumours in Laboratory Animals, Vol. I. Tumours of the Rat, Part 1*, pp. 151–167. IARC Scientific Publ. No.5.

CHESTERMAN, F.C., HARVEY, J.J., DOURMASHKIN, R.R. and SALAMAN, M.H. (1966): The pathology of tumors and other lesions induced in rodents by virus derived from a rat with Moloney leukemia. *Cancer Res.*, 26, 1759–1768.

CHOI, K.L. and SAUDER, D.N. (1987): Epidermal Langerhans cell density and contact sensitivity in young and aged BALB/c mice. *Mech.Ageing Dev.*, 39, 69–79.

COCCHIA, D., MICHETTI, F. and DONATO, R. (1981): Immunochemical and immunocytochemical localization of S-100 antigen in normal human skin. *Nature*, 294, 85–87.

COCKERELL, G.L. and SLAUSEN, D.O. (1979): Patterns of lymphoid infiltrate in the canine cutaneous histiocytoma. *J.Comp. Pathol.*, 89, 193–203.

COGGIN Jr. J.H., HYDE, B.M., HEATH, L.S., LEINBACH, S.S., FOWLER, E. and STADT-MORE, L.S. (1985): Papovavirus in epitheliomas appearing on lymphoma-bearing hamsters: Lack of association with horizontally transmitted lymphomas of Syrian hamsters. *J.N.C.I.*, 75, 91–97.

COHEN, I.S., MOSHER, M.B., O'KEEFE, E.J., KLAUS, S.N. and DE CONTI, R.C. (1973): Cutaneous toxicity of bleomycin therapy. *Arch. Dermatol.*, 107, 553–555.

COLEMAN, G.L. (1980): Four intrathoracic hibernomas in rats. *Vet. Pathol.*, 17, 634–637.

COTCHIN, E. (1984): Veterinary oncology: A Survey. *J.Pathol.*, 142, 101–127

COX, N.H., JONES, S.K., DOWNEY, D.J., TUYP, E.J., JAY, J.L., MOSELEY, H. and MACKIE, R.M. (1987) Cutaneous and ocular side-effects of oral photochemotheraphy:results of an 8-year follow- up study. *Br.J.Dermatol.*, 116, 145–152.

DARBY, T.D. (1987): Safety evaluation of polymer materials. *Ann.Rev. Pharmacol.Toxicol.*, 27, 157–167.

DENCKER S.J., ENOKSSON, P and PERSSON, P.S. (1969): Pigment deposits in various organs during phenothiazine treatment. *Acta Psychiatr. Scand.*, 43, 11–31.

DICTOR, M.R. (1987) Kaposi's sarcoma: A trifactorial model. *Med. Hypothesis*, 22, 429–441.

DRAIZE, J., WOODWARD, G., and CALVERY, H.O. (1944): Methods for the study of irritation and toxicity of substances applied topically to the skin and mucous membranes. *J.Pharmacol.Exp. Ther.*, 83, 377–390.

DUFRESNE, R.G. (1987): Skin necrosis from intravenously infused materials. *Cutis*, 39, 197–198.

DUPRÉ, A., ORTONNE, J.P., VIRABEN, R and ARFEUX, F (1985): Chloroquine-induced hypo-pigmentation of hair and freckles. Association with congenital renal failure. *Arch.Dermatol.*, 121, 1164–1166.

DUNNICK, J.K., FORBES, P.D., DAVIES, R.E. and IVERSON, W.O. (1987): toxicity of 8-metho-xypsoralen, 5-methoxypsoralen, 3-carbethoxypsoralen, or 5-methylisopsoralen with ultraviolet radiation in hairless (HRA/SKU) mouse. *Toxicol.Appl.Pharmacol.*, 89, 73–80.

EGAN, M.J., CROCKER, J., NEWMAN, J. and COLLARD M. (1986): Immunohistochemical localization of S100 protein in skin tumors. *Arch.Pathol.Lab.Med.*, 110, 765–767.

ENJOJI, M., HASHIMOTO, H., TSUNEYOSHI, M. and IWASAKI, H. (1980): Malignant fibrous histiocytoma. A clinicopathologic study of 130 cases. *Acta Pathol.Jpn.*, 30, 727–741.

ENTERLINE, H.T. (1981): Histopathology of sarcomas. *Semin.Oncol.*, 8, 133–155.

ENZINGER, F.M. and WEISS, S.W. (1983): General considerations In: *Soft Tissue Tumors,* Chap. 1, pp. 1–13. Mosby, St. Louis.

FLETCHER, C.D.M. (1987): Malignant fibrous histiocytoma? *Histopathology*, 11, 433–437.

FEINGOLD, K.R. and ELIAS, P.M. (1987): Endocrine-skin interactions. Cutaneous manifestation of pituitary disease, thyroid disease, calcium, and diabetes. *J.Am.Acad.Dermatol.*, 17, 921–940.

FITZHUGH, O.G., NELSON, A.A. and CALVERY, H.O. (1944): The chronic toxicity of ergot. *J.Pharmacol.Exp. Ther.*, 82, 364–376.

FLOTTE, T.J., SPRINGER, T.A. and THORBECKE, G.J. (1983): Dendritic cell and macrophage staining by monoclonal antibodies in tissue sections and epidermal sheets. *Am.J.Pathol.*, 111, 112–124.

FORD, H.G., EMPSON, R.N., PLOPPER, C.G. and BROWN, P.H. (1975): Giant cell tumor of soft parts: A report of an equine and a feline case. *Vet.Pathol.*, 12, 428–433.

FORTNER, J.G. (1957): Spontaneous tumors including gastrointestinal neoplasms and malignant melanomas, in the Syrian hamster. *Cancer*, 10, 1153–1156.

FURNESS, P.N., GOODFIELD, M.J., MACLENNAN, K.A., STEVENS, A. and MILLARD, L.G. (1986): Severe cutaneous reactions of captopril and enalapril; histological study and comparison with early mycosis fungoides. *J.Clin.Pathol.*, 39, 902–907.

GHADIALLY, F.N. (1961): The role of the hair follicle in the origin and evolution of some cutaneous neoplasms of man and experimental animals. *Cancer*, 14, 801–816.

GLAISTER, J.R. (1981): Rhabdomyosarcoma in a young rat. *Lab.Anim.*, 15, 145–146.

GLEISER, C.A., RAULSTON, G.L., JARDINE, J.H. and GRAY, K.N. (1979): Malignant fibrous histiocytoma in dogs and cats. *Vet.Pathol.*, 16, 199–208.

GLICK, A.D., HOLSCHER, M. and CAMPBELL, G.R. (1976): Canine cutaneous histiocytoma: Ultrastructural and cytochemical observations. *Vet.Pathol.*, 13, 374–380.

GOERTTLER, K., LOEHRKE, H., HESSE, B. and SCHWEIZER, J. (1984): Skin tumour forma-tion in the European hamster (Cricetus crictus, L.) after topical initiation with 7,12-dimethyl-benz(a)anthracene (DMBA) and promotion with 12-0-tetradecanoylphosbol-13-acetate (TPA). *Carcinogenesis*, 5, 521–524.

GOMEZ, E.C. (1985): Hamster flank organ: Assessment of drugs modulating sebaceous gland function. In: H.I. MAIBACH and- N.J. LOWE (Eds), *Models in Dermatology*, Vol. 2 pp. 100–111. Karger Basel.

GOUGH, A.W., BARSOUM, N.J., GRACON, S.I., MITCHELL, L and STURGESS, J.M. (1982): Poxvirus infection in a colony of common marmosets (Callithrix jaccus). *Lab.Anim.Sci.*, 32, 87–90.

GOUGH, A.W., HANNA, W., BARSOUM, N,J., MOORE, J and STURGESS, J.M. (1986): Morpho-logic and immunohistochemic at features of two spontaneous peripheral nerve tumors in Wistar rats. *Vet.Pathol.*, 23, 68–73.

GOWN, A.M., BOYD, H.C., CHANG, Y, FURGUSON, M., REICHLER, B and TIPPENS, D. (1988): Smooth muscle cells can express cytokeratins of 'simple' epithelium. Immunocytochemical and biochemical studies in vitro and in vivo. *Am.J.Pathol.*, 132, 223–232.

GRACON, S.I., MARTIN, R.A., BARSOUM, N.J., MITCHELL, L., STURGESS, J.M. and de la

IGLESIA, F.A. (1982): Hypopigmentary changes with a platelet aggregation inhibitor. *Fed.Proc.*, 41, 702.

GRASSO, P. (1987): Persistent organ damage and cancer production in rats and mice. *Arch.Toxicol.*, Suppl.11, 75–83.

GRASSO, P. and GOLDBERG, L. (1966)a: Early changes at the site of repeated subcutaneous injections of food colorings. *Food.Cosmet Toxicol.*, 4, 269–282.

GRASSO, P. and GOLDBERG, L. (1966)b: Subcutaneous sarcoma as an index of carcinogenic potency. *Food.Cosmet.Toxicol.*, 4, 297–320.

GREAVES, P. (1989) Fibrous histiocytoma, malignant, subcutis, rat. In: T.C. Jones., U. Mohr and R.D. Hunt (Eds), *Integument and Mammary Glands, Monographs on Pathology of Laboratory Animals*, pp. 106–112. Springer-Verlag, Berlin.

GREAVES, P. and BARSOUM, N. (1990): Tumours of soft tissues. In: V.S. Turusov (Ed.), *Pathology of Tumours in Laboratory Animals. Tumours of the Rat, 2nd Edition*, IARC Scientific Publ. In press.

GREAVES, P. and FACCINI, J.M. (1981): Spontaneous fibrous histiocytic neoplasms in rats. *Br.J.Cancer*, 43, 402–411.

GREAVES, P., MARTIN, J-M. and RABEMAMPIANINA, Y. (1985): Malignant fibrous histiocytoma in rats at sites of implanted millipore filters. *Am.J.Pathol.*, 120, 207–214.

GRIFFITH, J.F. and BUEHLER, E.V. (1977): Prediction of skin irritancy sensitizing potential by testing with animals and man. In: V.A. Drill and P. Lazar (Eds), *Cutaneous Toxicity*, pp. 155–173. Academic Press, New York.

GRIFFITH, R.W., GRAUWILER, J., HODEL, Ch., LEIST, K.H., MATTER, B. (1978). Toxicologic considerations. In: B. Berde and H.O. Schild (Eds), *Ergot Alkaloids and Related compounds*. Handbook of Experimental Pharmacology, Vol.49, Chap. 12, pp. 805–851. Springer-Verlag, Berlin.

GROSS, P. (1982): Man-made vitreous fibers: Present status of research on health effects. *Int.Arch.Occup. Environ.Health*, 50, 103–112.

HAIMOTO, H., HOSODA, S. and KATO, K. (1987): Differential distribution of immunoreactive S-100-α and S-100-β proteins in normal non-nervous human tissues. *Lab.Invest.*, 57, 489–498.

HAINES, K.A., FLOTTE, T.J., SPRINGER, T.A., GIGLI, I. and THORBECKE, G.J. (1983): Staining of Langerhans cells with monoclonal antibodies to macrophages and lymphoid cells. *Immunology*, 80, 3448–3451.

HAJDU, S.I. (1986) Histogenesis and classification. In: *Differential Diagnosis of Soft Tissue and Bone Tumours*, Chap. 1. pp. 3–34. Lea and Febiger, Philadelphia.

HALLIDAY, G.M., McARDLE, J.P., KNIGHT, B.A. and MULLER, H.K. (1986): New methodology for assessment of Langerhans cell network. *J.Pathol.*, 148, 127–134.

HAMERMAN, D., CHEN, F., DORFMAN, H. and ROJAS-CORONA, R. (1988): The distribution of S-100 protein in cartilage from osteoarthritic joints. *Calcif.Tissue Int.*, 42. A.31.

HARGIS, A.M., THOMASSON, R.W. and PHEMISTER, R.D. (1977): Chronic dermatosis and cutaneous squamous cell carcinoma in the Beagle dog. *Vet.Pathol.*, 14, 218–228.

HENDERSON, Jr J.D., MULLARKY, R.H. and RYAN, D.E. (1987): Tissue biocompatability of kevlar aramid fibers and polymethylmethacrylate composites in rabbits. *J.Biomed.Mater.Res.*, 21, 59–64.

HERLYN, M., CLARKE, W.H., RODECK, U., MANCIANTI, M.L., JAMBROSIC, J. and KOPROWSKI, H. (1987): Biology of tumor progression in human melanocytes. *Lab.Invest.*, 56, 461–474.

HEYWOOD, R., PALMER, A.K., GREGSON, R.L. and HUMMLER, H. (1985): The toxicity of beta-carotene. *Toxicology*, 36, 91–100.

HOOD, D.B. (1977): Practical and theoretical considerations in evaluating dermal safety. In: V.A. Driff and P. Lazar (Eds), *Cutaneous Toxicity*, pp. 15–30. Academic Press, New York.

HOOSON, J., GRASSO, P. and GANGOLLI, S.D. (1973): Injection site tumours and preceding pathological changes in rats treated subcutaneously with surfactants and carcinogens. *Br.J. Cancer*, 27, 230–244.

HOTTENDORF, G.H., and NIELSEN, S.W. (1966): Collagen necrosis in canine mastocytomas. *Am.J.Pathol.*, 49, 501–513.

41

INGRAM, A.J. and GRASSO, P. (1975): Patch testing in the rabbit using a modified patch test method. *Br.J.Dermatol.*, 92, 131–142.

INGRAM, A.J. and GRASSO, P. (1987): Nuclear enlargement produced in mouse skin by carcinogenic mineral oils. *J.Appl.Toxicol.*, 7, 289–295.

ITO, K., HANDA, J., MORI, M., EZURA, H., KUMAGAI, M., SUZUKI, A., MAKABAYASHI, Y., IRIE, Y., YAMASHITA, T., MIYAMOTO, K., TSUBOSAKI, M., MATSUDA, A. and KONOHA, N (1980): Toxicity test of bleomycin oil suspension. Chronic toxicity in Beagle dogs. *Jpn.J.Antibiot.*, 33, 29–72.

ITO, Y., and JIMBOW, K. (1987): Selective cytotoxicity of 4-S-cysteaminylphenol on follicular melanocytes of the black mouse: Rational basis for its application to melanoma chemotheraphy. *Cancer Res.*, 47, 3278–3284.

ITO, Y., JIMBOW, K. and ITO, S. (1987): Depigmentation of black guinea pig skin by topical application of cysteaminophenol, cysteinylphenol and related compounds. *J.Invest.Dermatol.*, 88, 77–82.

IWAKI, Y., TERASAKI, P.I., KINUKAWA, T., THAI, T.H., ROOT, T. and BILLING, R. (1983): Cross reactivity between human and canine Ia antigens using a mouse monclonal antibody (CIA). *Transplantation*, 36, 189–191.

KAHN, H.J., MARKS, A., THOM, H. and BAUMAL, R. (1983)a: Role of antibody to S-100 protein in diagnostic pathology. *Am.J.Clin.Pathol.*, 79, 341–347.

KAHN, H.J., MARKS, A., THOM, H. and BAUMAL, R (1983)b: Role of antibody to S-100 protein in diagnostic pathology. *Am.J.Clin. Pathol.*, 79, 341–347.

KANNO, J. (1989)a Melanocytic tumors, skin, mouse.In: T.C. Jones, U. Mohr and R.D. Hunt (Eds), *Integument and Mammary Glands, Monographs or Pathology of Laboratory Animals*, pp. 63–70. Springer-Verlag, Berlin.

KANNO, J. (1989)b Melanocytic tumors, skin, hamster. In: T.C. Jones, U. Mohr and R.D. Hunt (Eds), *Integument and Mammary Glands, Monographs on Pathology of Laboratory Animals*, pp. 70–75. Springer-Verlag, Berlin.

KAO, J., PATTERSON, F.K. and HALL, J. (1985): Skin penetration and metabolism of topically applied chemicals in six mammalian species including man: An in vitro study with benzo(a)pyrene and testosterone. *Toxicol.Appl.Pharmacol.*, 81, 501–516.

KATENKAMP, D. and NEUPERT, G. (1982): Experimental tumours with features of malignant fibrous histiocytomas. Light microscopic and electron microscopic investigations on tumours produced by cell implantation of an established fibrosarcoma cell line. *Exp. Pathol.*, 22, 11–27.

KIRBY, J.D. and MUNRO, D.D. (1976): Steroid-induced atrophy in an animal and human model. *Br.J.Dermatol.*, 94, Suppl. 12, 111–119.

KNOWLES, D.P. and HARGIS, A.M. (1986): Solar elastosis associated with neoplasia in two dalmations. *Vet.Pathol.*, 23, 512–514.

KOLDE, G. and KNOP, J. (1987): Different cellular reaction patterns of epidermal Langerhans cells after application of contact sensitizing, toxic and tolerogenic compounds. A comparative ultrastructural and morphometric time course analysis. *J.Invest.Dermatol.*, 89, 19–23.

KONISHI, Y., MARUYAMA, H., MII, Y., MIYAUCHI, Y., YOKOSE, Y. and MASUHARA, K. (1982): Malignant fibrous histiocytomas induced by 4-(hydroxyamino)quinoline 1-oxide in rats. *J.N.C.I.*, 68, 859–865.

KOSMA, V-M., COLLAN, Y., NAUKKARINEN, A., AALTO, M-L. and MÄNNISTÖ P. (1986): Histopathological and morphometrical analysis applied to skin changes in NMRI mice induced by dithranol (anthranil) and its acyl analogues. *Arch.Toxicol.*, Suppl. 9, 451–454.

KREBS, A. (1987): Medikamentösbedingte Hyper-und Depigmentierungen. *Schweiz Rundsch.Med. Prax.*, 76, 1069–1075.

KUZIEL, W.A., TAKASHIMA, A., BONYHADI, M., BERGSTRESSER, P.R., ALLISON, J.P., TIGELAAR, R.E. and TUCKER P.W. (1987). Regulation of T-cell receptor γ-chain RNA expression in murine Thy-1[+] dendritic epidermal cells. *Nature*, 328, 263–266.

LAVKER, R.M., SCHECHTER, N.M., and LAZARUS, G.S. (1986): Effects of topical corticosteroids on human dermis. *Br.J.Dermatol.*, 115, Suppl. 31, 101–107.

LAWSON, C.W., FISHER, C. and GATTER, K.C. (1986): An immunohisto-chemical study of differentiation in malignant fibrous histiocytoma. *Histopathology*, 11, 375–383.

LAZAR, P. (1977): What is a reaction: Factors in the interpretation of reporting of cometic data. In: V.A. Drill and P. Lazar (Eds.), *Cutaneous Toxicity*, pp. 5–14. Academic Press, New York.

LOWE, N.J. (1986): Cutaneous phototoxicity reactions. *Br.J.Dermatol.*, 115, Suppl. 31, 86–92.

LUDERSCHMIDT, C., BIDLINGMAIER, F. and PLEWIG, G. (1982): Inhibition of sebaceous gland activity by spironolactone in Syrian hamster. *J.Invest.Dermatol.*, 78, 253–255.

LUMB, G., MITCHELL, L. and DE LA IGLESIA, F.A. (1985): Regression of pathologic changes induced by long-term administration of contraceptive steroids to rodents. *Toxicol.Pathol.*, 13, 283–295.

MACKENZIE, I.C., and BICKENBACK, J.R. (1985): Label retaining keratinocytges and Langerhans cells in mouse epithelial. *Cell Tissue Res.*, 242, 551–556.

MAEKAWA, A. (1989) Trichoepithelioma, skin, rat. In: T.C. Jones, U.Mohr and R.D. Hunt (Eds), *Integument and Mammary Glands, Monographs on Pathology of Laboratory animals*, pp. 56–63. Springer Verlag, Berlin.

MADEWELL, B.R. (1981): Neoplasms in domestic animals: A review of experimental and spontaneous carcinogenesis. *Yale J.Biol.Med.*, 54, 111–125.

MAGNUSSON, B. and KLIGMAN, A.M. (1977): Usefulness of guinea pig tests for detection of contact sensitizers. In: F.N. Marzulli and H.I. Maibach (Eds), *Dermatotoxicity and Pharmacology*, pp. 551–560. Wiley, New York.

MARTINET, Y., ROM, W.N., GROTENDORST, G.R., MARTIN, G.R. and CRYSTAL, R.G. (1987): Exaggerated spontaneous release of platelet derived growth factor by alveolar macrophages from patients with idiopathic pulmonary fibrosis. *N.Engl.J.Med.*, 317, 20–209.

MAURER, Th. (1987): Phototoxicity testing: in vivo and in vitro. *Food Chem.Toxicol.*, 25, 407–414.

McCORMACK, P.C., LEDESMA, G.N. and VAILLANT, J.G. (1984): Linear hypopigmentation after intra-articular corticosteroid injection. *Arch.Dermatol.*, 120, 708–709.

McGRAE, J.D., and ZELICKSON, A.S. (1980). Skin pigmentation secondary to minocycline theraphy. *Arch.Dermatol.*, 116, 1262–1265.

McKILLOP, C.M., BROCK, J.A.C., OLIVER, G.J.A. and RHODES, C. (1987): A quantitative assessment of pyrethroid-induced paraesthesia in the guinea pig flank model. *Toxicol.Lett.*, 36, 1–7.

McMARTIN, D.N. (1979): Morphologic lesions in aging Syrian hamsters. *J.Gerontol.*, 34, 502–511.

McMILLAN, E.M., STONEKING, L., BURDICK, S., COWAN, I. and HUSAIN-HAMZAVI, S.L. (1985): Immunophenotype of lymphoid cells in positive patch tests of allergic contact dermatitis. *J.Invest.Dermatol.*, 84, 229–233.

MEDENICA, M. (1982): The skin. In: R.H. Riddell (Ed.), *Pathology of Drug Induced and Toxic Diseases*, Chap. 6, pp. 119–146. Churchill Livingstone, New York.

MIETTINEN, M., LEHTO, V-P., BADLEY, R.A. and VIRTANEN, I. (1982): Expression of intermediate filaments in soft tissue sarcomas. *Int.J.Cancer*, 30, 541–546.

MII, Y., MARUAMA, H., MIYAUCHI, Y., YOKOSE, Y., MASUHARA, K. and KONISHI, Y. (1982): Experimental studies on malignant fibrous histiocytomas in rats. I. Production of malignant fibrous histiocytomas by 4-hydroxyaminoquinoline 1-oxide in bone of Fischer 344 strain rats. *Cancer*, 50, 2057–2065.

MILITZER, K. and WECKER, E. (1986): Behavior associated alopecia areata in mice. *Lab.Anim.*, 20, 9–13.

MOORE, P.F. (1986)a: Characterization of cytoplasmic lysozyme immuno- reactivity as a histiocytic marker in normal canine tissues. *Vet.Pathol.*, 23, 763–769.

MOORE, P.F. (1986)b: Utilization of cytoplasmic lysozyme immunoreactivity as a histiocytic marker in canine histiocytic disorders. *Vet.Pathol.*, 23, 757–762.

MORHENN, V.B., NICKOLOFF, B.J. and MANSBRIDGE, J.A. (1985). Induction of the synthesis of triton-soluble proteins in human keratinocytes by gamma interferon. *J.Invest.Dermatol.*, 85, 275–295.

MURRAY, A.B. (1987): Weibel-Palade bodies are not reliable ultrastructural markers for mouse endothelial cells. *Lab.Anim.Sci.*, 37, 483–485.

43

NAKAMURA, K. and JOHNSON, W.C. (1968): Ultraviolet light induced connective tissue changes in rat skin: A histopathologic and histochemical study. *J.Invest.Dermatol.*, 51, 253–258.

NAKAMURA, S., NAKAMURA, T. and KAWAHARA, H. (1988): S-100 protein in human articular cartilage. *Acta Orthop. Scand.*, 59, 438–440.

NATIONAL ACADEMY OF SCIENCES (1977): Principles and procedures for evaluating the toxicity of household substances. NAS Publication 1138. National Academy of Sciences, Washington, D.C.

NIXON, G.A., TYSON, C.A. and WERTZ, W.C. (1975): Interspecies comparison of skin irritancy. *Toxicol.Appl.Pharmacol.*, 31, 481–490.

OPPENHEIMER, B.S.C, OPPENHEIMER, E.T., and STOUT, A.P. (1953): Carcinogenic effect of imbedding various plastic films in rat and mice. *Surg.Forum*, 4, 672–678.

PARKER, C.M., PATTERSON, D.R., VAN GELDER, G.A., GORDON, E.B., VALERIO, M.G. and HALL, W.C. (1984): Chronic toxicity and carcinogenicity evaluation of fenvalerate in rats. *J.Toxicol. Environ.Health*, 13, 83–97.

PARKINSON, E.K. (1985): Defective responses of transformed keratino- cytes to terminal differentiation stimuli. Their role in epidermal tumour promotion by phorbol esters and by deep skin wounding. *Br.J.Cancer*,52, 479–493.

PARRISH, J.A., FITZPATRICK, T.B., TANENBAUM, L. and PATHAK, M.A. (1974) Photochemotherapy of psoriasis with oral methoxsalen and longwave ultraviolet light. *N.Engl.J.Med.*, 291, 1207–1211.

PATRICK, E., BURKHALTER, A. and MAIBACH, H.I. (1987): Recent investigations of mechanisms of chemically induced skin irritation in laboratory mice. *J.Invest.Dermatol.*, 88, 24s-31s.

PATRICK, E., MAIBACH, H.I. and BURKHALTER, A. (1985): Mechanisms of chemically induced skin irritation. I. Studies of time course, dose response, and components of inflammation in the laboratory mouse. *Toxicol.Appl.Pharmacol.*, 81, 476–490.

PHILIPS, L., STEINBERG, M., MAIBACH, H.I. and AKERS, W.A. (1972): A comparison of rabbit and human skin responses to certain irritants. *Toxicol.Appl.Pharmacol.*, 21, 369–382.

PLEWIG, G. and LUDERSCHMITDT, C. (1977): Hamster ear model for sebaceous glands. *J.Invest.Dermatol.*, 68, 171–176.

PORT, C.D., NUNEZ, C. and BATTIFORA, H. (1979): An unusal neoplasm of adipose tissue in a rat. *Lab.Anim.Sci.*, 29, 214–217.

RABINOWITZ, J.L., FELDMAN, E.S., WEINBERGER, A. and SCHUMACHER, H.R. (1982): Comparative tissue absorption of oral 14C-aspirin and topical triethanolamine 14C salicylate in human and canine knee joints. *J.Clin.Pharmacol.*, 22, 42–48.

RAMSELAAR, C.G., RUITENBERG, E.J. and KRUIZINGER, W. (1980): Regression of induced keratocicanthomas in anagen (hair growth phase) skin grafts in mice. *Cancer Res.*, 40, 1668–1673.

REAL, F.X., KROWN, S.E. and KOZINER, B. (1986): Steroid-related development of Kaposi's sarcoma in a homosexual man with Burkitt's lymphoma. *Am.J.Med.*, 80, 119–122.

RENLUND, R.C. and PRITZKER, K.P.H. (1984): Malignant fibrous histiocytoma involving the digit of a cat. *Vet.Pathol.*, 21, 442–444.

RICHARDSON, B.P., TURKALJ, I. and FLÜCKIGER, E. (1984): Bromocriptine In: D.R. Laurence, A.E.M. Mclean and M. Weatherall (Eds), Safety Testing of New Drugs. Laboratory Predictions and Clinical Performance, Chap. 3, pp. 19–63. Academic Press, London.

RIGOR, V.U., GOLDSTONE, S.E., JONES, J., BERNSTEIN, R., GOLD, M.S. and WEINER, S. (1986): Hibernoma. A case report and discussion of a rare tumor. *Cancer*, 57, 2207–2211.

ROE, F.J.C. and CARTER, R.L. (1967): Iron-dextran carcinogenesis in rats: Influence of dose on the number of types of neoplasm induced. *Int.J.Cancer*, 2, 370–380.

ROE, F.J.C., HADDOW, A., DUKES, C.E. and MITCHLEY, B.C.V. (1964): Iron-dextran carcinogenesis in rats: Effects of distributing injected material between one, two, four or six sites. *Br.J.Cancer*, 18, 801–808.

ROHOLL, P.J.M., KLEIJNE, J., VAN BASTEN, C.D.H., VAN DER PUTTE, S.C.J. and VAN UNNIK, J.A.M. (1985): A study to analyse the origin of tumor cells in malignant fibrous histiocytoma. A multiparametric characterization. *Cancer*, 56, 2809–2815.

ROTHWELL, C.E., McGUIRE, E.J. and MARTIN, R.A. (1989): Chronic toxicity/oncogenicity studies of the β-blocker levobunolol. *Toxicologist*, 9, 213.

ROUGIER, A., LOTTE, C. and MAIBACH, H.I. (1987): The hairless rat: A relevant animal model to predict in vivo percutaneous absorption in humans? *J.Invest.Dermatol.*, 88, 577–581.

ROUSSEL, F. and DALION, J. (1988): Lectins as markers of endothelial cells: comparative study between human and animal cells. *Lab.Anim.*, 22, 135–140.

RYU, R.K.N., BOVILL, E.G., SKINNER, H.B. and MURRAY, W.R. (1987): Soft tissue sarcoma associated with aluminium oxide ceramic total hip arthroplasty. A case report. *Clin.Orthop.*, 216, 207–212.

SAKAMOTO, K. (1986): Malignant fibrous histiocytoma induced by intra-articular injection of 9,10-dimethyl-1,2-benzanthracene in the rat. Pathological enzyme histochemical studies. . *Cancer*, 57, 2313–2322.

SALTHOUSE, T.N. and WILLIGAN, D.A. (1972): An enzyme histochemical approach to the evaluation of polymers for tissue compatability. *J.Biomed.Mater.Res.*, 6, 105, 113

SANDUSKY, G.E. Jr., CARLTON, W.W. and WIGHTMAN, K.A. (1985): Immunochistochemical staining for S-100 protein in the diagnosis of canine amelanotic melanoma. *Vet Pathol.*, 22, 577–581.

SATO, S., MURPHY, G.F., BERNHARD, J.D., MIHM, M.C. and FITZPATRICK, T.B. (1981). Ultrastructural and X ray microanalytical observations of minocycline-related hyperpigmentation of the skin *J.Invest.Dermatol.*, 77, 264–271.

SAWADA, M., TERADA, N., TANIGUCHI, H., TATEISHI, R. and MORI, Y. (1987): Cyclosporin A stimulates hair growth in nude mice. *Lab.Invest.*, 56, 684–686.

SCHAEFER, H. (1986): Percutaneous absorption of topically-applied drugs in relation to their toxicity. *Brit.J.Dermatol.*, 115, Suppl. 31, 71–75.

SCHMIDT, D. (1983): Fatal toxic epidermal necrolysis following re-exposure with phenytoin. In: J. Oxley, D. Janz and H. Meinardi (Eds.), *Chronic Toxicity of Antiepileptic Drugs*, pp. 161–167. Raven Press, New York.

SCHMITT, G.M. and SCHMIDT, S.P. (1988): The effects of different fixations for immunofluorescent and immunoperoxidase localization of factor VIII-related antigen in canine carotid artery and vascular protheses. *Histochem.J.*, 18, 351–356.

SCHWEIZER, J., LOEHRKE, H. and GOERTTLER, K. (1982): 7,12-dimethylbenz(a)anthracene/1 2–0-tetradecanoyl-phorbol-13-acetate-mediated skin irritation and promotion in male Sprague-Dawley rats. *Carcinogenesis*, 3, 785–789.

SELLS, D.M. and GIBSON, J.P. (1987): Carcinogenicity studies with medroxalol hydrochloride in rats and mice. *Toxicol.Pathol.*, 15, 457–467.

SHAH, P.V., FISHER, H.L., SUMLER, M.R., MONROE, R.J., CHERNOFF, N and HALL, L.L. (1987): Comparison of the penetration of 14 pesticides through the skin of young and adult rats. *J.Toxicol.Environ. Health*, 21, 353–366.

SHER, S.P. (1982): Tumors in control hamsters, rats and mice: Literature tabulation. *CRC Crit.Rev.Toxicol.*, 10, 49–79.

SHIMADA, S. and KATZ, S.I. (1988): The skin as an immunologic organ. *Arch.Pathol.Lab.Med.*, 112, 231–234.

SNEDDON, I.B., (1976). Atrophy of the skin. The clinical problems. *Br.J.Dermatol.*, 94, Suppl. 12, 121–123.

SOBEL, R.A. and COLVIN, R.B. (1986): Responder strain-specific enhancement of endothelial and mononuclear cell Ia in delayed hyper-sensitivity reactions in (strain 2 x strain 13) F1. guinea pigs. *J.Immunol.*, 137, 2132–2138.

SONG, P.S. and TAPLEY, K.J. Jr. (1979): Photochemistry and photobiology of psoralens. *Photochem.Photobiol.*, 29, 1177–1197.

SPENCER, A.J. (1985): Subcutaneous nodules in rhesus monkeys. *Lab.Anim.Sci.*, 25, 79–80

STANTON, M.F., LAYARD, M., TEGERIS, A., MILLER, E., MAY, M., MORGAN, E. and SMITH, A. (1981): Relation of particle dimension to carcinogenicity in amphibole asbestoses and other fibrous minerals. *J.N.C.I.*, 67, 965–975.

STEFANSKI, S.A., ELWELL, M.R. and YOSHITOMI, K. (1987): Malignant hibernoma in a Fischer 344 rat. *Lab.Anim.Sci.*, 37, 347–350.

STEINBERG, M. (1984): Dermatotoxicology test techniques: An overview In: V.A. Drill and P. Lazar (Eds), Cutaneous Toxicity, pp. 41–53. Raven Press, New York.

STËNBACK, F. (1980): Skin carcinogenesis as a model system: Observations on species, strain and tissue sensitivity to 7,12-dimethylbenz(a)anthracene with or without promotion from croton oil. *Acta Pharm.Toxicol.*, 46, 89–97.

STERN, R.S., LAIRD, N., MELSKI, J., PARRISH, J.A., FITZPATRICK, T.B. and BLEICH, H.L. (1984): Cutaneous squamous-cell carcinoma in patient treated with PUVA. *N.Engl.J.Med.*, 310, 1156–1161.

STEWART, H.L. (1979): Tumours of the soft tissues. In: V.S. Turusov (Ed.), *Pathology of Tumours in Laboratory Animals*, Vol. 2, *Tumours of the Mouse*, pp. 487–525. IARC Scientific Publ. 23, Lyon.

STINGL, G., KATZ, S.I., SHEVACH, E.M., WOLFF-SCHREINER, E. and GREEN, I. (1978): Detection of Ia antigens on Langerhans cells in guinea pig skin. *J.Immunol.*, 120, 570–578.

STREILEIN, J.W. (1985): Circuits and signals of the skin-associated lymphoid tissues (SALT). *J.Invest.Dermatol.*, 85, 10s-13s.

SUNDBERG, J.P., JUNGE, R.E. and LANCASTER, W.D. (1984): Immunoperoxidase localization of papilloma viruses in hyperplastic and neoplastic epithelial lesions of animals. *Am.J.Vet.Res.*, 45, 1441–1446.

SUNDERMAN, F.W., Jr., (1989): Carcinogenicity of metal alloys in orthopedic prostheses: Clinical and experimental studies. *Fundam.Appl.Toxicol.*, 13, 205–216.

SYLVESTER, R.K., OGDEN, W.B., DRAXLER, C.A. and LEWIS, B. (1988): Vesicular eruption: A local complication of concentrated acyclovir infusions, *J.A.M.A.*, 255, 385–386.

SUZUKI, H., NAGAI, K., YAMAKI, H., TANAKA, N. and UMEZAWA, H. (1969): On the mechanism of action of bleomycin: Scission of DNA strands in vitro and in vivo. *J.Antibiot.*, (Tokyo), 22, 446–448.

SVENSON, O. and AAES-JÖRGENSEN, T. (1979): Studies of the fate of vegetable oil after intramuscular injection into experimental animals. *Acta Pharmacol. et Toxicol.*, 45, 352–378.

SZCZECH, G.M. and TUCKER, W.E. Jr. (1985): Nail loss and footpad erosions in beagle dogs given BW 134U, a nucleoside analog. *Toxicol.Pathol.*, 13, 181–184.

TAKASHI, M and MIYAKAWA, Y. (1989): Mast cell tumor, skin, mouse. In T.C.Jones, U.Mohr and R.D. Hunt (Eds), *Integument and Mammary Glands. Monographs on Pathology of Laboratory Animals*, pp. 112–117. Springer-Verlag, Berlin.

TAMAKI, K., STINGL, G., GULLINO, M., SACHS, D.H. and KATZ, S.I. (1979): Ia antigens in mouse skin are predominantly expressed on Langerhans cells. *J.Immunol.*, 123, 784–787.

TAYLOR, D.O.N., DORN, C.R. and LUIS, O.S. (1969): Morphologic and biologic characteristics of the canine cutaneous histiocytoma. *Cancer Res.*, 29, 83–92.

THOMAS R.H.M. and BLACK M.M. (1985): Corticosteroids. In: H.I.Maibach N.J. Lowe (Eds), *Models in Dermatology*, Vol. 2, pp 30–34. Karger, Basel.

THOMPSON, G.R., BAKER, J.R., FLEISCHMAN, R.W., ROSENKRANTZ, H., SCHAEPPI, U.H., COONEY, D.A. and DAVIS, R.D. (1972): Preclinical toxicologic evaluation of bleomycin (NSC 125 006), a new antitumor antibiotic. *Toxicol.Appl.Pharmacol.*, 22, 544–555.

THORNBURG, L.P., STOW, H.D. and PICK, J.R. (1973): The pathogenesis of the alopecia due to hair chewing in mice. *Lab.Anim.Sci.*, 23, 843–850.

TSCHACHLER, E., SCHULER, G., HUTTERER, J., LEIBL, H., WOLFF K and STINGL, G (1983): Expression of Thy-1 antigen by murine epidermal cells. *J.Invest.Dermatol.*, 81, 282–285.

TUCKER, W.E. Jr., KRASNY, H.C., de MIRANDA, P., GOLDENTHAL, E.I., ELION, G.B., HAJIAN, G. and SZCZECH, G.M. (1983): Preclinical toxicology studies with acyclovir: Carcinogenicity bioassays and chronic toxicity tests. *Fundam.Appl.Toxicol.*, 3, 579–586.

VAN HOOSIER, G.L. Jr. and TRENTIN, J.J. (1979): Naturally occurring tumors of the Syrian hamster. *Prog.Exp. Tumor Res.*, 23, 1–12.

VIRTANEN, I., LEHTO, V.P., LEHTONEN, E., VARTIO, T., STENMAN, S., KURKI, P.,

WAGER, O., SMALL, J.V., DAHL, D. and BADLEY, R.A. (1981): Expression of intermediate filaments in cultured cells. *J.Cell Sci.*, 50, 45–63.

VON GIALAMUS, J., HOGER, H. and ADAMIKER, D. (1985): Spontane Hautkalzinose bei der Ratte. *Z.Versuchstierkd.*, 27, 155–162.

WALSH, K.M. and GOUGH, A.W. (1989): Hypopigmentation in dogs treated with an inhibitor of platelet aggregation. *Toxicol.Pathol.*, 17, 549–553

WARD, J.M., GOODMAN, D.G., SQUIRE, R.A., CHU, K.C. and LINHART, M.S. (1979): Neoplastic and non-neoplastic lesions in aging (C57BL/6N x C3H/HeN) F1 (B6C3F1) mice. *J.N.C.I.*, 63, 849–854.

WEIBEL, E.R. and PALADE, C.E. (1964): New cytoplasmic components in arterial endothelia. *J.Cell.Biol.*, 23, 101–112.

WEICHBROD, R.H., PATRICK, D.H., CISAR, C.F. and HALL, J.E. (1987) Diagnostic exercise: Tail sloughing in mice. *Lab.Anim.Sci.*, 37, 644–645.

WEISS, E. and FRESE, K. (1974): Tumors of the skin. *Bull W.H.O.*, 50, 79–100

WEISS, S.W. and ENZINGER, F.M. (1978): Malignant fibrous histiocytoma. An analysis of 200 cases. *Cancer*, 41, 2250–2266.

WILCOCK, B.P., YAGER, J.A. and ZINK, M.C. (1986): The morphology and behaviour of feline cutaneous mastocytomas. *Vet.Pathol.*, 23, 320–324.

WINTER, G.D. and BURTON, J.L. (1976): Experimentally induced steroid atrophy in the domestic pig and man. *Br.J.Dermatol.*, 94, Suppl. 12, 107–109.

WINTER, G.D. and WILSON, L. (1976): The effect of clobetasone butyrate and other topical steroids on skin thickness of the domestic pig. *Br.J.Dermatol.*, 94, 545–550

WOLFF, K. and STINGL, G. (1983): The Langerhans cell. *J.Invest. Dermatol.*, 80, 17s-21s.

WOOD, G.S., VOLTERRA, A.S., ABEL, E.A., NICKOLOFF, B.J. and ADAMS, R.M. (1986): Allergic contact dermatitis: Novel immunohistologic features. *J.Invest.Dermatol.*, 87, 688–693.

YANG, H., JORIS, I., MAJNO, G. and WELSH, R.M. (1985): Necrosis of adipose tissue induced by sequential injections with unrelated viruses. *Am.J.Pathol.*, 120, 173–177.

ZURCHER, C and ROHOLL, P.J.M., (1989): Melanocytic tumors, rat. In: T.C. Jones, U. Mohr and R.D. Hunt (Eds), *Integument and Mammary Glands, Monographs on Pathology of Laboratory Animals*, pp. 76–86. Springer Verlag, Berlin.

47

II. Mammary Gland

The importance of the mammary gland in preclinical drug safety evaluation is largely the result of two facts. Firstly, the mammary gland, along with uterine tissue is a highly sensitive indicator of the functional activity of the hypothalamic pituitary-gonadal axis and its histological assessment can provide important information about compounds which modulate this activity. Secondly, in many mouse and rat strains, mammary neoplasms develop spontaneously or can be induced with relative ease by hormonal manipulation. Whilst this is of great interest in experimental oncology, it creates considerable problems in the safety evaluation of therapeutic agents which, at high doses, modulate the hypothalamic-pituitary-gonadal function to give rise to accelerated development of mammary neoplasms in carcinogenicity bioassays.

Assessment of drug-induced non-neoplastic and neoplastic changes in the mammary glands is complicated by considerable species differences in hormonal regulation of mammary gland development and function, perhaps compounded by the artificial physiological state of overfed laboratory animals (Roe, 1983).

It has been suggested that because the mammary gland is a recently evolved structure limited to mammals, the endocrine control of mammary gland development and function has developed in different ways among different species. This contrasts to more primitive biological processes which have similar control systems in a wider range of mammalian and non-mammalian species. (Neumann et al., 1985)

Another important general point about the mammary gland is that like the endometrium, it represents an example of a hormone dependent gland in which generation of new epithelial architecture from undifferentiated epithelium requires a complex interaction with mesenchymal cells or mesenchymal cell products (Cunha et al., 1983)

Endocrinology

The development and function of the mammary gland is under the control of a constellation of hormones which includes the sex steroids oestrogen and progesterone, prolactin and growth hormone, insulin, catecholamines and ACTH. In rodents, prolactin appears to be the most important pituitary hormone controlling mammary gland growth where it acts in synergy with oestrogen. By contrast, in dogs growth hormone is more important where it seems to act primarily in combination with progesterone. These differences perhaps explain why mammary neoplasia develops in rodents treated with oestrogenic compounds whereas in dogs progestagens appear more tumorigenic (Neumann et al., 1985)

As in other organs, the effects of steroid hormones are thought to be mediated through high-affinity receptor proteins situated on target cells. However, receptors are located on mammary mesenchymal cells as well as epithelial elements so that the effects of steroidal hormones may be regulated to some degree by epithelial stromal interactions (Cunha et al., 1983).

The pituitary gland contains several other hormones which act on the mammary gland and the relative roles and mechanism by which they affect normal and abnormal mammary growth are not only poorly understood but probably differ between experimental species and man. (Kleinberg, 1987)

It has also been shown that the mammary gland responds to catecholamines. In the rat, mammary tissues possess functional β-adrenergic receptors which have specificity and affinity characteristics similar to those found in other tissues. (Lavandero, 1985)

Anatomy

The basic microscopic anatomy of the resting mammary gland is similar among laboratory animals. It is composed of a system of alveolar buds or acini connected by a system of branching ducts to the main ducts which converge on the nipple.

The morphological details are less consistent between species and strains. Duct and alveolar tissues are not static structures but respond to hormonal changes of the oestrous cycle, pregnancy and lactation as well as those which accompany aging, changes in diet and environmental conditions.

The *rat* possesses six pairs of mammary glands. Glandular tissue of the resting mammary gland of the young virgin rat is composed of branching fine ductules, terminal end buds and alveolar buds within a connective tissue stroma embedded in adipose tissue. The primary proliferative compartment in the developing mammary gland of the rat is believed to be the terminal end bud which differentiates into the so-called alveolar bud and eventually into alveoli to form the lobule (Russo and Russo, 1980). This compartment is under the control of oestrogen and progesterone and the development of the terminal end bud to a lobular alveolar structure reflects the degree of serum prolactin, oestrogen and progesterone surges during the oestrous cycle (Sanz et al., 1988)

Ducts and ductules are lined by one or two layers of cuboidal epithelium surrounded by a layer of myoepithelial cells invested by basement membrane (Warburton et al., 1982). The long axes of myoepithelial cells are located at right

49

angles to those of epithelial cells and they are difficult to visualize in standard haematoxylin and eosin stained sections.

On the basis of immunocytochemical work using antibodies to cytokeratins and surface markers, Dulbecco and colleagues (1986) have demonstrated that some basal cells of rat mammary gland epithelium retain characteristics of primitive cells. They have suggested that these cells represent the pluripotential epithelial cell population which gives rise to differentiated epithelial and myoepithelial cells.

Immunocytochemical studies using antisera to myosin and prekeratin have shown that myoepithelial cells form a continuous layer around the epithelial cells in the resting mammary gland of the virgin rat (Warburton et al., 1982). Ultrastructural examination shows that myoepithelial cells contain only sparse amounts of myofilaments and poorly formed desmosomes in the resting gland (Joshi et al., 1986).

By about the fifth day of gestation, terminal end buds become replaced by alveolar buds and distinct alveoli. On the tenth day almost all the gland is composed of alveoli arranged in a lobular manner. There is a concurrent increase in the number of cytoplasmic ribosomes and lipid droplets which can be visualised at ultrastructural level. With the onset of lactation, alveoli become distended by lipid-rich secretions and glandular cells lose lipid droplets and develop abundant rough endoplasmic reticulum. Myoepithelial cells become stretched over the glandular cells and show increased numbers of cytoplasmic myofilaments and pinocytotic vesicles. (Joshi et al., 1986).

Using tritiated thymidine and immunocytochemical markers for keratin and actin, Joshi and colleagues (1986) demonstrated that the peak proliferative activity in both glandular and myoepithelial cells occurs at about day five of gestation with a smaller peak involving alveolar epithelium early in lactation. As pregnancy progresses myoepithelial cell division declines to insignificant levels as these cells acquire more abundant cytoplasmic filaments for their contractile function during lactation.

It is important to note that the degree of stromal fibroblast and vascular proliferation during pregnancy parallels that of the epithelial and myoepithelial cells. At the end of gestation pale-staining dendritic cells also show marked thymidine labelling, presumably a reflection of their proliferactive activity in preparation for their immunological role in lactation.

Three types of epithelial cell have been recognised in the adult rat (and human) mammary gland. These are light or clear cells, dark cells and intermediate cells (Ozzello., 1971, Russo et al., 1983). They are visualised best in semithin sections or by ultrastructural study. Dark cells are the smallest with dark electron dense cytoplasm, oval dark nuclei, moderate numbers of mitochondria, some rough endoplasmic reticulum, abundant ribosomes, well developed Golgi and numerous lipid droplets and secretory vacuoles. Intermediate cells show round or oval nuclei, moderately electron dense cytoplasm, numerous cytoplasmic organelles especially mitochondria but few lipid droplets. Light cells are the largest cells processing round nuclei, abundant electron-lucent cytoplasm, moderate numbers of mitochondria but little lipid (Russo et al., 1983).

Although the mammary glands of *mice* are arranged in five pairs, similar light and microscopic changes are found in the resting gland and during pregnancy and lactation (Rhodin 1974; Squartini 1979). As in the rat gland, immuno-cytochemical study of mouse mammary tissue using antisera to cell surface markers, basement membrane protein and cytokeratins has demonstrated the presence of several subtypes of epithelial cells, myoepithelial cells and a population of pluripotential basal cells (Sonnenberg et al., 1986).

Analogous, although less pronounced changes have also been described during the normal mouse oestrous cycle. During pro-oestrus, ducts and buds remain fairly poorly developed but during oestrus proliferative changes occur in the ductular epithelium and stroma. Usually marked lobular development of alveoli does not occur unless pregnancy supervenes although species and strain dif-ferencies in the degree of these changes in the oestrous cycle occur. (Squartini, 1979).

The cyclical changes which occur in the oestrous cycle in the beagle dog were characterised in a study based on histological examination of mammary tissue, ovaries and uterus in 40 females aged nine months to three years (Nelson and Kelly, 1974). The immature gland contains only rudimentary ductular struc-tures. Mild ductal and periductal stromal proliferation occurs in proestrus. In oestrus, ductal proliferation is more marked and ducts become better differenti-ated and lined by a single or two layers of epithelial cells. The stroma exhibits increased cellularity and interstitial oedema.

Early budding of alveolar structures characterised by small groups of epi-thelial buds arising from ductal structures are observed in early metoestrous. Alveolar proliferation becomes more marked and associated with slight secretion in metoestrous (60–90 days after oestrous) but subsequently this proliferation diminishes with involution of alveolar structures with further generalised involu-tion occurring in the anoestral phase (Nelson and Kelly, 1974).

The gross anatomy of the human mammary gland and that of non-human primates is quite similar. Study of the rhesus monkey has shown one pair of pectoral mammary glands although unlike the human gland the glandular tissue as more diffusely spread as a thin subcutaneous layer over the anterior chest wall and upper abdomen.

The histology of the normal resting human breast and the mammary gland of non-human primate is also similar and an identical terminology for the mammary duct system can be applied to both the human and rhesus monkey mammary gland (Ohuchi et al., 1986; Tavassoli et al., 1988). So called *ductules* (acini) open into *intralobular terminal ducts* which in turn connect to *extralobular ducts* and eventually *larger ducts*. The ductules and the terminal duct system are called the *terminal duct lobular unit*. Immunocytochemical study has shown that normal human mammary epithelium located in terminal duct lobular units demonstrates higher levels of ras p21 expression than that of the large ducts (Ohuchi et al., 1986). This is of interest because it has been suggested that the terminal duct lobular units of the human mammary gland (and the terminal end buds of the rat gland) contain the epithelial cell population which gives rsie to mammary carcinoma (Russo et al., 1982; Ohuchi et al., 1986).

The mammary changes which follow the natural alterations in endogeneous hormones in the oestrous and reproductive cycles form a baseline for the evaluation of the histological alterations which occur following administration of synthetic sex steroids and other xenobiotics which alter the hypothalamic-pituitary-gonadal axis.

Other important cells in the mammary gland include lymphoid cells. Mammary glands represent part of the mucosal immune system, important in the formation of immunological components of breast milk (Slade and Schwartz, 1987). Characterisation of cell surface markers of lymphoid cells in normal mammary glands of mice have shown that T cells (Thy 1.2 positive), are more common than B cells and that the helper subtype (L3T4 positive) forms a larger proportion than suppressor/cytotoxic T cells (Lyt 2 positive cells) (Wei et al., 1986). T cells have been shown to increase in number in favour of suppressor/cytotoxic T cell populations in preneoplastic and neoplastic states in mammary glands of both mouse and man (Wei et al., 1986).

Cytochemistry and immunocytochemistry

Immunocytochemical techniques used in the assessment of the mammary gland in man and laboratory animals have been alluded to previously. These include immunocytochemical staining of intermediate filaments, particularly cytokeratins for the study of glandular development, myofilaments, collagen type IV and laminin for basement membrane characterization, type I collagen and fibronectin as connective tissue markers and cytoplasmic milk fat globule membrane antigen (Warburton et al., 1982; Sonnenberg et al., 1986; Dulbecco et al., 1986; Molinolo et al., 1987).

Classical enzyme cytochemical techniques also have a place in the study of the mammary gland notably ATPase. Myoepithelial cells are characterised by a positive Na^+ K^+ ATPase reaction whereas epithelial cells show a positive reaction for Mg^{++} ATPase and are negative for Na^+ K^+ ATPase (Russo et al., 1982).

Another technique of application in the study of the mammary gland in man, rat and mouse is the demonstration of glycosylated cell components using lectin histochemistry (Vierbuchen et al., 1981; Walker 1984; Mori et al., 1986). Peanut lectin with affinity for βD-gal(1–3)gal NAc (see Digestive System 1, Chapter VII) appears to be particularly useful in the study of the rodent gland. Peanut lectin binding sites have been shown to be modulated by hormones in the rat mammary gland. Ovariectomy reduces the number of sites and administration of oestrogens increases them (Vierbuchen et al., 1981).

Mammary gland enlargement

Whereas mammary gland enlargement is frequently the result of pathological states particularly hyperplasia and neoplasia, drug-treatment may produce an increase in mammary gland size in a way analogous to the physiological changes seen in pregnancy or lactation.

Diffuse increase in mammary gland size accompanied by *lactation* have been described in rats, guinea pigs or rabbits treated with agents which influence hypothalamic function such as reserpine, phenothiazine derivatives, chlordiazepoxide (Librium) and haloperidol (Meites, 1957; Khazan et al., 1981; Leuschner et al., 1981).

Cystic change, cystic degeneration, 'milk cysts', galactocele, duct ectasia

Dilatation of ducts of ductules (acini) may occur in the mammary glands with or without evidence of epithelial proliferation. The lumina of dilated ducts contain proteinaceous eosinophilic material, lipid and scattered macrophages. Concentrically laminated, eosinophilic bodies or corpora amylacea found in dilated ducts in the rat mammary gland have been shown to possess histochemical and ultrastructural features of amyloid fibrils (Beems et al., 1978).

Cystic change is presumably the result of cyclical hormone-modulated activity with incomplete and uneven regression possibly a result of excessive hormone stimulation or an exaggerated response of unusually sensitive mammary tissue. For this reason, cystic change in the mammary gland of animals treated with xenobiotics may indicate an effect on the hypothalamic-pituitary-gonadal axis. The most striking examples of this phenomenon are found in studies with oral contraceptive steroids. Enhanced secretory activity and cystic dilatation of mammary ducts was reported in both male and female Sprague-Dawley rats and rhesus monkeys treated for long periods with the combination contraceptive steroid norlestrin (Schardein et al., 1970; Fitzgerald et al., 1982) or its oestrogenic or progestogenic components (Schardein et al 1980, a, b). It is nevertheless important to note that cystic dilatation of mammary ducts can occur spontaneously in aging rats where it may be associated with mammary gland hyperplasia and metaplasia (Barsoum et al., 1984). When cystic change is observed in the mammary gland of treated laboratory animals, it is important to record the degree of any hyperplasia of mammary glandular tissue which may be present.

Hyperplasia

A variety of different hyperplastic states are described in the mammary glands of laboratory animals and man. Although there are undoubtably species and strain differences in the histological characteristics of mammary hyperplasia, assessment is confounded by lack of consistent terminology. Terms such as epitheliosis, adenosis and lobular hyperplasia have been borrowed from human medicine where they are commonly applied to quite specific lesions and they may be used differently in veterinary pathology (see Hampe and Misdorp, 1974). Conversely, terms such as 'hyperplastic alveolar nodules' and 'pregnancy responsive tumours' have been coined specifically for use in experimental mouse mammary cancer models and may be quite misleading to medical reviewers not having detailed knowledge of the mouse mammary gland. Added to this is the common difficulty of histological classification, the greater the number of categories, the more they tend to overlap and the less reproducible they become.

Although hyperplasia of the mammary gland frequently occurs in man and animals in the presence of other changes including cystic change, fibrosis and atrophy, it is important to pay special attention to the degree and nature of mammary hyperplasia which occurs in preclinical safety studies. Some proliferative conditions have been associated with the development of mammary cancer in laboratory animals and the degree and nature of the proliferative component in human benign breast disease has also been recognised as an important risk factor for the development of mammary cancer (Page et al., 1985; Hutter, 1985).

Epithelial hyperplasia of the mammary gland can be divided into two main histological types, although mixed forms occur. The first type, characterised by epithelial proliferation within the extralobular ducts, is referred to as *duct hyperplasia (epitheliosis or papillomatosis*. The second type, is epithelial proliferation in the intralobular ductules (acini) and is termed *lobular hyperplasia*.

Duct hyperplasia

Duct hyperplasia is defined as the presence of increased numbers of epithelial layers (usually three or more) above the duct basement membrane. This form of hyperplasia has been best characterised in the human female breast where the terms *epitheliosis* or *papillomatosis* are also used. However, these terms epitheliosis and papillomatosis are not uniformly employed by pathologists. Usually epitheliosis refers to 'solid' hyperplasia in the ducts and papillomatosis to hyperplasia with papillary characteristics. Basement membrane immunocytochemistry using antibodies to type IV collagen may be useful in the distinction of the two types because papillary stalks are outlined well by this method (Willebrand et al., 1986).

Proliferating cells form focal, solid, cribriform or papillary structures within the duct lumen. These lesions show variable degrees of cellular atypia and mitotic activity but unless these features are marked, a benign diagnosis is usually preferred. Nevertheless, it needs to be remembered it has been recently shown that the presence or absence of cellular atypia is one of the most important histological features of human benign breast disease in the assessment of risk for developing mammary carcinoma (Dupont and Page, 1985).

Almost identical forms of duct hyperplasia with cellular atypia have been described in the mammary glands of rhesus monkeys teated with sex steroids. The study by Tavassoli and colleagues (1988) have demonstrated that similar criteria for the semiquantitative analysis used in the assessment of hyperplasia of the human breast are also applicable to the non-human primate model.

The degree of hyperplasia in the hormone-treated rhesus monkey was divided into four main groups, minimal, mild, moderate and severe hyperplasia:

Minimal duct hyperplasia

It was shown that the earliest indicator of epithelial proliferation in ducts of rhesus monkeys was characterised by loss of secretion, increased cellular basophilia, mild increase in the nuclear-cytoplasmic ratio and stratification of cells to three or four rather than the normal two layers. This minimal degree of duct hyperplasia is sometimes found in untreated control monkeys.

Mild duct hyperplasia

As the degree of hyperplasia increased it was associated with increasing atypia and the formation of epithelial tufts and micropapillae composed of monomorphic, rounded cells.

Moderate duct hyperplasia

Moderate degrees of epithelial proliferation were characterised by epithelial tufts, micropapillae and bridges of a degree comparable to *atypical hyperplasia* of the human mammary gland.

Severe duct hyperplasia

Severe changes were characterised by atypical micropapillary and cribriform growth patterns within the ducts, identical to the so-called *intraduct carcinomas* of the human gland. In the study by Tavassoli et al (1988) moderate and marked duct hyperplasias were only found in monkeys treated for 10 years with various synthetic oral contraceptives, raising the possibility of a carcinogenic effect of these agents when given at high doses to non-human primates.

Although proliferative duct lesions occur in the mammary glands of dogs and rodents, they are less well characterised in these species and it is not clear whether they are the exact counterparts of the hyperplastic duct lesions in man or non-human primates.

Intraduct epitheliosis and papillomatosis are found in dogs, although Hampe and Misdorp (1974) have suggested that these changes normally do not show the cellular atypia of analogous lesions in man.

Papillary and cystadenomatous intraduct proliferations are observed to arise spontaneously in aged rats and mice (Barsoum et al., 1984), although their relationship to the development of mammary neoplasia is less certain. Studies of mammary cancer development in the DMBA treated rat (see below) have suggested that early lesions which precede mammary carcinomas are intraduct hyperplasias occurring in the terminal end bud region and composed of six to ten epithelial cell layers (Russo et al., 1982).

Lobular hyperplasia

Hyperplasia of the intralobular ductules is usually termed lobular hyperplasia. In the human mammary gland, lobular hyperplasia is divided into two main histological types. One type results in an increase in the number of ductules in the lobule which is frequently referred to *adenosis*. The second type is a proliferation of epithelial cells within the intralobular ductule without an increase in the number of ductular profiles in the tissue section. The term *atypical lobular hyperplasia* is used to designate intralobular hyperplasia of the latter type in which the cells show atypical cytological feature but not of a degree of proliferation and expansion to merit the diagnosis of lobular carcinoma 'in situ'. Identical forms of proliferative lobular hyperplasia with and without cellular atypia have also been described in the mammary glands of rhesus monkeys treated for long periods with oral contraceptive steroids (Tavassoli et al., 1989).

Hyperplasia of the cells of the mammary lobular epithelium appears to be a more common phenomenon among laboratory rodents and beagle dogs than intraduct lesions. Histologically, these forms of lobular hyperplasia frequently resemble an inappropriate, exaggerated or focal physiological response similar to that found in pregnancy or lactation.

In dogs, lobular hyperplasia of the mammary gland is a well-documented phenomenon where it comprises an increase in the number of ductules similar to adenosis in man (Hampe and Misdorp, 1974). Epithelial proliferation may also be localised to pre-existing ductules. However, Hampe and Misdorp (1974) suggested that this form of lobular hyperplasia showed a much more uniform growth pattern and regular cytological features than this type of hyperplasia in the human female breast. They suggested that no conclusion could be reached with respect to its relationship to the development of mammary carcinoma. More recently lobular proliferation was found to develop one or two years earlier than mammary carcinoma in a large colony of beagle dogs (Moulton et al., 1986).

Burek (1978) described lobular hyperplasia in the mammary gland of aging Brown Norway and Wistar derived rat strains. This conditions was characterised by multifocal proliferation and increased secretion in acinar tissue, associated with dilatation of mammary ducts. This change occurred in nearly all aging females in his study despite considerable strain differences in the number of pituitary tumours. This lack of correlation with pituitary adenomas suggested that there was no direct relationship between the development of pituitary adenomas and mammary gland hyperplasia.

The hyperplastic alveolar nodule is also a form of lobular hyperplasia which occurs in high incidence in mammary cancer susceptible mouse strains harbouring milk-transmitted mammary tumour virus (MTV-positive).

Histologically, alveolar nodules are composed of groups of alveoli of variable size lined by a single layer of small basophilic cells showing variable mitotic and secretory activity. The lumens of the alveoli are frequently empty but they may also be distended by eosinophilic, PAS-positive secretions. These hyperplastic alveoli are surrounded by an increased amount of connective tissue with little or no inflammation. The lesions may be single or multiple but show no particular site of predilection in sensitive mouse strains (Squartini, 1979).

Although in experimental cancer models using mammary tumour virus bearing mice (MTV-positive) transformation appears to proceed through a stage of hyperplastic alveolar nodule formation, the evidence that all hyperplastic alveolar nodules should be considered preneoplastic is less convincing.

Hyperplastic alveolar nodules have morphologically more in common with localised forms of exaggerated physiological hyperplasia of the alveoli than the more atypical forms of lobular hyperplasia described in the non-human primate and man. This morphological resemblance to normal tissue is mirrored by their cytochemical characteristics. For instance, histochemical study of peanut lectin binding, usually considered to reflect the degree of differentiation and secretory function of normal and neoplastic mammary gland is similar in hyperplastic alveolar nodules and normal mouse mammary tissue but dissimilar to that of neoplastic mammary cells (Mori et al., 1986).

The relationship of the development of hyperplastic alveolar nodules to the presence of the mammary tumour virus is not clear. The transformation of the mouse mammary gland by the virus is a complex multistep process and a recent study of mammary tumour virus has shown that the virus is only one of two or more cooperating factors required to mediate transformation (Slagle et al., 1987). The hyperplastic alveolar nodules are also hormone-dependent and it has been suggested that the presence of the virus may increase the hormone sensitivity of the normal mammary gland (Squartini, 1979).

Hyperplastic nodules do not develop exclusively in MTV-positive mouse strains. In the study of MTV-positive and MTV-negative C3H mice by Highman and colleagues (1980), hyperplastic alveolar nodules developed spontaneously in both strains, although more commonly in MTV-positive animals. More interestingly was the fact that high doses diethylstilboestrol increased the incidence of hyperplastic alveolar nodules in both strains but not the incidence of adenocarcinoma in the MTV-negative strain.

The similar term, hyperplastic alveolar nodule has also been applied to proliferative alveolar lesions occurring in the mammary gland of carcinogen treated rats (see review by Young and Hallowes, 1973).

Mammary neoplasia

Although there is an immense body of information about experimental mammary neoplasia, it is often quite difficult to directly apply this information to the interpretation of treatment-related group differences in the prevalence of mammary neoplasia in drug safety studies. Much of the experimental data relates to neoplasms induced in rodents over short periods by powerful genotoxic carcinogens such as 7,12 dimethylbenz(a)anthracene (DMBA) whereas in drug safety assessment mammary neoplasms usually occur after longer periods in rodents already predisposed to the development of mammary neoplasms spontaneously with advancing age. Furthermore, spontaneous rodent mammary neoplasms are notorious for their variability in prevalence in control animals. Their prevalence may vary with time and between studies conducted at the same time in identical strains housed in the same laboratory under similar conditions. A further difficulty lies in the histological classification of mammary neoplasms. Not only is the classification applied to mammary tumours different between rodent and non-rodent species but also between pathologists studying the same species.

Classification

Considerable caution needs to be exercised in the categorisation of experimental mammary tumours and an over rigid application of detailed classifications is to be avoided. It has to be remembered that the various classifications applied to mammary tumours are based primarily on histological appearances rather than histogenesis. This is true for the various diagnostic categories of human mammary carcinomas (World Health Organisation, 1981), although unlike most experimental mammary neoplasms these categories have considerable significance to the physician in terms of potential biological behaviour, treatment and prognosis by virtue of many years of accumulated clinical experience.

Some authors have taken the view that the classification used for human mammary neoplasms is equally applicable to rodent neoplasms. The histological study of Barsoum and colleagues (1984) showed that there were common histological features between spontaneous mammary neoplasms in the Wistar rat and those in man and that the World Health Organisation (1981) classification of human tumours was also applicable to rat neoplasms. The risk of this approach is that rigid application of a classification of human neoplasms may lead to erroneous conclusions about biological behaviour of neoplasms in an animal species.

Others have taken the converse view, that rat mammary neoplasms bear so little histological resemblance to mammary tumours in man that a quite different classification is essential (Komitowski et al., 1982). For instance, a quite unique classification for mouse mammary tumours has also been devised by Dunn (1959) and later revised (Sass and Dunn, 1979). Even here, the categories are essentially descriptive in nature and frequently relate to a particular rodent strain or tumour model. Terms such as adenocarcinoma type A or B can be quite incomprehensible in an environment of drug safety evaluation where many reviewers are well-versed in human but not mouse pathology.

The tendency therefore in drug safety evaluation is to adopt a relatively simple classification, based on the common broad categories used in the pathological diagnosis of human tumours, notably benign and malignant neoplasms showing glandular, stromal or mixed glandular and stromal differentiation. In view of the close epithelial-stromal interactions which are important in mammary tissue (Cunha et al., 1983) it is perhaps not surprising that a considerable proportion of mammary neoplasias contain both epithelial and mesenchymal components.

Fibroadenoma

This is one of the most common categories of mammary neoplasms in many strains of rats. Fibroadenomas are characteristically well-delineated, lobulated or nodular masses composed of poorly cellular collageneous connective tissue interspersed with epithelial elements (Figs. 9 and 10). Epithelial elements comprise variable branching ducts lined by simple or stratified epithelium. Ducts sometimes contain eosinophilic secretions or concentric concretions similar to those found in other mammary conditions (Beems et al., 1978). Some glandular elements show compression by connective tissue components giving rise to typical intracanalicular or pericanalicular patterns seen in fibroadenomas found in women. Aggregates of vacuolated cells of acinar type are also found within rat fibroadenomas.

Although less common and less well recognised, fibroadenomas are also occasionally found in small numbers in the mammary gland of the ageing mouse, including strains commonly employed in drug safety evaluation (Haseman et al., 1984).

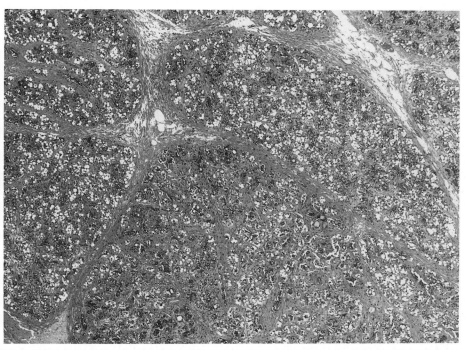

Fig. 9. Fibroadenoma from a 24-month-old female Sprague-Dawley rat showing a lobulated glandular pattern and fibrous septa. (He, ×50.)

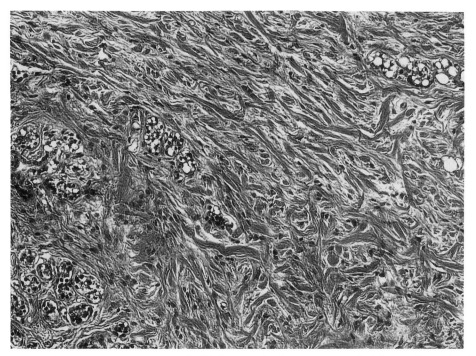

Fig. 10. Fibroadenoma from a 24-month-old Sprague-Dawley rat composed of dense collagen bands and small glandular remnants. (HE, ×200.)

Adenoma

Adenoma is a convenient term applied to a wide range of exclusively glandular neoplasms of the mammary gland in rodents which remain localised and show none of the histological and cytological features of malignancy. By definition, they are well demarcated from surrounding tissues by a connective tissue capsule or compressed non-neoplastic parenchyma with no evidence of local invasion. Tumour cells show low degrees of cellular pleomorphism and mitotic activity. Stroma is usually limited to fine strands of connective tissue forming a delicate supporting network. The glandular tissue is composed of a single or double layer of duct type epithelium or an orderly arrangement of cells acinar type. When the glandular epithelium is papillary in nature and localised within the duct lumen, the term, *intraduct papilloma* is usually used.

Adenomas are found in the mammary glands of both rats and mice used in carcinogenicity bioassays (Faccini et al., 1981; Schardein et al., 1970; Barsoum et al., 1984; Maita et al., 1988), although they are not termed adenomas in the classification of mouse mammary neoplasms of Dunn (1959).

Fibroma

The fibroma is occasionally reported in rats where it commonly represents a fibroadenoma in which there is attenuation and atrophy of the epithelial component (Barsoum et al., 1984). Histologically, this neoplasm is characterised by the presence of variable mixtures of active fibroblasts and thick collagen bands in which hyalinisation and mineralisation are common focal features. Residual normal mammary tissue may be found within these neoplasms (Barsoum et al., 1984).

Intraduct papilloma

These neoplasms represent proliferative papillary neoplasms which develop and remain localised within the ducts of mammary tissue. Papillary fronds are covered by one or two layers of fairly uniform cuboidal, duct-like cells which may show cytoplasmic vacuolation. The affected duct (or ducts) is usually dilated and lined by attenuated epithelium.

Carcinoma

In both rats and mice mammary carcinomas induced by xenobiotics as well as those arising spontaneously are usually well-differentiated adenocarcinomas which infiltrate local tissues but uncommonly produce distant metastasis. This contrasts with the common infiltrating ductal or lobular carcinomas of women which frequently infiltrate local lymph nodes and eventually produce distant metastatic deposits. However, the difference in metastatic potential may not always be quite so marked as some reported incidences suggest. Maita and colleagues (1988) reported an incidence of distant metastases, mostly to the lung in 14 out of 59 (23.7%) of spontaneous mammary carcinomas in CD-1 mice used as controls in two year carcinogenicity bioassays.

Nevertheless, the combination of well-differentiated histological appearances and relatively low-grade malignant potential make the separation of benign from malignant mammary neoplasms in rodents one of the main diagnostic difficulties.

Helpful histological features are the presence of multilayered glandular components, back to back arrangement of ducts and acini glands being separated, by only scantly stroma, cellular and nuclear pleomorphism, prominant mitotic activity and infiltration of local normal tissues. The latter feature is not without diagnostic difficulties as these neoplasms tend to expand in a manner more analogous to endocrine neoplasms rather than the infiltrating growth patterns commonly seen in human mammary cancer. It is of course axiomatic that for an adequate assessment of local tissue invasion, sufficient tissue sections with tumour margins are examined.

A variety of histological patterns are observed in mammary adenocarcinomas developing in the rat (Figs. 11 and 12). Frequently, extensive histological examination reveals mixed cellular appearances in single neoplasms so there seems generally little merit in defining separate subtypes of adenocarcinoma in routine carcinogenicity bioassays performed in the rat. Papillary, cribiform tubular, cystic and tubular glandular patterns are all seen. A lobular pattern similar to that observed in man appears also to be occasionally observed in the rat (Prejean et al., 1973; Barsoum et al., 1984). Poorly differentiated or anaplastic forms are also sometimes found. Various types of metaplastic alterations are also observed in otherwise unremarkable adenocarcinomas. These include squamous metaplasia (adenosquamous carcinoma, adenoacanthoma,) spindle cell differentiation (myoepithelioma or carcinosarcoma) and rarely other forms of mesenchymal differentiation such as cartilaginous or osseous metaplasia (Majeed and Gopinath, 1984).

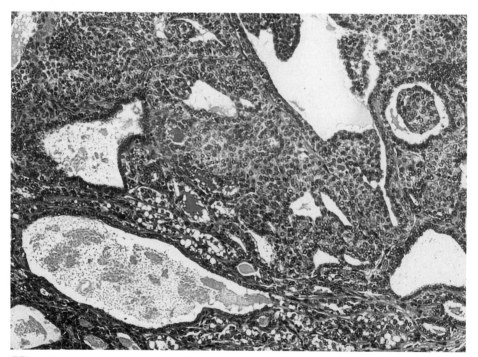

Fig. 11. Mammary gland adenocarcinoma in an aged, female Sprague-Dawley rat showing a glandular and myoepithelial pattern. (HE, ×200.)

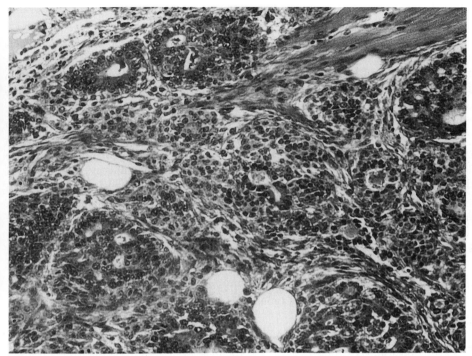

Fig. 12. Mammary adenocarcinoma in an aged, female Sprague-Dawley rat. This field shows a cribriform pattern and neoplastic glands infiltrating skeletal muscle and adjacent connective tissue (HE, ×260.)

Mammary carcinoma: mouse

In mouse mammary carcinomas a wide range of histological patterns are observed, the prevalence of each type dependent on strain and the presence or absence of the mammary tumour virus (MTV). These different patterns have been used to divide mammary adenocarcinomas of the mouse into a number of separate subtypes (Dunn, 1959, Sass and Dunn, 1979) although it is not common practice to apply this detailed classification to the diagnosis of mammary carcinomas in mouse strains employed in the assessment of carcinogenic potential of therapeutic agents.

Mouse mammary carcinomas, showing acinar differentiation, termed *type A* by Dunn, (1959) are characterised by the presence of acini lined by a single layer of cells sometimes showing secretory activity. This type appears to be more common in the CH3 MTV-positive strain than in a similar strain with a low titre to the virus (Highman et al., 1980). Pleomorphic, tubular, papillary, solid or comedo forms of adenocarcinoma, are usually termed *type B* (Squire et al., 1978).

Other patterns described include tubular and branching glandular structures (*Y type*) and a 'lace like' appearance of glandular cells with cytoplasmic vacuoles, luminal projections and a scanty fibrovascular stroma termed *type L* (Sass and Dunn, 1979).

As in the rat, some mouse mammary adenocarcinomas show squamous metaplasia. This category comprises neoplasms similar to typical adenosquamous carcinomas of the rat as well as the so-called pale cell carcinoma or *type P*. The pale cell carcinoma is a hormone-dependent neoplasm first described in the GR mouse strain (van Nie and Dux, 1971). Histologically, it is composed of cords, solid nests or islands of large pale eosinophilic cells with round or oval nuclei interspersed with clusters of basophilic cells containing oval nuclei and scanty cytoplasm. A characteristic feature is the radial arrangement of basophilic cells around cystic spaces (Sass and Dunn 1979). Ultrastructural study has shown that both the basophilic and pale cells are similar in nature, although pale cells more commonly show large desmosomes, aggregates of tonofilaments and keratohyaline granules (Strum, 1981).

Mammary carcinoma: hamster

In contrast to rats and mice mammary neoplasms are particularly uncommon in Syrian hamsters, although carcinomas are occasionally reported (Sher, 1982).

Mammary carcinoma: dog

A similar range of histological features can be recognised in dog mammary neoplasms including those in beagles. They represent one of the most common tumour categories in aged animals. (Hampe and Misdorp, 1974; Fowler et al., 1974; Frese 1985, Moulton et al., 1986). Tumour patterns which are seen in man such as lobular and scirrhous carcinoma are notable types in dogs although mixed epithelial and mesenchymal neoplasms are more common subtypes than in man (Frese, 1985).

Mammary carcinoma: primates

Such data that exists suggests that mammary carcinomas in non-human primates show a similar range of histological appearances to those found in mammary carcinomas in women and are also liable to develop metastic deposits in lymph nodes, liver and lungs (Squire et al., 1978). Histological appearances identical to those of intralobular 'in situ' carcinoma found in women have also been described in the mammary gland of rhesus monkeys treated for long periods with oral contraceptive steroids (Tavassoli et al., 1988).

Factors affecting development and growth of mammary neoplasms

A great variety of factors have been shown to modulate the develoment and growth of rat mammary neoplasms induced by the genotoxic carcinogens 7,12-dimethylbenzanthracene (DMBA), 3-methylcholanthrene (MCA), and methyl-nitrosourea (MNU). The carcinogen-induced rat mammary carcinoma, employing mostly DMBA, is the standard model for human breast cancer for which there is a large data base (see review by Welsch, 1985). Although these carcinogen-induced neoplasms are not always the exact counterparts of the mammary neoplasms observed in aged rodents in many carcinogenicity bioassays, it is important to be aware that many of our concepts of mammary cancer are based on the study of these models.

Studies of carcinogen-induced mammary neoplasms have shown that hormones of the anterior pituitary and ovary are key factors in neoplastic development and subsequent tumour growth, although the interactions of these hormones are complex. Hypophysectomy, pituitary stalk section, administration of anti-pituitary hormone antiserum and drugs which suppress pituitary function have all been shown to inhibit the development and growth of carcinogen-induced rat mammary carcinomas (Pierpaoli and Sorkin 1972; Welsch et al., 1973; Welsch, 1985). The mechanisms by which these hormones influence the growth of carcinogen-induced mammary carcinoma is not entirely clear although mammary tumour cells have been shown to possess receptors for prolactin, oestrogen and progesterone (Welsh, 1985).

Among pituitary hormones, the importance of prolactin in the carcinogen-induced rat tumour models has been demonstrated by numerous workers, who have shown that suppression of prolactin secretion by ergot alkaloids, ergoline derivatives or antiprolactin serum cause inhibition of tumour growth (Welsch, 1985). It is pertinent to note however that whereas elevation of prolactin may enhance growth of existing mammary carcinomas in these rat models, it has also been shown that an excess or deficiency of prolactin around the time of carcinogen administration can inhibit tumour development (Meites, 1980).

Ovarian steroids are also important modulators of the growth and development of carcinogen-induced mammary neoplasms in the rat. Oophorectomy, administration of antioestrogens such as tamoxifen and inhibitors of steroidogenesis have been shown to produce significant suppression of the development and growth of carcinogen-induced neoplasms (Nicholson and Golder, 1975; Jordan, 1976, Levin et al., 1976; Welsch, 1985).

Whereas moderate doses of oestrogens enhance growth of DMBA-induced rat carcinogens in the presence of an intact pituitary gland (Sterental et al., 1963), high doses of oestrogen have been shown to inhibit tumour development or growth, although this inhibition can be particularly overcome by the administration of prolactin (Meites et al., 1971). The effects of progesterone has been less well studied but work by Jabara and colleagues has shown that moderate doses of progesterone are also capable of enhancing carcinogen-induced tumorigenesis in the rat, particularly when given together with oestrogens (Jabara, 1967; Jabara et al., 1973).

The hormonal milieu which accompanies pregnancy, pseudo-pregnancy and lactation has also been shown to influence the growth of mammary carcinoma in the rat. Pregnancy and pseudo-pregnancy appear to accelerate the growth of carcinogen-induced mammary cancer in the rat, presumably by increasing the secretory rates of oestrogen and progesterone as well as prolactin (Sakamota et al., 1979). The reduction of mammary tumour growth which has been reported during lactation despite high levels of prolactin is possibly a result of deficiency of oestrogen and progesterone or increased adrenocortical activity (McCormick and Moon., 1967; Aylsworth et al., 1979; Sakamota et al., 1979).

The inhibitory effect of androgens on carcinogen-induced rat mammary tumours has been clearly demonstrated in intact rats. Although adrenocortical steroids can also influence the development of mammary cancer they do not appear to be a requirment for progressive growth of these neoplasms (Welsch, 1985).

Lesions of the median eminence, hypothalamic oestrogen implants and drugs which act on the hypothalamus also influence the development of carcinogen-induced mammary cancer. Drugs which tend to decrease hypothalamic dopaminergic activity such as reserpine, perphenazine, sulpiride, fluphenazine, methyldopa, pimozide, α-methylparatyrosine and haloperidol enhance the development of growth of mammary carcinomas after carcinogen administration. By contrast, administration of dopamine agonists such as L-dopa, iproniazid, pargyline, piribedil as well as ergot alkaloids and ergoline derivatives inhibit the development of growth of carcinogen induced mammary carcinomas (Welsch, 1985). It is possible that these treatments mediate their effects via prolactin since agents which increase hypothalamic dopaminergic activity also decrease serum prolactin levels and drugs which decrease dopaminergic activity increase serum prolactin (Welsch and Nagasawa, 1977).

Other factors which have been shown to increase the development or growth of carcinogen-induced mammary carcinomas in rats include insulin (Cohen and Hilf, 1974; Hilf et al., 1978) and high levels of dietary (unsaturated) fat (Welsch and Aylsworth, 1983). Underfeeding, administration of retinoids, selenium and antioxidants such as butylated hydroxytoluene (BHT) and butylated hydroxyanisol (BHA) have all been shown to reduce mammary carcinogenesis induced by DMBA in the rat (Ip 1981; Sylvester et al., 1982; McCormick et al., 1980, 1984).

Studies in which the mammary changes induced by agents such as DMBA have been correlated with structure at the time of carcinogen administration have suggested that it is the degree of differentiation of glandular cells at the time of exposure which make them appropriate targets in mammary carcinogenesis (Ciocca et al., 1982). Thus, the terminal end buds of the rat mammary gland, particularly when undergoing an active process of differentiation towards alveolar buds, are primary targets for a carcinogenic effect. It appears that as differentiation occurs towards more mature alveolar bud structures the number of induced benign lesions induced increases at the expense of carcinomas. Russo and colleages (1982) have suggested that the terminal end bud of the rat mammary gland is the equivalent of the terminal duct or intralobular terminal ducts believed to be site of origin of human mammary cancers.

Study of the proliferative characteristics of the dark light, intermediate and myoepithelial cells of the rat gland after DMBA administration has suggested that the intermediate cell is the primary target of the carcinogen and the cell of origin of mammary carcinoma in this model (Russo et al., 1983).

Although the data which relate to the influence of host factors on the development and growth of mammary neoplasms in other models are less complete, available evidence suggests that spontaneously developing rat and mouse mammary tumours are modulated by similar, although not always identical factors.

In strains of rats and mice that develop mammary neoplasms spontaneously with advancing age there is evidence that both prolactin and oestrogen are important in the development of mammary tumours. Spontaneous mammary tumours in predisposed strains of rat usually develop in the presence of increased levels of prolactin, decreased secretion of gonadotrophins and ovarian hormones accompanied by the loss of regular oestrous cycles. For this reason, it has been suggested that the requirements for prolactin are perhaps greater and ovarian steroids less in the development of spontaneous tumours than those induced in the rat by carcinogens (Meites, 1980). Elevated levels of prolactin produced by lesions in the median eminence or grafting of the pituitary under the renal capsule in Sprague-Dawley rats have been shown to increase the prevalence of mammary neoplasms, notably fibroadenomas (Welsch et al., 1968, 1969). Prolonged treatment of rats with reserpine also increases the total number of spontaneous mammary neoplasms whereas administration of L-dopa inhibits onset and development of spontaneous mammary tumours (Meites, 1980).

Oophorectomy almost totally eliminates the development of mammary tumours in the tumour-prone Sprague Dawley rat (Durbin et al., 1966; Solleveld et al., 1986). Conversely, administration of oestrogens to intact female rats has been shown to increase the incidence of mammary tumours. However, this effect is strain-dependent and is influenced by treatment-related reduction in life span as a result of concomitant treatment-induced pituitary adenomas and suppurative uterine infections (Solleveld et al., 1986). It appears, that highly susceptable strains are characterized by a more pronounced serum prolactin response to oestrogen administration than insensitive strains. (Blankenstein et al., 1984). Oestrogen treatment of sensitive female WAG/Rij rats not only increases the incidence of mammary tumours but also produces a raised number of mammary tumours per tumour-bearing animal, an increase in the proportion of malignant to benign tumours and an increase in the proportion of cribriform-comedo forms compared with the tubular tubulopapillary types found in untreated rats (Solleveld et al., 1986).

Dietary factors are also important modulators of the development of spontaneous rat mammary neoplasms. Food restriction alone is shown to reduce the incidence of spontaneous mammary tumours developing in aging female rats (Tucker, 1979). In a study which compared the relationship between bodyweight, survival and neoplastic disease in Sprague-Dawley rats, mammary fibroadenomas, adenomas and adenocarcinomas were more common in heavier than in lighter females and this correlation was highly significant statistically. (Turnbull et al., 1985).

In mice, there is also evidence that prolactin and oestrogen are important in the development of spontaneous mammary cancer. Prolactin administration, pituitary grafting, hypothalamic lesions and administration of reserpine have been shown to increase the prevalence of mammary cancer in mice (Welsch and Nagasawa,1977). Conversely chronic treatment of C_3H female mice with bromocryptine, a prolactin release inhibitor, results in inhibition of mammary tumour development (Welsch et al., 1977). However these hormonal manipulations appear not to alter the growth of well-developed or advanced mammary cancers in mice (Welsch and Nagasawa 1977).

In some mouse strains consideration has to be given to the contribution of the milk-transmitted mammary tumour virus (MTV) which is believed to be just one of the cooperating factors required to mediate mammary transformation (Slagle et al., 1987). However, the interaction of the virus with genetic, hormonal and other host factors is highly complex. Not all infected mice develop mammary tumours. Several strains of MTV are recognised each with different antigenic determinants and some showing different biological properties (Everett, 1984). Nevertheless, presence or absence of MTV accounts for much of the variation in incidence of mammary neoplasms among inbred strains of mice. Well-known high incidence strains infected with type B virus include A, CH3, DBA/2, and GR mice (Gross, 1983) although prevalence of neoplasms may be lower in some of the different substrains. See Squartini (1979) and Staats (1985), for a detailed review of substrains. Sher (1974, 1982) has reviewed mammary tumour prevalence in non-inbred strains.

The absence or presence of MTV may also be reflected in the anatomical location of mammary tumours in mice. In virus-infected mice the expected thoracic to inguinal ratio is about 6.4, whereas in virus free mice the mammary tumours occur more commonly in the thoracic glands (Prehn and Main 1954; Eaton et al., 1980). Adenocarcinomas situated in the thoracic region metastasize to the lungs more frequently that neoplasms situated in inguinal zones (Sheldon et al., 1982).

In the study in which oestrogens were administered for long periods to C3H/Hel and CBHeB/Fej mice with high and low titres to MTV respectively, Highman and colleagues (1980) demonstrated that mammary tumour prevalence was higher in the MTV-positive strain given oestrogen than the MTV negative strain. Although the distribution of histological types of mammary carcinomas (types A&B) were different between controls of the two strains, the ratios of tumour types were not influenced by hormone treatment. A subsequent study in C3H/HeN, MTV-positive female mice treated with diethylstilboestrol has shown that the time at which the first tumour occurs is largely dependent on duration of exposure rather than dose, whereas the rate of occurrence of subsequent tumours is more dependent on dose (Greenman et al., 1987). However, even in miceof a single inbred strain, exist that are highly insensitive to mammary tumour induction by oestrogens (Greenman and Delongchamp, 1986).

Other factors which influence the growth and development of rat mammary tumours also affect mouse mammary tumours and much of this was demonstrated by Tannenbaum and colleagues over 40 years ago. Restriction of diet or its caloric content reduces the incidence of mammary tumours in high incidence strains such as DBA and C3H (Tannenbaum, 1942a). High levels of dietary fat increases the prevalence of mammary neoplasms (Tannenbaum 1942b; Tinsley et al., 1981; Welsch and Aylsworth., 1983). A study by Gridley and colleagues (1983) showed that HVT positive C3H/HeJ mice fed a low fat, low milk protein diet were tumour free for longer periods than mice fed a diet containing beef or fish. Selenium added to the diet of MTV-positive C3H mice also lowers the incidence of spontaneous mammary carcinomas (Schrauzer et al., 1981).

A variety of endocrine alterations have been associated with the spontaneous development of canine mammary tumours. These include changes in oestrogens, progesterone, adrenal corticosteroids, thyroid hormones, prolactin and growth hormone. In the dog increased secretory activity of growth hormone appears more important than alterations in prolactin (El Etreby et al., 1980). Seven year studies in beagle dogs given combination oral contraceptive agents have demonstrated the importance of growth hormone in canine mammary tumorigenesis. All progestins including progesterone but particularly those of the 17-hydroxy-progesterone type are capable of stimulating the growth of focal mammary hyperplasia, benign and malignant mammary tumours if administered in an appropriate manner. The mechanism is related to the progestin stimulation of growth hormone released from the pituitary gland (Johnson, 1989).

The development and progression of human breast cancer is also influenced by endocrine factors. Endocrine manipulation can produce regression of the tumour in a proportion of patients although there is considerable individual variability. The protective effect of an early first pregnancy which has been demonstrated in a number of epidemiological studies may be mediated by a long-term decrease in serum prolactin levels (Musey et al., 1987).

Mammary tumours and safety assessment

In view of the variables which can influence the development and growth of mammary carcinomas in animals, considerable difficulty is experienced in the interpretation and risk assessment when high doses of potent therapeutic agents advance the appearance of or increase the numbers of mammary neoplasms in chronic toxicity or carcinogenicity studies. It is important to attempt to separate agents like DMBA which produce neoplasms principally as a result of direct DNA damage from those which induce neoplasms by indirect mechanisms, possibly of less relevance for man.

Characteristically, drugs which damage DNA produce mammary carcinomas rapidly and show activity in short term tests of mutagenic activity. For instance, a proposed neuroleptic drug, a pyrazole amine, was shown to produce mammary carcinomas in both male and female Wister rats within the period of a 13 week toxicity study (Gough et al., 1984). In this study, nodular intraduct carcinomas with a characteristic cribiform pattern were identified at 12 weeks. Tumour incidences were 20% of male and females in the high dose (100 mg/kg) group and

13% of males at a lower dose (50 mg/kg). A structural analogue was also shown to possess a similar tumorigenic effect (Fitzgerald et al., 1984, 1986).

This agent possessed a mechanism of action which did not involve prolaction stimulation. It was shown that these agents and their common chemical nucleus (5,amino-1,3-dimethy-pyrazol-4-yl) (2-fluorophenyl)-methanone were able to modify cellular DNA in assays of bacterial mutagenesis and sister chromatid exchange (Aust et al., 1984; Aust and Wold, 1986). It was proposed that the mechanism for this neoplastic effect resided in the common nucleus of this series of compounds and was probably related to an alteration of DNA in target mammary tissue (Aust and Wold, 1986; Fitzgerald et al., 1986).

By contrast, mammary neoplasms which developed in Sprague-Dawley rats following long term treatment with high doses (100-fold human dose) of the oral combination steroidal contraceptive agent, norlestrin only occurred after about an average of 500 days (Schardein et al., 1970). Treatment with norlestrin produced an increase of fibroepithelial mammary tumours in males and a greater number of adenomas and adenocarcinomas in females but latent periods for tumour development and survival of treated animals were somewhat longer than concurrent controls. Another example is provided by tolamolol, a β-adrenergic receptor blocking drug similar to propranolol. Tolamolol was withdrawn from clinical use when it was reported to produce mammary tumours in rat carcinogenicity studies (Food and Drug Administration, 1978; Jackson and Fishbein, 1988). The cause for the increase in tumour incidence was unclear, particularly as tolamolol was not mutagenic in any of the short-term tests. However there was a dose-dependent increase in prolactin reported in humans administered tolamolol, but not propanolol (Saxton et al., 1981), suggesting that this agent possessed the ability to modify pituitary hormone levels.

Whether these or other therapeutic agents which increase the incidence of mammary carcinomas in rodents after long-term, high dose administration increase the risk for the development of breast cancer in women when they are employed therapeutically is frequently uncertain. Rat and mouse tumours have much in common with human breast neoplasms but they are not identical. Although the pituitary gland is important in the development of both human and rodent mammary tumours, differences in the role of the pituitary are of a sufficient magnitude to preclude a direct extrapolation of findings in the rodent mammary gland to man. Although it has been shown that the protective effects of an early pregnancy in women is related to the subsequent long-term decrease in prolactin levels (Musey et al., 1987), there is still little evidence that patients with pathologically or pharmacologically elevated serum prolactin levels are at a higher risk for developing mammary cancer than the normal population (Keinberg et al., 1987). It is probable that other pituitary factors are of greater importance in man than prolactin in the genesis and development of mammary cancer. Therefore, it is not possible to conclude that a prolactin-mediated increase in rodent mammary tumours produced by a novel drug, would represent a significant additional risk for development of human mammary cancer if used therapeutically.

70

The finding of mammary neoplasms in dogs treated for seven years with various oral contraceptive steroid preparations and mammary duct hyperplasias in treated non-human primates also raised concerns about the possibility of oral contraceptive users being at an increased risk for developing mammary cancer. Extensive use of these agents for many years has, however, not demonstrated such a risk (Pasquale, 1989), suggesting that the findings in mammary glands in dogs, non-human primates and rodents treated with high doses of these contraceptive steroids are also poorly predictive for man. Nevertheless, the general and justified concern in society about breast cancer creates an environment in which even the slightest theoretical risk is sometimes considered unjustified.

REFERENCES

AUST, A.E., de la IGLESIA F.A and HEIFETZ, C. (1984): Comparative analysis of the mutagenic potential of two neuroleptic compounds that are carcinogenic in rats. *Environ.Mutagen.*, 6, 384

AUST, A.E. and WOLD, S.A. (1986): Induction of bacterial mutations by aminopyrazoles, compounds which cause mammary cancer in rats. *Carcinogenesis*, 7, 2019–2023.

AYLSWORTH, C.F., HODSON, C.A., BERG, G., KLEDZIK, G. and MEITES, J. (1979): Role of adrenals and estrogen in regression of mammary tumors during postpartum lactation in the rat. *Cancer Res.*, 39, 2436–2439.

BARSOUM, N.J., GOUGH, A.W., STURGESS, J.M. and de la IGLESIA, F.A. (1984): Morphologic features and incidence of spontaneous hyperplastic and neoplastic mammary gland lesions in Wistar rats. *Toxicol.Pathol.*, 12, 26–38.

BEEMS R.B., GRUYS, E. and SPIT, B.J. (1978): Amyloid in the corpora amylacea of the rat mammary gland. *Vet.Pathol.*, 15, 347–352.

BLANKENSTEIN, M.A., BROERSE, J.J., VAN ZWIETEN, M.J. and VAN DER MOLEN, H.J. (1984): Prolactin concentration in plasma and susceptibility to mammary tumors in female rats from different strains treated chemically with estradiol-17β. *Breast Cancer Res.Treat.*, 4, 137–141

BUREK, J.D. (1978) Age-associated pathology. In: *Pathology of Aging Rats*, Chap. 4, pp. 29–167. CRC Press, West Palm Beach, Fl.

CIOCCA, D.R., PARENTE, A. and RUSSO, J. (1982): Endocrinologic milieu and susceptibility of the rat mammary gland to carcinogenesis. *Am.J.Pathol.*, 109, 47–56.

COHEN, N.D. and HILF, R. (1974): Influence of insulin on growth and metabolism of 7, 12-dimethylbenz-anthracene-induced mammary tumors. *Cancer Res.*, 34, 3245–3252.

CUNHA, G.R., CHUNG, L.W.K., SHANNON, J.M., TAGUCHI, O. and FUJII, H. (1983): Hormone-induced morphogenesis and growth: Role of mesenchymal-epithelial interactions. *Rec.Prog.Horm.Res.*, 39, 559–598.

DULBECCO, R., ALLAN, W.R., BOLOGNA, M. and BOWMAN, M. (1986): Marker evolution during the development of the rat mammary gland: Stem cells identified by markers and the role of myoepithelial cells. *Cancer Res.*, 46, 2449–2456.

DUNN, T.B. (1959): Morphology of mammary tumors in mice. In: F. Homburger, (Ed.), *Physiopathology of Cancer*, 2nd Edition, pp., 38–84 Hoeber, New York.

DUPONT, W.D. and PAGE, D.L. (1985): Risk factors for breast cancer in women with proliferative breast disease. *N.Engl.J.Med.*, 312, 146–151.

DURBIN.P.W., WILLIAMS, M.H., JEUNG, N. and ARNOLD, J.S. (1966): Development of spontaneous mammary tumours over the lifespan of female Charles River (Sprague-Dawley) rat: The influence of ovariectomy, thyroidectomy, and adrenalectomy-ovariectomy. *Cancer Res.*, 26, 400–411.

EATON, G.J., JOHNSON, F.N., CUSTER, R.P. and CRANE, A.R. (1980): The Icr: Ha (ICR) mouse: A current account of breeding, mutations, diseases and mortality. *Lab.Anim.*, 14,17–24.

EL ETREBY, M.F., MULLER-PEDDINGHAUS, R., BHARGAVA, A.S., FATH EL BAB, M.R., GRAF, K-J. and TRAUTWEIN, G. (1980): The role of the pituitary gland in spontaneous canine mammary tumorigenesis. *Vet.Pathol.*, 17, 2–16.

EVERETT, R. (1984): Factors affecting spontaneous tumor incidence rates in mice: A literature review. *CRC Crit.Rev.Toxicol.*, 13, 235–251.

FACCINI, J.M., IRISARRI, E. and MONRO, A.M. (1981): A carcinogenicity study in mice of a β-adrenergic antagonist, primidolol; increased total tumour incidence with tissue specificity. *Toxicology*, 21, 279–290.

FITZGERALD, J., de la IGLESIA, F. and GOLDENTHAL, E.I. (1982): Ten year oral toxicity study with norlestrin in rhesus monkeys. *J. Toxicol.Environ.Health.*, 10, 879–896.

FITZGERALD, J.E., McGUIRE, E.J., ANDERSON, J.A. and de la IGLESIA, F.A. (1984): Structure-activity relationships of chemically induced mammary gland neoplasia in rats. Fed. Proc., 43, 592.

FITZGERALD, J.E., McGUIRE, E.J., ANDREWS, L.K. and de la IGLESIA, F.A. (1986): Structure-activity relationships in the induction of mammary gland neoplasia in male rats with substituted aminopyrazoles. *Am.J.Pathol.*, 124, 392–398

FOOD & DRUG ADMINISTRATION. (1978): Status report on beta-blocker. *FDA Drug Bulletin*, 8, 13.

FOWLER, E.H., WILSON, G.P. and KOESTNER, A. (1974): Biologic behaviour of canine mammary neoplasms based on a histogenetic classification. *Vet Pathol.*, 11. 212–229.

FRESE, K. (1985): Vergleichende Pathologie der Mammatumoren bei Haustieren. *Verh.Dtsch.Ges. Pathol.*, 69, 152–170.

GOUGH, A.W., BARSOUM, N.J., SMITH, G.S., STURGESS, J.M. and de la IGLESIA, F.A. (1984): Early development of mammary gland carcinomas in rats induced by a neuroleptic agents. Fed. Proc. 43, 592.

GREENMAN, D.L. and DELONGCHAMP, R.R. (1986): Interactive responses to diethylstilboestrol in C3H mice. *Food.Chem.Toxicol.*, 24, 931–934.

GREENMAN, D.L., KODELL, R.L., HIGHMAN, B., SCHIEFERSTEIN, G.J. and NORVELL, M.J. (1987): Mammary tumorigenesis in C3H/HEN-MTV + mice treated with diethylstilboestrol for varying periods. *Food.Chem. Toxicol.*, 25, 229–232.

GRIDLEY, D.S., KETTERING, J.D., SLATER, J.M. and NUTTER, R.L. (1983): Modification of spontaneous mammary tumours in mice fed different sources of protein, fat and carbohydrate. *Cancer Lett.*, 19, 133–146.

GROSS, L. (1983): The development of inbred strains of mice and its impact on experimental cancer research. In: *Oncogenic Viruses 3rd Edition*, Vol.1, Chap. 9, pp. 253–261, Pergamon, Oxford.

HAMPE, J.F. and MISDORP, W. (1974): Tumours and dysplasias of the mammary gland. *Bull.Wld.Hlth.Org.*, 50, 111–133.

HASEMAN, J.K., HUFF, J. and BOORMAN, G.A. (1984): Use of historical control data in carcinogenicity studies in rodents. *Toxicol.Pathol.*, 12, 126–135.

HIGHMAN, B., GREENMAN, D.L., NORVELL, M.J., FARMER, J. and SHELLENBERGER, E. (1980): Neoplastic and preneoplastic lesions induced in female C3H mice by diets containing diethylstilbestrol or 17β-estradiol. *J.Environ.Pathol.Toxicol.*, 4, 81–95.

HIGHMAN, B, NORVELL, M.J. and SHELLENBERGER, T.E. (1977): Pathological changes in female C3H mice continuously fed diets containing diethstilbestrol or 17 β-estradiol. *J.Environ.Pathol. Toxicol.*, 1, 1–30.

HILF, R., HISSIN, P.J., and SHAFIE, S.M. (1978): Regulatory interelationships for insulin and estrogen action in mammary tumors. *Cancer Res.*, 38, 4076–4085.

HUTTER, R.V.P. (1985): Goodbye to 'fibrocystic disease'. *N.Engl.J. Med.*, 312, 179–181.

IP, C. (1981): Prophylaxis of mammary neoplasia by selenium supplementation in the initiation and promotion phases of chemical carcinogenesis. *Cancer Res.*, 41, 4386–4390.

JABARA, A.G. (1967): Effects of progesterone on 9,12-dimethyl-1,2-benzanthracene-induced mammary tumours in Sprague-Dawley rats. *Br.J. Cancer.*, 21, 418–429.

JABARA, A.G., TOYNE, P.H. and HARCOURT, A.G. (1973): Effect of time and duration of progesterone administration in mammary tumours induced by 7, 12-dimethylbenzanthracene in Sprague-Dawley rat. *Br.J.Cancer.*, 27, 63–71.

JACKSON, C.D. and FISHBEIN, L. (1986): A toxicological review of beta-adrenergic blockers. *Fundam.Appl.Toxicol.*, 6, 395–422.

JOHNSON, A.N., (1989): Comparative aspects of contraceptive steroids: effects observed in beagle dogs. *Toxicol.Pathol.*, 17, 389–396.

JORDAN, V.C. (1976): Effect of tamoxifen (ICI 46,474) on initiation and growth of DMBA-induced rat mammary carcinomata. *Eur.J.Cancer.*, 12, 419–424.

JOSHI, K., ELLIS, J.T.B., HUGHES, C.M., MONAGHAN, P. and NEVILLE, A.M. (1986): Cellular proliferation in the rat mammary gland during pregnancy and lactation. *Lab.Invest.*, 54, 52–61.

KHAZAN, N., PRIMO C.H., DANON, A., ASSAEL, M., SULMAN, F.G. and WINNIK, H.Z. (1962): The mammotropic effect of tranquillizing drugs. *Arch.Int.Pharmacodyn.*, 136, 291–305.

KLEINBERG, D.L. (1987): Prolactin and breast cancer. *N.Engl.J.Med.*, 316, 269–271.

KOMITOWSKY, D., SASS, B. and LAUB, W. (1982): Rat mammary tumour classification: Notes on comparative aspects. *J.N.C.I.*, 68, 147–156.

LAVANDERO, S., PONOSO, E. and SAPAG-HAGAR, M. (1985): β-adrenergic receptors in rat mammary gland. *Biochem.Pharmacol.*, 34, 2034–2036.

LEVIN, J.M., GOLDMAN, A.S., RASATO, F.E. and RASATO, E.E. (1976): Therapy of dimethylbenzanthracene induced mammary carcinomas in the rat by selective inhibition of steroidogenesis. *Cancer*, 38, 56–61.

LEUSCHNER, F., NEUMAN, W. and HEMPEL, R. (1981): Toxicology of antipsychotic agents. In: Handbook of Experimental Pharmacology Vol. 55/1,Chap. 11, pp. 225–265.

MAITA, K., HIRANO, M., HARADA, T., MITSUMORI, K., YOSHIDA, A., TAKAHASHI, K., NAKASHIMA, N., KITAZAWA, T., ENOMOTO, A., INUI, K. and SHIRASU, Y. (1988): Mortality, may or cause of moribundity, and spontaneous tumors in CD-mice. *Toxicol.Pathol.*, 16, 340–349.

MAJEED, S.K., and GOPINATH, C. (1984): Mixed mammary tumour in a CD female rat. *J.Comp.Pathol.*, 94, 629–63.

McCORMICK, D.L., BURNS, F.J. and ALBERT, R.E. (1980): Inhibition of rat mammary carcinogenesis by short dietary exposure to retinyl acetate. *Cancer Res.*, 40, 1140–1143.

McCORMICK, D.L., MAJOR, N. and MOON, R.C. (1984): Inhibition of 7, 12-dimethylbenzanthracene-induced rat mammary carcinogens by concomitant or post carcinogen antioxidant exposure. *Cancer Res.*, 44, 2858–2863.

McCORMICK, G.M. and MOON, R.C. (1967): Hormones influencing postpartum growth of 7, 12-dimethylbenzanthracene induced rat mammary tumors. *Cancer Res.*, 27,629–631.

MEITES, J. (1957): Induction of lactation in rabbits with reserpine. *Proc.Soc.Exp.Biol.Med.*, 96, 728–730.

MEITES, J. (1980): Relation of neuroendocrine system to the development and growth of experimental mammary tumors. *J. Neural. Transm.*, 48, 25–42.

MEITES, J., CASSELL, E. and CLARK, J. (1971): Estrogen inhibition of mammary tumor growth in rats: Counteraction by prolactin. *Proc. Soc.Exp.Biol.Med.*, 137, 1225–1227.

MOLINOLO, A.A., LANARI, C., CHARREAU, E.H., SANJUAN, N. and PASQUALINI, C.D. (1987): Mouse mammary tumor induced by medroxyprogesterone acetate: Immunohistochemistry and hormonal receptors. *J.N.C.I.*, 79, 1341–1350.

MORI, T., OHMIYA, S. and NAGASAWA, H. (1986): Histochemical analysis by lectin in comparison with immunohistochemical prolactin staining of preneoplastic and neoplastic mammary glands in four strains of mice. *Acta. Histochem. Cytochem.*, 19, 421–428.

MOULTON, J.E., ROSENBLATT, L.S. and GOLDMAN, M. (1986): Mammary tumors in a colony of beagle dogs. *Vet.Pathol.*, 23, 741–749.

MUSEY, V.C., COLLINS, D.C., MUSEY, P.I., MARTINO-SALTZMAN, D. and PREEDY, J.R.K. (1987): Long term effect of a first pregnancy on the secretion of prolactin. *N.Engl.J.Med.*, 316, 229–234.

NELSON, L.W. and KELLY, W.A. (1974): Changes in canine mammary gland histology during the estrous cycle. *Toxicol.Appl.Pharmacol.*, 27, 113–122.

NEUMANN, F, ELGER, W. and EL ETREBY, M.F. (1985): Endokrinologie und Pathologie der Mammogenese im Experiment. *Verh.Dtsch.Ges.Pathol.*, 69, 1–19.

NICHOLSON, R.I. and GOLDER, M.P. (1975): The effect of synthetic anti-oestrogen on the growth and biochemistry of rat mammary tumours. *Eur.J.Cancer.*, 11, 571–579.

OHUCHI, N., THOR, A., PAGE, D.L., HORAN HAND, P., HALSTER, S.A. and SCHLOM, J. (1986): Expression of the 21,000 molecular weight *ras* protein in a spectrum of benign and malignant human mammary tissues. *Cancer Res.*, 46, 2511–2519.

OZZELLO, L. (1971): Ultrastructure of intraepithelial carcinomas of the breast. *Cancer*, 28, 1508–1515.

PAGE, D.L., DUPONT, W.D., ROGERS, L.W. and RADOS, M.S. (1985): Atypical hyperplastic lesions of the female breast. A long term follow up study. *Cancer*, 55, 2698–2708.

PASQUALE, S.A. (1989) Oral contraceptives: Significance of their effects in man and relationship to findings in animal models. *Toxicol. Pathol.*, 17, 396–400.

PIERPAOLI, W. and SORKIN, E. (1972): Inhibition of growth of methylcholanthrene-induced mammary carcinoma in rats by anti-adenohypophysis serum. *Nature*, 238, 58–59.

PREHN, R.T. and MAIN, J.W. (1954): Factors influencing tumour distribution among the mammary glands of the mouse. *J.N.C.I.*, 14, 895–904.

PREJEAN, J.D., PECKHAM, J.C., CASEY, A.E., GRISWOLD, D.P., WEISBURGER, E.K. and WEISBURGER, J.H. (1973): Spontaneous tumors in Sprague-Dawley rats and Swiss mice. *Cancer Res.*, 33, 2768–2773.

RHODIN, J.A.G. (1974): Female reproductive system. In: Histology. A Text and Atlas, Chap. 34, pp.703–747, Oxford University Press, New York.

ROE, F.J.C. (1983): Testing for carcinogenicity and the problem of pseudocarcinogenicity. *Nature*, 303, 657–658.

RUSSO, J. and RUSSO, I.H. (1980): Influence of differentiation and cell kinetics on the susceptibility of the rat mammary gland to carcinogens. *Cancer Res.*, 40, 2677–2687.

RUSSO, J., TAIT, L. and RUSSO, I.H. (1983): Susceptibility of the mammary gland to carcinogenesis. III. The cell of origin of rat mammary carcinoma. *Am.J.Pathol.*, 113, 50–66.

RUSSO, J., TAY, L.K. and RUSSO, I.H. (1982): Differentiation of the mammary gland and susceptibility to carcinogenesis. *Breast Cancer Res.Treat.*, 2, 5–73.

SAKAMOTA, S., IMAMVRA, Y, SASSA, S. and OKAMOTO, R. (1979): DMBA-induced mammary tumor and hormone environment in the rat during pregnancy, postpartum, and long term lactation. *Toxicol.Lett.*, 4, 237–240.

SANZ, M.C.A., LIU, J.M., HUANG, H.H. and HAWRYLEWICZ, E.J. (1986): Effect of dietary protein on morphologic development of rat mammary gland. *J.N.C.I.*, 77, 477–487.

SASS, B. and DUNN, T.B. (1979): Classification of mouse mammary tumors in Dunn's miscellaneous group including recently reported types. *J.N.C.I.*, 1287–1293.

SAXTON, C.A., FAULKNER, J.K. and GROOM, G.V. (1981): The effect of plasma prolactin, growth hormone and luteinising hormone concentrations of single oral doses of propranolol and tolamolol in normal man. *Eur.J.Clin.Pharmacol.*, 21, 103–108.

SCHARDEIN, J.L. (1980)a: Studies of the components of an oral contraceptive agent in albino rats. I. Estrogenic component. *J. Toxicol.Environ.Health.*, 6, 885–894.

SCHARDEIN, J.L. (1980)b: Studies of the components of an oral contraceptive agents in albino rats. II. Progestogenic component and comparison of effects of the components and the combined agent. *J. Toxicol.Environ.Health.*, 6, 895–906.

SCHARDEIN, J.L., KAUMP, D.H., WOOSLEY, E.T. and JELLEMA, M.MM (1970): Long-term toxicologic and tumorigenesis studies on an oral contraceptive agent in albino rats. *Toxicol.Appl.Pharmacol.*, 16, 10–23.

SCHRAUZER, G.N., KUEHN, K. and HAMM, D. (1981): Effect of dietary selenium and of lead of the genesis of spontaneous mammary tumours in mice. *Biol.Trac.Element Res.*, 3, 185–196.

SHELDON, W.G., OWEN, K., WEED, L. and KODELL, R. (1982): Distribution of mammary gland neoplasms and factors influencing metatases in hybrid mice. *Lab.Anim.Sci.*, 32, 166–168.

SHER, S.P. (1974): Tumors in control mice: Literature tabulation. *Toxicol.Appl.Pharmacol.*, 30, 337–359.

SHER, S.P. (1982): Tumors in control hamsters, rats, and mice: Literature tabulation. *CRC Crit.Rev.Toxicol.*, 10, 49–79.

SLADE, H.B. and SCHWARTZ, S.A. (1987): Mucosal immunity: The immunology of breast milk. *J.Allergy.Clin.Immunol.*, 80, 346–356.

SLAGLE, B.L., MEDINA, D. and BUTEL, J.S. (1987): Mammary cancer stages in BALB/CV mice: Mouse mammary tumor virus expression and virus-host interactions. *J.N.C.I.*, 79, 329–335.

SOLLEVELD, H.A., VAN ZWIETEN, M.J., BROERSE, J.J. and HOLLANDER, C.F. (1986): Effects of x-irradiation, ovariohysterectomy and estradiol-17β on incidence, benign/malignant ratio and multiplicity of rat mammary neoplasms: a preliminary report. *Leuk.Res.*, 10, 755–759.

SONNENBERG, A., DAAMS H., VAN DER VALK, M.A., HILKINS, J. and HILGERS, J. (1986): Development of mouse mammary gland: Identification of stages in differentiation of luminal and myoepithelial cells using monoclonial antibodies and polyvalent antiserum against keratin. *J.Histochem.Cytochem.*, 34, 1037–1046.

SQUARTINI, F. (1979): Tumours of the mammary gland. In: V.S. Turusov (Ed.) Pathology of Tumours in Laboratory Animals, Vol. 2, Tumours of the Mouse, pp. 43–90. IARC Scientific Publ. No 23, Lyon.

SQUIRE, R.A., GOODMAN, D.G., VALERIO, M.G., FREDRICKSON, T.N., STRANDBERG, J.D., LEVITT, M.H., LINGEMAN, C.H., HARSHBARGER, J.C. and DAWE, C.J. (1978): Tumors. In: K Benirsche, F.M. Garner and T.C. Jones (Eds). *Pathology of Laboratory Animals*, Vol. 2,Chap. 12, pp. 1051–1283. Springer-Verlag, New York.

STAATS, J. (1985): Standardised nomenclature for inbred strains of mice: Eight listing. *Cancer Res.*, 45, 945–977.

STERENTAL, A., DOMINGUEZ, J.M., WEISSMAN, C. and PEARSON, O.H. (1963): Pituitary in the estrogen dependency of experimental mammary cancer. *Cancer Res.*, 23, 481–484.

STRUM, J.M. (1981): Pale cell carcinoma. Ultrastructure of a hormone-dependent mammary tumor in GR mice. *Am.J.Pathol.*, 103, 283–291.

SYLVESTER, P.W., AYLSWORTH, C.F., VAN VUGT, D.A. and MEITES, J. (1982): Influence of underfeeding during the 'critical period' or thereafter on carcinogen-induced mammary tumors in rats. *Cancer Res.*, 42, 4943–4947.

TANNENBAUM, A. (1942)a: The genesis and growth of tumors. II. Effects of caloric restriction per se. *Cancer Res.*, 2, 460–467.

TANNENBAUM, A. (1942)b: The genesis and growth of tumors. III. Effects of a high fat diet. *Cancer Res.*, 2, 468–475.

TAVASSOLI, F.A., CASEY, H.W., and NORRIS, H.J. (1988): The morphologic effects of synthetic reproductive steroids on the mammary gland of rhesus monkeys. Mestranol, ethynerone, mestranol-ethynerone, chloroethynyl norgestrel-mestranol, and anagestone acetate-mestranol combinations. *Am.J.Pathol.*, 131, 213–234.

TINSLEY, I.J., SCHMITZ, J.A. and PIERCE, D.A. (1981): Influence of dietary fatty acids on the incidence of mammary tumours in the C3H mouse. *Cancer Res.*, 41, 1460–1465.

TUCKER, M.J., (1979): The effects of long-term food restriction on tumours in rodents. *Int.J.Cancer*, 23, 803–807.

TURNBULL, G.T., LEE, P.N. and ROE, F.J.C. (1985): Relationship of bodyweight gain to longevity and to risk of development of nephropathy and neoplasia in Sprague-Dawley rats. *Food Chem.Toxicol.*, 23, 355–361.

VAN NIE, R. and DUX, A. (1971): Biological and morphological characteristics of mammary tumors in GR mice. *J.N.C.I.*, 46, 885–897.

VIERBUCHEN, M., KLEIN, P.J., UHLENBRUCK, G. and FISCHER, R. (1981): Hormonabhängige Lektin-Bindungsstellen: I. Histochemischer Nachweis von Lektin-Bindungsstellen und ihre hormonelle Steuerung im Brustdrusengewebe der Ratte. *Tumor Diagnostik.*, 2, 235–239.

WALKER, R.A. (1984): The binding of peroxidase-labelled sections to human breast epithelium. I. Normal hyperplastic and lactating breast. *J. Pathol.*, 142, 279–291.

WARBURTON, M.J., MITCHELL, D., ORMEROD, E.J., and RUDLAND, P. (1982): Distribution of myoepithelial cells and basement membrane proteins in the resting, pregnant, lactating and involuting rat mammary gland. *J. Histochem. Cytochem.*, 30, 667–676.

WEI, W.Z., MALONE, K., MAHONEY, K. and HEPPNER, G. (1986): Characterisation of lymphocytic infiltrates in normal, preneoplastic, and neoplastic mouse mammary tissues. *Cancer Res.*, 46, 2680–2685.

WELSCH, C.W. (1985): Host factors affecting the growth of carcinogen-induced rat mammary carcinomas: A review and tribute to Charles Brenton Huggins. *Cancer Res.*, 45, 3415–3443.

WELSCH, C.W. and AYLESWORTH, C.F. (1983): Enhancement of murine mammary tumorigenesis by feeding high levels of dietary fat: A hormonal mechanism? *J.N.C.I.*, 70, 215–221.

WELSCH, C.W., CLEMENS, J.A. and MEITES, J. (1968): Effects of multiple pituitary homografts or progesterone on 7,12-dimethylbenz[a]anthracene-induced mammary tumors in rats. *J.N.C.I.*, 41, 465–471.

WELSH, C.W., CLEMENS, J.A. and MEITES, J.(1969): Effects of hypothalamic and amygdaloid lesions on development and growth of carcinogen-induced mammary tumors in the female rat. *Cancer Res.*, 29, 1541–1549.

WELSCH, C.W., GOODRICH-SMITH, M., BROWN, C.K., MACKIE, D. and JOHNSON, D. (1982): 2-Bromo-α-ergocryptine (CB-154) and tamoxifen (ICI 46,474) induced suppression of the genesis of mammary carcinomas in female rats treated with 7,12-dimethylbenzanthracene (DMBA): A comparison. *Oncology*, 39, 88–92.

WELSCH, C.W., ITURRI, G. and MEITES, J. (1973): Comparative effects of hypophysectomy, ergocornine and ergocornine-reserpine treatments on rat mammary carcinoma. *Int.J.Cancer.*, 12, 206–212.

WELSCH, C.W., LAMBRECHT, L.K. and HASSETT, C.C. (1977): Suppression of mammary tumorigenesis in C3H He mice by ovariectomy or treatment with 2-bromo-α-ergocryptine: A comparison. *J.N.C.I.*, 58, 1135–1138.

WELSCH, C.W. and NAGASWA, H. (1977): Prolactin and murine mammary tumorigenesis: A review. *Cancer Res.*, 37, 951–963.

WILLEBRAND, D., BOSMAN, F.T. and DE GOEIJ, A.F.P.M. (1986): Patterns of basement membrane deposition in benign and malignant breast tumours. *Histopathology*, 10, 1231–1241.

WORLD HEALTH ORGANISATION (1981): Histological Typing of Breast Tumours. International Histological Classification of Tumours, No. 2, Second Edition, pp. 15–25, Geneva.

YOUNG, S. and HALLOWES, R.C. (1973): Tumours of the mammary gland. In: V.S. Turusov (Ed): *Pathology of Tumours in Laboratory Animals*, Vol. 1, Tumours of the Rat, Part 1, pp 31–73. IARC Scientific Publ. No. 5, Lyon.

III. Haemopoietic and Lymphatic Systems

BLOOD / BONE MARROW

Damage to blood forming cells is one of the most feared drug reactions. Although these effects form about 10% of adverse reactions reported in man, they represent a high proportion of those with a fatal outcome, often as a result of aplastic anaemia and agranulocytosis (Bottiger et al., 1979). Although it is difficult to make an estimate of the true incidence of drug-induced blood dyscrasias, one survey from Sweden suggested that the mean annual incidence has not changed substantially in the last two decades, although the pattern of offending drug exposure has changed (Arneborn and Palmblad, 1982; Editorial, Lancet, 1983).

In the development of new drugs, it is necessary to avoid agents which possess the obvious potential to cause severe haematological abnormalities, although it is not always possible to predict those agents which will cause haematological reactions in man as a result of hypersensitivity. The importance of the haematological system in preclinical safety evaluation is widely recognized by the routine inclusion of standard haematological tests in toxicity studies, but there are few specific recommendations for the type of haematological investigation and considerable variation in the choice of tests exists between laboratories (Theus and Zbinden, 1984).

Like clinical chemistry, haematological study is of practical importance in safety evaluation for it allows sequential monitoring of a cellular system, both in preclinical and early clinical work with a new drug and forms a useful point of comparison between findings in laboratory animals and man. Furthermore, human leucocytes are easily available for comparative studies of metabolism and drug accumulation (Fig. 13) (Read et al., 1985).

A wide variety of drug-induced haematological reactions are described in man. These include aplastic anaemia, agranulocytosis, various red blood cell derangements such as hypochromic, sideroblastic, megaloblastic and haemolytic anaemias, methaemoglobinaemia, various thrombocytopenias and other bleeding disorders as well as leukaemia and lymphoma. In preclinical testing, drugs producing severe haematological changes at all dose levels would probably not be

77

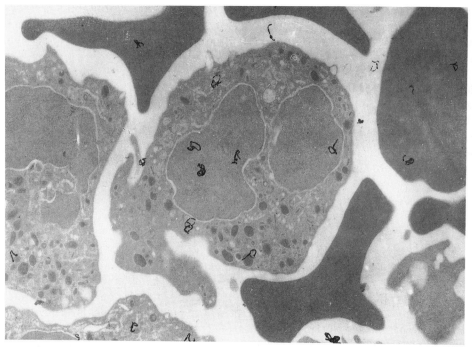

Fig. 13. Example of the electron microscopic autoradiograph technique reported by Read and colleges in 1985. This electron microscopic autoradiograph is of a preparation of human polymorphonuclear leukocytes incubated in vitro with tritiated 5-hydroxytryptamine. Silver grains are evident over the nuclei, granules and cytoplasm and quantitative analysis showed the cytoplasmic granules contained about 75% of the 5-hydroxytryptamine detected by this method in the cells. Illustration by courtesy of Dr. N.G. Read. (EM, ×5,500.)

developed unless for life-threatening conditions, such as cancer. Of more practical difficulty is the interpretation of the minor variations in haematological values which occur. This may be quite difficult in studies using small numbers of beagle dogs and primates prone to considerable individual variation in haematological values. The use of sensitive measuring equipment designed for use in man may also reveal mild treatment-related changes which have little or doubtful toxicological significance.

The preclinical assessment of anticancer drugs is a special case. As haematological toxicity is expected to occur with some anticancer agents in clinical use, haematological changes occurring in the test species need to be evaluated in this context. Although it has been demonstrated in a number of comparative studies that toxicity experiments with anticancer agents in rat and dog are reasonably predictive for bone marrow suppression occurring in man (Owens, 1962; Schein et al., 1970), a number of experimental variables need to be considered in the preclinical safety evaluation of cytotoxic drugs. The effect of repeated doses of cytotoxic agents on bone marrow cells is complex and depends on the stage in the generative cell cycle at which activity is optimal as well as the dosage regimen.

The differences in the life span and pool sizes of platelets, neutrophils and red cells also influence the blood picture which in turn may lag significantly behind morphological changes in the bone marrow. Drugs can also adversely affect the stromal microenvironment of the bone marrow. Cell damage in other organs and the subsequent inflammatory reaction may also have an impact on the haematological findings. Indeed, the evaluation of anticancer drugs is a complex matter which merits a sophisticated multidisciplinary approach (Chabner et al., 1984).

Nucleoside analogues with anti-viral activity represent another class of agents which is sometimes associated with adverse effects on blood forming cells in both laboratory animals and in humans. (Tucker et al., 1983; Luster, et al., 1989).

In man, therapeutic use of some drugs, notably β-lactam antibiotics (penicillins and cephalosporins) is sometimes associated with the development of immune-mediated haemolytic anaemia as well as neutropenia and thrombocytopenia, in the form of so called type II hypersensitivity reactions. Such reactions are believed to involve the binding of parent drug, metabolites or degradation products to endogenous proteins, followed by antibody production against these complexes, build up of the antibodies on blood cell surfaces and ultimately destruction or removal of affected cells from the circulation (Petz, 1980; Bang and Kammer, 1983).

Although immune-mediated haemolytic anaemia has been reported to occur in high incidence in both rhesus monkeys and rats treated intravenously with a modified β-lactam antibiotic or carbapenam for several weeks (Eydelloth, et al., 1987), this appears to be an unusual reaction in laboratory animals. In a study with a number of conventional β-lactam antibiotics associated with type II reactions in man, it was shown that neither rhesus monkeys or Sprague-Dawley rats developed immune-mediated haematological alterations, even though slight, non-immune mediated anaemias occurred in the primates at high doses (Kornbrust et al., 1989).

Although detailed discussion of haematological findings is outside the scope of this book, the following represents a brief account of haematological changes which may be found in toxicity studies. Details of haematological findings in laboratory animals have been described by Sanderson and Philips (1981).

Red blood cell values

Slight group differences and mild treatment-related trends in haemoglobin (Hb), packed cell volume (PCV) and red blood cell counts (RBC) observed in routine toxicity studies may not be associated with detectable changes in the bone marrow or spleen, reticulocytosis or increased red cell destruction. For instance, minor changes in haemoglobin values were reported in preclinical toxicity studies performed in rats with some benzodiazepines compounds (Owen et al., 1970), cimetidine (Brimblecombe et al., 1985) and omeprazole, a novel gastric acid inhibitor (Ekman et al., 1985). None of these changes appeared to have any clinical importance. In such studies, high doses of active agents are being administered and a variety of physiological and exaggerated pharmacological

79

changes can be expected. Alterations in circulation, and fluid and salt balance, food consumption and food utilization, in feeding patterns can be expected to indirectly influence red blood cell values. It has recently been shown in young Wistar rats that not only food restriction, but also rate of food consumption and feeding pattern may influence haemoglobin, packed cell volume and red blood cell counts (Pickering and Pickering, 1984).

In rats, both starvation and protein deficiency over periods of four or five weeks have been shown to reduce bone marrow progenitor cell activity which can lead to reduced numbers of erythrocytes, white cells and platelets in the peripheral blood (Brown, 1954; Fruhman and Gordon, 1955; Ito et al., 1964; Farnel and Maronpot, 1987). Protein malnutrition appears to produce a greater reduction in the normoblast population than caloric reduction alone (Brown, 1954; Ito et al., 1964).

Other experimental variables which influence the red blood cell values include venepuncture and blood sampling. Blood sampling in rats and mice can remove sufficient blood to cause a small depression in haemoglobin and a compensatory reticulocytosis lasting several days. Venepuncture alone may allow leakage of blood, particularly if drugs or vehicles with anticoagulant effects are also administered. The vehicles used for administration of drugs by parenteral routes may also adversely affect erythrocytes in the peripheral circulation.

In larger animals such as dogs, the effects of venepuncture are, by comparison with small rodents, of less significance. Nevertheless repeated sampling at frequent intervals can influence haematological findings. Even in human clinical practice, it has been shown that phlebotomy for diagnostic laboratory tests in adults can have adverse effects as a result of blood loss (Smoller and Kruskall, 1986). Nevertheless, the small number of dogs used per group, the considerable individual variation and fluctuation with time of red cell values in the same animals which occur in most colonies of dogs make interpretation of small group differences in red cell values less clear cut than might be supposed.

However, a clear dose-related decrease in haemoglobin, packed cell volume and red blood cell count may indicate an increased rate of red blood cell destruction caused by administration of an agent which injures the red cell membrane, causes oxidative damage to haemoglobin or suppresses the antioxidant defence system. It has been suggested that even if a compound has only weak haemolytic properties it represents a hazard for man, particularly in those patients with inherited erythrocytic metabolic defects (Beutler, 1969). When increased haemolysis occurs, decreased haemoglobin, red cell count and packed cell volumes are accompanied by raised reticulocyte counts, increased anisocytosis, increased red cell volumes and red cell distribution widths. Evidence of increased red cell turnover in the spleen is provided by increased splenic weight, changes in splenic pigmentation, presence of foam cells and intense erythropoiesis. Abnormal red cells may be seen in the blood smear preparations. Zbinden and his colleagues (1984) have elegantly shown how haematological study may be used in screening compounds for haemolytic effects in an in vivo system using small numbers of rats. Measurement of red cell counts and methaemoglobin levels, Heinz bodies and siderocytes appeared to be especially valuable. (Zbinden et al., 1984). Scanning and transmission electron microscopy of red blood cells can also be helpful in the characterization of the evolution in structural changes leading to drug-induced intravascular haemolysis and other forms of red cell damage (Fig. 14) (Jones et al., 1989).

However, some compounds which produced mild haemolytic effects when administered in high does to animals have been developed successfully for use in human therapy. For instance, a dose-related haemolytic effect characterized by reduction in haemoglobin values, erythrocyte count and haematocrit associated with increased erythropoiesis in bone marrow and spleen and haemosiderosis in splenic pulp and liver, was seen in dogs and rats treated for three months or longer with the angiotensin converting enzyme (ACE) inhibitor captopril (Hashimoto et al., 1981; Imai et al., 1981; Ohtaki et al., 1981). Haematological toxicity has only been rarely reported with captopril in human clinical practice and even this is more commonly neutropenia than effects on red blood cells (DiBianco, 1986).

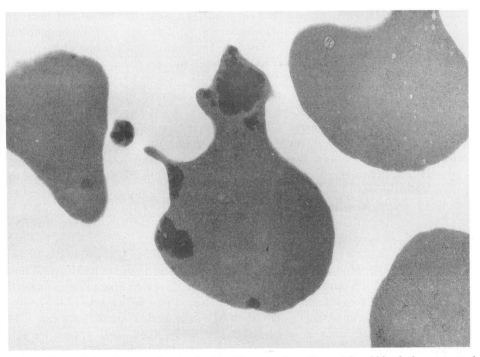

Fig. 14. Transmission electron micrograph of erytrhrocytes from the peripheral blood of a rat treated with phenylhydrazine which induced Heinz body anaemia. To avoid clumping of cells, the technique employed transferring blood to 0.1% glutaraldehyde in 0.1 M cacodylate buffer pH 7.2. After centrifugation, blood cells were transferred to 3% glutaraldehyde in 0.1 M cacodylate buffer. Illustration by courtesy of Dr. N.G. Read. (EM, ×18,000.)

Note: Several forms of macrocyte have been described in man, a true macrocyte, a pseudomacrocyte and a volumetric macrocyte (Burns et al., 1986). The true macrocyte is found in brisk reticulocytosis and is characterized by increased cell diameter, increased mean corpuscular volume (MCV) and increased corpuscular haemoglobin (MCH). The pseudomacrocyte shows increased diameter but normal MCV and MCH, a paradox caused by a membrane abnormality which allows the cell to expand along a rigid surface such as a microscope slide, thus appearing enlarged on microscopy. A third type of macrocyte appears normocytic on microscopy but possesses an increased haemoglobin content and is probably due to the adverse effect of agents such as hydroxyurea on erythropoiesis.

Platelet values

Platelet counts are quite commonly performed in industrial toxicology laboratories (Theus and Zbinden, 1984). However, even with additional measurements of platelet size and platelet distribution width now available on modern measuring equipment, platelet counts may not provide much information about platelet function. For instance, in the recent safety evaluation of dazoxiben, a highly specific inhibitor of thromboxane A2 synthetase, platelet counts were slightly raised in rats after only six months of treatment at many times the dose of dazoxiben needed for inhibition of thromboxane synthetase and thromboxane A2 production in rats (Irisarri et al., 1985). Yet, thromboxane A2 is one of the most potent platelet aggregants known and platelet function was altered at these doses.

The most common changes in platelet counts observed in toxicity studies are the result of spontaneous disease or tissue damage repair occurring in other organs. Nevertheless, decreased platelet counts are observed when there is significant treatment-related bone marrow suppression, such as produced by anticancer drugs. However, comparative studies with anticancer agents have suggested that although rodent and dog predict general bone marrow depression in man well, they are less good predictors of thrombocytopenia in man treated with these agents (Owens, 1962; Schein et al., 1970).

White blood cell and differential counts

Increases in neutrophil and lymphocyte counts occur under a variety of circumstances, usually related to spontaneous inflammatory disease or secondary to treatment-induced tissue damage in other organs. White cell counts vary considerably between individual dogs and with time in the same dogs. In both rats and mice the neutrophil count shows a tendency to increase with advancing age whereas the lymphocyte count tends to peak in the first few months of life and diminish with increasing age (Chvédoff et al., 1982). Although some immunosuppressive and anticancer agents depress the white cell counts in one or more of the preclinical test species, such alterations may be quite acceptable for some clinical indications. Indeed, serious granulocytopenia is closely associated with the treatment of cancer and frequently dictates the schedule of cancer treatment protocols (Pizzo, 1984). However, in the development of novel drugs intended for use in large populations for less life-threatening conditions, significant granulocytopenia or lymphocytopenia in preclinical toxicity studies may preclude further development in view of its potential consequences in man. Instances where this has occurred have been reported, notably with metiamide, an early histamine H2-receptor antagonist. The development of metiamide was terminated as a result of granulocytopenia in dogs (Brimblecombe et al., 1973) and in a small number of patients (Forrest et al., 1975). Similar observations were not made in man or animals during the development of the successful analogue, cimetidine (Brimblecombe et al., 1985).

A number of sulphur-containing drugs have been associated with granulocytopenia. These include penicillins, cephalosporins, thiazides, phenothiazines, sulphonamides, sulphones and sulphonylureas as well as a number of investigational drugs (Rosen et al., 1966; Finch, 1977; Bannerjee et al., 1979; Dawson, 1979; Martin et al., 1985). On the basis of dose-related granulocytopenia and bone marrow suppression found in both dogs and rats treated with a thiomopholine quinazosin antihypertensine agent, PD-88823, and the lack of similar effects with its analogue prazosin, it was suggested that the thiomorpholine group had a central role in its haemopoietic toxicity, possibly as a result of its sulphur moiety (Martin et al., 1985).

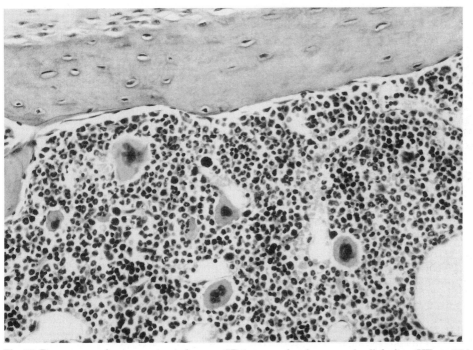

Fig. 15. Bone marrow from an untreated young CD-1 mouse showing normal cellularity. (HE, ×400.)

Bone marrow

The most important histological finding in the bone marrow is *atrophy* (hypocellularity, hypoplasia, aplasia) as a result of marrow suppression following administration of pharmaceutical agents. The use of tissue sections, particularly if embedded in methacrylate, is the method of choice in the assessment of bone marrow cellularity especially if assisted by semi-quantitative analysis, (Burkhardt et al., 1982; Krech and Thiele, 1985). Cytological detail is better evaluated in smear preparations.

However, decalcified, paraffin wax embedded sections are normally preferred in routine studies. The site of sampling should be consistent because considerable regional variation in the cellularity of bone marrow exists. Assessment of bone marrow cellularity at different sites in rats has suggested that the sternum, veterbrae or proximal femur show the most consistent cellularity (Cline and Maronpot, 1985; Wright, 1989). Considerable age-related variation in bone marrow cellularity has also been reported in untreated rats. In Fischer 344 rats, marrow cellularity was shown to be consistently higher in rats less than four months of age than in rats aged seven and sixteen months. Rats at 24 months of age showed the greatest inter-animal variation (Cline and Maronpot, 1985)

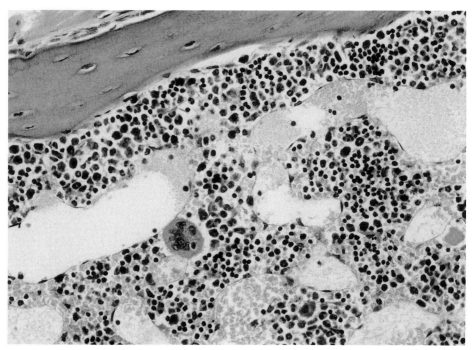

Fig. 16. Bone marrow from a young CD-1 mouse treated for two weeks with an antimitotic agent, similar site to that seen in Figure 15. Overall cellularity is reduced and there is increased prominence of blood-filled sinusoids. (HE, ×400.)

The histological appearance of bone marrow atrophy is not specific for particular drug types (Krech and Thiele, 1985). It is characterized in all species by a variable loss or reduction in cellularity of granulocytic and erythrocytic precursors (Figs. 15 and 16). Residual mature cells often include megakaryocytes. Dilatation of marrow sinusoids and extravasation of red blood cells into the marrow space are other striking features reported with antimitotic agents (Lévy and Raphaël, 1987).

Hyperplasia of the bone marrow occurs in a variety of reactive states, particularly when there is increased red cell or platelet turnover or destruction.

Most commonly, hyperplastic states in the bone marrow are observed in aged rodents as a result of a wide variety of spontaneous inflammatory and neoplastic conditions. Hyperplasia also occurs when administered xenobiotics increase destruction of formed blood cells in the peripheral circulation.

LYMPHOID SYSTEM

Immunotoxicology

There are understandable concerns about the potential adverse effects of drugs and chemicals on the immune system in view of the widespread use of chemicals in the environment, recent developments in our understanding of the immune system and the devastating effects of opportunist infections which result from severe immune depression in man. The unusually high occurrence rates of Kaposi sarcoma in the acquired immune deficiency syndrome (AIDS) has underscored the role of the immune system in the protection against malignant processes (Lane et al., 1985). The major success of organ transplantation have depended heavily on the use of non-specific immunosupppresive drugs. These not only prevent transplant rejection but unfortunately also lower the recipients response to bacterial and viral pathogens and predispose to the development of some types of neoplasia (Bach and Sachs, 1987).

Despite these concerns, uncertainty exists when considering how such effects of chemicals may be effectively detected in experimental work. This problem is highlighted by the large battery of tests studied in the National Toxicology Program (Dean et al, 1982; Luster et al., 1988)), the various screening regimens proposed by other workers notably Vos (1977) as well as the numerous discussion and review papers published by workers in the chemical and pharmaceutical industries, at university and within regulatory authorities (Davies, 1981; Norbury, 1982; Wachsmuth, 1983; Gardner et al., 1983; Loose, 1984; Dean and Thurmond, 1987; Koller, 1987).

More recently, guidelines for special testing batteries for the assessment of chemically induced immunotoxicity have been proposed by the National Toxicology Program (Luster et al., 1988) and the European Chemical Industry Ecology and Toxicology Centre (Trizio et al., 1988).

Although many special tests of immune function have a well accepted place in the study of mechanisms of immune toxicity and in the characteristics of the mode of action of immunosuppresive agents, they are usually not always appropriate for routine screens in the preclinical safety assessment of new pharmaceutical agents. Indeed, their use as screens rather than to study mechanisms can pose problems of interpretation. For instance, a battery of in vitro and in vivo tests of immune function in the mouse were added to the extensive preclinical toxicity studies performed with acyclovir, an acyclic analogue of a natural nucleoside with antiviral activity (Quinn et al., 1982; Tucker et al., 1983). Two of these tests proved to have positive results but despite extensive clinical experience including in immunocompromised patients, these positive experimental results appear to have little or no relevance for man.

It is tempting to conclude that detailed immune function studies should be performed in man, at an appropriate point in the development of a new drug, provided such studies are underwritten by reasonable amounts of conventional preclinical safety data. After all, careful observations in people exposed to drugs can give the only unequivocal evidence of an effect on the human immune system. One approach has been demonstrated recently by Marcoli et al., (1985) in which defects in humoral immunity and lymphocyte subpopulations were sought in patients on long term anticonvulsant therapy. Kelton (1985) elegantly demonstrated impaired reticuloendothelial function in patients treated with methyldopa by measuring the clearance of radiolabelled autologous red cells sensitized with anti-D alloantibody. However, these issues merit detailed discussion and collaboration between immunologists, toxicologists and physicians.

It is probable that conventional toxicity studies in two species are reasonably effective screening procedures for major effects of chemicals on the immune system, provided there is careful examination of the blood, blood forming organs, thymus, spleen, lymph nodes and mucosal-associated lymphoid tissues. If any finding in conventional studies suggests an effect on a particular component of the immune system, special studies can then be directed towards confirming a functional effect and exploring mechanisms involved.

Conventional toxicity studies allow examination of the lymphoid and blood forming organs concurrently with a wide range of other body systems. This is particularly important in the assessment of the immune system which is highly regulated and interacts with nervous, endocrine and other systems. Pertubations in the immune system may be manifest by secondary effects such as immune complex deposition in the renal glomerulus or blood vessels, development of autoimmune disorders, appearance of granulomas or other tissue infiltrates of lymphoreticular cells, development of lymphoid neoplasms, changes in the prevalence of spontaneous infectious disease or the development of opportunist infections (Taffs, 1974).

Conversely, it needs to be remembered that spontaneous or induced alterations in other body systems can lead to effects in the lymphoid organs and immune system. Effects on the immune system in both man and animals are reported following changes in endocrine or sex hormone status (Ahmed et al.,

1985; Ohtaki, 1988), under conditions of inanition (Farnel and Maronpot, 1987), in a number of stress states including surgery, trauma, anaesthesia, restraint, overcrowding and general ill health as a result of inflammatory disease and neoplasia. (Gisler, 1974; Riboli et al., 1984; Pollock et al., 1984; Blazer et al., 1986).

As always, extrapolation from animal models requires detailed metabolism and kinetic studies in the test species. This information is usually available for the conventional but not unusual species or special experimental models.

Immunocytochemistry of lymphoreticular cells

The toxicological pathologist, aided by cytochemistry, immunocytochemistry and the electron microscope, is particularly well situated to explain morphological effects on the immune organs in preclinical studies. Davis (1981) has made a convincing case for using immunocytochemistry and cytochemistry in this evaluation. The use of monoclonal antibodies to T cell subsets and immunoglobulins in laboratory animals, visualization and quantification of enzyme activities in various cell populations and ultrastructural autoradiography (Read et al., 1985), all possess considerable potential to help in the interpretation changes seen in immune organs and in the immune system in preclinical studies.

Immunocytochemistry using monoclonal antibodies against antigenic determinants of lymphoid subpopulations can readily be employed in the critical assessment of tissue sections and blood cells taken from conventional toxicity studies. Use of immunocytochemistry of lymphoid cells in spleen and lymph nodes in combination with image analysis represents a powerful tool for the pathologist in the characterization of drug-induced effects on lymphoid organs. Immunocytochemical techniques are available for the detection and characterization of specific antibody-forming cells in tissue sections, including those producing antibody directed against protein antigens and haptens (van Rooijen et al., 1984; van Rooijen and Classen, 1986).

A variety of monoclonal antibodies to cell surface antigens of lymphoid cells in laboratory animals are commonly available and can be used for the immunocytochemical demonstration of subpopulations of lymphoid cells in tissue sections). Although most of these cell surface markers do not resist routine fixation and paraffin embedding, they can be demonstrated on smear populations and frozen sections. A number of the monoclonal antibodies to rat T cell antigens notably MRC OX8, W3/13 and W3/25 and antibodies to Thy-1 in the mouse have been used in the study of the effects of immunosuppressive agents on the thymus, lymphoid tissue and peripheral blood (Beschorner et al., 1987; Hattori et al., 1987; Evans et al., 1988a). Some of the more important antigens and monoclonal antibodies are discussed below. Very few antibodies to human lymphocyte antigens cross react with the same cells in other animal species except for non-human primates (Greenlee et al., 1987).

Thy-1 (Thy-1.1 and Thy-1.2)

The theta isoantigen, more usually termed Thy-1, is the genetic nomenclature for the locus which codes for the antigen, which is found on the cell surface of thymocytes and mature T cells in the mouse. It was one of the first lymphocyte differentiation antigens to be described in the mouse and its homologues have been extensively studied in other species. Its function remains uncertain (Crawford and Barton, 1986). It is still regarded as one of the most convenient tools for the detection of mouse T cells, despite its distribution not being exclusive to lymphoid cells but also present on cells in the central nervous system, fibroblasts, foetal skeletal muscle, mammary carcinoma cells, epidermal cells (Ahmed and Smith, 1982), bone marrow cells including multipotent stem cells, prothymocytes, some B cell precursors and eosinophils (Raff, et al., 1971; Basch and Berman, 1982).

The Thy-1 locus consists of two alleles Thy-1.1 and Thy-1.2 and most strains of mice possess the Thy-1.2 allele. Therefore, antibodies to Thy-1.2 will label most mouse T-cells when employed in immunocytochemistry (Ermak and Owen, 1986). The intensity of Thy-1.2 labelling is generally higher on thymocytes than on peripheral T cells. This is different to the surface density of Lyt-1 (see following). The differences between thymocytes and more mature cells probably reflect the maturation sequence of these cells: cortical (immature) thymocytes → medullary (hydrocortisone resistant) → thymocytes → T lymphocytes (Ledbetter et al., 1980; Mansour et al., 1987). In the rat, peripheral T-lymphocytes are Thy-1 (OX7) negative (Barclay, 1981b) whereas in the dog Thy-1 is expressed on thymocytes, all peripheral T cells and some bone marrow cells (Dalchauand Fabre, 1981; McKenzie and Fabre, 1981a). A monoclonal antibody to canine Thy-1 has also been used effectively as a pan T-cell marker in this species (Krakowka, 1987; Evans et al., 1988b). In man, the distribution of Thy-1 appears different from that in the lymphoid tissues of mouse and rat. It is absent from blood lymphocytes and restricted to a halo around lymphatic nodules and in post capillary venules in lymph nodes, some peri-arteriolar lymphocytes in the spleen and the periphery of the thymic lobule, suggesting that Thy-1 is a marker for early T lymphocytes in man (MacKenzie and Fabre, 1981b).

Lyt-1, Lyt-2 and Lyt-3

These mouse antigens were the first series of alloantigens to be described which possessed a tissue distribution restricted to thymocytes and T cells (Ahmed and Smith, 1983). They have also been termed LyA, LyB and LyC and Ly-1, Ly-2 and Ly-3. Although their expression is more complex than originally realized, monoclonal rat antisera to these antigens are available and can be used to define subgroups of T cells in the mouse using immunocytochemical techniques.

These antigens are glycoproteins possessing molecular weights of about 35,000. The Lyt-1 alloantigen is expressed more equally between mature T cell and thymocytes (Ahmed and Smith, 1983), which is different to the expression of

Thy-1 (see previous). It seems generally agreed that helper cells are sensitive to the lytic effects of antisera to Lyt-1 but not Lyt-2/3 (Lyt-1 + 2/3-). Suppressor cells are either susceptible to the effects of anti-Lyt-2/3 (ie. Lyt-1-2/3 +) or both anti-Lyt-2/3 and anti-Lyt-1 (ie. Lyt-1 + 2/3 +). Cytotoxic cells are susceptible to lysis with the use of anti-Lyt-2 or Lyt-3 serum (Lyt-1-, 2/3 +) (Ahmed and Smith, 1983). Monoclonal antibodies to Lyt-1 stimulate the production of interleukin-2 by T cells, a function shared by anti-CD5 monoclonal antibodies to the human Lyt-1 counterpart (Ledbetter et al., 1985; Stanton et al., 1986).

These differences can be exploited to define mouse lymphocyte populations in tissue sections using immunocytochemical techniques. For instance antisera to Lyt-2 will label cytotoxic/suppressor T cells and Thy-1.2 most T cells (see Ermak and Owen, 1986). Flow cytometric analysis of spleen cells from C57BL/6 mice has shown that cells labelled Lyt-2 are the most susceptable to aging. In 24 month old mice splenic lymphocytes show a decrease density of Lyt-2 surface antigen as well as impaired PHA and Con A responsiveness (Utsuyama and Hirokawa, 1987). Rat T lymphocyte antigens comparable with mouse Lyt-1 and Lyt-2/3 have been also defined using monoclonal antibodies. MRC OX8 may define the rat homologue of Lyt-2/3.

Mac 1

M1/70.15 is a rat monoclonal antibody clone of 1gG2b class which recognises polypeptides of molecular weights 105,000 and 19000 (Mac 1) found on mouse macrophages and their precursors (Beller et al., 1982; Springer et al., 1978, 1979). This monoclonal antibody represents one of series of clones, all designated by the prefix M1, which were prepared following immunization of DA and AO in rat strains with spleen cells from B10 mice (Springer et al., 1978). This monoclonal antibody selectively inhibits both the mouse and human type three complement receptor (Beller et al., 1982).

L3T4 is a cell surface molecule of molecular weight about 52,000 present on mouse T cells recognised by a rat monoclonal antibody GK1.5 (YTS 191.5). Flow cytometric and biochemical data indicate that L3T4 is similar to the human Leu3/T molecule (Dialynas et al., 1983). L3T4 is expressed by about 80% of thymocytes and 20% of spleen cells in the mouse. Whereas the presence of L3T4 may correlate primarily with Class I MHC antigen, it seems to be expressed primarily by helper/inducer subsets of mouse T lymphocytes (Dialynas et al., 1983).

Asialo GM1

The glycolipid, asialo GM1 (ganglio-n-tetrosylceramide) is employed as a cell surface marker for murine natural killer (NK) cells, activated macrophages and some functionally activated lymphocyte subsets (Kasai et al., 1980, 1981; Stout et al., 1987). It has been suggested that expression of asialo GM1 may reflect changes in glycolipid sialation which is an early event associated with activation of effector cells (Stout et al., 1987).

A monoclonal antibody to asialo GM1, used to study the toxicity of inter-leukin-2 in mice, showed that activated, asialo GM1-positve lymphocytes were those responsible for the vascular leak syndrome induced by this agent (Anderson et al., 1988).

MRC OX1 is a mouse monoclonal antibody of the IgG1 class, specific for the rat leucocyte common antigen, a major glycoprotein of haemopoietic cells of approximate molecular weight 150,000 (Sunderland et al., 1979). Different molecular forms and antigenic heterogenicity of this antigen exist in different cell types (Woollet et al., 1985). This antigen is present on bone marrow cells, thoracic duct cells and over 95% of thymocytes. It is a thymocyte glycoprotein which results in intense PAS staining. Carbohydrate determinants of the leucocyte common antigen which are present in B lymphocytes also react with soyabean lectin, which probably accounts for the specific binding of this lectin with rat B lymphocytes (Brown and Williams, 1982).

MRC OX2 is a mouse IgG monoclonal antibody reactive against a glycoprotein of molecular weight of about 60,000 found in the thymus and brain (McMaster and Williams, 1979a). It labels B lymphocytes weakly but shows good imunocytochemical staining of follicular dendritic cells, endothelium of post capillary venules, thymocytes, peripheral nerves, brain and smooth muscle cells. (Barclay, 1981b).

MRC OX3 and OX4 are mouse monoclonal antibodies of IgG1 class which recognize rat Ia antigens. Ia antigens are polymorphic membrane glycoproteins coded for by the major histocompatability complex, MHC Class II (McMaster and Williams, 1979a,b).

Rat Ia antigen is homologous with mouse Ia antigen and human HLA-DR antigens. These antigens possess a similar molecular structure between species, being composed of two, non-covalently bound but strongly bonded polypeptide chains (α and β). The smaller chain possesses a molecular weight of about 25–32,000 daltons, the larger 32–36,000 daltons (McMaster and Williams, 1979b). In the mouse, the Ia antigens are coded for by two loci within the MHC complex notably in the I-A and the I-E/C subregions (Cullen et al., 1976) corresponding to DP, DQ and DR gene loci in man (Talal, 1987).

There is evidence that Ia antigens are involved in the recognition of foreign antigens by T cells in conjunction with the secretion of the macrophage product interleukin-1 (Talal, 1987). Study of the distribution of Ia antigens in several species including rat have shown that there are two categories of cells which express Ia antigens, those of bone marrow derivation and those of epithelial type (Mayrhofer et al., 1983).

The first group of cells are principally B cells, (Van der Valk and Meijer, 1987), some macrophages, Langerhans cells and dendritic or interdigitating cells. The second group comprise epithelial cells in the thymus, gut, kidney and mammary gland (Barclay and Mayrhofer, 1981; Mayrhofer et al., 1983). Monoclonal antibodies MRC OX3/4 can be used to demonstrate not only B cells in

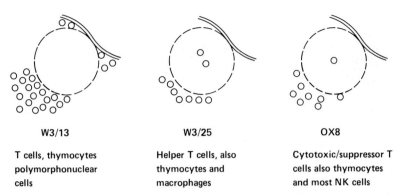

	W3/13	W3/25	OX8

T cells, thymocytes	Helper T cells, also	Cytotoxic/suppressor T
polymorphonuclear	thymocytes and	cells also thymocytes
cells	macrophages	and most NK cells

Figs. 17 and 18. Schematic diagrams of the immunocytochemical staining patterns of rat lymph node and thymus using monoclonal antibodies W/13, W3/25 and OX8.

the rat but also the level of Ia antigen expression in the rat thymic medullary epithelium which can be modified by xenobiotics (Beschorner, 1987). Ia antigens appear to be the receptors for lactate dehydrogenase virus in mice (Inada and Mims, 1984).

The structural similarity of Ia antigen between species is shown by the fact that the monoclonal antibodies to rat Ia antigen cross react between species. MRC OX3 and OX4 cross react with mouse allotypic determinants which can be mapped to the H-2 IA region. Furthermore, MRC OX3 cross-reacts with certain human lymphoblastoid cell lines (McMaster and Williams, 1979b). A mouse monoclonal antibody produced against human Ia antigens that reacts with 20–30% of human peripheral blood lymphocytes was also reported to cross react with more than 90% of lymphocytes in the dog (Iwaki et al., 1983). Ia antigens on canine interdigitating cells, follicular dendritic cells and Langerhans cells can also be demonstrated by this monoclonal antibody (Moore, 1986). Another monoclonal antibody against human HLD-DR antigens is also reported to stain canine lymphoid cells (Greenlee et al., 1987).

MRC OX7 This mouse monoclonal antibody of IgG1 class recognises the rat Thy1.1 molecule. Immunocytochemical study has shown that MRC OX7 stains a variety of cell types in rat lymphoid tissue. Stained cells include thymocytes, eosinophils, stem cells, immature B cells, mast cells, megakaryocytes, reticular cells (excluding those in germinal centres), a few peripheral lymphocytes, the pericyte sheath around post capillary venules and peripheral nerves (Barclay, 1981b)

MRC OX8 (Figs. 17 and 18) is also an IgG1 monoclonal antibody which recognizes a surface glycoprotein present on the majority of thymocytes, a T cell subset which mediates suppression of antibody formation, cytotoxic cell pre-

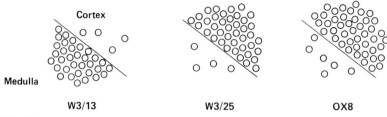

Fig. 18.

cursor (cytotoxic/suppressor T cells), most NK cells and granular intraepithelial leucocytes in the small intestine (Brideau et al., 1980)

On the basis of studies of molecular weight, tissue distribution of antigen and function of cells reactive with monoclonal antibodies, it is probable that the antigens labelled by MRC OX8 are homologous with Leu-2a, T8 (monoclonal OKT8) and Lyt-2. However MRC OX8 labels NK cells whereas anti-Leu-2a,

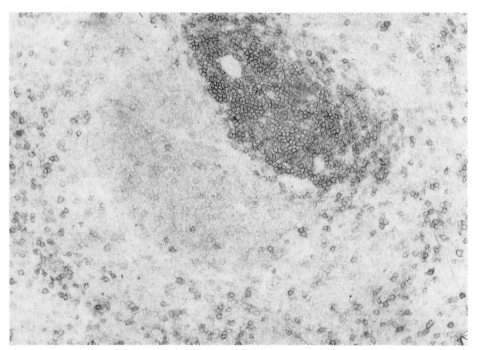

Fig. 19. Spleen from a young Wistar rat stained for T lymphocytes using monoclonal antibody W3/13. The periarteriolar lymphoid sheath is shown clearly. (Frozen section, immuno-alkaline phosphatase, ×250.)

anti-T8 (OKT-8) and anti-Lyt-2 antibodies label few, if any NK cells in man and mouse (Mason et al., 1983).

MRC OX19 is a monoclonal antibody against thymocyte glycoprotein of molecular weight 69,000 which binds to a determinant expressed on all thymocytes and peripheral T cells but not B cells, mast cells macrophages or NK cells. It is believed to be the homologue of T1 (OKT1) or Leu 1 in man and Lyt-1 in the mouse (Mason et al., 1983).

W3/13 is a monoclonal mouse IgG1 antibody which recognizes a heavily glycosylated glycoprotein of 95,000 molecular weight which has a high content of O-linked carbohydrate structures (Figs. 17, 18 and 19). This glycoprotein is also recognised by peanut lectin binding (Brown et al., 1981; Brown and Williams, 1982). This antigen is expressed on rat thymocytes, T but not B lymphocytes, immunoglobulin-secreting plasma cells, polymorphonuclear cells, stem cells and brain cells (Williams et al., 1977; Dyer and Hunt, 1981; Brown et al., 1981; Thomas and Green, 1983).

W3/25 is a monoclonal mouse IgG1 antibody which recognizes a surface glycoprotein 56,000 molecular weight found on a majority of thymocytes, the helper subset of rat peripheral T cells as well as macrophages (Figs. 17 and 18).

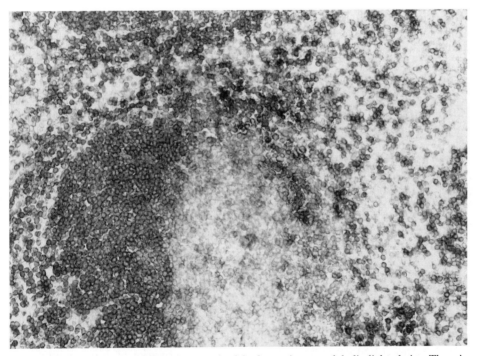

Fig. 20. Spleen from a young CD-1 mouse stained for kappa immunoglobulin light chains. There is a well-defined B-lymphocyte zone and lack of staining of the periarteriolar lymphoid sheath. (Frozen section, immunoperoxidase, ×140.)

These cells are not labelled by MRC OX8. This antigen is likely to represent the homologue of the human T4 (OKT4) and Leu 3a antigens (Williams et al., 1977; Brideau et al., 1980; Barclay, 1981a; Mason et al., 1983).

Immunoglobulins

Antibodies to immunoglobulins can be used to delineate B lymphocytes in tissue sections. As the individual B-lineage cells express only one of the two possible light chain classes, immunocytochemistry using antibodies to kappa or lamda light chains represents a common and convenient method for the assessment of the clonality of B-cell populations in the diagnosis of lymphoid neoplasms (Fig. 20). Although this methodology possesses some limitations, light chain analysis is considered to be the single most useful immunocytochemical procedure in the confirmation of neoplasm of B cell type (Picker et al., 1987).

It should be noted that in the mouse less than 5% of immunoglobulin contains the lamda chain due to paucity of the V-lamda gene in this species. Therefore, antibody to kappa light chain is the most appropriate reagent to demonstrate B cell lineage in this species.

Lectins

Other histochemical markers for lymphocyte populations are labelled lectins, particularly as many lectin receptors are resistant to paraffin embedding and can be demonstrated in routine paraffin embedded sections. For instance, labelled peanut lectin (Arachis hypogaea), specific for terminal β-galactose residues, stains activated lymphocytes (geminoblasts and centriblasts) in germinal centres of rat lymph nodes as well as cortical (immature) thymocytes and macrophages (Kabir et al., 1983). Peanut lectin probably binds to a 95,000 molecular weight leucocyte sialoglycoprotein present on thymocytes which is also bound by the W3/13 monoclonal antibody (Brown and Williams, 1982). The staining pattern of W3/13 on the rat thymus appears similar to that of labelled peanut lectin. The leucocyte common antigen present on B lymphocytes also binds soybean lectin (Glycine max) (Brown and Williams, 1982).

Systemic manifestations of immune derangements

The function of the immune system is undertaken by cells and molecules spread throughout the body and immune disorders can disrupt many organ systems. Its function can be divided into several different but interelated operations: encounter, recognition, activation, deployment, discrimination and regulation (Nossal, 1987).

The principle components of the immune system which undertake these operations are highly regulated but interelated networks of lymphocytes and their secretory products which, when activated, trigger responding cells throughout many organs in the body. Pivotal to the action of B and T lymphocytes are antigen presenting cells, notably macrophages but also dendritic reticulum cells, interdigitating cells, Langerhans cells which express high levels of class II histocompatability cell surface Ia antigens (DR in man). These Ia molecules are glycoproteins which are important for immune activation (Nossal,1987). They are known to be products of several IR gene loci in the major histocompatability complex (MHC): I-A and I-E in the mouse, DP, DQ and DR in man. The Ia antigens are functionally involved in T cell activation and release of the macrophage product, interleukin-1 (Talal, 1987). The helper T-cell responds to interleukin-1 and antigen, or antigen presenting cells to produce interleukin-2, a substance which interacts with receptors on T cells and NK cells to mediate lymphocyte proliferation, and interferon production and regulation of B cell growth and differentiation. Studies of Ia molecules at gene and cell surface level have shown immense polymorphism. This may explain the correlation of particular HLA types with increased susceptibility to autoimmune disorders (Talal, 1987).

It is the disruption of this delicately balanced system which leads to disorders of immune suppression, hypersensitivity, formation of immune complexes, development of autoimmune phenomena and lymphoreticular neoplasia (Krakowa, 1987). Some of these phenomena are discussed under other organs, notably skin, lung, kidney, liver, thyroid gland and gastrointestinal tract.

LYMPH NODES

Lymph nodes are routinely examined histologically in toxicity and carcinogenicity studies. In view of recent advances in our understanding of structure-function relationship in lymph nodes, careful histopathological examination of well-prepared sections of lymph nodes, aided where necessary by morphometric, enzyme and immunohistochemical techniques represents a powerful tool in the assessment of the effects of drugs and chemicals on the lymphoid system.

Although lymph node structure shows interspecies and strain variations (Bélisle and Sainte-Marie, 1981; Sainte-Marie et al., 1982; Sainte-Marie and Peng, 1983, 1985) and is influenced by exogeneous antigenic stimulation (Bélisle et al., 1982), the general architecture remains similar in most laboratory animal species. In resting lymph nodes the cortex is divided into discrete B cell areas called primary follicles and the T cell domain, the diffuse, deep or parafollicular cortex. Lymphocytes enter the lymph node via specialized post-capillary or high endothelial venules whereas other blood cells flow by without adhering to the lining cells of these specialized vessels. After traversing their specific cortical domains, recirculating T and B cells enter the medullary sinuses prior to entering lymphatic ducts (see Weissman et al., 1978; Sainte-Marie et al., 1982). The absolute size of deep cortex units varies little between the species, although nodes of larger species possess greater numbers of these units (Bélisle and Sainte-Marie, 1981).

Lymph nodes are exposed to various forms of antigen and their response to these antigens is reflected in lymph node histology. Immunological reactions can take place in one or more of the specific compartments of lymph nodes, the follicles, paracortex, medullary cords or sinuses.

Various descriptive, quantitative and semiquantitative methods have been employed in the assessment of lymph nodes, both in clinical and experimental histopathological studies (Gillman and Gillman, 1952; Tsakraklides et al., 1973; Patt et al., 1975; Hunter et al., 1975; Kaufman et al., 1977; Pihl et al., 1980; Ciocca, 1980). These methods are often based on the standardized system for reporting human lymph node morphology described by Cottier and colleagues (1972). One of the simpler methods based on this system which has been used in the assessment of lymphoid status in cancer patients (van Nagell et al., 1977; Nacopoulou et al., 1981), is of use in toxicology. In this method the principal histological pattern is defined, i.e. *lymphocyte predominance* when increased numbers of lymphocytes are present in the deep cortex and medulla, *germinal centre predominance* when the outer cortex shows large numbers of active germinal centres, *lymphocyte depletion* pattern when the cortex shows a paucity of lymphocyte often associated with fibrosis or hyalinization and *unstimulated pattern* when the cortex is thin, and germinal centres show little or no activity (see review by van der Valk and Maijer, 1987). Another effective method is the quantitative or semiquantitative analysis of the size of germinal centres, para-cortex and degree of sinus histiocytosis (Patt et al., 1975). In the use of these systems the tridimensional structure of the lymph node should be kept in mind. Tridimensional study may be necessary to obtain a complete view of the overall architecture of a node, particularly the organization of the deep cortex (Bélisle and Sainte-Marie, 1981).

Enzyme cytochemical study and the use of immunocytochemical techniques are also helpful in the evaluation of lymph node function, as well as in the diagnosis of hyperplastic and neoplastic states. The paracortex or T cell zone can be assessed in more detail in the rat by the use of monoclonal antibodies W3/13 for T cells, W3/25 for helper cell subsets and OX8 for suppressor cells (Mason et al., 1980; Barclay, 1981a), although unfixed frozen sections or specially fixed materials are usually necessary when using these particular monoclonal antibodies (Fig. 19).

The B cell populations are outlined by using antisera to the various immunoglobin classes. IgD may be particularly useful in outlining the germinal centres. Other important cells are the dendritic cells which trap antigens on their surface and present them to B lymphocytes and interdigitating cells important in the presentation of antigen to T cells. Dendritic cells stain immunocytochemically with antisera against C3b and C3d complement components and possess 5′-nucleotidase activity. Interdigitating cells can be recognised with antibodies to S-100 in paraffin sections. These are well-characterized in frozen sections by immunocytochemical demonstration of HLD-DR or Ia antigens (Barclay 1981b; Dijkstra, 1982; van derValk and Meijer, 1987). Tingible body and sinusoidal macrophages represent other prominant cells in lymph nodes. Immunocytochemical localization of lysozyme using antihuman urinary lysozyme anti-serum remains a valuable method for the demonstration of lymph node macro-phages in paraffin-embedded tissue sections from rats, mice and hamsters (Klockars and Osserman, 1974; Spicer et al., 1977). Macrophages also show acid phosphatase and non-specific esterase activity and may stain immunocytochemi-cally using antisera to Ia antigens (Dijstra, 1982).

Imprint preparations, plastic embedding and semi-thin sections also have their place in the morphological evaluation of lymphoid tissue (Beckstead, 1983; Wachsmuth, 1983; van der Valk and Meijer, 1987).

Atrophy, hypoplasia, aplasia, lymphocyte depletion, unstimulated pattern

Atrophy of lymphoid tissue or depletion of lymphocyte subpopulations occurs in preclinical safety studies under a variety of circumstances. Such changes are often observed in rodents in advancing age (Anver et al., 1982) although their extent is species, strain and environment-related. Burek (1978) has described the decrease in number of germinal centres which occurs with increasing age in both Brown Norway and Wistar rats as well as the increase in plasma cells which appear in the medullary sinuses. A wide range of morphological abnormalities such as atrophy of paracortex, germinal centres and medullary cords are found in aging CD-1, C3H, B10A and (B10AX A/J) F_1 mice (Sainte-Marie and Peng, 1987)

Germ-free animals also possess poorly developed cervical and mesenteric lymph nodes (Bélisle et al., 1982). Atrophy occurs after some viral infections (Biberfeld et al., 1985; Jaffe et al., 1985), stress and malnutrition (Wogan, 1984). Rapid lymphocyte depletion results from agonal changes in man and animals dying from spontaneous disease. Lymphocyte depletion (more correctly termed hypoplasia or aplasia rather than atrophy), is found in the deep cortex of athymic rodents (Fossum et al., 1980; Sainte-Marie and Peng, 1983; Sainte-Marie et al., 1984).

A number of chemical agents including drugs cause lymphocyte depletion or atrophy of lymph nodes in toxicity studies. The particular zone of the lymph nodes affected and the nature of the change is not only dependent on the type of agent, but the dose, the timing and duration of administration.

Following the administration of very high doses of corticosteroids, given when there is maximum germinal centre proliferation, cell necrosis in germinal centres has been observed (Durkin and Thorbecke, 1971). Under other conditions, lymphocyte lysis within germinal centres may not occur but simple depletion of lymphocytes may be seen in the coronas of follicles (van den Broek et al., 1983). As in the thymus, stress alone can produce similar changes to those produced in lymph nodes by corticosteroids, perhaps as a result of release of endogeneous steroids. It may, therefore, be difficult to separate stress-related lymphoid atrophy in toxicity studies from that produced by specific immunosuppressive agents, particularly at the end of toxicity studies when advanced, morphological changes are observed. The dose-response relationship of such effects on lymphoid and thymic tissue are helpful.

Immunosuppressive agents generally produce changes in lymphoid tissue at most dose levels including those doses which induce no signs of general toxicosis. By contrast, lymphoid changes as a result of stress can be expected to be limited to higher doses where there is also evidence of other stress-related phenomena.

Experience with immunosuppressants has shown that lymphoid hyperplasia can occur at low doses and atrophy of the cortex or paracortex at higher doses. This is not perhaps surprising for it has been shown with a number of immuno-suppressive agents that the nature of T cell suppression in laboratory animals is dose-dependent (Noble and Norbury, 1983). Selective T cell suppression can give rise to B cell hyperreactivity and subsequent lymphoid proliferation or hyper-plasia (Biberfeld et al., 1985; Jaffe et al., 1985). On this basis hyperplasia can occur at low doses and lymphoid atrophy in high-dose groups. In man prolifera-tive lymphoid disorders are also well recognised accompanied by post-transplant immunosuppression with cyclosporin A and prednisone where they have a close relationship to the presence of Epstein-Barr virus (Nalesnik et al., 1988).

Hyperplasia, lymphocyte predominance / hyperplasia of paracortex, germinal centre predominance / hyperplasia

Lymph nodes of mice, rats, hamsters and dogs undergo hyperplasia following a variety of stimuli. Different regions may be affected including the thymic dependent paracortex, germinal centres and medullary cords. In most normal rodents, germinal centres are not particularly prominent (Wogan, 1984) although this varies between laboratories. Beagle dogs generally show prominent germinal centres in lymph nodes.

Hyperplasia of germinal centres (follicular hyperplasia), occurs in rodents as a result of infective agents and administration of chemicals particularly if accom-panied by tissue damage. As noted above, follicular hyperplasia may occur in lymph nodes after administration of selective immunosuppressive agents. Elegant comparative studies between lymph nodes of man and mouse have shown that two types of germinal centre hyperplasia (follicular hyperplasia) can be dis-tinguished (Pattengale and Taylor, 1983). *Typical hyperplasia* is characterized by prominent active germinal centres which remain entirely normal in ap-pearances. By contrast, in *atypical hyperplasia* the prominent germinal centres show confluence, loss of marginal zones and partial effacement of normal node architecture. This form should be regarded with some care for it may indicate a pre-lymphomatous state (Pattengale and Taylor, 1983).

Typical follicular hyperplasia

This represents a normal humoral immune response. It is characterized in man and laboratory animals by the presence of prominant germinal centres in the cortex. These are composed of B cells of centrofollicular type with surface membrane immunoglobulin heavy chains, mu, light chains, kappa or lamda, receptors for C3b, the Fc receptor of IgG and class I and II histocompatability antigens (Audouin and Diebold, 1986). Germinal centres are characterized by a pale hemisphere on their capsular aspect composed of small and large centrocytes and some plasma cells and a deeper, darker staining hemisphere composed of centroblasts and immunoblasts. Tingible body body macrophages are more numerous in the dark zone whereas dendritic reticular cells are most dense in the clear zone. Follicles are surrounded by a rim of small lymphocytes most densely aggregated at the dark pole of the germinal centre. These are mostly polyclonal B cells containing IgM or IgD as well as receptors for C3b and Fc. Some cells of helper/inducer type are also found in this zone.

Atypical follicular hyperplasia

These follicles show atypical morphological features, including disruption of the normal architectural pattern of the germinal centre. Marker studies show disorganization of the normal immunostaining patterns. A key feature indicative of a pre-neoplastic or neoplastic state is the presence of antigenic monoclonality, e.g. cells positive for only *one* light chain, eiher kappa or lamda (van der Valk and Meijer, 1987).

Hyperplasia of the paracortex (deep cortex, T-cell zone) is characterized by an expansion of the zone by small dark lymphocytes often with a sprinkling of immunoblasts, plasma cells, clusters of interdigitating cells recognised by pale cytoplasm and ovoid or curved nuclei, and thickened post-capillary venules (Audouin and Diebold, 1986). These changes may be accompanied by plasma cell hyperplasia (medullary plasmacytosis) particularly in mice (Wogan, 1984).

It is important to recognise these different patterns of lymphoid hyperplasia when found in animals treated with xenobiotics because different patterns provide clues for a particular mechanism of action or type of changes in the immune system. For instance, subcutaneous injection of mice with the antiepileptic drug, diphenylhydantoin, was shown to produce lymphodenopathy which involved the T-cell dependent zones two days after injection. Four and six days after injection, numerous lymphoid cells and immunoblasts were noted in paracortical zones associated with enlargement of primary follicles and appearance of plasma cells in the medulla. Germinal centres developed at day eight and were prominant by day ten. Plasma cells showed mainly positive staining for IgM or IgG on day four but by day six, IgG-containing plasma cells were predominant. (Gleichmann et al., 1983). On the basis of these findings as well as functional studies Gleichmann and colleagues (1983) argued that the immune-mediated conditions associated with the use of diphenylhydantoin in man could be due to a similar T-cell dependent proliferation and functional activation of B cells. This could lead to a form of drug-induced graft-versus-host reaction. Various forms of atypical lymph node hyperplasia characterized by the presence of plentiful immunoblasts, plasma cells and prominant blood vessels have also been described in patients treated with this agent (Dorfman and Warnke, 1974).

Another instance of lymphoid hyperplasia was reported in the conventional subacute and chronic toxicity studies performed with muroctasin, a muramyl dipeptide derivative, a potent immunostimulatory agent and adjuvent. This was possibly a result of its ability to activate macrophages to produce interleukin-1. This agent also induced paracortical hyperplasia, hyperplasia of germinal centres and an increase in number of plasma cells in both mice and dogs (Ono et al., 1988). An analogous situation is the reported plasma cell hyperplasia in medullary cords of lymph nodes in mice treated with antilymphocytic serum (Krueger et al., 1971).

Lymph node hyperplasia, characterized by expansion of paracortical zones, prominance of germinal centres, presence of abundant plasma cells with round eosinophilic cytoplasmic inclusions (Russell bodies) and expansion of subcapsular sinuses by lymphocytes and eosinophils was also reported in BDF mice and Sprague-Dawley rats treated for several weeks with interleukin-1. This was postulated to be a reflection of its extensive effects on both T and B lymphocytes and haemopoietic cells (Anderson et al., 1988; Anderson and Hayes, 1989).

Sinus histiocytosis, histiocytic hyperplasia

Sinus histiocytosis is commonly seen in the lymph nodes of aging rodents and occurs as a non-specific reactive change in the presence of inflammatory lesions or large, necrotic or ulcerated neoplasms. Sinus histiocytosis is characterized by the presence of abundant, rounded macrophages possessing pale eosinophilic cytoplasm in the sinusoids, often associated with prominence of cells lining the sinusoids. In old rats, large histiocytic cells with pink, red or pigmented, granular cytoplasm are well described findings (Burek, 1978). In some instances the proliferation of histocytes may involve large areas of the lymph node and therefore the term *histiocytic hyperplasia* is merited.

SPLEEN

In man, the spleen has two primary functions, one of filtration and a second of immunological processing and destruction (Rosse, 1987). In adult humans, the bone marrow provides most of the erythropoietic activity under normal and hypoxic conditions, whereas in rats the spleen readily responds to increased demand. (Stutte et al., 1986). This difference can be explained on an anatomical basis by the larger capacity of the human bone marrow for increased erythropoiesis than that of small rodents (Seifert and Marks, 1985).

Although the spleen shows species and strain variations in structure, it is generally composed of the so-called white and red pulp. In rodents, dog and man extensive study has shown that the white pulp has a zonal structure comprising a central and peripheral periarteriolar lymphoid sheath (PALS) and a marginal or mantle zone (MZ) with marginal sinuses and germinal centres (Veerman and van Ewijk, 1975) (Figs. 19, 20 and 21). In addition to lymphoid cells, macro-

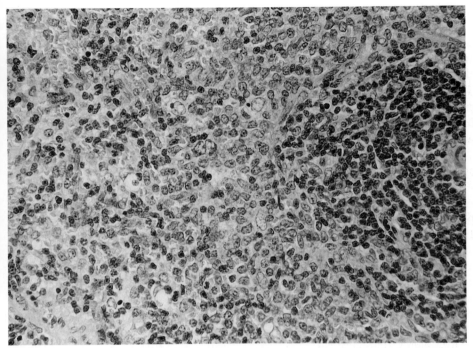

Fig. 21. Spleen from an untreated young Wistar rat showing a normal periarteriolar lymphoid sheath and a prominent mantle zone. (HE, X300.)

phages and dendritic cells are also found in the white pulp. Circulating B and T cells, traverse the walls of the marginal sinuses and migrate to their respective zones. The red pulp is composed of numerous sinusoids lined by macrophages ('littoral' phagocytes) enabling the disposal of senescent cells and cellular debris.

It is important that the pathologist be aware of the various functions and interactions which occur in these splenic zones. The effects of drugs and chemicals on the lymphoid and haemopoietic system may be manifested by quite subtle morphological alterations in the spleen. The central periarteriolar lymphatic sheath (PALS) is a T cell dependent area which is well labelled by various anti-T-cell antibodies such as W3/13 in the rat and anti-Thy-1 in the mouse (Barclay, 1981a) (Fig. 19). Most of these cells belong to the recirculating pool of T-lymphocytes (Veerman and Ewijk, 1975). Antigen activated T-lymphocytes proliferate and differentiate at this site in close association with interdigitating reticulum cells at the early stage of an immune response (Veerman and van Ewijk, 1975; Veerman and de Vries, 1978). The marginal zone (MZ) is the first site of antigen and immune complex deposition as well as the site of entrance of recirculating lymphocytes (van Rooijen, 1973, 1977). In this area, antigen-sensitive recirculating cells have an early contact with antigen. They are selected out of the cellular flow and are stimulated to proliferate. T and B cell cooperation probably starts in this part of the white pulp. Precursors of antibody producing cells also settle in the marginal zone, migrate into the follicles and proliferate following appropriate stimulation. Similarly, lymphocytes from the thymic cortex, probably suppressor cells, also colonize this area after antigenic stimulation. Indeed, the anti-T-cell antibody W3/13 labels a scattering of cells in the mantel zone of the rat spleen (Barclay, 1981a; Dijkstra and Döpp, 1983). Thus, activation of germinal centres can be regarded as the expression of antigen trapping followed by homing of specific antigen-binding B cells traversing the follicles which are then stimulated to proliferate in the germinal centres (Durkin and Thorbecke, 1971).

As in the lymph nodes, accessory cells are found among lymphoid cells of the spleen. It has been shown in the white pulp of the rat spleen that strongly Ia (OX-3) positive branching cells showing little or no acid phosphatase activity represent interdigitating cells. Conversely, rounded cells showing intense acid phosphatase activity and only sporadic Ia-staining are macrophages (Dijkstra, 1982).

Although the red pulp can alter as a result of immune stimulation, it also undergoes changes as a result of variations in circulation, extramedullary haemopoiesis, accumulation of macrophages, connective tissue and pigment as well as in response to increased demand for filtration of abnormal red blood cells (Rosse, 1987). All these changes may occur following the administration of drugs and chemicals.

Although weighing of the spleen is technically easy to perform, the interpretation of treatment-related splenic weight changes is more difficult in view of the complexity of the vascular, tissue and cellular responses which can occur. Although splenic weight is not reliable as a measure of cellular immune system changes in the dog, it is a better measurement in rodents (Wachsmuth, 1983). In addition, its small size and discrete morphology makes the rodent spleen relatively easy to orientate, embed and to cut standard sections for morphometric analysis. Furthermore, cutting unfixed frozen sections for application of monoclonal antibodies is technically easier than the production of unfixed frozen sections of lymph nodes. These factors serve to make the spleen an appropriate organ for quantitative or semiquantitative microscopic analysis. Simple morphometric analysis of the total cross-sectional area of the spleen in haematoxylin and eosin sections correlates well with splenic weight and provides a good basis for assessing the other compartments of the spleen. Furthermore, using a computerized image analysis system, these measurements are quick to perform and serve as a method for assessing spleen size retrospectively when the organ is not weighed at autopsy. Similarly, morphometric analysis of lymphocyte subsets using monoclonal antibodies on frozen sections of spleen is also a reliable technique which can be used in both mice and rats.

Congestion / haemorrhage

This is one of the most common findings in almost all species used in toxicity studies. It can be an agonal phenomenon related to mode of death or method of euthanasia. Severe congestion of the red pulp has also been described in the early phase of development of large granular cell leukaemia in the Fischer rat (Losco and Ward, 1984). Vasodilating drugs also influence the accumulation of blood in the splenic red pulp (Fort et al., 1984) as well as compounds which have primary or secondary effects on erythropoiesis. In the dog, congestion may be especially pronounced in view of the particular function of dog spleen and it, therefore, renders splenic weight an unreliable indicator of cellular changes in the lymphoid compartment.

Splenic congestion and haemorrhage accompanied by haemosiderin deposition, fatty change, extramedullary haemopoiesis and fibrosis (see following) is produced in rats by the administration of a variety of aniline-type compounds including the drug dapsone (Weinberger et al., 1985). It has been suggested that such changes result from methaemoglobinaemia produced by these compounds (Goodman et al., 1984) or the accumulation of potentially toxic metabolites in erythrocytes which are released in high concentrations in the spleen when red blood cells are broken down in the red pulp (Weinberger et al., 1985).

Extramedullary haemopoiesis

The degree of haemopoiesis occurring in the spleen varies between species, strains and conditions of diet and husbandry. In the normal adult rat evidence of haemopoiesis may be observed although this is less than in the mouse and hamster. In the dog, as in man, little or no splenic haemopoiesis is observed under normal conditions.

The red pulp may expand and develop marked haematopoiesis under a variety of circumstances. In rodents many of these stimuli are non-specific and are sporadically seen in carcinogenicity studies. Drugs and chemicals which affect blood cells may activate intense haemopoiesis in the spleen, the cytological nature of which varies with the type of cell affected.

The rapidity with which splenic erythropoiesis occurs in rats has been shown under hypoxic conditions. Exposure of 50 day and 120 day-old Wistar rats to hypoxic conditions corresponding to an altitude of 6000 m produced almost immediate but morphologically normal splenic erythropoiesis which reached a maximum between two and four weeks later (Stutte et al., 1986). It was shown to be associated with increased splenic weight and decrease in splenic haemosiderin. It reverted to normal within four weeks after return to sea level conditions.

Chemicals with effects on red blood cells produce large numbers of erythropoietic cells in the spleen (Weinberger et al., 1985). Increased erythropoiesis may be difficult to distinguish from plasma cell hyperplasia which also occurs in the red pulp. Careful cytological assessment of the red pulp in such instance can be of considerable help in the interpretation of toxicological findings. For instance, the presence of pigment-laden macrophages as well as numerous erythropoietic cells in the red pulp implies that there is increased red cell destruction.

Iron pigment is commonly seen in the spleen of the aged rat, largely in the red pulp. Similar changes are less striking in the aged mouse and hamster possibly because amyloid deposition is often an overriding feature in the spleen of these species. Accumulation of iron is sometimes observed in toxicity studies with novel drugs, but the reason for deposition of iron is not always very clear. However, increased iron deposition in the splenic red pulp of rats may indicate an adverse effect on red blood cells and be associated with decreases in haemoglobin levels. Of practical interest is that even in the normal rat spleen, sufficient iron pigment may be present for the Perl's stain for iron to be a useful stain for delineating red pulp clearly for morphometric study.

In addition to iron, *lipofuscin pigment* also accumulates in the spleen of aged rats (Ward and Reznik-Schuller, 1980). In certain strains of mice it is found in considerable quantities, typically in the upper pole of the spleen in young adults (Crichton et al., 1977). Hamsters also accumulate lipofuscin the splenic red pulp.

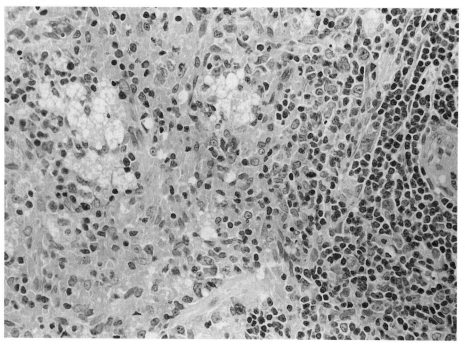

Fig. 22. Spleen from a young Wistar rat treated with a liposomal preparation by the intravenous route. The red pulp shows a loss of cellularity and an accumulation of foamy macrophages. (HE, ×500.)

Fatty change, clear cell change, foam cell accumulation

Clear cells or foam cells may be observed in the red pulp of the spleen in preclinical toxicity studies. The spleen, which acts as a filter for foreign substances circulating in the blood, can accumulate complex materials such as glycoproteins, phospholipids or liposomes injected repeatedly in toxicity studies. Endogeneous breakdown products also accumulate in the spleen under certain conditions and present a similar histopathological appearance.

It is well known that foam cell accumulation occurs in the splenic red pulp in man in a variety of haematological disorders including thalassaemia, idiopathic thrombocytopenic purpura and leukaemia probably as a result of the accelerated turnover of blood cells and the accumulation of their breakdown products in splenic histiocytes (Ishihara et al., 1985). Drugs and chemicals with adverse effects on blood cells may also produce an accumulation of foam cells in preclinical toxicity studies. Foam cells are described in the rat spleen following administration of aniline type compounds (Weinberger et al., 1985) and liposomes (Figs 22, 23 and 24). The precise mechanism involved may be difficult to elucidate for foam cells do not always accumulate when there is increased blood

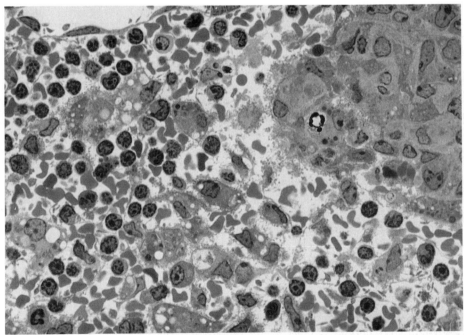

Fig. 23. High power view of the splenic red pulp from a male CD1 mouse following intravenous dosing for seven days with a drug-bearing liposome preparation. It shows details of the enlarged, vacuolated macrophages much more clearly than in Figure 22. Illustration by courtesy of Dr. N.G. Read. (Toluidine blue, plastic embedded, ×1200.)

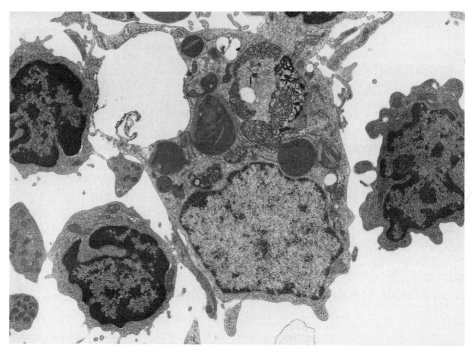

Fig. 24. Electron micrograph of a macrophage in the spleen illustrated in Figure 23 showing abundant cytoplasm and containing a number of secondary lysosomes, in some of which there are multilamellar bodies with appearences suggestive of liposomal debris. Illustration by courtesy of Dr. N.G. Read. (EM, ×10,000.)

cell turnover or destruction. Presumably as the macrophage is involved, factors influencing macrophage function also have a part to play in their development.

Macrophages in the marginal zones are the first cells to encounter injected particulate matter such as liposomes as the particles leave the white pulp capillaries (van Rooijen and Roeterink, 1980). Injected liposomes containing agents which damage macrophages also affect lymphocyte populations present in the marginal zones, probably be release of proteolytic enzymes or of the injected active agent from dying macrophages (van Rooijen et al., 1985).

Histochemical, enzyme cytochemical, immunocytochemical, and ultrastructural study may help in the elucidation of the nature of substances present in the clear cells (Ishihara et al., 1985).

Splenic atrophy

The lymphocyte population of the splenic parenchyma becomes depleted under a number of circumstances in rodents and dogs. This occurs with increasing age in rodents. In mice and hamsters lymphoid cells may be displaced by the accumulation of amyloid. Atrophy also occurs in all species as a non-specific reaction to

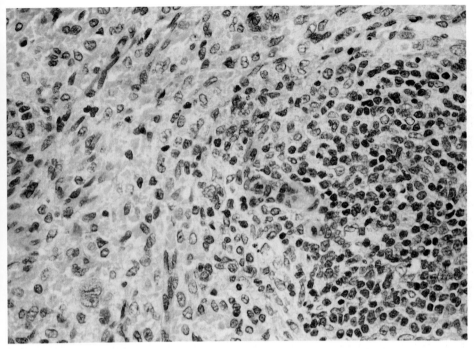

Fig. 25. Spleen from the same strain of Wistar rat to that seen in Figure 21, but treated for two days with cyclophosphamide. There is a major loss of cells from both the periarteriolar lymphoid sheath and the mantle zone. (HE, ×500.)

stress or severe weight loss. Loss of lymphocytes can also be a result of agonal change (see Thymus and Lymph Nodes).

Lymphocytes are also depleted as a result of treatment with xenobiotics, notably immunosuppressive and anticancer drugs. The precise lymphocytic populations affected and the degree of change depends on the nature of the drug, its dose, and length of administration, as in the thymus and lymph nodes.

The immunosuppressive agent, cyclosporin, has been shown to deplete lymphocyte populations in the periarterial lymphoid sheaths and marginal zones in rats, while lymph nodes remained unaffected undersome circumstances (Blair et al., 1982).

Cyclophosphamide also depletes the periarterial lymphoid sheaths. Initially, cell debris and increased numbers of macrophages are seen. Later, periarterial lymphoid sheaths contain only a few lymphocytes and prominent epithelioid cells (Fig. 25). Indeed, the atrophic process may extend into the red pulp which also shows a striking loss of nucleated cells, accumulation of red blood cells, prominent endothelial cells and a scattering of rounded cells with pale eosinophilic cytoplasm (Fig. 25).

The marginal zone was shown to be preferentially affected in the spleen of Lewis rats and albino Swiss mice treated with an otherwise non-toxic single dose of the antineoplastic anthracenedione derivative mitoxantrone (Levine and Gherson, 1986). Four to six hours following treatment there was evidence of a destructive process, largely limited to the marginal zone and characterized histologically by the presence of a pale zone of vacuolated macrophages containing nuclear debris. Subsequently, the marginal zone became atrophic, showing reduced cellularity with only a few residual macrophages and stromal cells. As slight changes were also described in the germinal centres and the periarterolar, lymphoid sheath remained essentially spared, it was postulated that the changes may have been a result of a primary effect of mitoxantrone on a B-lymphocyte subset, such as an IgM type which is prevalent in the marginal zone (Levine and Gherson, 1986). By contrast, the antimitotic drug, hydroxyurea, produced more diffuse changes in the mouse spleen involving most nucleated cells in both red and white pulp as well as the bone marrow (Lévy and Raphaël, 1987).

Lymphoid hyperplasia

As in the lymph node, reactive states are manifest by hyperplasia of the various lymphoid zones in the spleen. This may take the form of hyperplasia of the periarteriolar lymphoid sheath or marginal zone or follicular hyperplasia, each representing a particular functional state. These changes may be seen sporadically in untreated animals as a result of disease such as infection and neoplasia. Injections of foreign substances which are antigenic or immune stimulants also produce hyperplasia of lymphoid zone and spenomegaly.

Administration of purified human recombinant interleukin-2 to mice and rats produced increased splenic size accompanied by an increase in both red pulp and T and B zones, presumably as this agent induces changes in haemopoietic as well as the lymphoid system (Anderson et al., 1988; Anderson and Hayes, 1989).

Nodular hyperplasia, of mixed lymphocyte cells compressing, occur in the human spleen and may occasionally be seen in the rat spleen.

Plasma cell hyperplasia

Plasma cell hyperplasia, characterized histologically by an increase in the number of mature plasma cells in the red pulp of the spleen, is a well-described phenomenon related to stimulation of the immune system when it accompanies proliferation of splenic germinal centres (Veerman and de Vries, 1976).

Care has to be taken to distinguish plasma cells in the red pulp from erythroblasts which may also become increased in number with increased haemopoietic demands.

Fibrosis

Fibrosis occurs in the spleen following administration of a variety of agents including various aniline-type agents and the drug dapsone (Weinberger et al., 1985). It has been suggested that it may be the result of accumulation of metabolites in the splenic red pulp or a direct result of iron accumulation produced by these compounds (Goodman et al., 1984; Weinberger, 1985).

Amyloid

The spleen is an organ which is particularly predisposed to accumulate amyloid in untreated aged mice and hamsters as well as in mice and hamsters in which amyloidosis is produced by experimental procedures, such as the repeated injection of casein. Rats are resistant to the development of amyloid.

It is now apparent that amyloid accumulation is not a consequence of a single disease entity but the result of a variety of tissue processes which result in the deposition of characteristic twisted β-pleated sheet fibrils formed from various proteins. It is these arrays of rigid, non-branching fibrils 7.5 to 10 nm diameter, characteristic of both experimental and human amyloid, which stain with Congo red and show orange-green dichroism when viewed with polarized light. The characteristic appearance of amyloid fibrils under the electron microscopic make ultrastructural study the final arbiter in the tissue diagnosis of amyloid (Tribe and Perry, 1979).

There appear to be two major classes of amyloid fibrils, those composed of a homogeneous immunoglobulin light polypeptide chain designated AL and a similar group of proteins each with an almost identical N-terminal amino acid sequence which is designated AA (Glenner, 1980). Both these substances are believed to originate from precursor proteins found within circulating plasma.

It has been demonstrated that the major component of amyloid fibrils in experimental animals including mouse, guinea pig and monkey is a homologous AA-type protein (Cohen et al., 1978). Indeed, a high degree of immunological cross-reactivity between amyloid from different strains of mice regardless of whether spontaneous in type or of the method induction has been demonstrated (Isersky et al., 1971).

More recently it has been shown that antibody against murine amyloid is cross-reactive with human amyloid of AA-type (Livni et al., 1980). The potassium permanganate reaction, a histological method which is of use in distinguishing different chemical types of amyloid (Wright et al., 1977), also demonstrates that spontaneous amyloid in the hamster is likely to be of AA-type for it is sensitive to the permanganate reaction (Michel-Fouque, 1984).

In the mouse spleen, Dunn (1944, 1954) noted that amyloid deposition was often conspicuous in the marginal zone. Amyloid deposition appears to advance from the marginal zone into the red pulp and in advanced cases the entire red pulp becomes effaced by masses of dense pale eosinophilic amyloid. A similar picture is also observed in the aged hamster.

Recent studies using the murine model have suggested that the development of splenic amyloid starts around the arteriolar capillaries in the inner part of the marginal zone and that this distribution of amyloid is determined by arteriolar capillary injury rather than a result of inherent properties of the circulating precursor AA proteins (Schultz and Pitha, 1985; Schultz et al., 1985)

The prevalence of amyloid in mice and hamsters used in toxicity and carcinogenicity studies varies considerably between different strains, between males and females and with time in the same strain housed under identical conditions. Dietary factors may be important. The prevalence of spontaneous amyloid in the hamster was found to be greater in hamsters fed a flour diet than those fed the same diet in pelleted form (Michel-Fouque, 1984). However, such findings are difficult to interpret for, although our understanding of amyloid has advanced considerably, its precise pathogenesis remains uncertain However, it is worth mentioning that experimental data suggests that the deposition of amyloid can also be influenced by B and T lymphocyte reactivity and factors that influence the immune system such as thymic hormone administration (Cohen et al., 1978), oestrogens, and pituitary hormones (Russfield and Green, 1965). Renal amyloid has been reported in dogs treated with the anti-arthritic organic gold drug, auranofin, at high does for seven years (Bloom et al., 1987). This was associated with other derangements of the immune system including thrombocytopenia, haemolytic anaemia and lymphocytic thyroiditis.

Neoplasia

Lymphomas are the most frequently occurring neoplasms in the rodent spleen and these are discussed below. Other types of tumour are relatively uncommon but soft tissue neoplasms, particularly angiomas and angiosarcomas are occasionally found in the spleens of aged untreated rats, mice (Percy and Jonas, 1971) and hamsters (Pour et al., 1979).

Splenic sarcomas, principally of fibroblastic type have also been described in F344 rats following the administration of aniline and aniline-related aromatic amines, p-chloroaniline, D and C Red No.9, o-toluidine and the drug dapsone (National Cancer Institute, 1977; Weinberger et al., 1985). These neoplasms appear to arise following chronic tissue damage as shown histologically by vascular congestion, haemorrhage with pigment deposition and fibrosis, although the precise mechanism remains unclear (Weinberger, 1985).

In this context, dapsone (4,4′diamino-diphenylsulphone), a drug of importance in the treatment of leprosy and in malaria in combination with pyrimethamine, is of interest. In carcinogenicity bioassays undertaken with dapsone in the F344 rats and $B_6C_3F_1$ mice variably differentiated spindle cell sarcomas in the spleen and peritoneum were produced exclusively in male rats treated with 600 and 1,200 ppm of dapsone mixed in the diet. Fibrosis, congestion, haemorrhage, necrosis and osseous metaplasia were also present in the spleens of affected animals.

The histological appearances of these induced neoplasms were principally fibroblastic in type sometimes exhibiting a whorled appearance and focal osteoid differentiation (Weinberger et al., 1985).

The relevance of sarcomas developing in a single sex of one rodent species in a background of long standing chronic tissue damage remains uncertain. Dapsone is known to produce a metabolite in man which is implicated in the development of Heinz body haemolytic anaemia and methaemoglobinaemia, but despite widespread use dapson is not associated with the development of cancer.

Proliferative lesions of the splenic mesothelium (mesotheliomas) have also been described in untreated aged rats (Sass et al., 1975).

THYMUS

Histopathological examination of the thymus in toxicity studies is an appropriate method for assessment of the effects of chemicals and drugs on this organ. Wachsmuth (1983) has shown that the immunosuppressive effects of a number of different pharmaceutical agents are evident on histopathological examination of the thymus and that histological findings correlate well with thymic weight and peripheral lymphocyte counts in both rat and dog. Elegant studies in man using small thymic biopsies have also shown that histopathological examination supplemented by morphometric analysis is a sensitive method for the study of thymic function in certain clinical situations (Papaioannou et al., 1978). Pathologists can be aided in their interpretation of thymic changes by the use of immunocytochemistry using monoclonal antibodies specific for T cell subsets and thymocytes thymic hormones, cytokeratins, as well as mesenchymal elements (Bofill et al., 1985). Lymphocytes of the rat thymus can also be differentiated by cytochemical demonstration of cell surface enzymes such as aminopeptidases and γ-glutamyl transpeptidase (Grossrau et al., 1984).

Four stages of T lymphocyte maturation have been delineated in the thymus. These are subcapsular, cortical, medullary thymocytes and mature peripheral T cells (Bellanti, 1978). Subcapsular thymocytes, the most immature, are easily observed in foetal thymic tissue but not mature individuals. Cortical thymocytes are more mature than subcapsular thymocytes but less mature than medullary thymocytes and T cells. On the basis of reactivity with a battery of monoclonal antibodies against human T cell surface antigens, T cells and thymocytes have been separated into two main groups, immature cells in the thymic cortex and more mature medullary thymocytes and peripheral T cells (Hsu and Jaffe, 1985). A similar distribution of cell surface markers can be demonstrated in the rat thymus with monoclonal antibodies against rat T cells and thymocytes.

However, the thymus is subject to considerable variation in weight, morphology and function as a result of factors such as age and ill-health (Tak Cheung et al., 1981) as well as adrenal and gonadal steroid activity (Ahmed et al, 1985; Ohtaki, 1988). The thymus shows rapid involution with any form of stress (Goldstein and MacKay, 1969) which must always be considered in the interpretation of thymic changes in toxicity studies. The onset, rate and magnitude of age-related decline in thymus-dependent immunological function is to a certain extent genetically defined and this may be an important factor in the development of malignant lymphoma in the mouse (Hirokawa et al., 1984).

Atrophy, lymphocyte depletion

In the rat, mouse, hamster, dog and man atrophy of the thymus is a common, age-related change (McMartin, 1979; Tak Cheung et al., 1981; Kuper et al., 1986). As age progresses there is usually loss of lymphoid cells from both the cortex and the medulla and replacement by adipose tissue. In aged rodents, thymic lymphoid tissue may be quite difficult to find. Hassall's corpuscles become more prominent as lymphoid tissue is lost and they may show cystic change, epithelial proliferation and hyperplasia (Burek, 1978). In a detailed study of spontaneous thymic lesions in aging Wistar rats, Kuper and colleagues (1986) showed that the histological pattern of thymic involution differed between sexes. Severe thymic involution occurred more frequently in males although proliferation of thymic epithelium and formation of cystic structures was more pronounced in females. Despite these differences, survival was similar between sexes and the only histopathological finding which correlated with thymic involution was ovarian atrophy, emphasizing the influence of gonadal steroids on the thymus. Although the dog used in toxicity studies is usually quite young, thymic atrophy and epithelial proliferation is occasionally found in control dogs.

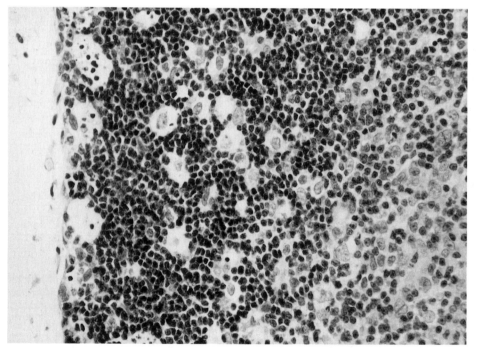

Fig. 26. Thymus from young Wistar rat treated for two days with cyclophosphamide. There is a loss of cortical thymocytes and an increase in the number of large, clear macrophages giving a "starry sky" appearance. (HE, ×500.)

After administration of immunosuppressive agents, depletion of lymphocytes or reduction in cellularity can occur in a diffuse manner or be limited to either the cortex or medulla. For example, cyclosporin causes a reduction in the overall cellularity of the thymic cortex and produces a 'starry-sky' appearance of scattered pale histiocytes when administered to rats (Fig. 26), but the medulla is particularly reduced in size (Blair et al., 1982; Beschorner et al., 1987). This effect of cyclosporin on the rat thymus has been shown to be extremely complex by the use of immunocytochemical techniques. The relative number of helper phenotype cells (W3/25 positive) are decreased compared to cytotoxic suppressor cells (OX 8 positive) in the medulla but not the cortex. In addition, Hassall's corpuscles and epithelial cells as shown by immunocytochemical staining for cytokeratin and Ia antigen (OX 4 positive cells) are also eliminated from the medulla but there is no detectable effect on cortical epithelial cells (Beschorner et al., 1987). Cyclophosphamide likewise produces a similar appearance although the cortex may be more strikingly affected (Fig. 26).

Other important modulators of thymic and T-cell function are the sex steroids which influence lymphocytes via effects on pre-T, pre-B cells, mature T cells, macrophages and thymic epithelium (Ahmed et al., 1985). Although these effects have been shown to be highly complex and dose-dependent, high doses of sex steroids result in thymic atrophy (Luster et al., 1987). Studies in mice have shown that cells in the thymus staining with Lyt-2 monoclonal antibody are particularly sensitive to sex hormone action. Generally oestrogen reduces and androgens maintain Lyt-2 cells (Ahmed et al., 1985). It is possible that some of the effects of sex steroids on the thymus are mediated by T-lymphokines. For this reason, it is of interest to note that mice treated with high doses of recombinant interleukin-2 showed severe lymphocyte depletion in the thymic cortex and loss of the demarcation between cortex and medulla in association with the vascular leak syndrome and lymphocytic infiltration of other organs (Anderson et al., 1988).

Unfortunately, it is sometimes difficult to make a clear distinction in routine toxicity studies from the thymic weight loss and atrophy produced by agents with immunomodulating properties from those compounds which produce similar morphological changes as a result of a generalized stress response at high doses. Indeed thymic involution, decreased responsiveness to Concanavalin A and lowered NK cell activity can be produced by a generalized stress response in a manner similar to that produced by the administration of glucocorticosteroids (Monjan and Collector, 1977; Smialowicz et al., 1985). At the end of conventional toxicity studies, advanced atrophy with fibrosis and epithelial proliferation may be seen which may give no morphological clues about the mechanism of action.

The dose-response relationship however is of some help in deciding whether thymic atrophy is a direct result of immunosuppression or a non-specific result of stress. Powerful immunosuppressive drugs such as cyclophosphamide appear to produce thymic (as well as lymph node and splenic) effects in a dose-related manner, with thymic weight loss and atrophy occurring at essentially non-toxic dose.

By contrast, atrophy which is a result of stress can be expected to be limited to high doses where there is other clear evidence of stress-related phenomena such as general clinical depression, weight loss or other overt evidence of intoxication (Smialowicz et al., 1985).

Thymic hypertrophy and hyperplasia

Under certain circumstance the thymus shows an increase in size a a result of increased numbers of lymphoid cells. Most commonly this is seen in aged rodents, particularly mice, as a well-defined localized focus or zone of lymphoid cells of mixed type compressing but not infiltrating the surrounding thymic tissue. In the absence of infiltration of surrounding thymus or connective tissue, a normal blood picture and normal lymphoid organs these focal thymic changes may be regarded as focal (nodular) hyperplasia.

Thymus weight, thymic cell content and cell proliferation are also affected by physiological alterations such as occur during pregnancy. In rats at least, the nature and degree of such change is strain dependent (Leeming et al., 1985). Orchidectomy, particularly when performed in immature animals, can bring about a delay in thymic involution and the development of thymic hyperplasia (Ahmed et al., 1985).

Species and strain differences in the evolution of thymic changes with age may be observed. For instance, female (NZB × SJL) F1 hybrid mice may develop an increase in thymic cell populations with increasing age. Morphologically, this hyperplasia is characterized by the presence of increased numbers of small lymphocytes and the development of lymphoid follicles in the medulla, associated with atrophy of the cortex (Dumont and Robert, 1980). Characterization of these cell populations suggests that there is an expansion of a sex-dependent subset of mature T cells as well as the emergence of B lymphocytes and plasma cells (Dumont et al., 1981).

Thymoma

The term thymoma is best reserved for a neoplasm of thymic epithelial cells, regardless of the presence or absence of a lymphoid component or its relevant abundance (Rosai and Levine, 1976). Thymomas are divided into three main histological groups; epithelial cell type, mixed epithelial and lymphoid cell type or composed predominently of lymphoid cells (lymphoid cell type). The latter type, however, also contains epithelial cells and should be distinguished from a lymphoma arising in the thymus, which is a more common finding in mice and rats.

The epithelial elements show a variety of patterns, including epidermoid (squamous), spindle cell, glandular, or rosette formations. They may be focal in nature or dispersed among lymphoid cells.

In conventional rat strains, thymomas are only very occasionally seen (Abbott and Cherry, 1982; Goodman et al., 1979; Maekawa et al., 1983; Ward et al., 1983;

114

Kuper et al., 1986). Similar neoplasms occur much more commonly in Buffalo rats where their light microscopic and ultrastructural appearances resemble thymomas occurring in man (Matsuyama et al., 1975).

Thymomas are also occasionally observed in aged mice and hamsters (Mc-Martin, 1979).

LYMPHORETICULAR NEOPLASMS

In studies designed to assess the long-term safety of potential new drugs, tumours of the haemopoietic system are quite commonly encountered, particularly in some mouse strains but also in certain types of rat. The hamster is also particularly prone to develop lymphomas (Coggin et al., 1983). The dog is not entirely free from haemopoietic neoplasms (Holmberg et al., 1976), although this is a rare occurrence in the young beagle dogs employed in conventional safety studies.

Classification

A variety of classifications of haemopoietic neoplasms have been described and are in use in safety assessment studies. Not only is the choice of classification often dependent on the particular species under study, but also on the background and experience of the particular pathologist, whether he or she be medical, veterinary or have a specific expertise in experimental pathology (Wogan, 1984).

The major recent advances in understanding of the function of the immune system and how this relates to morphology, the increased availability of methods such as immunocytochemistry and various hybridization techniques which allow a more objective assessment of lymphoid cells, have all rendered the older classifications of lymphoma and leukaemia obsolete. Although the newer classifications of lymphoma and leukaemia occurring in man may not be entirely satisfactory (Wintrobe et al., 1981 a,b), two classifications, that of Lukes and Collins (1974) and that from the Kiel group (Gerard-Marchant et al., 1974) have achieved widespread acceptance. Pattengale and Taylor (1983) have elegantly shown how these classifications are also applicable to murine lymphomas and similar findings have been reported by others for both the rat (Greaves and Faccini, 1984) and the hamster (Michel-Fouque et al., 1983).

Routinely, a simple morphological classification has much merit in studies conducted for the safety evaluation of drugs and chemicals in rodent species in view of the current practice of grouping lymphoid and haemopoietic neoplasms of the same type together in the assessment (Wogan, 1984). Whilst this is appropriate and effective when there are no particular problems associated with the findings in the lymphoid and haemopoietic tissues, it is important that the simple systems used are based on modern classifications and not older methods which leads to inappropriate grouping of tumours. In certain, cases a more

115

TABLE 1

Pattingale and Taylor (1983)	Rappaport (1966)	Wogan (1984)
Follicular centre cell types (B cell)		
Small cell	Poorly differentiated lymphocytic⎫	
Large cleaved cell	Mixed lymphocytic/histocytic ⎬	Pleomorphic (composite; mainly
Large non-cleaved cell	Histiocytic ⎭	Dunn type B in the mouse)
Mixed cell	Mixed lymphocytic/histiocytic	
Immunoblastic (B or T)	Histiocytic	Undifferentiated/stem cell (Dunn type B in the mouse)
Small lymphocyte/ lymphocytic (B or T)	Lymphocytic, well differentiated	Lymphocytic
Lymphoblastic (B or T)	Lymphoblastic	Undifferentiated/stem cell
Plasma cell (B)	Lymphocytic with plasmacytoid features	Plasma cell

Note: the classification of Pattengale & Taylor (1983) based on Lukes & Collins (1975) and that of Wogan (1984) were designed for the mouse but are applicable to rat and hamster. The classification of Rappaport (1966) is widely used for lymphoid tumours occuring in man and animals.

precise diagnosis is essential since each type of neoplasms may have a specific, although ill-understood biological significance (Della Porta, 1979). Thus, it is most appropriate to use a morphological classification for all rodent species based on that of Lukes and Collins or of the Kiel group which can be subsequently combined with immunological parameters, as shown for the mouse (Pattengale and Frith, 1983). This allows adequate correlation between the various species including man, and various strains of rodent. An overview of the various classifications of lymphoma are presented in Table 1. The classification of Rappaport (1966) is included in the table as it is in wide use in human pathology and has been applied to lymphomas in several animal species (Krueger and Konorza, 1979).

A useful additional technique in lymphoma classification in rodents is the cytochemical detection of immunoglobulins and cell surface markers, in view of the now widespread availability of reagents for use in both rat and mouse. A B-cell lymphoma may be defined as having easily detectable surface or cytoplasmic immunoglobulin, whereas a T cell lymphoma is defined as one possessing easily detectable surface T cell markers (Pattengale and Taylor, 1983). When using cytochemical methods a category of non-B, non-T cell lymphoma should be retained, defined as a lymphoma lacking easily detectable cell surface T/B cell markers or cytoplasmic immunoglobulin.

However, lymphomas and leukaemias of specific cell types may not express surface markers and for this reason the new DNA hybridization techniques are of considerable interest in the understanding of these neoplasms. Indeed, those pathologists who have just mastered the use of monoclonal antibodies for cell surface markers must now develop familiarity with the new DNA technology in the analysis of gene rearrangements, to stay abreast of developments in this field (Harris, 1985). The polymerase chain reaction (PCR), which can amplify and identify gene rearrangements, is a particularly relevant technique in pathology for demonstrating clonal origin of small numbers of cells for it can be applied to histopathological samples even when formalin fixed (Goudie, 1989).

Although identification of surface markers and DNA technology are useful in the diagnosis and classification of lymphomas, it is of note that these methods have demonstrated mixed or aberrant phenotypes on neoplastic haemopoietic cells. Marker studies of both human and murine haemopoietic neoplasms, including multiple myeloma, traditionally considered a cancer of mature plasma cells, have all tended to support the concept that lymphomas and leukaemias are derived from a stem cell or its immediate descendants as they differentiate into committed progenitor cells (Buchsbaum and Schwartz, 1990; Epstein et al., 1990).

Lymphomas are traditionally considered to be malignant neoplasms of lymphoid and histiocytic cells with localized but invasive growth patterns. *Leukaemias* are considered to be neoplasms of lymphoid and haemopoietic cells in which there is primary involvement of the bone marrow usually with malignant cells in the peripheral blood. However, lymphomas and leukaemias are not entirely separate entities and certain lymphomas and leukaemias of the same cell type should be grouped in a safety assessment.

Significance of lymphoma and leukaemia in safety studies

The interpretation of a treatment-related increase in the prevalence of lymphoma or leukaemia in preclinical safety studies and the subsequent risk assessment for man is fraught with difficulties. Although exhaustive study during the last few years has advanced our understanding of lymphoma and leukaemia quite remarkably in both man and animals, it has also served to demonstrate the immense complexity of the development of these neoplasms.

Although a recent literature survey suggested that chemicals which increased the incidence of leukaemia or lymphoma in mouse bioassays usually produce other types of cancer in the mouse or in other test species and are likely to be carcinogenic in man, this particular survey mainly involved known or suspected carcinogens (see Wogan 1984). The situation is quite different when an increased prevalence of lymphoma or leukaemia is observed in animal species following the long-term administration of high doses of potent pharmaceutical agents, in view of the great variety of factors which can influence the expression of neoplasms of the reticuloendothelial system.

Viruses are probably involved in the development of haemopoietic and lymphoid neoplasms in both man and rodents more commonly than previously believed (Gallo and Wong-Staal, 1982). Like chemicals, viruses can play the role of initiator in tumour promotion (Klein, 1979). Enhancement of virus specific cell transformation by chemical agents can also occur (Rapp, 1984). For instance, the

117

well-known association of lymphoproliferative disorders including lymphoma with immunosuppressed organ transplant recipients is closely related to Epstein-Barr virus infection (Nalesnik et al., 1988.)

Much of our knowledge of oncogenic viruses has been obtained from the study of murine lymphomas and leukaemias. Studies using inbred mice have shown marked variation in the incidence of leukemia and lymphoma. Strains such as C58 and AKR show a high incidences whilst in C3H relatively few are found (Wyke, 1981). Inbred strains used in toxicology such as C57BL and BALB/c as well as the outbred Swiss mouse, have somewhat more variable incidence of lymphoma and leukaemia (Rowlatt et al., 1976; Festing, 1979; Chvédoff et al., 1982; Everett, 1984). It is now known that several oncogenic RNA-containing viruses (retroviruses) [1] are integrated into the mouse host DNA as DNA proviruses and may be transmitted vertically from parent to offspring. Provirus expression as leukaemia or lymphoma depends not only on viral but also host genes which regulate transcription of proviral DNA and also determine susceptibility of host cells to the spread of viral infection (Wyke, 1981). Recent studies in the AKR mouse have suggested that the thymic epithelial cells are highly permissive for the replication of oncogenic viruses and that it is likely that virus-induced malignant transformation occurs when bone marrow derived prothymocytes home to the thymus and proliferate there (Kato and Hays, 1985). This perhaps explains the high prevalence of thymic or T cell leukaemia/lymphoma in many mouse populations and supports the view that the thymic microenvironment is important in leukaemogenesis (Boniver, 1981).

Comparable leukaemia viruses have been isolated from rats, hamsters and guinea pigs (Wyke, 1981). In the hamster, a horizontally transmitted DNA viroid-like agent has been described which produces lymphocytic, lymphoplasmocytic and immunoblastic lymphoma in hamster colonies (Coggin et al., 1983). However some authors have suggested that the responsible agent is more likely to be a hamster papova virus (Barthold et al., 1987).

It has been shown that retroviruses have a direct relevance to the understanding to tumorigenesis in man. This came about through the discovery of retroviruses as aetiological agents in certain human neoplasms (human T cell

---

[1] *Retroviruses:* The *mouse* carries genomic information for the production of at least three categories of endogeneous retroviruses, *Type C* virus particles are closely related with development of leukaemias and lymphomas as well as autoimmune diseases (Leiter, 1985; Gross et al., 1986). *Type B* particles and their immature precursors intracytoplasmic *Type A* particles are associated with mammary tumorigenesis. Both are shed from the cell surface to acquire an outer unit plasma membrane. The third type, the intracisternal *Type A* particle (IAP) are normally expressed in early embryogenesis but remain sequestered within the cisternae of the rough endoplasmic reticulum and do not bud from the plasma membrane. However, during embryogenesis a 73,000 dalton group specific antigen (p73) is expressed on the cell surface (Huang and Calarco, 1981). Why type C particles are detectable in mice with spontaneous leukaemias and lymphomas and not in rats such as Sprague-Dawley and Long-Evans which also develop leukaemia spontaneously, is uncertain. However, the apparent absence of formed C-type virus particles does not exclude a viral category for these rat neoplasms (Gross et al., 1986).

leukaemia/lymphoma virus) and through the discovery of a set of evolutionary conserved cellular genes, the oncogenes, which probably play an important part in cell growth by their association with retroviruses (Gallo and Wong-Staal, 1984). In this context the increasing availability of probes for the in-situ hybridization of viral nuclei acids which allow the detection of minute amounts of virus even in routinely fixed tissue sections (McAllister and Rock, 1985) clearly hold considerable promise for the future study of virally-induced lymphomas and leukaemias.

A variety of other factors are known to possess the potential to influence the prevalence of lymphoma and leukaemia in preclinical safety studies conducted in rodents. The prevalence of lymphoma can vary with time in control mice of the same strain housed under similar conditions (Clayson, 1984). Laboratory conditions, cage sizes, cage shelf level (Greenman et al., 1984), population density, quantity of diet (Roe and Tucker, 1974), aminoacid deficiencies (White et al., 1944), mineral (magnesium) deficiency (Gossrau et al., 1984), hormone status (Gardner et al., 1944), immune function (Hirokawa et al., 1984), and ionizing radiation (Major, 1979) can affect the prevalence of lymphoma and leukaemia in laboratory rodents (see reviews by Clayson, 1984; Everett, 1984). In a recent study of five control groups from carcinogenicity studies conducted between 1973 and 1980 with C57 B1/10J mice, Tucker (1985) found a high degree of variability in the prevalence of lymphoid neoplasms between the various groups, which suggested that environmental factors, particularly diet may override genetic characteristics of an inbred strain. This variation in prevalence of haemopoietic tissue neoplasms between control groups with time is not an unusual experience in laboratories undertaking drug safety evaluation. It has also been reported occurring in five carcinogenicity studies conducted between 1975 and 1979 with CD1 mice in another laboratory (Faccini et al., 1981).

A further complexity has been introduced by the establishment of a negative correlation between nodular liver lesions including hepatocellular carcinoma and malignant lymphoma in both mice and rats. It has been shown that even in controls, animals without malignant lymphoma are more likely to have hepatocellular carcinoma than those with lymphoma and that this is not entirely due to lymphoma-induced early deaths (Young and Gries, 1984). This factor also has to be considered during the interpretation of neoplasms in carcinogenicity studies.

A highly critical approach may be necessary in the assessment of immunosuppressive or anticancer agents and hormones. Prolonged immunosuppression in man as well as in laboratory animals may lead to the development of unusual lymphoproliferative states and lymphoreticular neoplasms, often of large B cell type (Metcalf, 1961; Krueger et al., 1971; Hanto et al., 1983; Hoover and Fraumeni, 1981; Starzl et al., 1984). Whether lymphoreticular neoplasms actually develop in laboratory animals on long-term immunosuppressive treatment is dependent on a number of experimental variables. Krueger et al., (1971) showed that BALB/c mice developed diffuse, poorly differentiated lymphocytic or lymphoblastic lymphomas when treated for long periods with azathioprine or antilymphocyte serum only when treatment was combined with persistent antigenic stimulation by administration of non-oncogenic antigens. In the same study, C57BL mice proved much more sensitive to the same immunosuppressive regime and did not survive long enough to develop malignant lymphomas.

Many antitumour agents produce cancer in rodents and some of the tumour types are lymphomas and leukaemias (Hottendorf, 1985; Schmähl and Habs 1979). This is not surprising with agents that interact with DNA and are mutagenic. Indeed, Hottendorf (1985) has suggested that antitumour agents that interact with DNA and are both mutagenic and teratogenic and should be considered as human carcinogens without confirmation in long-term rodent carcinogenicity bioassays. Not unexpectedly, anti-neoplastic agents have been associated with the development of second neoplasms in cancer patients treated with these agents and thus surviving for longer periods (Harris, 1979), although the second neoplasms reported do not generally appear to be the same types occurring in rodent bioassays.

In man, the type of neoplasm following anti-cancer therapy may be dependent not only on the therapy but the nature of the underlying neoplasm (Wintrobe et al., 1981b). Acute or non-lymphocytic leukaemia and its preleukaemic stages have been shown to be the principle types of cancer developing in man following anticancer therapy with alkylating agents (Hoover and Fraumeni, 1981; Pedersen-Bjergaard et al., 1987; Schmähl, 1987; Kaldor et al., 1990). The leukaemias are associated with consistent defects of chromosomes five and seven regardless of drug and are characteristically less responsive to conventional therapy than those arising de novo (Coltman and Dahlberg, 1990). The risk of this type of cancer appears to be dependent on cumulative dose and age of subject. It is of note that although alkylating agents produce a wide spectrum of tumours in laboratory animals, they induce predominantly a distinct cytogenetic subtype of an uncommon malignancy in man.

Lymphomas and leukaemias have been reported occurring in carcinogenicity bioassays of therapeutic agents of other types. Oestrogen therapy has been shown to enhance the appearance of leukaemia in C3H, CBA and PM strains of mice but not in A, C57B, JK or C121 strains (Gardner et al., 1944). Thymic lymphomas were observed in the Alderley Park strain of mouse in oncogenicity studies performed with the β-blocker, pronethanol, and this finding was thought sufficient to stop development of this agent (Cruickshank et al., 1984). However, studies with pronethanol in other strains of mice did not show this effect (Alcock and Bond, 1964; Newberne et al., 1977). Similar findings have been reported for the anti-infective agent metronidazole, particularly important in the treatment of anaerobic infection after abdominal surgery. Out of three mouse carcinogenicity studies performed in different Swiss strains with this agent, one showed an increased prevalence of malignant lymphoma among treated females compared with controls (Rustia and Shubik, 1972; Rust, 1981). However, there has been no evidence of any cancer occurring in patients treated with metronidazole despite widespread and continuing usage (Roe, 1983).

Follicular centre cell lymphoma

These lymphomas, believed to develop from cells of the B cell compartment of the lymphoid follicle have been described in considerable detail in the mouse by Pattengale and Taylor (1983) who showed that their cytological and immunocytochemical characteristics were strikingly similar to those found in man, thus confirming the applicability of the Lukes and Collins or Kiel classifications in murine neoplasms. In certain strains of mice, follicular centre cell lymphomas are some of the more common lymphoma types (Ward et al., 1975; Pattengale and Frith, 1983; Tucker, 1985). In view of their mixed cytological appearances these lymphomas have been designated *pleomorphic lymphomas* in the mouse lymphoma classification of Wogan (1984) and *composite lymphomas* in the classification of Della Porta et al (1979). They form the bulk of *reticulum cell sarcoma Type B* of Dunn, (1954).

The detailed immunomorphological study of lymphoreticular neoplasms in BABL/c mice, Pattengale and Frith (1983) demonstrated that follicular centre cell lymphoma was the most common cell type, comprising about 60% of all lymphomas occurring in this strain. Similar lymphomas occur spontaneously in other commonly used mouse strains including in the widely used Swiss (CrL CD-1, ICR BR) mouse.

Although lymphomas are much less frequently observed in rats, similar follicular centre cell lymphomas are seen, involving mainly abdominal, thoracic and cervical lymph nodes in the Sprague-Dawley and Long-Evans rats (Greaves and Faccini, 1984).

Some attempt has also been made to characterize the lymphoid neoplasms which occur in hamster colonies on an immunomorphological basis (Pour et al., 1976; McMartin, 1979; Coggin et al., 1983). Some of these neoplasms which commonly originate in Peyer's patches or abdominal lymph nodes, including those clearly induced by the DNA viroid-like agent, are of follicular centre cell type (Coggin et al., 1983; Michel-Fouque, 1983). Careful morphological classification of 130 lymphoid neoplasms occurring in two strains of Syrian hamster (LVG/LAK and Evic-Ceba, France) showed that 12% were of follicular centre cell type (Michel-Fouque, 1984, see Table 2).

Immunomorphological studies of random series of canine lymphomas have suggested that a major proportion are of follicular centre cell type, some of which possess a nodular growth pattern unlike those observed in rodents (Holmberg et al., 1976; Krueger and Konorza, 1979).

In all species, including man, follicular centre cell lymphomas are composed cytologically of monomorphic to mixed populations of small irregular and cleaved cells, larger cleaved or non-cleaved cells which infiltrate primarily spleen and lymph nodes but spread to adjacent organs such as liver, kidney and lungs. A follicular or nodular growth pattern, which is observed in the corresponding

Type	LVG/LAK		Evic Ceba		Total
	M	F	M	F	
Follicular centre cell types	10	9	4	7	30 (23%)
Immunoblastic	1	2	1	0	4 (3%)
Lymphocytic	15	14	12	7	48 (37%)
Lymphocytic/plasma cell	10	10	5	6	31 (24%)
Lymphoblastic	5	2	6	4	17 (13%)
	14	37	28	24	130

Note: Number of hamsters at risk 500 (LVG/LAK), 200 (Evic Ceba) equal numbers of males and females.

human and canine lymphomas, is seldom, if ever found in rodent neoplasms of this type, which remain diffuse in nature. As they are of B cell origin, the presence of surface immunoglobulin may be demonstrated with appropriate immunocytochemical techniques.

Lymphoblastic lymphoma

Lymphomas of this cell type may be of B or T cell type and are composed of fairly large rounded cells with scanty cytoplasm and immature rounded or irregular nuclei with finely dispersed chromatin and inconspicuous nucleoli. In the Kiel, Lukes and Collins, and Rappaport classifications, this lymphoma is uniformly called lymphoblastic lymphoma. The exception is in the mouse lymphoma classification of Wogan (1984) which groups this lymphoma as one of stem cell type. Lymphoblastic neoplasms of both T and B cells arise spontaneously in several mouse strains (Pattengale and Taylor, 1983). In their study of aged female BABL/c mice, Pattengale and Frith (1983) described 23 cases out of a total of 70 with morphological features of lymphoblastic lymphoma. Based on cytoplasmic pyrinophilia and the presence of immunoglobulin, seven of the 23 cases were classed as lymphoblastic lymphoma of B cell type. The remaining 16 neoplasms showed massive thymic and mediastinal involvement, were consistently negative for immunoglobulin and were regarded as T-lymphoblastic lymphoma, similar to Thy-1 positive thymic lymphomas observed spontaneously in AKR mice or induced by radiation in C57BL/6 mice (Pattengale et al., 1982) Similar clinicopathological patterns may be seen in other strains including the outbred Swiss mouse (personal observations) and occur in mice after prolonged immunosuppression (Krueger et al., 1971).

In Wistar, Sprague-Dawley and Long-Evans rats similar lymphoblastic lymphomas arising in peripheral lymphoid tissue or thymus may be observed (Kroes et al., 1981; Greaves and Faccini, 1984).

In the study by Michel-Fouque (1984), 17 cases of lymphoblastic lymphoma out of 130 (13%) were observed, arising mainly in abdominal lymphoid tissue and commonly (10 to 17) showing a 'Burkitt'-like or 'starry sky' appearance as a result of the presence of pale macrophages. Nevertheless, occasional cases appeared to be localized to the thymus and be composed of lymphoblasts with convoluted nuclei, possibly of T cell type.

Immunoblastic lymphoma

Immunoblasts are large, rounded cells possessing moderate amounts of cytoplasm and characteristic, large vesicular rounded nuclei containing conspicuous nucleoli. Immunoblasts of B cell type characteristically show amphiphilic or pyrinophilic cytoplasm. In their study of 70 lymphomas occurring in female BALB/c mice Pattengale and Frith (1983) found five immunoblastic lymphomas all of B cell type.

Lymphomas with similar cytological appearances are occasionally found in untreated aged rats (Greaves and Faccini, 1984). Immunoblastic neoplasms of probable B cell origin were also found in the abdomen of LVG/LAK and LSH/LAK Syrian hamsters infected with a viroid agent (Coggin et al., 1983). In the study by Michel-Fouque (1984) four immunoblastic lymphomas were found among 130 lymphomas (3%). Two cases appeared to be of B cell type localized to the abdomen and containing cytoplasmic immunoglobulin, with the further two being devoid of cytoplasmic immunoglobulin and localized to the thymus and probably of T cell origin. Occasional canine lymphomas also appear to be of immunoblastic B cell type (Holmberg et al., 1976).

Lymphocytic lymphoma

Lymphomas of lymphocytic type are composed of mature, small cells with scanty cytoplasm and small rounded nuclei possessing dense chromatin patterns. The cells form dense sheets which diffusely involve spleen and lymph nodes as well as other organs and frequently develop a leukaemic growth pattern (see also lymphocytic leukaemia). They are fairly common forms of lymphoma in some strains of mice (Ward et al., 1979), although they appear to be mainly of B cell origin (Pattengale and Taylor, 1983).

In the LVG/LAK and Evic Ceba strains of Syrian hamster over 35% of lymphomas found were of this cytological type, and mainly in abdominal lymphoid tissue (Michel-Fouque, 1984). Lymphoreticular neoplasms of this cytological type are found in most rat strains although appear commonly in a leukaemic form.

Plasma cell lymphoma

Plasma cell lymphomas, although generally uncommon in mice, rats and hamsters are quite characteristic, being composed of mature lymphoid cells which show plasmacytic differentiation, i.e. abundant amphiphilic cytoplasm, rounded nuclei with marginated dense chromatin patterns. In some mouse strains they occur spontaneously in the ileocaecal region (Dunn and Deringer, 1968; Rask-Nielsen and Ebbesen, 1969) and a similar form can occur in the hamster (Coggin et al., 1983). Plasma cell neoplasms are occasionally observed in untreated aged rats (Greaves and Faccini, 1984).

Histiocytic lymphoma (histiocytic sarcoma, malignant histiocytoma)

This neoplasm, thought to be derived from a true histiocyte, is relatively common in rodents and it should be generally considered separately from true lymphoid neoplasmas (Wogan, 1984). It should be distinguished from the so-called histiocytic lymphoma of the Rappaport classification which is of course a misnomer for large cell lymphomas of lymphoid cells (see Table 1).

In the mouse this histiocytic neoplasm was well described by Dunn (1954) under the term *reticulum cell sarcoma Type A*. It commonly involves abdominal organs of the mouse, particularly liver and uterus but it may be leukaemic in nature or form discrete subcutaneous or soft tissue masses. Neoplastic cells are quite variable in cytological appearance but they usually possess a fairly irregular nucleus with marginated chromatin pattern and occasional prominent nucleoli. Abundant eosinophilic cytoplasm may show erythrophagocytosis (Frith et al., 1980). In some tumours, spindle or fusiform cells are evident which may cause diagnostic difficulties and perhaps explains the use of the term *schwannoma* for certain subtypes of this tumour (Stewart et al., 1974; Frith et al., 1980).

Ultrastructural study has shown that the tumour cells possess deeply folded nuclei, electron-dense, marginated chromatin and cytoplasm containing variable numbers of mitochondria and profiles of smooth and rough endoplasmic reticulum. Certain cells contain numerous lysosomal bodies, although basement membranes and Langerhan's granules are lacking. Frith et al. (1980) have shown that these cells are highly phagocytic in culture.

The tumour cells are highly metastatic and deposits are often found in many organs but particularly lungs and liver. In the BALB/c strain bone marrow and lymph nodes are also commonly involved (Frith et al., 1980).

A strikingly similar clinicopathological pattern is observed in the rat usually termed *histiocytic sarcoma, histiocytic lymphoma* or *malignant histiocytoma*. Although this neoplasm may also present as a localized soft tissue mass it may also widely infiltrate the pelvis and abdominal organs in a lymphomatous manner as in the mouse (Greaves et al., 1982; Squire et al., 1981). These cells exhibit almost identical cytological and ultrastructural appearances to histiocytic lymphoma cells found in the mouse (Greaves et al., 1982) and show a similar distribution pattern in internal organs with liver and lungs being those mainly affected (Greaves and Faccini, 1981).

A similar tumour pattern may be observed occasionally in the hamster both as a locally invasive soft tissue mass (Fig. 5) or as a diffuse lymphomatous neoplasm.

Hodgkin's-like lymphomas

Lymphoreticular lesions with the histological features of Hodgkin's disease described in man have been recorded in the dog, mouse and rat but they are rare (Wells, 1974; Majeed and Gopinath, 1985).

Malignant mastocytoma

This is an extremely rare neoplasia but it is occasionally observed in mice where localized splenic, hepatic and disseminated forms have been described (Lewis and Offer, 1984). In all cases neoplastic cells appear well-differentiated with numerous metachromatic granules.

Leukaemia

Rats, mice and hamsters all develop leukaemia spontaneously although their prevalence, growth patterns and cell types differ markedly between species and strain. Leukaemia is a disease characterized by neoplastic proliferation of one of the blood forming cells and is usually classified according to the cell type involved: i.e. *lymphocytic, lymphoblastic, granulocytic, myeloblastic, myelo-monocytic,* and *erythroleukemia.*

In essence, classification follows that used in man which is appropriate for use in rodents provided smears and imprints stained with a Romanovski stain are available. It is probably prudent to avoid the prefixes acute and chronic as far less is known about the natural history of rodent leukaemias than those occurring in man. Even in man patients with acute lymphoblastic leukemia may live longer than those with chronic myeloid leukaemia such that the terms acute and chronic are no longer applicable to life span (Wintrobe et al., 1981 a,b).

Lymphocytic leukaemia

Lymphocytic leukaemia is a disseminated proliferation of small and medium sized mature lymphocytes with scant cytoplasm and rounded mature nuclei showing a dense chromatin pattern. In typical cases absolute lymphocyte counts in the peripheral blood increase markedly, and there is often associated anaemia and general ill-health of the affected animal. Bone marrow, spleen, lymph nodes are usually heavily infiltrated with lymphocytes. These organs achieve very large sizes by the time the animal is usually examined pathologically. This may make the distinction between a lymphocytic lymphoma and lymphocytic leukaemia difficult. A characteristic monomorphic infiltration pattern may also be seen in the hepatic portal tracts.

This type of leukaemia appears to occur in most rat strains including Sprague-Dawley (Chvédoff et al., 1982), Long-Evans (personal observations) and Wistar strains (Kroes et al., 1981). Total white cell counts range from 60 to 140,000 m^3 in the Sprague-Dawley rat (Chvédoff et al., 1982).

The heterogeneous leukaemia of *large granular lymphocyte* type occurring spontaneously in 10–35% of aged Fischer rats may perhaps also be regarded as a lymphocytic (chronic) leukaemia of T-cell type (Stromberg, 1985), although some cells are more immature (blasts) than typical small lymphocytes (Losco and Ward, 1984). Apart from general ill-health, anaemia and jaundice, this leukaemia is characterized by marked splenomegaly and diffuse infiltration of splenic red pulp, lymph nodes, bone marrow and other organs by a pleomorphic population of granular lymphocytes 10–15 mμ diameter with prominent azurophilic cytoplasmic granules and round to irregular shaped nuclei (Ward and Reynolds, 1983). White blood cell counts may vary from 5 to 370 mm^3 (Stromberg et al., 1983).

The cells show variable cytoplasmic activity of beta-glucuronidase, acid phosphatase, napthol AS-D acetate esterase sensitive to sodium fluoride and a fairly consistent positive immunoreactivity with monoclonal antibodies OX8 (suppressor/cytotoxic T cell antigen), OX7 (Thy-1.1 antigen) and W3/13 (rat thymocyte/T lymphocyte antigen) (Stromberg et al., 1983; Ward and Reynolds, 1983). They also show in vitro natural killer cell activity (Reynolds et al., 1984).

Lymphocytic leukaemias, in common with lymphomas of small lymphocytes, are quite common in several strains of mice including the Swiss mouse (Percy and Jonas, 1971) and B$_6$C$_3$F$_1$ mice (Ward et al., 1979). They may be either of B or T cell origin (Pattengale and Taylor, 1983).

A leukaemic form of a small lymphocytic neoplasm is only very rarely seen in the aged hamster (personal observations).

Lymphoblastic leukaemia

In lymphoblastic leukaemia, the peripheral blood and bone marrow contain large numbers of lymphoblasts which are characterized by high nuclear-cytoplasmic ratio, rounded nuclei with a finely dispersed chromatin pattern and one or two nucleoli. This leukaemia occurs less commonly in the Sprague-Dawley rat than lymphocytic leukaemia but somewhat higher white cell counts, up to over 200,000 per mm^3 may be seen (Greaves and Faccini, 1984).

In the mouse there is quite commonly a secondary leukaemia which develops in lymphoblastic lymphoma but pure leukaemic forms may be seen in the mouse and may be of B or T cell origin or of non-B, non-T cell type (Pattengale and Taylor, 1983).

A particularly well-studied B cell leukaemia which is decribed in BALB/c mice is the *BCL$_1$ leukaemia* (Slavin and Strober, 1978; Warnke et al., 1979). The chromatin structure of the BCL$_1$ cell is not exactly that of a typical small lymphocyte nor of a blast cell but can be regarded as an 'immature' lymphocyte which closely resembles human prolymphocytic leukaemia (Muirhead et al., 1981). In common with leukaemias of this morphological type found spontaneously in other strains of mice, animals affected with the BCL$_1$ leukaemia show massive splenic enlargement, large numbers of circulating leukaemia cells.

Granulocytic leukaemia

In all species this leukaemia is characterized by very high total white cell counts associated with heavy involvement of splenic tissue, such that, as in man with the same condition, enormous spleens can be seen. Cells are usually of intermediate maturity and mature granulocytic cells are also commonly observed. In the rat very high white cell counts may be observed (20,000 to 1 million cells per cubic mm^3) and similar values may be achieved in affected mice (Della Porta et al., 1979). Granulocytic leukaemia is uncommon, but occurs in hamsters (Mc-Martin, 1979), where particular care must be taken to distinguish it from a reactive leukaemoid reaction which is frequent.

An occasional but striking observation in rodents with this neoplasm is a characteristic green colour of infiltrated tissue (chloroleukaemia) due to a high concentration of myeloperoxidase in the neoplastic cells. This has been seen both in rats and mice. Occasionally a localized growth of these cells may also been seen (granulocytic sarcoma).

The distinction between granulocytic and other forms of leukaemia is not always clear in paraffin embedded tissue sections. If fresh material is available, enzyme cytochemistry of the cell population can be helpful, particularly the presence of naphthol AS-D chloroacetate esterase (Wolman et al., 1980).

As mentioned previously, the important differential diagnosis to be made is between granulocytic leukaemia and leukaemoid reaction, which may be quite difficult on a cytological basis without the benefit of smear preparations. Careful review of all the histopathological data for inflammatory conditions, necrotic or ulcerating neoplasms is of greatest importance here.

It is worth noting at this point that myeloid leukaemia is known to be a hazard of exposure to ionizing radiation in human populations (Ishimaru et al., 1971). Although in mice thymic lymphomas is the major type of neoplasms which follows radiation, myeloid (including granulocytic) leukaemia was shown to occur following single whole body x-irradiation in CBA mice (Major, 1979) and RF mice (Wolman et al., 1982). In RF mice at least, myeloid leukaemia occurs spontaneously and it appears that ionizing radiation increases its incidence, and advances its time of onset. This induction varies with radiation, dose, age, sex and physiological status of the irradiated mice (Wolman et al., 1982).

Myeloblastic leukaemia

In the rat, leukaemic cells of this type resemble normal myeloblasts. In the peripheral blood, cells are slightly more irregular with more abundant cytoplasm than in lymphoblasts and contain azurophilic granules. In addition, promyelocytes may be seen but few other more mature cells ('hiatus leucemicus') (Greaves and Faccini, 1984). These finer points of diagnostic detail of course may not be seen in routine paraffin wax sections. For this reason smear preparations can be of considerable diagnostic use in the distinction of this leukaemia from other immature cells. As in the differential diagnosis of acute leukaemia in man, naphthol AS or ASD acetate esterase activity is marked and unaffected by exposure to sodium fluoride. A leukaemia of similar morphological type is seen in the mouse (personal observations).

Other forms of leukaemia

Erythroleukaemia is an extremely rare spontaneous neoplasm in rodents but may be induced in Sprague-Dawley rats by administration of 7,8,12-trimethyl-benz[a]anthracene (Higgins et al., 1982). It is characterized by a heavy infiltration of spleen and liver by cells of the erythroid series.

Other types of leukaemia may also be observed (Kort et al., 1984) although pathologists may not be in close agreement in distinguishing various subtypes of large cell leukaemias such as myelomonocytic and monocytic leukaemia (Clarkson, 1980). Dissemination of malignant mastocytoma to involve the peripheral blood has been described in mice (Lewis and Offer, 1984).

REFERENCES

ABBOTT, D.P. and CHERRY, C.P. (1982): Malignant mixed thymic tumour with metastases in a rat. *Vet.Pathol.*, 19, 721–723.

AHMED, S.A., PENHALE, W,H., and TALAL, N. (1985): Sex hormones, immune responses, and autoimmune diseases. Mechanisms of sex hormone action. *Am.J.Pathol.*, 121, 531–551.

AHMED, A. and SMITH, A.H. (1983): Surface markers, antigens and receptorson murine T and B cells: Part 2. *CRC.Crit.Rev.Immunol.*, 4, 19–94.

ALCOCK, S.J. and BOND, P.A. (1964): Observations on the toxicity of 'Alderlin' (pronethalol) in laboratory animals. *Proc.Eur.Soc.Study Drug Toxicol.*, 4, 30–37.

ANDERSON, T.D. and HAYES, T.J. (1989): Toxicity of human recombinant interleukin-2 in rats. Pathologic changes are characterized by marked lymphocytic and eosinophilic proliferation and multisystem involvement. *Lab.Invest.*, 60, 331–346.

ANDERSON, T.D. and HAYES, T.J., GATELY, M.K., BONTEMPO, J.M., STERN, L.L.and TRUITT, G.A. (1988): Toxicity of human recombinant interleukin-2 in the mouse is mediated by interleukin-activated lymphocytes. Separation of efficacy and toxicity by selective lymphocyte subset depletion. *Lab.Invest.*, 59, 598–612.

ARNEBORN, P. and PALMBLAD, J. (1982): Drug induced neutropenia : survey from Stockholm, 1973–1978. *Acta.Med.Scand.*, 212, 289–292.

ANVER, M.R., COHEN, B.J., LATTUADA, C.P. and FOSTER, S.J. (1982): Age-associated lesions in barrier-reared male Sprague-Dawley rats : A comparison between Hap: (SD) and Crl COBS-CO(SD) stocks. *Exp.Aging Res.*, 8, 3–24.

AUDOUIN, J. and DIEBOLD, J. (1986): Modifications histologiques des ganglions lymphatiques au cours des réactions de stimulation immunitaire. *Ann.Pathol.*, 6, 85–98.

BACH, F.H. and SACHS, D.H. (1987): Transplantation immunology. *N.Engl.J.Med.*, 317, 489–492.

BANG, N.U. and KAMMER, R.B. (1983): Haematologic complications associated with β-lactam antibiotics. *Rev.Infect.Dis.*, 5. (Suppl 2), 380–393.

BANNERJEE, J.N., SOFIA, R.D., IVINS, N.J. and LUDWIG, B.J. (1979): Acute and subacute (30 day) toxicological investigations of 4-(p-chlorophenylthio) butanol (W-2719) in mice, rats and dogs. *Arzneimittelforschung*, 29, 1141–1145.

BARCLAY, A.N. (1981)a: The localization of populations of lymphocytes defined by monoclonal antibodies in rat lymphoid tissues. *Immunology*, 42, 593–600.

BARCLAY, A.N. (1981)b: Different reticular cells in rat lymphoid tissue identified by localization of Ia, Thy 1 and MRC OX2 antigens. *Immunology*, 44, 727–736.

BARCLAY, A.N. and MAYRHOFER, G (1981): Bone marrow origin of Ia-positive cells in the medulla of rat thymus. *J.Exp.Med.*, 153, 1666–1671.

BARTHOLD, S.W., BHATT, P.N. and JOHNSON, E.A. (1987): Further evidence for papovavirus as the probable etiology of transmissible lymphoma of Syrian hamsters. *Lab.Anim.Sci.*, 37, 283–288.

BASCH, R.S. and BERMAN, J.W. (1982): Thy-1 determinants are present on many murine haematopoietic cells other than T cells. *Eur.J.Immunol.*, 12, 359–364.

BECKSTEAD, J.H. (1983): The evaluation of human lymph nodes, using plastic sections and enzyme histochemistry. *Am.J.Clin.Pathol.*, 80, 131–139.

BÉLISLE, C. andSAINTE-MARIE, G. (1981): Topography of the deep cortex of the lymph nodes of various mammalian species. *Anat.Rec.*, 201, 553–561.

BÉLISLE, C., SAINTE-MARIE, G. and PENG, F-S (1982): Tridimensional study of the deep cortex of the rat lymph node. VI. The deep cortex units of the germ-free rat. *Am.J.Pathol.*, 107, 70–78.

BELLANTI, J.A. (1978): General immunobiology : Anatomic organization of the immune system. In: J.A. Bellanti (Ed.), *Immunology* II, pp. 60–65. W.B. Saunders, Philadelphia.

BELLER, D.I., SPRINGER, T.A., and SCHREIBER, R.D. (1982): Anti-Mac-1 selectively inhibits the mouse and human type three complement receptor. *J.Exp.Med.*, 156, 1000–1009.

BESCHORNER, W.E., NAMNOUM, J.D., HESS, A.D., SHINN, C.A. and SANTOS, G.W. (1987): Cyclosporin and the thymus. Immunopathology. *Am.J.Pathol.*, 126, 487–496.

BEUTLER, E. (1969): Drug-induced haemolytic anaemia. *Pharmacol.Rev.*, 21, 73–103.

BIBERFELD, P., PORWIT-KSIAZEK, A., BÖTTIGER, B., MORFELDT-MANSSON, L. and BIBERFELD, G. (1985): Immunohistopathology of lymph nodes in HLTV-III infected homosexuals with persistent adenopathy or AIDS. *Cancer Res.*, 45, 4665s–4670s.

BLAIR, J.T., THOMSON, A.W., WHITING, P.H., DAVIDSON, R.J.L. and SIMPSON, J.G. (1982): Toxicity of the immune suppressant cyclosporin A in the rat. *J.Pathol.*, 138, 163–178.

BLAZAR, B.A., RODRICK, M.L., O'MAHONY, J.B., WOOD, J.J., BESSEY, P.Q., WILMORE, D.W. and MANNICK, J.A. (1986): Suppression of natural killer-cell function in humans following thermal and traumatic injury. *J.Clin.Immunol.*, 6, 26–36.

BLOOM, J.C., THIEM, P.A. and MORGAN, D.G. (1987): The role of conventional pathology and toxicology in evaluating the immunotoxic potential of xenobiotics. *Toxicol.Pathol.*, 15, 283–293.

BOFILL, M., JANOSSY, G., WILLCOX, N., CHILOSI, M., TREJDOSIEWICZ, L.K. and NEWSOM-DAVIS, J. (1985): Microenvironments in the normal thymus and the thymus in myasthenia gravis. *Am.J.Pathol.*, 119, 462–473.

BONIVER, J. (1981): Pathogenesis of thymic lymphomas in C57BL mice. *Pathol.Res.Pract.*, 171, 268–278.

BOTTIGER, L.E., FURHOFF, A.R. and HOLMBERG, L. (1979): Fatal reactions to drugs. A study of 10 year material from the Swedish Adverse Drug Reaction Committee. *Acta.Med.Scand.*, 205, 457–461.

BRIDEAU, R.J., CARTER, P.B., McMASTER, W.R., MASON, D.W. and WILLIAMS, A.F. (1980): Two subsets of rat T lymphocytes defined with monoclonal antibodies. *Eur.J.Immunol.*, 10, 609–615.

BRIMBLECOMBE, R.W., DUNCAN, W.A.M. and WALKER, T.F. (1973): Toxicity of metiamide. In: C.J. Wood and M.A. Simkins (Eds.), *International Symposium on Histamine H2-Receptor Antagonists*, pp. 54–65. Excepta Medica, Oxford.

BRIMBLECOMBE, R.W., LESLIE, G.B. and WALKER, T.F. (1985): Toxicology of cimetidine. *Hum.Toxicol.*, 4, 13–25.

BROWN, J.W. (1954): A quantitative study of cellular changes occurring in bone marrow following protein deficiency in the rat. *Anat.Rec.*, 120, 515–533.

BROWN, W.R.A., BARCLAY, A.N., SUNDERLAND, C.A. and WILLIAMS, A.F. (1981): Identification of a glycophorin-like molecule at the cell surface of rat thymocytes. *Nature*, 289, 456–460.

BROWN, W.R.A. and WILLIAMS, A.F. (1982): Lymphocyte cell surface glyco-proteins which bind to soybean and peanut rectins. *Immunology*, 46, 713–726.

129

BUCHSBAUM, R.J. and SCHWARTZ, R.S. (1990): Cellular origins of hematologic neoplasms. *N.Engl.J.Med.*, 322, 694–695.

BUREK, J.D. (1978): Pathology of aging rats. In: *Age-associated Pathology*. Chap. 4, pp. 29–168. CRC Press, Boca Raton, Florida.

BURKHARDT, R., FIRSCH, B. and BARTL, R. (1982): Bone biopsies in haematological disorders. *J.Clin.Pathol.*, 25, 257–284.

BURNS, E.R., REED, L.J. and WENZ, B. (1986): Volumetric erythrocyte macrocytosis induced by hydroxyurea. *Am.J.Clin.Pathol.*, 85, 337–341.

CHABNER, B.A., FINE, R.L., ALLEGRA, C.J., YEH, G.W. and CURT, G.A. (1984): Cancer chemotherapy: Progress and expectations. *Cancer*, 54, 2599–2608.

CHVÉDOFF, M., CHIGNARD, G., DANCLA, J-L., FACCINI, J.M., LOYEAU, F., PERRAUD, J. and TARADACH, C. (1982): Le rongeur agé : observations recueillies au cours d'essais de carcinogénicite. *Sci.Tech.Anim.Lab.*, 7, 87–97.

CIOCCA, D.R. (1980): Immunomorphologic lymph node changes in rats bearing experimental breast tumours. *Am.J.Pathol.*, 99, 193–206.

CLARKSON, B. (1980): The acute leukemias. In: K.J. Isselbacher, R.D. Adams, E. Braunwald, R.G. Petersdorf and J.D. Wilson (Eds), Harrison's *Principles of Internal Medicine*, 9th Edition, Chap. 325, pp. 1620–1630. McGraw Hill, New York.

CLAYSON, D.B. (1984): Modulation of the incidence of murine leukemia and lymphoma. *CRC.Crit.Rev.Toxicol.*, 13, 183–195.

CLINE, J.M. and MARONPOT, R.R., (1985): Variations in the histologic distribution of rat bone marrow cells with respect to age and anatomic site. *Toxicol.Pathol.*, 13, 349–355.

COGGIN, J.H., BELLOMY, B.B., THOMAS, K.V., and POLLOCK, W.J. (1983): B-cell and T-cell lymphomas and other associated diseases induced by an infectious DNA viroid-like agent in hamsters (Mesocricetus auratus). *Am.J.Pathol.*, 110, 254–266.

COHEN, A.S., CATHCART, E.S. and SKINNER M., (1978): Amyloidosis: Current trends in investigation. *Arthritis Rheum.*, 21, 153–160

COLTMAN, C.A. and DAHLBERG, S. (1990): Treatment-related leukaemia. *N.Engl.J.Med.*, 322, 52–53.

COTTIER H., TURK, J., SOBIN L., (1972): A proposal for a standardized system of reporting human lymph node morphology in relation to immunological function. *Bull.WHO 47*, 375–408

CRICHTON D.N., BUSUTTIL, A. and PRICE W.H., (1977): Splenic lipofuscinosis in mice. *J.Pathol.*,126, 113–120.

CRAWFORD, J.M. and BARTON, R.W. (1986): Thy-1 glycoprotein: Structure, distribution and ontogeny. *Lab.Invest.*, 54, 122–135.

CRUICKSHANK, J.M., FITZGERALD, J.D. and TUCKER, M. (1984): Beta-adrenoceptor blocking drugs : pronethalol, propanolol and practolol. In: D.R. Laurence, A.E.M. McLean and M. Weatherall (Eds), *Safety Testing of New Drugs. Laboratory Predictions and Clinical Performance*, Chap. 5, pp. 93–123. Academic Press, London.

CULLEN, S.E., FREED, J.H. and NATHENSON, S.G. (1976): Structural and sero-logical properties of murine Ia allo-antigens. *Transplant.Rev.*, 30, 236–270.

DAVIES, G.E. (1981): Toxicology of the immune system. *Histochem. J.*, 13, 879–884.

DALCHAU, R. and FABRE, J.W. (1981): Studies with a monoclonal antibody on the distribution fo Thy-1 in the lymphoid and extracellular connective tissues of the dog. *Transplantation*, 31, 275–282.

DAWSON, A.A. (1979): Drug-induced haematological disease. *Br.Med.J.*, 1, 1195–1197.

DEAN, J.H., LUSTER, M.I. and BOORMAN, G.A. (1982): Methods and approaches for assessing immunotoxicity : An overview. *Environ.Health Perspect.*, 43, 27–29.

DEAN, J.H. and THURMOND, L.M. (1987): Immunotoxicology: An Overview. *Toxicol.Pathol.*, 15, 265–271.

DELLA-PORTA G., CHIECO-BIANCHI L. and PENNELLI N, (1979): Tumours of the haemopoietic system. In: V.S. Turusov (Ed.) *Pathology of Tumours in Laboratory Animals*, Vol.2, Tumours of the Mouse pp. 527–575. IARC Scientific Publ No 23, Lyon.

DIALYNAS, D.P., QUAN, Z.S., WALL, K.A., PIERRES, A., QUINTANS, J., LOKEN, M.R., PIERRES, M. and FITCH, F.W. (1983): Characterization of the murine T cell surface molecule designated L3T4, identified by monoclonal antibody GK 1.5: Similarity of L3T4 to the human Leu 3/T4 molecule. *J.Immunol.*, 131, 2445–2451.

DIBIANCO, R. (1986): Adverse reactions with angiotensin converting enzyme (ACE) inhibitors. *Med.Toxicol.*, 1, 122–141.

DIJKSTRA, C.D., (1982): Characterization of nonlymphoid cells in rat spleen, with special reference to strongly Ia-positive branched cells in T-cell areas. *J.Reticuloendoth.Soc.*, 32, 167–178.

DIJKSTRA C.D. and DÖPP E.A. (1983): Ontogenetic developement of T-and B-lymphocytes and non-lymphoid cells in the white pulp of the rat spleen.*Cell Tissue Res.*, 229, 351–363.

DORFMAN, R.F. and WARNKE, R. (1974): Lymphadenopathy simulating the malignant lymphomas. *Hum.Pathol.*, 5, 519–550.

DUMONT, F. and ROBERT, F. (1980): Age- and sex-dependent thymic abnormalities in NZB×SJL F1 hybrid mice. *Clin.Exp.Immunol.*, 41, 63–72.

DUMONT, F., ROBERT, F. and GERARD, H. (1981): Abnormalities of the thymus in aged female (NZB×SJF) F1 mice : Separation and characterization of intrathymic T cells, B cells and plasma cells. *J.Immunol.*, 126, 2450–2456.

DUNN T.B., (1944): Relationship of amyloid infiltration and renal disease in mice. *J.N.C.I.*,5, 17–28.

DUNN T.B. (1954): Normal and pathologic anatomy of the reticular tissue in laboratory mice, with a classification and discussion of neoplasms. *J.N.C.I.*, 14. 1281–1390.

DUNN, T.B. and DERINGER, M.K. (1968): Reticulum cell neoplasm, type B, or the 'Hodgkin's-like lesion' of the mouse. *J.N.C.I.*, 40, 771–820.

DURKIN, H.C. and THORBECKE, G.J. (1971): The relationship of germinal centres in lymphoid tissue to immunologic memory. The effect of prednisolone administered after peak of the primary response. *J.Immunol.*, 106, 1079–1085.

DYER, M.J.S. and HUNT S.V. (1981): Committed T lymphocyte stem cells of rats. Characterization by surface W3/13 antigen and radiosensitivity. *J.Exp.Med.*, 154, 1164–1177.

EDITORIAL (1983): Drug-induced neutropenia. *Lancet*, 1, 857–858.

EKMAN, L., HANSSON, E., HAVU, N., CARLSSON, E. and LUNDBERG, C.(1985): Toxicological studies on omeprazole. *Scand.J.Gastroenterol.*, 20, 53–69.

EPSTEIN, J., XIAO, H. and HE, X-Y. (1990): Markers of multiple haematopoietic-cell lineages in multiple myeloma. *N.Engl.J.Med.*, 322, 664–668.

ERMAK, T.H. and OWEN, R.L. (1986): Differential distribution of lymphocytes and accessory cells in mouse Peyer's patches. *Anat.Rec.*, 215, 144–152.

EVANS, G.O., FLYNN, R.M. and LUPTON, J.D. (1988)a: An immunogold labelling method for rat T lymphocytes. *Lab.Anim.* 22, 332–334.

EVANS, G.O., FLYNN, R.M. and LUPTON, J.D. (1988)b: An immunogold labelling method for enumeration of canine T-lymphocytes. *Vet.Q.*, 10, 273–275.

EVERETT, R. (1984): Factors affecting spontaneous tumor incidence rates in mice : A literature review. *CRC. Crit.Rev.Toxicol.*, 13, 235–251.

EYDELLOTH, R., KORNBRUST, D. and GARRATTY, G. (1987): Immune-mediated haemolytic anaemia and cytopenias associated with beta-lactam antibiotic administration. *Toxicologist*, 7, 26.

FACCINI, J.M., IRISARRI, E. and MONRO, A.M. (1981): A carcinogenicity study in mice of a beta-adrenergic antagonist, primidolol; increased total tumour incidence without tissue specificity. *Toxicology*, 21, 279–290.

FARNEL, D. and MARONPOT, R. (1987): Inanition in animals, an important consideration in evaluating pathologic effects of test substances. *Toxicol.Pathol.*, 15, 367.

FESTING, M.F.W. (1979): Inbred strains in biomedical research. *Inbred strains of mice*. Chap. 13, pp. 137–266. MacMillan, London.

FINCH, S.C. (1977): Granulocyte disorders: benign, quantitive abnormalities of granulocytes. In: W.J. Williams, E.Beutler, A.J. Erslev and R.W. Rundles (Eds), *Haematology*, pp. 717–746. McGraw-Hill, New York.

FORREST, J.A.H., SHEARMAN, D.J.C., SPENCE, R. and CELESTIN, L.R. (1975): Neutropenia associated with metiamide. *Lancet*, 1, 392–393.

FORT, F.L., TEKELI, S., MAJORS, K., HEYMAN, I.A., CUSICK, P.K. and KESTERSON, J.W. (1984): Terazasin: Intravenous safety evaluation in rats. *Drug Chem.Toxicol.*, 7, 435–449.

FOSSUM S., SMITH M.E., BELL E.B., FORD W.L. (1980): The architecture of rat lymph nodes. III. The lymph nodes and lymph-borne cells of the congenitally anthymic node rat (rnu). *Scand.J.Immunol.*, 12, 421–432.

FRITH, C.H., DAVIS, T.M., ZOLOTOR, L.A. and TOWNSEND, J.W. (1980): Histiocytic lymphoma in the mouse. *Leuk.Res.*, 4, 651–662.

FRUHMAN, G. and GORDON, A. (1955): Influence of starvation upon the formed elements of blood and bone marrow of the rat. *Anat.Rec.* 122, 492.

GALLO, R.C. and WONG-STAAL, F. (1982): Retroviruses as etiologic agents of some animal and human leukemias and lymphomas and as tools for elucidating the molecular mechanism of leukemogenesis. *Blood*, 60, 545–557.

GALLO, R.C. and WONG-STAAL, F. (1984): Current thoughts on the viral etiology of certain human cancers. The Richard and Hinda Rosenthal Foundation Award Lecture. *Cancer Res.*, 44, 2743–2749.

GARDNER, W.U., DOUGHERTY, T.F. and WILLIAMS, W.L. (1944): Lymphoid tumors in mice receiving steroid hormones. *Cancer Res.*, 4, 73–87.

GARDNER, D.E., SELGRADE, M.J.K. and GRAHAM, J.A. (1983): The use of immunotoxicological data in the environmental regulatory process. In: C.G. Gibson, R. Hubbard, D.V. Parks (Eds) *Immunotoxicology*, pp. 401–412. Academic Press, London.

GERARD-MARCHANT, R., HAMLIN, I., LENNERT, K., RILKE, F., STANSFELD, A.G. and VAN UNNIK, J.A.M. (1974): Classification of the non-Hodgkin's lymphoma. *Lancet*, 2, 406–408.

GILLMAN J. and GILLMAN T., (1952): The pathogenesis of experimentally produced lymphomata in rats (including Hodgkin's-like sarcoma). *Cancer*, 5, 792–846.

GISLER, R.H. (1974): Stress and the hormonal regulation of the immune response in mice. *Psychother. Psychosom.*, 23, 197–208.

GLEICHMAN, H.I.K., PALS, S.T. and RADASZKIEWICZ, T. (1983): T cell-dependent B-cell proliferation and activation induced by administration of the drug diphenylhydantoin to mice. *Hematol.Oncol.*, 1, 165–176.

GLENNER G.G. (1980): Amyloid deposits and amyloidosis The β-fibrilloses. *N. Engl. J.Med.*, 302, 1283–1292.

GOLDSTEIN, G. and MACKAY, R. (1969): The thymus and experimental pathology. In: *The Human Thymus*, Chap. 3, pp. 86–127. Heinemann, London.

GOODMAN, D.G., WARD, J.M. and REICHARDT, W.D. (1984): Splenic fibrosis and sarcomas in F344 rats fed diets containing aniline hydrochloride, p-chloroaniline, azobenzene, o-toluidine hydrochloride, 4,4'sulfonyldianiline, or D and C Red No.9. *J.N.C.I.*, 73, 265–273.

GOODMAN, D.G., WARD, J.M., SQUIRE, R.A., CHU, K.C. and LINHART, M.S. (1979): Neoplastic and non-neoplastic lesions in ageing F344 rats. *Toxicol.Appl.Pharmacol.*, 48, 237–248.

GOUDIE, R.B. (1989): A strategy for demonstrating the clonal origin of small numbers of T lymphocytes in histopathological specimens. *J.Pathol.*, 158, 261–265.

GREEN, J.R. (1984): Generation of cytotoxic T cells in the rat mixed lympho-cyte reaction in blocked by monoclonal antibody MRC OX-8. *Immunology*, 52, 253–260.

GREENLEE, P.G., CALVANO, S.E., QUIMBY, F.W. and HURVITZ, A.I. (1987): Investigation of cross-reactivity between commercially available antibodies directed against human, mouse and rat lymphocyte surface antigens and surface markers on canine cells. *Vet.Immunol.Immunopathol.*, 15, 285–296.

GREENMAN, D.L., KODELL, R.L. and SHELDON, W.G. (1984): Association between cage shelf level and spontaneous and induced neoplasms in mice. *J.N.C.I.*, 73, 107–113.

GREAVES, P. and FACCINI, J.M. (1981): Fibrous histiocytic neoplasms spontaneously arising in rats. *Br.J.Cancer*, 43, 402–411.

GREAVES, P. and FACCINI, J.M. (1984): Haemopoietic and lymphatic lymphatic systems. In: *Rat*

Histopathology. A Glossary for Use in Toxicity and Carcinogenicity Studies, Chapter II, pp. 35–56. Elsevier, Amsterdam.

GREAVES, P., MARTIN, J. and MASSON, M-T. (1982): Spontaneous rat malignant tumors of fibrohistiocytic origin. An ultrastructural study. *Vet.Pathol.*, 19, 497–505.

GREAVES, P. and RABEMAMPIANINA, Y. (1982): Choice of rat strain : A comparison of the general pathology and the tumour incidence in 2-year old Sprague-Dawley and Long-Evans rats. *Arch.Toxicol.*, S5, 298–303.

GROSS, L., FELDMAN, D. and DREYFUSS, Y. (1986): C-type virus particles in spontaneous and virus-induced leukemia and malignant lymphomas in mice and rats. *Cancer Res.*, 46, 2984–2987.

GROSSRAU, R., VORMANN, J. and GUNTHER, T. (1984): Enzyme histochemistry of malignant T cell lymphoma due to chronic magnesium deficiency in rats. *Histochemistry*, 80, 183–186.

HANTO, D.W., GAJL-PECZALSKA, K.J., FIRZZERA, G., ARTHUR, D.C., BALFOUR, H.H., McCLAIN, K., SIMMONS, R.L. and NAJARIAN, J.S. (1983): Epstein-Barr virus-induced polyclonal and monoclonal B-cell lymphoproliferative diseases occurring after renal transplantation : clinical pathologic and virologic findings and implications for therapy. *Ann.Surg.*, 198, 356–69.

HARRIS, C.C. (1979): A delayed complication of cancer therapy: cancer. *J.N.C.I.*, 63, 275–277.

HARRIS, N.L. (1985): The impact of molecular genetics on the study of lymphoid neoplasia. *Lab.Invest.*, 53, 509–512.

HASHIMOTO, K., IMAI, K., YOSHIMURA, S and OHTAKI, T. (1981): Experimental toxicity studies with captopril, an inhibitor of angiotensin 1-converting enzyme. 3. Twelve month studies of chronic toxicity of captopril in rats. *J.Toxicol.Sci.*, 6, Supp,2, 215–246.

HATTORI, A., KUNZ, H.W., GILL III, T.J. and SHINOZUKA, H. (1987): Thymic and lymphoid changes and serum immunoglobulin abnormalities in mice receiving cyclosporin. *Am.J.Pathol.*, 128, 111–120.

HELPAP, B., KAISER R (1981): The cellular response of T and B dependent areas of the spleen after focal thermocoagulation of liver and kidney. *Virchows Arch.*, [B] 36, 291–302.

HIGGINS, C.B., GRAND, L. and UEDA, N. (1982): Specific induction of erythro-leukemia and myelogenous leukemia in Sprague-Dawley rats. *Proc.Natl. Acad.Sci.*, USA, 79, 5411–5414.

HIROKAWA, K., UTSUYAMA, M., GOTO, H. and KARAMOTO, K. (1984): Differential rate of age-related decline in immune functions in genetically defined mice with different tumor incidence and life span. *Gerontology*, 30, 223–233.

HOLMBERG, C.A., MANNING, J.S. and OSBURN, B.I. (1976): Canine malignant lymphomas : Comparison of morphologic and immunologic parameters. *J.N.C.I.*, 56, 125–135.

HOTTENDORF, G.H. (1985): Carcinogenicity testing of antitumor agents. *Toxicol.Pathol.*, 13, 192–199.

HOOVER, R. and FRAUMENI, J.F., (1981): Drug-induced cancer. *Cancer*, 47, 1071–1080.

HSU, S-M. and JAFFE, E.S. (1985): Phenotypic expression of T lymphocytes in thymus and peripheral lymphoid tissues. *Am.J.Pathol.*, 121, 69–78.

HUANG, T.T.F. and CALARCO, A.G. (1981): Evidence for the cell surface expression of cell surface expression of intracisternal A particle-associated antigens during early mouse development. *Dev.Biol.*, 82, 388–392.

HUNTER, R.L., FERGUSON, D.J. and COPPLESON, L.W. (1975): Survival with mammary cancer related to the interaction of germinal center hyperplasia and sinus histiocytosis in axillary and internal mammary lymph nodes. *Cancer*, 36, 528–539.

IMAI, K., YOSHIMURA, OHIAKI, T. and HASHIMOTO, K. (1981): Experimental toxicity studies with captopril, an inhibitor of angiotensin 1-converting enzyme. 2. One month studies of chronic toxicity of captopril in rats. *J.Toxicol.Sci.*, 6, Suppl.2, 189–214.

INADA, T. and MIMS, C.A. (1984): Mouse Ia antigens are receptors for lactate dehydrogenase virus. *Nature*, 309, 59–61.

ISERSKY, C., PAGE, D.L., CUATRECASAS, P., DELELLIS, R.A. and GLENNER, G.G. (1971): Murine amyloidosis : Immunologic characterization of amyloid fibril protein. *J.Immunol.*, 107, 1690–1698.

IRISARRI, E., KESSEDJIAN, M.J., CHARUEL, C., FACCINI, J.M., GREAVES, P., MONRO, A.M., NACHBAUR, J. and RABEMAMPIANINA, Y. (1985): Dazoxiben, a prototype inhibitor of thromboxane synthesis, has little toxicity in laboratory animals. *Hum.Toxicol.*, 4, 311–315.

ISHIHARA, T., YAMASHITA, Y., OKUZONO, Y., YOKOTA, T., TAKAHASHI, M., KAMEI, T., UCHINO, F., MATSUMOTO, N., MIWA, S., FUJI, H. and KOZAKI, T. (1985): Three kinds of foamy cells in the spleen: Comparative histochemical and ultrastructural studies. *Ultrastruct.Pathol.*, 8, 13–23.

ISHIMARU, T., HOSHINO, T., ICHIMARU, M., OKAD, H., TOMIYASU, T., TSUCHIMOTO, T. and YAMAMOTO, T. (1971): Leukemia in atomic bomb survivers, Hiroshima and Nagasaki, October 1, 1950–September 30, 1966. *Radiat.Res.*, 45, 216–233.

ITO, K., SCHMAUS, J and REISSMAN, K (1964): Protein metabolism and erythropoiesis. III The erythroid marrow in protein-starved rats and its response to erythropoietin. *Acta Haematol.*, 32, 257–264.

IWAKI, Y., TERASAKI, P.I., KINUKAWA, T., THAI, T.H., ROOT, T. and BILLING, R. (1983): Cross-reactivity between human and canine Ia antigens using a mouse monoclonal antibody (CIA). *Transplatation*, 36, 189–191.

JAFFE, E.S., CLARK, J., STEIS, R., BLATTNER, W., MACHER, A.B., LONGO D.L. and REICHERT, C.M. (1985): Lymph node pathology of HTLV and HTLV-associated neoplasms. Cancer Res, 45, 4662s–4664s.

JONES, H.B., REID, P.G. and LUKE, J.S.H., (1989): Evolution of structural changes leading to haemolysis in human erythrocytes treated with SK and F 95018, an antihypertensive compound with combined vasodilator and β-adrenoceptor antagonist properties. *Toxicol.In Vitro*, 3, 299–309.

KABIR, A., WATANABE, M., TAKEDA, Z., KIZAKI, T. and URANO, Y. (1983): Distribution of peanut agglutinin binding sites in rat lymphatic organs. *Cell Struct.Funct.*, 8, 29–34.

KALDOR, J.M.,DAY, N.E., PETTERSSON, F., CLARKE, E.A., PEDERSEN, D., MEHNERT, W., BELL, J., HOST, H., PRIOR, P., KARJALAINEN, S., NEAL, F., KOCH, M., BAND, P., CHOI, W., POMPE KIRN, V., ARSLAN, A., ZARÉN, B., BELCH, A.R., STORM, H., KITTEL-MANN, B., FRASER, P. and STOVALL, M. (1990): Leukemia following chemotheraphy for ovarian cancer. *N.Engl.J.Med.* 322, 1–6.

KASAI, M., IWAMORI, M., NAGIA, Y., OKAMURA, K and TADA, T (1980): A glycolipid on the surface of mouse natural killer cells. *Eur.J.Immunol.*, 10, 175–180.

KASAI, M., YONEDA, T., HABU, S., MURUYAMA, Y., OKUMURA, K. and TOKUNAGA, T. (1981): In vivo effect of anti-asialo GM1 on natural killer cell activity. *Nature*, 291, 334–335.

KATO, A. and HAYS, E.F. (1985): Development of virus-accelerated thymic lymphoma in AKR mice. *J.N.C.I.*, 75, 491–497.

KAUFMAN, M., WIRTH, K., SCHEURER, J., ZIMMERMANN, A., LUSCIETI, P., and STJERNSWÄRD, J. (1977): Immunomorphological lymph node changes in patients with operable bronchogenic squamous cell carcinoma. *Cancer*, 39, 2371–2377.

KELTON, J.G. (1985): Impaired reticuloendothelial function in patients treated with methyldopa. *N.Engl.J.Med.*, 313, 596–600.

KLEIN, G. (1979): Lymphoma development in mice and humans : Diversity of initiation is followed by convergent cytogenetic evolution. *Proc.Natl. Acad.Sci.*, USA, 76, 2442–2446.

KLOCKARS, M., and OSSERMAN, E.F. (1974): Localization of lysozyme in normal rat tissue by an immunoperoxidase method. *J.Histochem.Cytochem.*, 22, 139–146.

KOLLER, L.D. (1987): Immunotoxicology today. *Toxicol.Pathol.* 15, 346–351.

KORNBRUST, D., EYDELLOTH, R. and GARRATTY, G. (1989): Investigations of the potential for five β-lactam antibiotics to elicit type II hypersensitivity reactions in rats and monkeys. *Fundam.Appl.Toxicol.*, 12, 558–566.

KORT, W.J., ZONDERVAN, P.E., HULSMAN, L.O.M., WEIJMA, I.M. and WESTBROEK, D.L. (1984): Incidence of spontaneous tumors in a group of retired breeder female Brown Norway rats. *J.N.C.I.*, 72, 709–713.

KRAKOWKA, S. In vitro and in vivo methods in immunotoxicology. *Toxicol.Pathol.* 15, 276–280.

KRECH, R. and THEILE, J. (1985): Histopathology of the bone marrow in toxic myelopathy. *Virchows Arch. [A].*, 405, 225–235.

KROES, R., GARBIS-BERKVENS, J.M., de VRIES, T. and van NESSELROOY, H.J. (1981): Histopathological profile of a Wistar rat stock including a survey of the literature. *J.Gerontol.*, 36, 259–279.

KRUEGER, G.R.F., MALMGREN, R.A. and BERARD, C.W. (1971): Malignant lymphomas and plasmacytosis in mice under prolonged immunosuppression and persistent antigenic stimulation. *Transplantation*, 11, 138–144.

KRUEGER, G.R.F. and KONORZA, G. (1979): Classification of animal lymphomas : The implications of applying Rappaport's classification for human lymphomas to experimental tumors. *Exp.Hematol.*, 7, 305–314.

KUPER, C.F., BEEMS, R.B. and HOLLANDERS, V.M.H. (1986): Spontaneous pathology of the thymus in aging Wistar (Cpb.WU) rats. *Vet.Pathol.* 23, 270–277.

LANE, H.C., DEPPER, J.M. GREENE, W.C., WHALEN, G., WALDMANN, T.A. and FAUCI, A.S. (1985): Qualitative analysis of immune function in patients with the acquired immunodeficiency syndrome. Evidence for a selective defect in soluble antigen recognition. *N.Engl.J.Med.*, 313, 79–84.

LANIER, L.L., LYNES, M., HAUGHTON, G. and WETTSTEIN, P.J. (1978): Novel type of murine B-cell lymphoma. *Nature*, 217, 554–556.

LEDBETTER, J.A., EVANS, R.L., LIPINSKI, M., CUNNINGHAM-RANDLES, C., GOOD, R. and HERZENBERG, L.A. (1981): Evolutionary conversation of surface molecules that distinguish lymphocyte-T helper-inducer and cytoxic-suppressor subpopulations in mouse and man. *J.Exp.Med.*, 153, 310–323.

LEDBETTER, J.A., MARTIN, P.G., SPOONER, C.E., WOFSY, D., TSU, T.T., BEATTY, P.G. and GLADSTONE, P. (1985): Antibodies to Tp67 and Tp44 augment and sustain proliferative responses of activated T cells. *J.Immunol.*, 135, 2331–2336.

LEDBETTER, J.A., ROUSE, R.V., MICKLEM, H.S. and HERZENBERG L.A. (1980): T cell subsets defined by expression of Lyt-1,2,3 and Thy-1 antigens. Two-parameter immunofluorescence and cytoxicity analysis with monoclonal antibodies modifies current views. *J.Exp.Med.*, 152, 280–295.

LEEMING, G., McLEAN, J.M. and GIBBS, A.C.L. (1985): The cell content and proliferative response of the rat thymus during first syngeneic and allogeneic pregnancy, and the effects of strain difference. *Thymus*, 4, 247–255.

LEITER, E.H. (1985): Type C retrovirus production by pancreatic beta cells. Association with accelerated pathogenesis in C3H-db/db ('diabetes') mice. *Am.J.Pathol.*, 119, 22–32.

LEVINE, S. and GHERSON, J. (1986): Morphologic effects of mitozantrone and a related anthracenedione on lymphoid tissues. *Int.J.Immunopharmacol.*, 8, 999–1007.

LÉVY, M., and RAPHAËL, M. (1987): Effects of antimitotic treatment on haematopoietic tissues in mice. *Ann.Inst.Pasteur Immunol.*, 138, 347–357.

LEWIS, D.J., and OFFER, J.M. (1984): Malignant mastocytoma in mice. *J.Comp.Pathol.*, 94, 615–620.

LIVNI, N., LAUFER, A., and LEVO, Y., (1980): Demonstration of amyloid in murine and human secondary amyloidosis by the immunoperoxidase technique. *J.Pathol.*, 132, 343–348.

LOOSE, L.D. (1984): Overview of progress in immunotoxicology: 1983. *Surv.Immunol.Res.*, 3, 238–240.

LOSCO, P.E. and WARD, J.M. (1984): The early stage of large granular lymphocyte leukemia in the F344 rat. *Vet.Pathol.*, 21, 286–291.

LUKES, R.J. and COLLINS, R.D. (1975): New approaches to the classification of the lymphomata. Symposium on non-Hodgkin's lymphomata. *Br.J.Cancer*, 31(S2), 1–28.

LUSTER, M.I., BLANK, J.A. and DEAN, J.H. (1987): Molecular and cellular basis of chemically induced immunotoxicity. *Ann.Rev. Pharmacol.Toxicol.*, 27, 23–49.

LUSTER, M.I., MUNSON, A.E., THOMAS, P.T., HOLSAPPLE, M.P., FENTERS, J.D., WHITE, K.L., LAUER, L.D., GERMOLEC, D.R., ROSENTHAL, G.J. and DEAN, J.H. (1988): Development of a testing battery to assess chemical induced immunotoxicity: National Toxicology Program's guidelines for immunotoxicity evaluation in mice. *Fundam.Appl.Toxicol.*, 10, 2–19.

LUSTER, M.I., GERMOLEC, D.R., WHITE, K.L., FUCHS, B.A., FORT, M.M., TOMASZEWSKI, J.E., THOMPSON, M., BLAIR, P.C., McCAY, J.A., MUNSON, A.E. and ROSENTHAL, G.J. (1989): A comparison of three nucleoside analogues with anti-retroviral activity on immune and haemopoietic functions in mice. In vitro toxicity to precursor cells and microstromal environment. *Toxicol.Appl.Pharmacol.*, 101, 328–339.

McALLISTER, H.A. and ROCK, D.L. (1985): Comparative usefulness of tissue fixatives for in situ viral nucleic acid hybridization. *J.Histochem. Cytochem.*, 33, 1026–1032.

McKENZIE, J.L. and FABRE, J.W. (1981)a: Studies with a monoclonal antibody or the distribution of Thy-1 in the lymphoid and extracellular connective tissues of the dog. *Transplantation*, *31*, 275–282.

McKENZIE, J.L. and FABRE, J.W. (1981)b: Human Thy-1 : unusual localization and possible functional significance in lymphoid tissues. *J.Immunol.*, *126*, 843–850.

McMARTIN, D.N. (1979): Morphological lesions in aging Syrian hamsters. *J.Gerontol.*, 34, 502–511.

McMASTER, W.R. and WILLIAMS, A.F. (1979)a: Identification of Ia glyco-proteins in rat thymus and purification from rat spleen. *Eur.J.Immunol.*, 9, 426–433.

McMASTER, W.R. and WILLIAMS, A.F. (1979)b: Monoclonal antibodies to Ia antigens from rat thymus: Cross reactions with mouse and human use in purification of rat Ia glycoproteins. *Immunol.Rev.*, 47, 117–137.

MAEKAWA, A., KUROKAWA, Y., TAKAHASHI, M., KOKUBO, T., OGIU, T., ONODERA, H., TANIGAWA, H., OHNO, Y. and FURUKAWA-HAYASHI, Y. (1983): Spontaneous tumors in F344/Du Crj rats. *Jpn.J.Cancer Res. (Gann)*, 74, 365–372.

MAJEED, S.K. and GOPINATH, C (1985): Hodgkin's disease-like lesion in a rat. *J.Comp.Pathol.*, 95, 123–126.

MAJOR, I.R. (1979): Induction of myeloid leukemia by whole-body single exposure of CBA male mice to X-rays. *Br.J.Cancer*, 40, 903–913.

MANSOUR, M.H., NEGM, H.I. and COOPER, E.L. (1987): Thy-l evolution. *Dev.Comp.Immunol.*, II, 2–15.

MARCOLI, M., GATTI, G., IPPOLITI, G., LOMBARDI, M., CREMA, A., ZOCCHI, M.T., DE PONTI, F., LECCHINI, S. and FRIGO, G.M. (1985): Effects of chronic anticonvulsant monotherapy on lymphocyte subpopulations in adult epileptic patients. *Hum. Toxicol.*, 4, 147–157.

MARTIN, R.A., BARSOUM, N.J., SURGESS, J.M. and de la IGLESIA, F.A., (1985): Leukocyte and bone marrow effects of a thiomorpholine quinazosin antihypertensive agent. *Toxicol.Appl.Pharmacol.*, 81, 166–173.

MASON, D.W., ARTHUR, R.P., DALLMAN, M.J., GREEN, J.R., SPICKETT, G.P. and THOMAS, M.L. (1983): Functions of rat T lymphocyte subsets isolated by means of monoclonal antibodies. *Immunol.Rev.*, 74, 57–82.

MASON, D.W., BRIDEAU, R.J., McMASTER, W.R., WEBB, M., WHITE, R.A.H. and WILLIAMS, A.F. (1980): Monoclonal antibodies that define T-lymphocytes subsets in the rat. In: R.H. Kennett, T.J. McKearn and K.B. Bechtol (Eds), *Monoclonal Antibodies*, Chap.15, p251–273. Plenum Publishing Corp, New York.

MATSUYAMA, M., SUZUKI, H., YAMADA, S., ITO, M. and NAGAYO, T. (1975): Ultra-structure of spontaneous and urethan-induced thymomas in Buffalo rats. *Cancer Res.*, 35, 2771.

MAYRHOFER, G., PUGH, C.W. and BARCLAY, A.N. (1983): The distribution, ontogeny and origin in the rat of Ia positive cells with dendritic morphology and of Ia antigen in epithelia, with special reference to the intestine. *Eur.J.Immunol.*, 13, 112–122.

METCALF, D. (1961): Reticular tumors in mice subjected to prolonged antigenic stimulation. *Br.J.Cancer*, 15, 769–779.

MICHEL-FOUQUE, M-C., GREAVES, P., MARTIN, J., and MASSON, M-T. (1983): Etude ultrastructurale des lymphomes malins non Hodgkiniens gastro-intestineaux spontanés chez le hamster Syrien (Mesocricetus auratus). *Biol.Cell.*, 48, 10a.

MICHEL-FOUQUE, M-C. (1984): Lymphomes malin non Hodgkiniens spontanés chez le hamster Syrien doré. Memoire pour l'obtention du diplôme d'études et de recherche en biologie humaine (D.E.R.B.H.). Faculté de Médecine, Marseille.

136

MONJAN, A.A. and COLLECTOR, M.I. (1977): Stress-induced modulation of the immune response. *Science*, 196, 307–308.

MOORE, P.F. (1986): Characterization of cytoplasmic lysozyme immunoreactivity as a histocytic marker in normal canine tissues. *Vet.Pathol.* 213, 763–769.

MUIRHEAD, M.J., HOLBERG Jr., J.M., UHR, J.W. and VITETTA, E.S. (1981): BCL1, a murine model of prolymphocytic leukemia. II Morphology and ultra-structure. *Am.J.Pathol.*, 105, 306–315.

NACOPOULOU, L., AZARIS, P., PAPACHARALAMPOUS, N., and DAVARIS, P. (1981): Prognostic significance of histologic host response in cancer of the large bowel. *Cancer*, 47, 930–936.

NALESNIK, M.H., JAFFE, R., STARZEL, T.E., DEMETRIS, A.J., PORTER, K., BURNHAM, J.A., MAKOWKA, L., HO, M. and LOCKER, J. (1988): The pathology of posttransplant lymphoproliferative disorders occurring in the setting of cyclosporin A-prednisone immunosuppression. *Am.J.Pathol.* 133, 173–192.

NATIONAL CANCER INSTITUTE (1977): Bioassay of dapsone for possible carcinogenicity. Carcinogenesis technical report series No.20, Washington DC, US Gov.Print.Off. [DHSS publication No (NIH) 77 –820].

NEWBERNE, J.W., NEWBERNE, P.M., GIBSON, J.P., HUFFMAN, K.K. and PALOLPOLI, F.P. (1977): Lack of carcinogenicity of oxprenolol, a beta-adrenergic blocking agent. *Toxicol.Appl.Pharmacol.*, 41, 535–542.

NOBLE, C. and NORBURY, K.C. (1983): The differential sensitivity of rat peripheral blood T cells to immunosuppressants : Cyclophosphamide and dexamethazone. *J.Immunopharmacol.*, 5, 341–358.

NOSSAL, G.J.V. (1987) Current Concepts: Immunology. The basic components of the immune system. *N.Engl.J.Med.*, 316, 1320–1325.

NORBURY, K.C. (1982): Immunotoxicology in the pharmaceutical industry. *Environ.Health Perspect.*, 43, 53–59.

OHTAKI, S. (1988): Quantitative interactions in weight of lymphoid organs and steroid hormonal organs in hamsters under several experimental conditions. *Br.J.Exp.Pathol.* 69, 1–16.

OHTAKI, T., IMAI, K., YOSHIMURA. and HASHIMOTO, K. (1981): Experimental toxicity studies with captopril, an inhibitor of angiotensin 1-converting enzyme. 4. Three months subacute toxicity of captopril in beagle dogs. *J.Toxicol.Sci.*, 6, Supp.2, 247–270.

ONO, Y., IWASAKI, T., SEKIGUCHI, M. and ONODERA, T. (1988): Subacute toxicity of muroctasin in mice and dogs. *Arzneimittelforschung*, 7, 1024–1027.

OWEN, G., SMITH, T.H.F. and AGERSBORG Jr., H.P.K. (1970): Toxicity of some benzodiazepine compounds with CNS activity. *Toxicol.Appl.Pharmacol.*, 16, 556–570.

OWENS Jr., A.H. (1962): Predicting anticancer drug effects in man from laboratory animal studies. *J.Chronic Dis.*, 15, 223–228.

PAPAIOANNOU, A.N., TSAKRALIDES, V., CRITSELIS, A.N., and GOOD, R.A. The thymus in breast cancer. Observations in 25 patients and controls. *Cancer*, 41, 790–796.

PATT, D.J., BRYNES, R.K., VARDIMAN, J.W., and COPPLESON, L.W. (1975): Mesocolic lymph node histology is an important prognostic indicator for patients with carcinoma of the sigmoid colon : An immunomorphologic study. *Cancer*, 35, 1388–1397.

PATTENGALE, P.K. and FRITH, C.H. (1983): Immunomorphologic classification of spontaneous lymphoid cell neoplasms occurring in female BALB/c mice. *J.N.C.I.*, 70, 169–179.

PATTENGALE, P.K. and TAYLOR, C.R. (1983): Experimental models of lymphoproliferative disease. The mouse as a model for human non-Hodgkin's lymphomas and related leukemias. *Am.J.Pathol.*, 113, 237–265.

PATTENGALE, P.K., TAYLOR, P., TWOMEY, P., HILL, S., JONASSON, J., BEARDSLEY, T. and HAAS, M. (1982): Immunopathology of B cell lymphomas induced iun C57BL/6 mice by dual-tropic murine leukemia virus (MuLV). *Am.J.Pathol.*, 107, 362–377.

PAUL, L.C., RENNKE, H.G., MILFORD, E.L. and CARPENTER, C.B. (1984): Thy-1.1 in glomeruli of rat kidneys. *Kidney Int.*, 25, 771–777.

PEDERSEN-BJERGAARD, J., SPECHT, L., LARSEN, S.O., ERSBOLL, J., STRUCK, J., HANSEN, M.M., HANSEN, H.H. and NISSEN, N.I. (1987): Risk of therapy-related leukaemia and preleukaemia after Hodgkin's disease, relative to age, cumulative dose of alkylating agents, and time from chemotherapy. *Lancet*, 2, 83–88.

PERCY, D.H. and JONAS, A.M. (1971): Incidence of spontaneous tumors in CD(R)-1 HaM/ICR mice. *J.N.C.I.*, 46, 1045–1065.

PETZ, L.D., (1980): Drug-induced immune haemolytic anaemia. *Clin.Haematol.*, 9, 455–482.

PICKER, L.J., WEISS, L.M., MEDEIROS, L.J., WOOD, G.S. and WARNKE, R.A. (1987): Immunophenotypic criteria for the diagnosis of non-Hodgkin's lymphoma. *Am.J.Pathol.* 128, 181–201.

PICKERING, R.G. and PICKERING, C.E. (1984): The effects of reduced dietary intake upon the body and organ weights, and some clinical chemistry and hematological variates of the young Wistar rat. *Toxicol.Lett.*, 21, 271–277.

PIHL, E., NAIRN, R.C., MILNE, B.J., CUTHBERTSON, A.M., HUGHES, E.S.R., and ROLLO, A. (1980): Lymphoid hyperplasia. A major prognostic feature in 519 cases of colorectal carcinoma. *Am.J.Pathol.*,100, 469–480.

PIZZO, P.A. (1984): Granulocytopenia and cancer therapy. Past problems, current solutions, future challenges. *Cancer*, 54, 2649–2661.

POLLOCK, R.E., BABCOCK, G.F., ROMSDAHL, M.M. and NISHIOKA, K. (1984): Surgical stress-mediated suppression of murine natural killer cell cytotoxicity. *Cancer Res.*, 44, 3888–3891.

POUR, P., ALTHOFF, J., SALMASI, S.Z. and STEPAN, K. (1979): Spontaneous tumors and common diseases in three types of hamsters. *J.N.C.I.*, 63, 797–811.

POUR, P., MOHR, U., ALTHOFF, J., CARDESA, A. and KMOCH, N. (1976): Spontaneous tumors and common diseases in two colonies of Syrian hamsters. IV Vascular and lymphatic systems and lesions at other sites. *J.N.C.I.*, 56, 963–974.

QUINN, R.P., WOLBERG, G., MEDZIHRADSKY, J. and ELION, G.B. (1982): Effect of acyclovir on various immune in vivo and in vitro immunologic assay systems. *Am.J.Med.*, 73, 1A, 62–66.

RAFF, M.C., NASE, S. and MITCHISON, N.A. (1971): Mouse specific bone marrow-derived lymphocyte antigen as a marker for thymus-independent lymphocytes. *Nature*, 230, 50–51.

RAPP, F. (1984): Current knowledge of mechanisms of viral carcinogenesis. *CRC Crit.Rev.Toxicol.*, 13, 197–204.

RAPPAPORT, H. (1966): Tumors of the Hemopoietic System. In: Armed Forces Institute of Pathology, *Atlas of Tumor Pathology*, Section 3, Fasc. 8, pp. 1–442, Washington, DC.

RASK-NIELSEN, R. and EBBESEN, P. (1969): Spontaneous reticular neoplasms in (CBA x DBA/2) F1 mice, with special emphasis on the occurrence of plasma cell neoplasms. *J.N.C.I.*, 43, 553–564.

READ, N.G., BEESLEY, J.E., BLACKETT, M.N. and TRIST, D.G. (1985): The accumulation of an aryloxylkylamidine (501C) and 5-hydroxytryptamine in human polymorphonuclear leucocytes : a quantitative electron microscopic study. *J.Pharm.Pharmacol.*, 37, 96–99.

REYNOLDS, C.W., BERE Jr., E.W. and WARD, J.M. (1984): Natural killer activity in the rat. III Characterization of transplantable large granular lymphocyte (LGL) leukemias in the F344 rat. *J.Immunol.*, 132, 534–540.

RIBOLI, E.B., TERRIZZI, A., ARNULFO, G. and BERTOGLIO, S. (1984): Immunosuppressive effects of surgery evaluated by the multitest cell-mediated immunity system. *Can.J.Surg.* 27, 60–63.

ROE, F.J.C. (1983): Toxicologic evaluation of metronidazole with particular reference to carcinogenic, mutagenic and teratogenic potential. *Surgery*, 93, 158–164.

ROE, F.J.C. and TUCKER, M.J. (1974): Recent developments in the design of carcinogenicity tests on laboratory animals. *Proc.Eur.Soc.Study Drug Toxicity*, 15, 171–177.

ROSAI, J. and LEVINE, G.D. (1976): Tumors of the Thymus, Armed Forces Institute of Pathology, Fascicle 13, 2nd Series, pp. 34–37, Washington, DC.

ROSEN, H., BLUMENTHAL, A., BECKFIELD, W.J. and AGERSBORG, H.P.K.Jr. (1966): Toxicity of a hypoglycaemic agent, 2-p-methoxybenzene-sulfonamido-5-isobutyl-1,3,4-thiadiazole. *Toxicol.Appl.Pharmacol.*, 8, 13–21.

ROSSE, W.F. (1987): The spleen as a filter. *N. Engl.J.Med.* 317, 704–706.

ROWLATT, C., CHESTERMAN, F.C. and SHERRIFF, M.U. (1976): Lifespan, age changes and tumour incidence in an aging C57BL mouse colony. *Lab.Anim.*, 10, 419–442.

RUSSFIELD, A.B., and GREEN, M.N. (1965): Serum protein patterns associated with amyloidosis in the Syrian hamster. *Am.J.Pathol.*, 46, 59–69.

RUST, J.R. (1981): An assessment of metronidazole tumorigenicity studies in mouse and rat. In: S.M. Finegold, J.A. McFadzean, F.J.C. Roe, (Eds), Metronidazole. *Proceedings of the International Metronidazole Conference, Montreal, Quebec, Canada.*

RUSTIA, M. and SHUBIK, P. (1972): Induction of lung tumors and malignant lymphomas in mice by metronidazole. *J.N.C.I.*, 48 721–729.

SAINTE-MARIE, G., PENG, F.S. and BÉLISLE, C. (1982): Overall architecture and pattern of lymph flow in the rat lymph node. *Am.J.Anat.*, 64, 275–309.

SAINTE-MARIE, G. and PENG, F.S. (1983): Structural and cell population changes in the lymph nodes of the athymic nude mouse. *Lab.Invest.*, 49, 420–429.

SAINTE-MARIE, G., PENG, F.S. and PELLETIER, M. (1984): Development of the lymph nodes in the very young and their evolution in the mature, nude rat. *Dev.Comp.Immunol.*, 8, 695–710.

SAINTE-MARIE, G. and PENG, F.S. (1985): Lymph nodes of the N:NIH(S)11-nu/nu mouse. *Lab.Invest.*, 52, 631–637.

SAINTE-MARIE, G. and PENG, F-S. (1987): Morphological anomalies associated with immunodeficiencies in the lymph nodes of aging mice. *Lab.Invest.* 56, 598–610.

SANDERSON, J.H. and PHILLIPS, C.E. (1981): *An Atlas of Laboratory Animal Hematology.* Clarendon Press, Oxford.

SASS, B., RABSTEIN, L.S., MADISON, R., NIMS, R.M., PETERS, R.L. and KELLOFF, G.J. (1975): Incidence of spontaneous neoplasms in F344 rats throughout the natural life-span. *J.N.C.I.*, 54, 1449–1456.

SATODATE, R., SASOU, S., KATSURA, S., YOSHIDA, M., and HIRATA, M. (1977): Vergleichende histologische-morphometrische Untersuchung der Marginalzone and des Keimzentrums den Milzfollikel der Ratte nach Endotoxininjektion. *Exp.Pathol.*, 14, 100–107.

SCHEIN, P.S., DAVIS, R.P., CARTER, S., NEWMAN, J., SCHEIN, D.R. and and RALL, D.P. (1970): The evaluation of anticancer drugs in dogs and monkeys for the prediction of qualitative toxicities in man. *Clin. Pharmacol.Ther.*, 11, 3–40.

SCHMÄHL, D. (1987): Zweittumoren uach chemotherapie maligner tumoren. *Arzneimittelforschung*, 37, 288–290.

SCHMÄHL, D. and HABS, M. (1979): Carcinogenic action of low-dose cyclophosphamide given orally to Sprague-Dawley rats in a life time experiment. *Int.J.Cancer.*, 23, 706–712.

SCHULTZ, R.T. and PITHA, J. (1985): Relation of hepatic and splenic micro-circulations to the development of lesions in experimental amyloidosis. *Am.J.Pathol.*, 19, 123–127.

SCHULTZ, R.T., PITHA, J., McDONALD, T. and DEBAULT, L.E. (1985): Ultrastuctural studies of vascular lesions in experimental amyloidosis of mice. *Am.J.Pathol.*, 119, 138–150.

SEIFERT, M.F. and MARKS, S.C. (1985): The regulation of haemopoiesis in the spleen. *Experientia*, 41, 192–199.

SLAVIN, S. and STROBER, S. (1978): Spontaneous murine B-cell leukemia. *Nature*, 272, 624–626.

SMIALOWICZ, R.J., LUEBKE, R.W., RIDDLE, M.M., ROGERS, R.R. and ROWE, D.G. (1985): Evaluation of the immunotoxic potential of chlordecone with comparison of cyclophosphamide. *J.Toxicol.Environ.Health*, 15, 561–574.

SMOLLER, B.R. and KRUSKALL, M.S. (1986): Phebotomy for diagnostic laboratory in adults. Pattern of use and effect on transfusion requirements. *N.Engl.J.Med.*, 314, 1233–1235.

SPICER, S.S., FRAYSER, R., VIRELLA, G. and HALL, B.J. (1977): Immunocytochemical localization of lysozymes in respiratory and other tissues. *Lab.Invest*, 36, 282–295.

SPRINGER, T., GALFRE, G., SECHER, D.S. and MILSTEIN, C. (1978): Monoclonal xenogeneic antibodies to murine cell surface antigens : identification of novel leucocyte differentiation antigens. *Eur.J.Immunol.*, 8, 539–551.

SPRINGER, T.A., GALFRE, G., SECHER, D.S., MILSTEIN, C. (1979): Mac-l: a macrophage differentiation antigen identified by monoclonal antibody. *Eur.J.Immunol.*, 9, 301–306.

139

SQUIRE, R.A., BRINKHOUS, K.M., PEIPER, S.C., FIRMINGER, H.I., MANN, R.B. and STRANDBERG, J.D. (1981): Histiocytic sarcoma with a granuloma-like component occurring in a large colony of Sprague-Dawley rats. *Am.J.Pathol.*, 105, 21–30.

STANTON, T., STEVENS, T.L., LEDBETTER, J.A. and WOFSY, D. (1986): Anti-Ly-1 antibody induces interleukin 2 release from T cells. *J.Immunol.*, 136, 1734–1737.

STARZL, T.E., NALESNIK, M.A., PORTER, K.A., HO, M., IWATSUKI, S., GRIFFITH, B.P., ROSENTHAL, J.T., HAKALA, T.R., SHAW Jr., B.W., HARDESTY, R.L., ATCHISON, R.W., JAFFE, R. and BAHNSON, H.T. (1984): Reversibility of lymphomas and lymphoproliferative lesions developing under cyclosporin-steroid therapy. *Lancet*, 1, 583–587.

STEWART, H.L., DERINGER, M.K., DUNN, T.B. and SNELL, K.C. (1974): Malignant schwannomas of nerve roots, uterus and epididymis in mice. *J.N.C.I.*, 53, 1749–1758.

STOUT, R.D., SCHWARTING, G.A. and SUTTLES, J. (1987): Evidence that expression of asialo-GM1 may be associated with cell activation. *J.Immunol.* 139, 2123–2129.

STROMBERG, P.C. (1985): Large granular lymphocyte leukemia in F344 rats. Model for human T lymphoma, malignant histiocytosis and T cell chronic lymphocytic leukemia. *Am.J.Pathol.*, 119, 517–519.

STROMBERG, P.C., ROJKO, J.L. VOGTSBERGER, L.M., CHENEY, C. and BERMAN, R. (1983): Immunologic, biochemical and ultrastructural characterization of the leukemia cell in F344 rats. *J.N.C.I.*, 71, 173–181.

STROMBERG, P.C., VOGTSBERGER, L.M., MARSH, L.R. and WILSON, F.D. (1983): Pathology of the mononuclear cell leukemia of Fischer rats. II Hematology. *Vet.Pathol.*, 20, 709–717.

STUTTE, H.J., SAKUMA, T., FALK, S. and SCHNEIDER, M. (1986): Splenic erythropoiesis in rats under hypoxic conditions. *Virchows Arch.*, [A] 409, 251–261.

SUNDERLAND, C.A., McMASTER, W.R. and WILLIAMS, A.F. (1979): Purification with monoclonal antibody of a predominant leukocyte-common antigen and glycoprotein from rat thymocytes. *Eur.J.Immunol*, 9, 155–159.

TAFFS, L.F., (1974): Some diseases in normal and immunosuppressed experimental animals. *Lab.Anim.*, 8, 149–154.

TAK CHEUNG, H., VOVOLKA, J. and TERRY, D.S. (1981): Age- and maturation-dependent changes in the immune system of Fisher F344 rats. *J.Reticuloendothelial.Soc.*, 30, 563–572.

TALAL, N. (1987): Autoimmune mechanisms in patients and animal models. *Toxicol.Pathol.* 15, 272–275.

THEUS, R. and ZBINDEN, G. (1984): Toxicological assessment of the haemostatic system. Regulatory requirements and industry practice. *Regul.Toxicol.Pharmacol.*, 4, 74–95.

THOMAS, M.L. and GREEN, J.R. (1983): Molecular nature of the W3/25 and MRC OX-8 marker antigens for rat T lymphocyte: Comparisons with mouse and human antigens. *Eur.J.Immunol.*, 13, 855–858.

TRIBE, C.R. and PERRY, V.A. (1979): Diagnosis of amyloid. Association of Clinical Pathologists. Broadsheet No. 92, p.9, British Medical Association, London.

TRIZIO, D., BASKETTER, D.A., BOTHAM, P.A., GRAEPEL, P.H., LAMBRÉ, C., MAGDA, S.J., PAL, T.M., RILEY, A.J., RONNENBERGER, H., VAN SITTER N.J. and BONTINCK, W.J. (1988): Identification of immunotoxic effects of chemicals and assessment of their relevance to man. *Food Chem.Toxicol.* 26, 527–539.

TSAKRAKLIDES, V., OLSON, P., KERSEY, J.H. and GOOD, R.A. (1974): Prognostic significance of the regional lymph node histology in cancer of the breast. *Cancer*,34, 1259–1267.

TUCKER, W.E. (1982): Pre-clinical toxicology profile of acyclovir : An overview. *Am.J.Med.*, 73, 1A, 27–30.

TUCKER, W.E., MACKLIN, A.W., SZOT, R.J., JOHNSTON, R.E., ELION, G.B., DE MIRANDA, P. and SZCZECH, G.M. (1983): Preclinical toxicity studies with acyclovir: Acute and subchronic tests. *Fundam.Appl.Toxicol.* 3, 573–578.

TUCKER, M.J. (1985): Effect of diet on spontaneous disease in the inbred mouse strain C57B1/10J. *Toxicol.Lett.*, 25, 131–135.

UTSUYAMA, M. and HIROKAWA, K. (1987): Age-related changes of splenic T cells in mice: a flow cytometric analysis. *Mech.Ageing Dev.* 40, 89–102.

VAN DEN BROEK, A.A., KEUNING, F.J., SOEHARTO, R., and PROP, N. (1983): Immune suppression and histophysiology of the immune response. I. Cortisone acetate and lymphoid migration. *Virchows Arch.* [B], 43, 43–54.

VAN DER VALK, P. and MEIJER, C.J.L.M. (1987): Histology of reactive lymph nodes. *Am.J.Surg.Pathol.*, 11, 866–882.

VAN NAGELL, J.R., DONALDSON, E.S., PARKER, J.C., VAN DYKE, A.H. and WOOD, E.G. (1977): The prognostic significance of pelvic lymph node morphology in carcinoma of the uterine cervix. *Cancer*, 39, 2624–2632.

VAN ROOIJEN, N. and CLAASSEN, E. (1986): Recent advances in the detection and characterization of specific antibody-forming cells in tissue sections. *Histochem.J.* 18, 465–471.

VAN ROOIJEN, N. (1973): Mechanism of follicular antigen trapping. Migration of antigen-antibody complexes from marginal zone toward follicle centres. *Immunology*,25, 847–852.

VAN ROOIJEN, N. (1977): Immune complexes in the spleen : Three concentric follicular areas of immune complex trapping, their inter-relationships and possible function. *J.Reticuloendothel.Soc.* 21, 143–151.

VAN ROOIJEN, J., KORS, N., BOORSMA, D.M., DE HAAN, P., and VAN NIEUWMEGEN, R. (1984): Peroxidase immunocytochemistry for the detection of specific anti-hapten (penicilloyl) antibody producing cells in the spleen, after injection of a hapten-carrier conjugate. *Immunol.Commun.*, 13, 29–34.

VAN ROOIJEN, N., VAN NIEUWMEGEN, R. and KAMPERDIJK, E.W.A. (1985): Elimination of phagocytic cells in the spleen after intravenous injection of liposome-encapsulated dichloromethylene diphosphonate. *Virchows Arch.*[B], 49, 375–383.

VAN ROOIJEN, J. and ROETERINK, C.H. (1980): Phagocytosis and lymphocyte migration : evidence that lymphocyte trapping in the spleen following carbon injection is not due to direct lymphocyte-macrophage adherence. *Immunology*, 39, 571–576.

VEERMAN, A.J.P, and EWIJK Van, W. (1975): White pulp compartments in the spleen of rats and mice. A light and electron microscopic study of lymphoid and non-lymphoid cell types in T- and B-areas. *Cell Tissue Res.*, 156, 417–441.

VEERMAN, A.J.P. and de VRIES, H. (1976): T- and B-areas in immune reactions. Volume changes in T and B cell compartments of the rat spleen following intravenous administration of a thymus-dependent (SRBC) and a thymus-independent (paratyphoid-vaccine-endotoxin) antigen. A histometric study. *Z.Immunol.Forsch.* 151, 202–218.

VOS, J.G. (1977): Immune suppression as related to toxicology. *CRC Crit. Rev.Toxicol.*, 5, 67–101.

WACHSMUTH, E.D. (1983): Evaluating immunopathological effects of new drugs. In: G.G. Gibson, R. Hubbard and D.V. Parke, (Eds) *Immunotoxicology*, pp 237–250. Academic Press, London.

WARD, J.M., WEISBURGER, J.H., YAMAMOTO, R.S., BENJAMIN, T., BROWN, C.A. and WEISBURGER, E.K. (1975): Long term effect of benzene in C57B1/6N mice. *Arch.Environ.Health*, 30, 22–25.

WARD, J.M., GOODMAN, D.G., SQUIRE, R.A., CHU, K.C. and LINHART, M.S. (1979): Neoplastic and non-neoplastic lesions in aging (C57BL/6N × C3H/HeN) F1 (B6C3 F1) mice. *J.N.C.I.*, 63, 849–854.

WARD, J.M. and REZNIK-SCHÜLLER, H. (1980): Morphological and histochemical characteristics of pigments in aging F344 rats. *Vet.Pathol.*, 17, 678–685.

WARD, J.M., HAMLIN II, M.H., ACKERMAN, L.J., LATTUADA, C.P., LONGFELLOW, D.G. and CAMERON, T.P. (1983): Age-related neoplastic and degenerative lesions in aging male virgin and ex-breeder AC1/seg Hap BR rats. *J.Gerontol.*, 38, 538–548.

WARD, J.M. and REYNOLDS, C.W. (1983): Large granular lymphocyte leukemia. A heterogeneous lymphocyte leukemia in F344 rats. *Am.J.Pathol.*, 111, 1–10.

WARNKE, R.A., SLAVIN, S., COFFMAN, R.L., BUTCHER, E.C., KNAPP, M.R., STROBER, S. and WEISSMAN, I.L. (1979): The pathology and homing of a transplantable murine B cell leukemia (BCl1). *J.Immunol.*, 123, 1181–1188.

WEINBERGER, M.A., ALBERT, R.H. and MONTGOMERY, S.B. (1985): Splenotoxicity associated with splenic sarcomas in rats fed high doses of D & C Red No.9 or aniline hydrochloride. *J.N.C.I.*, 75, 681–690.

WEISBROTH, S.H. (1979): Bacterial and mycotic diseases. In H.J.Baker, J.R.Lindsey and S.H. Weisbroth (Eds), *The Laboratory Rat*, Vol.1, Biology & Diseases, Chap.9, pp.193–241. Academic Press, New York.

WEISSMAN, I.L., WARNKE, R., BUTCHER, E.C., ROUSE, R. and LEVY, R. (1978): Lymphoid system: its normal architecture and potential for understanding through study of lymphoproliferative diseases. *Hum.Pathol.*, 9, 25–46.

WELLS, G.A.H. (1974): Hodgkin's disease-like lesions in the dog. *J.Pathol.* 112, 5–10.

WHITE, J., MIDER, G.B. and HESTON, W.E. (1944): Effects of amino acids on the induction of leukemia in mice. *J.N.C.I.*, 4, 409–411.

WILLIAMS, A.F., GALFRE, G. and MILSTEIN, C. (1977): Analysis of cell surfaces by xenogeneic myeloma-hybrid antibodies: Differentiation antigens of rat lymphocytes. *Cell*, 12, 663–673.

WINTROBE, M.M., LEE, G.R., BOGGS, D.R., BITHELL, T.C., FORESTER, J., ATHENS, J.W. and LUKENS, J.N. (1981)a: Lymphomas other than Hodgkin's disease. In: *Clinical Hematology*, 8th ed., Chap. 69, pp. 1681–1685. Lea and Febiger, Philadelphia.

WINTROBE, M.M., LEE, G.R., BOGGS, D.R., BITHELL, T.C., FORESTER, J., ATHENS, J.W. and LUKENS, J.N. (1981)b: Classification, pathogenesis and etiology of neoplastic diseases of the hematopoietic system. In: *Clinical Hematology*, 8th ed., Chap. 60, pp. 1449–1492, Lea & Febiger, Philadelphia.

WOGEN, G.N. (1984): Tumors of the mouse hematopoietic system : Their diagnosis and interpretation in safety evaluation tests. Report of a study group. *CRC.Crit.Rev.Toxicol.*, 13, 161–181.

WOLMAN, S.R., McMORROW, L.E. and COHEN, M.W. (1982): Animal model of human disease : Myelogenous leukemia in the R.F. mouse. *Am.J.Pathol.*, 107, 280–284.

WOLMAN, S.R., McMORROW, L.E., EDINGER, F.M. and COHEN, M.W. (1980): Histo-chemical identification of murine leukemia and lymphoma. *Proc.Am.Assoc.Cancer Res.*, 21, 45.

WOOLLETT, G.R., BARCLAY, A.N., PUKLAVEK, M. and WILLIAMS, A.F. (1985): Molecular and antigenic heterogeneity of the rat leukocyte common antigen from thymocytes and T and B lymphocytes. *Eur.J.Immunol.*, 15, 168–173.

WYKE, J.A. (1981): Oncogenic viruses. *J.Pathol.*, 135, 39–45.

WRIGHT, J.A. (1989): A comparison of rat femoral, sternebral and lumbar vetebral bone marrow fat content by subjective assessment and image analysis of histological sections. *J.Comp.Pathol.*, 100, 419–426.

WRIGHT, J.R., CALKINS, E. and HUMPHREY, R.L. (1977): Potassium permanganate reaction in amyloidosis. A histologic method to assist in differentiating forms of this disease. *Lab.Invest.*, 3 274–281.

YOUNG, S.S. and GRIES, C.L. (1984): Exploration of the negative correlation between proliferative hepatocellular lesions and lymphoma in rats and mice: establishment and implications. *Fundam.Appl.Toxicol.*, 4, 632–640.

ZBINDEN, G., ELSNER, J. and BOELSTERLI, U.A. (1984): Toxicological screening. *Regul.Toxicol.Pharmacol.*, 4, 275–286.

IV. Musculoskeletal System

BONE

Although the mechanical function of bone and cartilage is largely dependent on the physical nature of the extracellular matrix, the skeleton contains cell populations responsible for growth, repair and remodelling. These dynamic processes are modulated by a variety of factors including parathyroid hormone, vitamin D, calcium and phosphorus levels, gravity, work and load distribution and they may be affected adversely by administration of xenobiotics.

Long or tubular bones comprise a shaft or *diaphysis* composed mainly of *compact bone* which terminates at the metaphysis comprising a layer of a lighter framework of *cancellous bone*. Whereas compact bone possesses great tensile strength, cancellous or spongy bone provides mechanical strength without undue weight because its thickest trabeculae are arranged in directions subjected to the greatest mechanical forces. Cancellous bone possesses a high surface-volume ratio suitable for a high degree of metabolic activity and rapid turnover and it is also in close proximity to bone marrow cells. It therefore represents a site where pathological changes most frequently occur and where alterations in metabolic status are most easily vizualised.

Located between the metaphysis and the epiphysis lies the *growth plate*. The growth plate is composed of several different zones.

Immediately adjacent to the metaphysis is the *zone of provisional calcification*. Next to this is the *hypertrophic zone* which contains large chondrocytic cells. This gives way to the *proliferative zone* in which the only dividing cells of the growth plate are found. Adjacent to this is the *reserve zone* which typically contains more lipid and less acid and alkaline phosphatase, glucose-6-phosphate dehydrogenase, and lactic dehydrogenase activity than other zones (Revell, 1986).

As these growth centres in long bones are the zones from which metaphyseal and ultimately diaphyseal bone is formed, their histological examination can provide early evidence of the adverse effects of chemicals on bone.

The sternum, which is commonly examined histologically in rodent toxicity studies, develops from several ossification centres in a cartilagenous anlage. These sternal segments (sternebrae) do not usually fuse and remnants of the cartilageous anlage remain as synchrondroses. After sexual maturity, a bony subchrondral plate replaces the area of active enchondral ossification.

Collagen is the major organic component of bone which is laid down in parallel lamellae in mature compact and cancellous bone. These lamellae are observed in conventionally embedded sections in polarized light and can be used as a measure of the structural integrity of bone. When bone metabolism is accelerated as occurs in fracture repair or in the embryonic state, lamellar architecture is lost and becomes replaced by randomly arranged fibres, typical of so-called *woven bone*.

Mineral deposition is a complex process in which a carbonate-containing analogue of hydroxypatite [$Ca_{10}(PO_4)_6$ (OH_2)] is deposited in the collagen framework (Teitelbaum and Bullough, 1979). This process is believed to involve a combination of factors including changes in local ion concentration following enzymatic cleavage of organic phosphate esters, creation of nucleating sites and inactivation of naturally occuring inhibitors.

Ultrastructural study has consistently shown that extracellular matrix vesicles are present at the mineralisation front and that these represent the initial sites of mineral deposition. The vesicles probably derive from plasma membrane of adjacent cells and possess a complement of membrane alkaline phosphatase and other phosphatases capable of initiating mineralisation within the vesicle (Anderson, 1989). The rate of crystal deposition is promoted by the available calcium and phosphate ions and the presence of collagen. It is retarded by inhibitors such as proteoglycans and several non-collagenous, calcium binding proteins such as osteocalcin, phosphoproteins, osteonectin and α-2HS-glycoproteins (Anderson, 1989).

Initially, mineral is deposited in a relatively poorly crystalline form at the interface of previously mineralized tissue (osteoid) but more mature crystals of hydroxyapatite form subsequently. Tetracyclines and other autofluoerscent antibiotics bind stoichiometrically to the divalent cations of immature mineral, a characteristic which can be used to label the osteoid-mineralized bone interface (see below).

Osteoblasts are cuboidal or columnar cells lining osteoid seams, rich in rough endoplasmic reticulum, containing prominant Golgi and abundant alkaline phosphatase activity which are responsible for the synthesis of bone matrix. The osteoblast is believed to be derived from a primitive mesenchymal cell, closely related to other proliferating and differentiating mesenchymal cells of marrow stroma (Vaughan, 1981).

So called 'resting osteoblasts' which appear quiscent, flattened cells, are not inactive for they are capable of bone synthesis, although at a slower rate than active osteoblasts. They probably form part of the barrier separating the bone fluid compartment from the general extracellular space (Teitelbaum and Bullough 1979). Osteocytes represent a form of osteoblasts located within bone matrix which are some of the most numerous cells in bone, although their precise function is not well understood.

Osteoclasts are large multinucleated cells responsible for bone resorption of bone and calcified cartilage. They contain abundant lysosomal enzyme activity, notably acid phosphatases and collagenases. Active osteoclasts show a prominant ruffled border, a highly convoluted cell membrane which is visible at ultrastructural level or following light microscopy of high quality plastic or resin-embedded sections. Osteoclasts are believed to be derived from the same progenitors as circulating blood cells, namely pluripotent haemopoietic stem cells which first appear on the primitive yolk sac (Vaughan, 1981; Schneider et al., 1986).

Technical considerations

Appropriate laboratory processing of bone tissue is an important aspect of its good histological assessment in toxicity studies. Routine formalin fixation is usually adequate for most purposes. However, vital tetracycline labelling may be better preserved in 70% ethanol or methanol (Revell, 1986). Ice-cold buffered formalin is sometimes used for the preservation of acid phosphatase activity for histochemical demonstration of osteoclasts (Chappard et al., 1983). Undecalcified sections, usually employing methylcrylate embedding media, are necessary for adequate assessment of mineralised bone, using von Kossa, Goldner trichrome or solochrome cyanine staining to give good definition of mineralised tissue.

Wheras a descriptive approach to the study of bone is important, morphometric techniques have a key role in the assessment of metabolic bone alterations. Their application is a matter of careful judgement because they are not only time consuming, but require rigorous experimental design, careful sampling and measuring techniques. The remodeling rate and apposition rate may vary between different bones of the same animal, they can be different between males and females an they may change with age or duing periods of altered nutrition (Anderson and Danylchuk, 1978; Warren and Bedi 1985; Sontag, 1986). Undernutrition causes significant deficits on skeletal dimensions in rats which persist even following nutritional rehabilitation (Warren and Bedi, 1985).

Sampling is particularly important in morphometric analysis. Anderson and Danychuk (1978) showed that even in standardised, colony-raised normal beagle dogs, different ribs or different parts of the same rib showed statistically significant differences in ratios of cortical to total bone area, number of osteoid seams, number of resorption spaces, and bone formation rate.

A further difficulty relates to the confusion of terminology applied in bone histomorphometry although recent attempts have been made to overcome these semantic barriers (Parfitt et al., 1987).

Tetracyclines are the generally accepted fluorescent markers for the vital staining of sites of bone mineralisation although alizarin red S, calcein, procion and haematoporphyrin have also been used in experimental animals (Solheim, 1974).

In the following section bone lesions are divided into several histological categories, although it must be kept in mind that the divisions between the categories are not sharp and mixed histological features may be seen.

Osteonecrosis

Bone necrosis is a complication of damage to bone occurring as a result of infection (osteomyelitis), invasion by malignant cells, infiltration by other abnormal substances or infarction following disruption of bone vasculature. A primary vascular effect may be difficult to characterise in view of the inaccessability of the bone vasculature to dissection. In man, osteonecrosis is a well-recognised complication of corticosteroid therapy (Teitelbaum and Bullough, 1979).

Various forms of aseptic necrosis occur spontaneously in laboratory animals, including dogs and rodents although their pathogenesis remains poorly understood (Sokoloff and Habermann, 1958; Doige et al., 1986; Yamasaki and Itakura, 1988b). Necrosis may be localized or extensive, either within in the subarticular region or in the bone shaft. It may be associated with proliferation of surrounding connective tissue cells. The extent and distribution of bone necrosis in the tibia of aging ICR mice suggested that it was due to a disturbance of blood supply (Yamasaki and Itakura, 1988b). It has been associated with malignant bone tumours in the dog also probably a consequence of infarction (Dubielzig et al., 1981).

Osteoporosis

Osteoporosis is defined histologically as an abnormal decrease in the mass of mineralised bone. For a definitive histological diagnosis undecalcified sections are used to distinguish osteoporosis from conditions in which increased osteoid accompanies diminished skeletal mass (Teilelbaum and Bullough, 1979).

An unusual form of osteoporosis is induced in rats by administration of high doses of retinoic acid, a metabolite of vitamin A used in the therapy of severe skin diseases. The development of bone changes is dependent on the dose and duration of treatment but lesions are characterised by an unusual dissolution of bone substance in the shaft of long bones in the zone adjacent to the marrow cavity giving rise to a 'thread bare' appearance of the bone matrix. Woven bone, similar to that found in fracture callus, develops in subperiosteal zones (Dhem and Goret-Nicaise, 1984). Fractures occur at very high doses. The bone findings reported in rats appear similar to those observed in man and other species with vitamin A intoxication.

Osteoporosis is also a well-known consequence of glucocorticoid excess, either in association with Cushing's syndrome or following long-term glucocorticoid therapy notably in rheumatoid arthritis. However, our understanding of the mechanisms involved in glucocorticoid-induced osteoporosis is far from complete. Currently, it is believed that bone loss occurs as a result of a combination of factors including impairment of intestinal absorption and increased urinary excretion of calcium, secondary hyperparathyroidism and anti-anabolic or catabolic effects of glucocorticoids (Gennari, 1985).

Hyperosteoidosis

Hyperosteoidosis can be divided into two principle pathophysiological groups. In man, it is most commonly a result of *osteomalacia*, the consequence of an absolute deficiency in the rate of mineralisation, typically due to poor intake of vitamin D or abnormalities in vitamin D metabolism. Less commonly, hyperosteoidosis follows an increase in the rate of osteoid deposition in the face of a normal rate of mineralisation. These two types of hyperosteoidosis are morphologically similar in tissue sections but can be distinguished by the use of time-spaced, vital tetracycline staining (Teitelbaum and Bullough, 1979).

Osteomalacia also occurs in laboratory animals as a result of dietary deficiencies notably lack of vitamin D, calcium or phosphorus. It also occurs in the complex syndrome of renal osteodystrophy associated with chronic renal failure (Weisbrode, 1981). Osteomalacia can also be the direct result of exposure to xenobiotics. An important example of this in medical practice is the osteomalacia associated with exposure of patients on haemodialysis or in the uraemic state to excessive levels of aluminium. Risk factors here include contamination of the dialysate with aluminium, excessive or prolonged oral intake of aluminium salts, parathyroidectomy and diabetes mellitus (Andress et al., 1987). It is believed that parathyroidectomy and diabetes mellitus enhance aluminium-induced bone disease as a result of the low rate of bone formation which occurs in these conditions, with consequent increased accumulation of aluminium. Infants receiving prolonged intravenous therapy are also at risk of aluminium overloading from intravenous solutions contaminated with aluminium (Sedman et al., 1985). Similar changes have been induced in normal or uraemic rats administered excessive aluminium salts (Ellis et al., 1979; Robertson et al., 1983).

Aluminium-related bone disease is defined histologically by the presence of hyperosteoidosis together with deposition of aluminium at the osteoid-mineralised bone interface (Connor et al., 1986). In rats given high doses of aluminium salts, only minimal increase in the epiphyseal cartilage growth plate occurs but the cartilage septa are covered by excess thick woven osteoid. In addition, patchy excess of lamellar osteoid develops on diaphyseal and epiphyseal bone trabeculae (Ellis et al., 1979). In rats, it has been shown that chronic renal failure also increases the severity of the osteomalacia (Robertson et al., 1983). The presence of aluminium at the interface of osteoid and bone can be demonstrated in formalin-fixed, undecalcified sections by the use of triammonium aurine tricarboxylate staining (Maloney et al., 1982).

Mineral metabolism can be disturbed in epileptic patients treated for long periods by anticonvulsant medication. Affected patients show biochemical and bone biopsy alterations characteristic of osteomalacia and it has been suggested that this may occur as a result of altered vitamin D metabolism following

147

drug-induced hepatic enzyme induction (Dent et al., 1970, Richens and Rowe, 1970).

In vitro experiments have suggested that phenytoin inhibits parathyroid-induced calcium release from bone (Harris et al., 1974). In vivo studies in the rat have indicated that phenytoin can reduce bone growth in a manner characteristic of pseudohypoparathyroidism (Robinson et al., 1982).

The bone-resorption inhibiting properties of the bisphosphonates, compounds with the P-C-P chemical bond, form the basis for their clinical utility in the treatment of disorders characterised by increased bone degradation such as hypercalcaemia of malignancy and Paget's disease of bone. However, some of these compounds show little separation between doses which inhibit bone resorption from those which suppress bone growth and mineralisation, although this varies not only with dose but also duration of treatment, route of administration, age and species. Studies in rats have shown that these compounds may produce dose-related decreases in intestinal calcium absorption and longitudinal bone growth as well as increases in total plasma calcium concentration (Miller et al., 1985). Histologically, bones from animals treated with high doses of these agents show an accumulation of bone osteoid seams, (Flora et al., 1980; Fleisch 1987). Fractures are reported in dogs treated with biphosphonates. It has been suggested that such fractures can occur without impaired mineralisation. High doses of biphosphonates may only slow bone remodelling in the dog and limiting repair of microscopic cracks which normally develop in bone under everyday stresses (Flora et al., 1980).

A recent example is the biphosphonate, disodium pamidronate, which was shown to increase in the length of the primary spongiosa in the ribs, sternum and thoracic vertebrae at all doses when administered to dogs in conventional six or 12 month toxicity studies (Mertz et al., 1989). At the higher doses these were also thickened bony trabeculae and widened osteoid seams. Similar findings were reported in rats (Schenk et al., 1986).

However, toxicity of different agents of this class has been shown to vary considerably so that bone alternations in animals should be carefully analyzed before administering novel biophosphonates to man (Fleisch, 1989).

Osteosclerosis

Osteosclerosis is characterised by an increase in the volume of mineralised bone per unit volume in the marrow space. In man, osteosclerosis is a common form of uraemic osteodystrophy where it may be acccompanied by other bone changes including osteitis fibrosa. Various forms of osteosclerosis occur spontaneously in laboratory animals and can be induced by high doses of therapeutic agents, notably oestrogens and prostaglandins.

Osteosclerosis and myelofibrosis were reported in untreated F344/Du Crj rats by Yamasaki and Itakura (1988a). This condition developed in the tibia and sternum in both sexes at about the age of six months and subsequently increased in prevalence and severity with advancing age. Histologically, the changes

148

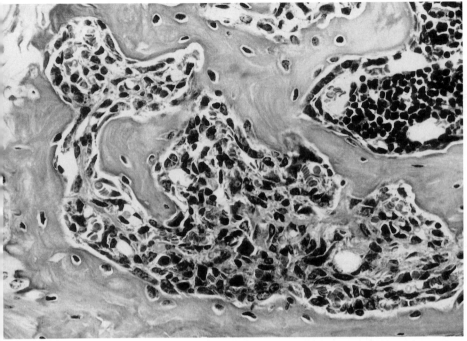

Fig. 27. Section from the sternum of an untreated, 78-week-old female B6C3F1 mouse showing fibro-osseous changes characterised by replacement of the bone marrow space by fibroblast-like cells and irregular bony trabeculae (HE, ×550.)

developed initially as a focal proliferation of fibrous tissue on the marrow surface of cortical bone and trabeculae. Subsequent thickening of bone trabeculae led to almost complete replacement of the marrow cavity by lamellar bone. Apart from the obvious age-relationship, the pathogenesis of the condition is unknown.

Similar alterations have been described in F344 rats affected with mono-nuclear cell leukaemia (Stromberg and Vogtsberger, 1983). Female rats were shown to be more commonly affected than males. The bones were characterised by myeloid hyperplasia, myelofibrosis and osteosclerosis. The osteosclerosis consisted of proliferation of trabecular bone at the inner cortex which extended to involve the entire marrow cavity. Similar changes have been reported in Sprague-Dawley rats affected with renal osteodystrophy (Itakura et al., 1977).

Analogous histological changes develop spontaneously in aging B6C3F1 mice, particularly females. The changes have been termed fibro-osseous lesions by Sass and Montali (1980). This condition is seen in the sternum as well as long bones and is characterised histologically by focal replacement of the bone marrow space at one or both ends by a dense infiltration of fibroblast-like cells, fibrous tissue, giant cells and eventually a network of bony trabeculae (Fig. 27). In addition, focal zones of thickening of the bone on the endosteal surface in the shaft of long bones also occurs (Fig. 28).

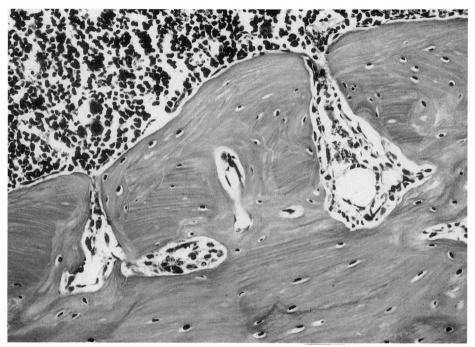

Fig. 28. Cortical bone from the femur of an untreated female, 78-week-old B6C3F1 mouse showing considerable thickening on the endosteal surface of the shaft by mature bone exibiting irregular cement lines. (HE, ×350.)

The cause of this condition in mice is uncertain. In view of its greater prevalence among female mice, particularly those showing evidence of sex hormone imbalance, Sass and Montali (1980) suggested that oestrogens may be involved in its development.

Analogous osteosclerotic changes can be induced by the administration of oestrogens (Figs. 29 and 30). When C57Bl/6J mice were treated with 0.1 mg of 17β-oestradiol cyclopentylproprionate, osteosclerosis of the tibial metaphyseal zone developed. This was characterised histologically by an increase in the thickness, length and number of the trabeculae to form a dense bony network in the metaphysis (Gaunt and Pierce, 1985). As these changes were associated with a depression in myelopoiesis, thymic atrophy and lymphopenia, it was suggested that the development of metaphyseal osteosclerosis may be linked to haematopoietic and lymphoid deficiencies (Gaunt and Pierce, 1985). Similar, oestrogen-inducing osteosclerosis has been reported in the metaphysis or in the medullary cavity of bones in mice other strains of (Urist et al., 1950; Highman et al., 1977). Proliferation of bony trabeculae was reported in the sternal and femoral medulla in both C3H/HeJ and C3HeJ and C3HeB/FeJ female mice treated with either dielthylstilboestrol or 17β-oestradiol for periods of over one year (Highman et al., 1977, 1981).

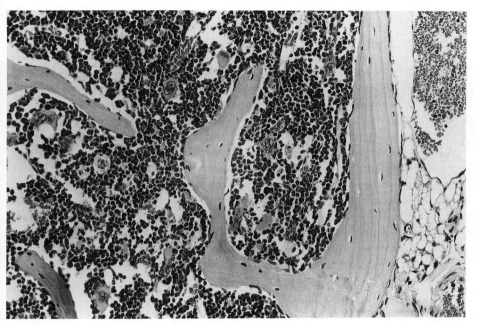

Fig. 29. Long bone from a 12-month-old B6C3F1 mouse showing the normal pattern of bone and bone marrow. For comparison with Figure 30. (HE, ×350.)

Analogous changes have been reported in Alderley Park strain mice treated with high doses of the antioestrogen, tamoxifen, for long periods (Tucker et al., 1984). After six months of treatment, mice showed kyphosis associated with marked increase in bone density accompanied by histological evidence of osteosclerosis. It was postulated that these bone changes were the result of an oestrogenic effect of tamoxifen in mice, in contrast to its antioestrogenic effects in primates where bone changes were not observed (Tucker et al., 1984).

An almost identical form of osteosclerosis (hyperostosis) has been reported in CD-1 mice treated orally with high doses of the synthetic prostaglandin E_1 analogue, misprostol, for 21 months (Dodd and Port, 1987). This change occurred in a dose-related manner mainly in females and was also characterised by a centripetal growth of fibroblastic tissue and lamellar bone starting at the epiphyseal growth plate in the femur and sternum, although not entirely obliterating the marrow space. The mechanism for this change remains unclear but as it occurred neither in dogs or rats, it was postulated to be a mouse-specific effect.

However, hyperostosis is described in dogs and rats treated experimentally with other prostaglandins (High, 1982; Jee et al., 1985). Histomorphometric analysis of the undecalcified tibia from young rats treated prostaglandin E_2 for 21 days showed depressed longitudinal bone growth, increased cartilage thickness in association with a striking increase in both endosteal bone apposition and

151

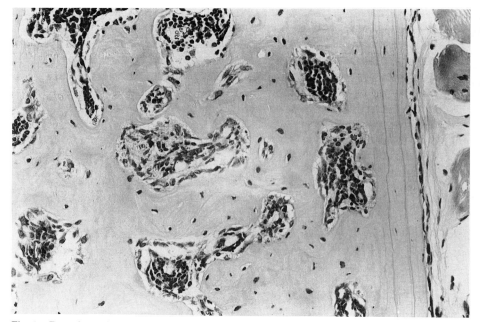

Fig. 30. Bone from the same site from that seen in Figure 29 but from a mouse treated for a long period with an oestrogenic agent. There is marked thickening of the bony trabeculae, typical of osteosclerosis. (HE, ×350.)

formation rates, giving rise to the growth of trabecular bone in the marrow cavity of the tibia shaft (Jee et al., 1985).

Little data exists about the effects of prostaglandins on human bone although long-term administration of low doses of prostaglandin E_1 to infants with cyanotic congenital heart disease has been reported to produce radiological evidence of periosteal thickening of long bones (Ueda et al., 1980)

Focal proliferative endosteal lesions were reported in the metaphysis and diaphysis of Wistar rats treated with anticancer drugs of several different classes (Morse et al., 1990). It was postulated that local bone marrow injury led to release of inflammatory mediators or growth factors which provoked the proliferative bone lesions.

Administration of calcitonin to rats and rabbits for periods of up to 25 days has also been shown to increase cortical bone thickness compared with untreated control animals (Wase et al., 1967).

Osteopetrosis

This condition is characterised by the replacement of the normal cortical and medullary bone by atypical trabeculae composed of calcified cartilage surrounded by poorly mineralized osseous matrix, which is believed to result from abnormal bone resorption. In man, it is an inherited condition. It has also been reported in mutant strains of rats, mice and dogs (Riser and Frankhauser, 1970; Walker 1973, 1975; Lees and Sautter, 1979; Minkin, 1981; Graf, 1985). The elegant studies of Walker (1973, 1975) showed that normal bone resorption could be restored in osteopetrotic mice by transfer of haemopoietic cells from phenotypically normal littermates. Conversely abnormal bone developed in normal littermates transplated with haemorpoietic cells from osteopetrotic mice. In addition, osteopetrotic mice are characterised by defective macrophage chemotaxis (Minkin, 1981).

Although the mechanisms responsible for the development of osteopetrosis are not entirely elucidated, they are clearly closely related to defective function of haemopoietic cells, macrophages and osteoclasts. However, a recent review could find no report of drug-induced osteopetrosis (Gopinath et al., 1987)

Osteitis fibrosa, fibrous osteodystrophy

Osteitis fibrosa is characterised by activation of large numbers of bone cells and rapid skeletal turnover which occurs in response to a number of different stimuli such as those which occur in hyperparathyroidism, hyperthyroidism, Paget's disease of bone and renal failure (Teitelbaum and Bullough, 1979). Histologically, this condition is characterised by an increase in the numbers of both osteoblasts and osteoclasts, the presence of irregular trabecular surfaces with increased surface to volume ratio. In addition hyperosteoidism may be evident either following increased collagen synthesis or osteomalacia.

Renal osteodystrophy

This diagnostic term is used to embrace a range of alterations in bone which accompany chronic renal failure. It occurs in both man and laboratory animals and there may be a wide range of histological changes including osteitis fibrosa, hyperosteoidosis, osteosclerosis and osteoporotic-like changes. It has been well-described in aged rats suffering from advanced glomerulosclerosis (Itakura et al., 1977).

Neoplasia

Primary bone neoplasms are uncommon in both man and laboratory animals. One of the most common bone neoplasms, osteosarcoma, or osteogenic sarcoma is however an important human neoplasm in view of its tendency to occur in younger age groups. In addition, increasing numbers of osteogenic sarcomas develop in extraosseous or in osseous locations as a direct consequence of therapeutic or incidental ionising radiation, as increasing numbers of cancer patients survive beyond the five or ten year period (Huvos et al., 1985). A recent study of childhood cancer patients has shown that in addition to ionising radiation, cancer chemotherapy with alkylating agents also increases the subsequent risk of developing bone cancer (Tucker et al., 1987).

Small numbers of bone neoplasms develop spontaneously in laboratory animals. Osteosarcoma appears to be the most commonly reported histological type of bone tumour although benign osteomas and chondroid neoplasms occasionally occur. Osteosarcomas have been described in aging rats of several different strains (MacKenzie and Garner, 1973; Goodman et al., 1980; Tucker 1986; Ruben et al., 1986) mice (Percy and Jonas 1971; Charles and Turusov, 1974) hamsters (Van Hoosier and Trentin, 1979), aging dogs (Misdorp, 1980) and occasionally in non-human primates (Pelfrène, 1985).

In view of the relatively rare spontaneous occurrence of bone tumours in laboratory animals, a number of different inducing agents have been employed in the search for a suitable animal model for bone sarcomas. Examples include the use of ionising radiation in a variety of animal species (Gossner, 1986) incluing the rat (Cobb, 1970) and intra-tibial inoculation of rats with the Moloney sarcoma virus (Olson and Capen, 1977). A wide range of chemicals have been reported to induce osteosarcomas as well as other histological types of sarcoma when administered locally into the bone of rats or mice. Chemicals include polycyclic hydrocarbons, N-hydroxy-2-acetylaminofluorene, vinyl chloride, nitrosamines, nitrosoureas and 4-nitroquinoline-1-oxide (Pelfrène, 1985). Occasionally, inert subcutaneous implants induce osteosarcoma as well as the more usual range of soft tissue sarcomas (Carter, 1973).

More directly related to therapeutic agents is the association of the development of osteogenic sarcoma with oestrogen-induced proliferative bone lesions in mice.

Classification

The classification of bone tumours, like those of other mesenchymal neoplasms is based on concepts of histogenesis (Fornasier, 1984). Neoplasms showing bone or osteoid differentiation patterns are conventionally regarded as osteomas or osteosarcomas whereas chondroid differentiation indicates one of the various forms of chondroma or chrondrosarcoma. Nevertheless, as in the case of other mesenchymal neoplasms, a particular differentiation pattern does not necessarily indicate that the neoplasm developed from the same type of mature tissue. It is far more likely that a differentiation pattern expressed by a bone neoplasm reflects a combination of cellular and local tissue factors which initiate and modulate the expression of primitive pluripotential mesenchymal stem cells (Fornasier, 1984). Only in this way can the observed mixed differentiation patterns and close morphological relationships between osteosarcoma and other mesenchymal neoplasms be adequately explained (Reddick et al., 1980; Brookes 1986). The close relationship between bone and other mesenchymal sarcomas is evident in experimental pathology. Both osteosarcomas and soft tissue tumour types may develop under similar conditions in mesenchymal cell tumour models. Studies of osteosarcomas in mice have demonstrated that when they invade a new tissue such as muscle there may be a change from osteoblastic to other cellular type (Highman et al., 1981).

Histological appearances

Most bone tumours reported in laboratory animals are *osteosarcomas* which are conventionally defined by the presence of tumour osteoid in tissue sections. As in man, they may arise in long bones, vertebrae or flat bones and they possess a highly variable range of histological appearances. In addition to the presence of neoplastic osteoid, stromal cells show considerable variation in shape and size ranging from cytologically malignant small spindle cells arranged in bundles as in fibrosarcomas, to highly pleomorphic and hyperchromatic cells with irregularly scattered multinucleated giant cells resembling osteoclasts. Chondroblast or vascular differentiation patterns have been described (Dahlin and Unni, 1977; Frith et al., 1982; Gössner, 1986; Ruben et al., 1986, Tucker, 1986). In man, about half of reported osteosarcomas produce large amounts of tumour osteoid and are frequently termed *osteoblastic osteosarcomas*. Smaller numbers of reported osteosarcomas show predominantly chondroid or spindle cell differentiation patterns (Dahlin and Unni, 1977). These subgroups occur in laboratory animals although their prevalence, biological behaviour and radiological appearances have been less well characterised. Some of these light microscopic appearances are common to these found in fibrosarcomas and malignant fibrous histocytomas and this may pose difficulties in their differential diagnosis.

Ultrastructural study of osteosarcomas in man has shown that most contain different cell types in addition to the osteoblast, (Reddick et al., 1980). The cell types described include variable proportions of chondroblasts, osteocytes, undifferentiated cells and myofibroblasts, analogous to the mixed cell populations found in soft tissue tumours at ultrastructural level. Enzyme cytochemical study of human bone neoplasms has suggested that tumour cells in osteosarcoma can also be characterised by their alkaline phosphatase activity for it has been shown that other neoplasms such as chondrosarcoma and fibrosarcoma are usually devoid of this enzymatic activity (Sanerkin, 1980).

Osteosarcomas typically infiltrate local tissues and eventually produce metastatic deposits, most commonly in the lungs, liver, kidney and lymph nodes.

Benign bone forming tumours or *osteomas* are also reported in both rats (Mackenzie and Garner, 1972) and mice (Charles and Turusov, 1974). They occur quite commonly in aged CF1 mice with a greater prevalence in females. The skull is involved in most cases in this strain but the osteomas are frequently multiple affecting limbs, vertebral bodies and pelvis. They are variable in size and are histologically characterised by trabeculae of dense compact bone with irregular lamellae with intratrabecular spaces containing bone marrow cells, blood vessels or connective tissue (Charles and Turusov, 1974).

Osteosarcomas: mice

In mice, osteosarcomas are uncommon but they occur predominantly in females and their development can be potentialed by exogenous oestrogen administration. Long term dietary administration of diethylstiboestrol or 17β-oestradiol to

C3H mice not only produced osteosclerosis (see above) but was also associated with the development of increased numbers of osteosarcomas (Highman et al., 1981). These osteosarcomas developed in mice fed oestrogenic diets for over one year were clearly shown to develop in areas of osteofibrosis at the ends of the intersternebral and costosternebral subchondral bony plates. This is analogous to the common involvement of the metaphysis of long bones in human osteosarcomas where active bone growth and cellular activity is most marked. It was postulated therefore that oestrogens may not have a primary role in the development of osteosarcoma in mice but only indirectly by increasing bone trabecular proliferation and osteofibrosis predisposing mice to osteosarcoma development (Highman et al., 1981).

JOINTS

Joints can either be formed of fibrocartilagenous tissue as represented by vertebral bodies or bone ends may be covered by a layer of hyaline cartilage and surrounded by a synovial capsule, as in diarthrodial joints.

The composition of hyaline cartilage matrix by weight is over 70% water with 10 to 15% of collagen and 10 to 15% of proteoglycans (Hamerman, 1989). Proteoglycans in cartilage are complex glycoconjugates formed from a protein core, molecular weight 180,000 to 370,000, to which glycosaminoglycan chains and N-linked and O-linked oligosaccharides are covalently attached (Hassell et al., 1986). Their synthesis takes place mainly in the endoplasmic reticulum of chondrocytes although most of the glycosylation is undertaken in the Golgi apparatus. Proteoglycans are then packaged into vesicles and secreted into the matrix. Proteoglycans found in cartilage consist of a core protein attached to glycosaminoglycan chains, keratan sulphate and chrondroitin sulphate although chondrocytes also elaborate a small glycoprotein called link protein and dermatan sulphate. Different types of proteoglycans are not uniformly distributed in cartilage matrix. For instance, small amounts of dermatan sulphate are found on the articular surface, whereas keratan sulphate-containing cartilage is situated in deeper zones (Hamerman, 1989).

Collagens in articular cartilage are predominantly type II, which contains three $\alpha 1$ chains in contrast to type I collagen with two $\alpha 1$ and one $\alpha 2$ chains (Mankin, 1974). It is the integrity of the glycoproteins in the collagen matrix which is the basis for the normal mechanical properties of articular cartilage.

Articular cartilage is generally divided anatomically into a superficial or *tangential zone* beneath which lies the *transitional zone*. The *radial zone* situated below the transitional zone is in continuity with the *epiphyseal cartilage*. In the superficial or tangential zone, collagen fibres possess a finer diameter and tighter weave than in the other layers and these fibres are firmly attached to the martins of the articular surface. This dense layer of collagen is believed to act as a barrier preventing leakage of proteoglycans and the entry of potentially harmful substances such as proteolytic enzymes (Teitelbaum and Bullough, 1979).

Chondrocytes represent the mature cells of cartilage. They possess abundant endoplasmic reticulum, a highly developed Golgi apparatus although only few mitochondria. They are capable of collagen matrix synthesis in a low oxygen environment. Differences exist in the metabolic and ultrastructural profiles of chondrocytes fromregions of the articular (and epiphyseal) cartilage complex. Enzyme cytochemical analysis of the chondrocytes from the femoral head of New Zealand rabbits has shown that the activity of the glycolytic enzyme, lactate dehydrogenase, was strong in all zones, compatable with the concept that articular cartillage can function predominantly anaerobically (Sampson and Cannon, 1986). By contrast, the activity of Krebs cycle enzymes (succinate and isocitrate dehydrogenase), cytochrome oxidase and enzymes of the hexomonophosphate shunt (glucose-6-phosphate dehydrogenase, diphosphopyridine and triphosphopyridine diaphorase) increased progressively in activity from the superficial tangential zone though to the epiphyseal cartilage (Sampson and Cannon, 1986). These data correspond to quantitative electron microscopic evidence of a progressive increase in the cell content of endoplasmic reticulum, Golgi apparatus, mitochondria and electron dense bodies (lyososomes) from the tangential zone through to the top half of the calcified zone (Brighton et al., 1984).

It has been suggested that low oxygen environments are conducive to cartilage differentiation and that high oxygen environments stimulates bone formation (Sampson and Cannon, 1986). It is important to note that the integrity and composition of cartilage is partly dependent on load bearing, because changes in load bearing may affect the thickness of articular cartilage as well as its glycosaminoglycan content. Immobilization of knee joints of young beagle dogs for 11 weeks was shown to produce nearly 50% reduction in glycosaminoglycan content in articular cartilage as assessed microspectrophotometrically using safranin O staining (Kiviranta et al., 1987). The actual thickness of the uncalcified cartilage did not diminish in immobilised joints in this particular study, although the contalateral joints which were under increased load, showed both an increase in glycosaminoglycan content and augmented cartillage thickness.

The joint space is surrounded by a strong fibrous capsule lined by synovial cells. Synovial cells are frequently considered to comprise two layers, the *synovial intima* and the *subintima* or subsynovial layer which merges with the connective tissue of the joint capsule. The subintima contains the vasculature, lymphatics and nerve fibres of the synovial lining. Cells lining the synovium form a discontinuous layer, one to three layers thick and comprise two principle morphological types, referred to as type A and type B cells.

Type A cells possess a prominant Golgi, numerous cytoplasmic vacuoles, small vesicles but little rough endoplasmic reticulum. They also show cytoplasmic processes or filopodia. Type B cells possess fewer vacuoles and vesicles but rough endoplasmic reticulum is more prominent. Type A and B cells have a close histogenetic relationship for they are both believed to arise from mesenchymal of the primordial skeletal blastema (Henderson and Pettipher 1985). Studies by Edwards and coworkers (Edwards, 1982; Edwards and Willoughby, 1982; Edwards et al., 1982) using radiation chimeras of normal and beige mice have suggested that type A synovial cells may be derived from bone marrow precursors and possess certain characteristics of macrophages where as type B cells may be of local mesenchymal cell origin (reviewed by Henderson and Pettipher, 1985).

It is generally agreed that synovial cells have two principle functions. One role is the removal of debris and other substances from the joint space by phagocytosis or pinocytosis. Data from experiments in which foreign substances have been injected into the joint suggests that the type A synovial cell is more active in ingestion of these materials than the type B cells. A second function is believed to be the synthesis of glycosaminoglycans although the degree to which this contributes to synovial fluid has not been well studied (Henderson and Pettipher, 1985).

Technical considerations

A number of histological and histochemical staining techniques can be used for the characterisation of cartilage glycosaminoglycans in tissue sections, notably metachromatic staining with toluidine blue or safranine O. Safranine O staining is widely used in experimental pathology for quantitative or semiquantitative assessment of glycosaminoglycans in cartilage. This cationic dye is bound stoichiometrically to glycosaminoglycan polyanions (Kiviranta et al., 1987).

Lectins, by virtue of their glycoconjugate-binding properties also represent useful reagents for histochemical characterisation of cartilage, particularly as lectin-binding affinity of extracellular glycoconjugates may relate to different functions within growth plate cartilage (Farnum and Wilsman, 1988).

Cartilage: spontaneous degeneration

A number of degenerative conditions are reported in the joints and articular cartilage of laboratory rodents, although their pathogenesis and prevalence is uncertain. Whereas there are species and strain differences, sampling procedures and orientation of tissue sections from joints among different laboratories greatly influence the reporting rates of joint lesions. Little work has been conducted in aging laboratory animals using carefully prepared resin-embedded, undecalcified sections.

In rats, focal degeneration of the deep zones of articular cartilage are quite commonly observed in some laboratories. These changes may involve the sternum as well as other joints. Histologically they are characterised by foci of degeneration, chondromucoid change or focal necrosis accompanied by a tissue reaction composed of fibroblasts, osteoblasts, ostoclasts and osteoid formation (Yamasaki and Inui, 1985, Jasty et al., 1986; Kato and Onodera, 1986, Tucker, 1986). Their aetiology is uncertain but foci may be seen in quite young rats.

Age-related degenerative joint changes have also been described in laboratory mice, although there is considerable interstrain variation in prevalence and degree of these changes. There appears to be some mild loss of articular cartilage and its proteoglycan content quite commonly in aging mice (Walton, 1977).

Cartilage: drug-induced degeneration

Although the transfer of systemically administered xenobiotics across the double diffusion system of the synovium is slow and cartilage itself is relatively resistant to agents which alter glucose utilisation or oxidative phosphorylation (Mankin, 1974), some systemically administered drugs are capable of damaging cartilage. However, once abnormal materials have gained access to articular cartilage, damage appears to develop with relative ease. In view of the relatively limited nature of the response of cartilage to injury, drug-induced damage is usually manifest histologically by degenerative alterations in cartilage rather than an inflammatory process.

The most striking example of degeneration of cartilage induced by systemic drug administration is provided by quinolone carboxylic acid compounds and analogues such as cinoxacin, nalidixic, pipemidic and oxolinic acids, norfloxacin and ciprofloxacin. These agents produce injury to articular cartilage in young animals and possibly also young human patients (Gough et al., 1979; Alfaham et al., 1987; Corrado et al., 1987).

The pathology of quinolone-induced articular changes has been well-documented in juvenile beagle dogs as these animals appear particularly susceptible. Treatment is rapidly followed by lameness which is associated with articular pathology in a number of joints (Gough et al., 1979).

Macroscopic examination of affected joints shows varying degrees of vesiculation, bullae development and detachment of a superficial layer from the surface of the articular cartilage. In severe cases, synovial fluid is tinged with blood and the synovial membrane appears yellowish and shows petechae. Histologically, the articular cartilage develops focal loss of matrix with varying degrees of cavitation (Figs. 31 and 32). Large cavities may be surrounded by fibrillar or laminated cartilage with clustering of chondrocytes. There may be erosion of cartilage down to the bone plate and in severe cases, bone spicules, tissue debris and inflammation may be seen. Reactive synovial alterations such as villous proliferation, fibrinoid or proteinaceous exudate, fibrinoid necrosis of small arteries, extravasation of fluid into the submembranous tissue may be seen (Gough et al., 1979).

An ultrastructural study of articular cartilage in young dogs treated with oxolinic acid showed loss of proteoglycan particles, reduced numbers and altered configuration of collagen fibrils in association with frank chondrocyte necrosis (Gough et al., 1985).

The pathogenesis of this change in juvenile dogs is obscuré, although it presumably represents a toxic action of these compounds on cartilage or on the metabolism of the chondrocyte of young animals.

159

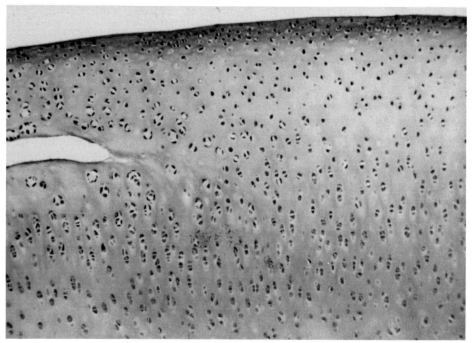

Fig. 31. Articular surface from the femur of a beagle dog treated with oxalinic acid showing the typical cavitation and the associated clustering of chondrocytes in the adjacent intact cartilage, as reported by Gough et al., 1979. (HE, ×140.)

The use of these agents as antibacterials is usually restricted to adult patients. Although humans may be less susceptible these effects on cartilage, young people treated with quinolone antibacterials have developed reversible articular symptoms (Alfaham et al., 1987).

Direct injections of chemical substances into the joint cavity can also produce degeneration of articular cartilage although this is often more closely associated with active inflammation and synovitis (See arthritis below). Some chemicals induce cartilage degeneration with little or no overt arthritis. For instance, injection of sodium iodoacetate into the knee joints of albino guinea pigs has been shown to produce cartilage degeneration characterised histologically by fibrillation and fissuring of the articular surface, loss of pericellular and interterritorial matrix glycoprotein, loss of chondrocytes and development of osteophytes (Williams and Brandt, 1985). Osteophytes were characterised by exophytic bone growth at the joint margins covered by a layer of hyaline cartilage.

Injection of anticancer cytotoxic drugs into the joints of laboratory animals has also been shown to produce degeneration of cartilage. Injection of nitrogen mustard into the knee joint of adult rabbits for periods of up to 12 weeks produced histological evidence of marked destruction of the articular cartilage

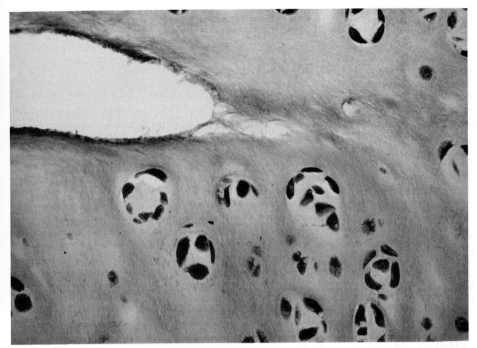

Fig. 32. Higher power view of the same section seen in Figure 29 showing the chondrocyte clustering in more detail. (HE, ×550.)

together with epiphyseal plates and underlying bone with inflammatory changes and fibrosis in the synovium (Steinberg et al., 1967). By contrast, a similar regimen of methotrexate or thiotepa produced relatively little change in articular cartilage under the same experimental conditions.

Of more general clinical importance is the potentially deleterious effects on cartilage of intra-articular injection of corticosteroids. Corticosteroids are quite frequently employed by this route to reduce synovial inflammation accompanying osteoarthritis, rheumatoid or other forms of arthritis (Mankin, 1974). Corticosteroids have been shown capable of reducing inflammation in experimental arthritis models (Williams and Brandt, 1985). However, degenerative changes in articular cartilage and underlying bone have also been ascribed to intra-articular injection of corticosteroids in patients although the pathogenesis for the alterations is not clear. Degeneration may be related to a number of different factors such as increased coagulability, vasculitis, local inhibition of pain sensation or decrease in cartilage matrix synthesis (Moskowitz et al., 1970; Mankin et al., 1972; Mankin, 1974).

Injection of rabbit knee joints with triamcinolone acetonide, a potent fluorinated corticosteroid for periods of up to six weeks produced degeneration of chondrocytes in tangential and transitional zones of articular cartilage, characterised by loss of nuclear staining, nuclear degeneration and the presence of empty lacunae (Moskowitz et al., 1970). In addition, numerous variably sized cysts containing degenerate chondrocytes and fibrillar debris were also found. The degree of changes was proportional to the number of injections given. The alterations to be localised in the medial tibial plateau of the rabbits in areas in which slight degenerative alterations were also noted in untreated controls, suggesting certain, perhaps more stressed zones of cartilage may be predisposed to degenerative alterations induced by corticosteroids (Moskowitz et al., 1970). However, these pathological lesions in rabbits are difficult to relate directly to man in view of the many variables involved in the intrarticular administration of corticosteroids to human patients with diseased joints.

In vitro studies have shown that a number of cytokines such as interleukin-1 and tumour necrosis factor are also capable of mediating breakdown of matrix glycoproteins in cartilage (Hamerman, 1989). The role of these cytokines in degeneration of cartilage in vivo is unclear although whole animal experiments have demonstrated that some cytokines cause degeneration of cartilage.

Interleukin-1, a polypeptide released by activated macrophages and a key mediator in host responses to infection, was shown to produce proteoglycan loss and histological changes similar to antigen-induced arthritis of about one week duration when injected into the joints of laboratory animals (Pettipher et al., 1986). This process was shown not to be the direct result of stimulation of polymorphonuclear cells and monocytes because endotoxin injection which produced a similar inflammatory response did not produce a similar alteration in cartilage.

Atrophy

In addition to disturbances in mineral metabolism, long term administration of anticonvulsant drugs can also produce atrophic changes in cartilage. Young rats treated either with diphenylhydantoin or sodium valproate for periods between six and seven weeks showed reduced chondrocyte numbers in both the femoral epiphysis and mandibular condylar cartilage as well as a reduction in cartilage thickness (Robinson et al., 1988). This suggested that these drugs may interfere with the regulation of chondrocyte proliferation and matrix synthesis. This effect on cartilage may contribute to the pathogenesis of abnormal skeletal growth reported in children treated with anticonvulsants for prolonged periods (Robinson et al., 1983).

Arthritis

Although degenerative changes develop spontaneously in the joints of laboratory animals, spontaneous inflammation of the joints is uncommon. However, in view of the importance of rheumatoid arthritis in man, a number of experimental models of arthritis have been developed. The most frequently employed models are of chronic immune arthritis employing antigens and adjuvents but non-immune arthritis is also induced by local administration of irritant substances such as zymosan (Schalkwijk et al., 1985).

Adjuvent arthritis is induced in laboratory rodents or rabbits by a single injection of certain heat-killed microorganisms notably Mycobacteria, Nocardia, Streptococci or their cell wall components within a suitable oily vehicle (Koga et al., 1973; Chang and Pearson, 1978). It has also been shown that a similar morphological form of arthritis can be induced by pure synthetic and apparently non-immunogenic adjuvents such as alkyldiamine [N,N-dioctadecyl-N',N'-bis(2-hydroxyethyl)propanediamine] or N-acetylmuramyl-L-alanyl-D-isoglutamine (MDP) and derivatives (Chang and Pearson, 1976; Kohashi et al., 1982).

Histologically, adjuvent arthritis is characterised intially by an acute exudative synovitis and pericarticular inflammation followed by hypertrophy of synovial villi, hyperplasia of synovial cells, development of granulation tissue in articular tissues and periosteal new bone formation (Kohashi et al., 1982). Resultant fibrous pannus develops at the joint margins and erodes articular cartilage.

Adjuvent arthritis is believed to result from a delayed hypersensitivity reaction involving T cells and bacterial wall components such as peptidoglycans although endogenous proteoglycan antigens and non-immune mechanisms may also be involved (Kohashi et al., 1982).

A similar form of immune arthritis can be induced in laboratory animals by sensitisation followed by intra-articular challenge by a number of antigens including homologous or heterologous fibrin, ovalbumin, bovine serum albumin, immunoglobulin, type II collagen and cartilage proteoglycans (Dumonde and Glynn, 1962; Mikecz et al., 1987; Kresina, 1987).

Mouse strains with certain major histocompatability haplotypes such as H2-q are susceptible to polyarthritic disease induced by intradermal immunisation using cartilage-derived type II collagen alone (Holmdahl et al., 1988).

As in the glomerulus, electrical charge of the injected antigen may be important in the development of articular damage. Intra-articular injection of cationic bovine serum albumin was shown to induce a chronic arthritis in immunised mice whereas when negatively changed it failed to produce protracted disease (Van den Berg and Van de Putte, 1985). It was postulated that positively changed antigen has a high affinity for negatively changed cartilage structures. Its subsequent deep penetration and retention provides a long lasting antigen supply, therefore sustaining inflammation. Conversly, negatively changed antigen is not retained in cartilage matrix.

Histologically, a similar chronic destructive inflammatory process usually develops in all these forms of arthritis although high dose antigen challenge may produce an acute destructive process with cartilage necrosis and vascular damage, features which are not usually evidence in human rheumatoid arthritis (Howson et al., 1986).

In the type II collagen-induced mouse arthritis model, the predominant cellular infiltrate is composed of Mac 1-positive macrophage-like cells with

163

relatively few T cells, suggestive of participation of an immune complex-mediated type III reaction (Hohmdahl et al., 1988).

A comparable process is also found in non-immune models of arthritis such as that which follows intra-articular injection of zymosan. However in a careful study in C57BL mice in which comparable degrees of joint inflammation were induced by bovine serum albumin or the non-immune stimulus of zymosan, histological differences were noted. Although both agents produced a chronic destructive process in the joints, the periarticular damage was greater in the immune model and periosteal bone apposition was more prominant (Schalkwijk et al., 1985). In addition, the immune mediated model, unlike zymosan, produced suppression of mitotic activity in bone marrow close to the inflammatory process during the first few days of of arthritis.

Similar types of immune and non-immune arthritis have been induced in laboratory animals by administration of therapeutic agents. Polyene antibiotics such as amphotericin and filipin produce both an acute and chronic non-immune form of arthritis in rabbits following intra-articular injection. After repeated injection, these antibiotics produce an early acute synovitis followed by a mononuclear and fibroblastic infiltration with hyperplasia and villous proliferation of the synovium (Weissmann et al., 1967). Pannus, consisting of layers of elongated fibroblasts covered by hyperplastic synovial cells, was found to extend over the peripheral margins of the articular surface. Articular cartilage not involved by pannus showed superficial loss of chondrocytes, chondrocyte clusters and loss of proteoglycan seen by loss of staining with safranin O or orthochromatic staining using toluidine blue. In severe cases, the articular surface developed fibrillation and vertical clefts or fissures. The pathogenesis of these changes is uncertain but it has been suggested that they are the result of the reactivity of polyenes with lipid structures in cell membranes because the degree of reactivity of these agents joints parallels their activity on isolated lysosomes and artificial membranes (Weissmann et al., 1967).

Arthritis similar to that induced by adjuvents has been induced in laboratory animals in conventional toxicity testing of immune modulators. Inflammation of the synovium, characterised by a diffuse infiltration by plasma cells and lymphocytes, development of germinal follicles and villous synovial hyperplasia was reported in dogs treated with an immunostimulant in toxicity studies (Gopinath et al., 1987). Likewise, muroctasin, a synthetic muramyl peptide, of potential clinical utility as an immune stimulant, also produced joint inflammation in conventional toxicity studies, perhaps not surprising in view of its close chemical relationship to substances found in classical adjuvants. Dogs treated daily with this agent for 28 days developed leucocytosis and cortical lymphoid hyperplasia. In the mid and high dose groups there was histological evidence of synovitis (Ono et al., 1988a). Similar changes were observed in rats but not in mice treated for 28 days. However treatment of mice for a longer period of 26 weeks did induce mild, reversible inflammation and hyperplasia of the synovium in the tarsal joints (Ono et al., 1988b).

SKELETAL MUSCLE

Although skeletal muscle forms about 40% of total body mass, drug-induced myopathy in man is uncommonly reported. However, minor degrees of drug-induced muscle damage are easily overlooked and its prevalence may be greater than generally realised (Mastaglia, 1982). Nevertheless, when severe, drug-induced muscle disease occurs, it can be disabling.

Drugs can cause derangement of the physiology and structure of skeletal muscle in a number of different ways. One of the most important results from a direct toxic effect on the muscle fibres, either following systemic exposure or more commonly due to localised effects of drugs administered by the intramuscular or subcutaneous routes. Damage to skeletal muscle also occurs secondary to other drug-induced effects such as electrolyte or metabolic disturbances, immunological reactions, ischaemia, compression of muscle in states of altered consciousness or in response to excessive neuronal activation at the neuromuscular junction (Mastaglia, 1982). Muscle changes are also an important component of motor neurone damage, whether of spontaneous nature or drug-induced.

Skeletal muscle fibres are heterogenous in nature and different types of muscle fibre respond differently to drugs and other stimuli. Skeletal muscle fibres of mature mammals fall into two main types based on their enzymatic and physiological characteristics and the nature of their contractile proteins. In practical terms, *slow twitch* or *type I fibres* are those which show the slow myosin ATPase activity in frozen sections incubated at pH 4.3 but not at pH 10.4. and have low glycolytic and high oxidative activity. *Fast-twitch or type II fibres* are those which contain the fast myosin isoform and show myosin ATPase activity at pH 10.4 but not at pH 4.3 and possess high glycolytic and low oxidative activity (Brooke and Kaiser, 1970; Brooke et al., 1971; Pierobon-Bormioli et al., 1980, 1981, Billeter et al., 1981). Type II fibres can be sub-divided into types A, B and C on the basis of their myosin ATPase activities and pH sensitivity. However, it should be remembered that the pH lability of this reactions is not identical between man, rat and rabbit (Brooke and Kaiser, 1970). Furthermore, detailed studies of the biochemical alterations which occur during development and in different metabolic states such as diabetes mellitus have suggested that the sub-division of muscle fibres into three or four distinct types is an oversimplification and that a much more heterogeneous population of muscle fibres exists (Lawrence et al., 1986; Abe et al., 1987).

Awareness of these fibre differences is relevant to toxicology for different fibre types have been shown to possess dissimilar sensitivities to metabolic alterations, workload and a variety of adverse stimuli including those produced by xenobiotics (Saltin et al., 1977, Lawrence et al., 1986; Abe et al., 1987; Helliwell 1988).

Although our understanding of hormonal factors involved in the development and growth of muscle has lagged considerably behind our knowledge of hormonal effects in other tissues, it is clear that pituitary growth hormone, thyroid hormones and insulin are major growth-promoting hormones and the glucocorticoids have catabolic effects in skeletal muscle. At an in vitro level, anabolic

165

hormones for cultured myoblasts are the somatomedins or insulin-like growth factors and fibroblast growth factor (Florini, 1987).

Histological techniques

In conventional toxicity studies, the skeletal muscle is usually examined histologically using well-orientated paraffin-embedded haematoxylin and eosin-stained sections, sometimes supplemented by PAS, silver impregnantion and trichrome stains. As in the diagnosis of human muscle disease by biopsy, use of cryostat sections and histochemical reactions such as myosin ATPase are of particular help in characterisation of muscle changes. Electron microscopy has proved of relatively limited use in muscle biopsy diagnosis (Weller, 1984) although it enables more precise characterisation of the subcellular alterations induced by drugs. Morphometric analysis of muscle fibre size is another useful tool in the characterisation of muscle alterations.

Immunocytochemical staining of muscle constituents such as myosin isoforms, myoglobin, desmin, collagens, fibronectin and laminin also have a place in the characterisation of alterations in muscle. Desmin staining is a particularly useful method for evaluating skeletal muscle regeneration in experimental studies (Helliwell, 1988). Lectin histochemistry, provides another method for the characterisation of muscle fibre changes in both man and rat (Pena et al., 1981; Capaldi et al., 1985; Yamagami et al., 1985; Helliwell, 1988). The lectin, Dolichos biflorus (DBA), selectively stains the neuromuscular junctions in several vetebrate species including rat, hamster and rabbit (Sanes and Cheney, 1982).

Inflammation and muscle necrosis

Review of the diverse forms of myositis in man has demonstrated that the inflammatory process within muscle tissue can show different morphological patterns. Inflammation in skeletal muscle can be primarily *interstitial* in type with little or no muscle fibre necrosis. Fibre *necrosis* may be the predominant component with little inflammatory infiltration (Peiffer, 1987). The inflammatory infiltrate may be composed of polymorphonuclear cells, macrophages or lymphocytes or be granulomatous in nature. The inflammation in muscle tissue can also be associated with either arteritis or small vessel vasculitis (Peiffer, 1987).

A similar range of inflammatory change is also possible within the context of preclinical drug safety evaluation, either as a result of spontaneous laboratory animal disease or following intramuscular, subcutaneous, intravenous or oral administration of chemical agents.

Localised, focal inflammation

Most inflammatory reactions found in skeletal muscle in preclinical studies result from local irritant effects of compounds administered by the intramuscu-

166

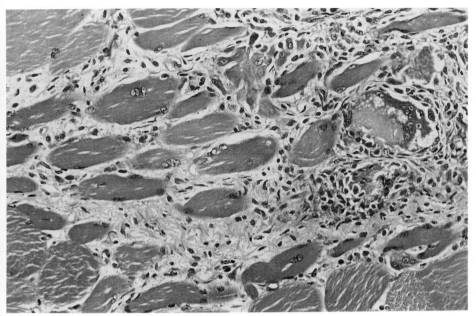

Fig. 33. Section of rabbit sacrospinalis muscle, ten days after a single local injection of a clinically employed, intramuscular formulation of an antibiotic. There is muscle fibre damage and a cellular response with foreign body type giant cells. (HE, ×250.)

lar or subcutaneous routes or following implantation of insoluble substances. Appraisal of the irritancy potential of intramuscular preparations is usually undertaken in the rabbit sacrospinalis muscles (Gray, 1981) but the dog, rat and other species are also sometimes employed. In these studies, clinical observations are made for several days or weeks after injection and this is followed by macroscopic and microscopic evaluation of the injection site after autopsy. The microscopic changes are assessed in a semiquantitative manner, particularly the extent of muscle necrosis, haemorrhage, degree and nature of the inflammatory response. Accompanying changes such mineralisation, microcyst formation, crystal deposition and foreign body giant cell reaction are recorded for these features may provide additional information about the nature of local effects in injected substances (Figs. 33 and 34). For instance, injection of calcium salts of antibiotics have been associated with increased mineralisation and foreign body giant cell reactions (Holbrook and Pilcher, 1950).

During the first two days following muscle injury it may be difficult to distinguish regenerating myoblasts from macrophages without the use of special stains. The detection of increased cytoplasmic RNA using acridine orange fluoresence is one technique for use in cryostat sections. Immunocytochemical staining for desmin has been shown to be a particularly reliable method for early identification of regenerating fibres in experimental studies (Helliwell, 1988).

167

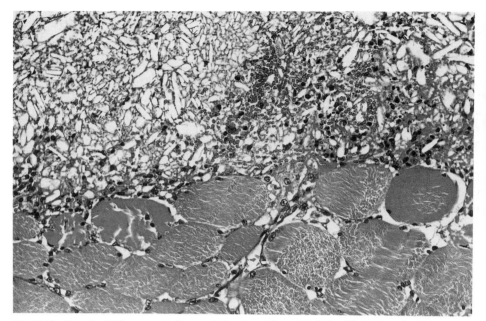

Fig. 34. Section of rabbit sacrospinalis muscle ten days after a single local injection of an intramuscular depot antibiotic preparation showing residual drug-related substances but little muscle fibre necrosis. (HE, ×250.)

As many agents induce some damage when injected into skeletal muscle, it is important that experimental studies with novel agents are carefully designed to allow comparison with clinically acceptable preparations and to show that any damage produced is capable of repair. Hence, the use of known positive controls and vehicle controls is important and it may be also necessary to conduct time-course studies over several weeks to assess the repair process. Careful fixation, slicing and selection of blocks from the injection site in order to provide a three-dimensional picture of the extent of any damage is also helpful. Usually, histological examination of the muscle after a single standard injection of the proposed formulation is usually sufficient for preclinical assessment of its local irritancy potential. It may be particularly difficult to assess the degree of damage or this effectiveness of the repair process in sites which have been injected on multiple occasions and single injections are usually to be preferred.

A certain degree of localised skeletal muscle damage can occur merely as a result of repeated needle insertion or injection of inocuous substances such as normal saline (Mastaglia, 1982). Muscle injury has also been demonstrated as a result of intramuscular injection of vehicles such as glycerol formol or propylene glycol (Steiness et al., 1974; Rasmussen and Svendsen, 1976).

A variety of drugs in current clinical use have been shown to be capable of inducing local tissue damage when injected by the intramuscular route in both man and animals. Examples include local anaesthetics, antibiotics, diazepam and

168

digoxin, many of which are lipid soluble or cationic amphiphilic molecules (Steiness et al., 1978; Benoit et al., 1980; Bergeson et al., 1982; Manor and Sadeh, 1989). Indeed it is probable that all intramuscular injections produce a certain degree of muscular damage.

The rapid necrosis and regeneration which occurs in muscle fibres following injection of local anaesthetic drugs makes these widely used agents for the experimental investigation of skeletal muscle damage. Repair appears to be rapid and complete with restoration of the original muscle fibre population after injection of local anaesthetics.

Using immunocytochemical methods, it has been shown that following injections of the local anaesthetic, bupivacaine, into the soleus (predominantly slow twitch type II fibres) and gastrocnemius (predominantly fast twitch type I fibres) muscles of rats, regeneration ultimately give rise to the original population of muscle fibres (Abe et al., 1987).

Although the mechanism for the particular liability of local anaesthetic agents to produce local muscle damage was originally believed to be an indirect effect of nerve block and denervation atrophy, it now appears that it occurs through a direct effect on muscle membrane systems. As verapamil, a calcium channel blocker, has been shown to almost completely inhibit local damage produced by mepivacaine, Benoit et al., (1980) have suggested that the myotoxicity is related to disturbance of intracellular calcium homeostasis rather that through their ability to alter sarcolemmal sodium conduction.

As some myotoxic agents are lipid soluble or cationic amphiphilic molecules it has been suggested that these properties may confer an ability to interfer with muscle cell membranes when injected locally (Manor and Sadeh, 1989). However, these properties themselves may also dictate the need for more complex vehicles which may themselves possess effects on muscle cells.

Measurement of serum enzymes of skeletal muscle origin such as creatine phosphokinase (CPK) 24 hours after injection is another value which relates to the degree of muscle fibre damage in these experimental models (Steiness et al., 1978; Gray, 1981). Measurement of CPK activity has enabled comparative studies of muscle damage following intramuscular injection of similar drug preparations in animals and humans. Steiness and colleagues (1978) showed intramuscular injections of lidocaine or diazepam may be followed by a small increase in CPK activity in human volunteers with similar but greater increase in pigs and rabbits following comparable injections. The degree of increase appeared to be primarily dependent on the total volume of distribution of CPK release from damaged muscle rather than major species difference in tissue sensitivity to the local effects of these drugs. Based on this evidence, drugs which are locally irritant to skeletal muscle in laboratory animals are also likely to produce similar effects in human muscle if given under comparable conditions.

Focal inflammation also occurs following implantation of solid materials within or in close proximity to skeletal muscle. For this reason, an implantation procedure is adopted in the evaluation of the tissue compatability of polymers used in medical devices. These materials are implanted in subcutaneous or

169

intramuscular sites in laboratory rodents or rabbits and the implantation sites subsequently removed several days or a week or two later, to be assessed histologically in a semiquantitative manner using known positive and negative control materials (Darby, 1987). The nature and extent of the tissue damage and inflammatory response is dependent on the type of implanted materials and time elapsed between implantation and examination. In general, during the first week following implantation, a polymorphonuclear and mononuclear cellular infiltrate with early formation of foreign body giant cells is the predominant pattern of response (Richardson et al., 1987). Over the second week, polymorphonuclear cells disappear but there is marked cellularity as a result of increased numbers of mononuclear cells, foreign body giant cells, fibroblasts and early capillary formation. In ensuing weeks there is increased fibrogenesis and angiogenesis frequently with a scattering of macrophages some of which may contain be pigment (haemosiderin).

In the evaluation of polymers for tissue compatability in muscle, enzyme histochemistry using unfixed frozen sections may be of additional help. For instance, loss of succinate dehydrogenase activity from muscle cells relates to the degree of muscle damage. Increase in, acid phosphatase activity is proportional to tissue damage and the contribution of macrophages and fibroblasts. Adenosine triphosphatase, normally confined to blood vessels, serves as a useful indication of the degree of vascularisation (Salthouse and Willigan, 1972).

Focal fibre necrosis and inflammation also occurs as a result of disruption and occlusion of the microcirculation of skeletal muscle either as a result of spontaneous vascular disease or experimental occlusion. Studies in rabbits in which a femoral artery was injected with dextran particles 20 μm and 80 μm diameter, showed foci of necrosis and regeneration and perivascular inflammation. This was followed by development of connective tissue around muscle fibres of variable size some of which contained central nuclei (Hathaway et al., 1970). Although the distribution of these focal lesions was inconsistent, they occurred more commonly towards the central zones of muscle fascicles with relative sparing of the peripheral muscle fibres.

Infections

Parasitic infestations also occasionally produce focal inflammation in skeletal muscle. This is reported in visceral larva migrans in laboratory beagle dogs in which larval nematodes can be found in skeletal muscle in association with focal chronic granulomatous inflammation (Barron and Saunders, 1966).

Sarcocystis, a coccidian parasite is also found in skeletal muscle, including that of the tongue, oesophagus and cardiac muscle in many non-human primates. Lesions are composed of rounded or oval aggregates of organisms usually devoid of inflammation (Fig. 35). They can be associated with inflammation and fibrosis (Toft, 1982).

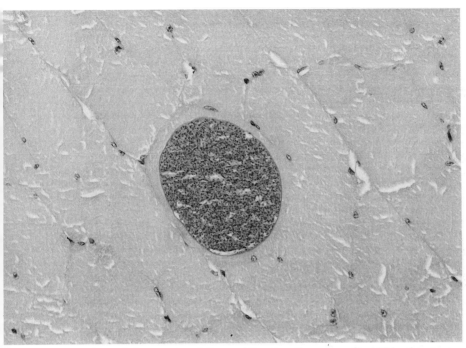

Fig. 35. The typical rounded aggregates of the coccidian parasite, sarcocystis, within almost normal skeletal muscle showing no cellular response. Cynomologus monkey. (HE, ×400.)

Diffuse inflammation

Diffuse necrotising myopathy can also be induced by systemic administration of therapeutic agents, although this is not commonly reported. Drugs which have been associated with this phenomenon in man include epsilon aminocaproic acid and clofibrate (Mastaglia, 1982). Analagous effects are not always reproducible in laboratory animals.

Clofibrate only rarely produces myopathy in man, but it has been reported to produce focal muscle fibre necrosis when particularly high levels of tissue exposure to the principle metabolite, chlorophenoxyisobutyric acid, occurs in patients with compromised renal function. The myopathy is characterised by muscle pain, high serum creative phosphokinase (CPK) and histological evidence of segmental fragmentation, hyalinisation, vacuolisation and phagocytosis of scattered single muscle fibres (Denizot et al., 1973).

Similar morphological changes have been described in rats treated with high doses of clofibrate following careful histological examination of skeletal muscle. Sprague-Dawley rats given 500 mg/kg/day for periods of up to six weeks developed focal degenerative changes in both type I and type II skeletal muscle fibres, characterised histologically by a ragged appearance due to fibres necrosis and phagocytosis (Teräväinen et al., 1977).

171

The biochemical basis for these muscular alterations following clofibrate administration remain unclear although they may be related to interference with lipid or carbohydrate metabolism or a result of a direct effect on sarcolemmal membrane.

In contrast, myopathy reported to occur in patients treated systemically with fibrinolytic agent, epsilon aminocaproic acid has not been reproduced in laboratory animals (Mastaglia, 1982). Following treatment, muscle fibre necrosis and regeneration associated with myoglobinuria develops over a few days. The mechanisms of this drug-induced muscle damage also remains uncertain but it has been suggested that it may be either the result of an effect on muscle membranes or intravascular coagulation (Mastaglia, 1982).

Malignant hyperpyrexia or *malignant hyperthermia* is a potentially life-threatening adverse reaction which occurs during general anaesthesia in susceptible individuals. It is characterised by muscular rigidity, myoglobinuria and a hypermetabolic state with metabolic acidosis (Mastaglia, 1982). Histological changes are not marked but comprise variability of muscle fibre size and increases in numbers of central nuclei and muscle cell necrosis in patients who survive an episode of hyperpyrexia (Weller, 1984).

Predisposition to this disorder appears to be familial with evidence of an autosomal dominant or polygenic inheritance (Ellis and Halsall, 1980). Agents most frequently involved are halothane and succinylcholine. Other halogenated anaesthetics, nitrous oxide, muscle relaxants and local anaesthetics can also precipitate the condition (Ellis and Halsall, 1980).

The precise cellular mechanism for the reaction is uncertain. The weight of evidence suggests that there is an acute rise intracellular calcium which leads to contracture of the myofibrillar apparatus, lowering of ATP and increased thermogenesis (Britt, 1979). The precise site or nature of the defect is also uncertain. Susceptible individuals can be identified by the presence of raised serum CPK levels or by the increased in vitro contractability of muscle fibres removed by biopsy (Moulds and Denborough, 1974).

The pig appears to be one of the few animal species susceptible to anaesthetic-induced malignant hyperthermia (Gallant et al., 1979). For this reason the pig was used in the preclinical assessment of the liability of a novel neuromuscular blocking agent, atracurium, to produce this reaction (Skarpa et al., 1983).

Other forms of myopathy: vacuolation

Although adriamycin (doxorubicin), an anthracene antibiotic used in the treatment of malignant disease, is well known for its cardiotoxic effects (see Cardiovascular System, Chapter VI), similar morphological alterations may also occur in skeletal muscle following therapy with agents of this class. Studies in rats to which adriamycin was administered by the intraperitoneal route showed that the severity of alterations in skeletal muscle were probably related to local tissue concentrations achieved because morphological alterations were more marked in diaphragmatic muscles adjacent to the site of administration than in the soleus (Doroshow et al., 1985).

Affected skeletal muscle showed variable degrees of interstitial vacuolation, presumably the result of interstitial oedema. There were also larger and greater numbers of cytoplasmic lipid vacuoles than in normal muscle. There was electron microscopic evidence of vesiculation of sarcoplasmic reticulum, myelin figures, distortion or loss of myofibrillar organisation and Z lines, fragmentation of the nucleolus and damage to mitochodria (Doroshow et al., 1985). Although fibres were only focally affected, there was apparently no preferential damage of particular fibre types. Overt lysis of individual muscle fibres and increased numbers of histocytes and fibroblasts was also seen in affected muscles.

Vacuolar or spheromembranous myopathy

Colchicine, used in the treatment of gout for over two centuries causes a characteristic myopathy in laboratory animals (Seiden 1973) and in man, particularly in patients with altered renal function (Kuncl et al., 1987). Similar changes are also produced by the anticancer drug vincristine, another agent which is capable of disaggregating microtubules (Slotwiner et al., 1966; Anderson et al., 1967; Bradley, 1970; Clarke et al., 1972).

This myopathy is characterised by irregular vacuolation in central zones of muscle fibres or in the peripheral subsarcolemmal zones. Vacuoles are filled with slightly basophilic material which stains for neutral lipid or phospholipid and possess marked acid phosphatase activity. These vacuoles have been termed spheromembranous bodies (Slotwiner et al., 1966). Electron microscopic examination shows that the vacuoles are essentially autophagocytic in nature containing heterogeneous membranous debris (Clarke et al., 1972; Seiden, 1973, Kuncl et al., 1987). Little or no frank cellular necrosis and inflammation is observed. Although these agents may also produce axonal polyneuropathy, this is mild and neuromuscular junctions in affected muscles remain essentially unaffected. Studies in rats treated with vincristine have shown that type II fibres are more frequently involved than type I fibres (Clarke et al., 1972).

It has been suggested that these agents disrupt the microtubule-dependent cytoskeletal system which normally interacts with lysosomes and autophagosomes to help in their extrusion from skeletal muscle (Kuncl et al., 1987).

Another agent which has been the cause of myopathy in man when taken in large amounts is emetine. Although clinical usage of emetine is now limited, it has been used in the management of amoebiasis and excessive amounts are sometimes ingested by patients with major eating disorders in order to self-induce vomiting (Palmer and Guay, 1985). This form of myopathy is characterised by weakness, aching, tenderness and stiffness in proximal muscle groups. Muscle biopsy obtained in a few patients has shown the presence of swollen core-targetoid fibres and amorphous eosinophilic intracytoplasmic rod-like inclusions in predominantly type I fibres, a slight decrease in fibre diameter, isolated necrotic granular basophilic fibres and a macrophage infiltrate (Palmer and Guay, 1985).

173

Similar alterations have been reported in rats treated with emetine. Rat treated with emetine for periods of up to about 30 weeks showed dose-related alterations in both extensor digitorum longus and soleus muscles. At high doses, these changes were characterised by loss of muscle weight, the presence of necrotic, hyaline or split muscle fibres and focal loss of myofibrillar adenosine triphosphatase (ATPase) activity (Bradley et al., 1976). The ultrastructural changes in skeletal muscles of treated rats included progressive Z line streaming, rod formation, myofilament loss, contraction clumping and extensive membrane proliferation affecting predominantly type I fibres. It was suggested that the changes were possibly a result of the effects of emetine on protein synthesis or mitochondrial oxidative phosphorylation (Bindoff and Cullen, 1978).

Vacuolation, vacuolar myopathy and phospholipidosis

Some amphiphilic cationic drugs which are capable of producing generalised phospholipidosis (See Respiratory System, Chapter V) also cause myopathy in man or laboratory rodents. Chloroquine is a well known example (Smith and O'Grady, 1966; Hughes et al., 1971; Mastaglia et al., 1977). Other drugs include amiodarone (Meier et al., 1979) perhexiline (Tomlinson and Rosenthal, 1977; Fardeau et al., 1979), the antioestrogen tamoxifen (Lüllmann and Lüllmann-Rauch, 1981) and a number of psychotropic drugs (Lüllmann-Rauch and Nassberger, 1983; Hruban, 1984).

This form of drug myopathy tends to occur in man only after prolonged or high doses are administered in the treatment of for chronic conditions. It is usually reversible after withdrawal of treatment for several months. The main clinical finding is muscle weakness but myasthesia-like symptoms have been recorded (Hughes et al., 1971; Sghirlanzoni et al., 1985). Electrophysiological findings are typically those of a myopathic disorder rather than a peripheral neuropathy (Sghirlanzoni et al., 1988).

The principal histological features in muscle biopsy samples taken from affected patients and in muscle taken from rats treated with these agents is vacuolation of muscle fibres. In haematoxylin and eosin-stained, paraffin embedded sections these vacuoles appear generally empty. In plastic embedded, toluidine blue-stained sections, the vacuoles appear more granular and basophilic. Enzyme cytochemical reactions show that the vacuoles are associated with high acid phosphatase activity and under the electron microscope membrane-bound, osmiophilic crystalloid or lamellated inclusions typical of phospholipidosis can be demonstrated (Drenkhahn and Lüllmann-Rauch, 1979; Sghirlanzoni et al., 1988).

A further electron-microscopic feature reported in skeletal muscle cytoplasm from patients with chloroquine myopathy is the presence of irregular, closely packed, curved profiles of membranous material surrounded by a unit membrane and referred to as curvilinear bodies (Neville et al., 1979; Sghirlanzoni et al., 1988).

Another histological component found in association with this form of phospholipidosis is degeneration of muscle fibres. Histologically, this is characterised

174

by marked variation in muscle fibre diameter, focal degeneration and frank necrosis of individual fibres, associated with branching of fibres, proliferation of myoblasts, with macrophage and fibroblastic infiltration (Hughes et al., 1971; Drenkhahn and Lüllmann-Rauch, 1979).

The precise cause of these degenerative changes is uncertain. Time-course studies in rats dosed with a number of cationic, amphiphilic drugs in rats have suggested that the muscle fibre damage occurs independently of the development of phospholipidosis (Drenkhahn and Lüllmann-Rauch, 1979). For this reason, Drenkhahn and Lüllmann-Rauch (1979) suggested that the phospholipidosis and the fibre necrosis were not causally related but developed independently, each as a result of drug effects on biomembranes.

Atrophy

Atrophy of skeletal muscle develops under a variety of different circumstances such as following disuse or denervation, nutritional or metabolic derangements, vascular insufficiency, after disturbance of hormonal growth control mechanisms and in advancing age. Although drugs and other xenobiotics produce atrophy in association with overt degeneration or necrosis of muscle fibres, simple muscle atrophy can be induced by some xenobiotics.

Studies in aging rats have shown that skeletal muscle atrophy tends to occur with advancing age, although this is not uniformly reported and can be retarded by food restriction and hypophysectomy (Everitt et al., 1985). Such age-related alterations are characterised by fall in muscle weight, reduced numbers of fibres, increased variability of muscle fibre size, the presence of increased numbers of lipid droplets and lipofuscin, frank fibre degeneration and ultrastructural evidence of myofibrillar breakdown and loss (Everitt et al., 1985). Although it is widely accepted that the decrease in fibre number which occurs in aging rats of many strains affects primarily type II fibres, this does not uniformly occur in all strains and in all muscle groups (Eddinger et al., 1985). Some of the reported changes in rat skeletal muscle, particularly in posterior muscle groups may be a response to spontaneous changes in spinal nerves and nerve roots (Fig. 36).

It is important, where possible, to distinguish the histological features of denervation atrophy because some drugs may produce primary peripheral nerve damage with secondary skeletal muscle atrophy. An example of this phenomenon has been reported in association with phospholipidosis in patients treated with perhexiline (Fardeau et al., 1979). Drugs which potentiate the development of age-related peripheral neuropathy in the rat may also accelerate the development of muscle atrophy in posterior muscle groups.

Denervation atrophy is characterised histologically by the presence of thin, angulated atrophic fibres of both type I and type II fibres with crowding of muscle fibre nuclei. As muscle fibres supplied by a single motor nerve are of the same histochemical type, the normal checkerboard pattern of fibres seen histochemically is lost. If reinervation occurs this normal checkerboard pattern is

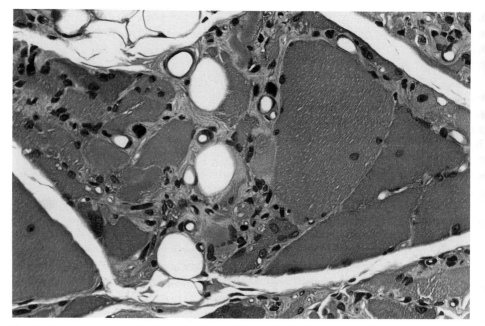

Fig. 36. Skeletal muscle (vastus lateralis) from a 24-month-old Wistar rat developing degeneration of spinal nerves and nerve roots. Muscle fibres are highly variable in size and shape, there is an increase in interstitial connective tissue and lipid droplets are prominent. (HE, ×250.)

not reconstituted but larger groups of uniform type I or type II fibres develop (Brooke et al., 1971).

The development of muscle weakness and atrophy as a complication of corticosteroid therapy is probably the most common drug-induced myopathy in clinical practice (Mastaglia, 1982). Usually this condition develops insidiously involving mainly proximal muscle groups. Serum levels of creatine kinase and other muscle enzymes are typically unaltered and muscle biopsy shows selective atrophy of type II fibres without destruction (Mastaglia, 1982).

Although results of animal experiments with corticosteroids are difficult to compare because of use of different agents and experimental designs, selective susceptability of type II fast twitch muscle fibres is well-established. It is associated with increased urinary secretion of methyl-histidine (Tomas et al., 1979; Livingstone et al., 1981; Florini 1987).

Studies in rats treated with dexamethasone showed that the mean weights of fast twitch muscles (extensor digitorum longus) were lower than slow twitch (soleus) muscles compared with controls. There was relatively severe impairment of type IIB (fast glycolytic) fibres compared to other fibre types, possibly due to their comparative inability to utilise alternative energy sources, particularly substrates derived from free fatty acids (Livingstone et al., 1981).

Histological and histochemical examination showed a similar decrease in the size of type II muscle fibres in rabbits treated with the synthetic corticosteroid, triamcinolone (Sheahan and Vignos, 1969). This change was reflected by a decrease in the weight of the gastrocnemius muscle, composed predominantly of type II fibres and a relative sparing of the soleus muscle, composed largely of type I fibres.

An agent which has been reported to produce muscle atrophy with little or no inflammation is 6-mercaptopurine. This is an immunosuppressive drug and purine antagonist, which interferes with the binding of adenine and hypo-xanthine and disrupts the synthesis of DNA and RNA (Jaweed et al., 1985). Examination of the soleus muscle in rats treated with 6-mercaptopurine showed fibre atrophy and variable degrees of fibre splitting in both type I and II fibres with increase in endomysial connective and fatty tissue (Alleva et al., 1981; Jaweed et al., 1985).

Hypertrophy

Enlargement of skeletal muscle occurs as a result of increased work load, although fibre type and metabolic potential also alters under these conditions (Saltin et al., 1977). Focal work hypertrophy of individual fibres is sometimes seen in association with chronic muscle damage or fibrosis, as a compensatory response.

Despite the widespread use of testosterone analogous as anabolic drugs and oestrogens in the enhancement of meat production relatively little experimental in vivo or in vitro work has been performed to show how these agents exert then effects on muscle (Florini, 1987).

Acromegaly is a well-known condition associated with a widespread increase in visceral size including an increase in muscle mass. Studies in rats have shown that the effects of administration of growth hormone are not uniform but that the increase in the size of muscle fibres occurs mainly in type I fibres with type II fibres remaining relatively unaffected (Prysor-Jones and Jenkins, 1980). Whether growth hormone can mediate this effect directly on skeletal muscle remains unclear but there is now considerable evidence that sometomedins or insulin-like growth factors are capable of mediating the effects of growth hormone on muscle (Florini, 1987).

Mineralisation

Dystrophic or metastatic calcification is sporadically observed a a spontaneous change in the skeletal muscle of laboratory animals. Certain strains of mice, notably BALB/c, C3H and DBA strains in which dystrophic calcification is particularly liable to occur in internal organs also develop mineralisation in skeletal muscle (Doi et al., 1985; Yamate et al., 1987). Various factors can influence the development of this form of mineralisation, such as diet and hormonal change. Administration of hydrocortisone or high endogeneous secre-tion of corticosteroids have also been postulated as contributing factors (Yamate et al., 1987).

Neoplasia

A variety of soft tissue neoplasms infiltrate skeletal muscle and a small number of sarcomas show skeletal muscle differentiation (See Integumentary System, Chapter I).

REFERENCES

ABE, J., FUTJII, Y., KUWAMURA, Y and HIZAWA, K. (1987): Fiber type differentiation and myosin expression in regenerating rat muscles. *Acta Pathol.Jpn.*, 37, 1537–1547.

ALFAHAM, M., HOLT, M.E. and GOODCHILD, M.C. (1987): Arthropathy in a patient with cystic fibrosis taking ciprofloxacin. *Br.Med.J.*, 295, 699.

ALLEVA, F.R., HABERMAN, B.H., SLAUGHTER, H.J and BALAZS, T. (1981): Muscular degeneration in rats after post-natal treatment with 6-mercaptopurine. *Drug Chem.Toxicol.*, 4, 133–146.

ANDERSON, H.C. (1989): Mechanism of mineral formation in bone. *Lab.Invest.*, 60, 320–330.

ANDERSON, C. and DANYLCHUCK, K.D. (1978): Bone-remodeling rates of the beagle: A comparison between different sites on the same rib. *Am.J.Vet.Res.*, 39, 1763–1765.

ANDERSON, P.J., SONG, S.K and SLOTWINER, P. (1967): The fine structure of spheromembranous degeneration of skeletal muscle induced by vincristine. *J.Neuropathol.Exp. Neurol.*, 26, 15–24.

ANDRESS, D.L., KOPP, J.B., MALONEY, N.A., COBURN, J.W and SHERRARD, D.J. (1987): Early deposition of aluminum in bone in diabetic patients on hemodialysis. *N.Engl.J.Med.*, 316, 292–296.

BARRON, C.N and SAUNDERS, L.Z. (1966): Visceral larva migrans in the dog. *Pathol.Vet.*, 3, 315–330.

BENOIT, P.W., YAGIELA, J.A and FORT, N.F. (1980): Pharmacologic correlation between local anaesthetic-induced myotoxicity and disturbances of intracellular calcium distribution. *Toxicol.Appl.Pharmacol.*, 52, 187–198.

BERGESON, P.S., SINGER, S.A. and KAPLAN, A.M. (1982): Intramuscular injections in children. *Pediatrics*, 70, 944–948.

BILLETER, R., HEIZMANN, C.W., HOWALD, H and JENNY, E. (1981): Analysis of myosin light and heavy chain types in single human skeletal muscle fibres. *Eur.J.Biochem.*, 116, 389–395.

BINDOFF, L and CULLEN, M.J. (1978): Experimental emetine myopathy. Ultrastructural and morphometric observations. *J.Neurol.Sci.*, 39, 1–15.

BRADLEY, W.G. (1970): The neuromyopathy of vincristine in the guinea pig. An electrophysiological and pathological study. *J.Neurol.Sci.*, 10, 133–162.

BRADLEY, W.G., FEWINGS, J.D., HARRIS, J.B and JOHNSON, M.A. (1976): Emetine myopathy in the rat. *Br.J.Pharmacol.*, 57, 29–41.

BRIGHTON, C.T., KITAJIMA, T and HUNT, R.M. (1984): Zonal analysis of cytoplasmic components of articular cartilage chondrocytes. *Arthritis Rheum.*, 27, 1290–1299.

BRITT, B.A. (1979): Etiology and pathophysiology of malignant hyperthermia. *Fed.Proc.*, 38, 44–48.

BROOKE, M.H and KAISER, K.K. (1970): Muscle fiber types: How many and what kind? *Arch.Neurol.*, 23, 369–379.

BROOKE, M.H., WILLIAMSON, E and KAISER, K.K. (1971): The behavior of four fiber types in developing and reinnervated muscle. *Arch.Neurol.*, 25, 360–366.

BROOKES, J.J. (1986): The significance of double phenotypic patterns and markers in human sarcomas. A new model of mesenchymal differentiation. *Am.J.Pathol.*, 125, 113–123.

CAPALDI, M.J., DUNN, M.J., SEWRY, C.A and DUBOWITZ, V. (1985): Lectin binding in human skeletal muscle: A comparison of 15 different lectins. *Histochem.J.*, 17, 81–92.

CARTER, R.L. (1973): Tumours of the soft tissues. In: V.S. Turusov, (Ed.) *Pathology of Tumours in Laboratory Animals, Vol. 1, Tumours of the Rat*, Part 1, pp. 151–167. IARC Scientific Publ No. 6, Lyon.

CHANG, Y-H and PEARSON, C.M. (1978): Pathogenesis of adjuvent arthritis in rats. *Arthritis Rheum.*, 21, 169–170.

CHAPPARD, D, ALEXANDRE, C and RIFFAT, G. (1983): Histochemical identification of oestoclasts. Review of current methods and reappraisal of a single procedure for routine diagnosis on undecalcified human iliac bone biopsies. *Basic Appl.Histochem.*, 27, 75–85.

CHARLES, R.T and TURUSOV, V.S. (1974): Bone tumours in CF-1 mice. *Lab.Anim.*, 8, 137–144.

CLARKE, J.T.R., KARPATI, G., CARPENTER, S and WOLFE, L.S. (1972): The effect vincristine on skeletal muscle in the rat. A correlative histochemical, ultrastructural and chemical study. *J.Neuropathol.Exp. Neurol.*, 131, 247–266.

COBB, L.M. (1970): Radiation-induced osteosarcoma in the rat as a model for osteosarcoma in man. *Br.J.Cancer*, 24, 294–299.

CONNOR, M.O., GARRETT, P., DOCKERY, M., DONOHOE, J.F., DOYLE, G.D., CARMODY, M and DERVAN, P.A. (1986): Aluminium-related bone disease. Correlation between symptoms, osteoid volume, and aluminum staining. *Am.J.Clin.Pathol.*, 86, 168–174.

CORRADO, M.L., STRUBLE, W.E., PETER, C., HOAGLAND, V and SABBAJ, J. (1987): Norfloxacin: Review of safety studies. *Am.J.Med.*, 82, Suppl. 6B, 22–26.

DAHLIN, D.C and UNNI, K.K. (1977): Osteosarcoma of bone and its important recognisable varieties. *Am.J.Surg.Pathol.*, 1, 61–72.

DARBY, T.D. (1987): Safety evaluation of polymer materials. *Ann.Rev.Pharmacol.Toxicol.*, 27, 157–167.

DENIZOT, M., FABRE, J., POMETTA, D and WILDI, E. (1973): Clofibrate, nephrotic syndrome and histological changes in muscle. *Lancet*, 1, 1326.

DENT, C.E., RICHENS, A., ROWE, D.J and STAMP (1970): Osteomalacia with long-term anticonvulsant therapy in epilepsy. *Br.Med.J.*, 4, 69–72.

DHEM, A. and GORET-NICAISE, M. (1984): Effects of retinoic acid on rat bone. *Food Chem.Toxicol.*, 22, 199–206.

DODD, D.C and PORT, C.D. (1987): Hyperostosis of the marrow cavity caused by misprostol in CD-1 strain mice. *Vet.Pathol.*, 24, 545–548.

DOI, K., MAEDA, N., DOI, C., ISEGAWA, N.K., SUGANO, S and MITSUOKA, T. (1985): Distribution and incidence of calcified lesions in DBA/2NCrj and BALB/c AnNCrj mice. *Jpn.J.Vet.Sci.*, 47, 479–482.

DOIGE, C.E., CROW, S and FARROW, C.S. (1986): Aseptic necrosis of bone in a dog. *Can.Vet.J.*, 27, 70–73.

DOROSHOW, J.H., TALLENT, C and SCHECHTER, J.E. (1985): Ultrastructural features of adriamycin-induced skeletal and cardiac muscle toxicity. *Am.J.Pathol.*, 118, 288–297.

DRENKHAHN, D. and LÜLLMANN-RAUCH, R. (1979): Experimental myopathy induced by amphilphilic cationic compounds including several psychotrophic drugs. *Neuroscience*, 4, 549–562.

DUBIELZIG, R.R., BIERY, D.N. and BRODEY, R.S. (1981): Bone sarcomas associated with multifocal medullary bone infarction in dogs. *J.Am.Vet.Med.Assoc.*, 179, 64–68.

DUMONDE, D.C. and GLYNN, L.E. (1962): The production of arthritis in rabbits by an immunological reaction to fibrin. *Br.J.Exp.Pathol.*, 43, 373–383.

EDDINGER, T.J., MOSS, R.L., CASSENS, R.G. (1985): Fiber number and type composition in extensor digitorum longus, soleus, and diaphragm muscles with ageing in Fischer 344 rats. *J.Histochem.Cytochem.*, 33, 1033–1041.

EDWARDS, J.C.W. (1982): The origin of the type A synovial lining cell. *Immunobiology*, 161, 227–231.

EDWARDS, J.C.W., SEDGWICK, A.D and WILLOUGHBY, D.A. (1982): Membrane properties and esterase activity of synovial living cells. Further evidence for a mononuclear phagocyte subpopulation. *Ann.Rheum.Dis.*, 41, 282–286.

EDWARDS, J.C.W and WILLOUGHBY, D.A. (1982): Demonstration of bone marrow derived cells in synovial lining by means of giant intracellular granules as genetic markers. *Ann.Rheum.Dis.*, 41, 177–182.

ELLIS, F.R and HALSALL, P.J. (1980): Malignant hyperpyrexia. *Br.J.Hosp.Med.*, 24, 318–327.

ELLIS, H.A., MCCARTHY, J.H and HERRINGTON, J. (1979): Bone aluminium in haemodialysed patients and in rats injected with aluminium chloride: relationship to impaired bone mineralization. *J.Clin.Pathol.*, 32, 832–844.

EVERITT, A.V., SHOREY, C.D and FICARRA, M.A. (1985): Skeletal muscle ageing in the hind limb of the old male Wistar rat: inhibitory effect of hyperphyectomy and food restriction. *Arch.Gerontol.Geriatr.*, 4, 101–115.

FARDEAU, M., TOME, F.M.S and SIMON, P. (1979): Muscle and nerve changes induced by perhexiline maleate in man and mice. *Muscle Nerve*, 2, 24–36.

FARNUM, C.E and WILSMAN, N.J. (1988): Lectin-binding histochemistry of intracellular and extracellular glycoconjugates of the reserve cell zone of growth plate cartilage. *J.Orthopaedic.Res.*, 6, 166–179.

FLEISCH, H. (1987): Bisphosphonates-History and experimental basis. *Bone*, 8, Suppl. 1, S23-S28.

FLEISCH, H. (1989): Bisphosphonates: A new class of drugs in diseases of bone and calcium metabolism. In: K.W. Brunner, H., Fleisch and H-J. Senn, (Eds). *Recent Results in Cancer Research*. Vol. 116, pp. 1–28. Springer Verlag, Berlin.

FLORA, L., HASSING, G.S., PARFITT, A.M and VILLANUEVA, A.R. (1980): Comparative skeletal effects of two diphosphonates in dogs. *Metab.Bone Dis.Relat.Res.*, 2, Suppl, 389–407.

FLORINI, J.R. (1987): Hormonal control of muscle growth. *Muscle Nerve*, 10, 577–598.

FORNASIER, V.L. (1984): Classification of bone tumors. In: H.K. Uhthoff and E. Stahl, (Eds). *Current Concepts of Diagnosis and Treatment of Bone and Soft Tissue Tumors*, pp. 23–27. Springer Verlag, Berlin.

FRITH, C.H., JOHNSON, B.P. and HIGHMAN, B. (1982): Osteosarcomas in BALB/c female mice. *Lab.Anim.Sci.*, 32, 60–63.

GALLANT, E.M., GODT, R.E and GRONERT, G.A. (1979): Role of plasma membrane defect of skeletal muscle in malignant hyperthermia. *Muscle Nerve*, 2, 491–494.

GAUNT, S.D and PIERCE, K.R. (1985): Myelopoiesis and marrow adherent cells in estradiol-treated mice. *Vet.Pathol.*, 22, 403–408.

GENNARI, C. (1985): Glucocorticoids and bone. In: W.A. Peck (Ed.), *Bone and Mineral Research*, 3, Chap 7, pp 213–231. Elsevier, Amsterdam.

GOODMAN, D.G., WARD, J.M., SQUIRE, R.A., PAXTON, M.B., REICHARDT, W.D., CHU, K.C and LINHART, M.S. (1980): Neoplastic and non-neoplastic lesions in aging Osborne-Mendel rats. *Toxicol.Appl.Pharmacol.*, 55, 433–447.

GOPINATH, C., PRENTICE, D.E and LEWIS, D.J. (1987): The musculoskeletal system and skin. In: *Atlas of Experimental Toxicological Pathology. Current Histopathology*, Vol. 13, Chap 11, pp. 156–166. MTP Press Lancaster.

GÖSSNER, W. (1986): Pathology of radiation-induced bone tumors. *Leuk.Res.*, 10, 897–904.

GOUGH, A., BARSOUM, N.J., MITCHELL, L., MCGUIRE, E.J and DE LA IGLESIA (1979): Juvenile canine drug-induced arthropathy: Clinicopathological studies on articular lesions caused by oxolinic and pipemidic acids. *Toxicol.Appl.Pharmacol.*, 51, 177–187.

GOUGH, A.W., BARSOUM, N.J., RENLUND, R.C., STURGESS, J.M and DE LA IGLESIA, F.A. (1985): Fine structural changes during reparative phase of canine drug-induced arthropathy. *Vet.Pathol.*, 22, 82–84.

GRAF, B. (1985): Etude morphologique de ostéopétrose congénitale du rat 'op'. *Pathol.Biol.*, 33, 82–89.

GRAY, J.E. (1981): Appraisal of the intramusclar irritation test in the rabbit. *Fundam.Appl.Toxicol.*, 1, 290–292.

HAMERMAN, D. (1989): The biology of osteoarthritis. *N.Engl.J.Med.*, 320, 1322–1330.

HARRIS, M., JENKINS, M.V and WILLS, M.R. (1974): Phenytoin inhibition of parathyroid hormone induced resorption in vitro. *Br.J.Pharmacol.*, 50, 405–408.

HASSELL, J.R., KIMURA, J.H and HASCALL, V.C. (1986): Proteoglycan core protein families. *Annu.Rev.Biochem.*, 55, 539–567.

HATHAWAY, P.W., ENGEL, K and ZELLWEGER, H. (1970): Experimental myopathy after microarterial embolization. Comparison with childhood x-linked pseudohypertrophic muscular dystrophy. *Arch.Neurol.*, 22, 365–378.

HELLIWELL, T.R. (1988): Lectin binding and desmin staining during bupivicaine: induced necrosis and regeneration in rat skeletal muscle. *J.Pathol.*, 155, 317–326.

HENDERSON, B and PETTIPHER, E.R. (1985): The synovial lining cell: Biology and pathology. *Semin.Arthritis Rheum.*, 15, 1–32.

HIGH, W.B. (1982): Prostaglandins and bone formation. Presented at the Thirty Third Annual meeting. *The American College of Veterinary Pathologists*, Atlanta.

HIGHMAN, B., NORVELL, M.J and SHELLENBERGER, T.E (1977): Pathological changes in female C3H mice continuously fed diets containing diethylstilbestrol or 17β-estradiol. *J.Environ.Pathol.Toxicol.*, 1, 1–30.

HIGHMAN, B., ROTH, I.R and GREENMAN, D.L. (1981): Osseous changes and osteosarcomas in mice continuous fed diets containing diethylbstilbestrol or 17β-estradiol *J.N.C.I.*, 67, 653–662.

HOLBROOK, T.J and PILCHER, C. (1950): The effect of injection of penicillin, peanut oil and beeswax, separated and in combination, upon nerve and muscle. *Surg.Gynecol.Obstet.*, 90, 39–44.

HOLMDAHL, R., JOHSSON, R., LARSSON, P. and KLARESKOG, L. (1988): Early appearance of activated CD4+T lymphocytes and class II antigen-expressing cells in joints of DBA/1 mice immunized with type II collagen. *Lab.Invest.*, 58, 53–60.

HOWSON, P., SHEPARD, N and MITCHELL., N. (1986): The antigen induced arthoritis models. The relevance of the method of induction to its use as a model of human disease. *J.Rheumatol.*, 13, 379–390.

HRUBAN, Z. (1984): Pulmonary and generalized lyosomal storage induced by amphiphilic drugs. *Environ.Health Perspect.*, 55, 53–76.

HUGHES, J.T., ESIRI, M., OXBURY, J.M AND WHITTY, C.W.M. (1971): Chloroquine myopathy. *Q.J.Med.*, 40, 85–93.

HUVOS, A.G., WOODARD, H.Q., CAHAN, W.G., HIGINBOTHAM, N.L., STEWART, F.W., BUTLER, A and BRETSKY, S.S. (1985): Postradiation osteogenic sarcoma of bone and soft tissues. A clinicopathologic study of 66 patients. *Cancer*, 55, 1244–1255.

ITAKURA, C., IIDA, M and GOTO, M. (1977): Renal secondary hyperparathyroidism aged Sprague-Dawley rats. *Vet.Pathol.*, 14, 463–469.

JASTY, V., BARE, J.J., JAMISON, J.R., PORTER, M.C., KOWALSKI, R.L., CLEMENS, G.R., JACKSON, G.E and HARTNAGEL, R.C (1986): Spontaneous lesions in the sternums of growing rats. *Lab.Anim.Sci.*, 36, 48–51.

JAWEED, M.M., ALLEVA, F.R., HERBISON, G.J., DITUNNO, J.F and BALAZS, T. (1985): Muscle atrophy and histopathology of the soleus in 6-mercaptopurine-treated rats. *Exp.Mol.Pathol.*, 43, 74–81.

JEE, W.S.S., UENO, K., DENG, Y.P and WOODBUTY, D.M (1985). The effects of prostaglandin E$_2$ in growing rats: Increased metaphyseal hard tissue and cortico-endosteal bone formation. *Calcif.Tissue Int.*, 37, 148–157.

KATO, M and ONODERA, T. (1986): Observations on the development of osteochondrosis in young rats. *Lab.Anim.*, 20, 249–256.

KIVIRANTA, I., JURVELIN, J., TAMMI, M., SÄÄMÄNEN A-M and HELMINEN, H.J (1987): Weight bearing controls glycosaminoglycan concentration and articular cartilage thickness in the knee joints of young beagle dogs. *Arthritis Rheum.*, 30, 801–809.

KOGA, T., PEARSON, C.M., NARITA, T. and KOTANI, S. (1973): Polyarthritis induced in the rat with cell walls from several bacteria and two streptomyces species. *Proc.Soc.Exp.Biol.Med.*, 143, 824–827.

KOHASHI, O., AIHARA, K., DZAWA, A., KOTANI, S. and AZUMA, I. (1982): New model of a synthetic adjuvent, N-acetylmuramyl-L-alanyl-D-isoglutamine-induced arthritis. *Lab.Invest.*, 47, 27–36

KRESINA, T.F. (1987): Immunotherapy of experimental arthritis. Analysis of the anticular cartilage of mice suppressed for collagen-induced arthritis by a T-cell hybridoma. *Am.J.Pathol.*, 129, 257–266.

181

KUNCL, R.W., DUNCAN, G., WATSON, D., ALDERSON, K., ROGWASKI, M.A. and PEPER, M. (1987): Colchicine myopathy and neuropathy. *N.Engl.J.Med.*, 316, 1562–1568.

LAWRENCE, G.M., WALKER, D.G. and TRAYER, I.P. (1986): Histochemical evidence of changes in fuel metabolism induced in red, white and intermediate fibres of streptozotocin-treated rats. *Histochem.J.*, 18, 203–212.

LEES, G.E. and SAUTTER, J.H. (1979): Anemia and osteopetrosis in a dog. *J.Am.Vet.Med.Assoc.*, 175, 820–824.

LIVINGSTONE, I., JOHNSON, M.A. and MASTAGLIA, F.L. (1981): Effects of dexamethasone on fibre subtypes in rat muscle. *Neuropathol.Appl.Neurobiol.*, 7, 381–398.

LÜLLMANN, H. and LÜLLMANN-RAUCH, R. (1981): Tamoxifen-induced generalised lipidosis in rats subchronically treated with high doses. *Toxicol.Appl.Pharmacol.*, 61, 138–146.

LÜLLMANN-RAUCH, R. and NASSBURGER, L. (1983): Citalopram-induced generalised lipidosis in rats. *Acta Pharmacol.Toxicol.*, 52, 161–167.

MACKENZIE, W.F. and GARNER, F.M. (1973): Comparison of neoplasms in six sources of rats. *J.N.C.I.*, 50, 1243–1257.

MALONEY, N.A., OTT, S.M., ALFREY, A.C., MILLER, N.L., COBURN, J.W., and SHERRARD, D.J. (1982). Histological quantitation of aluminum in iliac bone from patients with renal failure. *J.Lab.Clin.Med.*, 99, 206–216.

MANKIN, H.J. (1974): The reaction of articular cartilage to injury and osteoarthitis. *N.Engl.J.Med.*, 291, 1285–1291.

MANKIN, H.J., ZARINS, A. and JAFFE, W.L. (1972): The effect of systemic corticosteroids on rabbit articular cartilage. *Arthritis Rheum.*, 15, 593–599.

MANOR, D. and SADEH, M. (1989): Muscle fibre necrosis induced by intramuscular injection of drugs. *Br.J.Exp.Path.*, 70, 457–462.

MASTAGLIA, F.L. (1982): Adverse effects of drugs on muscle. *Drugs*, 24, 304–321.

MASTAGLIA, F.L., PAPADIMITRIOU, J.M., DAWKINS, R.L. and BEVERIDGE, B. (1977): Vacuolar myopathy associated with chloroquine, lupus erythematosis and thymoma. *J.Neurol.Sci.*, 34, 315–328.

MEIER, C., KAUER, B., MULLER, U. and LUDIN, H.P. (1979): Neuro-myopathy during chronic amiodarone treatment. A case report. *J.Neurol.*, 220, 231–239.

MERTZ.B., SPAET, R.H., PFANNKUCH, F. and GRAEPEL, P. (1989): Bone changes in a 6/12 month oral toxicity study in dogs following administration of disodium pamidronate, a bisphosphonate. *Presented 8th International Symposium of Society of Toxicologic Pathologists*, Cincinnati, Ohio.

MIKECZ, K., GLANT, T.T. and POOLE, A.R. (1987): Immunity to cartilage proteoglycans in BALB/C mice with progressive polyarthritis and ankylosing spondylitis induced by injection of human cartilage proteoglycan. *Arthritis Rheum.*, 30, 306–318.

MILLER, S.C., JEE, W.S.S., WOODBURY, D.D. and KEMP, J.W. (1985): Effects of N, N, N', N'-ethylenediaminetetramethylene phosphoric acid and 1-hydroxyethylidene-1, 1-bisphosphoric acid on calcium absorption, plasma calcium, longitudinal bone growth and bone histology in the growing rat. *Toxicol.Appl.Pharmacol.*, 77, 230–239.

MINKIN, C. (1981): Defective macrophage chemotaxis in osteopetrotic mice. *Calcif.Tissue.Int.*, 33, 677–678.

MISDORP, W. (1980): Canine osteosarcoma. Am.J.Pathol. 98, 285–288.

MORSE, C.C., KIM, S.N., WALSH, K.M., WATKINS, J.R. and DOMINICK, M.A. (1990): Proliferative bone lesions in rats given anticancer compounds. *Presented at the IXth International Symposium of the Society of Toxicological Pathologists, Ottawa.*

MOSKOWITZ, R.W., DAVIS, W., SAMMARCO, J., MAST, W. and CHASE, S.W. (1970): Experimentally induced corticosteroid arthropathy. *Arthritis Rheum.*, 13, 236–243.

MOULDS, R.F.W. and DENBOROUGH, M.A. (1974): Identification of susceptibility to malignant hyperpyrexia. *Br.Med.J.*, 2, 245–247.

NEVILLE, H.E., MAUNDER-SEWRY, C.A., McDOUGALL, J., SEWELL, J.R. and DUBOWITZ, V. (1979): Chloroquine-induced cytosomes with curvilinear profiles in muscle. *Muscle Nerve*, 2, 376–381.

OLSON, H.M. and CAPEN, C.C. (1977). Virus-induced animals model of osteosarcoma in the rat. Morphologic and biochemical studies. *Am.J.Pathol.*, 86, 432–458.

ONO, Y., IWASAKI, T., SEKIGUCHI, M. and ONODERA, T. (1988)a: Subacute toxicity of muroctasin in miceand dogs. *Arzneimittelforschung*, 38, 1024–1027.

ONO, Y., SEKIGUCHI, M., AIHARA, K. and ONODER, T. (1988)a: Chronic toxicity of muroctasin in mice. *Arzneimittelforschung*, 38, 1028–1030.

PALMER, E.P. and GUAY, A.T. (1985): Reversible myopathy secondary to abuse of ipecac in patients with major eating disorders. *N.Engl.J.Med.*, 313, 1457–1459.

PARFITT, A.M., DREZNER, M.K., GLORIEUX, F.H., KANIS, J.A., MALLUCHE, H., MEUNIER, P.J., OTT, S.M. and RECKER, R.R. (1987): Bone histomorphometry: Standardization of nomenclature, symbols and units. Report of the ASBMR histomorphometry nomenclature committee. *J.Bone Mineral Res.*, 2, 595–610.

PEIFFER, J. (1987): Classification of myositis. Correlations between morphological and clinical classifications ofinflammatory muscle disease. *Pathol.Res.Pract.*, 182, 141–156.

PELFRÈNE, A.F. (1985): A search for a suitable animal model for bone tumours: A review. *Drug Chem.Toxicol.*, 8, 83–99.

PENA, S.D.J., GORDON, B.B., KARPATI, G. and CARPENTER, S. (1981): Lectin histochemistry of human skeletal muscle. *J.Histochem. Cytochem.*, 29, 524–546.

PERCY, D.H. and JONAS, A.M. (1971): Incidence of spontaneous tumours in CD-1 Ham/ICR mice. *J.N.C.I.*, 46, 1046–1065.

PETTIPHER, E.R., HIGGS, G.A. and HENDERSON, B. (1986): Interleukin-1 induces leukocyte infiltration and cartilage proteoglycan degradation in the synovial joint. *Proc.Nat.Acad.Sci.USA*, 83, 8749–8755.

PIEROBON-BORMIOLI, S., SARTORE, S., VITADELLO, M. and SCHIAFFINO, S. (1980): 'Slow' myosins in vetebrate skeletal muscle. An immunofluorescene study. *J.Cell Biol.*, 85, 672–681.

PIEROBON-BORMIOLI, S., SARTORE, S., LIBERA, L.D., VITADELLO, M. and SCHIAFFINO, S. (1981): 'Fast' isomyosins and fibre types in mammalian skeletal muscle. *J.Histochem.Cytochem.*, 29, 1179–1188.

PRYSOR-JONES, R.A. and JENKINS, J.S. (1980): Effect of excessive secretion of growth hormone on tissues of the rat, with particular reference to the heart and skeletal muscle. *J.Endocrinol.*, 85, 75–82.

RASSMUSSEN,F. and SVENDSEN, O. (1976): Tissue damage and concentrations at the injection site after intramuscular injection of chemotherapeutics and vehicles in swine. *Res.Vet.Sci.*, 20, 55–60.

REDDICK, R.L., MICHELITCH, H.J., LEVINE, A.M. and TRICHE, T.J. (1980): Osteogenic sarcoma. A study of ultrastructure. *Cancer*, 45, 64–71.

REVELL, P.A. (1986): Normal bone. In: *Pathology of Bone*, Chap.1, pp. 1–34. Springer-Verlag, Berlin.

RICHARDSON, T.C., HUMPHRYES, J.A.H., and TOWNSEND, K.M.S. (1987): Subcutaneous implantation of double velour Dacron into the mouse: Infiltration and angiogenesis. *Br.J.Exp.Pathol.*, 68, 359–368.

RICHENS, A. and ROWE, D.J.F. (1979): Disturbance of calcium metabolism by anticonvulsant drugs. *Br.Med.J.*, 4, 73–76.

RISER, W.H. and FRANKHAUSER, R. (1970): Osteopetrosis in the dog: A report of three cases. *J.Am.Vet.Radiol.Soc.*, 11, 29–34.

ROBERTSON, J.A., FELSENFELD, A.J., HAYWOOD, C.C., WILSON, P., CLARKE, C. and LLACH, F. (1983). Animal models of aluminum-induced osteomalacia: Role of chronic renal failure. *Kidney Int.*, 23, 327–335.

ROBINSON, P.B., HARRIS, M., HARVEY, W. and PAPADOGEORGAKIS, N. (1982): Reduced bone growth in rats treated with anticonvulsant drugs: A type II pseudohyperparathyridism? *Metab.Bone Dis.Rel.Res.*, 4, 269–275.

ROBINSON, P.B., HARRIS, M. and HARVEY, W. (1983): Abnormal skeletal and dental growth in epileptic children. *Br.Dent.J.*, 154, 9–13.

183

ROBINSON, P.B., HARVEY, W. and BELAL, M.S. (1988): Inhibition of cartilage growth by the anticonvulsant drugs diphenylhydantoin and sodium valproate. *Br.J.Exp.Pathol.*, 69, 17–22.

RUBEN, Z., ROHBACHER, E. and MILLER, J.E. (1986): Spontaneous osteogenic sarcoma in the rat. *J.Comp.Pathol.*, 96, 89–94.

SALTHOUSE, T.M. and WILLIGAN, D.A. (1972): An enzyme histochemical approach to the evaluation of polymers for tissue compatability. *J.Biomed.Mater.Res.*, 6, 105–113.

SALTIN, B., HENRICKSSON, J., NYGAARD, E., ANDERSON, P. and JANSSON, E. (1977): Fibre types and metabolic potential of skeletal muscles in sedentary man endurance runners. *Ann.NY.Acad.Sci.*, 301, 3–29.

SAMPSON, H.W. and CANNON, M.S. (1986): Zonal analysis of metabolic profiles of articular-epiphyseal cartilage chrondocytes: A histochemical study. *Histochem.J.*, 18, 233–238.

SANERKIN, H.G. (1980): Definitions of osteosarcoma, chondrosarcoma and fibrosarcoma of bone. *Cancer*, 46, 178–185.

SANES, J.R. and CHENEY, J.M. (1982): Lectin binding reveals a synapse-specific carbohydrate in skeletal muscle. *Nature*, 300, 646–647.

SASS, B. and MONTALI, R.J. (1980): Spontaneous fibro-osseous lesions in aging female mice. *Lab.Anim.Sci.*, 30, 907–909.

SCHALKWIJK, J., VAN DEN BERG, W.B., VAN DER PUTTE, L.B.A., JOOSTEN, L.A.B. and VAN DER SLUIS, M. (1985): Effects of experimental joint inflammation on bone marrow and periarticular bone. A study of two types of arthritis, using variable degrees of inflammation. *Br.J.Exp.Pathol.*, 66, 435–444.

SCHENK, R., EGGLI, P., FLEISCH, H. AND ROSINI, S. (1986): Quantitative morphometric evaluation of the inhibitory activity of new aminobisphosphonates on bone resorption in the rat. *Calcif.Tissue Int.*, 38, 342–349.

SCHNEIDER, G.B., RELFSON, M. and NICOLAS, J. (1986): Pluripotent hemopoietic stem cells give rise to osteoclasts. *Am.J.Anat.*, 177, 505–511.

SEDMAN, A.B., KLEIN, G.L., MERRITT, R.J., MILLER, N.L., WEBER, K.O., GILL, W.L., ANAND, H. and ALFREY, A.C. (1985): Evidence of aluminum loading in infants receiving intravenous therapy. *N.Engl.J.Med.*, 312, 1337–1343.

SEIDEN, D. (1973): Effects of colchicine on myofilament arrangement and the lysosomal system in skeletal muscle. *Z.Zellforsch.*, 144, 467–473.

SGHIRLANZONI, A., MANTEGAZZA, R., MORA, A., PAREYSON, D. and CORNELIO, F. (1988): Chloroquine myopathy and myesthenia-like syndrome. *Muscle Nerve*, 11, 114–119.

SHEAHAN, M.G. and VIGNOS, P.J. (1969): Experimental corticosteroid myopathy. *Arthritis Rheum*, 12, 491–497.

SKARPA, M., DAYAN, A.D., FOLLENFANT, M., JAMES, D.A., MOORE, W.B., THOMSON, P.M., LUCKE, J.M., MORGAN, M., LOVELL, R. and MEDD, R. (1983): Toxicity testing of atracurium. *Br.J.Anaesth.*, 55, 275–295.

SLOTWINER, P., SONG, S.K. and ANDERSON, P.J. (1966): Spheromembraneous degeneration of muscle induced by vincristine. *Arch.Neurol.*, 15, 172–176.

SMITH, B. and O'GRADY, F. (1966): Experimental chloroquine myopathy. *J.Neurol.Neurosurg. Psychiat.*, 29, 255–258.

SOKOLOFF, L. and HABERMANN, R.T. (1958): Idiopathic necrosis of bone in small laboratory animals. *Arch.Pathol.*, 65, 323–330.

SOLHEIM, T. (1974): Pluricolor fluorescent labeling of mineralizing tissue. *Scand.J.Dent.Res.*, 82, 19–27.

SONTAG, W. (1986): Quantitative measurements of periosteal and cortical-endosteal bone formation and resorption in the midshaft of male rat femur. *Bone*, 7, 63–70.

STEINBERG, ME.E., COHEN, R.W. and COGEN, F.C. (1967): Effects of intra-articular anti-metabolites. *Arthritis Rheum.*, 10, 316–317.

STEINESS, E., RASMUSSEN, F., SVENDSEN, O. and NIELSEN, P. (1978): A comparative study of serum creatine phosphokinase (CPK) activity in rabbits, pigs and humans after intramuscular injection of local damaging drugs. *Acta Pharmacol.Toxicol.*, 42, 357–364.

STEINESS, E., SVENDSEN, O. and RASMUSSEN, F. (1974): Plasma digoxin after paranteral administration. Local reaction after intramuscular injection. *Clin.Pharmacol.Therap.*, 16, 430–434.

STROMBERG, P.C. and VOGTSBERGER, L.M. (1983): Pathology of the mononuclear cell leukemia of Fischer rats. 1. Morphologic Studies. *Vet.Pathol.*, 20, 698–708.

TEITELBAUM, S.L. and BULLOUGH, P.G. (1979): The pathoghysiology of bone and joint disease. *Am.J.Pathol.*, 96, 283–354.

TERÄVÄINEN, H., LARSEN, A. and HILLBOM, M. (1977): Clofibrate-induced myopathy in the rat. *Acta Neuropathol.*, 39 135–138.

TOMLINSON, I.W. and ROSENTHAL, F.D. (1977). Proximal myopathy after perhexiline maleate treatment. *Br.Med.J.*, 1, 1319–1320.

TOFT, J.D. (1982): The pathophysiology of the alimentery tract and pancrease of non-human primates. A review. *Vet.Pathol.* 19, Suppl.7, 44–92.

TOMAS, F.M., MONTRO, H.M. and YOUNG, V.R. (1979): Effect of glucortoid administration on the introduction of muscle protein breakdown in vivo in rats as measured by urinary execution of N-methylhistidine. *Biochem.J.*, 178, 139–146.

TUCKER, M.J. (1986): A survey of bone disease in the Alpk/Ap rat. *J.Comp.Pathol.*, 96, 197–203.

TUCKER, M.J., ADAM, H.K. and PATTERSON, J.S. (1984): Tamoxifen. In: D.R. Laurence, A.E.M. McLean and M. Weatherall, (Eds), *Safety Testing of New Drugs. Laboratory Prediction and Clinical Performance*. Chap. 6. pp. 125–161. Academic Press, London.

TUCKER, M.J., D'ANGIO, G.J. BOICE, J.D., STRONG, L.C., LI, F.P., STOVALL, M., STONE, B.J., GREEN, D.M., LOMBARDI, F., NEWTON, W., HOOVER, R.N., FRAUMENI, J.F. (1987): Bone sarcomas linked to radiotherapy and chemotherapy in children. *N.Engl.J.Med.*, 317, 588–593.

UEDA, K., SAITO, A., NAKANO, H., AOSHIMA, M., YOKOTA, M., MURAOKA, R. and IWAYA, T. (1980): Cortical hyperostosis following long-term administration of prostaglandin E, in infants with cyanotic congenital heart disease. *J.Pediatr.*, 97, 834–836.

URIST, M.R., BUDY, A.M. and MCLEAN, F.C. (1950): Endosteal bone formulation in estrogen-treated mice. *J.Bone Joint Surg.*, 32, 143–163.

VAN DEN BERG, W.B. and VAN DE PUTTE, L.B.A. (1985): Electrical charge of the antigen determines its location in the mouse knee joint. Deep penetration of cationic BSA in hyaline articular cartilage. *Am.J.Pathol.*, 121, 224–234.

VAN HOOSIER, G.L. and TRENTIN, J.J. (1979): Naturally occuring tumours of the Syrian hamster. *Prog.Exp.Tumor Res.*, 23, 1–12.

VAUGHAN, J. (1981): Osteogenesis and haematopoiesis. *Lancet*, 2, 133–136.

WALKER, D.G. (1973): Osteopetrosis in mice cured by temporary parabiosis. *Science*, 180, 875–876.

WALKER, D.G. (1975): Control of bone resorption by haematopoietic tissue. The induction an reversal of congenital osteopetrosis in mice through use of bone marrow and splenic transplants. *J.Exp.Med.*, 142, 651–663.

WALTON, M. (1977): Degenerative joint disease in the mouse knee: Histological observations. *J.Pathol.*, 123, 109–122.

WARREN, M.A. and BEDI, K.S. (1985): The effects of a lengthy period of undernutrition on the skeletal growth of rats. *J.Anat.*, 141, 53–64.

WASE, A.W., SOLEWSKI, J., RICKES, E. and SEIDENBERG, J. (1967): Action of thyrocalcitonin on bone. *Nature*, 214, 388–389.

WEISBRODE, S.E. (1981): short-term effects of vitamin D_3 and 1,25-dihydroxyvitamin D_3 on osteomalacia in uremic rats fed a low-calcium-low-phosporus diet. *Am.J.Pathol.*, 104, 35–40.

WEISSMANN, G., PRAS, M. and ROSENBERG, L. (1967): Arthritis induced by filipin and rabbits. *Arthritis Rheum.*, 10, 325–336.

WELLER, R.O., (1984): Muscle biopsy and the diagnosis of muscle disease. In: P.P. Anthony and R.N.M. Macsween, (Eds). *Recent Advances in Histopathology*, No. 12, Chap. 12, pp. 259–288. Churchill Livingston, Edinburgh.

WILLIAMS, J.M. and BRANDT, K.D. (1985): Triamcinolone hexacetonide protects against fibrillation and osteophyte formation following chemically induced articular cartilage damage. *Arthritis Rheum.*, 28, 1267–1274.

YAMAGAMI, T., HOSAKA, H. AND MORI, M. (1985): Classification of skeletal muscle fibers by comparison of enzyme histochemistry with lectin binding. *Cell Mol.Biol.*, 43, 241–249.

YAMASAKI, K. and INUI, S. (1985): Lesions of articular, sternal and growth plate cartilage in rats. *Vet.Pathol.*, 22, 46–50.

YAMASAKI, K. and ITAKURA, C. (1988)a: Osteosclerosis in F244/Du Crj. rats. *Lab.Anim.*, 22, 141–143.

YAMASAKI, K. and ITAKURA, C. (1988)b: Aseptic necrosis of bone in ICR mice. Lab.Anim., 22, 51–53.

YAMATE, J., TAJIMA, M., MARUYAMA, Y. and KUDOW, S. (1987): Observations of soft tissue calcification in DBA/2NCri mice in comparison with CRJ: CD-1 mice. *Lab.Anim.*, 21, 289–298.

YAMATE, J., TAJIMA, M., MARUYAMA, Y. and KUDOW, S. (1987): Observations of soft tissue calcification in DBA/2NCri mice in comparison with CRJ: CD-1 mice. *Lab.Anim.*, 21, 289–298.

V. Respiratory Tract

By far and away the most important pulmonary diseases in man are related to the smoking of tobacco. However, occupational lung diseases caused by inhalation of industrial chemicals, particulate matter and antigens are also important causes of morbidity and mortality. For this reason, considerable effort has been directed to the examination of airborne polluents over recent years, including study of their effects in laboratory animals when administered by the inhalation route. Extensive study has shown that a complex array of defensive mechanisms protect the lung against the adverse effects of airbone substances and pathogenic organisms. Aerodynamic factors prevent access of particles larger than 10 μm diameter for these are deposited on the walls of the nasal passages. Particles measuring between 2 and 10 μm diameter tend to be trapped by the mucus-covered ciliated epithelium lining the bronchial tree and removed by mucociliary transport aided by the cough reflex. Smaller particles may reach the alveoli where they are ingested and transported by pulmonary macrophages (Murphy and Florman, 1983).

In contrast to the adverse pulmonary effects of cigarette smoke and industrial polluents, therapeutic agents remain a relatively minor cause of pulmonary toxicity in man. Drug-induced toxicity usually occurs after exposure of lung tissue to parent drug or metabolite via the circulation. Nevertheless, an increasing number of pharmaceutical agents are being developed for therapeutic use by the nasal or inhalation route, particularly for pulmonary diseases (Ranney, 1986).

Therefore, the toxicologist is now faced with a need for a greater understanding of experimental inhalation toxicology than perhaps previously.

Drugs can affect the respiratory system in man in a number of quite different ways (Grant, 1979). Through their specific pharmacological action they can produce excessive effects on bronchial calibre or pulmonary function at high doses.

Drugs mediate allergic reactions in the bronchi or lungs and produce a variety of obscure, diffuse pulmonary alveolar conditions including a pulmonary syndrome resembling systemic lupus erythematosis. As the respiratory tract is a

187

major route by which micro-organisms gain entry into the body, opportunistic pulmonary infections with bacteria, viruses, fungi or protozoa are consequences of therapeutic immunosuppression or broad-spectrum antibacterial therapy. Recent data also indicate that treatment with antacids or histamine H_2 blockers can increase the risk of pneumonia developing in patients in intensive care units through increasing gastric pH which leads to an overgrowth of gram-negative bacteria in the stomach and retrograde pharangeal colonization (Craven et al., 1986). Mucociliary clearance is also sensitive to certain therapeutic agents which affect the secretion of mucus and fluid, ciliary activity and transport (Sturgess, 1985). Drugs which disturb coagulation may precipate pulmonary thromboembolism or haemorrhage. Localised lung lesions also result from accidental, diagnostic or therapeutic inhalation of xenobiotics.

Inhalation Toxicology

A complex science and technology has been developed to support the assessment of the adverse effects of inhaled substances in rodent and non-rodent species as well as in the extrapolation of the experimental findings to man.

In order to administer xenobiotics, including drugs, by inhalation, it is necessary to generate aerosols (suspensions of particles in a gas) with a well-defined composition, particle size and shape. They must be appropriately delivered to the respiratory tract of laboratory animals in a way which parallels the likely human exposure. In case of therapeutic agents, this should avoid non-respiratory pathways through the skin and food.

When aerosols are inhaled, various fractions of the particles are deposited at different locations in the respiratory tract. Site depends primarily on particle size, but variability in the sites of deposition occurs among different laboratory animal species and man by virtue of the differences in the shape and size of the respiratory passages.

For instance, the relative distribution of monodisperse aerosols in man and rat were found to be comparable when particles of 1 to 3 μm diameter were inhaled, but differed considerably above this size range (Raabe, 1980).

However, the subsequent fate of inhaled particles depends not only on their size but also their shape, chemical nature, and solubility in body fluids. Insoluble, inert particles will be removed primarily by the mucociliary transport system of the trachea and bronchi or through phagocytosis by macrophages. Soluble substances are absorbed into the blood stream and are removed by the pulmonary circulation. They may also undergo metabolism by enzymes present in the cell populations of the respiratory tract.

Mathematical models are useful in the prediction of deposition patterns of inhaled particles in different species. However, the accuracy of these models depends on the precision of anatomical measurements such as length, calibre and branching angle of airways. These measurements may be inaccurate, particularly for the nasopharangeal region (Patra, 1986).

As in conventional studies, a key component of the evaluation of the effects of inhaled substances is careful morphological assessment of the fixed tissues. However, measurements of respiration rate, tidal volume, airway resistance, pulmonary gas exchange and the disposition of the inhaled substances also have a place in the evaluation of chemically induced lung damage in laboratory animals (Nemery et al., 1987). Several variables in the respiratory pattern of rodents can be measured simultaneously with whole body plethysmography using only modest restraint (Coggins et al., 1981).

NOSE, NASAL SINUSES, NASOPHARYNX AND PHARYNX

The nasal chambers are the structures which are first subjected to the effects of inhaled substances, whether micro-organisms or chemical substances. Although these chambers are not usually examined in great detail in conventional toxicity studies in which substances are administered orally or by parenteral routes, it is important that they are carefully examined histologically when drugs are administered by inhalation.

In rodents, the relatively small size of the nose and nasal sinuses facilities histological examination. Usually this area is sectioned transversely into several standardised blocks following decalcification (Young, 1981). In larger species, particularly dogs and primates sectioning and blocking is more complex. Although dissection is required, a similar procedure following decalcification can be adopted (Levinski et al., 1981).

Study of nasopharangeal silicone rubber casts has shown considerable species differences in the anatomy of this part of the airway (Patra, 1986). Relative to total nasal length, the nasopharynx is longest in rat and shortest in man with the dog in an intermediate position. Maxilloturbinates are relatively simple structures in man and non-human primates but highly complex in dogs and rodents.

The anterior nares is lined by stratified squamous epithelium but in other zones the sinuses are covered either by respiratory or olfactory epithelium. *Respiratory epithelium* is similar to that found elsewhere in the respiratory passages being composed of ciliated cells, serous and mucous cells, brush cells, intermediate cells and progenitor basal cells. It represents a cellular system engaged in mucociliary clearance carrying surface secretions to the nasopharynx to be cleared by swallowing (Proctor, 1977). Although this epithelium is similar to that lining the other large airways, key differences are the particularly rich complement of secretory cells and the complex vasculature of the nose which can modulate capillary, arterial and venous blood flow through the mucosa (Proctor, 1977).

The proportion of the nose lined by *olfactory mucosa* is variable between species but it is structurally similar in man and rodents. It is located in more dorsal or posterior regions of the nasal passages out of the direct line of airflow during normal respiration.

Olfactory mucosa is a pseudostratified columnar epithelium composed of basal cells, sustentacular cells and sensory cells with mucus-secreting Bowman's glands situated in the lamina propria. *Basal Cells* are composed of two distinct types, light and dark cells. The light type represents the primitive, stem cell population. *Sustentacular* or *supporting cells* are non-ciliated, columnar cells possessing microvilli which extend into the overlying layer of mucus.

Cell bodies of *olfactory sensory neurons* are situated in the middle layer of the epithelium between sustentacular and basal cells. Their dendritic processes extend above the epithelial surface to end in a ciliated expansion referred to as the olfactory vesicle which is believed to be the receptor of odour perception. Olfactory axons extend from the cell body, penetrate the basement membrane in bundles to become surrounded by Schwann cells and eventually join with the olfactory bulb.

The olfactory system is of some importance in toxicology for it can be selectively damaged by inhaled xenobiotics such as methyl bromide (Hurtt et al., 1987). The superficial location of neural cells in the olfactory epithelium also provides a model system for the study of the effects of xenobiotic on neural cells.

A test system which relates to the innervation of the nasal mucosa is that proposed by Alarie (1966) for the detection of airborne sensory irritants and the prediction acceptable levels of exposure to the upper respiratory tract in man. The trigeminal nerve endings in the nasal mucosa of mice mediate the response to sensory irritants and this can be measured by a decrease in respiratory rate. It has been shown that a good correlation exists between the decrease in respiration rate in mice exposed to airborne chemicals and the nasal irritancy potential of the chemicals in man (Alarie, 1981).

Submucosal mucous glands have been well characterised in both the rat or hamster where they are divided into *lateral nasal glands* and *maxillary recess glands*. These are both situated in the posterior parts of the nasal cavity and composed of mucus-secreting cells (Vidic and Greditzer, 1971; Adams, 1982). Similar glands have also been characterised in the nasal cavity of the dog (Adams et al., 1981).

Immunocytochemical study using antisera raised against the major isoenzymes of rat hepatic microsomal cytochromes P450 induced by β-napthoflavone, 3-methylcholanthrene, phenobarbitone and pregnenolone-16-α-carbonitrile as well as NADPH-cytochrome P450 reductase, epoxide hydrolase and glutathione S-transferases B, C and E has shown the presence of these immune-reactive enzymes in the rat nasal mucosal cells (Baron et al., 1988). This suggests that the nasal mucosa not only has a capacity for metabolising and activating xenobiotics by oxidation, but also forhydration and inactivation of potentially toxic epoxides and conjugating electrophilically reactive metabolites with reduced glutathion. In addition, it has been shown that the distribution of immune-reactive enzymes is different in olfactory and respiratory mucosa and the differences correlate with activity shown by enzyme histochemical methods. Therefore, xenobiotics can be metabolised within both olfactory and respiratory mucosa, but the olfactory regions appear to possess greatest capability for oxidative metabolism.

Another feature of this metabolising activity is its inducability by sytemically administered inducers. This occurs in a way which alters the *distribution* of enzyme activity in the nasal mucosa. (Baron et al., 1988).

Inflammation, ulceration, (rhinitis, sinusitis)

Infective agents cause inflammation in the nose and nasal sinuses and this may be associated with inflammation in the conjunctiva, middle ear and oral cavity. In rats, microbiological agents implicated in the development of rhinitis and sinusitis include Corynebacterium kutscheri (pseudotuberculosis), Streptococcus pneumonia, Pasteurella pneumotropica, Klebsiella pneumoniae, Mycoplasma pulmonis and sialodacryoadenitis virus or rat corona virus (Greaves and Faccini, 1984).

Rats exposed to ammonia, a common pollutant of the air in laboratory animal cages, have also been shown to develop lesions of the dorsal meatus, dorsal nasal septum and prominances of the turbinates. These lesions are characterized histologically by swelling or mild degeneration of the epithelium (Pinson et al., 1986). Furthermore, ammonia exposure can potentiate the acute inflammation response of the nasal cavity to microbiological pathogens (Pinson et al., 1986).

Another variable which has been shown to influence the severity of the rhinitis produced by Mycoplasma pulmonis is the strain of rat. Following housing of LEW and F344 strains together to eliminate microbial and environmental differences, Davis and Cassell (1982) showed that the LEW strain developed a more severe rhinitis following inoculation with Mycoplasma pulmonis than F344 rats, although the reason for the difference was unclear.

A micro-organism reported in the nasal cavity of rhesus monkeys employed in inhalation studies is the nematode of the genus Anatrichosoma (Klonne et al., 1987). Sections of this nematode are found in the squamous epithelium of the nasal vestibule and are associated with acanthosis and hyperkeratosis of the epithelium and a multifocal or diffuse granulomatous inflammation in the submucosa.

Administration of toxic or irritant substances to laboratory animals by the inhalation route produces degenerative, inflammatory and reactive changes in the nasal mucosa with a range of histological features similar to those found in mucosal surfaces damaged by other exogenous agents.

An example of the type and distribution of the degenerative and inflammatory conditions which can be induced by inhaled irritants is provided by the study in which Swiss-Webster mice were given various irritants by inhalation for periods of 6 hours per day for five days at concentrations which produced a 50% decrease in respiratory rate (Alarie test). Although the degree of histological changes varied with different agents, the changes were broadly similar in type and distribution (Buckley et al., 1984).

Most agents examined produced little or no alteration in the squamous mucosa lining the anterior part of the noses apart from some mild increase in thickness of the squamous epithelium. Principle sites of damage were shown to be the anterior respiratory epithelium adjacent to the vestibule and the olfactory epithelium of the dorsal meatus. There was a distinct decrease in severity more posteriorly.

Histologically, the lesions in respiratory epithelium ranged from mild loss of cilia and small areas of epithelial exfoliation to frank erosion, ulceration and necrosis of the epithelium and underlying tissues including bone. Variable polymorphonuclear cell infiltration was also found. In some cases, early squamous metaplasia developed on the free margins or the naso-maxillo-turbinates. Changes to the olfactory epithelium varied from focal to extensive loss of sensory cells associated with damage to sustentacular cells. In severe case, complete loss of olfactory epithelium occurred.

Although the degree of histological change was shown to vary with different agents, lesions induced by the more water soluble chemicals tended to remain localised in the anterior part of the nasal cavity whereas agents with relatively low water solubilities produced lung lesions in addition. It was suggested that these findings demonstrated the powerful 'scrubbing' action of the nasal cavity for water soluble, airborne xenobiotics (Buckley et al., 1984).

Similar inflammatory alterations can be induced in the nasal cavity of rodents treated with therapeutic agents by inhalation. However, the precise relevance of such changes for human therapy by the inhalation route are sometimes questionable when the nasal damage is limited to high doses and it is not associated with alterations in other parts of the respiratory tract. In the case of tulobuterol, a β2-adrenergic receptor agonist, it was argued that the nasal inflammation induced in rats in a one month inhalation toxicity study was the result of a particulary high exposure of the nasal epithelium to drug, not representative of the likely human exposure to tulobuterol by inhalation, where little or no nasal exposure would occur (Dudley et al., 1989).

A particular response of the rodent nasal mucosa to some irritant substances, including pharmaceutical agents, is the formation of rounded eosinophilic inclusions in the cytoplasm of sustentacular cells of the olfactory epithelium and to a lesser extent in respiratory and glandular epithelial cells (Buckley et al., 1985; Gopinath et al., 1987). These inclusions are PAS-negative and ultrastructurally comprise membrane-bound, ellipsoid bodies containing homogenous electron dense matrix. Their significance remains uncertain.

LARYNX AND TRACHEA

The mucosa lining the larynx and trachea becomes involved as part of an upper or lower respiratory tract infection.

For instance, in rats, an acute laryngitis or tracheitis has been shown to accompany experimental infection with Mycoplasma pulmonis and the sialo-dycroadenitis virus (Davis and Cassell, 1982; Wojcinski and Percy, 1986).

The larynx of rodents is particularly susceptible to the effect of inhaled substances, notably tobacco smoke but also pharmaceutical agents (Coggins et al., 1980; Gopinath et al., 1987). Lesions tend to occur in the ventrolateral region which is covered by respiratory epithelium and the inner aspect of the arytenoid processes which is lined by squamous mucosa. The larynx (and tracheal mucosa) responds to inhaled irritants by inflammatory, degenerative and regenerative changes. These include disruption of the epithelial cells, inflammatory cell exudatation and infiltration, goblet cell hyperplasia and squamous metaplasia (Coggins et al, 1980). It is important to note that these changes are not specific to inhaled irritants but also occur as a response to natural respiratory tract pathogens in conventionally housed rats (Lewis, 1982).

Neoplasia

Neoplasms of the nasal cavity develop spontaneously in rats and mice, although focal proliferative polypoid squamous lesions and olfactory carcinomas forming glands, follicles and rosettes are occasionally reported in aged Syrian hamsters (Pour et al., 1976, 1979).

BRONCHI AND LUNGS

In man and laboratory animals, the trachea terminates at the bifurcation giving rise to two main bronchi which serve left and right lungs. Depending on species, the main bronchi subdivide into further branches which enter the different lobes. Various forms of branching are recognized.

Bronchi may arise as side-branches from a parent or stem bronchus (*monopodial*). The parent bronchus can divide into two equal daughter bronchus (*dichotomous*) or several daughter bronchi (polychotomous) (Yeh, 1979). Study of silicone rubber casts of the respiratory tract has shown that the bronchial trees of man and non-human primates are essentially dichotomous, in contrast to the monopodial pattern of rodents (Patra, 1986). The comparatively long trachea of the dog gives rise to dichotomous upper airways but monopodial branching develops peripherally within each lobe.

The size of the lungs is dependent on size and weight of the different species, although the dog has comparatively smaller body mass and higher airway dimensions compared to man (Patra, 1986). The number of lobes is species-dependent. The human lung possesses an upper and lower left lobe and an upper, middle and lower right lobe. This contrasts with the upper, middle and lower left lobes and a fourth, azygos right lobe in rhesus monkeys and baboons (Hartman and Straus, 1965; Patra, 1986). The dog has three lobes on both right and left sides. Rats, mice and hamsters show cranial, middle, candal and postcaval right lobes with a single, left lobe in mice and rats and a superior and inferior lobe on the left side in hamsters.

Cell types lining the bronchi are generally similar between species although not all subtypes have been clearly determined in every species (reviewed by Sturgess, 1985). The majority of cells are the ciliated cells which are accompanied by variable but relatively smaller proportions of basal cells, intermediate cells, mucous or goblet cells, serous cells, neuroendrocrine and brush cells. In addition, mucous cells line the adjacent bronchial glands. (Dormans, 1983).

Ciliated cells are tall, columnar cells attached to basal and intermediate cells by desmosomal junctions. Tight junctions exist between adjacent specialised cells at the apex. Each cell possesses 200 or more cilia that are engaged in mucociliary clearance (Serafini and Michaelson, 1977). The superficial cell surface also shows a pronounced glycocalyx. The cytoplasm of ciliated cells contains scattered profiles of rough endoplasmic reticulum, a supranuclear Golgi, numerous mitochondria particularly near the apex where a prominent cytoskeleton is also found. *Mucous or goblet cells* are typical mucus-secreting cells representing about 10% of the bronchial mucosa cell population in man but less than 1% in pathogen-free rats (Sturgess, 1985). *The serous cell* is a cylindrical or pyramidal cell containing small, round, closely packed serous granules (Dormans, 1983).

Basal Cells are compact, pyramidal cells resting on the basement membrane, believed to be progenitor stem cells with the *intermediate cells* representing an intermediate stage of cell differentiation.

The mucus-secreting and ciliated cells form the cellular basis for the mucociliary clearance mechanism of the main conducting airways. The epithelium is covered by a mucous blanket which is fairly complete in man and rabbit but more patchy in the rat (Sturgess, 1985). The mucous layer is segregated into an upper layer or gel phase separated from epithelial cells by a serous layer or sol phase. The complex carbohydrates of the glycocalyx and secreted mucosubstances show species-related differences in their sugar residues which can be demonstrated histochemically by the use of labelled-lectins (Geleff et al., 1986).

Mucociliary clearance mechanisms are sensitive to the effects of many therapeutic agents, particularly those that influence mucins, fluid or electrolyte balance and ciliary activity. Anaesthetic gases, barbiturates, narcotics and alcohol depress clearance function. By contrast, topical, oral or parenteral administration of β-adrenergic agonists, isoprenaline and adrenaline, produce a dose-dependent stimulation of mucociliary transport by an effect on ciliary beat frequency, probably mediated by increasing levels of cyclic adenosine monophosphate in ciliated cells rather than through vascular changes. Although basal mucociliary function is dependent of normal vagal tone, mucociliary transport can be affected by parasympathomimetic agents. Acetylcholine and cholinergic agents stimulate ciliary activity whereas anticholinergic drugs, atropine and hyoscine, inhibit ciliary activity and mucociliary transport. These substances may alter deposition on inhaled particles in the lung (Sturgess, 1985).

Clara cells or non-ciliated bronchiolar cells located in the bronchiolar epithelium, first described by Clara (1937), are small and cylindrical in shape with highly infolded nuclei, surface microvilli, well developed Golgi, abundant endoplasmic reticulum and characteristic oval, homogeneous electron-dense granules in the apical cytoplasm. In rat, rabbit and man the granules are PAS-positive, although they are usually considered PAS-negative in hamster and mouse (Dormans, 1983).

On the basis of ultrastructural cytochemistry using frozen thin sections, in order to preserve Clara cell granules, surfactant-type proteins with partial or complete identity to those secreted by type II pneumocytes have been identified in Clara cells of the rat (Walker et al., 1986). Immune-reactivity was greatest in the cytoplasmic granules but was also shown in the Golgi and endoplasmic reticulum suggesting that surfactant-type apoproteins are synthesised and secreted by Clara cells. Clara cells also are highly active metabolically and contain cytochrome P450-dependent enzymes.

In most laboratory rodents, the conducting airways terminate abruptly at the non-cartilaginous and non-alveolarized *terminal bronchiole* which opens directly into an alveolarized airway, the *alveolar duct*. This in turn communicates with the alveoli (Bal and Ghoshal, 1988). Squamous epithelial or *type I cells* form only about 10% of all lung cells but they line over 90% of the alveolar surface, by virtue of extremely long cytoplasmic extensions. The principle gas exchange takes place across this cell. In the rat, the typical thickness of this barrier is 20 nm for a cytoplasmic extension of a type I pneumocyte, 90 nm for basal lamina and 90 nm for an endothelial cell (Dormans, 1983). The type I cell contains juxtanuclear mitochondria and the long smooth cytoplasmic extensions contain many ribosomes and pinocytotic vesicles. The anatomical configuration and function of type I cells render them highly vulnerable to inhaled gases and particles.

The other main alveolar lining cell is the *granular pneumocyte* or *type II cell* which constitutes about 10% of all lung cells, but which covers only about 5% of the alveolar surface (Pinkerton et al., 1982). This cell does not possess the long cytoplasmic processes typical of type I cells and it shows many microvilli at its luminal surface. The cell cytoplasm contains rough endoplasmic reticulum, Golgi apparatus, some mitochondria and characteristic oval, osmiophilic lamellar inclusions. Surfactant, or pulmonary surface active material, a microaggregate of phospholipid and protein which modifies alveolar surface tension at low inflation volumes, is secreted by type II alveolar cells. Ultrastructural immunocytochemistry has shown the presence of surfactant apoproteins in the synthetic organelles and in the lamellar bodies of these cells, in agreement with the concept that the surfactant apoproteins are synthesized in the rough endoplasmic reticulum, glycosylated in the Golgi and are stored in lamellar bodies (Walker et al, 1986).

Type II cells are more resistant to the damaging effects of xenobiotics and unlike type I cells, they retain the ability to undergo mitotic division. Following damage to type I cells, increased numbers of mitoses are evident in type II cells which results in the appearance of large undifferentiated epithelial cells which ultimately differentiate into type I and type II cells (Dormans, 1983).

The *alveolar brush cell* (type III cell) is a cell of disputed function. It is described in rodents and man and constitutes only 1 to 5% of all lung cells. It is a pyramidal cell located principally at the junction of septa with a microvillous brush border on the surface.

Neurosecretory cells (Kultschitsky or APUD cells) are located in the epithelial surface of the larynx, trachea bronchi, bronchioles and alveoli (Becker and

Gazdar, 1985). These cells are oval or cuboidal with oval nuclei, argyrophilic cytoplasm which electron microscopic examination shows to contain dense core granules. The role of neuroendocrine cells in the lung is uncertain but immunocytochemical study has shown them to contain neurone-specific enolase and a variety of peptides similar to vasoactive intestinal peptide, bombesin, calcitonin, serotonin, leu-encephalin, β-endorphin and ACTH (Becker and Gazdar, 1985; Sturgess, 1985).

Cells lining the bronchi, bronchioles and alveolar walls are also capable of metabolising xenobiotics.Immunocytochemical study has shown the presence of immune-reactive cytochromes P450, NADPH cytochrome P450 reductase, epoxide hydroxylase and glutathione S-transferase in bronchial epithelial cells, ciliated bronchiolar cells, Clara cells, type II and possibly type I pneumocytes in the rat lung (Baron et al., 1988). Baron and colleagues showed that the different cell populations contained different amounts of enzymes, Clara cells containing the greatest concentrations of the phenobarbitone-inducible isoenzyme of cytochrome P450, NADPH-cytochrome P450 reductase and epoxide hydrolase. Furthermore, enzymes were inducible in some, but not all cells. Pulmonary microsomal mixed function oxidases have been shown to be induced to different degrees by cigarette smoke in various mouse strains (Abramson and Hutton, 1975).

Other important cells are the pulmonary alveolar macrophages and lymphocytes. Lymphocytes are found in the epithelium of the airways, in the interstitium of alveoli and as part of follicles in bronchial walls.

Pulmonary macrophages form part of the specific human immune defence system of the lung, involving, as elsewhere in the body, the complex role of antigen presentation. In the rat and mouse, distinctive populations of pulmonary macrophages have been described based on enzyme activities and reactivities to monoclonal antibodies against monocyte and macrophages surface determinates (van de Brugge-Gamelkoorn et al., 1985a; Breel et al., 1988). Bronchus associated macrophages in rat and mouse have more acid phosphatase and less non-specific esterase activity than the populations found in the pulmonary alveoli and interstitial tissues.

An important anatomical region of the immune system is the *bronchus-associated lymphoid tissue* or BALT, which forms part of the mucosal lymphoid system found in other epithelia, notably the gastrointestional tract. The morphology of BALT can be a useful guide to the nature and degree of immune stimulus reacting in the lung.

Structurally, the BALT is organised in a way which is characteristic of other peripheral lymphoid organs. Its organisation and function has been particularly well studied in the laboratory rat where it closely resembles the BALT in other laboratory animal species including the mouse, rabbit, guinea pig as well as man (Bienenstock et al., 1973; van der Brugge-Gamelkoorn and Kraal, 1985; Breel et al., 1988). Its size and prominance is species and strain-dependent as well as a function of the degree of antigenic stimulus. Bienenstock and colleagues (1973) were unable to demonstrate the presence of BALT in their strain of golden hamsters.

In the rat, the BALT is composed of lymphoid aggregates or follicles located mostly between a bronchus and artery with a zone of lymphocytes situated immediately under the bronchial epithelium. As in other peripheral lymphoid tissue, BALT is organised into B and T-cell zones but in no predetermined manner. Immunocytochemical staining has shown that B and T lymphocyte zones differ in location from one aggregate to another.

In the rat BALT, it has been shown that there are about two T lymphocytes for every three B cells compared with a ratio of 2:5 in rat Peyer's particles (van der Brugge-Gamelkoorn and Sminia, 1985). The ratios may be different in other species. In the rabbit equal percentages of B and T cells have been found in both BALT and Peyers patches (Rudzik et al., 1975).

Quantitative observations of T-cell subsets using monoclonal antibody clones W3/13, W3/25 and OX8 have also shown that rat BALT contains twice as many T-helper as T-suppressor/cytotoxic lymphocytes (van der Brugge and Sminia, 1985). The T cells are confined to one or two discrete zones with a light scattering of T cells within the B-cell zones and immediately under the bronchial epithelium.

These numbers appear to correlate with the different numbers of B and T lymphocytes which enter these lymphoid aggregates through the high endothelial venules. Binding assays have shown that there are differences in the adherence specificity of high endothelial venules in rat BALT compared with those in mesenteric lymphoid tissue (van der Brugge-Gamelkoorn and Kraal, 1985).

In common with lymph nodes, Ia-positive interdigiting cells are found in T cell zones of BALT which, in view of their expression of Ia antigen, can be demonstrated in the rat using the mouse monoclonal antibody MRC OX4 (van der Brugge-Gamelkoorn et al., 1985a). In B cell zones, interdigiting cells are also found and they can be demonstrated in rat BALT as in lymph nodes using mouse monoclonal MRC OX2 (van der Brugge-Gamelkoorn et al., 1985a).

The epithelium overlying BALT shows anatomical modifications. It is composed of ciliated and non-ciliated cells covered by microvilli. Cells express the Ia-antigen and are probably involved in immune recognition.

The conventional, untreated laboratory rats, BALT shows little activity and germinal centres are usually absent. BALT is also present in germ free animals although it is less pronounced than in conventional rats (Bienenstock et al., 1973).

In the young Wistar rats studied by van der Brugge-Gamelkoorn and colleagues (1985b, 1986) germinal centres were not seen in BALT in untreated animals but they developed following the administration of a single intratracheal dose of lipopolysaccharide, a T-cell-independent antigen. Single intratracheal doses of T-cell dependent antigens such as horseradish peroxidase, bovine serum albumin and BCG, only produced minor morphological changes which included expansion of the zone of lymphocytes immediately under the epithelium and infiltration of the bronchial epithelium overlying BALT by lymphocytes. In addition, perivascular, peribronchial or alveolar infiltrates of small and large lymphocytes and macrophages were observed in the lungs of rats given BCG.

Immunocytochemical study of the rat BALT following intratracheal challenge with horseradish peroxidase showed that the majority of cells which infiltrated the bronchial epithelium were T helper (W3/25 positive) lymphocytes (van der Brugge-Gamelkoorn et al., 1986). Furthermore, the Ia expression of the epithelial cells overlying the BALT was shown to increase, associated with electron microscopic evidence of an increase in the number and size of microvilli, a more pronounced glycocalyx and a decrease in number and size of cilia.

Immunocytochemical study of the BALT tissue in C57B1/6 mice using monoclonal antibodies to lymphoid and macrophage populations has demonstrated quite similar arrangements of cells to those in the rat with the majority of T cells belonging to the L3T4 positive (T helper) class (Breel et al., 1988).

Ultimately the pulmonary lymphatic system drains into mediastinal or cervical lymph nodes. Although among rat strains, differences in the location of lymph nodes and their drainage pattern occur, tracer studies in the Fischer 344 rat using colloidal carbon have shown that the lung lymphatics drain mainly into posterior mediastinal lymph nodes and those in the tracheal wall drains primarily to the internal jugular and posterior cervical nodes (Takahashi and Patrick, 1987).

The mechanisms by which lung damage occur in man are not always clear, particularly interstitial lung diseases, including those related to drug therapy. Under certain circumstances, an initial insult may trigger a whole cascade of immune-mediated phenomena leading to chronic lung disease. Experimental evidence suggests that complement is an important source of mediator for the induction of acute pulmonary inflammation (Johnson et al., 1979). Stimulation of alveolar macrophages or neutrophils during phagocytosis or by chemotaxic factors increases production of enzymes which have the potential to hydrolyse elastin and collagen. It is probable that the neutrophil is an important effector cell in IgG immune complex-induced lung injury. IgA immune complexes appear capable of producing lung injury in the rat by stimulating oxygen radical formation by macrophages (Johnson et al., 1988).

It has been shown that T lymphocytes are capable of inducing vascular injury in the lung (Anderson et al., 1988). T lymphocytes are important in the development of granulomatous pneumonitis induced in the mouse by BCG (Takizawa et al., 1986).

Structural evaluation

Although a variety of fixation, embedding and staining procedures are available for light and electron microscopic examination of lung tissue, there is no substitute for initial, careful visual inspection of the lungs at autopsy. Uneven collapse of lungs on opening the thoracic cavity, discolouration or alteration in texture of the pleural or cut surface, congestion and presence of fluid in the larger airways may indicate structural damage. In rodent lungs, small pulmonary adenomas may be detectable by inspection in good light.

Fresh lung weight is also a helpful measure in lung assessment, although passive vascular engorgement can significantly affect this value. Nevertheless, studies in the normal Fischer 344 rat have shown that after exsanguination, wet lung weights show a close relationship to body weight and that dry weight of lungs consistently represent about 20% of the wet weights regardless of age or body weight (Tillery and Lehnert, 1986a). It has been suggested that an increase in wet weight over dry weight is a good index of pulmonary oedema. However as pulmonary transudate or exudate is protein rich, dry lung weight may also increase to a variable extent when there is an increase in pulmonary fluid (Nemery et al., 1987).

Various methods of fixation have been employed although simple immersion fixation in formalin for conventional light microscopy has the virtue of simplicity and it avoids the risk of translocating or removing exudates from airways and alveoli. Mixtures of formaldehyde, paraformaldehyde and glutaraldehyde are used in initial fixation for electron microscopy (Tyler et al., 1985). Better appreciation of lung architecture is achieved by instillation of fixative via the trachea under an appropriate constant pressure or by perfusion fixation of the pulmonary arteries which is less liable to dislodge intraalveolar exudate. However, even with care, significant artefact can result from airway instillation or vascular perfusion fixation (Michel, 1985).

The sampling procedure is an important aspect of histological examination of the lungs, particularly for examination of lungs from large laboratory animals. The extent of histological sectioning in conventional toxicity studies should be modulated to take account of lesions found by macroscopic examination, the type of study and the nature of the test substance. Morphometric analysis represents a sensitive tool which can be of great value in the evaluation of drug-induced lung changes, but it requires a particularly rigorous sampling procedure. A tiered or multiple stage sampling technique is normally considered the most appropriate for morphometric studies (Barry and Crapo, 1985). This involves dividing the lung into a series of homogeneous compartments or strata from which randomly selected samples can be examined by appropriate light or electron microscopic techniques.

As in other tissues, immunocytochemistry or enzyme cytochemistry are useful additional techniques but they are particularly helpful in the study of the heterogeneous cell population of the lung. Xenobiotic metabolising activity can be studied both by enzyme cytochemical methods as well as by immunocytochemical techniques using antisera specific for pulmonary monooxygenases and related enzymes. Important structural components, particularly collagens and laminin can be studied both at light and ultrastructural level with immunocytochemical methods (Gil and Martinez-Hernadez, 1984).

Endothelial cells of the Fischer 344 rat pulmonary vasculature may be demarcated immunocytochemically by some antisera to factor VIII-related antigens and this can be helpful in the study of changes in lung endothelium (Tillery and Lehnert, 1986b), although this may not be a reliable stain for endothelial cells in all organs (see Integumetary System, Chapter I). Other antigens which can be usefully demonstrated in the lung include surfactants, lysozyme, immunoglobulins, T lymphocyte surface markers as well as a variety of microorganisms which infect the lung (Linniola and Petrusz, 1984).

Inflammation due to infections and infestations

Lower respiratory tract infection is generally not a major health hazard among laboratory animals but it is nevertheless an ever present threat which can cause overt respiratory disease within a colony or develop following administration of xenobiotics. Subclinical pulmonary infections and infestations can also produce histological alterations in the bronchial airways or pulmonary parenchyma which mimic changes induced by inhaled irritants or systemically administered drugs. Furthermore, some respiratory pathogens alter immune defences and exacerbate the effects of inhaled substances (Jakab, 1981).

Typically, bacterial pathogens such as Steptococcus pneumoniae produce acute bronchitis associated with a variable degree of acute inflammation of the lung parenchyma (*bronchopneumonia)* or a confluent *lobar pneumonia*. Viral agents are generally associated with histological features of *bronchiolitis* and *interstitial pneumonia*, characterised by an increase in mononuclear cells in the respiratory bronchioles and alveolar septa. However, the histological features are variable for they depend on the particular pathogen, species and strain, immune status, presence or absence of secondary infection and the particular stage at which the infection is examined. In addition, respiratory infections are frequently mixed. Changes due to secondary bacterial infection are frequently superimposed on those induced by viruses.

Nevertheless, sequential histopathological examination of the lungs of laboratory animals following inoculation with respiratory tract pathogens have been able to characterise changes produced by individual oganisms.

An example of this is provided by studies of rats infected with *Mycoplasma pulmonis*, one of the more important intercurrent respiratory pathogens among laboratory rodents. Following inoculation, LEW and F344 rats were shown to develop an upper and lower respiratory tract inflammatory process. In the LEW strain this was characterised after 28 days by a variable acute inflammatory exudate in bronchi and bronchioles with focal bronchiectasis, inflammation and hyperplasia of the epithelium with a predominately macrophage infiltration of the alveoli and aveolar walls (Davis and Cassell, 1982). These changes were associated with marked hyperplasia of the bronchus-associated lymphoid tissue (BALT) which extended further down the airways and blood vessels towards the periphery of the lungs. Although the lymphoid hyperplasia was also found in inoculated F344 rats, it was less marked and accompanied by little or no mucopurulent exudate or active inflammation of the bronchial walls.

Similar studies have been conducted in both rats and mice infected with another important respiratory pathogen of laboratory rodents, *Sendai Virus* (parainfluenza type 1). Sequential studies have shown that the initial damage to bronchial and bronchiolar epithelium is associated with polymorphonuclear and lymphocytic inflammation (bronchiolitis) which immunocytochemical and ultra-structural studies show is accompanied by the presence of viral antigen in the mucosa (Jakab, 1981). Hyperplastic and multinucleated syncytial epithelial cells develop in the hyperplastic terminal bronchiolar epithelium. Subsequently, the inflammatory process extends to involve peribronchial or peribronchiolar parenchyma with infiltration of alveolar walls by mononuclear cells, macro-phages and neutrophils. A similar cell population accompanied by cell debris and oedema fluid develops in air spaces. Pulmonary arteries show only modest involvement with mild infiltration by inflammatory cells and focal reactive hyperplasia of the endothelium. Immunocytochemistry and ultrastructural ex-amination has suggested that virus replication take place in alveolar type I and type II epithelial cells and macrophages but not in endothelial or interstitial cells of the alveolar septae (Castleman et al., 1987).

Subsequently, repair occurs but there may be residual distortion of bronchio-lar and alveolar walls by collagen. Hyperplastic cuboidal epithelium may line thickened alveolar septa and air spaces contain enlarged macrophages with pale vacuolated cytoplasm (Castleman, 1983).

The *Corona virus* which causes *sialodacryoadenitis* in many rat colonies also produces lower respiratory tract inflammation. This is characterised by acute bronchitis and bronchiolitis with focal extension into lung parenchyma. This is shown by thickened oedematous, hypercellular alveolar walls infiltrated by monocytic cells (Wojcinski and Percy, 1986). Immunocytochemistry has shown the presence of viral antigen in bronchial and bronchiolar epithelial cells. There is also peribronchial lymphocytic infiltration and increased prominance of BALT but ultimately complete resolution occurs.

Castleman (1985) has also shown a similar evolution of histological changes and antigen localisation in the lungs of young beagle dogs experimentally inoculated with canine adenovirus type 2. It is of note that viruses remain a potential source of spontaneous respiratory disease in laboratory dogs. Canine adenovirus type 2, parainfluenza SV5, canine herpes virus, coronavirus and parvovirus have all been isolated from laboratory dogs developing respiratory disease (Binn et al., 1979).

The syndrome of *visceral larva migrans* also incites focal inflammation, granulomas and fibrosis in the lungs of species such as dog and primate in which parasites are prevalent. The syndrome of visceral larva migrans is usually defined as that which results from the migration of nematode larvae into the viscera.

It has been well-described in the beagle dog lung where it results from the larvae of toxocara species or metastrongyloid nematodes (Barron and Saunders, 1966; Hirth and Hottendorf, 1973). The precise identification of parasites is not always possible in tissue sections. Histological appearances of infested lungs are highly variable. Nematodes surrounded by granulomas and granulomatous in-flammation, mostly in a subpleural location, may be visible in sections. In affected lungs there may be perivasculitis and active arteriolitis, bronchiolitis and peribronchiolitis. Pleural involvement by the inflammatory process can be marked, particularly in regions overlying granulomas. Scarring develops and pleural and subpleural fibrosis is frequently associated with epithelial hyperplasia and squamous metaplasia of the associated airways (Hirth and Hottendorf, 1973). The lesions may sufficiently marked to resemble those induced by high doses of anticancer drugs such as bleomycin (see below).

Pulmonary acariasis is a common infestation of many species of non-human primates caused by various species of the mite Pneumonyssus. Although it is most prevalent in wild caught primates, the disease is not easily eliminated during breeding in captivity (Joseph et al., 1984). As the mite can produce significant destructive pulmonary pathology and render animals susceptible to secondary pulmonary bacterial infections, pulmonary acariasis possesses considerable potential to disrupt or confound the interpretation of toxicity studies performed in primates.

Macroscopically, lesions are characterised by the presence of bullae distending the pleural surface, parenchymal cysts, nodules and scar tissue located most frequently in cranial lobes (Joseph et al., 1984; Kim, 1988). Histologically, there is a wide range of inflammatory activity. Fully developed lesions are characterised by granulomatous bronchiolitis and peribronchiolitis with involvement of immediately adjacent alveoli. Cystic lesions involving the bronchiolar walls develop around the parasites giving rise to the appearance of walled-off cysts composed of highly cellular granulation tissue, associated with neutrophils, lymphocytes, macrophages, multinucleated giant cells and various pigments (see below). In less active lesions, cystically dilated airways composed of walls with thick bands of smooth muscle and lined by squamous or cuboidal epithelium are found (Joseph et al., 1984).

Reproduction of the mites appears to take place in the terminal bronchioles. Pneumonyssus simicola is the recognised form found in rhesus monkeys (Kim, 1988).

Pneumocystis carinii is an important cause of pneumonia in patients with the acquired immunodeficiency syndrome (AIDS) as well as in other immunocompromised patients including those treated with immunosupressive drugs (Walzer, 1986). The natural habitat of *Pneumocystis carinii* is pulmonary alveoli and it is widely encountered in the human population without being associated with overt disease. Both clinical and experimental evidence suggests that impaired cellular immunity is much more important as a predisposing factor than impaired humoral immunity (Walzer, 1986).

As in man, laboratory animals may have latent pneumocystis infection which becomes clinically evident following immunosuppression. It has been shown in the rat that chronic administration of various regimens of adenocorticosteroids, low protein diets, cyclophosphamide and other immunosuppressive drugs with concomitant antibiotic administration to prevent other infections gives rise to typical pneumocystis pneumonia (Chandler et al., 1979). Rodents with genetically deficient cellular immunity also develop pneumocystis pneumonia (Fig. 37).

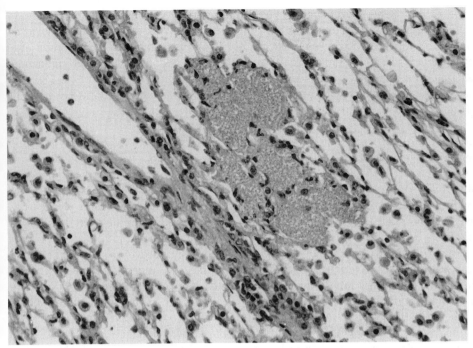

Fig. 37. Lung from an immune deficient ('nude') mouse showing the typical granular eosinophilic appearances of pneumocystis within the air spaces. (HE, ×500.)

In haematoxylin and eosin stained sections, pneumocystis pneumonia is characterised in both man and rodents by the presence of alveoli filled with foamy eosinophilic material containing a few macrophages and indistinct nuclei of pneumocystis (Fig. 37). Ovoid or crescent-shaped structures of the organisms become clearly visible with Gomori methenamine silver or toluidine blue stains.

Ultrastructural study of rats with pneumocystis pneumonia shows that trophozoites attach themselves most frequently to type I pneumocytes by altering their morphology to the contours of the pneumocytes rather than by a process of invasion (Long et al., 1986).

The importance of pneumocystis pneumonia in toxicology is that it can be considered as a sentinal of chronic immune depression.

Drug-induced inflammation

Systemically administered therapeutic agents may produce histological changes within the lung parenchyma which mimic components of the normal response to respiratory pathogens. A prime example of this phenomenon occurs following the administration of interleukin-2.

Interleukin-2 is a glycoprotein lymphokine, molecular weight 15000, which is normally produced by activated T cells and mediates immunoregulatory responses. It has been produced in large quantities by recombinant DNA technology for use in tumour immunotherapy where high doses have been associated with a number of adverse effects notably the *vascular leak syndrome*. This syndrome is characterised clinically by pulmonary oedema, pleural effusions and ascites (Rosenberg et al., 1987).

A similar vascular leak syndrome has been reported in laboratory animals given high doses of this agent. Histological examination of the lungs of B6D2F, mice developing this syndrome following administration of the interleukin-2 showed infiltration of the alveolar walls with large lymphocytes and intra-alveolar proteinaceous exudate containing large lymphocytes, macrophages and red blood cells (Anderson et al., 1988). In addition, pulmonary venules and arterioles showed the presence of lymphocytes attached to or lying beneath the endothelium, infiltrating vessel walls or in a perivascular location where they were accompanied by oedema fluid or red blood cells. Similar, but less severe changes have been demonstrated in rats given interleukin-2 (Anderson and Hayes, 1989). In addition, treated rats showed an infiltration of pulmonary vasculature with eosinophils probably secondary to an eosinopoietic cytokine produced by interleukin-2 stimulated lymphocytes.

Immunocytochemical evaluation of the lymphoid infiltrate in mice showed that most of the cells were Thy 1.2-positive lymphocytes. Furthermore, co-administration of asialo GM1 (ganglio-n-tetrosyl-ceremide) with interleukin-2 not only abrogated the clinical signs but reduced the number of asialo GM1-positive lymphocytes in the tissue sections.

As lymphoid cells expressing Lyt-2 (suppressor/cytotoxic T cells) were unaffected by asialo GM1 treatment, it was postulated that the vascular leak syndrome (but not antitumour efficacy) in these mice was mediated by an endogenous subset of interleukin-2 stimulated lymphocytes or lymphokine-activated killer cells (Anderson et al., 1988). Corresponding changes were also observed in liver and lymphoid tissue (see Liver, Chapter VIII, and Haemopoietic and Lymphatic Sytems, Chapter III).

As in man, severe chronic pulmonary inflammatory disease in laboratory animals may compromise pulmonary function and lead to secondary alterations in other organs. Although the mechanisms were not explored in detail, a diffuse interstitial pulmonary inflammatory process with lung haemorrhage was induced in rats treated for two years with prizidilol (SK and F 92657-A2), an antihypertensive agent with both vasodilatory and β-adenoceptor blocking properties (Sutton et al., 1986). Affected animals developed dyspnoea associated with reduction in lung volume, deformity of the thoracic spinal column and marked cardiac hypertrophy.

Granuloma, granulomatous inflammation

Inflammation with a granulomatous component develops in the lungs of laboratory animals under a variety of different circumstances which have been alluded to above. A common cause in rodents is the response to accidently inhaled

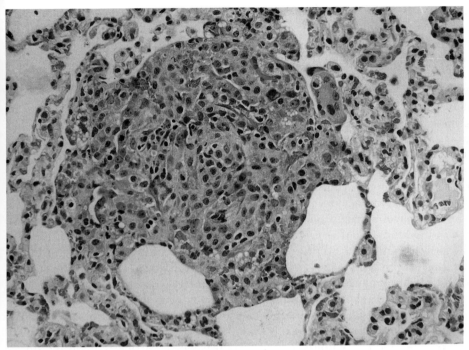

Fig. 38. Granuloma of uncertain cause found in the lung of an untreated, aged Sprague-Dawley rat. It is composed mainly of macrophages with occasional giant cells. (HE, ×500.)

foreign bodies and they may also be found without obvious causation (Fig. 38). Lipid granulomas with cholesterol clefts and fibrosis develop focally in response to lipid released from foamy macrophages which accumulate in rats with increasing age or in drug-induced phospholipidosis. As dogs and primates are more liable to be infested by parasites, granulomatous inflammation in response to pulmonary larvae is more common in these species.

Another form of granulomatous pulmonary inflammation results from aspiration of stomach contents or food particles (*aspiration pneumonia*). This is sporadically observed in aged rats where it is associated with general ill-health, particuarly resulting from pressure effects of large pituitary adenomas and subsequent disturbance of pharangeal or laryngeal reflex mechanisms (Dixon and Jure, 1988). Histologically, the lungs show peribronchial and peribronchiolar granulomatous inflammation with macrophages and foreign body cells associated with fragments of refractile vegetable matter. Bronchial mucosa also shows goblet cell hyperplasia in long-standing cases.

Pulmonary tuberculosis represents a potential problem among non-human primate colonies in view of its insidious onset and its liability for transmission from monkeys to man (Wolf et al., 1988). Pathological findings are similar to those so well known in the human disease. The disease is characterised by the presence of granulomas in lung parenchyma and lymph nodes. In florid cases there may be caseation surrounded by epitheloid and multinucleated giant cells and variable numbers of lymphocytes, plasma cells and fibroblasts. Diffuse granulomatous pneumonia as a result of tuberculosis is also reported in non-human primates (Wolf et al., 1988).

Granulomatous pneumonitis is produced in laboratory animals by the intravenous injection of BCG. Twenty eight days following intravenous injection of BCG, the lungs of C57B1/6 mice contained numerous granulomas composed of histiocytes and round cells which were surrounded by alveoli with thickened walls and associated with mild interstitial pneumonitis (Takizawa, 1986). These histological changes were associated with an increase in the number of Thy 1.2 positive cells, especially Lyt-1 positive lymphocytes. The histological changes were abrogated by treatment with cyclosporin A suggesting an important role for Lyt-1 positive lymphocytes in the development of the granulomas. Methotrexate is an example of a drug which is believed to produce a granulomatous inflammation in the lungs of patients (Gutin et al., 1976).

Discrete granulomas occur in the lungs of experimental animals in response to intratracheal or intravenous injection of certain relatively insoluble substances. Intratracheal administration of insoluble polymerised dextran and latex microparticles to mice showed that the morphology and the systemic effects of granulomas depended on the nature of the injected substances. Large granulomas rapidly developed in the pulmonary parenchyma around dextran particles which subsequently regressed quite quickly, whereas latex particles produced small, discrete stable granulomas (Allred et al., 1985). Although both forms of granulomas were of foreign body or non-immunological in type, those produced by dextran but not latex beads, were associated with anergy-like immunosuppression probably caused by release of soluble factors from the granulomas.

Localised, *angiocentric granulomas* of foreign body type, clustered around pulmonary arteries and arterioles and occasionally alveolar capillaries and venules also develop following intravenous injection of relatively insoluble polysaccarides or other polymers (Jonson et al., 1984). Characteristic epithelioid and large, foreign body type giant cells efface the smaller vessels although overt necrosis is not usually observed.

Oedema

Pulmonary oedema is a component of many inflammatory conditions of the lung including those induced by infections agents. However, the term oedema is reserved for a poorly cellular exudate characterised by the presence of pale, homogenous eosinophilic material in the alveoli, sometimes associated with a similar exudate in the lung septae and perivascular connective tissue, rather than inflammatory exudate. It occurs in congestive cardiac failure, it may accompany metastatic pulmonary neoplasms or be found as an agonal change in association with pulmonary congestion and haemorrhage. Inhalation of toxic chemicals also produces an acute pulmonary oedema. Some substances such as phenylthiourea and α-naphlythiourea produce massive pulmonary oedema in laboratory animals when administered orally, principally as a result of damage to the endothelium of pulmonary capillaries and venules (Keher and Kacew, 1985).

Another potentially important form of pulmonary oedema is that which involves the main airways. Precipitation of allergic reactions reactions in sensitised airways of asthmatic individuals is believed to result from cross-linking of IgE and activation of mast cells which degranulate and release inflammatory mediators (Holgate et al., 1986).

This has been shown to occur in the main airways of rats sensitised to ovalbumin and then challenged with ovalbumin by the intratracheal route (Lebargy et al., 1987). This treatment leads to rapid accumulation of bronchial exudate, degranulation of mast cells and the development of mucosal oedema, most marked immediately below the respiratory epithelium.

Congestion and haemorrhage

Congestion and haemorrhage is a frequent finding in the lungs of laboratory animals where it is usually related to certain modes of death. It can be associated with administration of drugs and chemicals which have adverse effects on cardiac function or on the coagulation system. Administration of heparin to rats produces a characteristic extravasation of blood into the air spaces (Larsen et al., 1986).

Pigment

Haemosiderin-laden macrophages accumulate in the alveoli of laboratory animals in association with chronic pulmonary congestion and haemorrhage. Similar changes occur in man particularly in congestive cardiac failure where the haemosiderin-laden macrophages are frequently termed 'heart failure' cells.

The lungs of non-human primates are especially liable to contain alveolar, perivascular and peribronchial aggregates of macrophages laden with various brown pigments. Iron-containing pigments have been associated with the inflammatory changes produced by simian lung mites (Pneumonyssus simicola) which are prevalent in many non-human primates. In addition, primate lungs commonly contain perivascular and peribronchial collections of brown-grey macrophages containing highly refractile spicules and plates composed of high concentrations of silica (Dayan et al., 1978; Kim and Cole, 1987). It has been shown that in Old World primates including rhesus and cynomologous monkeys, this pigment contains fossil diatomaceous material, compatable with the concept that the animals inhale dusts containing diatoms and other silicon fragments to which they are exposed in their semi-arid, natural habitats (Dayan et al., 1978).

Emphysema

Emphysema is characterised by abnormal, permanent enlargment of airspaces distal to terminal bronchioles, accompanied by destruction of their walls without obvious fibrosis.

Three principle types, *centriacinar*, *panacinar* and *distal acinar* emphysema are recognised in man. Enlargement of air spaces as a result of congenital factors or fibrous scarring are grouped separately and not regarded as true emphysemas (Snider et al., 1986).

Although emphysema is occasionally observed as an age-related spontaneous change in laboratory rodents (Levame, 1980), several experimental rodent emphysema models have been developed, using intratracheal instillation of proteolytic enzymes papain, pancreatic and neutrophil elastase. This gives rise to histological appearances resembling panacinar emphysema in man. Elastase enters the alveolar wall via type I pneumocytes and spreads through the lung interstitium producing degradation of elastin fibres with associated oedema and cellular exudate. Elastase finally enters the blood where it is inactivated and cleared by the pulmonary circulation. Eventually the alveolar exudate clears and air space enlargement occurs (See review Snider et al., 1986). Intravenous administration of elastase may also induce emphysema but higher doses are required.

Irritant gases notably oxides of nitrogen are also capable of inducing changes in the lungs of laboratory rats and hamsters following long term exposure which resemble mild human, centrilobular emphysema (Juhos et al., 1980; Lam et al., 1985).

Fibrosis

Pulmonary fibrosis is a common sequelae of chronic lower respiratory tract inflammation. It may be associated with, or preceded by interstitial pneumonitis, characterised by infiltration by lymphocytes, plasma cells and macrophages with scattered polymorphonuclear cells (Singer et al., 1986).

In man, conditions leading to pulmonary fibrosis vary widely. They include infections, shock lung syndrome, ionizing radiation, exposure to antigens or excessive amounts of oxygen as well as the results of the toxicity of paraquat and some therapeutic agents (Johnson et al., 1979) Focal pulmonary fibrosis occurs spontaneously in laboratory animals, although this is usually most prevalent in dogs and non-human primates as a response to chronic infestation by parasites which are not easily eliminated during breeding.

The principle therapeutic agents which produce pulmonary fibrosis in man and laboratory animals are anticancer drugs. Bleomycin, a glycopeptide preparation derived from Streptomyces verticillus is the best known example but pulmonary fibrosis is also associated with the clinical use of 1,3-bis-(2-chloroethyl)-1-nitrosourea (BCNU or carmustine), cyclophosphamide, busulphan, mitomycin C and methotrexate (Weiss and Muggia, 1980; Kehrer and Kacew, 1985).

The mechanisms involved in the induction of pulmonary fibrosis by antineoplastic drugs in man are poorly understood. The fibrosis can be accentuated by concomitant administration of several antineoplastic agents, radiation therapy, hyperoxia, pre-existing pulmonary damage and age of the patient. Severity is related total dose of drug received (Kehrer and Kacew, 1985).

Bleomycin was first associated with the development of interstitial pneumonia and pulmonary fibrosis in its early clinical use and this was subsequently shown to occur in experimental animals. Beagle dogs given cycles of bleomycin by the intravenous route for periods of up to 26 weeks developed anorexia, weight loss, a variety of epithelial lesions as well as focal interstitial pneumonia and fibrosis (Thompson et al., 1972). In the dog study reported by Thompson and colleagues (1972), pulmonary lesions were restricted to pleural and subpleural surfaces. Histologically, the lesions were those of a focal interstitial pneumonia and fibrosis characterised by increased elastic fibres, reticulin, collagen and acid mucosubstances. The lesions were situated predominantly in the pleural and subpleural zones, suggestive of a potentiating effect of friction between the pleural surfaces. Histologically the lesions resembled those produced by larvae migrans in the dog. Similar histological changes have also been described in both rats and mice treated with bleomycin by both the intravenous and intratracheal route (Thrall et al., 1979; Lindenschmidt et al., 1986). As fibrosis is such a consistent change, bleomycin-treated rodents have been extensively employed as a model for pulmonary fibrosis. Early changes include mild, diffuse increase in interstitial lymphocytes, macrophages, a few polymorphonuclear cells and perivascular or interstitial oedema. After about a week, interstitial infiltrates also comprise fibroblasts with early collagen deposition, associated with proliferation of macrophages and type II pneumocytes (Thrall et al., 1979; Lindenschmidt et al., 1986). Subsequently, the amount of interstitial collagen increases, with eventual scarring and collapse of lung tissue which appears to be proportional to the culmulative dose given (Brown et al, 1988). Immunohistochemical and ultrastructural study of rats and mice treated with bleomycin shows large accumulation of immune-reactive laminin and reduplication of the basement lamina within the thickened alveolar walls (Singer et al., 1986).

Other findings in bleomycin-treated rats which have been demonstrated by three dimensional scanning electron microscopy have been changes in pulmonary capillary structure. Treatment produces irregular alveolar and pleural capillaries with increased diameter and decreased branching (Schraufnagel et al., 1986).

It is also of interest that certain strains of mice have been shown to respond to bleomycin with a greater degree of fibrosis. The C57BL/6 strain produces a greater fibroblastic response than DBA/2 and Swiss mice. The BALB/C strain demonstrates a particularly poor fibroblastic response (Schrier et al., 1983).

Although it is difficult to critically compare the histopathological appearances of bleomycin induced pulmonary fibrosis in animals with findings in patients treated with this agent because of confounding factors of the primary neoplastic disease, multiple drug and radiation therapy as well as secondary pulmonary infections, interstitial pneumonitis and fibrosis are clearly associated with bleomycin therapy in cancer patients (Luna et al., 1972).

Therapeutic use of cyclophosphamide is also occasionally associated with the development of pulmonary interstitial fibrosis (Weiss and Muggia, 1980) although typical interstitial changes have been less easy to reproduce in laboratory animals. When mice were sequentially examined for periods of up to one year after a single intravenous dose of 100 mg/kg of cyclophosphamide, only slight pulmonary interstitial thickening and hypercellularity was observed in association with progressive multifocal accumulation of intra-alveolar macrophages (Morse et al., 1985). However, these changes were also accompanied by a progressive increase in pulmonary hydroxyproline content and a decrease in pulmonary compliance with time in treated animals compared with controls. The changes were amplified by exposure to 70% ambient oxygen.

Phospholipidosis (lipidosis)

A variety of different names have been applied to membrane-bound, acid phosphatase-positive cytoplasmic inclusions with lamellated or crystalloid ultrastructural matrix. These include *myeloid bodies, myelinoid bodies, myelin figures* or *myelinosomes*. These lysosomal inclusions are seen in small numbers in a variety of normal cell types, but they accumulate in various organs following administration of a wide variety of xenobiotics. A characteristic and generalised accumulation of these cytoplasmic inclusions is reported in laboratory animals following repeated administration of a number of amphiphilic, cationic drugs. Examples include the anorectic drug chlorphentermine, tricyclic antidepressants, inhibitors of cholesterol biosynthesis such as triparanol, the antihistamine, chlorcyclizine and its analogues and the antioestrogen, tamoxifen (Lüllmann et al., 1975; Lüllmann and Lüllmann-Rauch, 1981). Furthermore, similar findings have been reported in man as well as in laboratory animals following therapy with chloroquine. The cardiovascular drugs amiodarone, 4, 4'-diethylaminoethoxyhexestrol and perhexiline (Lüllmann-Rauch, 1979). Generalised accumulation of lysosomal cytoplasmic bodies is generally called *phospholipidosis*, a term coined to describe the tissue accumulation of phospholipids (Shikata et al, 1972). Many tissues and organs develop the cytoplasmic inclusions including lymphoid cells, liver, pancreas, endocrine tissue, nervous system, muscle cells and eyes but it is frequently the lungs which are prominantly affected in laboratory rodents treated with these agents (Figs. 39 and 40).

It has been suggested that the lungs are especially vulnerable to drug-induced phospholipidosis because macrophages are in very close proximity to blood-borne agents (Reasor, 1981). The continuous uptake of phospholipid-rich surfactant material from the alveoli by macrophages leads to excessive accumulation of phospholipids when their catabolism is impaired (Lüllmann et al., 1975).

The fact that lungs are commonly affected is a potentially useful diagnostic feature because in many organs phospholipidosis can be extremely difficult to recognize by light microscopy of haematoxylin and eosin-stained sections. Although the changes in the lungs are not specific for drug-induced phospholipidosis, an increase in the number of lipid-contain lung macrophages in treated animals compared with controls is relatived easy to detect and provides a simple way for the pathologist to screen for this effect.

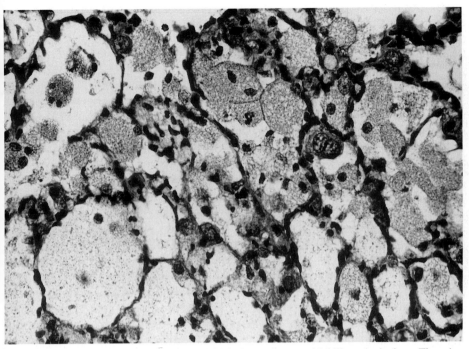

Fig. 39. Lung from a Wistar rat treated with high doses of an amphiphilic cationic drug. There is an accumulation of foamy macrophages in the alveolar spaces. (HE, ×550.)

It should be noted that peripheral lymphocytes are also sensitive to phospholipidosis and cytoplasmic vacuoles representing cytoplasmic myelinoid inclusions may be visualized in routine peripheral blood smears by light microcospy. (Lüllmann et al., 1975). In other organs, phospholipidosis also presents as cellular vacuolization. This may be associated with the presence of neutral lipid and therefore stain with oil red O. This can give the misleading impression of an accumulation of neutral fat (fatty change) rather than phospholipid.

In severe generalised phopholipidosis in rats, the lungs show irregular pale grey or yellowish patches of discolouration of the pleura and parenchyma. This is a result of patchy or confluent aggregrates of large, pale, foamy macrophages, free lying or packed in alveoli and commonly accompanied by granular, extracellular material (Fig. 39). Their abundant cytoplasm shows a vacuolated appearance in which fine eosinophilic granules are sometimes visible. The nuclei are rounded and centrally located structures of variable size. Multilaminated cells are also occasionally seen, as are vacuolated cells firmly attached to alveolar walls, probably pneumocytes. These foamy cells stain typically for phospholipids (eg. acid haematin), although neutral lipid may also be present and stain with oil red O.

In semi-thin plastic embedded sections stained with toluidine blue, the phospholipidosis is better characterized in all organs including the lungs (Fig. 40).

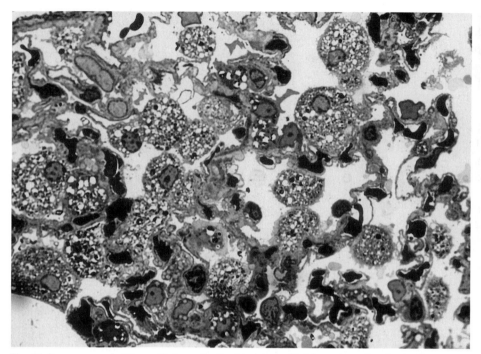

Fig. 40. Same case as in Figure 39, formalin fixed but embedded in resin and stained with toluidine blue. Dark cytoplasmic droplets characteristic of phospholipidosis are visible in the macrophages. (Toluidine blue, ×1400.)

The macrophages in the air spaces contain unmistakable dense, dark round cytoplasmic inclusions of variable size, some over 5 mm diameter (Heath et al., 1985). Plastic embedded sections also show the inclusions in other pulmonary cells including pneumocytes attached to the alveolar walls from which they can be seen discharging into the alveolar spaces.

As in other organs affected by phospholipidosis, ultrastructural examination reveals dense, multilamellated membranes and numerous heterogeneus dense bodies of lysosomal origin. These bodies need to be distinguished from membranous bodies which form as a result of fixation for ultrastructural study. Lipids tend to leach out and become hydrated to form myelinoid membranes during glutaraldehyde fixation. These structures are subsequently fixed by osmium to give rise to electron-dense membranous figures both outside and inside cells particularly in mitochondria where they may be mistaken for pathological lesions (Ghadially, 1980; Lullmann-Rauch, 1979; Costa-Jussà et al., 1984; Robinson et al., 1985).

The laminated patterns seen in phospholipidosis may be simple alternating dense and clear lines spaced at 4–5 nm, or more complex arrangements of clear and dense lines. (Lüllmann-Rauch, 1979). The other typical crystalloid inclusions of hexagonal aggregates of tubular subunits seen in other organs, are not usually found in the lungs. The significance of these various forms is uncertain but they probably represent the various phases in which phospholipids exist and which are influenced by proportions of lipids present. (Lüllmann-Rauch, 1979). Electron microscopic examination reveals that not only are pulmonary macrophages affected by these changes but that inclusions may be present in pneumocytes types I and II, pulmonary capillary endothelial cells, smooth muscle cells, bronchiolar epithelium and occasionally neutrophils (Lüllmann-Rauch and Reil, 1974; Costa-Jussà et al., 1984; Robinson et al., 1985). The changes are typically still visible several weeks after withdrawal from treatment with the offending agent.

The accumulation of foamy macrophages in the alveolar spaces also occurs as a spontaneous change in aging rats (Yang et al., 1966). In contrast to drug-induced changes, the spontanous lipidosis occurs sporadically in older rats and is observed in both controls and treated animals. Drug-induced phopholipidosis occurs within a period of several months, during which lungs of control animals remain fairly free of spontaneous, foam-cell accumulation.

Although the extent of pulmonary phospholipidosis in the lungs may vary between therepeutic regimen and species, studies with chlorphentermine, 4, 4'-diethylaminoethoxyhexestrol and amiodarone have indicated that similar cytological and ultrastructural changes occur in most laboratory animal species studied including rats, mice, hamsters, guinea pigs, rabbits, dog and man (Lüllmann-Rauch and Reil, 1974; de la Iglesia et al., 1975; Costa-Jussà et al., 1984; Mazué et al., 1984).

Drugs which cause generalised phosopholipidosis in laboratory animals have been reviewed in the papers by Lüllmann and collegues (1975) and Reasor (1981). Inducing agents are of quite different therapeutic classes but they usually share structural features including a hydrophilic cationic side chain, a primary, secondary or tertiary amine and a hydrophobic region which is usually an aromatic ring or ring system. As this structural pattern renders these molecules amphiphilic, these drugs probably bind with polar lipids by means of electrostatic and hydrophobic forces (Lüllmann et al., 1975).

This leads to formation of drug-lipid complexes which are poorly degraded by lysosomal enzymes and which accumulate in the cell cytoplasm to form the inclusions described above.

As the binding is not covalent, its reversibility depends on the dissociation rate constant under the particular intracellular conditions and drug concentration achieved.

Predictions of this activity based on molecular structure have shown reasonably good correlation with the ability of compounds to produce phospholipidosis in cultured rat peritoneal macrophages (Lüllmann-Rauch, 1979). These correlations have been less good when whole animal data are evaluated, presumably because of differences in drug disposition in blood and tissues.

Although not all agents which produce phospholipidosis in animals have been studied in man, only some of these drugs are capable of inducing phospholipidosis in human clinical practice. Agents such as chloroquine, 4,4'-diethylamin-dethoyhexestrol and amiodarone which are capable of producing phospholipido-sis in man also induce frank cellular damage in the same organs. Although it is not always clear whether the phenomena are causally related, these findings have implications for the safety assessment of novel drugs which produce phospholiposis in animals.

An example of this problem is the iodinated benzofuran derivative amiodarone, an antiarrhymic drug effective against ventricular arrythmias. Phospholipidosis occurs in a wide variety of organs in laboratory animals treated with amiodarone (Mazué et al., 1984; Riva et al., 1987) and is reported to occur in man at therapeutic doses in liver, peripheral nerve cells, skin, lymphoid cells and lungs (Costa-Jussà et al., 1984; Shepherd et al., 1987; Fan et al., 1987). Whereas phospholipidosis induced by amiodarone in the lungs of rodents is not associated with fibrosis or significant functional alterations (Riva et al., 1987; Heath et al., 1985), pulmonary interstitial fibrosis may occur in association with phospholi-pidosis in man (Costa-Jussà et al., 1984). It is not certain that the accumulation of lipid-laden histiocytes and interstitial fibrosis are casually related. However, an immune-mediated mechanism has been postulated which is possibly favoured by the binding of drug to components of pulmonary tissue (Fan et al., 1987).

Despite undoubted differences in tissue and species sensitivity to development of phospholipidosis, the degree of tissue exposure to drug which relates to dose, drug disposition, metabolism and elimination are undoubtably important consid-erations. Although phospholipidosis is more likely to occur at high doses em-ployed in toxicity studies than at lower therapeutic doses used in man, this may be offset by faster elimination of the drug, characteristic of small laboratory animals (Lüllmann et al., 1975).

The potential for drugs to accumulate in critical tissues such as eye and heart are especially important when drugs are administered for long periods of time particularly as tissue/plasma ratios of some amphiphilic drug may exceed 100, following repeated administration (Lüllmann et al., 1978).

The fact that lymphocytes are predisposed to develop phospholipidosis is of interest for peripheral blood lymphocytes are relatively easily monitored for these morphologial effects in man.

It is important to underline that the mechanisms for the development of these morphological changes are complex and similar morphological changes can also result from treatment with compounds which are not considered to be cationic amphiphilic structures. An example of this is the induction of lysosomal inclu-sions in the lungs of rat and dogs by the antibiotic, erythromycin (Gray et al., 1978).

Hyperplasia

Various forms of hyperplasia are found in the lungs of laboratory animals. *Goblet cell hyperplasia* is a well recognised response of the conducting airways to chronic inflammation and inhalation of irritant substances such as cigarette smoke and sulphur dioxide (Reid, 1963; Jones et al., 1973; Coggins et al., 1980). It has also been reported to occur in the hamster emphysema model in which human neutrophil elastase is instilled by the intratracheal route (Christensen et al., 1987).

The degree of goblet cell hyperplasia is dictated by the severity and duration of the irritation or inflammatory process. However, species differences exist because the airways of laboratory animals are variably endowed with goblet cells and submucosal mucous glands. For instance, the normal rat has more goblet cells lining the airways than either mouse or hamster (Reid, 1963).

Florid cases of goblet cell hyperplasia are characterised histologically by thickening and pseudostratification of the tracheal or bronchial mucosa by a population of tall, mucus-secreting cells with abundant pale cytoplasm. In addition, goblet cells extend further down the airways than in normal animals and mucus may fill or distend the airways or impact in the alveoli (Reid, 1963). In less florid cases, a simple increase in the number of goblet cells may be found without other structural change (Coggins et al., 1980).

The factors controlling these alterations are uncertain but is has been suggested that increased mitotic activity as well as cell conversion, probably by metaplasia of serous or Clara cells to mucous cells is involved (Bolduc et al., 1981; Christensen et al., 1987).

This type of goblet cell hyperplasia of the lining epithelium may be accompanied by an increase in size of the underlying submucosal glands. This has clearly been demonstrated in patients with chronic bronchitis and in rats where submucosal glands are normally quite prominant (Reid, 1960, 1963).

Similar morphological changes can be induced by pharmacological agents. Rats given 6 or 12 daily injections of isoprenaline, a non-selective β-receptor agonist showed a dose and time-dependent increase in the number and size of alcian blue-positive goblet (mucous) cells as well as serous cells in the tracheal and bronchial mucosa. This was associated with an increase in length, width and depth of submucosal glands (Sturgess and Reid, 1973). Similar changes were produced by pilocarpine, although both alcian blue and PAS positive cells were increased in number following this agent, suggesting that pilocarpine induced both acid and neutral glycoprotein secretion.

Critical comparison of the distribution of these changes in the rat following isoprenaline, with those of salbutamol, pilocarpine and tobacco smoke showed that there were regional differences in the distribution of these changes in the airways (Reid and Jones, 1983). Isoprenaline produced a greater increase in secretory cells in peripheral airways than tobacco smoke which itself produces a greater increase in mitotic activity. Isoprenaline and pilocarpine produced a more diffuse change than the more selective β-agonist, salbutamol.

The changes induced by these therapeutic agents are presumably the result of their pharmacological activity, although the mechanisms are not clear (Reid and Jones, 1983). The changes in the rat were shown to be accompanied by hypertrophy of the pancreas, submaxillary and parotid salivary glands (Sturgess and Reid, 1973). See Digestive System, Chapter VII.

Unlike the rat and mouse, the hamster appears predisposed to develop minor multifocal epithelial hyperplasia of the tracheal and bronchial mucosa spontaneously with advancing age. These changes are flat or polypoid in nature and are composed of clear cells and goblet cells. There may be evidence of early squamous metaplasia (Pour et al., 1976, 1979).

Another form of hyperplasia which is well described in hamsters is *neuroendocrine hyperplasia*. Although small aggregates of neuroendocrine cells (neuroepithelial bodies) are found at various levels of the bronchi and bronchioli in the normal hamster, administration of nitrosamines and 4-nitroquinoline 1-oxide can produce neuroendocrine hyperplasia (Reznik-Schüller, 1977; Linnoila et al., 1981; Ito et al., 1986). Hyperplastic lesions are recognizable as groups of non-ciliated cuboidal, oval or columnar cells located in the bronchial or bronchiolar epithelium. They contain argyrophilic granules which show immunoreactivity for corticotrophin (ACTH) and neurone-specific enolase (Ito et al., 1986; Linnoila et al., 1981). Ultrastructural examination reveals the presence of dense-core cytoplasmic granules of APUD type (Reznik-Schüller, 1977; Linnoila et al., 1981; Ito et al., 1986).

Another form of hyperplasia involves the lining epithelium of the alveoli and may be termed *alveolar hyperplasia, adenomatosis, alveolar bronchiolization* or *epithelialization*. In rats, this form of hyperplasia occurs spontaneously. It can be induced by infections and administration of xenobiotics in rats (Coleman et al., 1977; Goodman et al., 1979; Kroes et al., 1981; Greaves and Faccini, 1984), mice (Ward et al., 1974, 1979) and hamsters (Rehm et al., 1989).

Whether alveolar hyperplasia results from hyperplasia of type II cells or bronchiolar cells migrating into alveoli is disputed (Rehm et al., 1989). Histologically, the lesions consist of localized but unencapsulated foci of hyperchromatic regular, cuboidal or columnar cells investing airspaces without appreciable distortion of alveolar walls.

Neoplasia

The common lung neoplasm in man, bronchogenic squamous carcinoma is only occasionally observed as a spontaneous pulmonary neoplasm in laboratory rodents including rats (Goodman et al., 1979). There is no good experimental model for small cell (oat cell) cancer which comprises about 25% of all lung cancers in man and which believed to be of neuroendocrine derivation (Becker and Gazder, 1985).

By far the most common primary pulmonary neoplasms found in laboratory rats, mice and hamsters are *adenomas and adenocarcinomas*. These appear to develop from the bronchiolar or alveolar epithelium although their precise histogenesis is somewhat disputed.

Rat

In most *rat* strains alveolar or bronchiolar neoplasms occur spontaneously in relatively small numbers, but morphologically identical neoplasia can be induced by administration of chemical carcinogens (Reznik-Schüller and Reznik, 1982). Histologically, they are mostly small, discrete, rounded nodules located in the lung parenchyma and composed of fairly uniform cells with moderately hyperchromatic nucei arranged in *solid* (alveolar), *tubular, papillary* or *mixed* growth patterns. They usually compress surrounding tissues without infiltration or metastatic spread (*adenoma*) although loss of differentiation, infiltration and spreadto adjacent tissues can occur (*adenocarcinoma*).

Ultrastructural study of bronchiolar-alveolar neoplasia in Fischer 344 rats has shown the presence of osmiophilic, lamellated inclusion bodies similar to those found in alveolar type II cells. Therefore it has been suggested that the neoplasms are derived from this cell type. (Reznik-Schüller and Reznik, 1982). However, lamellated inclusions can occur in cells of other types, including Clara cells (Rehm et al., 1989).

Mice

Analogous neoplasms are found more commonly in most strains of laboratory *mice* used in carcinogenicity bioassays although there is considerable reported variation in incidence. They are common in strain A mice where they are observed in low frequency at three to four months of age and incidences reach nearly 100% by 24 months of age (Stoner and Shimkin, 1982). Fewer, but significant numbers are found in B6C3F1 mice, although considerable interlaboratory variation in the presence of these neoplasms is reported (Tarone et al., 1981). Even in the same laboratory, mice housed under similar conditions show variation in incidence in these neoplasms with time. The incidence of lung adenomas and adenocarcinomas occurring in CD-1 mice used as controls in 18-month carcinogenicity bioassays in the same laboratory under similar conditions for a period of three years varied from between 19 to 36% in males and from 6 to 16% in females (Faccini et al., 1981). By contrast, some strains of mice such as the C5781/10J strain show a very low predisposition to lung adenomas (Tucker, 1985).

Histologically, pulmonary tumours of this type in mice are generally small, sharply circumscribed nodules composed of fairly uniform, closely packed columns of cuboidal or columnar cells arranged in tubular or papillary structures with scanty fibrovascular stroma (Figs. 41 and 42). Dedifferentation with invasion of lung parenchyma, intrabronchial growth, cellular pleomorphism and metastatic spread also occur (Stewart et al., 1979).

The precise histogenesis of mouse pulmonary adenomas and adenocarcinomas is disputed. On the basis of sequential light and electron microscopic study of pulmonary adenomas induced in Bagg-Webster Swiss mice by transplacental exposureto ethylnitrosourea, it has been suggested that they develop from either alveolar type II cells or Clara cells (Kauffman et al., 1979; Kauffman, 1981).

Careful, stepwise analysis using light microscopic and electron microscopic examination showed that adenomas fell into three principle groups. Some were composed of solid growths of uniform cuboidal cells with expanding margins

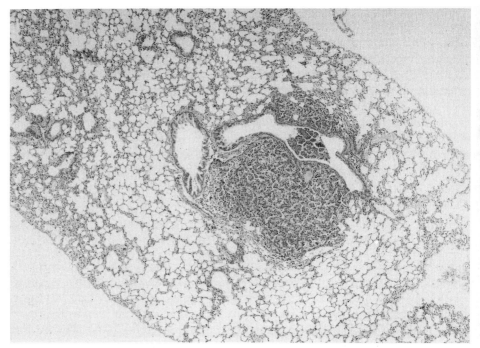

Fig. 41. Typical, small lung adenoma developing spontaneously in an aged CFLP mouse. It shows a papillary arrangement of eosinophilic cuboidal cells extending into a small airway and showing early compression of adjacent parenchyma. (HE, ×75.)

limited to alveolar septae (*alveolar pattern*). These cells contained concentrically arranged cytoplasmic lamellar bodies and abundant, large mitochondria similar to mitochondria found in alveolar type II cells. Other patterns were *tubular* or *papillary* in type, each being composed of cuboidal cells showing histological and ultrastructural features of Clara cell differentation. Based on the time sequence of development, it was suggested that tumours with a tubular arrangement evolved into papillary adenomas in this experimental model (Kauffman, 1981).

More recently, immunocytochemical studies of chemically-induced and spontaneous pulmonary neoplasia in B6C3F1, BALB/c or A strain mice have shown that the majority of adenocarcinomas, including those showing papillary patterns, contained immune-reactive surfactant apoprotein, typical of type II Clara cell antigens suggesting that most neoplasms are of alveolar type II derivation (Ward et al., 1985). Perhaps, these differences are not suprising in view of the pluripotential nature of lung precursor cells and the fact that differentiation may proceed along different pathways during tumour progression so that different antigens are expressed.

The usual high incidence and the inherent variability of pulmonary adenomas and adenocarcinomas in conventional mouse carcinogenicity bioassays sometimes gives rise to statistically significance differences between control and treatment

218

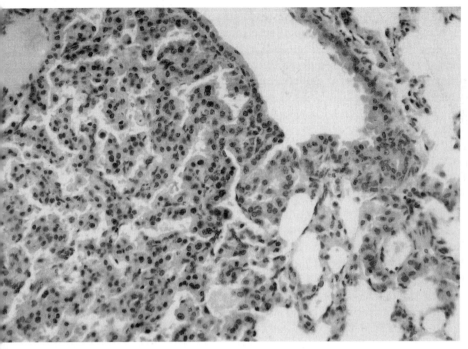

Fig. 42. Higher power view of the adenoma seen in Figure 41. (HE, ×500.)

groups. As frank genotoxic carcinogens also increase the prevalance of similar neoplasms in strain A mice, there is considerable risk in over-interpretation of such group differences in conventional mouse bioassays. In the analysis of group differences, it is important that consideration is given to tissue sampling procedure, age-standardisation, historical control incidence, effects on food intake, and the results of mutagenicity studies and carcinogenity bioassays in other rodent species.

For instance, in a carcinogenicity bioassay in which CF1 mice were treated for 80 weeks with the synthetic analgesic tilidine fumarate, a statistically significant difference (p < 0.01) was reported in the incidence of lung adenocarcinomas between the top dose female group (24%) and concurrent controls (10%) (McGuire et al., 1986). It was argued that group differences did not indicate tumorigenic potential of tilidine fumarate on the basis that the incidence in the high dose group was within the historical control range (27%) and that there was no tumorigenic effect evidence in an analogous 104 week rat carcinogenicity study.

A more difficult evaluation concerned metronidazole, a nitroimidazole, which is an important therapeutic agent active against anaerobic organisms and trichomonas species. Administration of this compound led to an increased incidence of pulmonary adenomas and carcinomas in three separate mouse carcinogenicity bioassays (Rustia and Shubik, 1972; Roe, 1983).

219

The analysis of these findings was complicated by evidence that metronidazole shows mutagenic activity in bacterial assays using some strains of Salmonella typhimurium. Roe (1983) argued that the risk to man was slight because the increase in prevalence in pulmonary tumours was likely to be a result of changes in nutritional status of the mice through the effect of metronidazole on gut flora, as similar differences could occur between ad libitum fed mice and those fed the same but restricted diet. He also suggested that the positive findings in bacterial mutagenesis assays were an inherent part of the antibacterial activity of metronidazole as a result of nitroreduction which does not occur in normal mammalian tissues. This conclusion was supported by lack of a positive effect in hamster carcinogenicity bioassays, other assays for genotoxic activity and lack of excess cancer risk in women followed up for 10 years or more (Roe, 1983).

Strain A mouse pulmonary tumour bioassay

The common occurrence of lung adenomas in strain A mice has been utilized in the development of a quantitative bioassay for carcinogenic activity. This followed the demonstration that administration of carcinogens such as 3-methylcholanthrene to this strain could significantly increase the incidence of pulmonary adenomas within periods of up to six months (Shimkin, 1940). Over many years the strain A mouse pulmonary tumour assay has been used to test a large number of chemicals of different classes including polycyclic hydrocarbons, nitrosamines, food additives, alkyl halides, metals and chemotherapeutic agents (Stoner et al., 1973). However, as with many biological systems, interlaboratory agreement in the strain A test system and correlation with two-year carcinogenicity study data and genotoxicity results have been shown to be poor, so particular care is needed in the interpretation of this test (Maronpot et al., 1986). Nevertheless, it may serve to help in the ranking of tumorigenic activity of some anticancer drugs provided cognizance is given to drug stability, route of administration and vehicle as well as species differences in metabolism and drug disposition.

Hamsters

Hamsters develop lung adenomas spontaneously in small numbers with advancing age. They are composed of uniform cylindrical cells similar to those found in bronchial epithelium or goblet cells showing distinct mucus production (Pour et al., 1976, 1979; Mohr and Ketkar, 1980). An immunohistochemical study of similar pulmonary neoplasms induced in hamsters by N-nitrosodiethylamine has shown the presence of Clara cell antigen in early phase of development but as the tumours developed they became more squamous in type and showed immunoreactivity for cytokeratins (Rehm et al., 1989). A predominantly Clara cell origin was suggested for these neoplasms.

REFERENCES

ABRAMSON, R.K. and HUTTON, J.J. (1975): Effects of cigarette smoking on aryl hydrocarbon hydroxylase activity in lungs and tissues of inbred mice. *Cancer Res.*, 23–29.

ADAMS, D.R. (1982): Hamster nasal glands: Their structure, sialic acid content, and vulnerability to actinomycin D. *J. Morphol.*, 174, 79–94.

ADAMS, D.R., DEYOUNG, D.W. and GRIFFITH R. (1981): The lateral nasal gland of the dog, its structure and secretory content. *J. Anat.*, 132, 29–37.

ALARIE, Y. (1966): Irritating properties of airborne materials to the upper respiratory tract. *Arch. Environ. Health*, 13, 433–449.

ALARIE, Y. (1981): Bioassay for evaluating the potency of airborne sensory irritants and predicting acceptable levels of exposure in man. *Food Cosmet. Toxicol.*, 19, 623–626.

ALLRED, D.C., KOBAYASHI, K. and YOSHIDA, T. (1985): Anergy-like immunosuppression in mice bearing pulmonary foreign body granulomatous inflammation. *Am. J. Pathol.*, 121, 466–473.

ANDERSON, T.D. and HAYES, T.J. (1989): Toxicity of human recombinant interleukin-2 in rats. Pathologic changes are characterised by marked lymphocytic and eosinophilic proliferation and multisystem involvement. *Lab. Invest.*, 60, 331–346.

ANDERSON, T.D., HAYES, T.J., GATELY, M.K., BONTEMPO, J.M., STERN, L.L. and TRUITT, G.A. (1988): Toxicity of human recombinant interleukin-2 in the mouse is mediated by interleukin-activated lymphocytes. Separation of efficacy and toxicity by selective lymphocytes subset depletion. *Lab. Invest.*, 59, 598–612.

BAL, H.S. and GHOSHAL, N.G. (1988): Morphology of the terminal bronchiolar region of common laboratory mammals. *Lab. Anim.*, 22, 76–82.

BARON, J., BURKE, J.P., GUENGERICH, F.P., JAKOBY, W.B. and VOIGT, J.M. (1988): Sites for xenobiotic activation and detoxication within the respiratory tract: Implications for chemically induced toxicity. *Toxicol. Appl. Pharmacol.*, 93, 493–505.

BARRON, C.N. and SAUNDERS, L.Z. (1966): Visceral larva migrans in the dog. *Pathol. Vet.*, 3, 315–330.

BARRY, B.E. and CRAPO, J.D. (1985): Application of morphometric methods to study diffuse and focal injury in the lung caused by toxic agents. *CRC Crit. Rev. Toxicol.*, 14, 1–32.

BECKER, K.L. and GAZDAR, A.F. (1985): What can the biology of small cell cancer of the lung teach us about the endocrine lung? *Biochem. Pharmacol.*, 34, 155–159.

BIENENSTOCK, J., JOHNSTON, N. and PEREY, D.Y.E., (1973): Bronchial lymphoid tissue. 1. morphologic characteristics. *Lab. Invest.*, 28, 686–692.

BINN, L.N., ALFORD.J.P., MARCHWICKI, R.H., KEEFE, T.J., BEATTIE, R.J. and WALL, H.G. (1979): Studies of respiratory disease in random source laboratory dogs: Viral infections in unconditioned dogs. *Lab. Anim. Sci.*, 29, 48–52.

BOLDUC, P., JONES, R. and REID, L. (1981): Mitotic activity of airway epithelium after short exposure to tobacco smoke and the effect of the anti-inflammatory agent phenylmethyloxadiazole. *Br. J. Exp. Pathol.*, 62, 461–468.

BREEL, M., VAN DER ENDE, M., SMINIA, T. and KRAAL, G. (1988): Subpopulations of lymphoid and non-lymphoid cells in bronchus-associated lymphoid tissue (BALT) of the mouse. *Immunology*, 63, 657–662.

BROWN, R.F.R., DRAWBAUGH, R.B. and MARRS, T.C. (1988): An investigation of possible models for the production of progressive pulmonary fibrosis in the rat. The effects of repeated intraatracheal instillation of bleomyin. *Toxicology*, 51, 101–110.

BUCKLEY, L.A., JIANG, X.Z., JAMES, R.A., MORGAN, K.T. and BARROW, C.S. (1984): Respiratory tract lesions induced by sensory irritants at the RD 50 concentrations. *Toxicol. Appl. Pharmacol.*, 74, 417–429.

BUCKLEY, L.A., MORGAN, K.T., SWENBERG, J.A., JAMES, R., HAMMTE and BARROW, C.S. (1985): The toxicity of diethylamine in F-334 rats and $B_6C_3F_1$ mice following 1 year inhalation exposure. *Fundam. Appl. Toxicol.*, 5, 341–352.

CASTLEMAN, W.L. (1983): Respiratory tact lesions in weanling outbred rats infected with Sendai virus *Am. J. Vet. Res.*, 44, 1024–1031

CASTLEMAN, W.L. (1985): Bronchiolitis obliterans and pneumonia induced in young dogs by experimental adenovirus infection. *Am. J. Pathol.*, 119, 495–504.

CASTLEMAN, W.L., BRUNDAGE-ANGUISH, L.J., KREITZER, L. and NEUENSCHWANDER, S.B. (1987): Pathogenesis of bronchiolitis and pneumonia induced in neonatal and weanling rats by parainfluenza (Sendai) virus. *Am. J. Pathol.*, 129, 277–286.

CHANDLER, F.W., FRENKEL, J.K. and CAMPBELL, W.G. (1979): Animal model:Pneumocystis carinii pneumonia in the immunosuppressed rat. *Am. J. Pathol.*, 95, 571–574.

CHRISTENSEN, T.G., BREUER, R., HORNSTRA, L.J., LUCEY, E.C., STONE, P.J. and SNIDER, G.L. (1987): An ultrastructural study of the response of hamster bronchial epithelium to human neutrophil elastase. *Exp. Lung. Res.*, 13, 279–297.

COGGINS, C.R.E., DUCHOSAL, F., MUSY, C. and VENTRONE, R. (1981): Measurement of respiratory patterns in rodents using whole-body plethysmography and a pneumotachograph. *Lab. Anim.*, 15, 137–140.

COGGINS, C.R.E., FOUILLET, X.L.M., LAM, R. and MORGAN, K.T. (1980): Cigarette smoke induced pathology of the rat respiratory tract: A comparison of the effects of the particulate and vapour phases *Toxicology*, 16, 83–101.

COLEMAN, G.L., BARTHOLD, S.W., OSBALDISTON, G.W., FOSTER, S.J. and JONAS, A.M. (1977): Pathological changes during aging in barrier-reared Fischer 344 male rats. *J. Gerontol.*, 32, 258–278.

COSTA-JUSSA, F.R., CORRIN, B. and JACOBS, J.M. (1984): Amiodarone lung toxicity: A human and experimental study. *J. Pathol.*, 143, 73–79.

CRAVEN, D.E., KUNCHES, L.M., KILINSKY, V., LICHTENBERG, D.A., MAKE, B.J. and McCABE, W.R. (1986): Risk factors for pneumonia and fatality in patients receiving continuous mechanical ventilation. *Am. Rev. Respir Dis.*, 133, 792,796.

DAVIS, J.K. and CASSELL, G.H. (1982): Murine respiratory mycoplasmosis in LEW and F344 rats: Strain differences in lesion severity. *Vet. Pathol.*, 19, 280–293.

DAYAN, A.D., MORGAN, R.J.I., TREFTY, B.T. and PADDOCK, T.B.B. (1978): Naturally occurring diatomaceous pneumoconiosis in subhuman primates. *J. Comp. Pathol.*, 88, 321–327.

DE LA IGLESIA, F.A., FEUER, G., McGUIRE, E.J. and TAKADA, A. (1975): Morphological and biochemical changes in the liver of various species in experimental phospholipidosis after diethyl-aminoethoxyhexestrol. *Toxicol. Appl. Phamacol.*, 34, 28–44.

DIXON, D. and JURE, M.N. (1988): Diagnostic exercise: Pneumonia in a rat. *Lab. Anim. Sci.*, 38, 727–728.

DORMANS, J.A.M.A. (1983): The ultrastructure of various cell types in the lung of the rat. *Exp. Pathol.*, 24, 15–33.

DUDLEY, R.E., PATTERSON, S.E., MACHOTKA, S.V. and KESTERSON, J.W. (1989): One-month inhalation study of tulobuterol hydrochloride in rats and dogs. *Fundam. Appl. Toxicol.*, 13, 694–701.

FACCINI, J.M., IRISARRI, E. and MONRO, A.M. (1981): A carcinogenicity study in mice of a β-adrenegic antagonist, primidolol; increased total tumour incidence without tissue specificity. *Toxicology*, 21, 279–290.

FAN, K., BELL, R., EUDY, S. and FULLENWIDER, J. (1987): Amiodarone-associated pulmonary fibrosis. Evidence of an immunologically mediated mechanism. *Chest*, 92, 625–637.

GELEFF, S., BOCK, P. and STOCKINGER, L. (1986): Lectin-binding affinities of the respiratory tract. A light microscopical study of ciliated epithelium in rat, guinea pig and hamster. *Acta Histochem.*, 78, 83–95.

GHADIALLY, F.N. (1980): Collecting and processing tissues for diagnostic electron microscopy. In: *Diagnostic Electron Microscopy of Tumours*, Chap. 1, pp 3–12 Butterworths, London.

GIL, J. and MARTINEZ-HERNANDEZ, A. (1984): The connective tissue of the rat lung: Electron immunohistochemical studies. *J. Histochem. Cytochem.*, 32, 230–238.

GOODMAN, D.G., WARD, J.M., SQUIRE, R.A., CHU, K.C. and LINHART, M.S. (1979): Neoplastic and nonneoplastic lesions in aging F344 rats. *Toxicol. Appl. Pharmacol.*, 48, 237–248.

GOPINATH, C., PRENTICE, D.E. and LEWIS, D.J. (1987): The respiratory system. In: *Atlas of Experimental Toxicological Pathology*, Chap. 2, pp 22–42. M T P Press, Lancaster.

GRANT, I.W.B. (1979): Drug-induced diseases. Drug-induced respiratory disease. *Br. Med. J.*, 1, 1070–1071.

GRAY, J.E., WEAVER, R.N., STERN, K.F. and PHILLIPS, W.A. (1978): Foam cell response in the lung and lymphatic tissues during long-term high-level treatment with erythromycin. *Toxicol. Appl. Pharmacol.*,45, 701–711.

GREAVES, P. and FACCINI, J.M. (1984): Respiratory Tract. In: Rat *Histopathology. A Glossary for Use in Toxicity and Carcinogenicity Studies*, Chap. 4, pp 62–69. Elsevier, Amsterdam.

GUTIN, P.H., GREEN, M.R., BLEYER, W.A., BAUER, V.L., WIERNIK, P.H. and WALKER, M.D. (1976): Methotrexate pneumonitis induced by intrathecal methotrexate therapy. A case report with pharmacokinetic data. *Cancer,* 38, 1529–1534.

HARBECK, R.J., LAUNDER, T.L. and STASZAK, C. (1986): Mononuclear cell pulmonary vasculitis in NZB/W mice. II Immunohistochemical characterization of the infiltratingcells. *Am. J. Pathol.*, 123, 204–211.

HARTMAN, C.G. and STRAUS, W.L. (1965): The Anatomy of the Rhesus Monkey. pp 189–191, Hafner, New York.

HEATH, M.F., COSTA-JUSSA, F.R., JACOBS, J.M. and JACOBSON, W. (1985): The induction of pulmonary phospholipidosis and the inhibition of lysosomal phospholipases by amiodarone. *Br. J. Exp. Pathol.*, 66, 391–397.

HIRTH, R.S. and HOTTENDORF, G.H. (1973): Lesions produced by a new lung worm in beagle dogs. *Vet. Pathol.*, 10, 385–407.

HOLGATE, S., HARDY, C., HAWARTH, P., ROBINSON, C., CHURCH, M. and AGIUS, R. (1986): Bronchial mucosal mast cells and their implications in the pathogenesis of asthma. *Bull. Eur. Physiopathol. Respir.*, 22, Suppl. 7, 39–47.

HURTT, M.E., MORGAN, K.T. and WORKING, P.K. (1987): Histopathology of acute toxic responses in selected tissues from rats exposed by inhalation to methyl bromide. *Fundam. Appl. Toxicol.*, 9, 352–365.

ITO, T., KITAMURA, H., INAYAMA, Y. and KANISHAWA (1986): 4-Nitroquinoline 1-oxide-induced pulmonary endocrine cell hyperplasia in Syrian golden hamsters. *Jpn. J. Cancer Res. (Gann)*, 77, 441–445.

JAKAB, G.J. (1981): Interactions between Sendai virus and bacterial pathogens in the murine lung: A review. *Lab. Anim. Sci.*, 31, 170–177.

JOHNSON, K.J., CHAPMAN, W.E. and WARD, P.A. (1979): Immunopathology of the lung. A review. *Am. J. Pathol.*, 95, 795–844.

JOHNSON, K,J., GLOVSKY, M., SCHRIER, D. (1984): Animal model: Pulmonary granulomatous vasculitis induced in rats by treatment with glucan. *Am. J. Pathol.*, 144, 515–516.

JOHNSON, K.J., WARD, P.A., KUNKEL, R.G. and WILSON, B.S. (1988): Mediation of IgA induced lung injury in the rat. Role of macrophages and reactive oxygen products. *Lab. Invest.*, 54, 499–506.

JONES, R., BOLDUC, P. and REID, L. (1973): Goblet cell glycoprotein and tracheal gland hypertrophy in rat airways: The effect of tobacco smoke with or without the anti-inflammatory agent phenylmethyloxadiazole. *Br. J. Exp. Pathol.*, 54, 229–239.

JOSEPH, B.E., WILSON, D.W., HENRICKSON, R.V., ROBINSON, R.T. and BEINRSCHKE, K. (1984): Treatment of pulmonary acariasis in rhesus macaques with ivermectin. *Lab. Anim. Sci.*, 34, 360–364.

JUHOS, L.T., GREEN, D.P., FURIOSI, N.J. and FREEMAN, G.A. (1980): A quantitative study of stenosis in the respiratory bronchiole of the rat in NO_2-induced emphysema. *Am. Rev. Respir. Dis.*, 121, 541–549.

KAUFFMAN, S.L. (1981): Histogenesis of the papillary Clara cell adenoma. *Am. J. Pathol.*, 103, 174–180.

KAUFFMAN, S.L., ALEXANDER, L. and SASS, L. (1979): Histologic and ultrastructural features of the Clara cell adenoma of the mouse lung. *Lab. Invest.*, 40, 708–716.

KEHRER, J.P. and KACEW, S. (1985): Systemically applied chemicals that damage lung tissue. *Toxicology*, 35, 251–293.

KIM, J.C.S. (1988): Diagnostic exercise: Macaque with dyspnoea. *Lab. Anim. Sci.*, 38, 77–78.

KIM, J.C.S. and COLE, R. (1987): Ultrastructural and micropulse analysis of simian lung mite pigments. *Am. J. Vet. Res.*, 48, 511–514.

KLONNE, D.R., ULRICH, C.E., RILEY, M.G., HAMM, T.E., MORGAN, K.T. and BARROW, C.S. (1987): One year inhalation toxicity study of chlorine in rhesus monkeys. (Macaca mulatta). *Fundam. Appl. Toxicol.*, 9, 557–572.

KROES, R., GARBIS-BERKVENS, J.M., DE VRIES, T. and VAN NESSELROOY, J.H.J (1981): Histopathological profile of a Wistar rat stock including a survey of the literature. *J. Gerontol.*, 36, 259–279.

LAM, C., KATTAN, M., COLLINS, A. and KLEINERMAN, J. (1983): Long-term sequelae of bronchiolitis induced by nitrogen dioxide in hamsters. *Am Rev. Res. Dis.*, 128, 1020–1023.

LARSEN, A.K., NEWBERNE, P.M. and LANGER, R. (1986): Comparative studies of heparin and heparin fragments: Distribution and toxicity in the rat. *Fundam. Appl. Toxicol.*, 7, 86–93.

LEBARGY, F., LENORMAND, E., PARIENTE, R. and FORNIER, M. (1987): Morphological changes in rat tracheal mucosa immediately after antigen challenge. *Bull. Eur. Physiopathol. Respir.*, 23, 417–421.

LEVAME, M. (1980): Lung scleroproteins in young and adult rats and in ratswith spontaneous emphysema: Comparative studies by biochemicaland histochemical approach. *Bull. Eur. Physiological. Respir.*, 16 (Suppl), 115–123.

LEVINSKY, H.V., BRECKENRIDGE, C., LOUGH, R., GONCI, D.A., McILHENNY, H.M. and QURESHI, S. (1981): Six month inhalation studies of pirbuterol acetate aerosol in the beagle dog and squirrel monkey. *Fundam. Appl. Toxicol.*, 1, 426–431.

LEWIS, D.J. (1982): A comparison of the pathology of the larynx from SPF, germ-free, conventional, feral and myoplasma-infected rats. *J. Comp. Pathol.*, 92, 149–160.

LINDENSCHMIDT, R.C., TRYKA, A.F., GODFREY, G.A., FROME, E.L. and WITSCHI, H., (1986): Intratracheal versus intravenous administration of bleomycin in mice: Acute effects. *Toxicol. Appl. Pharmacol.*, 85, 69–77.

LINNOILA, R.I., NETTESHEIM, P. and DIAUGUSTINE, R.P. (1981): Lung endocrine-like cells in hamsters treated with diethylnitrosamine: Alterations in vivo and in cell culture. *Proc. Natl. Acad. Sci. USA*, 78, 5170–5174.

LINNOILA, I. and PETRUSZ, P. (1984): Immunohistochemical techniques and their applications in the histopathology of the respiratory system. *Environ. Health Perspect.*, 56, 131–148.

LONG, E.G., SMITH, J.S. and MEIER, J.L. (1986): Attachment of Pneumocystis carinii to rat pneumocytes. *Lab. Invest.*, 54, 609–615.

LÜLLMANN, H and LULLMANN-RAUCH, R. (1981): Tamoxifen-induced generalized lipidosis in rats subchronically treated with high doses. *Toxicol. Appl. Pharmacol.*, 61, 138–146.

LÜLLMANN-RAUCH, R. (1979): Drug-induced lysosomal disorders. In: J.T. Dingle, P.J., Jaques and I.H. Shaw (Eds), *Lysosomes in Applied Biology and Therapeutics*, 6, Chap. 3, pp 49–130, North Holland, Amsterdam.

LÜLLMANN, H., LÜLLMANN-RAUCH, R. and WASSERMANN, O. (1975): Drug-induced phospholipidoses. *CRC Crit. Rev. Toxicol.*, 4, 185–218.

LÜLLMANN, H., LÜLLMANN-RAUCH, R. and WASSERMANN, O. (1978): Lipidosis induced by amphiphilic cationic drugs. *Biochem. Pharmacol.*, 27, 1103, 1108.

LÜLLMANN-RAUCH, R. and REIL, G.H. (1974): Chlorphentermine-induced lipidosis like ultrastructural alterations in lungs and adrenal glands of several species. *Toxicol. Appl. Pharmacol.*, 30, 408–421.

LUNA, M.A., BEDROSSIAN, C.W.M., LICHTIGER, B. and SALEM, P.A. (1972): Interstitial pneumonitis associated with bleomycin therapy. *Am. J. Clin. Pathol.*, 58, 501–510.

MARONPOT, R.R., SHIMKIN, M.B., WITSCHI, H.P., SMITH, L.H. and CLINE, J.M. (1986): Strain A mouse pulmonary tumor test results for chemicals previously tested in the National Cancer Institute carcinogenicity tests. *J.N.C.I.*, 76, 1101–1112.

MAZUE, G., VIC, P., GOUY, D., REMANDET, B., LACHERETZ, F., BERTHE, J., BARCHE-WITZ, G. and GAGNOL, J.P. (1984): Recovery from amiodarone-induced lipidosis in laboratory animals. A toxicological study. *Fundam. Appl. Toxicol.*, 4, 992–999.

McGUIRE, E.J., DIFONZO, C.J., MARTIN, R.A. and DE LA IGLESIA, F.A. (1986): Evaluation of chronic toxicity and carcinogenesis in rodents with the synthetic analgesic, tilidine fumarate. *Toxicology* 39, 149–163.

MICHEL, R.P. (1985): Lung microvascular permeability to dextran in α-naphthylthiourea-induced edema. *Am. J. Pathol.*, 119, 474–484.

MOHR, U. and KETKAR, M.B. (1980): Animal model: Spontaneous carcinoma of the lung in hamsters. *Am. J. Pathol.*, 99, 521–524.

MORSE, C.C., SIGLER, C., LOCK, S., HAKKINEN, P.J., HASCHEK, W.M. and WITSCHI, H.P. (1985): Pulmonary toxicology of cyclophosphamide: A 1-year study. *Exp. Mol. Pathol.*, 42, 251–260.

MURPHY, S and FLORMAN, A.L. (1983): Lung defenses against infection: a clinical correlation. *Pediatrics*, 72, 1–15.

NEMERY, B., DINSDALE, D. and VERSCHOYLE, R.D. (1987): Detecting and evaluating chemical-induced lung damage in experimental animals. *Bull. Eur. Physiopathol. Respir.*, 23, 501–528.

PATRA, A.L. (1986): Comparative anatomy of mammalian respiratory tracts: The nasopharangeal region and the tracheobronchial region. *J. Toxicol. Environ. Health*, 17, 163–174.

PINKERTON, K.E., BARRY, B.E., O'NEIL, J.J., RAUB, J.A., PRATT, P.C. and CRAPO, J.D. (1982): Morphological changes in the lung duringthe life span of Fischer 344 rats. *Am. J. Anat.*, 164, 155–174.

PINSON, D.M., SCHOEB, T.R., LINDSEY, J.R. and DAVIS, J.K. (1986): Evaluation by scoring and computerized morphometry of lesions of early Mycoplasma pulmonis infection and ammonia exposure in F344/N rats. *Vet. Pathol.*, 23, 550–555.

POUR, P., ALTHOFF, J., SALMASI, S.Z. and STEPAN, K. (1979): Spontaneous tumors and common diseases in three types of hamsters. *J.N.C.I.*, 63, 797–811.

POUR, P., MOHR, U., CARDESA, A., ALTHOFF,J. and KMOCH, N. (1976): Spontaneous tumors and common diseases in two colonies of Syrian hamsters. II Respiratory tract and digestive system. *J.N.C.I.*, 56, 937–948.

PROCTOR, D.F. (1977): The upper airways. 1. Nasal physiology and defence of the lungs. *Am. Rev. Respir. Dis.*, 115, 97–129.

RAABE, O.G. (1980): Deposition and Clearance of Inhaled Aerosols. Part V, pp 24–34, Laboratory for Energy Related Health Research, Report UCD 472–503, University of California, Davis.

RANNEY, D.F. (1986): Drug targetting to the lungs. *Biochem. Pharmacol.*,35, 1063–1069.

REASOR, M.J. (1981): Drug-induced lipidosis and the alveolar macrophage. *Toxicology*, 20, 1–23.

REHM, S., TAKAHASHI, M., WARD, J.M., SINGH, G., KATYAL, S.SL. and HENNEMAN, J.R. (1989): Immunohistochemical demonstration of Clara cell antigen in lung tumors of bronchiolar origin induced by N-nitrosodiethylamine in Syrian golden hamsters. *Am. J. Pathol.*, 134, 79–87.

REID, L. (1960): Measurement of the bronchial mucous gland layer: a diagnostic yarkstick in chronic bronchitis. *Thorax*, 15, 132–141.

REID, L. (1963): An experimental study of hypersecretion of mucus in the bronchial tree. *Br. J. Pathol.*, 44, 437–445.

REID, L. and JONES, R. (1983): Experimental chronic bronchitis. *Int. Rev. Exp. Pathol.*, 24, 335–382.

REZNIK-SCHÜLLER, H. (1977): Sequential morphologic alterations in the bronchial epithelium of Syrian golden hamsters during N-nitrosomorpholine-induced pulmonary tumorigenesis. *Am. J. Pathol.*, 89, 59–66.

REZNIK-SCHÜLLER, H.M. and REZNIK, G. (1982): Morphology of spontaneous and induced tumors in the bronchiolo-alveolar region of F344 rats. *Anticancer Res.*, 2, 53–58.

RIVA, E., MARCHI, S., PESENTI, A., BIZZA, A., CINI, M., VERERONI, E., TAVBANI, E., BOERI, R., BERTANI, T. and LATINI, R. (1987): Amiodarone induced phospholipidosis. Biochemical, morphological and functional changes in the lungs of rats chronically treated with amiodarone. *Biochem. Pharmacol.*, 36, 3209–3214.

ROBINSON, R., VBISSCHER, G.E., ROBERTS, S.A., ENGSTROM, R.G., HARTMAN, H.A. and BALLARD, F.H. (1985): Generalized phospholipidosis induced by amphiphilic cationic psychycotropic drug. *Toxicol. Pathol.*, 13, 335–348.

ROE, F.J.C. (1983): Toxicologic evaluation of metronidazole with particular reference to carcinogenic, mutagenic, and teratogenicpotential. *Surgery*, 93, 158–164.

ROSENBERG, S.A., LOTZE, M.T., MUUL, L.M., CHANG, A.E., AVIS,F.P., LEITMAN, S., LIREHAN, W.M., ROBERTSON, C.N., LEE, R.E., RUBIN, J.T., SEIPP, C.A., SIMPSON, C.G. and WHITE, D.E. (1987): A progress report on the treatment of 157 patients with advanced cancer using lymphokine-activated killer cells and interleukin 2 or high-dose interleukin 2 alone. *N. Engl. J. Med.*, 316, 889–897.

RUBEN, Z. (1987): The pathobiologic significance of intercellular drugstorage. *Hum. Pathol.*, 18, 1197–1198.

RUDZIK, R., CLANCY, R.L., PEREY, D.Y.E., DAY, D.P. and BIENENSTOCK, J. (1975): Repopulation with IgA-containing cells of bronchial and intestinal lamina propria after transfer of homologous Peyer'spatch and bronchial lymphocytes. *J. Immunol.*, 114, 1599–1604.

RUSTIA, M. and SHUBIK, P. (1972): Induction of lung tumors and malignant lymphomas in mice by metronidazole. *J.N.C.I.*, 48, 721–729.

SCHRAUFNAGEL, D.E., MEHTA, D., HARSHBARGER, R., TREVIRANUS, K., and WANG, N.S. (1986): Capillary remodeling in bleomycin-induced pulmonary fibrosis. *Am. J. Pathol.*, 125, 97–106.

SCHRIER, D.J., KUNKEL, R.G. and PHAN, S.H. (1983): The role of strain variation in murine bleomycin-induced pulmonary fibrosis. *Am. Rev. Respir. Dis.*, 127, 63–66.

SERAFINI, S.M. and MICHAELSON, E.D. (1977): Length and distribution ofcilia in human and canine airways. *Bull. Eur. Physiopathol. Respir.*, 13, 551–559.

SHEPHERD, N.A., DAWSON, A.M., CROCKER, P.R. and LEVISON, D.A. (1987): Granular cells as a marker of early amiodarone hepatotoxicity: a pathological and analytical study. *J. Clin. Pathol.*, 40, 418–423.

SHIKATA, T., KANETAKA, T., ENDO, Y. and NAGASHIMA, K. (1972): Drug-induced generalized phospholipidosis. *Acta Pathol. Jpn.*, 22, 517–531.

SHIMKIN, M.B. (1940): Induced pulmonary tumors in mice. II. Reaction of lungs of strain A mice to carcinogenic hydrocarbons. *Arch. Pathol.*, 29, 239–255.

SINGER, I.I., KAWKA, D.W., McNALLY, S.M., EIERMANN, G.J., METZGER, J.M. and PETERSON, L.B. (1986): Extensive laminin and basement membrane accumulation occurs at the onset of bleomycin-induced rodent pulmonary fibrosis. *Am. J. Pathol.*, 125, 258–268.

SNIDER, G.L., LUCEY, E.C. and STONE, P.J. (1986): Animal models of emphysema. *Am. Rev. Respir. Dis.*, 133, 149–169.

STEWART, H.L., DUNN, T.B., SNELL, K.C. and DERINGER, M.K (1979): Tumours of the respiratory tract. In:V.S. Turusov (Ed.). *Pathology of Tumours in Laboratory Animals, Vol. 2 Tumours of the Mouse.* pp 251–267. IARC Scientific Publ. No 23, Lyon.

STONER, G.D. and SHIMKIN , M.B. (1982): Strain A mouse lung tumor bioassay. *J. Am. Coll. Toxicol.*, 1, 145–169.

STONER, G.D., SHIMKIN, M.B., KNIAZEFF, A.J., WEISBURGER, J.H., WEISBURGER, E.K. and GORI, G.B. (1973): Tests for carcinogenicity of food additives and chemotherapeutic agents by the pulmonary tumor response in strain A mice. *Cancer Res.*, 33, 3069–3085.

STURGESS, J.M. (1985): Mucociliary clearance and mucus secretion in the lung. In: H.P. Witschi and J.D. Brian (Eds), *Toxicology of Inhaled Materials. General Principles of Inhalation Toxicology*, Chap. 12, pp 319–367. Springer-Verlag, Berlin.

STURGESS, J. and REID, L (1973): The effect of isoprenaline and pilocarpine on (a) bronchial mucus-secreting tissue and (b) pancreas, salivary glands, heart, thymus, liver and spleen. *Br. J. Exp. Pathol.*, 54, 388–403.

SUTTON, T.J., DARBY, A.J., JOHNSON, P., LESLIE, G.B. and WALKER, T.F. (1986): Dyspnoea and thoracic spinal deformation in rats after oral prizidilol (SK&F 92657-A2). *Hum. Toxicol.*, 5, 183–187.

TAKAHSHI, S. and PATRICK, G. (1987): Patterns of lymphatic drainage to individual thoracic and cervical lymph nodes in the rat. *Lab. Anim.*, 21, 31–34.

TAKIZAWA, H., SUKO, M., SHOJI, S., OHTA, K., HORIUCHI, T., OKUDAIRA, H MIYAMOTO,

T. and SHIGA, J. (1986): Granulomatouspneumonitis induced by bacille Calmette-Guérin in the mouse and its treatment with cyclosporin A. *Am. Rev. Respir. Dis.*, 134, 296–299.

TARONE, R.E., CHU, K.C. and WARD, J.M. (1981): Variability in the rates of some common naturally occuring tumors in Fischer 344 rats and)C57BL/6NxC3H/HeN)F1 (B6C3F1) mice. *J.N.C.I.*, 66, 1175–1181.

THOMPSON, G.R., BAKER, J.R., FLEISCHMAN, R.W., ROSENKRANTZ, H., SCHAEPPI, U.H., COONEY, D.A. and DAVIS, R.D. (1972): Preclinical toxicologic evaluation of bleomycin (NSC 125 066), a new antitumor autibiotic. *Toxicol. Appl. Pharmacol.*, 22, 544–555.

THRALL, R.S., McCORMICK, J.R., JACK, R.M., McREYNOLDS, R.A. and WARD, P.A. (1979): Bleomycin-induced pulmonary toxicity in the rat. *Am. J. Pathol.*, 95, 117–127.

TILLERY, S.I. and LEHNERT, B.E. (1986)a: Age-body weight relationships to lung growth in the F344 rat as indexed by lung weight measurements. *Lab. Anim.*, 20, 189–194.

TILLERY, S.I. and LEHNERT, B.E. (1986)b: Immunohistochemical identification of factor VIII related antigen in frozen sections of rat lung. *Lab. Anim. Sci.*, 36, 65–67.

TUCKER, M.J. (1985): Effect of diet on spontaneous disease in the inbred mouse strain C57B1/10J. *Toxicol. Lett.*, 25, 131–135.

TYLER, W.S., DUNGWORTH, D.L., PLOPPER, C.G., HYDE, D.M. and TYLER, N.K (1985): Structural evaluation of the respiratory system. *Fundam. Appl. Toxicol.*, 5, 405–422.

VAN DER BRUGGE-GAMELKOORN and KRAAL, G. (1985): The specificity of the high endothelial venule in bronchus-associated lymphoid tissue (BALT). *J. Immunol.*, 134, 3746–3750.

VAN DER BRUGGE-GAMELKOORN, G.J., DIJKSTRA, C.D. and SMINIA, T. (1985)a: Characterization of pulmonary macrophages and bronchus-associated lymphoid tissue (BALT) macrophages in the rat. An enzyme-cytochemical and immunocytochemical study. *Immunobiology*, 169, 553–562.

VAN DER BRUGGE-GAMELKOORN, G.J., PLESCH, B.E.C., SMINIA, T. and LANGEVOORT, H.L. (1985)b: Histological changes in rat bronchus-associated lymphoid tissue after administration of five different antigens. *Respiration*, 48, 29–36.

VAN DER BRUGGE-GAMELKOORN, G.J. and SMINIA, T. (1985): T cells and T cell subsets in rat bronchus associated lymphoid tissue (BALT) in situ and in suspension. In: G.G.B Klaus (Ed.) *Microenvironments in the Lymphoid System*, pp 323. Plenum, New York.

VAN DER BRUGGE-GAMELKOORN, G.J., VAN DER ENDE, M.B. and SMINIA, T. (1985)c: Non-lymphoid cells of bronchus associated lymphoid tissue of the rat in situ and in suspension with special reference to interdigitating and follicular dendritic cells. *Cell Tissue Res.*, 239, 177–182.

VAN DER BRUGGE-GAMELKOORN, G.J., VAN DER ENDE, M. and SMINIA, T. (1986): Changes occurring in the epithelium covering the bronchus-associated lymphoid tissue of rats after intracheal challenge with horseradishperoxidase. *Cell Tissue Res.*, 245, 439–444.

VIDIC, B. and GREDITZER, H.G. (1971): The histochemical and microscopical differentation of the respiratory glands around the maxillary sinus of the rat. *Am. J. Anat.*, 132, 491–514.

WALKER, S.R., WILLIAMS, M.C. and BENSON, B (1986): Immunocytochemical localization of the major surfactant apoproteins in type II cells, Clara cells and alveolar macrophages of rat lung. *J. Histochem. Cytochem.*, 34, 1137–1148.

WALZER, P.D. (1986): Attachment of microbes to host cells: Relevance of Pneumocystis carinii. *Lab. Invest.*, 54, 589–592.

WARD, J.M. (1974): Naturally occuring Sendai disease of mice. *Lab. Anim. Sci.*, 24, 938–945.

WARD, J.M., GOODWIN, D.G., SQUIRE, R.A., CHU, K.C. and LINHART, M.S. (1979): Neoplastic and nonneoplastic lesions in aging (C57BL/6NxC3H/HeN)F1 (B6C3F1) mice. *J.N.C.I.*, 63, 849–854.

WARD, J.M., SINGH, G., KATYAL, S.L., ANDERSON, L.M. and KOVATCH, R.M. (1985): Immunocytochemical localization of the surfactant apoprotein and Clara cell antigen in chemically induced and naturally occurring pulmonary neoplasms of mice. *Am. J. Pathol.*, 118, 493–499.

WEISS, R.B. and MUGGIA, F.M. (1980): Cytotoxic drug-induced pulmonary disease: Update 1980. *Am. J. Med.*, 68, 259–266.

WOJCINSKI, Z.W. and PERCY, D.H. (1986): Sialodacyoadenitis virus-associated lesions in the lower respiratory tract of rats. *Vet. Pathol.*, 23, 278–286.

WOLF, R.H., GIBSON, S.V., WATSON, E.A.and BASKIN, G.B. (1988): Multidrug chemotherapy of tuberculosis in rhesus monkeys. *Lab. Anim. Sci.*, 38, 25–33.

YANG, Y.H., YANG, C.Y. and GRICE, H.C. (1966): Multifocal histiocytosis in the lungs of rats. *J. Pathol. Bacteriol.*, 92, 599–561.

YEH, H.C. (1979): Modelling of biological tree structures. *Bull. Math. Biol.*, 41, 893–898.

YOUNG, J.T. (1981): Histopathologic examination of the rat nasal cavity. *Fundam. Appl. Toxicol.*, 1, 309–312.

VI. Cardiovascular System

HEART AND PERICARDIUM

The recognition of drug-induced structural changes in cardiac tissues in man has been hampered by the problems of differentiating drug-induced injury from naturally occurring cardiovascular disease, so common in Western Societies. This difficulty is compounded by the fact that different drugs produce morphologically similar patterns of injury in man (McAllister and Mullick, 1982). These patterns may be quite unlike those produced in animal models which frequently employ high doses of drugs, well above the therapeutic dose range (Billingham, 1980). Nevertheless, as some of the most common cardiotoxic reactions of drugs in man are believed to be the result of inappropriate dosing (Balazs, 1986), the liabilities resulting from any drug-induced cardiovascular alterations occurring in high dose toxicity studies in animals are important and must be assessed with considerable care.

It is important to remain aware of the limitations of animal experiments to accurately predict certain forms of cardiac toxicity such as that associated with antidepressant drugs. Only after extensive clinical use over many years, was the nature and degree of the adverse cardiac effects of drugs such as the tricyclic antidepressants fully appreciated, particularly their ability to produce orthostatic hypotension and cardiac arrhythmias in normal clinical use. These effects were associated with potentially serious sequelae in a selected population of aged patients or patients with pre-existing cardiac disease (Glassman, 1984a). It is now clear that these drugs, because of their effects on ion channels in electrically active membranes of neurones, also exhibit similar activity in the closely related specialised conducting tissue of the heart. Newer antidepressant agents may, for similar reasons, also have effects on the cardiac conducting tissues. However, the prediction of the nature and the degree of risk in certain categories of patients may not be possible on the basis of animal experiments or clinical work in a few normal human subjects and young patients, but requires extensive clinical experience in large patient populations (Glassman, 1984b).

Whereas histopathological examination of the myocardium is a key component of cardiovascular assessment, histological examination of blood vessels, measurements of heart weight, blood pressure and heart rate as well as electrocardiography and blood chemistry are also of considerable importance (Osborne and Dent, 1973; Zbinden, 1981; Detweiler, 1981). These data allow construction of a complete picture of any cardiovascular effects which helps towards the elucidation of the mechanisms involved in the development of drug-induced structural changes in cardiac or vascular tissues.

Furthermore, drug-induced alterations in blood pressure, heart rate or cardiac conduction in animal studies may have important implications for safety of a novel drug, even if they are devoid of any morphological correlate. For drugs to be used in some clinical conditions, it may also be important to consider their effects on cardiac conducting tissue under special circumstances such as hypokalaemia or in combination with other drugs (Osborne et al., 1985). Zbinden (1986) has shown how monitoring of physiological parameters in pre-clinical studies is highly sensitive and capable of the early detection of cardiotoxic effects of agents such as emetine and allylamine. Electrocardiographic monitoring of rats has also been shown to be useful for determining the cardiotoxic potential of anti-cancer drugs (Figueroa et al., 1986).

Fundamental to pathological assessment of the heart, is the manner in which it is sampled for histological examination, especially as the heart is a complex organ and some parts are at particular risk for certain types of drug-induced damage. It is important that representative sections of each cardiac chamber are examined with attention being paid to the papillary muscles and subendocardial zones for effects of ischaemia. The endocardium may also show the effects of alterations in blood flow (jet effects). Sampling procedures have been reviewed in detail by Piper (1981).

A number of other techniques including morphometric analysis, enzyme cytochemistry, immunohistochemistry and electron microscopy are also useful aids in the study of structural changes in cardiac tissues in pre-clinical toxicity studies. Conventional special stains for collagen and elastic tissue are helpful for depicting myocardial fibrosis and endocardial thickening. Polarised light microscopy using formalin-fixed sections stained with picrosirius red is a powerful technique for the assessment of the orientation and size of collagen fibres within myocardial scar tissue (Pick et al., 1989; Whittaker et al., 1989).

Other techniques applicable to the detection of early myocardial damage in formalin fixed material include immunohistochemical demonstration of the loss of myosin, tropomyosin ATPase, creatine kinase or lactate dehydrogenase from muscle fibres (Block et al., 1983; Hayakawa et al., 1984; Spinale et al., 1989). Damaged fibres also stain red with the haematoxylin basic fuchsin-picric acid method or show fluorescence in haematoxylin and eosin stained sections (Al-Rufai et al., 1983).

It should not be forgotten that the results of the effects of drugs on the heart may be manifest in blood vessels and organs such as the skin, liver and spleen and histological findings in these tissues can be helpful in the overall interpretation of drug-induced cardiac changes.

Cardiac weight changes, cardiac hypertrophy

In both man and laboratory animals, heart weight varies with body weight, body length, age, sex and other genetic factors as well as with circulatory demands (Zeek, 1942; Payling Wright, 1976; Tanase et al., 1982).

Comparison of heart weight from different strains of rats has shown considerable interstrain variation (Tanase et al., 1982) as well as differencies in the same strain obtained from different suppliers (Cambell and Gerdes, 1987). The study by Tanase and colleagues (1982) comparing 23 different strains of rats calculated that the effect of genetic factors on cardiac enlargement was larger than that of blood pressure. Furthermore, it has been shown that there are normally regional differences in myocyte size in the hearts of adult rats, hamsters and guinea pigs (Gerdes et al., 1986; Campbell et al., 1987). For instance, in the rat, myocyte cross sectional areas and volumes are larger in the endomyocardium than in the epimyocardium of the left ventricle and right ventricular myocytes are smaller than those in the left ventricle (Gerdes et al., 1986).

Although the factors controlling cardiac size are undoubtably very complex, there is a considerable body of evidence to support the concept that cardiac hypertrophy develops in response to increased haemodynamic loading and subsequent abnormal systolic and diastolic stresses at the myocardial fibre level (Grossman, 1980). The pattern of hypertrophy is characteristic of the initiating stress.

For instance, volume overload results in *eccentric hypertrophy* which resembles the pattern in normal growth. When the primary stimulus is pressure overload, there is a disproportionate increase in ventricular wall thickness with normal or reduced chamber volume, so called *concentric hypertrophy* (Grant et al., 1965). Studies of ventricular wall stresses have suggested that pressure overload produces increased wall stresses during systole which lead to the addition of new myofibrils in parallel, wall thickening and concentric hypertrophy (Grossman et al., 1975). This increase in wall thickening tends to normalise the wall stresses during systole. Conversely, ventricular volume overload produces increased wall stresses during diastole, leading to addition of new sarcomeres, fibre elongation and chamber enlargement. Chamber enlargement is followed by an increase in systolic pressure which produces wall thickening of a degree to normalise systolic stress (Grossman et al., 1975; Grossman, 1980).

It is important to note that whilst systemic hypertensive states lead to left ventricular hypertrophy, increased pulmonary circulatory demands primarily affect the right ventricle (see below).

Experimental myocardial hypertrophy is also reported to occur as a compensatory response to myocardial infarction (Rubin et al., 1983), following chronic exposure to catecholamines (Rona, 1985), thyroxine (Craft-Cormney and Hansen, 1980), growth hormone (Gilbert et al., 1985) or alterations in cardiac muscle energy metabolism (Greaves et al., 1984).

On the basis of studies in which noradrenaline can produce a significant degree of left ventricular hypertrophy when administered to dogs in subhypertensive and non-necrogenic doses and the finding of increased cardiac noradrenaline concentrations in physiological myocardial hypertrophy, it has been suggested that noradrenaline may play an important role in the development of myocardial hypertrophy (Laks and Morady, 1976). These workers have proposed that noradrenaline may be the hormone which initiates myocardial hypertrophy in response to an increase in ventricular wall tension.

In toxicity studies employing high doses of cardiac drugs, dose-related increases in cardiac weight are sometimes observed. Reported examples include sympathomimetic agents, vasodilating antihypertensive drugs, α- and β- blocking agents, antiarrhythmics and calcium channel blockers, some of which are in widespread use in clinical practice (Whitehead et al., 1979; Womble et al., 1982; French et al., 1983; Case et al., 1984; Cruickshank et al., 1984; Hoffman, 1984; Gomi et al., 1985; Sutton et al., 1986). When weight increases are unassociated with adverse cellular or subcellular alterations in myocardial tissue and are accompanied by evidence of increased cardiac work in treated animals, it is usually considered that the changes are adaptive in nature, a hypothesis which has been advanced in the literature for a number of cardiac drugs (Whitehead et al., 1979; Hoffman, 1984).

Whilst this is a useful working hypothesis, it may be a considerable over simplification. Further mechanisms may involve hormones or other cellular mediators and disruption of energy metabolism. It is important to assess the myocardium carefully for any microscopic alterations, using supplementary techniques to exclude deleterious effects on cardiac muscle cells.

For instance, it was shown that the agent oxfenicine (S-4-hydroxyphenyl glycine), a cardioselective inhibitor of long chain fatty acid oxidation in man and laboratory animals, produced marked increase in cardiac weight in both dog and rat when administered at high doses for long periods (Greaves et al., 1984). Although small foci of subendocardial damage in the largest hearts of dogs and slight accumulation of cardiac lipid were found, there was no ultrastructural evidence of cell damage. Furthermore, no cytochemical alterations such as loss of mitochondrial enzymes or increases in lysosomal activity suggestive of a degenerative process were observed (Greaves et al., 1984). It was therefore argued that the increased cardiac weights were an adaptive hypertrophy as a result of inhibition of fatty acid oxidation by oxfenicine (Greaves et al., 1984; Higgins et al., 1985).

By contrast, another inhibitor of long chain fatty acid oxidation, methyl-2-tetradecylglycidate, also produced increased cardiac weights in rats but in contrast to oxfenicine treated rats, the hearts were greyish and flabby in appearance with dilated ventricles (Bachmann et al., 1984). It was postulated that this latter agent had a direct and potentially noxious effect on heart energy metabolism.

Subsequent metabolic studies confirmed that progressive, dose-dependent damage to mitochondrial membranes and loss of function occurred during treatment (Zbinden, 1986).

Another striking example was reported in rats treated with an investigational antiallergy drug, CI-959, a tetrazole, designed to block response-coupling mecha-

232

nisms in leukocytes to prevent the generation of inflammatory mediators and oxygen free radicles (Dominick et al., 1990; Metz et al., 1990). Intravenous administration of CI-959 to rats for periods of up to 14 days produced an increase in height weight of about 20%, with the free wall of the left ventricle showing the greatest increase in thickness. In perfusion-fixed material, there was histological evidence of fibre hypertrophy but no interstitial oedema, fibre necrosis or subcellular degeneration. However, individual myocytes showed increased intracellular glycogen and a loss of α-glucosidase activity. The hypertrophy was fully reversible two weeks following cessation of treatment and could not be reproduced in the rat by oral treatment with CI-959. The mechanism involved was not elucidated, although the changes in glycogen suggested that it may have been the result of a disturbance of energy metabolism.

Reduced heart weight has been reported in toxicity studies in which dogs and rats were treated with high doses of angiotensin-converting enzyme (ACE) inhibitors. This appears to be a result of the reduced circulatory demand under these circumstances (see kidney).

Reductions in total ventricular weight, left ventricular weight and right ventricular weight, normalised for body weight and reductions in mean arterial blood pressure were also reported in Sprague-Dawley rats receiving continuous infusions of the synthetic atriopeptin III (Spokas et al., 1987). It was postulated that the reductions in heart weight were the result of the effect of atriopeptin III on fluid volume by an enhanced passage of fluid from the intramuscular to extramuscular compartment, or diuresis with subsequent alterations to cardiac work load.

Spontaneous focal myocardial inflammation and fibrosis, myocarditis

Although the myocardium can be damaged by a variety of different insults produced by anoxia, ischaemia, infectious agents, physical and chemical agents, its pattern of response remains relatively limited. Myocardial fibre damage can take the form of a cytoplasmic alteration such as vacuolation (see below) but the irreversible consequence of myocyte damage is *necrosis*. Necrosis is accompanied by a variable inflammatory exudation which depends to some extent on the injurious agent. However, unlike many other tissues which can heal by either restoration or scar tissue formation, the myocardium appears to be limited to healing by scar tissue alone by a process which appears to be guided by the physical forces of continuing myocyte contractions (Vracko et al., 1989).

Whereas the term, necrosis, is applicable to many different types of myocardial damage, including irreversible drug-induced injury, the terms infarction and myocarditis have more limited application. Myocardial *infarction* implies necrosis secondary to ischaemia, whereas the diagnosis of *myocarditis* should only be made if myocyte necrosis or degeneration is associated with an inflammatory infiltrate adjacent to damage myocytes (Aretz, 1987).

Beagle dog The myocardium of the young beagle dog may contain small foci of degenerate or necrotic myocardial fibres, with or without inflammatory cells, foci of chronic inflammation or small fibrous scars. Some lesions may also be associated with mineral deposition. The lesions usually show no particular regional distribution and may be regarded as non-specific inflammatory lesions for which no causative agent is demonstrable (Hottendorf and Hirth, 1974). They have also been associated with stenosing lesions in small intramyocardial vessels of the dog heart and they can be associated with lesions in the large branches of the coronary arteries (Lüginbuhl and Detweiler, 1965). Focal cardiac inflammation, followed by fibrosis has also been associated with canine parvovirus infection in young dogs (Thompson et al., 1979; Robinson et al., 1980) and its sequelae may be observed in older dogs used in toxicity studies. Other infective agents may also be responsible (Ayers and Jones, 1978; Van Vleet and Ferrans, 1986).

Rat Small foci of necrosis, focal inflammation and fibrosis are occasionally observed in young untreated rats and become more common with increasing age (Greaves and Faccini, 1984). Apart from small microabscesses which are usually infective in origin (eg Tyzzer's disease), it is generally believed that these foci are due to focal ischaemia as a result of myocardial vascular disease (Ayers and Jones, 1978). This hypothesis is supported by the fact that the distribution of these lesions is predominantly in the subendocardial zones and papillary muscles, regions most at risk for ischaemia. In addition, they increase in prevalence and severity with increasing age and are more common in hypertensive rats which are generally more liable to develop vascular disease (Yamori and Okomoto, 1976). Detailed studies with hypertensive rats have suggested that changes in the cardiac microvasculature are particularly important in the development of these lesions rather than changes to large branches of the coronary arteries (Factor et al., 1984).

It has also been suggested that these myocardial changes in the rat are due to chronic renal disease, although this type of fibrosis can undoubtably be found in rats unaffected by significant renal disease (Van Vleet and Ferrans, 1986).

Nevertheless, there is an association between long-standing uraemia and focal myocardial necrosis, although the mechanisms involved are unclear. For instance, focal, but disseminated cardiac necrosis as well as calcification has been shown to develop in normotensive rats made uraemic by partial nephrectomy or by injection with mercuric chloride (Rhodes et al., 1987).

Histologically, this type of cardiac necrosis is characterised by the presence of dense eosinophilic staining of muscle fibres, nuclear pyknosis or total loss of nuclei with a variable but mild inflammatory response, infiltration by macrophages and eventually interstitial fibrosis. Pigment-laden macrophages and mineral deposits are also occasionally seen in older lesions.

Hamster Certain strains of hamsters are particularly notable in that they develop a striking but complex cardiac myopathy characterised histologically by multifocal myocardial necrosis, accompanied by inflammation, fibrosis and

234

mineralisation which eventually leads to dilatation of the cardiac chambers and overt heart failure (Jasmin and Eu, 1979). These cardiac changes are paralleled by similar histological changes in skeletal muscle in this species (see Muscoloskeletal System, Chapter IV). Cardiac enzymes may be raised in the serum of affected animals and histochemical studies show that the activity of acid phosphatase and other lysosomal enzymes are increased in muscle fibres (Karliner et al., 1981). Affected cardiac muscle shows raised responsiveness to noradrenaline (Karliner et al., 1981).

Similar histopathological changes are seen in the usual strains of hamster employed in toxicology, although they occur less frequently and in older animals than in cardiomyopathic strains. However, there is considerable variation in the prevalance of cardiac disease in the different strains of hamster (Pour et al., 1979).

As in the myopathic hamster, the cardiac lesions are characterised histologically by focal necrosis, inflammation and fibrous scarring, affecting both subendocardial and other zones of all chambers of the heart. Diffuse inflammation is also seen and lesions can be associated with atrial thrombosis, valvular mucoid degeneration, valvulitis, massive valvular fibrosis and calcification.

Such lesions naturally influence the outcome of toxicity and carcinogenicity studies performed with cardiovascular agents in the hamster. Certainly, sudden 'cardiac' death is an important cause of mortality in untreated aged hamster (personal observations).

Mouse The untreated, aging mouse also develops foci of myocardial degeneration, inflammation and fibrosis although this generally is less common than in the rat (Ward et al., 1979; Chvédoff et al., 1982). Its distribution and histopathology is often quite similar to that found in the rat heart with involvement of endocardial zones and papillary muscles. In the aged mouse, the lesions comprise focal fibrous replacement of myocardial cells rather than fresh necrosis and inflammation. A particularly striking phenomenon is the propensity for inflammatory cell damage and fibrosis to develop in the ventricular myocardium immediately below the insertion of the mitral valve ring.

Focal coagulation necrosis with a prominent lymphoid infiltrate (myocarditis) has been reported in mice infected with coxsackie B3 or murine cytomegalovirus (Gang et al., 1986; Godeny and Gauntt, 1987). In some strains of mice with inherited cardiomyopathies, focal necrosis of myocardial fibres is also a component of the cardiac alterations (Van Vleet and Ferrans, 1986).

Induced myocardial necrosis, inflammation and fibrosis

Although the mechanism by which many drugs produce myocardial cell damage remain unclear, drugs which produce myocardial damage fall broadly into two main groups. There are a large number of cardioactive agents such as antihypertensive drugs, bronchiodilators, inotropic drugs as well as the catecholamines themselves which appear at least in part to produce their effects by disruption of cardiac perfusion as a result of exaggerated pharmacological activity at excessive doses. The other groups of agents, exemplified by anthracyclines, produce myocardial damage by a more direct disruption of subcellular systems within cardiac myocytes (Godfraind, 1984).

In the context of cardioactive drugs, it is important to be aware of the large body of older literature concerning the myocardial necrosis induced in experimental animals, notably rats, rabbits and dogs by catecholamines. Much work has been performed with isoprenaline but studies have also been conducted with adrenaline, noradrenaline, salbutamol, terbutaline, ephedrine as well as allylamine, a highly reactive unsaturated alkylamine with a number of industrial applications (Van Vleet and Ferrans, 1986; Boor, 1987; Boor and Hysmith, 1987).

In experimental animals, these amines typically produce multifocal myocardial necrosis, predominantly in the left ventricular subendocardial zones and papillary muscles. This type of damage is characterised histologically by focal myocardial fibre necrosis, often with contraction bands and infiltration by macrophages but with a notable absence of polymorphonuclear cells. Ultimately, fibrosis occurs. This pattern of fibre damage is quite unlike that seen in man or laboratory animals following occlusion of a large coronary artery which is typically transmural in type and associated with an intense neutrophilic response in the first few days (infarction).

Although the relevance of catecholamine-induced myocardial necrosis in laboratory animals as a model for the common form of transmural myocardial infarction following coronary artery occlusion can be questioned, there has been renewed interest in experimental catecholamine-induced myocardial damage because of the discovery of similar, focal 'contraction band' myocardial necrosis in several forms of human disease in which there are high circulating or tissue levels of endogenous catecholamines (Boor, 1987). Clinically significant subendocardial necrosis has been reported in patients with high circulating levels of catecholamines due to pheochromocytomas (Kline, 1961), head injury, other causes of raised intracranial pressure and drowning which is also associated with high endogenous catecholamine levels (Lunt and Rose, 1987; Boor, 1987). Cocaine abuse, possibly through its effects on neuronal reuptake of noradrenaline has also been associated with myocardial contraction band necrosis (Karch and Billingham, 1988).

Whilst there is uncertainty about the precise cellular mechanisms involved in catecholamine-induced myocardial injury as well as the damage to blood vessels which can also occur (see systemic blood vessels), it has been postulated that the key factor is the exaggerated pharmacological activity at excessive doses which leads to myocardial ischaemia and ischaemic damage. It has been suggested that ischaemia results from intense spasm of coronary arteries, hypotension and reflex tachycardia which leads to lowered perfusion pressure and reduced perfusion time in diastole, in the face of increased myocardial oxygen demand, pertubations in transmural blood flow or subendocardial steal phenomena (Rona et al., 1959; Windsor et al., 1975; Balazs and Bloom, 1982; Simons and Downing, 1985).

236

In view of the diverse pharmacological actions of catecholamines, different agents may mediate cardiac damage by different haemodynamic mechanisms. Comparative pharmacological and morphological studies have shown that the pure vasodilator, isoprenaline, is more cardiotoxic than either noradrenaline, a pure vasoconstrictor, or adrenalin which possesses both activities (Rona, 1985).

The complexity of myocardial perfusion has been emphasized by important recent observations that adrenergic coronary vasoconstriction, as well as vasodilation, occurs during exercise and other forms of generalised sympathetic activation. It has been shown that although during exercise the net effect of sympathetic activation is an increase in coronary blood flow, paradoxical coronary vasoconstriction also occurs and this retards metabolic vasodilation by 20 or 30% (Feigl, 1987). It has been shown that this vasoconstriction is mediated by α-receptors and affects principally smaller intramural resistance vessels, helping to maintain an average distribution of myocardial blood flow during exercise (Huang and Feigl, 1988). Experimental studies have shown that vasoconstriction can occur in both large and small coronary arteries but it is mediated predominantly by α_1 receptors in large vessels and both α_1 and α_2 receptors in smaller resistance vessels. In addition, coronary arteries also posses β-receptors which subserve vasodilation (Feigl, 1987). Excessive activation of these receptors by high doses of catecholamines and other cardiovascular agents may have therefore potential to produce cardiac ischaemia either through inappropriate vasodilation or excessive vasoconstriction.

Other mechanisms of potential importance include alterations in cellular calcium or magnesium, generation of toxic metabolites or free radical injury (Singal et al., 1983; Noronha-Dutra et al., 1984; Balazs, 1986; Bloor, 1987).

Beagle dog The beagle dog appears to be particularly liable to develop focal myocardial necrosis following administration of high doses of a variety of cardiovascular drugs. Such agents not only include catecholamines and their synthetic analogues (Waters and de Suto-Nagy, 1950; Ferrans et al., 1969; Balazs, 1981) but also vasodilating antihypertensive drugs (Balazs and Payne, 1971; Carlson and Feenstra, 1977) cardiac glycosides (Teske et al., 1976) non-glycoside inotropic agents (Alousi et al., 1985; Harleman et al., 1986; Sandusky and Means, 1987) and calcium channel blockers (Kazda et al., 1983; Schlüter, 1986).

Although it is difficult to make close comparisons between cardiac pathology produced by such a wide variety of drugs in different laboratories using a variety of experimental protocols, several general patterns of injury can be defined (Fig. 43).

Drugs such as vasodilating antihypertensive drugs and calcium channel blockers, which when given to dogs at high doses, induce severe hypotension and reflex tachycardia, produce myocyte necrosis in papillary muscles and subendocardial zones of the left ventricle (Fig. 44). Lesions typically develop early during the course of treatment. They are characterised histologically by focal myocyte necrosis or eosinophilic degeneration of individual muscle fibres, particularly in the posterior papillary muscle but also in other subendocardial zones of the left

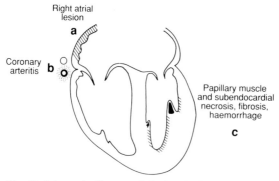

Fig. 43. Schematic diagram of the beagle dog heart showing distribution of the principle spontaneous and drug-induced lesions. (a) Right atrial lesion; (b) coronary arteritis; (c) myocardial damage produced by high doses of vasodilating, antihypertensive drugs and analogous agents.

ventricle including the outflow tract (Schneider et al., 1981). Necrosis is sometimes accompanied by haemorrhage but infiltration by polymorphonuclear cells, common in myocardial infarction due to coronary occlusion, is typically not seen. As these lesions tend to occur early during the course of treatment with high

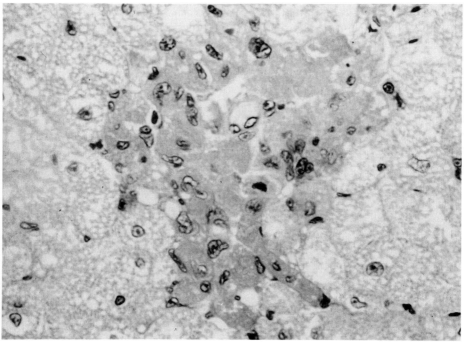

Fig. 44. Papillary muscle necrosis in beagle dog heart. There is a characteristic focus of degenerate muscle fibers without evidence of an acute inflammatory response. (HE, ×400.)

238

doses of these drugs, it is believed than an adaption or tolerance to continued treatment occurs (Herman et al., 1979). For this reason, the lesions seen in conventional toxicity studies of one month or longer duration are generally those of fibrous scarring rather than fresh necrosis. There may be focal aggregates of macrophages, sometimes containing iron pigment, and a variable degree of fibrosis. The endocardium may also be thickened by fibrous and elastic tissue and contain iron pigment as sequelae of endocardial haemorrhage and associated damage (Harleman et al., 1986).

At least some of the agents which produce these left ventricular alterations also provoke segmental necrosis in branches of the coronary arteries, and haemorrhagic lesions in the right atrium (see below).

It is widely thought that these subendocardial and papillary muscle lesions occurring in the dog after the administration of high and therefore unphysiological doses of these cardiovascular agents are primarily ischaemic in orgin (Lehr, 1981). The observations that gradients of tissue pressure, blood flow and oxygen pressure exist between the endo- and epicardium as well as the fact that the innermost layers of the myocardium may only be effectively perfused in diastole when local intracoronary pressure exceeds intramyocardial pressure, form the basis for the common occurrence of myocardial ischaemic change in the papillary muscles and subendocardial zones (De Busk and Harrison, 1969). It is believed that many of these cardiovascular agents, by virtue of their various abilities at high doses to reduce systemic and coronary artery pressure, increase heart rate, augment myocardial oxygen demand and reduce the interval for diastolic perfusion of the subendocardial zones, are factors which underlie the development of these lesions (Balazs, 1981). However, in many cases the precise interplay of hypotension, reflex tachycardia, vasodilatation and inotropism remains unclear.

An interpretative difficulty which relates to papillary muscle damage is its variability between individual animals given similar doses of these agents. Whilst differences in drug disposition and pharmacological response may partly account for this, the high variability of papillary muscle abnormalities in ischaemic states is a well recognised phenomenon in both man and dogs (Bailas, 1965; De Busk and Harrison, 1969). This is probably due to anatomical variability in blood supply to papillary muscles, notably the degree of collateral circulation within the subendocardial plexus and through trabecular muscle bridges (De Busk and Harrison, 1969; Allwork, 1987).

Despite the evident liability of the dog to develop cardiac necrosis in response to administration of high doses of these cardioactive agents, similar lesions can be reproduced in other species and in man if the appropriate combination of hypotension and tachycardia is achieved (Billingham, 1980). In man, therapeutic objectives are aimed at restoring normal cardiac function, so that severe hypotension and reflex tachycardia is not a normal result of therapy. Nevertheless, different species appear to respond in different ways to the hypotensive, inotrophic and chronotrophic effects of these agents.

For instance, the positive inotropic and vasodilating drug milrinone produced papillary muscle necrosis and fibrosis in both beagle dog and rat but not

239

cynomologus monkeys when administered at similar high doses (Alousi et al., 1985). Although the metabolic fate of milrinone was shown to be similar in beagle dog, non-human primate and man, it appeared that doses which caused both hypotension and tachycardia with associated ECG and histological evidence of ischaemia in the dog, produced hypotension without tachycardia and subsequent myocardial necrosis in primates (Alousi et al., 1985). Other cardiotoxic agents have been shown to produce myocardial damage in dogs and primates but not rats (Gracon et al., 1984; De Wit et al., 1985).

Undoubtably, some cardioactive drugs produce ischaemic muscle damage under quite different haemodynamic circumstances. An example is provided by digoxin and other cardiac glycosides, which when administered to dogs at high doses, not only produce subendocardial changes but also more scattered focal myocyte necrosis throughout the myocardium in association with extensive segmental vascular damage. These alterations occur in the absence of severe hypotension and tachycardia and are probably the result of intense, localised vasoconstriction (Bourdois et al., 1982).

Cardiac hypertrophy, by virtue of increasing muscle mass, oxygen demand and distance for perfusion may also predispose to the development of cardiac ischaemia, particularly as capillary growth may not keep pace with cardiac enlargement which occurs in adults (Anversa et al., 1986). This was reported in dogs given high doses of the cardiovascular drug, oxfenicine, for periods of up to one year.

In oxfenicine treated dogs, foci of necrosis were observed in papillary muscles and subendocardial regions of enlarged hearts. However, in contrast to lesions observed after administration of vasodilatory antihypertensive agents, changes were of various ages with fresh necrosis occurring throughout the test period, implying a continuous effect.

Rat As in the dog, cardiac necrosis with subsequent fibrosis is also produced in the rat by the administration of a range of cardioactive agents, particularly vasodilating antihypertensive drugs. Lesions also occur primarily in papillary muscles and subendocardial zones and they are believed to be ischaemic in origin, developing in a similar way to those produced by these drugs in the dog (Balazs, 1973; Balazs and Bloom, 1982).

Nevertheless, there are additional interpretational difficulties, particularly in longer term studies, because similar lesions develop spontaneously with advancing age and this can make it difficult to define a no-effect dose. It may not be clear whether fibrosis occurring in longer term studies is due to the initial insult to the myocardium following the early doses, or is an exaggeration of spontaneous disease following a prolonged, treatment-related increase in circulatory demand. Studies in hypertensive rats have demonstrated that the degree of fibrous replacement in cardiac muscle is not only correlated with the severity of haemodynamic stress but also its duration (Lawler et al., 1981).

These uncertainties may be compounded by the frequent lack of detailed haemodynamic monitoring in rodent toxicity studies and paucity of drug disposition data in older animals. This can be important in the interpretation of drug-induced myocardial damage appearing in long term rat studies, particularly for cardioactive drugs with a narrow therapeutic index. It has been shown that significant changesin cardiac function occur in the rat with advancing age (Yates and Hiley, 1979; Capasso et al., 1983) as well as alterations to drug disposition and metabolism (Yacobi et al., 1982).

Histologically, these induced cardiac lesions are similar to the necrosis and fibrosis found spontaneously in the aged rat, being distributed largely in subendocardial zones and papillary muscles.

Mineralisation

Myocardial mineralisation is found sporadically in most strains of aged rats, mice and hamsters particularly following myocardial injury, but it is a frequent finding in some inbred mice strains such as DBA/2, C, C3H, BALB/C, A, CBA and CH1 strains where it is believed a genetic susceptibility exists (Van Vleet and Ferrans, 1986). Its distribution in the heart varies between strains but its frequency and severity is dependent on age, sex, number of pregnancies, dietary factors and corticosteroid levels (Van Vleet and Ferrans, 1986; Yamate et al., 1987). It may also be associated with mineralisation in other organs.

Dystrophic cardiac calcification involving the outer myocardial layers and pericardium was reported to occur in BALB/C mice several months after acute myopericarditis induced by murine cytomegalovirus infection (Gang et al., 1986).

Subendocardial proliferation, endomyocardial fibrosis, endomyocardial disease of rats

Whereas localised fibrous thickening of the endocardium may follow ischaemic subendocardial damage, endocarditis, or the effects of abnormal cardiac blood flow (jet effects), rats appear particularly predisposed to the development of a proliferative type of subendocardial fibrosis. This condition was reported in the hearts of aged untreated rats by Boorman and colleagues (1973) who described a spectrum of appearances ranging from minimal proliferation of fibroblast-like spindle cells, to massive nodular growths of mesenchymal cells which were undoubtably neoplastic.

The proliferation is variable in its thickness and depth of penetration into the underlying myocardium. It is usually limited to the left ventricle, notably over the interventricular septum, although other cardiac chambers are occasionally involved (Naylor et al., 1986). Typically, the proliferation is composed of rather featureless spindle cells with plump oval or elongated nuclei and indistinct pale cytoplasm. Nuclei may exhibit features of Anitschkow cells (Fig. 48) and occasional mitoses can be found (Hoch-Ligeti et al., 1986).

The cells are surrounded by delicate collagen fibres but not the dense fibrosis usually associated with other forms of myocardial scarring seen in the aged rat. Elastic tissue is minimal or absent. Cells may be arranged in a herringbone pattern but pallisading of nuclei and Verocay bodies, characteristic of schwannoma, are typically not seen. At ultrastructural level, cells are fibroblast-like mesenchymal cells with no specific morphological features to suggest Schwann cell, smooth or skeletal muscle differentiation (Lewis 1980; Naylor et al., 1986).

The distinction of the benign form of endocardial proliferation from a malignant tumour is not clear cut. It can only be made using criteria such as the extent of proliferation, presence or absence of fine tissue invasion, degree of cellular pleomorphism and mitotic activity. Indeed, this lack of sharp distinction between benign and malignant subendocardial proliferation and the progressively increasing cell dedifferentiation which occurs in quite small lesions, has led to a proposal that all examples of subendocardial proliferation of this type should be considered neoplastic (Hoch-Ligeti et al., 1986).

The histogenesis of subendocardial proliferation in the rat as well as related endocardial neoplasms (see below) remains a matter of speculation. The histological features of the condition, notably the presence of Anitschkow cells, have much in common with the characteristic reaction of the myocardium to experimental injury (Rubenstone and Saphir, 1962). It has been suggested that it is a reactive process, possibly resulting from infection, or involving immunological or metabolic factors (Boorman et al., 1973).

However, it should be noted that the subendocardial proliferation in the rat appears morphologically quite distinct from the various forms of endocardial fibrosis and fibroelastosis described in man which are characterized by excessive deposition of collagen and poorly cellular connective tissue (Naylor et al., 1986).

Subendocardial proliferative lesions, similar to those reported occurring spontaneously in aged rats, can also be induced in rats by administration of chemical agents including carcinogens (Frith et al., 1977; Berman et al., 1980; Mayer and Bannasch, 1983) as well as by intrapleural implantation of durable fibrous materials (Hoch-Ligeti et al., 1983). On the basis of their studies with N-nitrosomorpholine, Mayer and Bannasch (1983) suggested that the lesions could be a direct result of carcinogen on the subendocardial mesenchymal cells.

The proliferation associated with durable fibres was postulated to be either a direct effect of the fibres which had migrated through the myocardium, perhaps transported by macrophages or spread through blood vessels or lymphatics, or possibly due to some indirect mechanism such as chronic lymphatic obstruction (Hoch-Ligeti et al., 1983).

Vacuolar degeneration (anthracyclines and other anticancer drugs)

Anthracyclines are potent chemotherapeutic agents effective against a number of human malignancies such as acute leukaemia, lymphoma, breast cancer and sarcomas but their use has been hampered by the development of cardiotoxicity. Von Hoff and colleagues (1977, 1979) have shown in cancer patients that there is an abrupt increase in the risk of developing cardiac toxicity at high cumulative doses of the two most widely used drugs in this class, doxorubicin and daunorubicin. Although the exact mechanism for anthracycline-induced cardiac damage is uncertain, a particularly favoured theory is a free radical effect on myocytes, as there is abundant evidence to support the generation of free radicals by anthracyclines (Green et al., 1984; Singal et al., 1987).

Studies in a variety of animal species including rat, mouse, guinea pig, rabbit, dog and monkey have demonstrated that the anthracyclines produce a similar form of chronic cardiotoxicity to that observed in cancer patients (Solcia et al., 1981; Villani et al., 1985; Van Vleet and Ferrans, 1986). The principle light microscopic changes, seen particularly well in 1 to 2 μm thick plastic embedded sections, is a widespread vacuolar cytoplasmic degeneration which may be associated with myocytolysis and frank necrosis of individual fibres. Unlike changes with cardioactive drugs, alterations produced in animals by anthracyclines have been shown to increase in severity as dosing continues (Paulus et al., 1988). Ultrastructural examination reveals sarcoplasmic vacuolation as a result of distension of sarcoplasmic reticulum, myofibrillar loss, dispersion of Z-band material, enlargement or swelling of mitochondria with disruption of cristae, an increase in lysosomes and residual bodies as well as a loss of specific cytoplasmic vacuoles of atrial myocytes (Solchia et al., 1981; Van Vleet and Ferrans, 1986; Paulus et al., 1988). These findings correlate with changes in enzyme activity as shown by loss in activity in mitochondrial or respiratory chain enzymes and increases in lysosomal enzymes (Aversano and Boor, 1983; Paulus et al., 1988). Immunocytochemical study of the right atrium of rats treated with doxorubicin has shown a loss in immunoreactive atrial natriuretic peptide (Jobit and Paulus, 1988).

The degree and distribution of these cardiac changes vary with the treatment schedule and the test species. Solcia and colleagues (1981) have suggested that the rat is more resistant to the cardiotoxic effects of anthracyclines compared with man, rabbit, monkey and mouse. However, spontaneously hypertensive rats are more sensitive to the cardiac effects of anthracyclines than their normotensive counterparts (Herman et al., 1985).

Scanning electron microscopy of the myocardium of rats treated with doxorubicin has shown that there is also focal but progressive loss of the normal interstitial collagen matrix with deposition of abnormal collagen fibres and fibrosis around individual muscle fibres (Caulfield and Bittner, 1988). This suggests that the cardiotoxicity of these agents may be partly due to effects on collagen matrix.

Serial recording of the ECG is also a sensitive way of detecting early cardiac damage produced by anthracyclines in the rat (Zbinden, 1981; Jensen et al., 1984).

Although less well studied, other types of anti-cancer drugs such as mitoxanthrone, cyclophosphamide, 5-fluorouracil, vincristine and amsacrine have been associated with analogous cardiac toxicity in man and experimental animals (Lang-Stevenson et al., 1977; Leone et al., 1985; Van Vleet and Ferrans, 1986; Lindpainter et al., 1986; Thyss et al., 1987). The anti-tumour antibiotic, mitomycin C and derivatives, have also been shown to produce cardiac changes in rats comparable to those associated with anthracyclines (Bregman et al., 1987, 1989).

Lipidosis, phospholipidosis

Cardiac muscle cells can be affected in the generalized form of drug-induced phospholipidosis and in appropriately prepared sections, the typical lamellated or crystalloid, membrane-bound inclusions are seen.

The antimalarial agent chloroquine and its derivatives, often used for long periods in the treatment of collagen vascular disorders, have been shown to produce phospholipidosis in the myocardium of both humans and laboratory animals, in addition to retinopathy and skeletal myopathy.

Affected patients develop symptoms of congestive cardiac failure. Endomyocardial biopsy samples show light and electron microscopic features of phospholipidosis which are diagnostic of chloroquine cardiomyopathy (Hughes et al., 1971; McAllister et al., 1987; Ratliff et al., 1987). Myocytes become swollen and contain numerous vacuoles which appear empty in paraffin wax embedded sections. In frozen sections, vacuoles contain faintly basophilic granular material. Plastic sections reveal the presence of complex osmiophilic membranes which appear as electron-dense concentric and parallel lamellae and large secondary lysosomes (Ratliff et al., 1987). Distinctive, curvilinear bodies consisting of numerous, regular curved profiles, similar to those described in the skeletal muscle of affected patients, are found (McAllister et al., 1987). Membrane-bound structures have also been described in the myocardium of laboratory animals treated with chloroquine, although animal studies have been relatively short and typical curvilinear bodies have not been described (Smith and O'Grady, 1966; Hendy et al., 1969).

These features are consistent with the findings that chloroquine accumulates in lysosomes, inhibits lysosomal enzymes directly and raises lysosomal pH above the point at which lysosomal enzymes are inactivated (de Duve et al., 1974; Homewood et al., 1972; Ratliff et al., 1987).

Neutral lipid droplet accumulation occurs in the myocardium of animal species after short periods of fasting (Adams et al., 1981). In fasted rats, lipid droplet accumulation was shown to reach a peak after about two days fasting and was maximal in the right ventricle followed by the left ventricle predominantly in the superior parts of the ventricles close to the atria (Adams et al., 1981). Metabolic derangements found in experimental diabetes mellitus and hypothyroidism are also associated with lipid droplet accumulation in myocardial muscle (Van Vleet and Ferrans, 1986). Furthermore, isoprenaline administration is reported to produce lipolysis as well as an increase in the fractional volume of neutral lipid droplets in rodent myocardial cells (Jodalen et al., 1982).

Oxfenicine, an agent which modifies cardiac lipid metabolism, was also shown to produce lipid droplet accumulation in rats and dogs accompanied by marked hypertrophy (Greaves et al., 1984). Lipid droplets are found in association with cell damage produced by cardiotoxic compounds such as allylamine (Van Vleet and Ferrans, 1986).

Atrial lesions: beagle dog

Characteristic lesions of the right atrium were first described in dogs following repeated administration of high doses of the vasodilating antihypertensive agent, minoxidil (Carlson and Feenstra, 1977) but they have also been reported after treatment with agents such as theobromide (Gans et al., 1980), nicorandil and hydralazine (Mesfin et al., 1987).

Fully developed lesions are usually visible at necropsy as well-delineated, focally thickened, haemorrhagic or pale yellowish segments within the free wall of the right atrium extending to involve the epicardial surface. Histologically, the thickened zones are composed of proliferating fibroblasts, small blood vessels sprinkled with chronic inflammatory cells, extravasated red blood cells and pigment-laden macrophages among which essentially intact muscle fibres can be seen (Figs. 43, 45 and 46). The lesions tend to involve the epicardium and extend

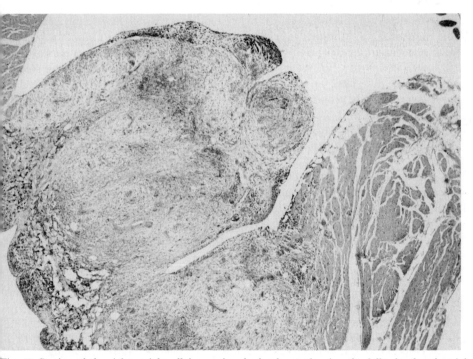

Fig. 45. Section of the right atrial wall from a beagle dog heart showing the fully developed atrial lesion which follows chronic treatment with the vasodilating antihypertensive drug, minoxidil and other agents with similar haemodynamic effects in dogs. There is focal, but full-thickness replacement of the atrial muscle by proliferating fibrovascular tissue. (HE, ×50.)

245

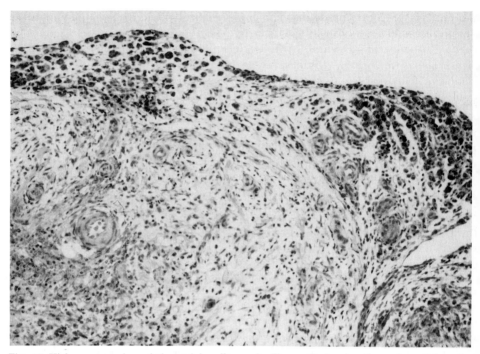

Fig. 46. Higher power view of the atrial wall seen in Figure 45 showing the endocardial surface infiltrated by numerous pigment-laden macrophages. There is diffuse involvement of the atrial wall by loose connective tissue containing prominent blood vessels and interstitial red blood cells. (HE, ×200.)

in a perivascular fashion towards the endocardium. Early lesions are less florid with apparent separation of fairly intact muscle fibres by ground substance, fresh extravasated erythrocytes and some chronic inflammatory cells. Muscle fibre necrosis is not a characteristic feature, although associated penetrating branches of the right coronary artery may show mild medial thickening, swelling of smooth muscle cells or fibrinoid necrosis. In common with vascular fibrinoid necrosis induced in the beagle dog right atrium by other agents, vessels involved tend to be medium-sized branches of the right coronary artery penetrating the right atrial wall, rather than the large extramural coronary arteries typically involved by the spontaneous form of beagle dog arteritis (see below).

The atrial alterations may extend to involve the endocardial surface (Fig. 46) although endocardial damage and mural thrombosis is uncommon.

The pathogenesis of this right atrial lesion is uncertain. Carlson and Feenstra (1977) originally suggested that the lesions developed as an exaggerated physiological response to high doses of minoxidil. Herman and colleagues (1979) postulated that it may be directly related to the vasodilating properties of minoxidil and prolonged hyperaemia in the right atrial wall. The principle haemodynamic changes produced by minoxidil in the dog include hypotension, lowered peripheral resistance, raised heart rate, coronary vasolidation and increased coronary blood flow. However, no appreciable differences in blood flow to left and right atria have been observed to explain the unilateral development of the lesion (Humphrey and Zins, 1984).

A more recent study with hydralazine, another vasodilating antihypertensive agent, has tended to support the concept that atrial lesions develop as a result of an exaggerated pharmacological, high dose effect. It has been shown in short-term studies in the beagle dog that hydralazine can also produce atrial changes, provided that the dose and dosage regimen are pharmacologically equivalent to doses of minoxidil capable of producing atrial lesions (Mesfin et al., 1987).

These authors were also able to show that the degree or distribution of the atrial changes did not correlate with coronary artery medial injury produced by hydralazine, suggesting that the actual mechanisms for the two phenomena are different (see below).

These factors support the hypothesis that the atrial changes result from interstitial haemorrhage or extravasation of blood cells from capillaries following intense hyperaemia, which ultimately leads to the florid chronic lesion with accumulation of iron-laden macrophages. Despite uncertain mechanisms involved in the development of the atrial lesions in the dog, a prospective study in which pathological examination of the hearts from patients who died as a result of the effects of severe hypertension, but who were also receiving minoxidil, showed no evidence of the right atrial pathology of the type observed in beagle dogs (Sobota et al., 1980). On balance, therefore, the right atrial lesion appears to represent a specific response of the dog atrium to drugs like minoxidil which at high doses are capable of producing marked coronary hyperaemia.

The atrium may develop haemorrhagic changes after administration of high doses of digoxin. However, the typical minoxidil type lesions have not been reported and therefore this form of acute haemorrhage may possess a different pathogenesis.

Cardiac thrombosis

Laminated thrombus is occasionally found in the beagle dog heart, attached to the endocardium. It may occur following endocardial damage as a result of treatment with cardiovascular agents or trauma due to indwelling catheters (Mesfin et al., 1988). It has been described in the right ventricle in dogs receiving repeated treatment with corticosteroids (Bertens et al., 1982) and the right atrium may be involved in severe cases of spontaneous coronary arteritis when the inflammatory process is extensive and extends to the endocardial surface.

Massive atrial thrombosis is also observed in the aged rodent heart. Both the rat and mouse may occasionally develop this condition, although it occurs most frequently in aged hamsters (Van Vleet and Ferrans, 1986; Doi et al., 1987) and spontaneously hypertensive rats (Wexler et al., 1981). Microscopically, the atria (one or both) are dilated and partially or completely filled by thrombus which can be fresh or organized and show typical lamination on histological examination. It may be a cause of death, particularly in the hamster (McMartin and Dodds, 1982).

The actual cause of atrial thrombosis is not clear from the findings in the histological sections. However, in the aged rodent there are often associated myocardial lesions such as degeneration and focal inflammation, mineralization or degenerative myxoid lesions in the valves.

Atrial thrombosis has been described after the administration of cardiotoxic drugs. Solcia and co-workers, (1981) described atrial thrombosis in association with atrial endothelial hypertrophy and desquamation with atrial myocyte damage in mice treated with anthracyclines. In mice, atrial thrombosis has also been associated with administration of thrombogenic or semipurified diets and following multiple pregnancies (Everitt et al., 1986; Van Vleet and Ferrans, 1988).

Neoplasia

Primary cardiac neoplasms are uncommon in rodents. In rats, most primary neoplasms are usually poorly differentiated mesenchymal neoplasms composed of spindle cells which form one extreme of the spectrum of appearances of subendocardial proliferation (see above).

These rat neoplasms are composed of infiltrating, nodular growths of spindle cells showing moderate cellular pleomorphism and considerable mitotic activity. Nuclei may show the characteristic owl eye features of Anitschkow cells (Figs. 47

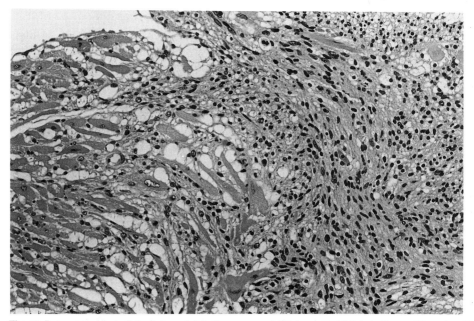

Fig. 47. Low power view of the left ventricle from an aged Wistar rat which is infiltrated by a locally developing sarcoma. (HE, ×100.)

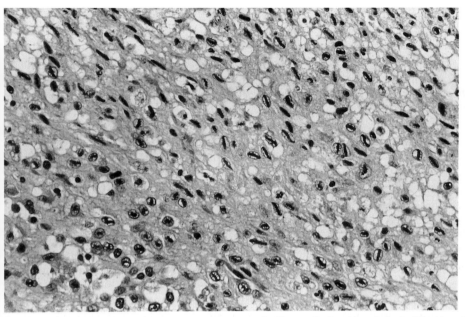

Fig. 48. Higher power view of the same sarcoma seen in Figure 47 showing cytological features in detail. Note the presence of Anitschkoff cells showing nuclei with the characteristic, centrally condensed nuclear chromatin pattern. (HE, ×250.)

and 48). Some whorling and palisading may be seen, but this is not of the degree or nature typical of schwannoma. Elastic fibres are sparse and collagen formation is minimal.

These spindle cell neoplasms have been regarded as schwannomas (Berman et al., 1980) and this view has been reinforced by the demonstration of positive staining for S100 protein by some workers Other authors have been unable to demonstrate the presence of this antigen (Naylor et al., 1986). As S100 can be expressed by a variety of cell types, S100 protein expression alone cannot be regarded as conclusive evidence of Schwann cell differentiation. These tumours are probably best regarded as sarcomas derived from primitive cardiac mesenchymal.

Other differentiation patterns are only occasionally reported in cardiac neoplasms in the rat. In the mouse and hamster, primary cardiac neoplasms appear to be even less common than in the rat although similar mesenchymal neoplasms occur. Those reported in the mouse have been associated with exposure to ionizing radiation (Hoch-Ligeti and Stewart, 1984). Cardiac neoplasms occurring in man and rodents have been reviewed by Hoch-Ligeti and colleagues (1986).

SYSTEMIC BLOOD VESSELS

Vasculitis

The classification of vasculitis both in man and laboratory animals is complicated by considerable overlap between different clinical syndromes, its association with a variety of inducing agents and the confusion in terminology which frequently accompanies morphological descriptions of the lesions. It is widely believed that most of the vasculitis which occurs in man are closely associated with, if not caused by, the deposition of immune complexes in blood vessel walls (Fauci et al., 1978). However, as with other immune-complex disorders, there is no completely satisfactory explanation for many of the clinical syndromes of vasculitis. Factors which can influence pathogenicity include duration of antigenaemia, type and size of immune complexes and the degree of impairment of clearing of formed complexes.

In man, most drug-induced vasculitis appears to be of the *hypersensitivity type*, characterized histologically by an inflammatory infiltrate of mononuclear cells, eosinophils, scattered polymorphonuclear cells in the walls of arterioles, capillaries, venules and small veins, with sparing of large arteries. A clinico-pathological study of drug-induced vasculitis in man by Mullick and colleagues (1979) showed a complete absence of necrotizing arterial lesions *(necrotizing arteritis)* of the type usually observed in polyarteritis nodosa. It was, therefore, suggested that necrotizing arteritis reported in association with drug therapy or in serum sickness in man is probably a secondary phenomenon due to hypertension, vasoconstriction, or precipitation of drug within blood vessel walls.

A form of necrotizing angiitis, indistinguishable from polyarteritis nodosa is, however, reported in drug abusers (Citron et al., 1970). Immunological mechanisms have been proposed for the development of this type of drug-induced damage because of its polymorphic character and the frequently delayed onset of symptoms such as stroke which can occur after cessation of drug abuse (Caplan et al., 1982). However, any study of drug abusers is complicated by unreliable information about the use of drugs which are frequently used in combination or are contaminated with other substances (Citron et al., 1970). For this reason, other factors of possible importance in this type of drug-induced vascular disease include infections, notably bacterial endocarditis, embolization of particulate foreign matter, direct toxic injury or pharmacologically mediated damage (Caplan et al., 1982).

Pharmacologically-mediated vascular damage is undoubtably a potential hazard of inappropriate dosing with vasoactive agents, as illustrated by the vascular changes reported in humans following excessive localized exposure to ergotamine (Eigler et al., 1986).

Vasculitis which occurs in laboratory animals is usually a necrotizing form of arteritis, although its characterization and classification is also complicated by the variety of circumstances under which it can be found and the different procedures which can initiate or accelerate its development.

Necrotizing arteritis of unknown aetiology occurs sporadically in untreated rodents and beagle dogs used in conventional toxicity studies. Certain strains of mice such as the (NZBxNZW)F$_1$ hybrid and MRL/Mp mice predisposed to autoimmune disorders, develop inflammatory vascular disease which may be of necrotizing type (Hicks, 1966; Alexander, 1985; Hewicker and Trautwein, 1987). Inflammatory vascular alterations are also a component found in animal models of serum sickness (Germuth et al., 1953; Wilens, 1965).

Spontaneously hypertensive rats, particularly if salt-loaded, renal hypertensive rats or normotensive rats in renal failure also develop necrotizing arteritis (Zimmerman et al., 1977; Wexler 1978; Limas et al., 1980). Other experimental procedures which have been associated with the development of necrotizing vasculitis in laboratory animals include the injection of particulate matter or viable bacteria, (Shinomiya and Nakato, 1985) ionizing radiation, chronic sodium chloride excess (Watanabe et al., 1987) and renal failure (Zimmerman et al., 1977, Rhodes et al., 1987).

Vasculitis can also been induced in laboratory animals by administration of a wide range of xenobiotics including therapeutic agents. Some of these, notably anti-cancer drugs and immunosuppressive agents, may have a direct toxic effect on components of the vascular wall (Bregman et al., 1987). Of particular importance in drug safety evaluation is the association of necrotizing vasculitis in rodents, dogs and non-human primates with the administration of high doses of compounds with pharmacological activity on the cardiovascular system.

The mechanisms involved in the development of arterial damage following administration of cardiovascular agents are complex. There is a close relationship in both man and laboratory animals between severe or rapidly progressive systemic hypertension and arterial medial necrosis. It has been shown in severely hypertensive rats that the distribution of vascular destruction is within those segments of arteries showing vasoconstriction alternating with vasodilation, suggesting that medial necrosis may be a response to excessive vasoconstriction or vasodilation (Byrom, 1954; Thorball and Olson, 1974). In experiments in which L-norepinephrine was applied locally to blood vessels, it was shown that smooth muscle cells are particularly susceptible to damage during the course of their contractile activity and when contraction is excessive, medial necrosis can occur (Joris and Majno, 1981).

However, studies of blood vessels in rats in renal failure or after infusion of angiotensin II have shown that medial necrosis of a similar type and distribution to that occurring in hypertensive rats, can also occur in normotensive states (Zimmerman et al., 1977; Nemes et al., 1980; Rhodes et al., 1987).

Based on these and other investigations, Nemes and colleagues (1980) postulated that medial necrosis could follow *either* intense vasoconstriction in which metabolic capacity of smooth muscle cells is exceeded *or* as a result of local overdilation in which there is breakdown of autoregulation, development of excessive tension within the vessel wall leading to damage of smooth muscle cells.

Whilst experimental models demonstrate that pertubation of immune system, infections, particulate matter, hypertension, renal failure as well as administra-

251

tion of cytotoxic drugs and cardiovascular drugs are all capable of leading to necrosis of blood vessels, several different mechanisms may act in combination to increase the prevalence or severity of the damage. For instance, pressor drugs have been shown capable of potentiating arteritis of the autoimmune type induced in rabbits (Wilens, 1965). Acute hypertensive damage to arterial walls induced by intravenous injection of rats with hypertension has been shown to be followed by autoimmunity against arterial wall antigens (Drivsholm et al., 1985).

Despite the variety and complexity of factors which may lead to vascular damage, the vasculature can respond in only a limited number of ways to injury and different insults lead to quite similar morphological expression of vascular insults.

Spontaneous polyarteritis: dog

Over recent years it has become increasingly apparent that the young beagle dog has a liability to develop necrotizing arteritis or polyarteritis spontaneously. This condition is liable to affect the coronary vasculature in a manner similar to polyarteritis nodosa and Kawasaki's disease in man (Lie, 1987) as well as involve arteries in other organs, notably meningeal and vertebral arteries. This was first reported in Beagles in the pharmaceutical industry by Harcourt (1978) in England. Harcourt described a particular constellation of clinical features, notably meningeal irritation, associated with segmental necrotizing arteritis involving a number of vascular beds but especially meningeal and extramural coronary vessels. The lesions described were similar to those seen in polyarteritis nodosa in man, i.e. a focal or nodular necrotizing inflammatory process with a variable degree of inflammatory activity, repair and fibrous scarring (Figs. 49 and 50).

Lesions found comprise a perivascular infiltrate of lymphoid cells and macrophages with focal muscle fibrinoid degeneration associated with a neutrophilic infiltration, nuclear debris and intimal thickening (Figs. 51 and 52). The internal elastic lamina is frequently broken or fragmented and forms a useful indicator of previous active inflammation when healing has taken place. Surprisingly,

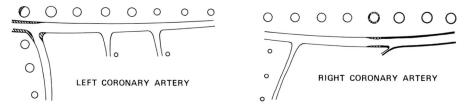

Fig. 49. Figs. 49 and 50. Schematic diagrams of the distribution of beagle dog coronary arteritis as reported by Spencer and Greaves in 1987. Most commonly and most severely affected zone is the proximal segment of the right coronary artery (dark area). Less frequently or less severely affected are more distal parts of the right coronary artery and the left coronary artery (cross-hatched area).

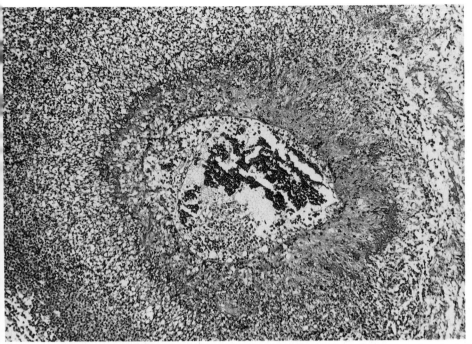

Fig. 51. Proximal part of the main branch of the right coronary artery from a young beagle dog. There is intense, active arteritis characterised be focal, intramural fibrin deposition and infiltration of the entire vessel wall and adjacent tissues by polymorphonuclear cells. (HE, ×150.)

thrombosis of the vessel lumen is not a common occurrence even in very active lesions, although recanalized arteries are sometimes encountered.

This disease has since been reported in a number of other European beagle dog colonies (Stejskal et al., 1982; Brooks, 1984; Spencer and Greaves, 1987) as well as in North America (Hartman, 1987; Albassam et al., 1989). The arteritis reported in the dogs from the Pfizer colony, Sandwich, England (Spencer and Greaves, 1987) is of particular interest in view of its high prevalence (in over 30% of dogs) in the main extramural branch of the right coronary artery (Figs. 49 and 50). Its causation remains unknown.

High doses of cardioactive drugs of different classes can potentiate the development of arteritis of this type and distribution. Potentiation of the spontaneous arteritis has also been reported in dogs following administration of immune modulators (Stejskal et al., 1982).

Vasculitis associated with vasodilating antihypertensive agents: dog

The pathological features of this necrotizing vascular process is exemplified by minoxidil but it has also been reported in dogs following treatment with theo-

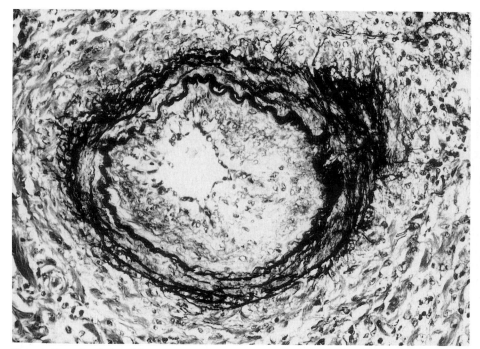

Fig. 52. Branch of the right coronary artery from a young beagle dog showing more chronic involvement by arteritis. Although there is less active inflammation, fragmentation of the internal elastic lamina and marked subendothelial thickening is evident. (Trichrome stain, ×350.)

bromine and other vasodilating antihypertensive agents (Carlson and Feenstra, 1977; Gans et al., 1980; Mesfin et al., 1987). The lesions typically associated with administration of high doses of minoxidil are characterized by segmental necrosis of coronary arteries, primarily located over or in the wall of the right atrium with an inflammatory process variably extending into the surrounding muscle and fatty connective tissue. These vascular lesions may be associated with the development of a focal reactive process in the right atrial wall after repeated administration. This is characterized histologically by separation of myocardial cells by oedema fluid, extravasated red blood cells, fibroblasts, lymphocytes and macrophages with relatively little acute active inflammation. After longer-term treatment the atrium typically develops an accumulation of many haemo-siderin-laden macrophages (see above).

The precise pathogenesis of the medial damage is uncertain although it appears to develop independently of the atrial change (Mesfin et al., 1987). Nevertheless, it may also be related to marked arterial vasodilation and subsequent excessive intramural tension.

Administration of high doses of digoxin or other cardiac glycosides to dogs produces an acute, widespread segmental necrosis of intra- and extramural branches of the coronary arteries (Figs. 53 and 54). The lesions may be found within the atria as well as in the ventricular myocardium. They are associated with necrosis of myocardial fibres, haemorrhage of the right atrial wall, perivascular necrosis in other chambers, and papillary muscle and subendocardial haemorrhage in the left ventricle (Bourdois et al., 1982; Teske et al., 1976). The typical atrial lesions and focal papillary muscle necrosis associated with minoxidil treatment in the dog are however not seen.

A further salient pathological feature found in the dog treated with high doses of digoxin is the presence of renal tubular dilatation and degeneration.

Haemodynamic changes associated with these lesions are unlike those produced by vasodilating antihypertensives. Digoxin does not produce profound hypotension and reflex tachycardia but it is generally associated with only modest falls in systolic blood pressure and decreased heart rates. In contrast to minoxidil, digoxin *reduces* myocardial blood flow in dogs (Steiness et al., 1978).

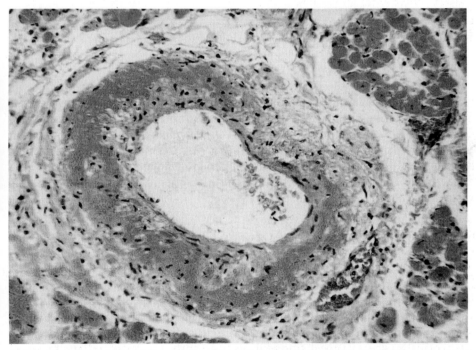

Fig. 53. Intramural branch of the right coronary artery from a beagle dog treated for several days with a high dose of digoxin. There is necrosis of the artery wall with little or no inflammation. (HE, ×300.)

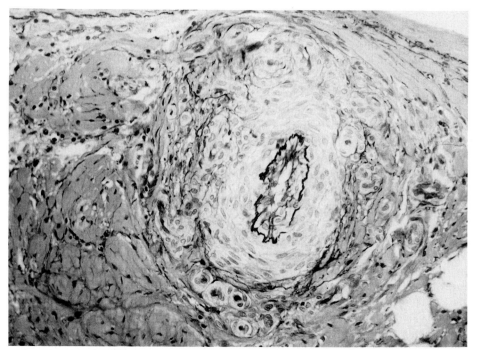

Fig. 54. Branch of the right coronary artery of a young beagle dog treated for several weeks with digoxin showing disruption of the internal elastic lamina and thickening of the media. (Elastic van Gieson, ×300.)

The cause of digoxin-related vascular damage is unclear, but the effect on blood vessels appears unrelated to the inotropic effects of digoxin. These effects may partly be related to the marked electrolyte disturbances produced by digoxin. However, the general pattern of vascular changes has given rise to the suggestion that different vascular beds respond in different ways to the effects of digoxin and that damage may result from intense local vasoconstriction (Bourdois et al., 1982). Renal changes may also result from lowered perfusion of the renal vasculature.

Spontaneous necrotizing vasculitis: rodents

Necrotizing vasculitis occurs spontaneously in most strains of rat, mouse and hamster used in toxicology although there is considerable variation in its prevalence and anatomical distribution in the different species and strains and with the same strains in different laboratories. This condition appears generally as a necrotizing polyarteritis affecting the small and medium sized muscular arteries. Histologically, there is focal fibrinoid necrosis with associated inflammation of variable age, endothelial proliferation and disruption or duplication of the elastic lamina. Various vessels can be affected depending on species and strain but the lesions usually remain sporadic. In the aged rat, pancreatic, testicular and mesenteric vessels are most often affected although a variety of organs may be involved (Anver et al., 1982; Greaves and Faccini, 1984). Affected arteries may rupture and cause the death of the animal. In the mouse, lesions are histologically similar to those occurring in the rat but distributed more frequently in renal blood vessels in some strains. A true necrotizing arteritis is observed in the aged hamster where renal, testicular and coronary arteries may be affected.

The precise cause or causes of this sporadic form of necrotizing arteritis remains quite obscure, although it possesses some features in common with polyarteritis nodosa in man and in some inbred mouse strains an autoimmune mechanism is believed to be important. However, its prevalence can be modulated by a number of experimental variables. Dietary levels of fat and protein may affect the incidence of polyarteritis in mice (Tucker, 1985) and food restriction has been shown to markedly reduce the incidence of polyarteritis in rats (Yu et al., 1982). In some colonies of rats the incidence of polyarteritis shows a male sex predominance (Goodman et al., 1980; Richardson et al., 1984). Wexler (1978) has shown how the severity of polyarteritis can be markedly increased in breeder rats by desoxycorticosterone and saline treatment. A remarkable reduction in the incidence and severity of polyarteritis was found in a two year carcinogenicity bioassay in which rats were treated with bromocriptine, an agent shown to inhibit prolactin secretion (Richardson et al., 1984). It was postulated that prolactin may also be important in the aetiology of arteritis in rats.

Treatment-related necrosis and vasculitis: rodent

Vascular damage is described in the rodent following the administration of a number of different pharmaceutical agents including cardiovascular drugs of various types, antibiotics, immunosuppressants and foreign proteins (Johansson, 1981; Nemes et al., 1980; Joris and Majno, 1981; Yuhas, 1985; Ryffel et al., 1983). In view of the complex nature of the pathogenesis of vasculitis and vascular necrosis and the fact that rodents may develop vascular inflammatory lesions spontaneously, care needs to be taken by the pathologist when assessing vascular changes believed due to therapy. The distribution and the histopathological characteristics of the vasculitis or necrosis should be evaluated in the light of the spontaneous vascular pathology, haemodynamic changes, uptake and distribution of drug and metabolites as well immunological factors such as the presence of circulating immune complexes.

Cardioactive agents are capable of producing medial necrosis and inflammation in small and medium sized arteries when administered in high doses to rats. For instance, continuous infusion but not repeated injection of the selective, post synaptic dopaminergic vasodilator, fenoldopam mesylate, produced medial necrosis and haemorrhage in small and medium sized arteries in rats (Yuhas et al., 1985).

Microscopic examination after 24 hours continuous infusion of rats with fenoldopam mesylate showed a dose-related increase in incidence and severity of

257

focal smooth muscle necrosis and haemorrhage involving the entire circumference of the arterial wall. Interlobular arteries of the pancreas and subserosal arteries of the stomach, characterised by a media of four to five layers of smooth muscle cells, were most frequently and severely affected but lesions were also seen in hilar, interlobar and arcuate arteries of the kidney at the highest dose and less commonly in the arteries of the mesentery and subserosa of the small intestine and colon. Ultrastructural examination of early lesions showed primary damage to the smooth muscle cells of the media characterized by formation of pseudovacuoles and autophagocytic vacuoles without evidence of damage to the endothelium, internal or external elastic lamina or collagen fibres (Bugelski et al., 1989). It was therefore postulated that fenoldopam mesylate produced arterial necrosis primarily though its pharmacological activity in which smooth muscle cells were damaged by excessive intramural tension developing from excessive vasodilation.

Other vasodilating agents have also been reported to produce medial necrosis and periarteritis in rats. LY 195115, an investigational inotropic agent with vasodilator activity, produced arteritis in small and medium sized arteries in the pancreas, stomach and kidney in rats treated orally with high doses for three months (Sandusky and Means, 1987). It was also suggested that the changes were the result of the pharmacological activity of LY 195115, although other confounding alterations were seen, notably renal damage.

Necrotizing arteritis of the mesenteric arteries has also been reported in rats treated with the inotropic vasodilator and phosphodiesterase inhibitor, ICI 153,110 (Westwood et al., 1990) and the dopamine receptor agonist, Abbott-68979 (Weltman et al., 1990).

Infusions of vasopressor and vasoconstrictor substances also produce medial necrosis of medium sized arteries in the rat. For instance, repeated injections or infusion of angiotensin has been shown to produce smooth muscle injury and medial necrosis in pancreatic, intestinal and renal vessels in rats, which is believed to be at least partly due to excessive or sustained vasoconstriction (Thorball and Olsen, 1974; Nemes et al., 1980).

The reason for the particular predisposition of medium sized arteries in mesenteric and pancreatic vascular beds in the rat in response to many cardiovascular drugs is unclear. Vascular morphology may play a part, for it has been shown that tension achieved in a vessel wall is a function of pressure and internal radius, inversely related to vessel wall thickness and influenced by the physical properties of the supporting tissues (Nordborg et al., 1985). It is of note that these vessels in the rat also show a liability to develop spontaneous polyarteritis with advancing age as well as medial necrosis in hypertension and renal failure.

By contrast, ergotamine and related alkaloids produce their principle vascular manifestations in the tails of rats when they are administered systemically in high doses. Changes are characterized by intense constriction of the central muscular artery of the tail, swelling of the intima and intimal proliferation, thrombosis in associated veins and ultimately gangrene of the tail itself (Lund,

1951). Adrenaline appears to be able to induce similar changes if it is injected locally into the tail (Lund, 1951).

Some anti-cancer and immunomodulatory drugs have been shown to produce vascular damage in rats and in other species including man. The mechanisms involved are not clear although they may possibly produce damage by a direct cytotoxic effect on components of the blood vessel wall or through derangement of the immune system. However, the nature and distribution of the vascular lesions induce by these agents may be quite unusual and are frequently associated with significant adverse effects in a number of organs including the myocardium, as well as suppression of bone marrow and immune function.

A well described recent example is the arteritis developing in rats treated with single or multiple intravenous doses of BMY-25282, one of a novel series of amidino mitomycin derivatives (Bregman et al., 1987). Arteritis was found in medium sized vessels in the lungs and also in a wide range of other organs including caecum, colon, pancreas, kidneys and testes and was accompanied by myocardial and renal tubular degeneration, renal glomerular pathology, myelosuppression and splenic lymphoid depletion. Arteritis was characterized by focal endothelial destruction and proliferation, subintimal infiltration by neutrophil

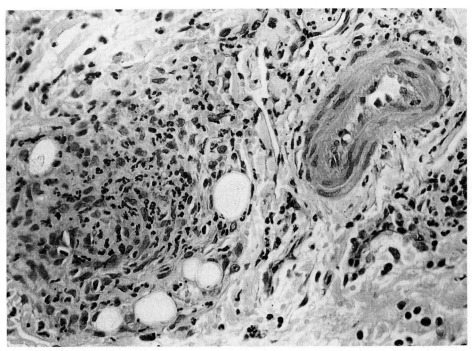

Fig. 55. Vasculitis produced by antibody-antigen reaction. This sample was taken one day after local injection of ovalbumin into the tissues of a rabbit previously sensitised using ovalbumin and Freund's adjuvent. There is an intense inflammation involving a thin-walled vessel with complete sparing of the adjacent small artery. (HE, ×250)

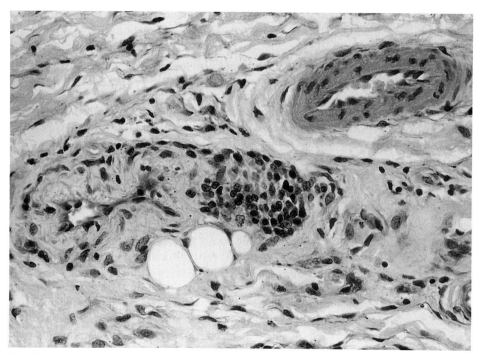

Fig. 56. Rabbit treated similarly to that seen in Figure 55. This sample, taken four days after local injection of ovalbumin, shows residual changes in the thin walled vessel but a similarly unaffected artery. (HE, ×250.)

and mononuclear cells and occasionally subintimal deposits of fibrin. Focal disruption of the internal elastic lamina, fibrinoid necrosis of the media, perivascular oedema, inflammation and haemorrhage also occurred.

Analogous arteritis involving the pancreas, kidney, intestinal mesentery, heart and skeletal muscle has been reported in female Sprague-Dawley rats within periods of up to one year following a single intravenous injection of the anthracycline daunomycin (Sternberg et al., 1972). However, treated rats also developed advanced renal disease and secondary hyperparathyroidism later in the study, confounding interpretation of the vascular changes.

The fibrinoid necrosis which has been recorded in renal arterioles in rats treated with cyclosporin A, is unusual, for this effect appears limited to spontaneously hypertensive rats, not being found in Sprague-Dawley, Fischer 344, Lewis or Wistar strains (Ryffel et al., 1983; Ryffel and Mihatsch, 1986). Fibrinoid necrosis is followed by a proliferative endarteritis and obliteration of the vessel lumen. It may be related to the increase in blood pressure which occurs in hypertensive rats treated with cyclosporin A.

Injection of complex substances such as polysaccharides into the circulation may give rise to a granulomatous lesions in and around blood vessels although these lesions are found notably in the lungs. Antigen-antibody reactions may give rise to an immune-type vasculitis of small, thin walled vessels, sparing the muscular arteries (Figs. 55 and 56).

Vasculitis in primates

A *granulomatous arteritis* has been described in feral rhesus monkeys infested with the nematode oesophagostomum (Lumb et al., 1985). The lesion is characterized by endothelial proliferation with scattered foreign body giant cells and associated exudate composed of plasma cells, lymphocytes and granulocytic cells. Birefringent material probably from the parasite cuticle is found in these lesions, which can be found scattered in the walls of the gastrointestinal tract and oesophagus, pancreas, kidney, myocardium and prostate.

A variable pattern of obliterative arteritis and endarteritis, characterized by infiltration of intima and media with eosinophils and proliferation of vascular smooth muscle cells, occurred in a variety of tissues in a dose-dependent manner in cynomolgus monkeys treated for one month with recombinant human interleukin-4 (Barbolt and Cornacoff, 1990).

Hypertrophy and hyperplasia

Thickening of the media of muscular arteries as a result of hypertrophy or hyperplasia of smooth muscle fibres is a hallmark of hypertension. It is believed to be an adaptive response of the vessel wall to increased intramural stresses, for according to the formula of Laplace, increased wall thickness and reduced luminal diameter bring about a lowering of wall tension (Limas et al., 1980). However, the mechanisms involved in the development of medial hypertrophy and hyperplasia and the role of such vascular alterations in the development and maintenance of hypertensive states both in the systemic and pulmonary circulation are complex.

Current concepts of vessel wall remodelling suggest that cell proliferation of the vessel wall can also occur as a response to endothelial injury or denudation with enhanced interaction of inflammatory cells, platelets and vasoactive mediators with components of the vessel wall or as direct metabolic effects of catecholamine (Fried and Reid, 1985; Coflesky et al., 1988).

Medial thickening is observed in hypertensive states in both humans and animals. The evolution of medial hypertrophy and hyperplasia in response to hypertension have probably been best evaluated in the spontaneously hypertensive (SHR) rat, where the disease process resembles the more slowly evolving hypertensive states more commonly observed in man than some of the rapidly evolving forms of experimental hypertension seen in renovascular, aortic constriction and salt-DOCA rodent and dog models which are characterized by a more destructive picture (Limas et al., 1980; Cimprich et al., 1986).

Studies in SHR rats have shown that medial thickening predominates in peripheral muscular arteries whereas both intimal and medial thickening develop in the aorta. In the aorta, the number of elastic laminae remains unchanged although the interlamellar spaces are thickened by smooth muscle fibres and the subendothial space is expanded by acid mucosubstances (Limas et al., 1980). Muscular arteries and arterioles show increased numbers of concentric smooth muscle cells. Ultrastructural study shows that these possess greater amounts of cell cytoplasm and cytoplasmic organelles, features suggesting that both hypertrophy and hyperplasia contribute to medial thickening.

A notable feature is the individual variability of the morphological response of muscular arteries in different vascular beds to hypertension (Limas et al., 1980; Ibayashi et al., 1986). This implies that the degree of cellular reorganization depends on the capacity of individual cells to proliferate or undergo hypertrophy, as well as the influence of local humoral, toxic or neurogenic factors (Limas et al., 1980). Studies of the internal carotid and vertebral arteries in SHR rats and their normotensive counterparts have suggested that the physical properties of supporting tissues may modify the outcome of increased arterial pressure on the vessel wall. Arteries well supported within bony canals were shown to have less medial thickening following increases in systemic blood pressure than unsupported vessels (Nordborg et al., 1985).

This individual variability makes accurate assessment of medial thickening difficult unless large numbers of vessels are studied by morphometric methods using perfusion fixation at appropriate pressure. The problem of perfusion fixation may be circumvented to a certain extent by the use of planimetric methods which calculate ideal vascular diameter from measurement of the length of contracted internal elastic lamina in non-perfused small and medium sized muscular arteries (Lowe, 1984).

Although medial thickening is characteristic of hypertension, similar morphological alterations have been reported in rats treated with novel drugs, without an apparent increase in systemic blood pressure. Pronounced arterial and venous wall thickening as a result of smooth muscle mass was reported in rats treated for periods of up to six months with the orally active inotropic vasodilator ICI 153,110 (Westwood et al., 1990). As systemic hypertension was not detected in this study, it was postulated that the medial hypertrophy was an adaptive response to marked vessel wall tension being achieved by excessive vasodilation.

Catecholamines may also be able to induce medial hypertrophy in the absence of hypertension (see pulmonary circulation).

Another form of smooth muscle hypertrophy involves longitudinal smooth muscle fibres in the intima of muscular arteries. This has been well-described in bronchial arteries in man and has also been induced in systemic blood vessels in laboratory rats. Histologically, there is a non-concentric increase in smooth muscle mass composed of longitudinally arranged fibres surrounded by a split elastic lamina (Weibel, 1958). These changes can be induced in mesenteric arteries in rats by local surgical damage or rhythmic longitudinal stretching in respiration produced by suturing mesenteric vessels to the diaphagm (Weibel, 1958; Wagenaar and Wagenvoort, 1978).

Amyloid develops spontaneously in some strains of mice and in hamsters and quite commonly involves small blood vessels where it needs to be distinguished from other fibrinoid changes. Amyloid deposition can also be induced in the mouse and hamster, although the rat appears to be a resistant species (Gruys et al., 1979; Schultz and Pitha, 1985). Although the immune system is important in the genesis of amyloid (Cohen et al., 1978), it has been suggested that vascular injury may be a factor in the deposition and distribution of amyloid within the tissues (Schultz and Pitha, 1985).

By allowing circulating amyloid precursors access to certain tissues, vascular damage may be partly responsible for the deposition of amyloid in particular organs (see spleen for full review, Chapter III).

PULMONARY BLOOD VESSELS

The pulmonary circulation is characterized by high blood flow and low resistance which is normally capable of accommodating large increases in cardiac output such as those occurring during exercise, with little or no increase in arterial pressure. This capability resides in the ability of open microvessels to undergo further distension, closed microvessels to open, and in the low tone of the thin muscularis of pulmonary arterioles (Rounds and Hill, 1984).

Determinants of pulmonary arterial pressure are cardiac output, atrial or pulmonary venous pressure, blood viscosity and the luminal area of the pulmonary artery bed. Thus, increases in pulmonary blood flow, left atrial or pulmonary venous pressure or reduction in luminal area can each result in increased pulmonary arterial pressure which will eventually be accompanied by structural alterations in pulmonary vessels.

Examples of increased pulmonary blood pressure in man include pulmonary hypertension occurring as a result of increased venous pressure in mitral stenosis, increased blood flow accompanying congenital, left to right cardiac shunts and increased blood viscosity of polycythaemia. Pulmonary hypertension also accompanies decreased effective area in the pulmonary arterial circulation as a result of destructive lung conditions, vascular obstruction and embolization as well as the vasoconstriction typically associated with hypoxia. A number of drugs and toxins have also been associated with pulmonary hypertension in man. Use of the anorectic drug, aminorex fumarate, was associated with an epidemic of pulmonary hypertension in young women in Germany, Switzerland and Austria two decades ago (Follath et al., 1971). Other reports have implicated chlorphentermine and fenfluramine (Douglas et al., 1981), chemically related to aminorex, phenformin (Fahlén et al., 1973) and oral contraceptives (Kleiger et al., 1976). However, the mechanisms involved remain unclear, particularly as consistent changes have not been produced in animal models by these agents.

Although Wagenvoort and Wagenvoort (1970) have suggested that certain histopathological alterations in the pulmonary vasculature are diagnostic for particular types of pulmonary hypertension in man, there is considerable overlap in the pathological appearances among various forms of hypertension which render precise histopathological diagnosis difficult (Rounds and Hill, 1984). Nevertheless, it is important in toxicologic pathology that any changes in the pulmonary vasculature are accurately characterized, along with any changes in the weight of the right ventricle for this may provide some clues to haemodynamic alterations in the pulmonary circulation.

Vasculitis

Although pulmonary vessels are frequently uninvolved when necrotizing vascular processes develop in systemic blood vessels, vasculitis can develop in the lungs of laboratory animals or in man under a number of different circumstances, analogous to those associated with vasculitis in the systemic circulation.

Fibrinoid necrosis of muscular pulmonary arteries is a component of the plexogenic arteriopathy associated with severe hypertensive pulmonary vascular disease which is likely to result from intensive or excessive vasoconstriction of the relatively thin muscular coat (Wagenvoort and Wagenvoort, 1981; Yamaki and Wagenvoort, 1981).

As in some syndromes of pulmonary vasculitis found in man, some forms of vasculitis occurring in laboratory animals which have similar patterns of vascular involvement are believed to have an auto-immune pathogenesis. A notable example is the pulmonary vasculitis which has been reported in New Zealand (NZB × NZW) F_1 hybrid mice with disordered immunoregulation.

Sequential pathological studies with mice of this strain have shown that at about four months of age, mild perivascular and peribronchial lymphoid hyperplasia develops, composed of a mixture of B and T cells (Staszak and Harbeck, 1985; Harbeck et al., 1986). This becomes more marked with advancing age. At about eight months of age pulmonary vasculitis involving arterioles, veins and venules with only occasional involvement of muscular arteries, develops. Affected vessels show transmural infiltration by lymphoid cells which immunocytochemical study shows are mostly Thy-1 and Lyt-1 positive T lymphocytes with a notable absence of Lyt-2 positive cells (Harbeck et al., 1986). Although narrowing of the vascular lumen and fragmentation of the limiting elastic lamina is reported, necrosis of the vessel walls is not seen, despite the intense lymphoid infiltrate (Staszak and Harbeck, 1985).

It is believed that the disordered regulation of the immune system is important in the development of this condition but mechanisms remain unclear. It has been suggested that the lymphoid hyperplasia which precedes vasculitis is the result of chronic antigenic stimulation in the context of defective immunoregulation. The subsequent development of vasculitis represents failure of Lyt-2 positive T (suppressor) cells to regulate inflammatory lymphokine production with persistence of inflammation and uncontrolled proliferation of antigen-reactive cells (Harbeck et al., 1986).

Analogous vasculitis affecting small pulmonary vessels has also been reported in laboratory mice and rats following administration of immunomodulating agents. A notable example is provided by studies in which high doses of human recombinant interleukin-2 (T-cell growth factor), a cytokine normally produced by activated T cells, were administered to mice and rats. In mice, high doses of interleukin-2 produced a vascular leak syndrome (see lungs) part of which comprised lymphocytic infiltration of pulmonary venules and arterioles as well as within the perivascular interstitium. Cells were predominantly Thy Lyt-2 and asialo GM1 positive lymphocytes (Anderson et al., 1988). Likewise, marked infiltration of pulmonary arterioles, capillaries and venules by lymphocytes as well as eosinophils was reported in rats given high doses of interleukin-2 (Anderson and Hayes, 1989). It was suggested that the tissue infiltration by eosinophils was secondary to an eosinopoietic cytokine produced by interleukin-2 stimulated lymphocytes (Anderson and Hayes, 1989). Both rat and mouse appear to be appropriate models for the toxicity of high dose interleukin-2 therapy in man. Perivascular eosinophilic infiltration without vessel damage has also been reported in small pulmonary vessels in rats treated with an immunosuppressive agent FK 506 (Nalesnik et al., 1987).

Pulmonary arteritis, characterised histologically by focal endothelial destruction and proliferation, subintimal infiltration by neutrophils and mononuclear cells, subintimal deposits of fibrin and marked adventitial fibrosis and mononuclear cell infiltration was also reported in rats treated with high doses of the anti-cancer mitomycin derivative BMY-25282 (Bregman et al., 1987).

Injection of substances with large molecular weights, particularly polysaccharides, can give rise to vasculitis which is characterised by small, angiocentric non-necrotising granulomas clustered mainly around small pulmonary arteries, arterioles and capillaries. There is no evidence of an immune mediated mechanism for this type of lesion which may simply result from the deposition of the injected material in small vessels (Johnson et al., 1984; Greaves and Faccini, 1984).

Fragments of skin, hair or keratin may be punched out by the needle used during intravenous toxicity studies, enter the circulation to form small pulmonary emboli. This phenomenon can occur in both rodents and larger animals and although functional derangement is not usually evident, thrombi, focal inflammation and foreign body granulomas may form in and around small pulmonary blood vessels (Tekeli, 1974; Schneider and Pappritz, 1976).

Hypertrophy and hyperplasia

As in the systemic circulation, medial thickening of pulmonary arteries is characteristic of pulmonary hypertension. Whilst pulmonary hypertension occurs in association with a variety of pathological states, evolution of medial hypertrophy and the accompanying vascular remodelling associated with hypoxia have been particularly well studied experimentally and forms a useful basis for the analysis of drug-induced changes in the pulmonary circulation in experimental animals. Hyperoxia has also been shown to produce similar alterations in the pulmonary circulation of experimental animals (Coflesky et al., 1988).

Studies in rats have shown that hypoxia causes an acute rise in pulmonary arterial pressure. This is initially reversible and believed to be due to vasoconstriction (Fried and Reid, 1985). Within a few days however, hypoxia produces structural changes in pulmonary arteries, principally an increase in medial thickness of pre-acinar muscular arteries due to both hypertrophy of smooth muscle cells and cytoplasmic organelles and an increase in mitotic activity (Meyrick and Reid, 1979, 1980). In addition, there is an increase in the proportion of muscular arteries which are observed in the periphery of the lung accompanying respiratory bronchioles, alveolar ducts and walls (Meyrick and Reid, 1981). In the normal rat lung, intra-acinar arterial segments, usually up to 0.5 cm in length, quickly loose their muscle fibres before reaching the capillary bed (Hislop and Reid, 1978). In hypoxic states, these vessels become muscularised presumably by proliferation and differentiation of undifferentiated precursor smooth muscle cells such as pericytes and intermediate cells (Meyrick and Reid, 1979; Langleben et al., 1987).

Whereas the general pulmonary response to hypoxia is similar among different mammalian species, age, strain and species-related susceptibility to hypoxia is variable (Tucker et al., 1975; Weir et al., 1979; Meyrick and Reid, 1981, 1982; Langleben et al., 1987). Studies in cattle have suggested that the medial thickness of undistended, normal pulmonary arteries may predict for the degree of pulmonary hypertension and arterial medial thickening which can develop under hypoxic conditions at high altitude or in response to administration of agents such as prostaglandins $E_2\alpha$, E_1 and 5-hydroxytryptamine (Tucker et al., 1975; Weir et al., 1979).

Langleben and colleagues (1987) have demonstrated different susceptibilities of two colonies of Sprague-Dawley rats to chronic hypobaric hypoxia. Although Sprague-Dawley rats from the Hilltop Colony were shown to normally possess more muscular intra-acinar arteries and a lesser vasoconstrictive response to acute hypoxia than Sprague-Dawley rats from the Madison Colony, they showed a greater response to chronic hypoxia. Chronic hypoxia caused a greater degree of pulmonary hypertension as well as more polycythaemia, vasoconstriction, muscularisation of intra-acinar arteries and medial thickening of pre-acinar arteries.

Hyperoxia has also been shown to produce medial thickening of muscular pulmonary arteries and a higher proportion of muscular intra-acinar and pre-acinar arteries in rats as well as right ventricular hypertrophy (Jones et al., 1985; Coflesky et al., 1988). The mechanism for this response in unclear, but it may be a response to increase pressure in the distal pulmonary bed, or a response to endothelial injury and enhanced action of inflammatory cells, platelets or vasoactive mediations on the vessel wall (Coflesky et al., 1988). Oxygen excess also injuries small veins in the alveolar region of the lung and enhances their muscularisation (Hu and Jones, 1989).

Medial hypertrophy of a similar morphological type can also be induced in laboratory animals by administration by vasoactive drugs. This has been demonstrated in a study by Fried and Reid (1985) in which modest doses of isoprenaline were administered to rats for two weeks by continuous intravenous infusion using osmotic minipumps. Treated rats showed similar alterations in the pulmonary vasculature to those found in rats maintained in a hypobaric hypoxic environment for a few days, notably an increase in the thickness of the media of muscular arteries and muscularisation of more peripherally situated vessels. These changes were associated with an increase in heart weight relative to body weight, affecting the right more than the left ventricle. Haemodynamic studies showed no increases in pulmonary arterial pressure. However, the systemic arterial pressure decreased, the cardiac index (cardiac output per square meter of body surface) increased, there was a marked reduction in systemic vascular resistance with only mild falls in pulmonary vascular resistance.

As the haemodynamic changes in the pulmonary circulation were slight, it was argued that the medial hypertrophy may have been a metabolic effect of isoprenaline administration (Fried and Reid, 1985).

REFERENCES

ADAMS, M.G., BARER, R., JOSEPH S. and OM'INIABOHS, F. (1981): Fat accumulation in the rat heart during fasting. *J.Pathol.*, 135, 111–126.

ALBASSAM, M.A., HOUSTON, B.J., GREAVES, P. and BARSOUM, N. (1989): Polyarteritis in a beagle. *J.Am.Vet.Med. Assoc.* 194, 1595–1597.

ALOUSI, A.A., FABIAN, R.J., BAKER, J.F. and STROSHANE, R.M. (1985): Milrinone. In: A. Scriabine (Ed.), *New Drugs Annual*: Cardiovascular Drugs, Vol. 3, 245–283. Raven Press, New York.

ALEXANDER, E.L., MOYER, C., TRAVLOS, G.S., ROTHS, J.B. and MURPHY, E.D. (1985): Two histopathologic types of inflammatory vascular disease in MRL/MP autoimmune mice. *Arthritis Rheum.*, 28, 1146–1155.

AL-RUFAIE, H.K., FLORIO, R.A. and OLSEN, E.G.J. (1983): Comparison of the haematoxylin basic fuchsin picric acid method and the fluorescence of haematoyxlin and eosin stained sections for the identification of early myocardial infarction. *J.Clin.Pathol.*, 36, 646–649.

ALLWORK, S.P. (1987): The applied anatomy of the arterial blood supply to the heart in man. *J.Anat.*, 153, 1–16.

ANDERSON, T.D. and HAYES, T.J. (1989): Toxicity of human recombinant interleukin-2 in rats. Pathologic changes are characterized by marked lymphocytic and eosinophilic proliferation and multisystem involvement. *Lab.Invest.*, 60, 331–346.

ANDERSON, T.D., HAYES, T.J., GATELY, M.K., BONTEMPO, J.M., STERN, L.L. and TRUITT, G.A. (1988): Toxicity of human recombinant interleukin-2 in the mouse is mediated by interleukin-activated lymphocytes. Separation of efficacy and toxicity by selective lymphocyte subset depletion. *Lab.Invest.*, 59, 598–612.

ANVER, M.R., COHEN, B.J., LATTUADA, C.P. and FOSTER, S.J. (1982): Age-associated lesions in barrier-reared male Sprague-Dawley rats: A comparison between Hap: (SD) and Crl: COBS CD (SD) stocks Exp. *Aging Res.*, 8, 3–24.

ANVERSA, P., RICCI, R. and OLIVETTI, G. (1986): Quantitative structural analysis of the myocardium during physiological growth and induced cardiac hypertrophy: A review. *J.Am.Coll.Cardiol.*, 7, 1140–1149.

ARETZ, H.T. (1987): Myocarditis: The Dallas Criteria. *Hum.Pathol.*, 18, 619–624.

AVERSANO, R.C. and BOOR, P.J. (1983): Histochemical alterations of acute and chronic doxorubicin cardiotoxicity. *J.Mol.Cell Cardiol.*, 15, 543–553.

AYERS, K.M. and JONES, S.R. (1978): The cardiovascular system. In: K. Benirschke, F.M. Garner and T.C. Jones (Eds), *Pathology of Laboratory Animals*, Vol. 1, Chap. 1, 1–69. Springer-Verlag, New York.

BACHMAN, E., WEBER, E. and ZBINDEN, G. (1984): The effect of methyl-2-tetradecyglycidate (McNeil 3716) on heart mitochondrial metabolism in rats. *Biochem.Pharmacol.*, 33, 1947–1950.

BAILAS, N. (1965): Functional mitral insufficiency in acute myocardial ischemia. *Am.J.Cardiol.*, 16, 807–812.

BALAZS, T. (1973): Cardiotoxicity of sympathomimetic bronchodilator and vasodilating antihypertensive drugs in experimental animals. In: Duncan, W.A. (Ed.), Experimental Model Systems in Toxicology and Their Significance in Man. Vol. 15, 71–82. Excerpta Medica, Amsterdam.

BALAZS, T. (1981): Cardiotoxicity of adrenergic bronchodilator and vasodilating antihypertensive agents. In: T. Balazs (Ed.), *Cardiac Toxicology*, Vol. 2, Chap. 6, 61–73. CRC Press, Boca Raton, Florida.

BALAZS, T. and BLOOM, S. (1982): Cardiotoxicity of adrenergic bronchodilator and vasodilating antihypertensive drugs. In: E.W. Van Stee, (Ed.), *Cardiovascular Toxicology*, pp.199–220. Raven Press, New York.

BALAZS, T. and PAYNE, B.J. (1971): Myocardial papillary muscle necrosis induced by hypotensive agents in dogs. *Toxicol.Appl.Pharmacol.*, 20, 442–445.

BALAZS, T. (1986). Cardiotoxicity mechanisms from the safety point of view of preclinical or premarketing safety evaluation. *Arch.Toxicol.*, Suppl. 9, 171–177.

BARBOLT, T.A. and CORNACOFF, J.B. (1990): Dose-dependent arteritis in cynomolgus monkeys after exposure to recombinant human interleukin-4. Presented at IX International Symposium of

BERMAN, J.J., RICE, J.M. and REDDICK, R. (1980): Endocardial Schwannomas in rats. *Arch.Pathol.Lab.Med.*, 104, 187–191

BERTENS, A.P.M.G., VAM CAMPEN, G.J. and MIKX, F.H.M. (1982): Thrombosis of the right ventricle in dogs after frequent administration of corticosteroids. *Z. Versuchstierkd*, 24, 237–240.

BILLINGHAM, M.E. (1980): Morphologic changes in drug-induced heart disease. In: M.R. Bristow (Ed.), Chap. 6, pp.127–149. Elsevier, Amsterdam.

BLOCK, M.I., SAID, J.W., SIEGEL, R.J. and FISHBEIN, M.C. (1983): Myocardial myoglobin following coronary artery occlusion. An immunohistochemical study. *Am.J.Pathol.*, 111, 374–379.

BOOR, P.J. (1985): Allylamine cardiovascular toxicity: V. tissue distribution and toxicokinetics after oral administration. *Toxicology,* 35, 167–177.

BOOR, P.J. (1987). Amines and the heart. *Arch.Pathol.Lab.Med.*, 111, 930–932.

BOOR, P.J. and HYSMITH, R.M. (1987): Allylamine cardiovascular toxicity. *Toxicology*, 44, 129–145.

BOORMAN, G.A., ZURCHER, C., HOLLANDER, C.F. and FERON, V.J. (1973): Naturally occurring endocardial disease in the rat. *Arch.Pathol.*, 96, 39–45.

BOURDOIS, P.S., DANCLA, J-L., FACCINI, J.M., NACHBAUR, J. and MONRO, A.M. (1982): The subacute toxicology of digoxin in dogs: Clinical chemistry and histopathology of heart and kidneys. *Arch.Toxicol.*, 51, 273–283.

BREGMAN, C.L., COMERESKI, C.R., BUROKER, R.A., HIRTH, R.S., MADISSOO, H. and HOTTENDORF, G.H. (1987): Single dose and multiple-dose intravenous toxicity studies of BMY-25282 in rats. *Fundam.Appl.Toxicol.*, 9, 90–109.

BREGMAN, C.L., BUROKER, R.A., BRADNER, W.T., HIRTH, R.S. and MADISSOO, H. (1989): Cardiac, renal and pulmonary toxicity of several mitomycin derivatives in rats. *Fundam.Appl. Toxicol.*, 13, 46–64.

BROOKS, P.N. (1984): Necrotizing vasculitis in a group of Beagles. *Lab.Anim.*, 18, 285–290.

BUGELSKI, P.J., WALSH VOCKLEY, C.M., SOWINSKI, J.M., ARENA, E., BERKOWITZ, B.A. and MORGAN, D.G. (1989): Ultrastructure of an arterial lesion induced in rats by fenoldopam mesylate, a dopaminergic vasolidator. *Br.J.Exp.Pathol.*, 70, 153–165.

BYROM, F.B. (1954): The pathogenesis of hypertensive encephalopathy and its relation to the malignant phase of hypertension. *Lancet*, 2, 201–211.

CAMPBELL, S.E. and GERDES, A.M. (1987): Regional differences in myocyte dimensions and number in Sprague-Dawley rats from different suppliers. *Proc.Soc.Exp.Biol.Med.*, 186, 221–217.

CAMPBELL, S.E., GERDES, A.M. and SMITH, T.D. (1987): Comparison of regional differences in cardiac myocyte dimensions in rats, hamsters and guinea pigs. *Anat.Rec.*, 219, 53–59.

CANTIN, M., GUTKOWSKA, J., THIBAULT, G., MILNE, R.W., LEDOUX, S., MINLI, S., CHAPEAU, C., GARCIA, R., HAMET, P. and GENEST, J. (1984): Immunocytochemical localization of atrial natriuretic factor in the heart and salivary glands. *Histochemistry*, 80, 113–127.

CAPASSO, J.M., REMILY, R.M. and SONNENBLICK, E.H. (1983): Age-related differences in excitation-contraction in rat papillary muscle. *Basic Res.Cardiol.*, 78, 492–504.

CAPLAN, L.R., HIER, D.B. and BANKS, G. (1982): Current concepts of cerebrovascular disease. Stroke: stroke and drug abuse. *Stroke*, 13, 869–872.

CARLSON, R.G. and FEENSTRA, E.S. (1977): Toxicologic studies with the hypotensive agent minoxidil. *Toxicol.Appl.Pharmacol.*, 39, 1–11.

CASE, M.T., SIBINSKI, L.J. and STEFFEN, G.R. (1984): Chronic oral toxicity and oncogenicity studies of flecanide, an antiarrhythmic, in rats and mice. *Toxicol.Appl.Pharmacol.*, 73, 232–242.

CAULFIELD, J.B. and BITTNER, V. (1988): Cardiac matrix alterations induced by adriamycin. *Am.J.Pathol.*, 133, 298–305.

CHVÉDOFF, M., CHIGNARD, G., DANCLA, J.L., FACCINI, J.M., LOYEAU, F., PERRAUD, J. and TARADACH, C. (1982): Le rongeur agé: observations recueillies au cours d'essais de carcinogénicité. *Sci.Tech.Lab.*, 7, 87–97.

CIMPRICH, R.E., ZIEMBA, L.J., KUTZ, S.A., ROBERTSON, J.L. and COCKRELL, B. (1986): Experimentally induced malignant hypertension in beagle dogs. *Toxicol.Pathol.*, 14, 183–187.

CITRON, B.P., HALPERN, M., McCARRON, M., LUNDBERG, G.D., McCORMICK, R., PINCUS, I.J., TATTER, D. and HAVERBACK, B.J. (1970): Necrotizing angiitis associated with drug abuse. *N.Engl.J.Med.*, 283, 1003–1001.

COFLESKY, J.T., ADLER, K.B., WOODCOCK-MITCHELL, J. MITCHELL, J. and EVANS, J.E. (1988): Proliferative changes in the pulmonary arterial wall during short-term hyperoxic injury to the lung. *Am.J.Pathol.*, 132, 563–573.

COHEN, A.S.., CATHCART, E.S. and SKINNER, M. (1978): Amyloidosis. Current trends in its investigation. *Arthritis Rheum.*, 21, 153–160.

CRAFT-CORMNEY, C. and HANSEN, J.T. (1980): Early ultrastructural changes in the myocardium following thyroxine-induced hypertrophy. *Virchows Arch.* [B], 33, 267–273.

CRUICKSHANK, J.M., FITZGERALD, J.D., and TUCKER, M. (1984): Beta-adrenoceptor blocking drugs: pronethalol, propanol and practolol. In: D.R. Lawrence, A.E.M. McLean, M. Weatheral (Eds), Safety Testing of New Drugs, Laboratory Predictions and Clinical Performance, Chap.5, 93–123. Academic Press, London.

DE BUSK, R.F. and HARRISON, D.C. (1969): The clinical spectrum of papillary muscle disease. *N.Engl.J.Med.*, 281, 1458–1467.

de DUVE, C., de BARSY, T., POOLE, B., TROUET, A., TULKENS, P. and VAN HOOF, F. (1974): Lysosomotropic agents. *Biochem.Pharmacol.*, 23, 2495–2531.

DETWEILER, D.K. (1981): The use of electrocardiography in toxicological studies with Beagle Dogs. In: T. Balazs, (Ed.), *Cardiac Toxicology*, Vol. 3, pp.33–38. CRC Press, Boca Raton, Florida.

DETWEILER, D.K., BISHOP, S.P., TESKE, R.H. and FILLMORE, G.E. (1981): Experimental subchronic digoxin toxicosis in the dog. In: T. Balazs (Ed.), *Cardiac Toxicology*, Vol. 2, Chap. 4, 43–53. CRC Press, Boca Raton, Florida.

DE WIT, R.H., PETER, G.K., FITZGERALD, J.E. and DE LA IGLESIA, F.A. (1985): Preliminary toxicologic evaluation of a novel cardiotonic agent. *Toxicologist*, 5, 94.

DOI, K., YAMAMOTO, T., ISEGAWA, N., DOI, C. and MITSUOKA, T. (1987): Age-related non-neoplastic alterations in the heart and kidneys of Syrian hamsters of the APA strain. *Lab.Anim.*, 21, 241–248.

DOMINICK, M.A., METZ, A.L. and GOUGH, A.W. (1990): Reversible cardiac morphologic alterations following intravenous administration of CI-959, an antiallergy compound, to rats. Presented at IX International Symposium of Society of Toxicologic Pathologists, Ottawa.

DOUGLAS, J.G., MONRO, J.F., KITCHIN, A.H., MUIR, A.L. and PROUDFOOT, A.T. (1981): Pulmonary hypertension and fenfluramine. *Br.Med.J.*, 283, 881–883.

DRIVSHOLM, L., LAYBOURN, C. and OLSEN, F. (1985): Further evidence of the development of delayed-type autoimmunity against arterial vessel-wall antigens following acute hypertensive damage to arterial vessels in rats. *Acta Pathol.Microbiol.Immunol.* [C], 93, 105–110.

EIGLER, F.W., SCHAARSCHMIDT, K., GROSS, E. and RICHTER, H.J. (1986): Anorectal ulcers as a complication of migraine therapy. *J.R.Soc.Med.*, 24–428.

EVERITT, J.I., ROSS, P.W., MANGUM, J.B., OLSON, L.M. and VISEK, W.J. (1986): Severe myocardial disease in C3H/Ouj mice associated with feeding of a semipurified diet containing soybean oil. *Lab.Anim.Sci.*, 70.

FACTOR, S.M., MINASE, T., CHO, S., FEIN, F., CAPASSO, J.M. and SONNENBLICK, E.H. (1984): Coronary microvascular abnormalities in the hypertensive-diabetic rat. A primary cause of cardiomyopathy? *Am.J.Pathol.*, 116, 9–20.

FAHLÉN, M., BERGMAN, H., HELDER, G., RYDÉN, L., WALLENTIN, I. and ZETTERGREN, L. (1973): Phenformin and pulmonary hypertension. *Br.Heart J.*, 35, 824–828.

FAUCI, A.S., HAYNES, B.F. and KATZ, P. (1978): The spectrum of vasculitis. Clinical, pathologic, immunologic and therapeutic considerations. *Ann.Int.Med.*, 89, 660–676.

FEIGL, E.O. (1987): The paradox of adrenergic coronary vasoconstrictuion. *Circulation*, 76, 737–745.

FERRANS, V.J., HIBBS, R.G., WALSH, J.J. and BURCH, G.E. (1969): Histochemical and electron microscopical studies on the cardiac necrosis produced by sympathomimetic agents. *Ann.N.Y.Acad.Sci.*, 156, 309–332.

FIGUEROA, I.C., PEGG, D.G., KIM, S.N. and DE LA IGLESIA, F.S. (1986): Assessment of methodology for determining acute cardiotoxic potential of anticancer drugs. *Toxicologist*, 6, 199.

FILLMORE, G.E. and DETWEILER, D.K. (1973): Maintenance of subacute digoxin toxicosis in normal beagles. *Toxicol.Appl.Pharmacol.*, 25, 418–429.

FOLLATH, F., BURKART, F. and SCHWEIZER (1971): Drug-induced pulmonary hypertension? *Br.Med.J.*, 1, 265–266.

FRENCH, W.J., ADOMIAN, G.E., AVERILL, W.K., GARNER, D. and LAKS, M.M. (1983): Chronic infusion of verapamil produces increased heart weight in conscious dogs. *Clin.Res.*, 31, 184A.

FRIED, R. and REID, L.M. (1985): The effect of isoproterenol on the development and recovery of hypoxic pulmonary hypertension. A structural and haemodynamic study. *Am.J.Pathol.*, 121, 102–111.

FRITH, C.H., FARRIS, H.E. and HIGHMAN, E. (1977): Endocardial fibromatous proliferation in a rat. *Lab.Anim.Sci.*, 27, 114–117.

GANG, D.L., BARRETT, L.V., WILSON, E.J., RUBIN, R.H. and MEDEARIS, D.N. (1986): Myopericarditis and enhanced dystropic cardiac calcification in murine cytomegalovirus infection. *Am.J.Pathol.*, 124, 207–215.

GANS, J.H., KORSON, R., CATER, M.R. and ACKERLY, C.C. (1980): Effects of short-term and long-term theobromine administration to male dogs. *Toxicol.Appl.Pharmacol.*, 53, 481–496.

GERDES, A.M., MOORE, J.A., HINES, J.M., KIRKLAND, P.A. and BISHOP, S.P. (1986): Regional differences in myocyte size in normal rat heart. *Anat.Rec.*, 215, 420–426.

GERMUTH, F.G. (1953): A comparative histologic and immunologic study in rabbits of induced hypersensitivity of the serum sickness type. *J.Exp.Med.*, 97, 257–282.

GILBERT, P.L., SIEGEL, R.J., MELMED, S., SHERMAN, C.T. and FISHBEIN, M.C. (1985): Cardiac morphology in rats with growth hormone-producing tumours. *J.Mol.Cell Cardiol.*, 17, 805–811.

GLASSMAN, A.H. (1984)a: Cardiovascular effects of tricyclic antidepressants. *Ann.Rev.Med.*, 35, 503–511.

GLASSMAN, A.H. (1984)b: The newer antidepressant drugs and their cardiovascular effects. *Psychopharmacol.Bull.*, 20, 272–279.

GODENY, E.K. and GAUNTT, C.J. (1987): In situ immune autoradio-graphic identification of cells in heart tissues of mice with coxsackievirus B3-induced myocarditis. *Am.J.Pathol.*, 129, 267–276.

GODFRAIND, T. (1984): Drug-induced cardionecrosis. *Arch.Toxicol.*, *Suppl.* 7, 1–15.

GOMI, T. YAMAMOTO, H., OZEKI, M., FUJIKURA, M., HIRAO, A., KOBAYASHI, M., TATEISHI, T., YUMOTO, S. and OKUMURA, M. (1985): Acute and subacute toxicity of 2,6-dimethyl-3,5-dimethoxycarbonyl-4-(o-difluoromethoxyphenyl)-1,4- dihydropyridine (PP-1466), *Arzneimittelforschung*, 35, 915–922.

GOODMAN, D.G., WARD, J.M., SQUIRE, R.A., PAXTON, M.B., REICHARDT, W.D., CHU, K.C., and LINHART, M.S. (1980): Neoplastic and non-neoplastic lesions in ageing Osborne-Mendel Rats. *Toxicol.Appl.Pharmacol.*, 55, 433–447.

GRACON, S.I., DIFONZO, C.J., FITZGERALD, J.E., STURGESS, J.M. and DE LA IGLESIA (1984): Oral toxicity evaluation of a novel cardiotonic. *Toxicologist*, 4, 7.

GRANT, C., GREENE, D.G. and BUNNELL, I.L. (1965): Left ventricular enlargement and hypertrophy. A clinical and angiocardiographic study. *Am.J.Med.*, 39, 895–904.

GREAVES, P. and FACCINI, J.M. (1984): Cardiovascular system. In: A Glossary for use in Toxicity and Carcinogenicity Studies. Chap. 5, pp.74–81. Elsevier, Amsterdam.

GREAVES, P., MARTIN, J., MICHEL, M.C. and MOMPON, P. (1984): Cardiac hypertrophy in the dog and rat induced by oxfenicine, an agent which modifies muscle metabolism. *Arch.Toxicol.*, *Suppl.* 7, 488–493.

GREEN, M.D., SPEYER, J.L. and MUGGIA, F.M. (1984): Cardiotoxicity of anthracyclines. *Eur.J. Cancer Clin.Oncol.*, 20, 293–296.

GROSSMAN, W., JONES, D. and McLAURIN, L.P. (1975): Wall stress and patterns of hypertrophy. *J. Clin.Invest.*, 56, 56–64.

GROSSMAN, W. (1980): Cardiac hypertrophy: Useful adaption or pathological process? *Am.J.Med.*, 69, 576–584.

GRUYS, E., TIMMERMANS and van EDEREN, A.M. (1979): Deposition of amyloid in the liver of hamsters: an enzyme-histochemical and electron-microscopical study. *Lab.Anim.*, 13, 1–9.

HARBECK, R.J., LAUNDER, T. and STASZAK, C. (1986): Mononuclear cell pulmonary vasculitis in NZB/W mice. X Immunohistochemical characterization of the infiltrating cells. *Am.J.Pathol.*, 123, 204–211.

HARCOURT, R.A. (1978): Polyarteritis in a colony of beagles. *Vet.Rec.*, 102, 519–522.

HARLEMAN, J.H., JOSEPH, E.C., EDEN, R.J., WALKER, T.F., MAJOR, I.R. and LAMB, M.S. (1986): Cardiotoxicity of a new inotrope/vasodilator drug (SK & F 94120) in the dog. *Arch.Toxicol.*, 59, 51–55.

HARTMAN, H.A. (1987): Idiopathic extramural coronary arteritis in Beagle and mongrel dogs. *Vet.Pathol.*, 24, 537–544.

HAYAKAWA, B.N., JORGENSEN, A.O., GOTLIEB, A.I., ZHAO, M-S. and LIEW, C.C. (1984): Immunofluorescent microscopy for the identification of human necrotic myocardium. *Arch.Pathol.Lab.Med.*, 198, 284–286.

HENDY, R.J., ABRAHAM, R. and GRASSO, P. (1969): The effect of chloroquine on rat heart lysosomes. *J.Ultrastructure Res.*, 29, 485–495.

HERMAN, E.H., BALAZS, T., YOUNG, R., EARL, F.L., KROP, S. and FERRANS, V.J. (1979): Acute cardiomyopathy induced by the vasodilating antihypertensive agent minoxidil. *Toxicol.Appl.Pharmacol.*, 47, 493–503.

HERMAN, E.H., EL-HAGE, A.N., FERRANS, V.J. and ARDALAN, B. (1985): Comparison of the severity of the chronic cardiotoxicity produced by doxorubicin in normotensive and hypertensive rats. *Toxicol.Appl.Pharmacol.*, 78, 202–214.

HEWICKER, M. and TRAUTWEIN, G. (1987): Sequential study of vasculitis in MRL mice. *Lab.Anim.*, 21, 335–341.

HICKS, J.D. (1966): Vascular changes in the kidneys of NZB mice and FI NZBxNZW hydrids. *J.Pathol.Bacteriol.*, 91, 479–486.

HIGGINS, A.J., FACCINI, J.M. and GREAVES, P. (1985): Coronary hyperemia and cardiac hypertrophy following inhibition of fatty acid oxidation. Evidence of a regulatory role for cytosolic phosphorylation potential. In: N.S. Dhalla, D.J. Hearse, (Eds), *Advances in Myocardiology*, Vol. 6, 329–338. Plenum Press.

HISLOP, A. and REID, L. (1978): Normal structure and dimensions of the pulmonary arteries in the rat. *J.Anat.*, 125, 71–83.

HOCH-LIGETI, C., SASS, B., SOBEL, H.J. and STEWART, H.L. (1983): Endocardial tumours in rats exposed to durable fibrous materials. *J.N.C.I.*, 71, 1067–1077.

HOCH-LIGETI, C. and STEWART, H.L. (1984): Cardiac tumours of mice. *J.N.C.I.*, 72, 1449–1456.

HOCH-LIGETI, C., RESTREPO, C. and STEWART, H.L. (1986): Comparative pathology of cardiac neoplasms in humans and in laboratory rodents: A review. *J.N.C.I.*, 76, 127–142.

HOFFMAN, K. (1984): Toxicological studies with nitrendipine. In: A. Scriabine, S. Vanov and K. Deck, (Eds), *Nitrendipine*, Chap. 3, 25–31. Urban and Schwarzenberg, Baltimore.

HOMEWOOD, C.A., WARHURST, D.C., PETERS, W. and BAGGALEY, V.C. (1972): Lysosomes, pH and the antimalarial action of chloroquine. *Nature*, 235, 50–52.

HOTTENDORF, G.H. and HIRTH, R.S. (1974): Lesions of spontaneous subclinical disease in beagle dogs. *Vet.Pathol.*, 11, 240–258.

HU, L-M. and JONES, R. (1989): Injury and remodelling of pulmonary veins by high oxygen. A morphometric study. *Am.J.Pathol.*, 134, 253–262.

HUANG, A.H. and FEIGL, E.O. (1988): Adrenergic coronary vasoconstriction helps maintain uniform transmural blood flow distribution during exercise. *Circ.Res.*, 62, 286–298.

HUGHES, J.T., ESIRI, M., OXBURY, J.M. and WHITTY, C.W.M. (1971): Chloroquine myopathy. *Q.J.Med.*, 40, 85–93.

HUMPHREY, S.J. and ZINS, G.R. (1984): Wholebody and regional haemodynamic effects of minoxidil in the conscious dog. *J.Cardiovasc.Pharmacol.*, 6, 979–988.

IBAYASHI, S.. OGATA, J., SADOSHIMA, S., FUJII, K., YAO, H. and FUGISHIMA, M. (1986): The effect of long-term anti-hypertensive treatment on medial hypertrophy of cerebral arteries in spontaneously hypertensive rats. *Stroke*, 17, 515–519.

JASMIN, G. and EU, H.Y. (1979): Cardiomyopathy of hamster dystrophy. *Ann.N.Y.Acad.Sci.*, 317, 46–58.

JENSEN, R.A., ACTON, E.M. and PETER, J.H. (1984): Doxorubicin cardiotoxicity in the rat. Comparison of electrocardiogram, transmembrane potential and structural effects. *J.Cardiovasc.Pharmacol.*, 6, 186–200.

JOBIT, C. and PAULUS, G. (1988): La cardiotoxicité de la doxorubicine. Une étude immunocytochimique du facteur natriurétique atrial (FNA) chez le rat. *Rev.Fr.Histotechnol.*, 1, 11–15.

JODALEN, H., LIE, R. and ROTEVATN, S. (1982): Effect of isoproterenol on lipid accumulation in myocardial cells. *Res.Exp.Med.*, (Berl), 181, 239–244.

JOHANSSON, S. (1981): Cardiovascular lesions in Sprague-Dawley rats induced by long-term treatment with caffeine. *Acta Pathol.Microbiol. Scand.* [A], 89, 185–191.

JOHNSON, K.J., GLOVSKY, M. and SCHRIER, D. (1984): Pulmonary granulomatons vasculitis induced in rats by treatment with glucan. *Am.J.Pathol.*, 114, 515–516.

JONES, R., ZAPOL, W.M. and REID, L. (1985): Oxygen toxicity and restructuring of pulmonary arteries: a morphometric study. The response to 4 weeks' exposure to hyperoxia and return to breathing air. *Am.J.Pathol.*, 121, 212–223.

JORIS, I. and MAJNO, G. (1981): Medial changes in arterial spasm induced by L-norepinephrine. *Am.J.Pathol.*, 105, 212–222.

KARCH, S.B. and BILLINGHAM, M.E. (1988): The pathology and etiology of cocaine-induced heart disease. *Arch.Pathol.Lab.Med.*, 112, 225–230.

KARLINER, J.S., ALABASTER, C. STEPHENS, H. BARNES, P. and DOLLERY, C. (1981): Enhanced noradrenaline response in cardiomyopathic hamsters: Possible relation to changes in adrenoceptors studied by radioligand binding. *Cardiovasc.Res.*, 15, 296–304.

KAZDA, S., GARTHOFF, B., RAMSCH, K-D. and SCHLÜTER, G. (1983): Nisoldipine. In: A. Scriabine (Ed.), *New Drugs Annual*, Cardiovascular Drugs, pp.243–258. Raven Press, New York.

KLEIGER, R.E., BOYER, M., INGHAM, R.E. and HARRISON, D.C. (1976): Pulmonary hypertension in patients using oral contraceptives: A report of six cases. *Chest*, 69, 143–147.

KLINE, I.K. (1961): Myocardial alterations associated with pheochromocytomas. *Am.J.Pathol.*, 38, 539–551.

LAKS, M.M. and MORADY, F. (1976): Norepinephrine: the myocardial hypertrophy hormone? *Am.Heart J.*, 91, 674–675.

LANGLEBEN, D., JONES, R.C., ARONOVITZ, M.J., HILL, N.S., OU, L-C and REID, L.M. (1987): Pulmonary artery structural changes in two colonies of rats with different sensitivity to chronic hypoxia. *Am.J.Pathol.*, 128, 61–66.

LANG-STEVENSON, D., MIKHAILIDIS, D.P. and GILLETT, D.S. (1977): Cardiotoxicity of 5-fluorouracil. *Lancet*, 2, 406–407.

LAWLER, J.E., BARKER, G.F., HUBBARD, J.W. and SCHAUB, R.G. (1981): Effects of stress on blood pressure and cardiac pathology in rats with borderline hypertension. *Hypertension*, 3, 496–305.

LEHR, D. (1981): Studies on the cardiotoxicity of α- and β-adrenergic amines. In: T. Balazs, (Ed.), *Cardiac Toxicology.*, Vol. 3, Chap. 7, pp.75–112. CRC Press, Boca Raton, Florida.

LEONE, B., RABINOVICH, M., FERRARI, C.R., BOYER, J., ROSSO, H. and STRAUSS, E. (1985): Cardiotoxicity as a result of 5-fluorouracil therapy. *Tumori*, 71, 55–57.

LEWIS, D.J. (1980): Sub-endocardial fibrosis in the rat: A light and electron microscopic study. *J.Comp.Pathol.*, 90, 577–583.

LIE, J.T. (1987): Coronary vasculitis: a review of the current scheme of classification of vasculitis. *Arch.Pathol.Lab.Med.*, 111, 224–233.

LINDPAINTER, K., LINDPAINTER, L.S., WENTWORTH, M. and BURNS, C.P. (1986): Acute myocardial necrosis during administration of amsacrine. *Cancer*, 57, 1284–1286.

LIMAS, C., WESTRUM, B. and LIMAS, C.J. (1980): The evolution of vascular changes in the spontaneously hypertensive rat. *Am.J.Pathol.*, 98, 357–384.

LOWE, J. (1984): Method for the morphometric analysis of arterial structure. *J.Clin.Pathol.*, 37, 1413–1415.

LUGINBÜHL, H. and DETWEILER, D.K. (1965): Cardiovascular lesions in dogs. *Ann.N.Y.Acad. Sci.*, 127, 517–540.

LUMB, G.D., BEAMER, P.R. and RUST, J.H. (1985): Oesophagostomiasis in feral monkeys (Macaca mulatta). *Toxicol.Pathol.*, 13, 209–214.

LUND, F. (1951): Vasodilator drugs against experimental peripheral gangrene. A method of testing the effect of vasodilator drugs on constricted peripheral vessels. *Acta Physiol.Scand.*, 23, Suppl. 82, 4–79.

LUNT, D.W.R. and ROSE, A.G. (1987): Pathology of the human heart in drowning. *Arch.Pathol.Lab.Med.*, 111, 939–942.

MAYER, D. and BANNASCH, P. (1983): Endomyocardial fibrosis in rats treated with N-nitrosomorpholine. *Virchows Arch.* [A], 401, 129–135.

McALLISTER, H.A., FERRANS, V.J., HALL, R.J., STICKMAN, N.E. and BOSSART, M.I. (1987): Chloroquine-induced cardiomyopathy. *Arch.Pathol.Lab.Med.*, 111, 953–956.

McALLISTER, H.A. and MULLICK, F.G. (1982): The cardiovascular system. In: R.H. Riddell (Ed.), *Pathology of Drug-induced and Toxic Diseases*, Chap. 10, pp.201–228. Churchill Livingston, New York.

McMARTIN, D.N. and DODDS, W.J. (1982): Atrial thrombosis in aged Syrian hamsters. *Am.J.Pathol.*, 107, 277–279.

MESFIN, G.M., SHAWARYN, G.G. and HIGGINS, M.J. (1987): Cardiovascular alterations in dogs treated with hydralazine. *Toxicol.Pathol.*, 15, 409–416.

MESFIN, G.M., HIGGINS, M.J., BROWN, W.P. and ROSNICK, D. (1988): Cardiovascular complications of chronic catheterization of the jugular vein in the dog. *Vet.Pathol.*, 25, 492–502.

METZ, A.L., ROBERTSON, D.G., GOUGH, A.W. and DOMINICK, M.A. (1990): Reversible cardiac biochemical alterations following intravenous administration of CI-959, an antiallergy compound, to rats. Presented at IX International Symposium of Society of Toxicologic Pathologists, Ottawa.

MEYRICK, B. and REID, L. (1979): Hypoxia and incorporation of ^{3}H-thymidine by cells of the rat pulmonary arteries and alveolar wall. Am.J.Pathol., 96, 51–70.

MEYRICK, B. and REID, L. (1980): Hypoxia-induced structural changes in the media and adventitia of the rat hilar pulmonary artery and their regression. Am.J.Pathol., 100, 151–178.

MEYRICK, B. and REID, L. (1981): The effect of chronic hypoxia on pulmonary arteries in young rats. Exp.Lung Res., 2, 257–271.

MEYRICK, B. and REID, L. (1982): Normal postnatal development of the media of the rat hilar pulmonary artery and its remodelling by chronic hypoxia. Lab.Invest., 46, 505–514.

MULLICK, F.G. McALLISTER, H.A., WAGNER, B.M. and FENOGLIO, J.J. (1979): Drug-related vasculitis: clinicopathologic correlations in 30 patients. Human Pathol., 10, 313–325.

NALESNIK, M.A., TODO, S., MURASE, N., GRYZAN, S., LEE, P-H., MAKOWKA, L. and STARZL, T.E. (1987): Toxicology of FK-506 in the Lewis rat. Transplant.Proc., 19, Suppl. 6, 89–92.

NAYLOR, D.C., KRINKE, G. and ZAK, F. (1986): A comparison of endomyocardial disease in the rat with endomyocardial fibrosis in man. J.Comp.Pathol., 96, 473–483.

NEMES, Z., DIETZ, R., MANN, J.F.E., LÜTH, J.B. and GROSS, F. (1980): Vasoconstriction and increased blood pressure in the development of accelerated vascular disease. Virchows Arch. [A], 386, 161–173.

NORDBORG, C., FREDRIKSSON, K. and JOHANSSON, B.B. (1985): Internal carotid and vertebral arteries of spontaneously hypertensive and normotensive rats. Acta Pathol.Microbiol. Immunol.Scand. [A], 93, 153–158.

NORONHA-DUTRA, A.A., STEEN, E.M. and WOOLF, N. (1984): The early changes induced by isoproterenol in the endocardium and adjacent myocardium. Am.J.Pathol., 114, 231–239.

OSBORNE, B.E. and DENT, N.J. (1973): Electrocardiography and blood chemistry in the detection of myocardial lesions in dogs. Food Cosmet.Toxicol., 11, 265–275.

OSBORNE, R.J., SLEVIN, M.L., HUNTER, R.W. and HAMER, J. (1985): Cardiac arrhythmias during cytotoxic chemotherapy: Role of domeridone. Hum.Toxicol., 4, 617–623.

PAULUS, G., MASSON, M.T. and MOMPON, P. (1988): Cardiotoxicity of doxorubicin: A histochemical and morphometric approach. Arch.Toxicol., Suppl. 12, 410–412.

PAYLING-WRIGHT, G. Revised by CRAWFORD, T. (1976): The heart. In: W.St. C. Symmers (Ed.), Systemic Pathology, 2nd Ed., Vol. 1, Chap. 1, pp.1–72, Churchill Livingstone, Edinburgh.

PICK, R., JALIL, J.E., JANICKI, J.S. and WEBER, K.T. (1989): The fibrillar nature and structure of isoproterenol-induced myocardial fibrosis in the rat. Am.J.Pathol., 134, 365–371.

PIPER, R.C. (1981): Morphologic evaluation of the heart in toxicology studies. In: T. Balazs, (Ed.), Cardiac Toxicology, Vol. 3, Chap. 5, pp.111–136. CRC Press, Boca Raton, Florida.

POUR, P., ALTHOFF, J., SALMASI, S.Z. and STEPAN, K. (1979): Spontaneous tumours and common diseases in three types of hamsters. J.N.C.I., 63, 797–811.

RATLIFF, N.B., ESTES, M.L., MYLES, J.L., SHIREY, E.K. and McMAHON, J.T. (1987): Diagnosis of chloroquine cardiomyopathy by endomyocardial biopsy. N.Engl.J.Med., 316, 191–193.

RHODES, G.C., BLINKHORN, S.A. and YONG, L.C.J. (1987): Cardiovascular lesions in experimental acute and chronic renel failure in the rat. Exp.Pathol., 31, 221–229.

RICHARDSON, B.P., TURKALJ, I. and FLÜCKINGER, E. (1984): Bromocriptine. In: D.R. Laurence, A.E.M. McLean and M. Weatherall (Eds), Safety Testing of New Drugs. Laboratory Predictions and Clinical Performance, Chap. 3, pp.19–63. Academic Press, London.

ROBINSON, W.F., HUXTABLE, C.R. and PASS, D.A. (1980): Canine parvovirus myocarditis: A morphologic description of the natural disease. Vet.Pathol., 17, 282–293.

RONA, G., CHAPPEL, C.I., BALAZS, T. and GAUDRY, R. (1959): An infarct-like myocardial lesion and other toxic manifestations produced by isoproterenol in the rat. Arch.Pathol., 67, 443–459.

RONA, G. (1985): Catecholamine cardiotoxicity. J.Mol.Cell Cardiol., 17, 291–306.

ROUNDS, S. and HILL, N.S. (1984): Pulmonary hypertensive diseases. Chest, 85, 397–405.

RUBENSTONE, A.I. and SAPHIR, O. (1962): Myocardial reactions to induced necrosis and foreign bodies, with particular reference to the role of the Anitschkow cell. *Lab.Invest.*, 11, 791–807.

RUBIN, S.A., FISHBEIN, M.C., SWAN, H.J.C. and RABINES, A. (1983): Compensatory hypertrophy in the heart after myocardial infarction in the rat. *J.Am.Coll.Cardiol.*, 1, 1435–1441.

RYFFEL, B., DONATSCH, P., MADÖRIN, M., MATTER, B.E., RÜTTIMAN, G., SCHÖN, H., STOLL, R., WILSON, J. (1983): Toxicological evaluation of cyclosporin A. *Arch.Toxicol.*, 53, 107–141.

RYFFEL, B. and MIHATSCH, M.J. (1986): Cyclosporin nephrotoxicity. *Toxicol.Pathol.*, 14, 73–82.

SANDUSKY, G.E. and MEANS, J.R. (1987): Acute and subchronic toxicity of LY-195115 in rats and dogs. *Toxicol.Lett.*, 38, 177–186.

SCHLÜTER, G. (1986): Toxicological investigations with nimodipine. Summary of relevant studies. *Arzneimittelforschung*, 36, 1733–1735.

SCHNEIDER, P. and PAPPRITZ, G. (1976): Hairs causing pulmonary emboli. A rare complication in long-term intravenous studies in dogs. *Vet.Pathol.*, 13, 394–400.

SCHNEIDER, P., BAUER, M., ECKENFELS, A., LEHMANN, H., LÜTZEN, L. and UEBERBERG, H. (1981): Tierexperimentelle Untersuchung zur Verträglichkeit von AR-L115 BS. *Arzneimittelforschung*, 31, 226–232.

SCHULTZ, R.T. and PITHA, J. (1985): Relation of hepatic and splenic micro-circulation to the development of lesions in experimental amyloidosis. *Am.J.Pathol.*, 119, 123–127.

SHINOMIYA, K. and NAKATO, H. (1985): An experimental model of arteritis: Periarteritis induced by Erysipelothrix rhusiopathiae in young rats. *Int.J.Tissue React.*, 7, 267–271.

SIMONS, M. and DOWNING, S.E. (1985): Coronary vasoconstriction and catecholamine cardiomyopathy. *Am.Heart J.*, 109, 297–304.

SINGAL, P.K., BEAMISH, R.E. and DHALLA, N.S. (1983): Potential oxidative pathways of catecholamines in the formation of lipid peroxides and genesis of heart disease. *Adv.Exp.Med.Biol.*, 161, 391–401.

SINGAL, P.K., DEALLY, C.M.R. and WEINBERG, L.E. (1987): Subcellular effects of adriamycin in the heart. A concise review. *J.Mol.Coll.Cardiol.*, 19, 817–828.

SMITH, B. and O'GRADY, F. (1966): Experimental chloroquine myopathy. *J.Neurol.Neurosurg. Psychiat.*, 29, 255–258.

SOBOTA, J.T., MARTIN, W.B., CARLSON, R.G. and FEENSTRA, E.S. (1980): Minoxidil: Right atrial cardiac pathology in animals and man. *Circulation*, 62, 376–387.

SOLCIA,E., BALLERINI, L., BELLINI, O., MAGRINI, V., BERTAZZOLI, C., TOSANA, G., SALA, L., BALCONI, F. and RALLO, F. (1981): Cardiomyopathy of doxorubicin in experimental animals. Factors affecting the severity, distribution and evolution of myocardial lesions. *Tumori*, 67, 461–472.

SPENCER, A. and GREAVES, P. (1987): Periarteritis in a Beagle colony. *J.Comp.Pathol.*, 97, 122–128.

SPINALE, F.G., SCHULTE, B.A. and CRAWFORD, F.A. (1989): Demonstration of early ischemic injury in porcine right ventricular myocardium. *Am.J.Pathol.*, 134, 693–704.

SPOKAS, E.G., SULEYMANOV, O.D., BITTNER, S.E., CAMPION, J.G., GORCZYNSKI, R.J., LENAERS, A. and WALSH, G. (1987): Cardiovascular effects of chronic high-dose atriopeptin III infusion in normotensive rats. *Toxicol.Appl.Pharmacol.*, 91, 305–314.

STASZAK, C. and HARBECK, R.J. (1985): Mononuclear-cell pulmonary vasculitis in NZB/W mice. 1. Histopathologic evaluation of spontaneously occurring pulmonary infiltrates. *Am.J.Pathol.*, 120, 99–105.

STEINESS, E., BILLE-BRAHE, N.E., HANSEN, J.F., LOMHOLT, N. and RING-LARSEN, H. (1978): Reduced myocardial blood flow in acute and chronic digitalization. *Acta Pharmacol.Toxicol.*, 43, 29–35.

STEJSKAL, V., HAVU, N. and MALMFORS, T. (1982): Necrotizing vasculitis as an immunogical complication in toxicity study. *Arch.Toxicol.*, *Suppl.* 5, 283–286.

STERNBERG, S.S., PHILIPS, F.S. and CRONIN, A.P. (1972): Renal tumors and other lesions in rats following a single intravenous injection of daunomycin. *Cancer Res.*, 32, 1029–1036.

SUTTON, T.J., DARBY, A.J., JOHNSON, P., LESLIE, G.B. and WALKER, T.F. (1986): Dyspnoea and thoracic spinal deformation in rats after oral prizidilol (SK & F 92657-A2). *Hum.Toxicol.*, 5, 183–187.

TANASE, H., YAMORI, Y., HANSEN, C.T. and LOVENBERG, W. (1982): Heart size in inbred strains of rats. Part 1. Genetic determination of the development of cardiovascular enlargement in rats. *Hypertension*, 864–872.

TEKELI, S. (1974): Occurrence of hair fragment emboli in the pulmonary vascular system of rats. *Vet.Pathol.*, 11, 482–485.

TESKE, R.H., BISHOP, S.P., RIGHTER, H.F. and DETWEILER, D.K. (1976): Subacute digoxin toxicosis in the beagle dog. *Toxicol.Appl.Pharmacol.*, 35, 283–301.

THOMPSON, H., McCANDLISH, I.A.P., CORNWELL, H.I.C., WRIGHTER, N.G. and ROGERSON, P. (1979): Myocarditis in puppies. *Vet.Rec.*, 104, 107–108.

THORBALL, N. and OLSEN, F. (1974): Ultrastructural pathological changes in intestinal submucosal arterioles in angiotensin induced acute hypertension in rats. *Acta Pathol.Microbiol.Immunol.Scand.* [A], 82, 703–713.

THYSS, A., FALEWEE, M.N., LEBORGNE, L., VIENS, P., SCHNEIDER, M. and DEMARD, F. (1987): Cardiotoxicité du 5 fluorouracile. Spasme ou oxicité myocardique directe? *Bull.Cancer*, 74, 381–385.

TUCKER, M.J. (1985): Effect of diet on spontaneous disease in the inbred mouse strain C57B1/10J. *Toxicol.Lett.*, 25, 131–135.

TUCKER, A., McMURTRY, I.F., REEVES, J.T., ALEXANDER, A.F., WILL, D.H. and GROVER, R.F. (1975): Lung vascular smooth muscle as a determinant of pulmonary hypertension at high altitude. *Am.J.Physiol.*, 228, 762–767.

VAN VLEET, J.F. and FERRANS, V.J. (1986): Myocardial diseases of animals. *Am.J.Pathol.*, 124, 98–178.

VILLANI, F., COMAZZI, R., GENITONI, V., LACAITA, G., GUINDANI, A., CRIPPA, F., MONTI, E., PICCININI, F., ROZZA, A., LANZA, E. and FAVALLI, L. (1985): Preliminary evaluation of myocardial toxicity of 4'-deoxydoxorubicin: Experimental and clinical results. *Drugs Expt.Clin.Res.*, 11, 223–231.

VON HOFF, D.D., LAYARD, M.W., BASA, P., VON HOFF, A.L., ROZENWEIZ, M. and MUZIO, M. (1979): Risk factors for doxorubicin-induced congestive heart failure. *Ann.Intern.Med.*, 91, 710–717.

VON HOFF, D.D., ROZENCWEIG, M., LAYARD, M., SLAVIK, M. and MUGGIA, F.M. (1977): Daunomycin-induced cardiotoxicity in children and adults. A review of 110 cases. *Am.J.Med.*, 62, 200–208.

VRACKO, R., THORNING, D. and FREDERICKSON, R.G. (1989): Connective tissue cells in healing rat myocardium. A study of cell reactions in rhythmically contracting environment. *Am.J.Pathol.*, 134, 99–1006.

WAGENAAR, SJ. SC. and WAGENVOORT, C.A. (1978): Experimental production of longitudinal smooth muscle cells in the intima of muscular arteries. *Lab.Invest.*, 39, 370–374.

WAGENVOORT, C.A. and WAGENVOORT, N. (1970): Primary pulmonary hypertension. A pathologic study of the lung vessels in 156 clinically diagnosed cases. *Circulation*, 42, 1163–1184.

WARD, J.M., GOODMAN, D.G., SQUIRE, R.A., CHU, K.C. and LINHART, M.S. (1979): Neoplastic and non-neoplastic lesions in ageing (C57BL/6NX C3H/HeN) F_1 (B6C3F$_1$) mice. *J.N.C.I.*, 63, 849–854.

WATANABE, H. NAKAGAWA, Y., ITO, A. and KAJIHARA, H. (1987): Periarteritis nodosa in rats treated with chronic excess sodium chloride (NaCl) after X-irradiation (42548). *Proc.Soc.Exp.Biol.Med.*, 185, 297–304.

WATERS, I.L., DE SUTO-NAGY, G.I. (1950): Lesions of the coronary arteritis and great vessels, of the dog following the injection of adrenaline. *Science*, 111, 634–635.

WATERS, L.L. and DE SUTO-NAGY, G.I. (1950): Lesions of the coronary arteritis and great vessels of the dog following injection of adrenalin. Their prevention by dibenamide. *Science*, 111, 634–635.

WEIBEL, E. (1958): Die Entstehung der Längsmuskulatur in den Ästen der A. bronchialis. *Z. Zellforsch.*, 47, 440–468.

WEIR, E.K., WILL, D.H., ALEXANDER, A.F., McMURTRY, I.F., LOOGA, R., REEVES, J.T. and GROVER, R.F. (1979): Vascular hypertyrophy in cattle susceptible to hypoxic pulmonary hypertension. *J.Appl.Physiol.*, 46, 517–521.

WELTMAN, R.H., TEKELI, S., FRIEDMAN, M.B., KRASULA, R.W., CUSICK, P.K. and PATTERSON, D.R. (1990): Arteritis in rats given a dopamine receptor agonist. Presented at IX International Symposium of Society of Toxicologic Pathologists, Ottawa.

WESTWOOD, F.R., ISWARAN, T.J. and GREAVES, P. (1989): Pathologic changes in blood vessels following administration of an inotropic vasodilator (ICI 153,110) to the rat. *Fundam.Appl.Toxicol.*, 14, 797–809.

WEXLER, B.C. (1978): Corticotropin stimulation of hypertensive rats with and without arteriosclerosis. *Am.Pathol.Lab.Med.*, 102, 587–591.

WEXLER, B.C., McMURTRY, J.P. and IAMS, S.G. (1981): Histopathologic changes in aging male vs female spontaneously hypertensive rats. *J.Gerontol.*, 36, 514–519.

WHITEHEAD, P.N., CHESTERMAN, H., STREET, A.E., PRENTICE, D.E., HEYWOOD, R. and SADO, T. (1979): Toxicity of nicardipine hydrochloride, a new vasolidator, in the beagle dog. *Toxicol.Lett.*, 4, 57–59.

WHITTAKER, P., BOUGHNER, D.R. and KLONER, R.A. (1989): Analysis of healing after myocardial infarction using polarized light microscopy. *Am.J.Pathol.*, 134, 879–893.

WILENS, S.L. (1965): Enhancement of serum sickness lesions in rabbits with pressor agents. *Arch.Pathol.*, 80, 590–603.

WINSOR, T., MILLS, B., WINBURY, M.M., HOWE, B.B. and BERGER, H.J. (1975): Intramyocardial diversion of coronary blood flow: Effects of isoproterenol-induced subendocardial ischaemia. *Microvasc.Res.*, 9, 261–278.

WOMBLE, J.R., LARSON, D.F., COPELAND, J.G. and RUSSELL, D.H. (1982): Low-dose oral terbutaline therapy rapidly induces significant cardiac hypertrophy. *Clin.Pharmacol.Ther.*, 31, 283.

YACOBI, A., KAMATH, B.L. and CHII-MING, L. (1982): Pharmacokinetic studies in chronic animal toxicity studies. *Drug Metab.Rev.*, 13, 1021–1051.

YAMAKI, S. and WAGENVOORT, C.A. (1981): Plexogenic pulmonary arteriopathy. Significance of medial thickness with respect to advanced pulmonary vascular lesions. *Am.J.Pathol.*, 105, 70–75.

YAMATI, J., TAJIMA, M., MARUYAMA, Y. and KUDOW, S. (1987): Observations on soft tissue calcification in DBA/2NCrj mice in comparison with CRJ:CD-1 mice. *Lab.Anim.*, 21, 289–298.

YAMORI, Y. and OKOMOTO, K. (1976): The Japanese spontaneously hypertensive rat (SHR). *Clin.Exp.Pharmacol.Physiol.*, Suppl. 3, 1–4.

YATES, M.S. and HILEY, C.R. (1979): The effect of age on cardiac output and its distribution in the rat. *Experientia*, 35, 78–79.

YU, B.P., MASORO, E.J., MURATA, I., BERTRAND, H.A. and LYND, F.T. (1982): Life span study of SPF Fischer 344 male rats fed ad libitum or restricted diets: Longevity, growth, lean body mass and disease. *J.Gerontol.*, 37, 130–141.

YUHAS, E.M., MORGAN, D.G., ARENA, E., KUPP, P., SAUNDERS, L.Z. and LEWIS, H.B. (1985): Arterial medial necrosis and haemorrhage induced in rats by intravenous infusion of fenoldopam mesylate, a dopaminergic vasodilator. *Am.J.Pathol.*, 119, 83–91.

ZBINDEN, G. (1981): Assessment of cardiotoxic effects in subacute and chronic rat toxicity studies. In: T. Balazs (Ed.), *Cardiac Toxicology* Vol. 3, Chap. 2, pp.7–32. CRC Press, Boca Raton, Florida.

ZBINDEN, G. (1986): Detection of cardiotoxic hazards. *Arch.Toxicol.*, Suppl. 9, 178–187.

ZEEK, P.M. (1942): Heart weight. 1. The weight of the normal human heart. *Arch.Pathol.*, 34, 820–832.

ZIMMERMAN, H.D., MAYKEMPER, B. and DICKER, D. (1977): Intra- and extra renal vascular charges in acute renal failure of the rat caused by high dose folic acid injection. *Virchows Arch.* [A], 376, 47–73.

VII. Digestive System 1

MOUTH AND OROPHARYNX

Inspection of the oral mucosa in clinical practice or during the in-life phase of toxicity studies may reveal manifestations of local or systemic disease or evidence of systemic derangements produced by therapeutic agents. Excessive local trauma from foreign materials, hard fragments in food, and damaged teeth may produce ulceration of the mucosa with subsequent infection. Excessive contact by therapeutic agents such as aspirin, potassium supplements and corticosteroids have also been reported to produce local ulceration in the mouth (Zentler-Monro and Northfield, 1979). Systemic disorders produced by anticoagulants or chemotherapeutic drugs may also be evident by bleeding or ulceration in the oral cavity (Goepp, 1982). Buccal ulceration is also described as part of a generalized hypersensitivity reaction to drugs (Zentler-Monro and Northfield, 1979).

The major and minor salivary glands and their secretions also represent and integral part of the protective mechanism of the oral cavity and derangement of saliva production may lead to loss of integrity of the oral mucosa.

Drugs that effect motor coordination can give rise to drooling and disruption of cricopharyngeal coordination (Wyllie et al., 1986). Drug-induced abnormalities of taste sensation are also well-described phenomena occurring in man although human studies are necessary for the detection of these effects. Indeed, many alterations in the oral mucosa are those which are more readily detected by careful clinical and macroscopic observation rather than exhaustive histopathological examination of the buccal mucosa in laboratory animals.

Oral mucosa irritation studies

Oral irritation studies are used in the testing of products intended for use in the oral cavity, mainly for surgical and dental purposes. They may also be necessary for therapeutic agents intended for administration by the sublingual route. This route may be selected for substances that are broken down in the stomach or show a rapid first pass effect. As it is technically difficult to perform full preclinical toxicity studies by the sublingual route, conventional oral or parenteral routes may be preferred for systemic toxicity studies on such compounds. The choice of the best route will to a large extent be dictated by pharmacokinetic considerations. However, it may still be necessary to assess local irritancy potential to oral mucosa using a laboratory animal model.

Test species for oral irritation studies are usually rats, hamsters (cheek pouch), guinea pigs, dogs or primates and gross and histopathological assessment of the mucosa is used for final assessment. A similar scheme to that employed in the histological assessment of skin irritancy is appropriate.

Inflammation

Inflammation of the oral cavity (stomatitis) may involve the buccal mucosa, the gingiva (gingivitis), the tongue (glossitis) and the peridontal tissues (peridontitis). Although inflammatory lesions of all these types are found sporadically in untreated labortory rodents, dogs and primates, stomatitis can be induced by systemic administration of high doses of therapeutic agents in toxicity studies. Anticancer and antimitotic agents are particularly liable to induce stomatitis. A notable example is bleomycin which is capable of producing stomatitis as part of its general effect on squamous cells (Thompson et al., 1972).

Diuretics and other agents which are capable of producing severe electrolyte disturbances at excessive doses can also produce stomatitis when then are administered in high doses to laboratory animals (Garthoff et al., 1982). These particular lesions may be analogous to the well-described association of ulcerative stomatitis and uraemia in man and laboratory animals (Boyd, 1978; Barker and Van Dreumel, 1985). The dog appears very sensitive to the ulcerogenic effects of uraemia in the oral cavity, although as there is a poor correlation between actual levels of blood urea and stomatitis, other biochemical factors are undoubtably involved in its pathogenesis (Barker and Van Drumel, 1985).

Pigmentation

Compounds which effect pigmentation of the skin can produce similar changes in pigmented oral mucosa. A number of drugs including chlorpromazine, quinacrine, chloroquine, amodiaquine and pyrimethamine cause pigmentation of the oral mucosa in man notably over the hard palate. Chloroquine and pyrimethamine have also been shown to significantly increase numbers of active melanocytes within the palatal mucosa of pigmented DA rats when treated orally for 12 weeks (Savage et al., 1986). Melanocytes in treated rats were shown to be enlarged and packed with melanin pigment and show extensive arborization of cell processes between squamous cells.

An experimental inhibitor of platelet aggregation which produced pigment loss in the dark hair of Long-Evans rats and the skin of beagle dogs, also induced pallor of the normally pigmented oral mucous membranes in dogs (Gracon et al.,

1982; Walsh and Gough, 1989). Apart from loss of pigment, the histology of the mucous membranes and skin was within normal limits.

Tongue

The tongue is conveniently sectioned for histological study, although this is not performed in all laboratories. Often reliance is placed on careful visual inspection, because the usefulness of systematic histological examination of the tongue in routine preclinical safety studies has not been clearly established. A few lesions occur which are fairly specific to the tongue. Amyloid may become deposited in the muscular and connective tissue of the tongue in amyloid-prone species, particularly mice (Dunn, 1967). Mice, especially DBA and DBA/2NCrj strains, are liable to develop *calcification* in the lingual muscle spontaneously, even at a young age (Imaoka et al., 1986). Calcified lesions are seen in the longitudinal muscle under the dorsolateral epithelium and the central part of the tongue, which, when severe, are associated with inflammation, granulation tissue, polypoid change, hyperplasia of the overlying squamous epithelium and ulceration. The histogenesis of this lesion is uncertain. In the DBA/2NCrj mice, mineralization of the tongue is associated with myocardial and aortic mineralization (Doi et al., 1985).

Teeth

Teeth are usually only inspected by naked eye in conventional toxicity studies and this is appropriate for the assessment of a mature dentition. However, with increasing numbers of children surviving malignant disease, physicians are becoming aware that damage to dentition can occur as a result of cytotoxic therapy during the development phase of dentition which starts in utero and lasts into the second decade.

Clinical study of the teeth of children treated for malignancy have shown increased incidence of enamel hypoplasia and missing teeth (Welbury et al., 1984). Histological examination of teeth from children treated with vincristine or combination chemotherapy for malignant disease has demonstrated prominent incremental lines in dentine correlating with the number of times the intravenous cytotoxic agents were administered (MacLeod et al., 1987). It has also been shown that vincristine, a drug which interferes with the assembly of microtubules and reduces secretory activity in a number of cells including osteoblasts and chondroblasts, also has an effect on dentine formation in the rat incisor (Stene and Koppang, 1976). Two weeks following a single intravenous dose of vincristine to young adult rats, a faint incremental line in the dentine was observed, probably a reflection of a direct effect of the drug on the entire dentinogenic tissue at the time of injection. At higher doses, focal niche-like or punched out defects in dentine were observed, expression of more severe injury to highly sensitive dentinogenic populations at the time of injection (Stene and Koppang, 1976). The precise mechanism of damage is not fully understood although decreased secretion of dentine matrix by odontoblasts has been demonstrated. Calcification appears unaltered (Stene and Koppang, 1980).

Administration of cyclophosphamide, an alkylating anticancer agent or a single exposure to ionizing radiation, produces localized niche-like or punched out defects in the rat incisor, rather than the more diffuse changes induced by vincristine. This presumably reflects more localized injury to a sensitive subpopulation of dentinogenic cells (Koppang, 1973).

Anticonvulsant drugs also produce changes in the dentition of man and experimental animals. In man, reported alterations include tooth root resorption, small teeth, delayed shedding of deciduous teeth and retarded eruption of permanent teeth, features similar to those found in hypoparathyroid or pseudohypoparathyroid conditions (Robinson et al., 1983). Tooth root alterations were also reported in a study in which young male Wistar rats were treated with diphenylhyantoin for one month. Treated rats showed evidence of molar root resorption lacunae which penetrated the cementum and involved the dentine (Robinson and Harvey, 1989).

The lacunae contained a dense infiltrate of cells contiguous with similar cells in the surrounding periodontal ligament. The mechanism involved was not clear but Robinson and Harvey (1989) showed that the changes were similar to those occurring in parathyroidectomized rats but not to those occurring in rats made hypocalcaemic with a calcium deficient diet. They suggested that the changes induced by diphenylhydantoin in rats were similar to those in pseudohypoparathyroidism in which resistance of tooth roots to resorption is reduced. Discolouration of teeth and bone is a well described side-effect of tetracycline administration and it has also been reported in patients treated with the semisynthetic derivative, minocycline (Cale et al., 1988).

Periodontitis

Periodontitis is a common and important disease in man and animals although overt cases are not usually seen in toxicity studies. However, periodontitis of a degree sufficient to disrupt chronic rat toxicity and carcinogenicity studies has been reported. Robinson (1985) described periodontitis in Alpk/AP rats in which there were erosive granulomatous cavities adjacent to molar teeth with fistulas opening into the nasal cavity. These changes were associated with penetrating food fibres in the gingival sulcus and it was suggested that the presence of long pointed food fibres in the powdered diet was the main reason for occurrence of periodontitis.

Gingival overgrowth, hyperplasia

Drug-induced overgrowth of the gingival tissues is a well described phenomenon in both man and laboratory animals including dogs, cats, and rats. In man, these changes have been associated with diphenylhydantoin (phenytoin) (Beghi et al, 1986) nifedipine, a calcium channel blocker (Ledermann et al., 1984), cyclosporin

281

A (Barthold, 1987) and valproic acid (Syrjamen and Syrjamen, 1979). Cyclosporin A and diphenylhydantoin have been associated with similar changes in laboratory animals (Latimer et al., 1986; do'Nascimento et al., 1985). Recently, gingival hyperplasia has been reported in beagle dogs treated with a novel calcium channel blocker oxodipine (Waner et al., 1988). These reports suggest that drug-induced gingival hyperplasia is common to both man and laboratory animals. In most instances there is swelling of the gingiva by firm nodular overgrowths around the teeth. Histologically, these overgrowths are characterized by marked acanthosis of the squamous epithelium overlying connective tissue which is infiltrated by large numbers of chronic inflammatory cells. Fibrovascular proliferation may be marked. In patients treated with cyclosporin, myxomatous degeneration is described in association with dense infiltration of plasma cells and lymphocytes (Barthold, 1987). Secondary acute inflammation in association with food debris and hair shafts is described in dogs treated with oxodipine (Waner et al., 1988).

The forces behind the development of these changes are unclear. Studies with nifedipine-and hydantoin-induced changes have shown increases in extracellular ground substance and increased numbers of fibroblasts containing sulphated acid mucopolysaccharides (Kantor and Hassel, 1983; Lucas et al., 1985). It has been suggested that these drugs alter fibroblastic proliferative and synthetic activity, possibly by selection of a subpopulation of fibroblasts (Hassel et al., 1976). It has also been suggested that an underlying mechanism in phenytoin-induced gingival hyperplasia involves the decrease in salivary IgA which develops in some patients (Beghi et al., 1986). Study of cyclosporin A-induced changes have suggested that impairment of T lymphocyte function may permit overgrowth of oral bacteria and bacterial products which in turn may influence fibroblast function (Barthold, 1987).

Neoplastic lesions

Papillomas of the oral cavity

Sessile or pedunculated squamous papillomas or infiltrating squamous carcinomas are occasionally found in the oral cavity of most laboratory animals including rodents (Odashima, 1979; Emminger and Mohr, 1982), rabbits (Sundberg et al., 1985; Sundberg and Everitt, 1986), and beagle dogs (Watrach et al., 1970). Although the structure of these neoplasms resembles those occurring in squamous epithelium in other sites, the oral papillomas occurring in rabbits and dogs are of note because they can occur in quite young animals, apparently as a result of infection with viruses of the papilloma group.

In rabbits, the prevalence of oral papillomas varies considerably but they are quite common in some laboratory strains. They are overlooked because of their small size and a distribution limited to the ventral surface of the tongue (Sundberg et al., 1985). Microscopically, they are typical squamous papillomas composed of irregular acanthotic squamous epithelium and a fibrovascular stalk of variable size. Squamous cells at the margins of papillomas at the junction with normal mucosa, often show large, oval nuclei, marginated chromatin and central, basophilic, intranuclear inclusions, which electron microscopic examination shows to contain viral particles. Oral papillomas in dogs develop as multiple growths, regressing spontaneously after a few months. They are also caused by a virus of the papilloma group which possesses a high degree of specificity for the mucosa of the oral cavity and adjacent skin (Watrach et al., 1970). Histologically, they are composed of proliferative masses of epithelial cells, keratinized on the surface and resting on an irregular connective tissue stroma or pedicule. Large vesicular cells with basophilic intranuclear inclusions are also found in the granular cell layer, identifiable as virus arrays by electron microscopy (Cheville and Olson, 1964). Malignant change has been described in these canine lesions and this can occur in young beagle dogs (Watrach et al., 1970).

Although many types of papilloma viruses have been identified in both man and animals (Pfister, 1984), common antigenic determinants exist between viruses in different species. This immunological cross-reactivity can be exploited in the immunocytochemical localization of papilloma viruses in epithelial lesions of many animal species. Papilloma virus antigen has been demonstrated in oral papilloma of dogs and rabbits using antisera to bovine papilloma virus type I (Sundberg et al., 1984). Cells positive for virus are located in the upper layers of the epithelium, especially within cells of the granular layer, where viral inclusions are most commonly found.

The presence of papilloma viruses in laboratory species should be kept in mind in toxicology in view of the fact that the progression of virally induced papillomas to malignant squamous carcinomas can be accelerated by non-viral factors including application of chemicals (Howley et al., 1986). Recent studies have also revealed a strong association of some of the many distinct genotypes of human papilloma viruses with genital cancer development in man (MacNab et al., 1986).

Odontogenic neoplasms

Spontaneously developing odontogenic tumours are rare in rodents but have been induced in rats treated with powerful carcinogens such as aflatoxins, methylnitrosourea or related compounds. Those developing in Fischer rats treated with aflatoxin, were located in the upper jaw associated with the incisor teeth and were composed of proliferating fibroblast-like cells within which ovoid calcified bodies resembling cementum were seen (Cullen et al., 1987). Occasional inclusions of solid epithelial nests were also seen. No metastatic deposits were found although the neoplasm were locally aggressive.

SALIVARY GLANDS

The stratified squamous mucosa of the oral cavity is covered by a protective layer of mucus, a slimy visco-elastic material containing high molecular weight glycoproteins produced by the major and minor salivary glands. These mucins usually contain more than 50% carbohydrate in the form of neutral and acidic oliosaccharide chains, O-glycosidically linked to threonine or serine. They are believed to possess several roles including physico-mechanical flushing of the oral cavity, protection and lubrication of soft and hard tissues, modulation of oral microbial flora, buffering activity, regulation of calcium/phosphate equilibrium, digestion and extracellular post translational processing of molecules present in saliva (Levine et al., 1987). The heterogeneity of salivary glycoproteins suggests that they act as a defense against pathogenic micro-organisms by competing with microbial binding sites of similar structure on the surface of cells lining the digestive tract (Schulte, 1987). Minor salivary glands may also play an important part in the local immuno-surveillance of the oral cavity for their ducts are anatomically closely associated with lymphoid tissue (Nair and Schroeder, 1986; Nair et al., 1987). Salivary secretions also possess digestive enzyme activity although in herbivores and carnivors, it is usually low in contrast to high digestive enzyme activity in omnivorous species (Junqueira et al., 1973).

The phylogenetic association of the salivary glands with the thyroid gland is evident functionally by the fact that salivary glands are capable of concentrating iodide in their secretions, although this is not under control of thyroid stimulating hormone (Ingbar, 1985). It has been shown that thyroxine accelerates the differentiation of the granular convoluted tubule cells and the appearance of epidermal growth factor in the submandibular gland of the neonatal mouse (Chabot et al., 1987).

Although salivary glands may not represent vital organs in the same sense as the kidneys or heart, severe derangement of their secretions can alter both the quality and quantity of saliva. Depending on the particular glands and cells affected, dry mouth, mucositis, and dental caries may develop which can be severely debilitating (Stephens et al. 1986a).

In toxicity studies, the main salivary glands are routinely examined by light microscopy. Both the macroscopic and microscopic structure of the salivary glands differ remarkably between species and between different glands in the same species. It is usually considered that there are three major salivary glands, the parotid, the sublingual and submandibular (submaxillary) glands. Minor salivary glands are scattered in other locations throughout the mouth and oropharynx. In dogs and other carnivors, the zygomatic (infraorbital) glands, located just below the zygomatic arch and the buccal (molar) gland are also often referred to as major salivary glands.

Microscopically, salivary glands are composed of secretory glands or 'end-pieces' of variable morphology, attached to a connecting system of intralobular and extralobular (secretory) ducts. Beyond this basic description, the complexity of microscopic structure is remarkable. Secretory endpieces may be acinar or tubulo-acinar in nature. The secretory cells have been subdivided into serous, mucous, seromucous and special serous types. Unfortunately, controversy remains about the precise nature of the secretory cells found in the various salivary glands of different species and this makes critical interspecies comparisons difficult (see detailed discussion of this problem by Pinkstaff, 1980). For instance, the well-studied human parotid gland is most commonly considered to be purely serous in type but some authors class it as seromucous on the basis that it also secretes some mucosubstances. Differences of opinion also exist about the salivary glands in laboratory animal species, underlining the need for caution in the use of terminology when salivary tissue is being assessed in experimental studies.

Less controversy exists about the duct system. This comprises an *intercalated duct* which leads from the secretory endpiece into a *striated* (secretory or intralobular) duct, so termed because their lining cells are striated by delicate eosinophilic cytoplasmic rods. The striated ducts converge into interlobular ducts and a main excretory duct system.

Rodent salivary glands

In rats, mice and hamsters, an overall similarity in gross and microscopic anatomy of the various salivary glands exists although there are histochemical differences (Munhoz, 1971; Glucksmann and Cherry, 1973; Dawe, 1979; Pinkstaff, 1980; Emmiger and Mohr, 1982). The *sublingual gland* in rats, mice and hamsters is composed principally of mucous acini, with indistinct serous demilunes. Acini open into fairly long intercalated ducts lined by flat or cuboidal cells devoid of granules. The *parotid gland* is composed of serous-type secretory cells containing zymogen granules and prominant hyperchromatic basal cytoplasmic poles. Acini open into intercalated ducts lined by cells which contain PAS-positive secretory granules.

The *submandibular gland* is anatomically the most complex salivary gland in rodents. Secretory endpieces are composed of small or moderately sized cells with foamy cytoplasm and basophilic basal poles. The most striking feature is the presence of an additional duct segment interposed between the intercalated and striated ducts. This segment is lined by cylindical epithelium with basal nuclei and eosinophilic cytoplasm containing secretory granules. This duct segment is termed the *granular duct* or *granular convoluted tubule*. These granular cells are of special interest because they contain a large number of heterologous biologically active peptides including nerve growth factor, epidermal growth factor, renin, and kallikrinins (Barka, 1980; Mori et al., 1983). The precise physiological role of many of these peptides in salivary gland remains uncertain. Epidermal growth factor was originally isolated from the mouse salivary gland. It initiates premature eyelid opening and incisor eruption when injected into the neonatal mouse (Cohen, 1962). It is believed to act on the proliferation and differentiation of cells in many different tissues which possess an epidermal growth factor-receptor.

Epidermal growth factor synthesis is of course not limited to mouse salivary tissue because immunocytochemical study and analysis of cellular sites of synthesis of prepro-epidermal growth factor mRNA has shown it to be also synthesized in the distal renal tubules (Rall et al., 1985). Homologues are found in other species including man (Damjanov et al., 1986).

Study of the mouse submandibular gland has shown that both epidermal growth factor and nerve growth factor are released into saliva following the administration of phenylephrine, a sympathomimetic amine acting mainly on α-receptors and isoprenaline (isoproterenol), a β-adrenergic agent (Murphy et al., 1980). Immunohistochemical study also demonstrates that epidermal growth factor becomes depleted in mouse salivary tissue following administration of phenylephrine and similar agents (Tsukitani and Mori, 1987). Phenylephrine has been shown to cause marked secretory activity accompanied by loss of granules from granular cells, as well as loss of immune reactive carbonic anhydrase, an enzyme which participates both in membrane transport of bicarbonate ions into saliva and glandular secretion (Noda, 1986). Morphological studies have shown that both acinar and granular tubular cells participate in this response to adrenergic agents (Murphy et al., 1980). This is in contrast to the effects of pilocarpine, a cholinergic agent, which elicits the secretion of saliva deficient in serous proteins with little or none of the growth factors, as its effects are more limited to acinar cells (Murphy et al., 1980).

The complexity of the glycoprotein secretions of rodent salivary glands has stimulated histochemical study using both conventional mucin histochemical techniques and labelled lectins which possess affinity for specific sugars or sugar sequences (Tables 1 and 2).

Studies of rat, mouse and hamster salivary glands using batteries of labelled lectins have shown a greater heterogeneity of oligosaccharides in salivary glands

TABLE 1 *Lectins of use in histochemistry* [a]

Lectin	Inhibitory saccharide
Arachis hypogaea (peanut) PNA	β-D-Gal- (1-3)-D-GalNAc
Ricinus communis (castor bean) RCA1	β-D-Gal > α-D-Gal
Bandeirea simplicifolia	
BSA 1-B	α-D-Gal
BSA II[4]	β-D-GlcNAc = A-D-GlcNAc
Dolichos biflorus (horse gram) DBA	α-D-GalNAc
Glycine max (soybean) SBA	α-D-GalNAc > β-D-GalNAc ≫ D-gal
Lotus tetragonolobus (asparagus pea) LTA	α-L-Fuc
Ulex europeus (gorse seed) UEA 1	α-L-Fuc
Lens culinaris (lentil) LCA	α-D-Man > α-D-Glc > α-D-GlcNAc
Canavalia ensiformis (jackbean) Con A	α-D-Man, α-D-Glc
Tritium vulgaris (wheat germ) WGA	$(D-GlcNAc)_2$, sialic acid
Limulus polyphemus (horseshoe crab) LPA	sialic acid

Key: Gal, galactose; Glc, D-glucose; Man, D-mannose; Fuc, L-fucose; GalNAc, N-acetyl-D-galactosamine; GlcNAc, N-acetyl-D-glucosamine; Sialic acid, N-acetylneuraminic acid.

Saccharide binding specifications are much more complex than the inhibition by simpler sugars outlined above suggests. See review by Nicholson (1974).

[a] Goldstein and Hayes, 1978; Nicholson, 1974; Schulte and Spicer, 1983.

286

TABLE 2   *Histochemical methods for the visualization of epithelial mucins in the gastrointestinal tract (adapted from Filipe, 1979)*

Diastate-Periodic Acid Schiff, D-PAS (Pearse, 1968)	*Magenta*:	All mucosubstances containing hexoses and deoxyhexoses with vicinal glycol groups. Neutral mucosubstances. Some non-sulphated acid mucosubstances.
Periodate-borohydride/ saponification/PAS, PB/KOH/ PAS (Reid et al., 1973; Culling et al., 1974; 1976)	*Magenta*:	PAS activity following periodate borohydride/potassium hydroxide indicates presence of O-acylated sialic acids. Periodate borohydride: reduces periodate generated aldehydes. Potassium hydroxide: removes O-acylesters from potential vicinoldiols and sialic residues linked glycosidically to a potential vicinoldiol.
Alcian blue pH 2.5 (Pearse, 1968)	*Basophilia*:	Weakly sulphated mucins. Carboxyl groups of sialomucins.
Alcian blue pH 1.0 (Lev & Spicer, 1964)	*Basophilia*:	Sulphated mucins.
Alcian blue pH 2.5 – periodic acid	*Magenta*:	Neutral mucins.
Schiff, AB/PAS	*Basophilia*:	Acid mucins.
(Mowry & Morard, 1957)	*Purple-Blue*:	Neural and periodate reactive acid mucins.
High iron-diamine, HID	*Brown-Black*:	Sulphated mucins.
(Spicer, 1965)	*Unstained*:	Sialomucins.
High iron-diamine-alcian blue pH 2.5,	*Brown-Black*:	Sulphated mucins (sialomucins).

than seen by classical histochemical techniques. There are considerable species differences and variations between murine strains as well as heterogeneity among morphologically similar cells within one gland (Schulte and Spicer, 1983, 1984; Schulte, 1987). The results of histochemical studies are in excellent agreement with studies using biochemical methods but suggest a greater degree of genetic and hormonal influence on the synthesis of salivary glycoproteins than previously recognized (Schulte, 1987).

Dog salivary gland

Less attention has been paid to the structure and cytochemistry of the dog salivary glands. There appears to be little variation between the structure of salivary tissues between beagles and other strains although variation with age has been reported (Reifel and Travill, 1972; Nagoyo and Tandler, 1986). Histochemistry of the dog parotid gland has been studied by Munhoz (1971). The dog parotid is of seromucinous type secreting both acidic and neutral mucosubstances, in contrast to the more neutral mucosubstances secreted by rodent glands.

Primate salivary glands

The salivary glands of non-human primates are similar to those in man. They possess parotid glands of serous or seromucous type, submandibular glands with both serous and mucous acini and sublingual glands of mainly mucous type. It appears that the salivary glands of the non-human primate react to certain adverse stimuli such as ionizing radiation in a similar manner to human salivary tissue (Stephens et al., 1986a,b).

Non-neoplastic lesions

Inflammation and necrosis

Focal chronic inflammation of the salivary glands occurs sporadically in unteated rats, mice, hamsters dogs or primates employed in toxicology although severity and prevalence is variable.

Sialoadenitis as a result of a corona virus, the sialodacryoadenitis virus, is a well-known and fairly ubiquitous condition in rats, first described by Innes and Stanton (1961). The condition is characterized histologically by oedema and congestion of submandibular and parotid salivary glands as well as extra-orbital lacrymal and harderian glands. It is accompanied by inflammation of variable severity and chronicity in both glandular and connective tissue. Degeneration and necrosis of duct epithelium also takes place. The regenerative hyperplasia of the duct epithelium may be quite intense about a week after infection but all changes regress after about two weeks and glands are essentially normal after three or four weeks (Carthew and Slinger, 1981; Percy and Wojcinski, 1986). There appears to be no change in the nature and intensity of the disease in rats treated with immunosuppressive agents during the course of the disease, nor is there evidence of reactivation or persistence of viral infection. There may be a delay in the appearance of inflammatory cells and the onset of repair in rats immunosuppressed with cyclophosphamide (Hanna et al., 1984). Depletion of salivary gland epidermal growth factor also occurs during the infection (Percy et al., 1988).

Suppurative infections in the neck region of the rat such as those produced by Klebsiella aerogenes also cause acute and chronic inflammation of salivary glands with fibrosis and glandular proliferation of salivary tissue (Arseculeratne et al., 1981).

In the mouse, intralobular periductular lymphoid aggregates and germinal centers can be found in some strains (Dawe, 1979). The reasons for these minor sporadic foci are unclear. In the non-obese diabetic strain derived from JcL-ICR mice, a periductal chronic inflammatory infiltrate is found in the submandibular gland at about the same time that immune-mediated insulitis is most marked. This suggests that there is an extension of the autoimmune process to salivary tissue (Fujino-Kurihara et al., 1985).

288

Sialadenitis also occurs spontaneously in autoimmune-prone strains of mice such as the NZB/NZW and SL/Ni strains, and it has been recently reported in aging female, but not male BDF1 mice (Hayashi et al., 1988). In ageing BDF1 females the submandibular gland was shown to be involved by a destructive inflammatory process characterized by an intense infiltration by small and medium sized lymphocytes, associated with mild inflammation in other organs such as the parotid, and sublingual glands, pancreas and kidney. Immunocytochemistry showed that most of the lymphocytes were T cells (Thy-1.2 and Lyt-1 positive) of the helper/inducer subset (L3T4 positive) and less than 10% were of suppressor/cytotoxic (Lyt-2) type (see Haemopoietic and Lymphatic Systems, Chapter III). Circulating anti-salivary duct antibody of IgG was also detected in afflicted mice. It was suggested that Lyt-1 and L3T4 positive T cells played a key role in the production of this change, unlike induced autoimmune sialodenitis in which Lyt-2 subsets may directly destroy glandular tissue. Although the cause was uncertain, it is possible that the development of this process in aging females is related to the decline in the number of splenic Lyt-2 cells in mice with advancing age (Hayashi et al., 1988).

An autoimmune type of sialoadenitis can also be experimentally induced certain strains of mice. CRJ:CD1 mice, thymectomized at three days, a time point at which Lyt-2 + cells (suppressor T lymphocytes) can be maximally reduced, followed by immunization at 28 and 42 days after birth with homogenates of salivary gland and complete Freund's adjuvent, develop a distinctive sialoadenitis in the submandibular and to some extent the parotid glands (Hayashi et al., 1985). This sialoadenitis is characterized by degenerative changes in salivary glandular tissue associated with an extensive and intense infiltrate composed of small and medium sized lymphocytes. These cells appear shortly after immunization but increase in numbers with time. Immunocytochemical study has shown that many of these cells are reactive to antisera to Thy-1.2 and Lyt-2, features of suppressor/cytotoxic T lymphocytes. Cells appearing later in the process show features of plasmacytoid lymphocytes and contain immunoglobulin of mainly IgG class (Hayashi et al., 1985). These authors therefore suggested the sialadenitis appeared as both a result of cytotoxic/suppressor T cell activity and an antibody-dependent cell-mediated cytotoxicity.

In the hamster salivary glands, interstitial infiltrates of lymphocytes and plasma cell are quite common and may become more marked with advancing age (McMartin, 1979).

Whereas necrosis of the parotid gland of uncertain aetiology sometimes occurs in the dog, mild focal chronic inflammation is quite a common incidental finding in canine salivary glands and has been reported in about 5% of normal beagle dogs (Kelly et al., 1982).

Although the inflammation in salivary tissue which results from ionizing radiation is only indirectly relevant to drug safety evaluation, it is of interest in view of the notable species differences in sensitivity to this form of insult. Serous acinar cells in man and rhesus monkey appear least resistant to the effects of ionizing radiation, where damage is characterized by widespread degranulation and degeneration of acini, infiltration by polymorphonuclear cells followed by lymphocytes, plasma cells and subsequent atrophy and fibrosis (Stephens et al., 1986a,b). These changes contrast with the lesser effects of ionization radiation on the rodent salivary glands in which there is little or no acute inflammatory response.

Lymphoid bodies

Lymphoid bodies are sharply circumscribed collections of lymphoid cells generally located between the parotid and sublingual glands close to a cervical lymph node in mice. They are apparently normal aggregates of lymphoid tissue (Dawe, 1979).

Atrophy

Like many other glandular organs, the size of the secretory tissue of the salivary gland is responsive to functional demand and is subject to age-related changes. In man, the gland parenchyma frequently becomes atrophic and replaced by connective tissue or fat with advancing age, possibly partly related to vascular changes (Waterhouse et al., 1973; Scott, 1977). In aging rats, the extent and height of granular ducts and their content of mature secretory granules has also been shown to decrease with age (Sashima, 1986).

Dietary factors influence salivary gland size. Decreased food consumption or protein starvation can reduce the weight of salivary glands in rats. There is shrinking of mucous and serous glands and loss of zymogen granules associated with decreased RNA but unchanged DNA content, attributable to the reduced requirements for protein synthesis (Boyd et al., 1970, McBride et al., 1987).

As salivary gland function is responsive to adrenergic stimulation, it is not surprising that atrophy occurs following adrenergic blockade. The weights of the submandibular gland in mice were shown to decrease following administration of the β-adrenergic blocking agent, propranolol (Smith and Butler, 1977). This was associated with a reduction in stainable neutral mucins and a decrease in the thickness of the acinar cells making the gland lumens appear larger than normal.

The cytotoxic agent, alloxan, known primarily for its specific effect on pancreatic B cells, has also been shown to produce weight loss of the rat submandibular gland, associated with lipid inclusions in the acinar cells, capillary basement membrane thickening and reduced salivary flow (Reuterving et al., 1987). It is probable that alloxan exerts a cytotoxic effect on the acinar cells of the rat submandibular gland (Sagström et al., 1987). Methotrexate, a folic acid antagonist, has also been reported to cause vacuolization of acinar and ductular cells with reduction of secretory granules in rat salivary glands (McBride et al., 1987).

Enlargement of salivary glands may occur as a result of spontaneous inflammatory disease or neoplasia. A number of therapeutic agents are reported to increase salivary gland size in man, although the scarcity of biopsy data precludes a critical assessment of the precise mechanism in many cases. Drugs reported to produce salivary gland enlargement in man include iodide-containing radiological contrast media, isoprenaline and anti-inflammatory agents phenylbutazone and oxyphenbutazone. Enlargement may also occur after endotracheal anaesthesia and upper gastrointestinal tract endoscopy in man (Riddell, 1982). Some of these agents and procedures may occur as a result of spasm of large salivary ducts and retention of secretions.

Several pharmacological agents, particularly sympathomimetic amines, have been shown to produce increases in salivary gland size in rodents following repeated dosing (Brenner and Stanton, 1970). This is perhaps not surprising in view of the intimate relationship of sympathomimetic amines to the control of the secretory process in salivary tissue. Whereas a single injection of isoprenaline (isoprotorenol) in the range of 20–200 mg/kg induces discharge of preformed secretory granules followed by gradual resynthesis and reconstitution, repeated injections produces an increase in the size of salivary glands (Simson et al., 1974). Histologically, the enlarged glands are composed of secretory cells of increased size that contain increased amounts of secretory substances in the cytoplasm (Simson et al., 1974). Although these histological features are principally those of diffuse cellular hypertrophy, an increase in DNA content and radioactive thymidine uptake has also been described in the salivary tissue following repeated administration of isoprenaline, suggestive of a degree of cell replication (hyperplasia) (Barka et al., 1972). There is also elevated membrane phospholipid content in the parotid and submandibular glands of rats treated with isoprenaline for ten days (Yashiro et al., 1987).

These effects do not depend on the integrity of the autonomic nerves because they occur after ablation of the autonomic ganglia (Barka et al., 1972). They appear to be mediated by an effect on adrenergic β-receptors. The effects can be blocked by propranalol, a β-receptor antagonist but not by phenoxybenzamine, an α-receptor antagonist (Brenner and Stanton, 1970). As theophylline and caffeine also elicit salivary gland enlargement in rats, a role for cyclic 3′,5-adenosine monophosphate (cAMP) in salivary gland enlargement has been postulated (Brenner and Stanton, 1970).

Detailed study of hypertrophy, protein synthesis, and intracellular cAMP activity in the salivary glands of rats treated for ten days with isoprenaline (isoproterenol), a series of β-adrenergic receptor agonists and the phosphodiesterase inhibitors, theophylline and caffeine, showed that similar effects occurred with all agents althoug differences in the degree of hypertrophy, the nature of protein and glycoprotein synthesis and activity of Golgi membrane enzyme, UDP-galactose : N-acetylglucocosamine 4β-galactosyltransferase, were recorded (Wells and Humphreys-Beher, 1985). The parotoid gland showed the most pronounced hypertrophy followed by the submandibular gland but the sublingual gland appeared to be unaffected by treatment. The degree and nature of the changes induced by the various $\beta 1/\beta 2$ receptor agonists suggested that most of these effects were mediated through $\beta 1$ receptors which are present in greatest numbers on the parotid and salivary cells. It was suggested that the effects of β-adrenergic agonists on salivary gland are produced by a receptor-mediated stimulation of adenylate cyclase activity causing an increase in levels of intracellular cAMP. However, other factors may be important for Wells and Humphreys-Beher (1985) also showed that although isoproterenol and caffeine increased salivary cell cAMP to comparable levels, the hypertrophy was greater with isoproterenol.

Recently, a series of cardiotonic phosphodiesterase inhibitors were shown to produce submaxillary hypertrophy in rat subacute toxicity studies (Rogers et al.,1985; Jayasekara et al 1986; Smith et al., 1988). As the agents produced their positive inotropic action via selctive inhibition of cardiac phosphodiesterase subfraction III, the enzyme fraction requiring specifically cAMP as its substrate, it was suggested that the salivary gland hypertrophy was also a result of phosphodiesterase inhibition (Smith et al., 1988).

Other classes of drugs can also produce salivary gland enlargement in rats in repeated dose studies. Doxylamine, a representative of the widely used ethanolamine group of antihistamines, has been reported to produce marked cytomegaly in the Fischer 344 rat parotid gland. Enlarged cells were characterized by a basophilic and coarsely granular or vacuolated cytoplasm (Jackson and Blackwell, 1988). The B6C3F1 mouse did not develop these changes after a similar treatment schedule.

Eosinophilic (oncocytic, oxyphil) cells, oncocytes of the salivary glands

Epithelial cells characterized by abundant granular eosinophilic cytoplasm as a result of the accumulation of mitochondria are often referred to as oncocytes, a term used by Hamperl (1950) to describe similar cells in Hürthle tumours of the thyroid gland. They may be found in various focal nodular and neoplastic states of the salivary glands in both man and laboratory animals.

The precise significance of these cells is uncertain. The mitochondria usually appear unremarkable except for lack of dense granules and it has been suggested that the mitochondrial changes represent an adaptive phenomenon or compensatory hyperplasia (Ghadially, 1982).

In human salivary tissue their prevalence seems to increase with advancing age and they can be associated with hyperplasic lesions or neoplasms such as oxyphil adenomas and adenolymphomas.

Eosinophilic cells also occur in the salivary glands of certain strains of aged rats (Bogart, 1970) and in mice with experimentally induced autoallergic sialadenitis (Takeda et al., 1985). In the study of Takeda and his colleagues (1985), the eosinophilic cells appeared to arise predominantly in the secretory (glandular) ducts of the submandibular glands, although eosinophilic cells can apparently develop from either duct or acinar cells.

Hypertrophic foci (foci of cellular alteration, basophilic foci, giant acini)

Well-defined, unencapsulated foci of enlarged acinar cells occur spontaneously in the salivary glands, particularly the parotid of rats, mice (Chiu and Chen, 1986), and hamsters (personal observations) although their reported incidence varies between laboratory. The enlarged cells possess greatly expanded cytoplasmic volume which retains a vesicular, vacuolated or foamy appearance or possesses a pale eosinophilic granular texture. The basal parts of the cells usually stain intensely blue in heamatoxylin and eosin stained sections and contain large, dense, irregular hyperchromatic or pyknotic nuclei showing little evidence of mitotic activity. Although there has been little ultrastructural study of these foci, the cytoplasmic alterations appear to be distinct from those of so-called oncocytes which characterized by granular eosinophilic cytoplasm packed with mitochondria.

The biological nature of these foci is uncertain. The lack of any prominant mitotic activity, cell proliferation or expansive growth suggests that they are most aptly regarded as hypertrophic lesions (Chiu and Chen, 1986). Although they increase in prevalence with increasing age in certain strains of rat, there is no evidence to suggest that they represent pre-neoplastic lesions or possess any relationship with development of neoplasia in salivary tissue (Dawe, 1979).

Duct hyperplasia and metaplasia

Hyperplasia and squamous metaplasia of the salivary ducts are common features of many inflammatory and reactive conditions in the salivary glands of rodents, dogs, non-human primates and man and can be associated with the presence of stones and calculi with the duct system.

Squamous metaplasia and regenerative change in the ducts occurs in rats afflicted with sialodacryoadenitis (Carthew and Slinger, 1981). It is also described specifically located in the ducts of the sublingual glands in the Wistar rat in the absence of obvious sialodacryoadenitis or evidence of any specific disease. Similar regenerative hyperplastic duct changes are also seen in necrotic and inflammatory conditions in the dog salivary gland (Kelly et al., 1979).

Detailed morphological examination of the rat salivary gland after arterial ligation with immunocytochemical study of epidermal cytokeratins has shown that the acinar units can also undergo squamous metaplasia (Dardick et al., 1985). It appears that the acinar-intercalated duct complexes can rapidly reprogram to produce epidermal cytokeratin filaments in ischaemic or inflammatory states.

Neoplasia

Primary neoplasms of the rodent salivary glands are uncommon. Although, carcinomas showing squamous or glandular differentiation are sometimes observed infiltrating the salivary gland, they usually originate in other local structures of the head and neck region. Occasionally, salivary gland neoplasms show adenomyomatous differentiation. Mixed glandular and lymphoid tissue patterns resembling Wartin's tumor in man are also sometimes observed. Neoplasms of soft tissues also develop in and around the major salivary gland in rodents (see Integumentary System Chapter I).

OESOPHAGUS

Although the oesophagus is not considered a common site for drug-induced injury in man, recent studies have suggested that medication-induced changes are much more prevalent than previously supposed (Bonavina et al., 1987). Severe damage can occur following prolonged contact between mucosa and ingested tablets or capsules which results in local high concentrations of potentially irritant substances (Bott and McCallum, 1986; Brors, 1987). Damage as a result of local contact tends to be more common in elderly subjects as the amplitude of oesophageal contractions decrease with age and capsules more liable to lodge in the lumen of the oesophagus (Bonavina et al., 1987). The shape and surface coating of tablets may influence their tendancy to adhere to the mucosa and lodge in the oesophagus (Marvola et al., 1983). Bonavina and colleagues (1987) have suggested that the well-known, but poorly understood, oesophageal web of the Plummer-Vinson syndrome in iron-deficient patients may be a result of local injury from ferrous sulphate medication. Some of the causative agents such as potassium chloride and aspirin are also implicated in ulceration lower in the gastrointestinal tract. Oesophagitis due to *Candida albicans* is a well-described complication of antibiotic therapy. Administration of immunosuppressive drugs may predispose to viral infections in the oesophagus. A number of agents affecting neuromuscular coordination may also predispose to gastro-oesophageal regurgitation and reflux oesophagitis (Bott and McCallum, 1986).

The relative infrequency of drug-related oesophageal injury in man is reflected in the low level of oesophageal pathology found generally in preclinical toxicity studies. One of the most common pathological findings in rodents is perforation of the oesophagus as a result of a gavage accident. Under these circumstances there is a variable inflammatory and often purulent exudate localized around the perforation or spread within the pleural or occasionally the pericardial cavities.

Spontaneous lesions of the oesophagus are very occasionally seen in laboratory rodents. *Oesophageal impaction* has been described in untreated SrL:BHE rats. This is characterized by massive dilatation of the oesophagus with food or bedding (Ruben et al., 1983). Histologically, the muscle fibres in the wall of the oesophagus show varying degrees of degeneration including swelling or shrinking of fibres, myofibrillar fragmentation, cytoplasmic vacuolation and mineralization. So-called *megaoesophageous*, characterized by enlargement of the oesophagus, degeneration of muscle fibres and ganglion cells in the myenteric plexus has also been described in certain strains of rats and mice (Harkness and Ferguson, 1979; Randelia and Lalitha, 1988). Its cause is unknown. A commonly occurring lesion reported in Fischer 344 rats is oesophageal hyperkeratosis, which occurs at all ages (Maeda et al., 1985). In the study by Maeda and colleagues (1985), it occurred more commonly in rats fed a protein-restricted, calorie unrestricted diet than in rats fed ad libitum with normal diet. It was suggested that the particular high prevalence of oesophageal hyperkeratosis observed in all groups in this particular study was related to acidification of drinking water (Maeda et al, 1985).

Oesophageal lesions are uncommon in laboratory beagles, even though emesis and vomiting are frequent responses of this species following dosing in toxicity studies.

Various special animal models for the assessment of local oesophageal irritancy potential of drugs have been used, notably the cat and pig (Carlborg and Densert, 1980; Olovson et al., 1983). In these models, the test drugs are placed in the upper oesophagus using endoscopic techniques for periods of several hours to allow dissolution of the preparation. Subsequently, the animals are followed for 3–6 days, then sacrificed and histopathological assessment performed on the oesophagus. The degree of inflammation, erosion of mucosa or deep ulceration is recorded in a semiquantitative manner. The degree of ulcerogenic activity of drugs in these models seems to correlate with reported ulcerogenic activity in the human oesophagus (Carlborg et al., 1983).

Drugs with radiomimetic or antimitotic activity can cause hypoplastic changes in the oesophageal mucosa as well as the remaining gastrointestinal tract mucosa (Tucker et al., 1983). Conversely, hyperplasia with increased keratinization has been reported in the oesophagus of the rat following chronic high dose administration of alcohol (Mascrès et al., 1984). Acanthosis with hyperkeratosis and parakeratosis has been reported in the oesophagus but not stomach of rats treated for up to 18 months with mesuprine hydrochloride, a β-adrenergic receptor stimulator (Nelson et al., 1972).

Finally, it should be noted that agents which produce changes in the rodent forestomach are also liable to produce similar alterations in the oesophagus.

FORESTOMACH

The stomach of small rodents, including the rat, mouse and hamster, is characterized by the presence of the forestomach which occupies about two-thirds of the proximal stomach area and is lined by cornified stratified squamous epithelium. The limiting ridge is a distinct elevated mucosal fold at the junction between the forestomach and the mucosa of the glandular part of the stomach. The relevance of changes produced by drugs and chemicals in the rodent forestomach for man is debated, as man lacks a forestomach. However, there is some evidence to suggest that the squamous mucosa lining the oesophagus in species without a forestomach may react to xenobiotics in a similar way to the forestomach mucosa of rodents if equivalent exposure levels are attained. Hence, interpretation of forestomach changes should take into account the various physiological factors and differences exposure to drugs between the rodent forestomach and human oesophagus.

Non-neoplastic lesions

Inflammation, erosions, ulceration

Inflammation and ulceration of the forestomach mucosa are some of the commonest spontaneous gastrointestinal lesions in laboratory rats, mice and hamsters. The prevalence of these gastric lesions is variable between species and strains of laboratory rodents. Considerable inter-laboratory variation is also reported in the incidence of forestomach ulceration within the same laboratory rodent strains. For instance, the B6C3F1 mouse usually develops forestomach ulceration only sporadically but in one laboratory up to 50% of these mice developed forestomach ulcers at about 100 weeks of age (Yoshitomi et al., 1986). The precise causes of forestomach ulceration remain unclear although a variety of factors have been associated with forestomach ulceration in animals including advanced age, infection, parasitism, dietary factors, feeding regimens and stress. In rats, conflict-induced ulceration occurs in the forestomach and there is an age-related susceptability, older rats developing more ulcers than younger rats (Sawrey and Sawrey, 1966). In rats and mice dying of spontaneous disease, ulceration of the forestomach is also quite frequently observed. Protein restriction or starvation alone has also been shown to produce forestomach ulceration in rats (Boyd et al, 1970).

In toxicity studies, the prevalence of forestomach ulceration is sometimes higher in treated groups. In view of the number of factors which can influence the expression of gastric ulceration, such findings are frequently difficult to interpret. They are often considered incidental in nature, if the lesions are few and show no clear relationship to dose. They can be stress-related if they are limited to high dose groups. However, administered chemicals may have direct local effects of sufficient severity to cause focal damage to the forestomach mucosa.

Histological features of ulcers and inflammatory lesions of the forestomach are similar in rats, mice and hamsters. In mild cases, a scattering of acute inflammatory cells are seen in the intact squamous mucosa. Ulcers can be single or multiple and are characterized by loss of squamous epithelium with a variable accumulation of neutrophils, mononuclear cells, cellular debris, fibrin and hair fragments in the ulcer crater. The inflammatory process may extend deeply into the stomach wall wall and be associated with intramural inflammation, oedema, endarteritis and fibrosis. Haemosiderin pigment is also found in the ulcer margins. Profuse haemorrhage may follow erosion of large blood vessels and complete perforation of the stomach wall with peritoneal involvement also

296

occurs (Greaves and Faccini, 1984). In long standing cases of ulceration, hyperplasia of the adjoining squamous epithelium occurs, characterized by irregular acanthosis and downgrowths of squamous epithelium into the submucosa (Yoshitomi et al., 1986).

Xenobiotics may produce inflammatory changes in the forestomach mucosa following initial dosing but subsequently, repair occurs even though treatment continues. An example of this phenomenon is illustrated by butylated hydroxyanisole. After one week of administration of this agent in a 2% mixture in diet to rats, a vesicular inflammatory reaction, characterized histologically by the presence of subepithelial vesicles containing inflammatory cells and exudate was seen (Altmann et al., 1985). After further treatment, only hyperplasia of the squamous epithelium was evident.

Hyperplasia (hyperkeratosis, parakeratosis, acanthosis, papillomatosis)

Hyperkeratosis associated with varying degrees of hyperplasia in the squamous epithelium is seen sporadically in untreated aged rodents. These changes may be localized to the margins of chronic forestomach ulcers or they can be associated with diffuse inflammation of the mucosa. Occasionally, the forestomach mucosa of untreated aged rodents exhibits hyperkeratosis with hyperplasia without inflammation. Such changes may be diffuse or focal, but they are often localized to the zone adjoining the glandular stomach mucosa. Histologically, the changes are characterized by hyperkeratosis, parakeratosis with varying degrees of acanthosis and papillomatosis (Greaves and Faccini, 1984). The changes can be florid and it may be difficult to make a clear distinction between hyperplasia and neoplasia.

Dietary factors also influence the thickness of the forestomach mucosa. Vitamin A deficiency, known to produce squamous metaplasia in glandular tissues may produce forestomach hyperplasia and hyperkeratosis in rats. When SPF Fischer 344 rats were maintained in a vitamin A deficient state for over three months, hyperplasia with hyperkeratosis, not unlike that produced by known carcinogens was reported (Klein-Szanto et al., 1982).

Administration of certain chemicals also produces hyperkeratosis and hyperplasia of the forestomach epithelium. Some of the difficulties in the assessment of human risk from the finding of treatment-induced hyperplasia of the rodent stomach are well illustrated by studies with butylated hydroxyanisole (BHA), an important food antioxidant in widespread use. When administered to rats for two years as a 2% mixture in the diet, it produced squamous hyperplasia, squamous papillomas and squamous carcinomas although a level of 0.5% in the diet induced only hyperplasia (Ito et al., 1983). It also produces proliferative lesions in the forestomach of both mouse and hamster (Ito et al., 1986). The mechanism for the development of this neoplasia remains unknown, particularly as butylated hydroxyanisole possesses little or no mutagenic activity in vitro.

Feeding studies in which butylated hydroxyanisole was fed in the diet to rats for shorter periods have shown that squamous epithelial hyperplasia occurs after only one week of treatment, although sometimes associated with some inflammatory changes (Altmann et al., 1985). The site of predeliction for hyperplasia in these studies was over the lesser curvature, the site at which carcinomas also developed in the two year studies.

After 13 weeks treatment, mucosal hyperplasia was histologically evident only in rats given 2% butylated hydroxyanisole in diet and not in rats given 0.5, 0.25 and 0.1% mixtures (Iverson et al., 1985a). The lesions were characterized by pronounced hyperkeratosis. Parakeratosis was evident over the lesser curvature where the lesions were most marked. The squamous epithelial layer showed marked acanthosis with elongated and widened rete pegs, interspersed by narrow papillae. Abundant mitoses were found in the basal cells layers. The underlying submucosa was increased in thickness over the lesser curvature and it contained a sparse scattering of lymphocytes. Examination of the tritiated-thymidine labelling index confirmed that the changes were accompanied by a high rate of cell proliferation. Following cessation of administration of butylated hydroxyanisole after 13 weeks, the tritiated-thymidine labelling index rapidly reverted to control levels, within about one week. Despite a rapid decrease in labelling however, the hyperplasia took far longer to regress. After one week of normal diet the mucosa assumed a saw-tooth appearance with shorter rete pegs spaced further apart. After about 9 weeks of normal diet, nearly complete regression of the hyperplasia had occurred (Iverson et al., 1985a).

The distribution of squamous hyperplasia induced in the rodent stomach by butylated hydroxyanisole was shown to be influenced by the mode of administration. Whereas following feeding of rats with butylated hydroxyanisole mixed in the diet lesions tended to be located near the limiting ridge, Altmann and his colleagues (1985) showed that gavage of butylated hydroxyanisole in corn oil produced similar changes at the apex of the forestomach. It was suggested that this difference was due to incomplete mixing of butylated hydroxyanisole in the stomach lumen when given by gavage and prolonged contact of the gavage mixture with the upper segment of the forestomach (Altmann et al., 1985).

Residence time of administered compounds with local effects on the forestomach may be a key factor in the development of lesions. Although it has been demonstrated that butylated hydroxyanisole does not produce hyperplasia in the oesophagus of animals without a forestomach, Iverson and colleagues (1985b) have shown that high-doses given to primates are capable of producing an increase in mitotic activity in the lower end of the oesophagus similar to that occurring at equivalent exposure levels in the rat. The implication is that these interspecies differences may simply be a question of differences in exposure of the squamous mucosa to compound. This underlines the fact that mechanisms of action and exposure levels of xenobiotics attained in the gastrointestinal tract of rodent and non-rodent species as well as of man need to be carefully assessed when hyperplastic changes are induced in the forestomach mucosa of rodents. Such information can be helpful in facilitating regulatory decisions (Moch, 1988). In view of the low levels of exposure to butylated hydroxyanisole which occurs with the usual use of this agent, carcinogenic hazard for the human stomach is, on balance, probably very small.

Further complexity of the response of the rodent forestomach to xenobiotics has also been revealed by studies of phenols and acids which are structurally related to butylated hydroxyanisole. Marked acanthosis and hyperkeratosis with oedema and infiltration of the lamina propria with eosinophils and lymphocytes was observed along the lesser curvature in rats treated with 4% n-butyl and 4% n-propyl-4-hydroxybenzoic acid esters mixed in the diet for nine days but similar changes only took place after 21 or 27 days of treatment with 4% propionic acid (Rodrigues et al., 1986). By contrast, a similar treatment regimen with 4-methoxyphenol produced changes in both the lesser and greater curvatures. These histopathological differences corresponded to the differences in the tritiated thymidine labelling index of the forestomach mucosa following treatment with these different agents. These studies suggested that various areas of the forestomach epithelium react differently to structurally related chemicals, possibly due to the variable levels of activating enzymes within different zones of the forestomach epithelium. Co-administration of acetylsalicylic acid was shown to abrogate some of these effects, suggesting that prostaglandin synthetase may be involved in the hyperplastic response (Rodrigues et al., 1986).

This is of interest as hyperkeratosis has also been reported in the forestomach of rats treated with gastric cytoprotective agents of the prostaglandin type (Levin, 1988). Rats treated with high doses of misprostol, a synthetic prostaglandin E1 methyl ester analogue with gastric anti-secretory and anti-ulcer activity, showed thickening of the superficial keratin layers of the forestomach mucosa (Kotsonis et al., 1985). Histologically the underlying squamous epithelium was unremarkable. Hyperplasia of the forestomach mucosa over the limiting ridge has also been described in rats treated with a synthetic analogue of prostaglandin E1 type (+)-[11α,13E,15R]-11,16-dihydroxy-1-(hydroxymethyl)-16-methylpros-13-ene-1,9-dione (CL115,574), for six months by both gavage or mixed in the diet (Kramer et al., 1985). Histologically hyperkeratosis, acanthosis with irregular infolding of the thickened epithelium and cytological evidence of increased proliferation in the basal cell layers were observed. The hyperplasia was largely reversible after one month without drug and completely after cessation of treatment for two months (Kramer et al., 1985).

Forestomach mucosa also became thickened in rats treated orally with 100 µg/kg of 16, 16-dimethyl prostaglandin E2 for 21 days (Reinhart et al., 1983). Histologically, the forestomach mucosa in treated rats showed acanthosis of the squamous epithelium and hyperkeratosis. This change was diffuse but also appeared particularly prominent at the forestomach corpus ridge which developed a polypoid or nodular appearance. These changes were not associated with changes in maximal acid output or marked changes in circulating gastrin levels suggesting that the effects were not mediated via gastrin.

A different distribution of hyperplasia was observed in rats following the administration by gavage of the histamine H2 receptor antagonist SK&F 93479 for one year (Betton and Salmon, 1984). Dose-related hyperkeratosis, dyskeratosis, marked and irregular acanthosis with prominant mitotic activity was observed in the squamous mucosa of forestomach but this was most severe in the upper part of the forestomach away from the limiting ridge. Despite the atypical cytological features, neoplasia was not observed after one year of treatment and endoscopy revealed regression after cessation of treatment for 22 weeks (Betton and Salmon, 1984). The mechanism for this change was unclear but appeared unrelated to the inhibition of the H2 receptor which was complete even at dosage levels at which hyperplasia did not occur.

Inflammation, ulceration with acanthosis and hyperkeratosis were also observed in mice but not rats treated for two years with high doses of the extensively used antibiotic, ampicillin (National Toxicology Program Technical Report, 1987). In the context of extensive and generally safe clinical use of this drug, the relevance of this finding for man is doubtful but emphasizes the uncertainties in extrapolation of such findings for man.

A contrasting example is provided by aristolochic acid, a nitrophenanthrene derivative of the ancient medicinal plant Aristolochia clematis. This agent, which was used as an anti-inflammatory component in a number of medicinal preparations in Germany until 1982, is a direct acting mutagen in Salmonella Typhimuriun (Göggelmann et al., 1982, Schmeiser et al., 1988). When fed to rats at doses of 1.0 and 10 mg/kg/day, aristolochic acid produced severe papillomatosis of the entire forestomach within a period of three months. This was characterised histologically by the presence of branched squamous papillomas up to 6 mm high with focal dysplastic features. Invasive squamous carcinomas with metatsases werefound subsequently, three or six months later without further treatment (Mengs et al., 1982). Even at a low dose of 0.1 mg/kg/day papillomas and sqamous carcinomas developed nine months after a three month period of treatment.

Quite clearly the complexity of the hyperplastic response of the rodent stomach to xenobiotics, the association of hyperplasia induced by non-mutagenic compounds with the development of forestomach carcinomas, and the similarity of response in the forestomach to that of the oesophagus, dictates the need for a careful analysis of hyperplasia induced by novel drugs in the forestomach. The prelude to this assessment is careful histopathological characterization of the changes.

Neoplasia

See Glandular Stomach.

STOMACH (Glandular)

Unlike the mouth and oesophagus through which tablets, capsules, gavage fluids and drug/diet mixtures pass relatively rapidly, the human stomach mucosa remains in contact with high local concentrations of administered compounds for much longer periods of time. This may result in localized adverse effects on the glandular mucosa. The residence time of a drug in the stomach depends on a number of different factors. Administration in liquid or solid form, particle size, fasting and feeding all affect the gastric motility pattern. In the fasted state there is a cyclical pattern of motility consisting of three main phases. The first is a quiescent phase, followed by a phase of irregular contractions which increase in amplitude and frequency to reach a maximum, designated phase III activity. Feeding results in the replacement of this cyclic pattern by regular tonic contractions which move food towards the antrum and mix it with gastric secretions. These patterns have been well studied in both dog and man and appear to be qualitatively similar in the two species (Sarna, 1985). These motility patterns may have an impact on the length of time drugs remain in contact with stomach mucosa. For instance, the residence time of large non-disintegrating capsules or tablets administered in the fasting state is more dependent on the frequency of powerful phase III contraction than if drugs are given as fluids or mixed with diet. For dosage forms released in the stomach, gastric residence time will influence drug supply to the main absorptive surfaces in the small intestine which in turn may affect drug absorption (Dressman, 1986). These factors may alter the expression of toxic damage to the mucosal cells.

Gastric acid is also be important in the solublisation of ingested salts. However it should be noted there are other sources of acid in the gastrointestinal tract. These sources include food, itself acid secretions from the jejunum, the acid microclimate adjacent to small intestinal cells and acid produced by colonic bacteria.

Although the presence of food in the stomach is a stimulus of acid production, the pH in the forestomach of rats is highest in full stomachs and lowest when empty, presumably as a consequence of the buffering action of food (Ward and Coates, 1987).

General morphology

The glandular stomach is conveniently divided into the fundus characterized by mucosal folds or rugae and the smoother antrum which opens into the pylorus and duodenum. In species devoid of a forestomach, the proximal stomach mucosa or cardia is also lined by glandular mucosa.

The glandular mucosa is covered by surface epithelium of regular columnar cells which extends downwards to form small gastric pits or foveolae. The gastric glands are simple tubular structures usually considered to comprise three segments. The base is the deepest part, the neck the mid-region, and the most superficial is the isthmus, continuous with the gastric pit. The gastric pits are not usually considered integral parts of the gastric glands.

The upper part of the gastric gland contains mucous neck cells. Parietal or zymogenic cells which secrete pepsinogen and stain blue or purple in haematoxylin and eosin sections are located in deeper parts of the gland. The eosinophilic-staining chief cells which produce hydrochloric acid are distributed more randomly throughout the gastric glands.

The gastric glands which are situated near the limiting ridge in rodents, show a modified structure. In species not endowed with a forestomach, the mucosa near the cardia is composed of simplified branched glands lined by columnar epithelium. The antral mucosa is covered by a surface epithelium with gastric pits similar to that of the fundus but the glands themselves are lined by mucous secreting columnar glands.

The stomach mucosa is richly endowed with endocrine cells, many of which have not been well characterized with respect to the hormones they produce. Enterochromaffin cells are usually quite numerous in the basal parts of the gastric glands of the fundus, particularly in the rat (Håkanson et al., 1986a,b). They are generally argyrophilic, staining with silver staining techniques such as that of Grimelius (1968) which utilize exogenous reducing agents. These cells contain histamine and histamine-related enzymes such as histidine decarboxylase in the rat and other species (Håkanson et al., 1986a,b). Gastric enterochromaffin cells can be demonstrated in the rat by immunocytochemical techniques using antisera to histamine and histidine decarboxylase as well as to non-specific enolase and chromogranin A. (Watanabe et al., 1984b; Sundler et al., 1986; Betton et al., 1988). Immunocytochemical study of the rat fundus using a battery of antisera to a variety of gastrointestinal peptides has shown some somatostatin containing (D) cells and glucagon staining cells but no cells with gastrin (G cells) or serotonin reactivity (Bishop et al., 1986). Somatostatin containing cells are closely associated with fundal parietal cells suggesting that these cells may be involved in the control of acid secretion (Larsson, 1980). Ultrastructurally, these cells are characterized by the presence of numerous rounded or oval, vesicular, electron-luscent granules frequently containing a small eccentric electron dense core (Håkanson et al., 1986a,b).

Endocrine cells which are argentaffin in type stain with silver stains such as that of Masson (1914) because of the presence of endogeneous reducing substances such as 5-hydroxytyptamine or catecholamines. These occur in the mucosa of the fundus of some species including man but apparently not in the rat (Håkanson et al., 1986a).

Gastrin or G cells are found in the rat antral and pyloric mucosa, concentrated preferentially towards the base of the glands where they can be clearly demonstrated by immunocytochemical techniques using antisera to gastrin (Bishop et al., 1986). These cells possess an apical process which reaches the stomach lumen which is believed to be important in stimulation of gastrin release as a result in increases in antral lumen pH or the presence of amino acids or peptides (Håkanson et al., 1986a). Although neural control is also important in gastrin release, the actual mediators involved are not well characterized. Morphological studies have demonstrated a close association of somatostatin-containing D cells with antral gastrin secreting cells suggesting somatostatin may also possess a role in gastrin release (Larsson, 1980). Glucagon and serotonin containing endocrine cells have also been described in the rat antral mucosa (Bishop et al., 1986).

Kinetics of the gastric mucosa

Generative cells in the gastric mucosa as shown by uptake of tritiated thymidine for DNA synthesis are distributed principally in the isthmus (Inokuchi et al., 1983). Tracing of cells using thymidine-labelling have shown that most of the cells in the generative zone migrate in a successive manner to the mucosal surface to form columnar epithelium. The life span of surface epithelium in the stomach of rats, mice and hamsters has been calculated to be about three to four days. Studies of cell cycle and DNA synthesis time in the proliferative zones in the stomach of rat, hamster and man have suggested that the generative cells in the isthmus undergo mitoses at about 30 hour intervals in rodents and 40 hour intervals in man (Inokuchi et al., 1983).

Although surface epithelial cells are renewed frequently by this process of migration from the proliferating cell zone of the isthmus, cell migration to the lower parts of the gastric glands is much slower and more complex. Morphological studies have clearly show that undifferentiated cells in the region of the isthmus represent a common source for surface mucous cells and mucous neck cells, but morphological evidence of their differentiation to chief and parietal cells is equivocal (Kataoka, 1970). Nevertheless, electron microscopic study avoiding the use of osmium post-fixation for better delineation of cytoplasmic granules and ultrastructural cytochemistry has suggested that chief cells in the adult rat stomach also develop from undifferentiated stem cells in the isthmus (Suzuki et al., 1983). Graft experiments in mice have also suggested that immature cells of the isthmus differentiate into chief cells as well as parietal cells (Matsuyama and Suzuki, 1970). Thus, current evidence supports the origin of chief and parietal cells, surface mucous cells and mucous neck cells from the same undifferentiated precursors situated in the isthmus.

Labelling experiments in the hamster stomach have shown that both chief and parietal cells possess a similar but quite long life span of about 200 days (Hattori, 1974; Hattori and Fujita, 1976). It has been suggested that the relative distribution of chief and parietal cells in the gastric gland represents an expression of their different migration patterns downwards from the proliferative zones in the isthmus. This type of migration pattern in which cells are able to overtake each other has been termed a 'stochastic flow system' (Inokuchi et al., 1983).

Proliferating cells in the antral mucosa and the cardiac glands are also located in the isthmus and migrate to form the mucous cells in these zones.

The origin and kinetics of endocrine cells of the stomach has also been the subject of debate but the available morphological, cytochemical and kinetic evidence suggests that the majority of these cells develop from the same stem cells as the other non-endocrine cells of the gastric mucosa, although self replication also occurs (Matsuyama and Suzuki, 1970; Inokuchi et al., 1983; Solcia et al., 1986).

Mucin histochemistry

Much of our knowledge about mucins produced by the epithelial cells lining the gastrointestinal tract, has been obtained using histochemical techniques and these approaches continue to be helpful in the understanding of spontaneous and drug-induced gastrointestinal disease (Sheahan and Jarvis, 1978; Filipe, 1979; Tsiftsis et al., 1980). Techniques commonly employed are presented in Table 2.

The physiochemical properties of gastrointestinal mucins are dependent on their glycoprotein constituents. These glycoproteins are high molecular weight compounds with large numbers of sugar chains attached to a polypeptide backbone by 0-glycosidic linkages between N-acetylgalactosamine and serine or threonine (Berger et al., 1982). The principle monosaccharides present are fucose, galactose, N-acetylgalactosamine, N-acetylglucosamine and sialic acid. Traces of mannose may be present and ester sulphate residues are common (Filipe, 1979).

Terminal sugars or sugar sequences can be demonstrated histochemically by the use of labelled lectins, mostly plant proteins which combine non-enzymatically with particular sugar molecules (Table 1) (Goldstein and Hayes, 1978; Debray et al., 1981; Rüdiger, 1982).

There are considerable regional variations in glycoprotein constituents in the gastrointestinal tract and these differences are probably related to physiological and functional factors. Furthermore, synthesis and segretion of glycoproteins alter with changes in cell differentiation. Alterations also occur in mucins in various inflammatory and neoplastic disease states as well as following administration of certain drugs and chemicals (Ishihara et al., 1984).

For these reasons, mucin histochemical techniques represent useful tools for the characterization and elucidation of experimentally or drug-induced changes in the glandular mucosa of gastrointestinal tract.

Stomach mucins

When gastrointestinal mucins were studied in several species using histochemical techniques under uniform conditions, species differences were most obvious in the stomach and duodenum (Sheahan and Jarvis, 1976). In general terms however, neutral mucins predominate in the stomach, contrasting with acid mucins in the small intestine, and sulphated mucins in the colon.

In the stomach neutral mucins staining purple with the PAS/alcian blue stain, predominate in the surface and foveolar mucosa, whereas mucous neck cells and antral glands contain acidic mucins which stain blue with PAS/alcian blue procedure. Sulphated mucins, as shown by the high iron diamine technique (HID) are also found in the deep glandular mucosa of the antrum in rat, mouse and man (Filipe, 1979; Jass, 1980; Greaves and Boiziau, 1984). Extremely heterologous staining patterns are seen in the gastric mucosa with labelled lectins, each lectin staining quite different cell populations. There are considerable interspecies differences in staining patterns with the same labelled lectins (Kuhlmann et al., 1983; Suganuma et al., 1984).

Non-neoplastic lesions

Inflammation, erosions and ulceration of the gastric glandular mucosa

Although gastric erosions and ulcers in the glandular mucosa occur quite commonly in laboratory animals in the context of toxicity studies, it is often difficult to determine whether such lesions in treated animals indicate a real ulcerogenic risk for the test compound when administered to man.

This difficulty is partly related to the complex nature of the pathophysiology of gastric ulceration. In man, formation of gastric and duodenal ulcers is critically dependent on the presence of both acid and peptic activity in gastric juice because acid without pepsin appears to have little digestive power. Important predisposing factors in human patients with peptic ulceration include Campylobacter pylori (now Helicobacter pylori) infection of the antrum, cigarette smoking and ingestion of non-steroidal anti-inflammatory drugs (Soll, 1990).

Erosions and ulcers also develop following stress, reflux of intestinal contents and bile, changes in acid secretion and hypoxia, all of which may develop under the conditions occuring in high-dose toxicity studies. The requirement to give the test compound in high doses may also dictate the need to administer exceedingly high concentrations of test agent. This may produce damaging high local concentrations on the mucosa not relevant to therapeutic doses used in clinical practice. It has been demonstrated that hyperosmolar solutions of quite inocuous substances such as glucose can cause haemorrhage, erosions and ulcers of the rat gastric mucosa (Puurunen et al., 1980). The well-known association of gastric erosions and haemorrhage with uraemia may also be manifest following administration of high doses of drugs such as diuretics which severely derange fluid and electrolyte balance (Garthoff et al., 1982).

The potential of stress to disrupt the balance between cellular resistance and insults from exposure to hydrogen ions, digestive enzymes and exogeneous substances should also not be underestimated. A major cause of stress ulceration appears to be a temporary ischaemia of the mucosa (Dubois, 1987). This may also confound the interpretation of studies performed with classes of compounds possessing ulcerogenic potential because synergism between the ulcerogenic action of drugs and stress is a well-described phenomenon (Rainsford, 1975; Beattie, 1977). Protein depletion and starvation is also capable of inducing gastric ulceration in rats (Boyd et al., 1970).

The difficulty in the prediction of the degree of ulcerogenic potential of novel agents in man based on animal data is illustrated by the complexity which surrounds the ulcerogenic activity of non-steroidal anti-inflammatory drugs. Although gastric pathology represents the largest cause of morbidity and mortality in man following therapy with non-steroidal anti-inflammatory agents (Fowler, 1987), the reasons for this are probably multifactorial. The acidic properties of some of these drugs may cause direct local damage of gastric epithelial cells, demonstrable by the fact that appropriate formulation can reduce gastric toxicity of these agents in man (Brors, 1987). Anti-inflammatory agents are capable of decreasing synthesis of glycoproteins and this may adversely influence protective mucus production of gastric mucosa (Azuumi et al., 1980; Ishihara et al., 1984).

It has also been suggested that non-steroidal anti-inflammatory agents cause cellular damage to the gastric mucosa by back-diffusion of gastric acid into mucosal tissues (Davenport, 1964) or by causing damage to the gastric capillary bed with subsequent mucosal infarction (Robins, 1980).

The theory which has gained widespread acceptance is that the ulcerogenic potential of non-steroidal anti-inflammatory drugs is related to their pharmacological activity. Vane (1971) proposed that the ulcerogenic potential of these agents was largely a result of their ability to inhibit prostaglandin synthetase, thereby reducing the protective effects of prostaglandins.

Pharmacokinetic factors also require consideration. For instance, it has been proposed that anti-inflammatory agents such as BW755C are likely to possess lesser ulcerogenic potential in man because their inhibition of prostaglandin production is more limited to sites of inflammation, sparing gastric mucosa (Whittle et al., 1980; Whittle and Vane, 1984). However, the low ulcerogenic potential of BW755C in that rat has also been explained on the basis of pharmacokinetic factors. BW755C can exist in a lipid-insoluble form in the low pH environment of the stomach precluding local penetration into the mucosa (McCormack and Brune, 1987).

It has also been demonstrated that factors altering the enterohepatic circulation of drugs can influence the expression of gastric damage (Overvold et al., 1987). Recent comparative studies of the ulcerogenic activity of indomethacin in beagle dogs and domestic pigs has suggested that the dog may be an excessively sensitive species for reliable prediction to man as a result of extensive enterohepatic circulation of indomethacin in this species (Hanhijärvi et al., 1986).

Unfortunately, prediction of ulcerogenic potential for man based on data from animal models is clouded by the fact lack of good comparative data on the relative ulcerogenic potential of even widely used non-steroidal anti-inflammatory agents in man (Fowler, 1987). Proper comparison in man between such agents requires not only equivalent therapeutic doses but also optimal dosage forms (Brors, 1987). There are also extensive geographical differences in side effect reporting which have also important implications when attempts are made to compare the results from different centers (Fowler, 1987).

There is little that is histologically specific to drug-induced ulceration of the gastric glandular mucosa. Mucosal haemorrhage, depletion of mucin, erosions and ulcers with or without inflammation may all be found. Erosions represent mucosal breaks superficial to the muscularis mucosa. Ulcers are lesions which extend through the muscularis mucosa. In man, biopsy data suggests that drug-induced ulceration is characteristically devoid of an inflammatory component, but the most usual histological appearances are those of underlying gastric pathology (Riddell, 1982).

In laboratory animals, a variety of different patterns of drug-induced gastric damage have been described. The study by Shriver and colleagues (1975) in which a wide variety of different anti-inflammatory drugs were administered to fasted Sprague-Dawley rats under identical conditions, suggested the drugs could be divided into three groups based on their profiles of gastrointestinal toxicity. Immunological agents such as azathiaprine, cyclophosphamide, methotrexate and d-penicillamine produced gastric mucosal haemorrhage whereas aspirin and related agents produced gastric mucosal haemorrhage and ulcers. The powerful non-steroidal anti-inflammatory drugs indomethacin and phenylbutazone produced gastric mucosal erosion and ulcers as well as small intestinal damage.

Comparative single oral dose studies of several different non-steroidal anti-inflammatory agents at three different dose levels by Suwa and colleagues (1987) in the rat using histology and measurement of faecal blood loss with 51Cr-labelled blood cells have also shown that different patterns of ulceration can be produced by different agents when administered under identical conditions. Single oral doses of some non-steroidal anti-inflammatory drugs including aspirin produced widespread superficial damage and desquamation of gastric epithelium with little or no inflammation at six hours following dosing which completely healed two weeks later. This damage was associated with transient faecal blood loss. By contrast, indomethacin and ibuprofen produced both gastric damage and circumscribed, penetrating ulcers along the mesenteric border of the jejunum and ileum. Furthermore, ulcers were still present after two weeks and were associated with prolonged or biphasic blood loss (see Small Intestine).

The distribution of erosions and ulcers in laboratory animals has been shown to be partly dependent on feeding conditions. In fasted rats, erosions due to indomethacin treatment are found in the body of the stomach whilst in conventionally fed rats they are most prominent in the small intestine. Detailed studies by Satoh and his colleagues (1981) showed that rats fed for one hour after a 24 hour fast and given a single dose of indomethacin within two hours of refeeding developed erosions and ulcers in the antrum primarily along the lesser curvature. Indomethacin given to fasted rats produced erosions in the body mucosa.

Single dose experiments have also clearly showed the time-dependency of the histological features of gastric damage. Six hours after indomethacin, there was extensive but superficial degeneration of the mucosa (erosions) with pyknosis and cytoplasmic shrinkage of parietal and chief cells with mononuclear and polymorphonuclear leukocytes infiltration. At 24 hours, the mucosa appeared completely necrotic with involvement of the muscularis mucosa (ulcers) and submucosal oedema and inflammation. By three days, lesions penetrated to the muscularis externa (Satoh et al., 1981).

A further factor which needs to be kept in mind when interpreting the effects of repeated-dose toxicity studies is that chronic administration of ulcerogenic compounds may produce quite different pathological appearances to those found following single dose administration. Administration of aspirin to rats for four weeks has been shown to stimulate epithelial proliferation of the gastric body but not antral mucosa, possibly by an effect on cyclic adenosine $3',5'$ monophosphate (cyclic AMP) or though increasing the rate of epithelial exfoliation (Eastwood and Quimby, 1982). Such a response may be the basis for increased resistance of the gastric mucosa to the chronic affects of these agents. It also may explain the tendancy for ulcers to occur in the antrum following chronic administration of aspirin-like drugs as the proliferative response and presumably the adaptive potential appears less in this part of the gastric mucosa.

Both interspecies variations and strain differences have been reported in the response to ulcerogenic compounds. Rainsford and colleagues (1982) showed that extravasation of red blood cells and greater vascular damage was observed in rats treated with aspirin or benoxprofen than in pigs given similar doses. Sprague-Dawley rats appear less susceptible to the ulcerogenic effects of cold-restraint stress than Wistar rats (Goldenberg, 1973).

Diuretics and some angiotensin converting enzyme (ACE) inhibitors have been associated with the development of gastric erosions and ulceration when administered in high doses to laboratory animals (Imai et al 1981, Garthoff et al, 1982). However, these effects appear related to the severe electrolyte disturbances produced by excessive doses of these drugs. This is perhaps analogous to the well-known association of gastrointestinal tract erosion and haemorrhage with uraemia. Dogs appear to have a particular predisposition to this effect where it may be associated with deposition of basophilic ground substance and mineral in connective tissues and blood vessels in the mucosa (Barker and Van Dreumel, 1985).

Although inflammatory conditions due to micro-organisms are generally uncommon in the stomach, gastritis is reported in laboratory rhesus monkeys in association with the presence of Campylobacter (Helicobacter) organisms (Reed and Berridge, 1988). As in the analogous condition in man, the stomach of affected animals shows an infiltration of the central mucosa by small lymphocytes and plasma cells, associated with reactive or atrophic changes in the mucosa and the presence of small curved bacteria in glands, visualized best with the Warthin-Starry stain.

Infiltration of the stomach by lymphocytes in rats treated with human recombinant interleukin-2 without ulceration was reported as part of a multisystems involvement induced by this agent (Anderson and Hayes, 1989).

Mucus depletion

Decrease in gastric mucus secretion may accompany both spontaneous inflammatory conditions and drug-induced lesions in the stomach of man and experimental animals. Mucus depletion is characterized histologically by the presence of an intact epithelial layer in which cells show loss of the normal clear cytoplasm replete with mucous substances by more basophilic cells which contain little or no mucin.

Qualitative changes in mucus composition can also accompany mucus depletion. Gastric epithelium in man may show decreases in sulphated mucosubstances following stress, high alcohol consumption or after aspirin administration (Filipe, 1979). Similar changes occur in laboratory animals subjected to ulcerogenic regimens. Stress ulceration in the rat is accompanied by decreased sulphation of gastric glycoproteins, presumably an expression of the changes in gastric cellular activity accompanying stress (Lambert et al., 1969). Administration of aspirin and other anti-inflammatory agents including adrenocortical steroids to laboratory animals also reduces the content of sulphomucins in the gastric mucosa, probably by reducing their synthesis (Denko, 1958; 1964; Gerard, 1965; Ishihara et al., 1984). As it has been suggested that the ulcerogenic property of these chemicals may be partly related to their effects on the synthesis and sulphation of glycoproteins, consideration needs to be given to the study of mucin changes in the safety evaluation of ulcerogenic compounds.

Intestinal metaplasia

Intestinal metaplasia of the stomach is characterized by the presence of differentiated epithelium which resembles small intestine on the basis of light microscopic and ultrastructural morphology, mucin patterns and enzyme histochemistry (Morson, 1955; Lev, 1966; Goldman and Ming, 1968; Planteydt and Willighagen, 1960; Watanabe et al., 1984a). It develops in man in gastric mucosa altered by chronic atrophic gastritis and its significance is due to the fact that there is an association between intestinal metaplasia and gastric cancer. Although intestinal metaplasia is found much less commonly in laboratory animals, it has also been reported to occur in association with gastric cancer induced by polychlorinated biphenyls (Ward, 1985). In view of this association with gastric cancer, it has been suggested that intestinal metaplasia represents a pre-neoplastic lesion. However, over recent years prospective clinical studies and experimental data have suggested that it is an epiphenomenon, coexisting with, but unrelated to the development of cancer.

In man, several forms of intestinal metaplasia have been described. These varients fall into two main groups, an incomplete type and a complete form (Teglbjaerg and Nielson, 1978; Jass and Filipe, 1979; Jass, 1980).

Complete intestinal metaplasia is characterized by the presence of goblet cells, Paneth cells and absorptive cells with brush borders and variably developed intestinal villi. Incomplete forms are more heterogeneous characterized by goblet and mucous columnar cells but no absorptive cells. Mucin histochemical study also reveals variable patterns. The routine alcian blue: pH 2.5, periodic acid-Schiff stain (AB/PAS) (Table 2) distinguishes between the intestinal acid mucins (blue) from the neutral mucins of gastric type. However, variable sialomucin and sulphomucin staining patterns are seen in intestinal metaplasia in man with the high iron-diamine/alcian blue stain (HID/AB) (Jass, 1980). The incomplete form of intestinal metaplasia, showing marked sulphomucin secretion, has been found more commonly in association with gastric cancer in man and for this reason it has been considered a premalignant subtype (Jass and Filipe, 1979; Jass, 1980; Wells et al., 1982). However, this association with cancer has not been based on aged-matched material. Prospective studies have tended to indicate that intestinal metaplasia with sulphomucin secretion may be an age-related form of chronic atrophic gastritis and not a premalignant lesion (Ectors and Dixon, 1986). It has been suggested that intestinal metaplasia represents an adaptive response to long-standing chronic inflammation and reduced acid secretion. It may also represent an adaptative defensive response to long-standing Campylobacter infection as intestinal mucosa appears to be more resistant to such organisms (Steer, 1984; Ectors and Dixon, 1986).

These factors parallel those in the development of intestinal metaplasia in laboratory animals. Although not characterized in such detail, intestinal metaplasia has been found in association with gastric cancer in laboratory animals. Fischer 344 rats treated with the polychlorinated biphenyl, Aroclor 1254, mixed in the diet for two years developed foci of intestinal metaplasia in the stomach epithelium in association with gastric adenocarcinomas (Ward, 1985). These lesions were characterized by abundant mucin-containing cells and alkaline phosphatase activity typical of the small intestine (Morgan et al., 1981; Ward, 1985). Similar, but more diffuse intestinal metaplasia was reported in the stomach of primates treated with polychlorinated biphenyls, although unassociated with gastric neoplasia (Allen, 1975; McConnell et al., 1979). However, intestinal metaplasia does not appear to be a common finding in the stomach of laboratory animals treated with powerful gastric carcinogens. Studies in rats after administration of N-methyl-N-nitro-N-nitroguanidine have shown hyperplasia and foci of atypical changes (dysplasia) but little or no intestinal metaplasia (Tsiftsis et al., 1980). By contrast, intestinal metaplasia can be induced in rodents by a variety of different procedures which are not associated with the development of gastric cancer. Intestinal metaplasia can be induced in the glandular stomach of rodents by fractionated, localized, ionizing radiation (Watanabe, 1978; Watanabe et al., 1980), injection of xenogenic stomach antigens (Watanabe et al., 1984a) as well as propantheline bromide and the non-carcinogen, iodoacetamine (Watanabe et al., 1984a; Shirai et al., 1985).

The characteristics of intestinal metaplasia in laboratory rodents are similar to those seen in man with early increases in intestinal enzyme activity (alkaline phosphatase, lactase, trehalase, sucrose and maltase), development of goblet cells containing neutral, sialo-, or sulphomucins, and intestinal crypts with or without Paneth cells. Both the fundus or antrum can show changes although as in man, males appear more prone to develop intestinal metaplasia than females (Watanabe et al., 1984a).

Based on these experimental findings, Watanabe and his colleagues (1984a) have proposed that intestinal metaplasia is not a precancerous condition but an adaptive response to a chronic elevation in pH in gastric secretion due to the early loss of parital cell mass brought about by these various procedures.

On balance therefore, the evidence to date suggests that although intestinal metaplasia is associated with cancer and may consequently be considered a helpful morphological feature in the evaluation of human gastric biopsies, the finding of isolated intestinal metaplasia in safety studies does not indicate a preneoplastic state.

Mineralisation

The gastric glandular epithelium shows a particular predisposition to the deposition of calcium possibly as it is a site at which marked ion exchange normally takes place. Focal aggregates or concretions of densely blue-staining mineral are fairly commonly observed in haematoxylin-stained sections from the stomachs of aged rats where they are associated with cystic dilatation of the gastric glands (Greaves and Faccini, 1984). Mice and hamsters may occasionally show similar changes. Small concretions are also observed in gastric glands in the beagle dog. These appear to represent aggregates of calcium around mucoid material.

Gastric mineralization may become marked in rodents and dogs when there is disturbance of mineral metabolism, particularly in association with renal pathology. This has been well described in rats with severe renal disease (renal glomerulosclerosis) and parathyroid hyperplasia (Snell, 1967).

A similar phenomenon has been described in the stomach of dogs in uraemic states (Cheville, 1979). Identical changes result from the administration of drugs which induce prolonged azotemia or electrolyte disturbances. These changes are characterized by diffuse deposition of mineral in the intestinal tissue of the

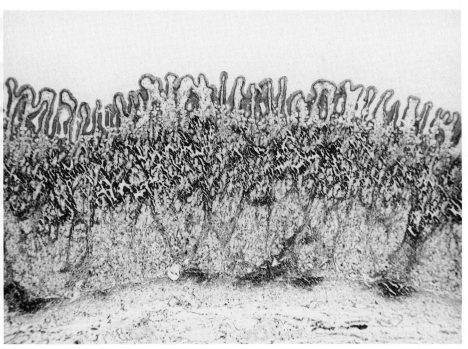

Fig. 57. Mineralization of beagle dog stomach body mucosa. There is a diffuse granular deposit principally involving the submucosa. (von Kossa, ×55.)

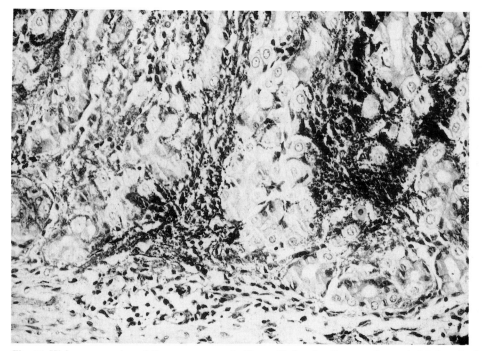

Fig. 58. Higher power view of the same case as in Figure 57 showing the granular material deposited around gastric glands in more detail. (von Kossa, ×350.)

mucosa of the gastric body but not cardia, antrum or pylorus (Figs. 57 and 58). Mineral deposits develop around basement membranes surrounding epithelium and blood vessels. The lamina propria becomes expanded by oedema and fibroplasia of the interstitium also develops. The gastric glands themselves become distorted with swelling and degeneration of parietal cells and atrophy of chief cells. Erosion of the glandular epithelium with haemorrhage occurs presumably as a result of the ischaemia caused by diffuse vascular injury and altered parietal cell function (Cheville, 1979).

Atrophy

Focal atrophy of the gastric glandular mucosa is a sporadic occurrence in laboratory rodents, usually as a result of previous focal gastric inflammation, ulceration, mineralization or vascular occlusion. These changes, characterized histologically by focal fibrosis of the mucosa, gastric glandular dilatation and atrophy variably accompanied by polymorphonuclear cells and mast cells are common in certain strains of rats when two years or more in age (Anver et al., 1982).

312

Whereas diffuse mucosal atrophy occurs following severe inflammatory insult, diffuse atrophy of the stomach glandular mucosa without inflammation can be a result of a surgically or drug-induced reduction in trophic factors necessary for the maintainence of normal gastric morphology and function. This is most strikingly observed both in man and experimental animals following antrectomy which removes the peptide-producing cells of the antrum (Gjurldsen et al., 1968; Neilsen et al., 1972). In the rat, antrectomy is accompanied by hypogastrinaemia, reduced weight and height of the oxyntic mucosa and a reduced number of argyrophil cells (Håkanson et al., 1976; 1986b). This is in contrast to procedures such as antral exclusion which lead to hypergastrinemia and increased thickness of the oxyntic mucosa.

The complexity of trophic control of the stomach glandular mucosa is illustrated by the findings following vagotomy. Although bilateral vagotomy produces profound functional changes in the stomach, notably reduction of gastric acid secretion, morphological changes in the fundal mucosa are not striking either in experimental animals or in man (Crean et al., 1969; Aase and Roland, 1977). Sequential morphological studies in the rat have shown that diffuse atrophy of the gastric glands with a decrease in the number and size of parietal, chief and mucous cells occurs transiently following truncal vagotomy but histological features return to normal by about one month after surgery (Nakamura, 1985).

By contrast, unilateral vagotomy in the rat leads to marked and persistent atrophy of the oxyntic zone on the denervated side. This is characterized histologically by reduced height of the mucosa and reduced numbers and staining intensity of argyrophil cells (Håkanson et al., 1984). It was argued by Håkanson and his colleagues that this was due to the removal of the trophic action or the vagus. The lack of lasting atrophy after bilateral vagotomy was explained by the action of counteracting forces. The rise in gastrin which occurs subsequent to bilateral vagotomy presumably as a result of lack of acid feedback inhibition of gastrin release does not occur following unilateral vagotomy. It is probably this rise in gastrin which counterbalances the antitrophic effects of bilateral vagotomy (Håkanson et al., 1984).

Removal or reduction in extra-gastric trophic factors or hormones may also bring about reduction in the thickness of the gastric mucosa. This is clearly demonstrated in the rat by hypophysectomy. This causes a reduction in thickness of oxyntic and antral mucosa, compared with pair-fed controls (Bastie et al., 1985). Morphometric study showed little or no change in peptic : parietal cell ratios following hypophysectomy but a significant decrease in cell volume and secretory activity of gastric glandular cells, findings which suggested a widespread disturbance of synthesis and secretory mechanisms (Bastie et al., 1985).

Therapeutic agents which are able to mimic these effects, especially by feedback-inhibition of trophic factors may produce a range of similar atrophic changes in the gastric mucosa in toxicity studies.

Although the gastric effects of the inhibitors of gastric acid secretion are complex, atrophic changes in the chief cells were observed in rats treated for six

313

months with high doses of omeprazole, an inhibitor of acid secretion. The findings were considered to represent disuse atrophy secondary to the inhibition of acid secretion (Hansson et al., 1986).

Another inhibitor of gastric acid secretion, the tricyclic agent pirenzepin, also produced atrophy of the fundic mucosa of rats following three months but not one month of treatment (Lehy et al., 1978). The atrophy was characterized by reduced numbers of parietal cells associated with lower numbers of gastrin-containing cells in the antrum, features unlike those following prolonged treatment with histamine H_2 antagonists.

Gastric hypertrophy, hyperplasia, dysplasia and neoplasia

An increase in the thickness of the gastric mucosa can be the result of hypertrophy or hyperplasia of the mucosal cells and this occurs both spontaneously or following administration of drugs and chemicals. In view of the different cell populations in the gastric mucosa and the variety of morphological alterations that occur, it may be difficult to make a clear distinction between hypertrophy and hyperplasia without morphometric techniques. Indeed, morphometric techniques have shown that hypertrophy of some mucosal cells can coexist with hyperplasia of other gastric cell populations. It is therefore important in the evaluation of hypertrophy and hyperplasia of the gastric mucosa that the cell types involved and the nature of the changes are clearly characterized, where necessary using special stains, immunocytochemistry, ultrastructural and morphometric techniques. A distinction also needs to be made between diffuse or uniform hyperplasia involving one or more of the cell populations from the hyperplasia associated with proliferative or adenomatous overgrowth. Adenomatous forms of hyperplasia also need to be evaluated for atypical cytological features (dysplasia) which may predispose to the development of gastric carcinoma.

Diffuse hypertrophy and hyperplasia of glandular mucosa

Cells of gastric glandular mucosa undergo increases in size or number in response to the effects of gastrointestinal trophic hormones or their synthetic analogues. Similar changes also follow administration of compounds which inhibit gastric acid secretion. Although results from studies with agents of the same type however are not always comparable because of the different doses or dose-schedules employed, different species or variation in the manner in which histological or morphometric examination is undertaken, certain general morphological responses can be defined.

When gastrin or its synthetic analogue, pentagastrin is administered subcutaneously to rats and mice for several weeks, there is both an increase in the number and size of parietal cells without concomitant increase in zymogenic chief cells, when assessed morphometrically (Willems and Lehy, 1975; Crean et

314

al., 1978; Balas et al., 1985). In addition, diffuse hyperplasia of enterochromaffin cells also occurs.

By contrast, cholecysokinin, a trophic peptide found in the duodenum and sharing the same C-terminal tetrapeptide sequence as gastrin, increases in the number of chief cells but not parietal cells when administered to mice under similar conditions (Balas et al., 1985).

Drugs which inhibit or neutralize gastric acid secretion such as histamine H2 antagonists and antacids also induce hypertrophy or hyperplasia of the parietal cell population (Witzel et al., 1977; Crean et al., 1978; Mazzacca et al., 1978; Kaduk and Haüser, 1980). These agents are associated with a rise in serum gastrin levels, probably as a result of loss of feedback inhibition of low antral pH on gastrin producing G cells (Witzel et al., 1977). Cessation of treatment with histamine H2 antagonists may lead to rebound hypersecretion of gastric acid from the increased parietal cell mass.

However, not all histamine H2 antagonists consistantly produce this effect. Other cytological changes have been reported with famotidine, another H2-receptor antagonist. This agent produced a dose-related increase in the prevalence and degree of eosinophilic granularity in chief cells of the stomach in toxicity studies in rats but not dogs (Burek et al., 1985). Electron microscopy showed an increase in electron density of zymogen granules and it was argued that these effects were the result of secondary inhibition of pepsin secretion or turnover due to inhibition of acid secretion.

Potential cytoprotective agents of prostaglandin type produce different forms of diffuse gastric hyperplasia. Rats treated with 16,16-dimethyl prostaglandin E2 hourly for three weeks, not only developed forestomach alterations (see above) but also thickening of both the body and antral mucosa. The small and large bowel walls were also thickened (see below). In the body mucosa, these changes were the result of a proportional increase in the total mass of surface and foveolar mucous cells, mucous neck cells, chief cells, parietal and endocrine cells as well as connective tissue. This was largely as a result of increase in cell number, although parietal cells also increased in size (Reinhart et al., 1983). Unlike treatment with gastrin and gastrin analogues there was an increase in number of surface and foveolar mucous cells associated with increase in mucus content.

Misprostal, a synthetic prostaglandin E1 methyl ester analogue also produced diffuse glandular hyperplasia, characterized by lengthening of gastric pits and increased mucous secretion in the preclinical safety studies in dogs and rats (Kotsonis et al., 1985). This glandular hyperplasia not only affected the body but also the antral mucosal. Studies with tritiated thymidine showed that the labelling index was reduced in rats treated with misprostal, suggesting hyperplasia following administration of prostanoids is a result of an increase in cell survival and decrease in cell shedding rather than an increase in cell proliferation (Fich et al., 1988).

The effects of prostaglandins of the E series on the gastrointestinal tract of dogs and rodents has been reviewed by Levin (1988).

315

Gastric hyperplasia with proliferative or adenomatous features (adenomatous hyperplasia, giant hypertrophic gastritis, hypertrophic gastropathy)

Thickening of the gastric glandular mucosa as a result of an irregular proliferation and cystic dilatation of gastric glands associated with inflammation, characterizes a number of non-neoplastic conditions in the stomach of man and laboratory animals. Cystic change with chronic inflammation and foveolar hyperplasia is observed in biopsies taken from the edge of chronic gastric ulcers in man (Franzin and Novelli, 1981). Although the pathogenesis of Ménétriers disease in man remains elusive, it is also characterized by hypertrophy and hyperplasia of mucous glands with cystic features (Berenson et al., 1976).

Similar changes have been observed in animals in association with infestation of the gastrointestinal tract by parasites (Jubb and Kennedy, 1970; Cook et al., 1981). Laboratory rodents may develop a similar pattern of changes spontaneously with advancing age, although the cause of this change remains uncertain. For convenience, changes in rat and mouse are discussed separately.

Gastric hyperplasia: mouse

Proliferation of the gastric glandular mucosa has been well characterized in the laboratory mouse because certain strains have a particular tendency to develop this condition spontaneously with advancing age (Stewart and Andervont, 1936; Rowlatt et al, 1969). Hyperplasia also occurs spontaneously in conventional laboratory strains employed in carcinogenicity bioassays and its prevalence in such studies can be influenced by environmental factors such as housing (Chvedoff et al, 1984), food restriction (Rehm et al., 1987), and the administration of xenobiotics (Poynter et al., 1985; Betton et al., 1987). Similar gastric changes have also been reported to occur in mice thymectomized shortly after birth (Suzuki et al., 1981).

Histologically, these changes in mice are characterized by hyperplasia of the foveolar and neck regions of the body mucosa. In advanced cases this is accompanied by elongated, tortuous, or dilated glands lined by simple columnar or cuboidal epithelium, devoid of parietal or chief cells (Figs. 59 and 60). The abnormal cells show only mild cellular pleomorphism and mitotic activity. The abnormal glands displace normal glandular tissue and even penetrate through the muscularis mucosa to reach the muscularis externa and serosa. Step sections however demonstrate continuity between these glandular elements and a total absence of metastatic spread in the adjacent tissues and lymph nodes. The lamina propria also shows increased amounts of smooth muscle and collagen accompanied by variable numbers of lymphocytes and other chronic inflammatory cells. Oedema may be observed and blood vessels are often dilated. The antral mucosa remains relatively unaffected.

Histochemistry has shown variable mucin secretion of the altered glands. Some glands are devoid of mucin, others show an increase in sulphomucin as revealed by the high-iron diamine technique (Greaves and Boiziau, 1984).

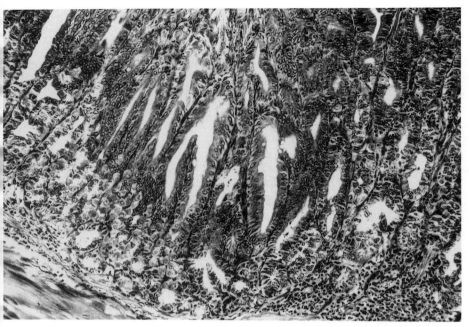

Fig. 59. Stomach from an untreated 18-month-old CD-1 mouse showing moderate hyperplasia of the gastric glands of the body mucosa. (HE, ×200.)

The aetiology of this spontaneous condition in the mouse is uncertain. As a high prevalence of these changes was observed among densely housed mice in one long term study, it was argued that stress-induced gastric damage may be a factor in its development (Chvédoff et al., 1980). The occurence of similar lesions in thymectomized mice has also given rise to the suggestion that autoimmune damage to the gastric mucosa may be responsible (Kojima et al., 1980). The presence of circulating anti-parietal antibodies and the decrease in the number of parietal cells in thymectomized mice suggested that autoimmune damage can occur to parietal cells with compensatory chronic stimulation and proliferation of the generative zones (Suzuki et al., 1981).

However, based on findings in female Han NMRI mice, Rehm and colleagues (1987) showed that this proliferative condition can develop in mice in the absence of antiparietal antibodies. They demonstrated that the prevalence of this change can be reduced by food restriction and that it is associated with an increase in the number of antral gastrin cells, raising the possibility of a hormonally-related pathogenesis.

It is, therefore, of interest to note that similar changes occur with increased prevalence in CD-1 mice treated with the novel histamine H2 receptor antagonist SK&F 93479 for 21 months (Betton et al., 1987; 1988). Although treated mice developed hyperplasia of gastric neuroendocrine cells similar to that observed in rodents treated with other antisecretory agents, they also showed an increase in

317

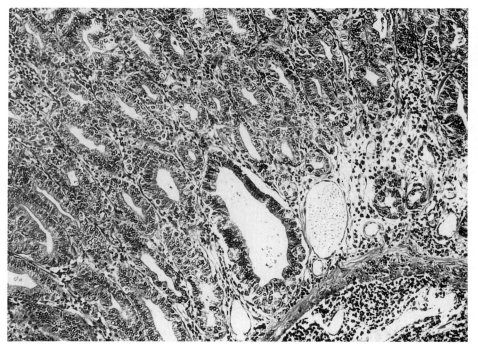

Fig. 60. Another example of gastric glandular hyperplasia found in the gatric body mucosa in an 18-month-old CD-1 mouse in which hyperplastic glands extend down to the muscularis mucosae. (HE, ×200.)

the severity of glandular hyperplasia. Like the spontaneous condition, these changes were characterized by thickening of the mucosa by hyperplasia of the foveolar and neck regions, and downward proliferation of glandular elements into gastric glands (Betton et al., 1988). Poynter and colleagues (1985) have also reported similar glandular hyperplasia in the mouse stomach associated with histamine H_2 blockade with the agent ioxtidine. These findings were similarly associated with hyperplasia of neuroendocrine cells.

Although the histological features and mucin histochemical characteristics of this condition in the mouse indicates incomplete maturation of gastric glandular cells (Greaves and Boiziau, 1984), the rarity of gastric carcinoma in the mouse suggests that it is not a preneoplastic state. However, it is important to note that this hyperplasia possesses histological features in common with the proliferative lesions which procede the development of experimental gastric carcinoma in rodents or atypical hyperplasia (dysplasia) associated with gastric cancer in man. Therefore, careful characterization of such changes are necessary when their prevalence is greater in treated mice. It is necessary to assess the degree of cellular pleomorphism, mitotic activity and glandular growth disturbances. The distribution of the lesions within the stomach may be helpful. This spontaneous

318

condition affects principally the body mucosa whereas carcinogens usually also produce proliferative effects in the antral mucosa.

Gastric hyperplasia: rat

Although usually less prevalent and less exhuberent than in mice, the aged rat also develops proliferative gastric glandular changes spontaneously. These changes are characterized by hyperplasia of the foveolar and mucin-secreting cells of the body mucosa, development of cystic glands lined by simple mucous or flattened cells, accompanied by chronic inflammatory cells, prominant blood vessels and smooth muscle in the lamina propria (Greaves and Faccini, 1984). The antrum remains relatively unaffected.

A proliferative condition of the gastric mucosa has also been shown to develop following long-term treatment of rats with an ulcerogenic regimen of aspirin. Female Sprague-Dawley rats given 250 mg/kg of asiprin in 1% methylcellulose once daily orally by gavage for six months followed for periods of up to 18 months without treatment, developed focal proliferative changes at the sites of healed ulcers, mainly in the mucosa of antrum or antral-body junction (St John et al., 1977). These lesions were characterized by the presence of proliferating gastric glands lined by columnar, cuboidal or flattened epithelial cells in the mucosa which also extended through the muscularis mucosa. Mucus content of these glands was variable but when present was principally acidic in type, as shown by staining with alcian blue at pH 2.5. The lesions were accompanied by increased collagen in the lamina propria, endarteritis and an infiltration of lymphocytes, plasma cells and mast cells. The lesions were not associated with the development of carcinoma following 18 months observation and it is probable that they were the result of the chronic damage and repair induced by aspirin treatment.

Hyperplasia of the gastric glandular mucosa also occurs in rats following the administration of powerful genotoxic carcinogens, although characteristically in association with of atypical histological changes and ultimately carcinoma. These changes have been best characterized in sequential studies with the rat using the carcinogen N-methyl-N′-nitro-N-nitrosoguanidine at doses low enough to avoid overt gastric ulceration and regenerative hyperplasia. It was shown that hyperplasia developing under these conditions occurrs diffusely both in the body and antral mucosa. Furthermore, the changes occurred earlier in the antrum than in the body and were focal or polypoid in character (Tsiftsis et al., 1980). Involvement of the antrum in this way is quite unlike the spontaneous hyperplasia of the rat gastric mucosa. Histologically, this form of hyperplasia is characterized by lengthening of the foveolae and neck regions both in the antrum and body. Hyperplastic pits or foveolae show increased secretion of sialomucins and sulphomucins with a concomitant loss of neutral mucins.

Polychlorinated biphenyls such as Arochlor 1254 which produce intestinal metaplasia and adenocarcinoma in the stomach of rats also induce proliferative alterations characterized by proliferative cystic lesions in the mucosa associated with inflammation and fibrosis (Morgan et al., 1981). In common with lesions induced by genotoxic agents, these proliferative features are found primarily in the antrum and pyloric regions, zones of predilection for the development of gastric carcinoma in man and experimental animals.

Gastric dysplasia

It is important to distinguish between the various hyperplastic and adenomatous conditions found in the gastric glandular mucosa in laboratory animals which are not associated with neoplasia from those which precede the development of carcinoma. This distinction is complicated by the fact that some of the proliferative changes associated with the development of cancer both in man and laboratory animals possess features in common with lesions not associated with cancer development. However, a key distinctive feature is the degree of epithelial dysplasia.

Dysplasia is considered to be the lesion common to the gastric conditions in man such as atrophic gastritis and gastric polyps which have been linked with a significantly increased risk of gastric cancer. Although the term dysplasia may be less widely employed in experimental pathology, similar dysplastic changes to those occurring in man have been characterized in laboratory animals in which precancerous gastric lesions have been studied (Tsiftsis et al., 1980). It therefore represents a useful unifying concept in the assessment of proliferative changes in the gastric glandular mucosa of laboratory animals.

As defined by an international group concerned with the diagnosis of preneoplastic conditions in the stomach of man, the principle features of dysplasia are i) cellular atypia; ii) abnormal differentiation; and iii) disorganized mucosal architecture (Morson et al., 1980; Nagayo, 1981). Cellular atypia is characterized by nuclear pleomorphism, hyperchromasia, stratification of nuclei, increased nuclear-cytoplasmic ratio and loss of cellular and nuclear polarity. Abnormal differentiation is shown by reduction or alteration in the normal secretory products of the mucosa. Disorganized mucosal architecture comprises irregularity of crypt structure, back to back glands, budding and branching of crypts and intraluminal and surface papillary growths.

It is important to assess gastric mucosa very carefully for the features of dysplasia when hyperplastic gastric changes are found in treated animals. In the rat gastric cancer model employing the carcinogen N-methyl-N'-nitro-N-nitrosoguanidine, dysplastic changes were shown to start in the proliferating neck region of hyperplastic zones (Tsiftsis et al., 1980). These changes were characterized histologically by irregular growth patterns of glandular cells showing reduced mucin secretion, numerous mitoses and enlarged pleomorphic nuclei. These atypical glands were observed to extend downwards, eventually replacing normal gastric glands and ultimately penetrating the muscularis mucosa forming infiltrating adenocarcinomas of variable differentiation. The antrum developed these changes earlier than the body mucosa (Tsiftsis et al., 1980).

Such considerations were important in the safety evaluation of the histamine H2 receptor antagonist, tiotidine (1C1 125,211) a guanidino-thiazole derivative which also produced proliferative gastric lesions in the stomach of rats in a 24 month carcinogenicity study (Streett et al., 1984; 1988). These changes were found mainly in the pyloric region and were characterized histologically by superficial erosions and irregular pyloric glands lined by cells with basophilic cytoplasm and enlarged hyperchromatic nuclei. Some atypical glands penetrated the muscularis mucosae. Dysplastic lesions situated primarily in the pyloric region were also associated with the development of invasive carcinoma in some rats. Extensive histological sectioning of the stomach in rats treated with tiotidine for only six months also revealed evidence of early proliferative changes (Streett et al., 1988). Therefore, these lesions produced by tiotidine possessed more in common with those induced by powerful carcinogens such as N-methyl-N'-nitro-N-nitrosoguanidine than the benign, species-specific proliferative change of little or no relevance for human safety. Interestingly, mice treated for 18 months with tiotidine were devoid of dysplastic changes in the gastric mucosa (Streett et al. 1988).

Hyperplasia and neoplasia of gastric endocrine cells: carcinoid tumors

One of the most remarkable examples drug-induced gastric alterations in rodent bioassays reported in recent years is the hyperplasia of enterochromaffin cells and development of carcinoid-like neoplasms in the stomach of rats treated with omeprazole (Havu, 1986). Omeprazole is a substituted benzimidazole which inhibits gastric acid secretion by blocking the enzyme H + , K + -ATPase, the proton pump of the parietal cells, in a specific and dose-dependent manner (Fellenius et al., 1981).

Although in rats there is a increase in number of gastric argyophilic cells with increasing age, rats treated with omeprazole for 104 weeks showed a marked, dose-related and diffuse increase of argyophilic, non-argentaffin cells in the basal half of the oxyntic fundal mucosa (Havu, 1986). These changes were more marked in female than in male rats but were not observed in the bioassay in which CD-1 mice were treated with similar doses of omeprazole for 78 weeks.

These diffuse changes in the rat stomach were associated with focal hyperplasia of argyrophilic cells. These focal lesions were also associated with a dose-related increase in larger focal nodular lesions of argyrophilic cells, some of which were undoubtably locally infiltrating carcinoid tumors. Unfortunately, these nodular argyrophil lesions posed the usual problems of differential diagnosis of endocrine hyperplasia and neoplasia (see Endocrine System, chapter XIII) and distinction of hyperplasia from neoplasia was uncertain.

Histologically, nodular lesions were composed of multifocal anastomosing solid or pseudoacinar cords of proliferating, regular cells with uniform nuclei and moderately abundant fine granular pale cytoplasm. These nodules showed little or no cellular pleomorphism or mitotic activity but clear evidence of submucosal infiltration without involvement of the muscularis externa was observed in some cases. Thus, the overall light microscopic features of some nodules were similar to those of gastrointestinal carcinoid tumours reported in man. The incidence of gastric carcinoids was reported to be as high as 40% in females in the high dose group but only a few cases observed in similarly treated males (Ekman et al, 1985; Havu, 1986). Similar tumours are not usually observed spontaneously in rats.

Electron microscopy of the altered argyophil cells confirmed the presence of electron-luscent, vesicular granules, frequently with small irregular dense cores characteristic of enterochromaffin cells of the stomach. Immunocytochemical study showed that these cells contained histidine decarboxylase which is found normally in gastric enterchromaffin cells which produce and store histamine (Sundler et al., 1986).

Other findings reported in rats treated with omeprazole have been a proportional increase in the number and size of non-endocrine cells of the fundus (Blom, 1986), an increase in the number and immunostaining properties of the antral gastrin-containing G cells and hypergastrinaemia (Bishop et al., 1986; Creutzfeldt et al., 1986). All functional and morphological changes following treatment for 60 days were fully reversible after 42 days drug withdrawal (Creutzfeldt et al., 1986).

As a result of these treatment-related increases of these normally rare gastric carcinoids in the rat bioassay with omeprazole, clinical trials with this agent were suspended until it was successfully argued that the endocrine alterations were not a totally unexpected result of prolonged drug-induced achlorhydria. It was postulated that omeprazole causes a prolonged inhibition of acid secretion in the rat which causes activation and subsequently hyperplasia of antral gastrin cells and marked hypergastrinaemia. Hypergastrinaemia in turn stimulates enterochromaffin cells of the fundus which in time results in enterochromaffin hyperplasia. The development of nodular hyperplasia and neoplasia of endocrine cells was argued to be the consequence of a sustained hypergastrinaemia for a prolonged period of time (Håkanson et al., 1986a,b). This argument is supported by the fact that similar morphological findings are reported in chronic atrophic gastritis and other achlorhydric states in man (Solchia et al., 1986; Müller et al., 1987) and that antrectomy in the rat prevents the appearance of enterochromaffin hyperplasia following treatment with omeprazole (Larsson et al., 1986).

Although mild dose-related gastric argyrophil cell hyperplasia was noted in dogs treated with omeprazole for one year, neoplasms of the stomach were not observed during this time period. Why mice neither developed neither argyrophil hyperplasia nor gastric carcinoids with a similar treatment regimen is not entirely clear, as the mechanism of action of omeprazole is similar in rat, dog and mouse. However, as the duration of action of omeprazole is shorter in the mouse, it was postulated that sustained inhibition of gastric acid secretion over 24 hours is necessary to activate increased gastrin secretion from antral cells (Havu, 1986). It has also been suggested that the mouse possesses fewer gastric enterochromaffin cells than the rat and shows a much lower serum gastrin response to omeprazole treatment (Ekman et al., 1985).

322

Duration of action or potency may also be the explanation for the lack of reports of carcinoid neoplasms in rats following inhibition of gastric acid secretion by the histamine H2-blockers cimetidine and ranitidine, neither of which completely inhibit gastric acid secretion in the rat for 24 hours (Leslie and Walker, 1977; Larsson et al., 1986), although mild gastric neuroendocrine hyperplasia has been recently described in cimetidine-treated rats (Hirth et al., 1988).

By contrast, the long acting H2 receptor antagonist SK&F 93479 produced gastric carcinoid neoplasms when administered at a high dose (1000 mg/kg) to rats for two years (Betton et al., 1987; 1988). Although this dose level of SK&F 93479 did not entirely suppress gastric acid secretion and control gastric pH over 24 hours, plasma gastrin levels remained elevated at three to four times control values over this period. In a 21 month oral carcinogenicity study in CD-1 mice at the same dose level (1000 mg/kg), a diffuse neuroendocrine cell hyperplasia and multifocal glandular hyperplasia or neoplasia was also observed (Betton et al., 1987). Similarly, loxitidine, a potent, non-competitive, unsurmountable histamine H2 antagonist produced hyperplasia of neuroendocrine cells and carcinoid tumors in the gastric fundus of both rats and mice after two years treatment in diet and drinking water, respectively (Poynter et al., 1985, 1986). Other histamine antagonists BL-6341 and ICI 162846 have been reported to produce neuroendocrine neoplasms in the stomach of rats and rats and mice, respectively (Hirth et al., 1988; Streett et al., 1988).

The salient features of the safety assessment of drugs designed for the long-term treatment of peptic ulcers has been reviewed in detail by Wormsley (1984).

Drugs of other classes also cause hyperplasia of gastrin-containing cells. Immunocytochemical study using antigastrin antibody revealed increased gastrin cell numbers in the antral mucosa of dogs given high doses of adrenocorticosteroids for four weeks and these changes were accompanied by enhanced serum and tissue gastrin levels (Delaney et al., 1979). These results suggest that adreno-corticosteroids also have an important trophic effect on gastrin-containing cells.

In human patients hypergastrinaemia is also produced by pharmacologically induced hypochlorhydria although thisis usually only slight and hyperplasia of enterochromaffin cells has not been observed (Soll, 1990). The development of high gastrin levels in treated patients would initiate investigation for endocrine cell pathology by some physicians using antisecretory therapy (Soll, 1990).

Gastric carcinoma and nitrosation

The development of primary gastric cancer spontaneously in laboratory species used in toxicology is uncommon. However, carcinomas of the forestomach and glandular stomach can be induced by administration of a number of aromatic hydrocarbons and N-nitroso compounds. Furthermore, at least two types of gastric neoplasms have been reported in laboratory animals following administration of potential therapeutic agents, notably potent inhibitors of gastric secretion.

Long term treatment of rats with agents which inhibit gastric secretion may induce gastric carcinoids (see above). Administration of the histamine H2 antagonist tiotidine, a guanidinolthiazol derivative, produced gastric antral adenocarcinomas in the rat, similar to those produced by N-methyl-N'-nitro-N-nitrosoguanidine (Streett et al., 1984).

A complicating factor in drug safety evaluation is the association of gastric cancer in both man and laboratory animals with N-nitroso compounds. Some of the most effective stomach carcinogens in laboratory animals have proved to be N-nitroso compounds particularly since Sugimura and Fujimura (1967) induced gastric adenocarcinomas in rats with N-methyl-N'-nitro-N-nitrosoguanidine dissolved in drinking water. Furthermore, epidemiological evidence associating N-nitroso compounds with human cancer is also fairly strong for the stomach (Corea et al., 1975; Pocock, 1985).

The formation of N-nitroso compounds is theoretically possible with a variety of compounds which contain amino groups. It has been suggested that the formation of nitrosamines occurs in vivo under the acidic conditions in the stomach following dietary ingestion of nitrite, nitrates and secondary amines (Mirvish, 1975; 1983). Low levels of preformed nitrosamines are also present in some commercial pelleted diets for laboratory animals, principally derived from fish meal (Edwards et al., 1979). Calculations based on dietary intake and nitrosatability of precusors and carcinogenicity of derivatives have suggested that the risk which arises from endogeneous nitrosation is highly variable but highest from ureas and aromatic amines (Shephard et al., 1987).

A number of drugs in widespread clinical use have been shown to produce N-nitroso products in acidic aqueous media, although the extent to which this occurs in actual therapeutic use is unclear (Gillatt et al., 1985). Nevertheless, some clinical evidence exists to suggest that nitrosation of therapeutic agents can occur in clinical practice. For instance piperazine, a cyclic secondary amine, widely used as an antihelmintic drug, has been shown to form small quantities of N-mononitrosopiperazine in the human stomach as measured by gas chromatography-thermal energy analysis (Bellander et al., 1985). However, N-mononitrosopiperazine has not been shown to be carcinogenic in rodents (Love et al., 1977). N,N'-dinitrosopiperazine, carcinogenic to the upper gastrointestinal tract in rodents (Lijinsky and Taylor, 1975), was not detected in man after administration of piperazine under the same circumstances (Bellander et al., 1985).

The possibility of nitrosation occurring is not usually taken into account in the testing of carcinogenic potential of novel drugs as bioassays are usually only performed with parent compound. However, concerns about nitrosation may develop in subsequent clinical practice. An example of this was the proposal that a few gastric cancers found in patients whilst being treated with the histamine H2-receptor antagonist cimetidine, were the result of treatment (Elder et al., 1979; Reed et al., 1979; Hawker et al., 1980). It now seems likely that all those observed cancers associated with cimetidine were incidental (Penston and

Wormsley, 1986). However, the concerns were increased by the theoretical possibility that cimetidine may be nitrosated in vivo with carcinogenic consequences (Elder et al., 1982). A further factor was the concept that the treatment-induced gastric secretory inhibition with subsequent bacterial colonization of the stomach rendered the conditions conducive to the generation of N-nitroso compounds from normal dietary constituents (Reed et al., 1981; Penston and Wormsley, 1986).

To date these concerns appear to be unfounded. Long-term surveillance studies with cimetidine have shown no causal link between its clinical usage and gastric malignancy (Colin-Jones et al., 1965; Langman, 1985). In addition, carcinogenicity bioassays performed with cimetidine, cimetidine plus nitrite and nitrosocimetidine have not shown any tumorigenic effect in the gastric mucosa (Anderson et al., 1985). A seven-year study in dogs in which multiple gastric biopsies were taken at intervals of approximately six months have also shown no indication of gastric hyperplasia, dysplasia, intestinal metaplasia or neoplastic change (Walker et al., 1987). Thus, the available evidence does not indicate that the widely used histamine H2 antagonist possesses a carcinogenic risk for man. Although complacency is certainly not warranted with respect to the nitrosation of therapeutic agents in vivo, the risks of this being a significant risk for the development of gastric malignancy from drugs which are administered on a short term basis are probably very small (World Health Organization, 1978). Even for gastric antisecretory agents which may be administered for longer periods of time, the balanced view would also permit development of novel agents provided they are not obviously mutagenic or carcinogenic in the usual preclinical studies and non possess molecular structures which are particularly liable to undergo rapid nitrosation.

Gastric carcinoma: histological appearances

Neoplasms arising in the forestomach of rodents are usually squamous carcinomas although basaloid features are seen (Fukushima and Ito, 1985). Squamous carcinomas, as at other sites, show variable differentiation being composed of proliferating squamous epithelium with moderate to marked cellular atypia, pleomorphism and mitotic activity with clear evidence of invasion into the muscularis.

Adenocarcinomas, whether induced by the classical genotoxic carcinogens or potential therapeutic agents tend to develop in the antral region in rodents (Streett et al., 1984; Szentirmay and Sugar, 1985). These neoplasms are variably differentiated. They range from those with well differentiated tubular or papillary features to poorly differentiated forms with trabecular, mucoid or signet ring features. Squamous metaplasia within adenocarcinoma can also be observed. Stroma may be abundant with pronounced chronic inflammatory infiltration and hyalinization. Metaplastic cartilage and bone has also been described (Szentirmay and Sugar, 1985). Gastric adenocarcinomas induced in dogs by N-methyl-

N'-nitro-N-nitrosoguanidine show similar histological features although their reported distribution in the stomach appears more variable (Fujita et al., 1974).

It is important to note that the histological criteria for the diagnosis of invasive adenocarcinoma in experimental animals may vary between individual pathologists. Some retain the criteria of Stewart and coworkers (1961) who defined invasive cancer as a neoplastic lesion reaching the serosa. It is now more appropriate to apply criteria of use in human diagnostic pathology, that is unequivocal invasion of the submucosa is sufficient evidence of an invasive and therefore malignant process (Greaves and Faccini, 1984).

SMALL INTESTINE

The small intestine is of major importance in drug safety evaluation for it represents the primary site of drug absorption. In view of its length and the presence of villi, it possesses an enormous surface area of specialized absorptive epithelium. Furthermore, ingested substances have an extended residence time in this part of the gastrointestinal tract.

The canine model has been one of the most popular for the study of drug absorption because the dimensions of the canine gastrointestinal tract permit administration of dosage forms intended for clinical use in man. For this reason, factors which influence drug absorption have been better studied in dog and man than many other species. However, data from dog and man not only suggest that many factors influence drug absorption from the small intestine but that there are considerable species differences.

Residence time is of particular importance for drugs which are incompletely absorbed because differences in mucosal contact time can be expected to result in differences in the fraction absorbed. Dressman (1986) has shown using the Heidelberg capsule technique, that small intestine transit time in dogs is varies from between 15 to over 200 minutes whereas in man equivalent times are between 180 and 300 minutes. These results suggest that absorption of poorly absorbable drugs is likely to be less although more variable in dogs than in man. However, these differences do not explain why some poorly lipophilic drugs such as chlorothiazine, acyclovir and phosphalinic acid are more extensively absorbed in dogs than in man. Intestinal pH is consistently higher in dogs than in man so that drugs with half maximal absorption pH in the range pH 5 to 7 may also be expected to be absorbed at different rates in man and dog (Dressman, 1986). Physiological and anatomical differences between the small intestine of other test species particularly rodents and man are also likely to have an impact on drug absorption although many of these factors are still poorly understood.

In addition to the small intestine acting as an absorptive surface, it is becoming increasingly obvious that it plays an important part in the metabolism of drugs (Breckenridge, 1987). Although monoxygenase activity is relatively low in the gut compared with the liver, conjugation mechanisms are efficient and activities of UDP-glucuronosyltransferase and glutathione-S-transferase are as high or even higher than in the liver (Hänninen et al., 1987). In addition, the gastrointestinal microflora not only possesses metabolic capacity itself but also can influence the turnover rate of mucosal cells and subsequent exfoliation and release of enzymes into the lumen (Hänninen et al., 1987). Gastrointestinal metabolising activity is important because that the mucosa is exposed to high concentrations of xenobiotics in toxicity studies, and this can influence their overall bioavailability (Chhabra and Eastin, 1984).

Studies in untreated rats have shown that the concentration of total cytochrome P450 in small intestinal microsomes is only about 10% of that found in liver microsomes (Bonkovsky et al., 1985). However, it exists in at least two forms and as in the liver, its activity can be induced by xenobiotics. It has been shown that in the rat, the concentration of cytochrome P450 and drug metabolizing enzyme activity increases in intestinal epithelial cells as they move from crypt to villous tips and they are found in greater concentration in the proximal two thirds of the small intestine than in the distal third (Hoensch et al., 1976; Bonkovsky et al., 1985). Bonkovsky and colleagues (1985) also showed that the phenobarbital-inducible form of cytochrome P450 represents less than 5% of total P450 in the small bowel, but as in the liver, phenobarbital treatment can increase this form to about 50% of total cytochrome P450 in small intestine cells. Furthermore, it has been shown that drug metabolizing activity in the tips of the villi in the duodenum is greater in rats fed a conventional diet than a semisynthetic diet and that the activity depends critically on the absorption of iron from the intestine (Hoensch et al., 1976).

Glutathione is also present throughout the entire mucosa, although in rats, cells at the tips of the villi contain less than cells located more basally, whereas related enzymes gamma-glutamyl transpeptidase and glutathione-S-transferase show highest activity in the villous tip region (Ogasawara et al., 1985). The fact that these enzyme activities are highest in the duodenum and lowest in the terminal ileum suggests that detoxification systems for exogenous compounds are greater in the proximal small intestine.

Histological and histochemical characteristics

The small intestinal mucosa is constructed not only to act as an absorptive surface but also as a barrier to potentially pathogenic substances and microorganisms. Although the main cell population of the epithelium is composed of absorptive cells, other major epithelial cell types, the mucous (goblet) cells, Paneth cells and endocrine cells have important protective functions. In addition, specialized epithelial cells, the microfold (membranous or M) cells are located in the epithelium over Peyer's patches. These cells form part of the other important protective system of the intestine, the gut associated lymphoid tissue (GALT) or mucosal associated lymphoid tissue (MALT).

The mucosal lining is in a constant state of renewal. Enteric epithelium possesses the fastest rate of turnover of any tissue exceeded only by a few

327

rapidly growing neoplasms (Williamson, 1978a). In normal circumstances, the constant turnover of small bowel mucosa is maintained by an equilibrium between cell production in the crypts and cell loss at the tips of the villi. The regulation of this process is highly complex and not completely understood. There are intrinsic controls within the mucosa itself. Exogeneous substances, intraluminal secretions, mechanical and neural factors as well as alterations in blood flow all possess potential to influence mucosal cell kinetics (Williamson, 1978b).

All main epithelial cell types are believed to arise from undifferentiated columnar cells at the crypt base (Cheng and Leblond, 1974), although mucous cells may also arise by proliferation of partly differentiated mucous cells in the crypts. As cell division is limited to crypts, the cell population in the crypts have high activities of enzymes such as thymidine kinase which are involved in nucleic acid synthesis (Imondi et al., 1969).

The complete cell cycle lasts about 10 to 17 hours in rodents and at least 24 hours in man. Enteric epithelium is completely replaced within two to three days in mice and rats and within three to six days in man (Williamson, 1978a).

After two or more divisions in the crypt cells migrate to the villus, lose ability to incorporate thymidine and differentiate into mature cells equipped with enzymes associated with nutrient absorption (Imondi et al., 1969). Cell migration in the rat is completed more rapidly in the ileum than in the jejunum principally as a result of the lower villous height in the ileal mucosa (Altman and Enesco, 1967). Migration terminates by loss of cells from the tip of the villi.

Surrounding the crypt is a sheath of fibroblastic cells. These cells also undergo synchronous division and migration with the epithelial cells, maintaining the intimate relationship between the epithelium and supporting tissues (Parker et al., 1974).

Mature absorptive cells are important in the active and passive transport of nutrients as well as in the endocytosis of macromolecules. They are characterized by the presence of a striated or brush border which is seen in haematoxylin and eosin-stained sections as a refractile bilamina band. The inner, wider lamina corresponds to the microvillous region which is associated with the presence of neutral mucosubstances in most species. The outer, thinner band corresponds to the glycocalyx which is composed principally of acidic mucosubstances (Sheahan and Jarvis, 1976). This outer band of the brush border shows histochemical staining predominantly for sulphomucins in most species including mouse, hamster, dog and rhesus monkey, although in the duodenum of the rats and in the entire human small bowel sialomucins predominate in this layer.

Electron microscopy of the absorptive cells shows that the surface of absorptive cells is covered by tightly packed and well developed microvilli approximately 1 μm long and 0.1 μm wide. These are considered the first site of entry of food substances into the cell. The plasma membrane of microvilli is associated with fine filamentous projections which probably represent the polysaccharide chains of the glycocalyx (Bennett, 1969). As the glycocalyx is composed of a network of polysaccharides, it has been suggested that it may behave like an ion-exchange resin, be able to bind certain lectin-like molecules or trap substances in its matrix so providing a site for efficient intraluminal digestion (Bennett, 1969; Goldberg et al., 1969; King et al., 1986).

The plasma membrane shows a trilamina structure at ultrastructural level. Freeze fracture replicas from the microvilli which cleave this membrane through the plane of apposed non-polar groups of the lipid bilayer, demonstrate smooth complementary surfaces studded with small particles. These particles represent integral globular proteins of the plasma membrane. Some of these intramembranous particles, mostly those of 10 nm diameter show irregular outlines with a central pit and are believed to represent gap junctions or transport channels (Yamamoto, 1982).

A particularly important aspect of the absorptive cell membrane is its high concentration of disaccharidases such as sucrase, maltase and lactase, related to the absorption of sugars. Alkaline phosphatase activity is also abundant on the surface of absorptive cells, although its precise role here uncertain (Owen and Bhalla, 1983). Immunocytochemical demonstration of alkaline phosphatase provides a useful tool to examine the effects of xenobiotics on intrinsic membrane glycoproteins in the small intestine (Hasegawa et al., 1987).

Enterokinase, the glycoprotein enzyme which initiates the activation of pancreatic zymogens by converting trypsinogen to trypsin is also present in the brush border and glycocalyx of the small intestinal epithelium, both in man and animals. Immunocytochemical studies have demonstrated that in man this enzyme is located in the duodenum and proximal jejunum but not ileum, colon and stomach (Hermon-Taylor et al., 1977).

These enzymes constitute integral structural proteins of the cell membrane with active sites protruding from the cell surface. They are synthesized by the absorptive cells (Blok et al., 1984).

The lateral surfaces of absorptive cells are in direct contact with neighbouring cells and firmly attached to each other by terminal bars or junctional complexes. A terminal bar comprises an apically situated tight junction or zonula accludens, a central zone, the zonula adherens, below which is situated a desmosome or macula adherens. The junctional complexes are relatively impermeable to macromolecules. Studies with labelled tracers in the rat jejunum have shown that horseradish peroxidase (molecular weight 40,000, diameter 5 nm) and ferritin (molecular weight 100,000, diameter 10 nm) do not penetrate junctional complexes (Yamamoto, 1982).

Below the junctional complexes, the cell membranes interdigitate and the intercellular space widens towards the cell base, a feature that may be important in the movement of electrolytes and water across the intestinal epithelium (Rhodin, 1974).

The cytoplasm of absorptive cells contains smooth and granular endoplasmic reticulum, free ribosomes and mitochondria. The Golgi apparatus is located above the nucleus. The apical part of the cytoplasm is devoid of organelles except for a tight meshwork of filaments called the terminal web. Filaments of actin within the microvilli are linked to the terminal web and this is believed to be important in the movement of microvilli (Moosker and Tilney, 1975; Moosker et al., 1978).

Goblet cells are much fewer in number than absorptive cells in the small intestine but they increase in number from the duodenum to the lower ileum. They are important in the production of mucus which remains on the surface of the mucosa as a viscous layer and acts as the first line of defense against intestinal pathogens. Goblet cells are characterized by the presence of abundant mucous droplets formed by the Golgi complex and which accumulate in the apical part of the cell cytoplasm. Histochemical study shows that neutral mucrosubstances are present in the goblet cells found in crypts and on the villi in the entire small bowel mucosa of most species including man but there is an interspecies variation in the population of sialo- and sulphomucins (Sheahan and Jarvis, 1976). In the mouse sulphomucins predominate but among rats considerable individual variation in the proportion of sialo- and sulphomucins is reported. In the hamster, sulphomucins are more prominant in the proximal and sialomucins in the distal small bowel. In the dog, both sulphomucins and sialomucins are found with predominance of one or other in individual animals. Staining for acidic mucins is less intense in the goblet cells of the small intestine in man compared with non-human primates but sialomucins are predominant in both species. A few goblet cells in the distal ileum in man also contain sulphated mucins (Sheahan and Jarvis, 1976).

Although it is now generally believed that Paneth cells also form by differentiation from undifferentiated cells, they remain located near the crypt base throughout the small intestine. They are found in rodents and man but not in carnivors such as dog and cat (Rhodin, 1974; Satoh et al., 1986). They are characterized by the presence of numerous eosinophilic cytoplasmic secretory granules between about 1.0 and 2 μm diameter that contain various enzymes and mucosubstances.

Particular care is needed in fixation and staining for optimal demonstration of Paneth cells for they rapidly degranulate after death and granules are destroyed by acetic acid fixation. Formalin and mercuric fixatives appear appropriate methods and they permit staining with methylene blue, Lendrum's phloxine-tartrazine and Masson's trichrone (Lewin, 1969). The apical parts of Paneth cells show glucose-6-phosphatase, carbonicanhydrase and monoamine oxidase activity and they have been shown to contain lysozyme and immunoglobulins, particularly IgA (Riecken and Pearse, 1966; Speece, 1964; Ghoos and Vantrappen, 1971). Their precise function remains uncertain. A number of different theories have been proposed but technical problems with older staining techniques and fixation have undoubtably been the cause of much confusion (Sandow and Whitehead, 1979). However, in view of the fact that the Paneth cell granules contain lysozyme and show immunoreactivity for IgA it has been recently suggested that they may possess a role in the regulation of the microbiological milieu of the intestine by release of these substances into the lumen (Satoh et al., 1986). It has been shown that these substances are released from Paneth cells when germ free rats are dosed with the intestinal flora from specific pathogen free rats (Satoh et al., 1986; Satoh and Vollrath, 1986).

Endocrine cells are also scattered throughout the small intestinal mucosa. They are of both argentaffin and argyrophil types and are situated predominatly in crypts. Immunocytochemical study shows that they contain a variety of different peptides although gastrin, secretion and serotonin-containing cells have been those most extensively studied (Inokuchi et al., 1983).

In addition to the barrier formed by mucus and epithelial cells, lymphocytes, plasma cells, macrophages, dendritic cells and mast cells also form part of the protective function of the small intestine. Some lymphocytes are located within the epithelium mostly, above the basal lamina but below epithelial nuclei (Pabst, 1987). These lymphocytes are termed intraepithelial lymphocytes and are predominantly of T-suppressor/cytotoxic type in man and laboratory animals (Selby, 1981; Martin et al., 1986; Pabst, 1987).

Most lymphocytes in the lamina propria are also T cells but T helper cells outnumber the T suppressor/cytotoxic phenotype (Hirata et al., 1986; Pabst, 1987). Mature small B lymphocytes are uncommon in the lamina propria but plasma cells are present in large numbers. Many of the plasma cells produce IgA, the major immunoglobulin of mucosal secretions (Michalek et al., 1975). IgA represents another important component of the mucosal barrier between the gastrointestinal mucosa and intraluminal antigens. The main function of IgA is to effect immune exclusion by intimate cooperation with non-specific defence mechanisms (Brandtzaeg et al., 1985). Plasma cells in the lamina propria produce dimeric IgA with two dimeric molecules joined by a joint (J) piece. A secretory component (SC), a glycoprotein expressed on the basolateral surface of epithelial cells acts as a receptor for dimeric IgA and as a transport system for IgA to the gut lumen where monomeric IgA is secreted (Brandtzaeg et al., 1985). Morphometric analysis of IgA-containing immunocytes in the rat ileal mucosa using immunocytochemical staining has shown that the number of these cells varies with alterations in the microbiological status of intestinal contents (Rodning et al., 1983). A significant reduction in IgA-containing lymphocytes and plasma cells was observed following microbial reduction associated with gnotobiosis, probably reflecting decreased microbial antigenic stimulation. A decrease in IgA containing cells was also observed in self-filling intestinal blind loops in which microbial proliferation occurred, suggesting that there was an increased population of lymphoid cells producing other immunoglobulin types (Rodning et al., 1983). Experimental studies using labelled mesenteric lymphocytes also suggests that local microenvironments are important in the distribution of there cells in the intestinal wall (McDermott et al., 1985).

Peyer's patches are the most prominent aggregates of lymphoid tissue in the gastrointestinal tract and constitute important sites at which antigens from the gut lumen encounter immune competent cells which are responsible for the initiation of immune responses. Peyer's patches are located on the antemesenteric wall of the small bowel and consist principally of collections of lymphoid follicles. There are species differences of importance in the pre- and post-natal development of Peyer's patches and in their distribution in the intestine and these differences may possess considerable functional significance (Pabst, 1987). In man, Peyer's patches are more common in the ileum (Cornes, 1965) but in mice they are more uniformly distributed (Owen and Neumanic, 1978). In rats they are also more numerous in the distal than in the proximal small intestine and the number of follicles in patches usually varies from 2 to 6 but sometimes many more may be seen in any particular section (Martin et al., 1986). Particular care in selection and orientation of tissue blocks is therefore essential for any form of quantitive or semi-quantitiative assessment of Peyer's patches.

Peyer's patches are more than simple aggregates of lymphoid follicles. They consist of lymphoid follicles surrounded by a corona of small lymphocytes principally of B cell type. The interfollicular area contains post-capillary venules with specialized cobble-stone type epithelium (Yamaguchi and Schoefl, 1983) and many T lymphocytes. Beneath the epithelium, over the bulging follicles (dome area), mixtures of T and B lymphocytes, plasma cells and macrophages can be seen (Pabst, 1987). Immunohistochemical study in rats demonstrates the presence of W3/13-positive T cells in the interfollicular area. In the rat, many cells with macrophage morphology also stain with the W3/25 monoclonal antibody in the interfollicular zone (Bland and Warren, 1985; Martin et al., 1986). Immunocytochemical study of the Peyer's patches in the mouse has also shown considerable heterogeneity of staining patterns, particularly under the dome epithelium (Ermak and Owen, 1986). Similar patterns have been observed following immunohistochemical study of Peyer's patches in man (Spencer et al., 1986).

Few of these lymphoid cells can be considered sessile cells and a population of small circulating lymphocytes migrating mostly through gut associated lymphoid tissue has been demonstrated. Furthermore, it has also been shown that lymphocyte traffic also occurs between the gut and other organs lined by mucous membrane and associated with lymphoid tissue such as the bronchus and salivary, lacrymal and mammary glands (Pabst, 1987). Therefore, lymphoid cells in a fixed histological section of bowel only represent the situation at one specific time point, following which many cells would have circulated through this zone within a few hours.

The epithelium overlying the Peyer's patch follicles (dome area) contains specialized epithelial cells, called microfold, membranous or simply M cells. These cells have been identified in many species including rats, mice, hamsters, dogs, monkeys and man (Owen and Bhalla, 1983; Wolf and Bye, 1984). These cells differ functionally from other enterocytes by their ability to transport large molecules such as ferritin and horseradish peroxidase and particulate matter from the lumen to the underlying lymphoid tissue (Owen, 1977; Jeurissen et al., 1985). They have also been shown to be the site of penetration of reoviruses into the epithelium and they can transport Vibrio cholerae and other organisms (Wolf and Bye, 1974; Smith et al., 1987). M cells therefore form weak points in the intestinal wall which transport intact antigen and macromolecules to the follicles where they can be processed and be transported to lymph nodes with consequent IgA immune responses. This contrasts with the uptake of soluble antigens which can be taken up by ordinary epithelial cells and transported in the circulation of the villi to be ultimately trapped in the spleen possibly to evoke an IgM/IgG response (Jeurissen et al., 1985). It has been recently shown that M cell production in mice can be selectively increased within the follicle-associated epithelium in response to changes in the bacterial flora of the intestine (Smith et al., 1987).

Unfortunately, M cells cannot be easily identified in routine histological sections. They were originally characterized as the basis of their ultrastructural characteristics. The M cell shares tight junctions and desmosomes with adjacent epithelial cells but it has fewer and shorter microvilli than absorptive cells. There is lack of a well organized terminal web. Vesicles are abundant in the apical cytoplasm but lysosomes are reduced in number. Attenuated cytoplasmic processes may be seen embracing lymphocytes (Owen and Nemanic, 1978; Wolf and Bye, 1984).

With care, these attenuated microvilli can be seen at light microscopy in semi-thin plastic sections (Wolf and Bye, 1984). Cytochemical analysis has also demonstrated that they can be distinguished at light microscopic level by markedly reduced alkaline phosphatase activity on their terminal surface, in contrast to the dense reaction product produced by other enterocytes (Owen and Bhalla, 1983).

Mucosal mast cells also appear to be involved in the immunological defense of the gastrointestinal tract. They respond by proliferation, migration and discharge of granules during nematode infestations (Miller, 1980). It has been shown in the rat that mucosal mast cells of the gut differ in several ways from connective tissue mast cells. These differences result in poor preservation of mast cells of the gut if the usual metachromatic staining techniques employed for the demonstration of mast cells in tissue sections and used (Wingren and Enerbäck, 1983). Histochemical study suggests that mucosal mast cells differ from connective tissue mast cells by a lower degree of sulphation of glycosaminoglycans and different spatial relationships of protein and glycosaminoglycans in their granules. These cross link following formalin fixation in a way which is sufficient to prohibit cationic dye binding. Wingren and Enerback (1983) showed that these staining difficulties can be surmounted in tissues fixed in formaldehyde by staining in toluidine blue for prolonged periods of time (5–7 days), a procedure which allows adequate penetration of the toluidine blue molecule.

Histological techniques

Optimal histopathological study of the small intestine is complicated by its great length and mucosal fragility. It is exceedingly important to avoid vigorous washing procedures or any form of excessive manipulation of the unfixed bowel, as artefact caused by washing may confound interpretation of changes induced by xenobiotics (Roe, 1984). Combination of artefact due to washing, autolysis and the presence of neurophils can produce a histological appearance which mimics in vivo damage and trap the unwary pathologist.

Although careful visual inspection of the intestine and sampling of appropriate segments for histological examination is usually quite sufficient for routine examination, various forms of 'Swiss roll' techniques are helpful for more complete study. Rolling the unfixed, opened rodent intestine around a wooden stick prior to freezing or fixation is one proposed method (Moolenbeck and Ruitenberg, 1981), although this method risks undue manipulation of the unfixed tissue. Another more versatile technique applicable to rodent, large animal and human intestine can be performed after fixation. The unfixed opened bowel is pinned flat on a cork or board and fixed in a bath of formal saline. After fixation, the full thickness of rodent intestine can be rolled, transfixed by a pin and embedded in paraffin wax. Likewise the mucosa of the intestine of large animal species or man can be rolled after fixation by separating it from the muscularis externa (Filipe and Branfoot, 1974).

Non-neoplastic lesions

Inflammation and ulceration of the small intestine (duodenitis, jejunitis, ileitis)

Inflammation and ulceration of the mucosa occurs as a result of stress, infection with bacteria, infestation by parasites or as a direct result of the effects of xenobiotics or ionizing radiation. Antimitotic or radiomimetic agents as well as ionizing radiation itself are particularly liable to adversely effect the rapidly dividing cells of the small intestine with resulting breakdown of the mucosal barrier. The ulcerogenic activity of non-steroidal anti-inflammatory drugs may also be expressed in the small bowel as well as in the gastric mucosa.

Different agents also act synergistically to enhance damage to the small bowel mucosa. An important example is the effect of drugs which depress the immune system and thus permit the development of pathological infections by microorganisms of the opportunistic type in the small intestine.

The histological features of the inflammatory process in the small intestine are not usually specific for a particular agent. However, it is important that the pathologist searches for evidence of microbiological organisms and viral inclusions which can indicate the cause of intestinal inflammation and ulceration. Associated features in non-ulcerated mucosa such as morphology of the villi, accumulation of abnormal cells or foreign substances and changes in blood vessels are also be important in the assessment of these changes.

Infections and infestations

A number of organisms including those which are normal residents of the gastrointestinal tract cause inflammatory changes in the intestinal mucosa of laboratory animals. With the notable exception of non-human primates, inflammatory bowel disease caused by microbiological organisms is not usually

334

evident or of concern in most toxicity or carcinogenicity studies. However, when animals are treated with antibiotics, immuno-suppressive agents or other drugs which alter the normal intestinal flora, conditions may favour the proliferation of potentially pathogenic organisms in sufficient quantities to cause overt damage to the mucosa. Certain bacterial flora may also act synergistically with intestinal protozoans to produce pathological changes (Boorman et al., 1973).

In non-human primate colonies, gastrointestinal disease remains one of the most important causes of death (Holmberg et al., 1982a). In contrast to other laboratory species, histological evidence of intestinal infectious disease is relatively common and may confound the interpretation of gastrointestinal alterations occurring in toxicity studies. Although the majority of potentially pathogenic organisms affect the primate colon, a number of bacteria, protozoa and metazoa occur in the small intestine. A detailed review of the protozoa and metazoa occurring in the primate gastrointestinal tract has been published (Toft, 1982) and the key reference for identification of metazoa in tissue sections remains that of Chitwood and Lichtenfels (1973).

Organisms which can cause inflammatory disease in the small bowel but which are primarily agents which cause colonic inflammation are reported under 'Colon' (see following).

Bacterial infections

Bacillus piliform, is the agent responsible for Tyzzer's disease produces intestinal inflammation and ulcers in rats, mice and hamsters. Susceptability of different species and strains to experimental infection with *Bacillus piliformis* is variable. For instance, C57BL, BALB mice and F344 rats appear more resistant to infection than outbred Syrian hamsters (Waggie et al., 1987). Lesions of variable severity usually occur in the ileum but may also extend into the caecum and colon. Severe infections are characterized histologically by ulceration of the mucosa, associated with oedema and acute inflammation of the submucosa and muscle coats. Muscle may also show focal necrosis. Non-ulcerated mucosa is typically infiltrated by polymorphonuclear cells, with crypt abscess. There is blunting and fusion of villi with reactive hyperplasia and mucin depletion of the overlying epithelium (Ganaway, 1985a). Mucosal lymphoid tissue may also show reactive changes or hyperplasia.

Filamentous bundles of *Bacillus piliformis* can usually be found in the cytoplasm of both epithelial cells and smooth muscle cells at the edges of necrotic zones. Methylene blue, Giemsa or silver inpregnation techniques such as Warthin-Starry or Levaditi stains are the best stains for the demonstration of these organisms although with care they can be visualized in haematoxylin and eosin stained sections (Weisbroth, 1979). They are also PAS positive and gram negative.

Intestinal infections due to salmonella species are relatively common in the mouse but also occur in the hamster and rat (Ganaway, 1985b). *Salmonella typhimurium* and *Salmonella enteritidis* are regarded as the organisms typical of murine salmonellosis (Weisbroth, 1979). Lesions occur in the ileum and may extend into the jejunum and caecum. They are characterized by the presence of ulcers covered by fibrinous exudate and associated with diffuse infiltration of the adjacent mucosa by macrophages, neutrophils and lymphocytes. Intact crypt epithelium shows mucin loss and reactive proliferative changes. A characteristic feature is the presence of poorly defined granulomatous lesions composed of macrophages mainly in associated lymphoid tissue or Peyer's patches.

Clostridia species, especially *Clostridia difficile* which cause a pseudomembranous colitis in man and laboratory animals (especially hamsters) may also produce inflammation and ulceration in the terminal ileum with histological features similar to those found in the colon (see following).

Proliferative ileitis (transmissible ileal hyperplasia) is a striking lesion of hamsters affecting the distal segment of the ileum which is associated with intracellular invasion of the intestine mucosa epithelium by bacteria. The organism has not been cultivated, but has been suggested that it is a campylobacter (Jacoby, 1985).

Although it is characterized by hyperplasia of the ileal mucosa in its early stages, subsequently an inflammatory phase intervenes in which there is focal necrosis and haemorrhage of the mucosa, crypt abscesses and infiltration of the lamina propria by acute inflammatory cells and macrophages. The histological features of the associated hyperplasia are characteristic. The mucosa is covered by immature, mucin-depleted pseudostratified hyperchromatic epithelium with mitoses extending to the tips of villi and densely basophilic intracytoplasmic inclusions (Jacoby, 1985).

Campylobacter jejuni (*Helicobacter jejuni*) is a common cause of diarrhoea in man and may be the causative agent in small intestinal inflammation in laboratory dogs and primates. Campylobacter species may be more prevalent in beagle dogs and primates than commonly appreciated. It is important to recognize that dogs colonized with these agents may be susceptible to stress-induced, acute onset gastroenteritis (Fox et al., 1988; Reed and Berridge, 1988). In man this form of bacterial disease is characterized histologically by mucin-depletion, flattening and reactive changes in the small bowel epithelium, crypt abscesses, oedema and infiltration of the mucosa by neutrophils, lymphocytes and plasma cells. Similar histological findings have been reported in dogs infected with this organism (Prescott and Monroe, 1982). The organisms are gram-negative curved, slender rods which can be visualized in tissue sections with the Warthin-Starry stain, a recognized technique for spiral bacteria. The carbol fuchsin technique of Gimenez (1964), first used for the identification of Ricketsiae in yolk sac culture and a cresyl fast violet technique have also been shown to be useful methods for the identification of Campylobacter species in paraffin sections (Burnett et al., 1987; McMullen et al., 1987). Another Campylobacter like organism, *Campylobacter-pyloridis* (*Helicobacter pylori*) has been identified in human patients with gastritis, gastric and duodenal ulcers. It is an aetiological or predisposing factor in these forms of gastrointestinal disease (Marshall and Warren, 1984; Rouvroy et al., 1987).

Spironucleus muris (Hexamitis muris) is also a cause of inflammation in the small bowel of rats, mice and hamsters. During overt infestation, organisms are seen extracellularly in crypts and intervillous spaces associated with blunting of intestinal villi, epithelial degeneration and mucin-depletion, reactive epithelial hyperplasia, oedema and leukocyte infiltration (Boorman et al., 1973; Wagner et al., 1974). The morphological expression of damage is accompanied by decreased levels of disaccharidases such as maltase, sucrase and lactase which may represent a direct effect of the trophozoites on the brush border enzymes (Gillon et al., 1982). Trophozoites are characteristically elongated symmetrical flagellates approximately 2–5 μm wide, 12–20 μm long.

Giardia species represent marginally pathogenic flagellates which are found in the upper gastrointestinal tract. They are opportunistic agents that can become important in both animals and man with depressed immune function. However, the interaction between host and parasites is complex and not entirely understood. Although variable virulence of different strains may explain the variability of response to giardia infestation, host factors are also important. Studies in mice infected experimentally with Giardia muris have shown that an early response is an increased infiltration of the epithelium by lymphocytes, predominantly T cells (Gillon et al., 1982). This has led to the suggestion that the response to infection by these parasite is primarily a cell-mediated immune reaction similar to experimental graft versus host reaction in the small intestine of mice (Mowat and Furguson, 1981; Gillon et al., 1982).

Depression of the immune response by treatment with corticosteroids has been shown not only to increase parasite numbers in murine giardiasis but also cause recrudescence of occult infections (Nair et al., 1981). It has also been suggested that decreased gastric acidity can predispose to giardiasis in man (Nalin et al., 1978).

Giardia muris (Lamblia muris) is the species sometimes found in the small intestine of rat and mouse but it is common in the hamster. Trophozoites appear in histological sections as crescent-shaped structures on the brush border of the intestinal mucosa or in the adjacent lumen (Fig. 61). Mucosal lesions may be totally absent or there may be blunting of villi, reactive epithelial hyperplasia. A typical feature is increased infiltration of the epithelium and lamina propria by mononuclear cells (Boorman et al., 1973). Another important finding is that lactase, sucrase and maltase levels have been shown to decrease in the small intestine in mice infested with *Giardia muris* (Gillon et al., 1982).

Giardia lamblia may colonize the small intestine of non-human primates and of man and produce similar morphological appearances to those found with infestations in rodents by Giardia muris. Other flagellates such as *Tritrichomonas muris* are also be found in the small intestine of mice, rats and hamsters.

The coccidian protozoan parasite *Cryposporidium* represents a striking example of the close relationship between some human and animal diseases. This

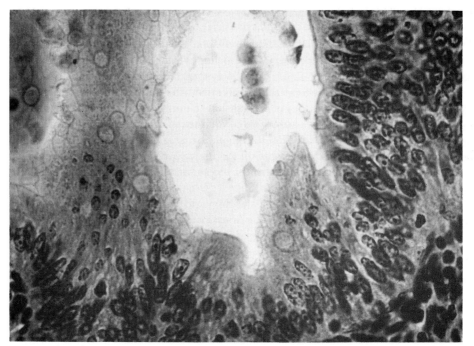

Fig. 61. Section through the duodenal mucosa of an untreated aged Syrian hamster showing the presence of Lamblia muris free lying in the lumen just above the epithelial surface. (HE, ×400.)

organism was first recognized in the gastric glands of mice by Tyzzer in 1907 and has since been confirmed as a cause of diarrhea in animals. Only recently has it been recognized as a human pathogen. It causes mild diarrhoea in normal subjects especially children and young adults but it can produce severe intestinal disease in immunocompromized individuals (Casemore et al., 1985). There are several species of *Cryptosporidium* but as there is uncertainty regarding their specificity for a particular host, most workers continue to employ the term '*Cryptosporidium species*' (Casemore et al., 1985).

Histological examination of the small intestine of laboratory animals infested by Cryptosporidium species reveals the presence of organisms attached to the mucosal surface, often associated, as in man, with other parasites or infections. They are rounded, weakly basophilic structures 1–4 μm diameter in haematoxylin and eosin stained sections but are strongly basophilic following Romanowsky staining. Transmission electron microscopy reveals the detailed internal structure of Cryptosporidium attached to the microvillous surface of the epithelial cells. The various stages in the life cycle have been visualized by light and electron microscopy. Infection starts with ingestion of an oocyst containing four sporozoites which are probably released by the action of digestive enzymes. These attach themselves to the intestinal mucosa and undertake their life cycle attached to the epithelial cells (Casemore et al., 1985). These organisms have been demonstrated in laboratory species including mice, hamsters, rabbits, dogs and non-human primates (Cockrell et al., 1974; Rehg et al., 1979; Toft, 1982; Fukushima and Helman, 1984; Davis and Jenkins, 1986).

Metazoa

Hymenolepis nana (dwarf tapeworm) and *Hymenolepis diminuta* (rat tapeworm) are described in the intestine of rats, mice, hamsters, non-human primates and man (Hsu, 1979). A variety of other metazoan patients are found in the small intestine of non-human primates, see review by Toft (1982).

Viruses

Certain viruses produce inflammatory small bowel changes in mice. Mouse hepatitis virus (lethal intestinal virus of infant mice) can cause mucosal epithelial necrosis and inflammation with characteristic compensatory epithelial hyperplasia and the formation of epithelial syncytia (Barthold, 1985a).

Murine rotavirus (epidermic diarrhea of infant mice) produces swollen enterocytes of small and large bowel with fine cytoplasmic vesiculation with little or no inflammation but dilated lymphatics and vascular congestion. Cytoplasmic acidophilic inclusions, $1-4$ μm diameter, are also characteristic findings (Barthold, 1985b). Electron microscopic examination shows cytoplasmic vesicles arising from the rough endoplasmic reticulum which contain virus particles and electron dense granular material (Barthold, 1985c). A mouse adenovirus may also produce large basophilic intranuclear inclusions in the epithelial cells of the small intestine and caecum.

K virus infection produces lesions in the jejunal and ileal mucosa of mice. Histological features are characterized by mild polymorphonuclear infiltration, with ballooning of occasional endothelial cells within intestinal villi. Intranuclear inclusions can be demonstrated in these endothelial cells by light microscopy using appropriate fixation (Greenlee, 1985).

A great variety of viruses have been isolated from the gastrointestinal tract of non-human primates including viruses of man (Kalter, 1982). However, they appear to be relatively infrequent causes of gastrointestinal disease and when disease is caused by these viruses it usually affects other organs.

Drug-induced inflammation and ulceration

Not only can non-steroidal anti-inflammatory agents such as indomethacin and phenylbutazone produce gastric ulceration but also penetrating ulcers of the small bowel of laboratory animals (Shriver et al., 1975). Recent imaging studies with indium 111-labelled leukocytes in man have also suggested that subclinical intestinal inflammation is associated with long-term therapy with non-steroidal anti-inflammatory drugs (Bjarnason et al., 1987).

It has been postulated that indomethacin-induced intestinal ulcers in rats and dogs are produced by a prostaglandin-independent mechanism, different from the manner in which gastric ulceration is induced (Whittle, 1981; Tabata and Okabe, 1980). Satoh and colleagues (1981) have however suggested that similar mechanisms are responsible for both gastric and intestinal ulceration. They showed that indomethacin-induced gastric ulceration developed in the body mucosa in fasted rats but in the antrum and small intestine in rats given indomethacin 30 minutes after a one hour period of refeeding following a 24 hour fast. There was good temporal correlation between the development of intestinal ulcers and inhibition of prostaglandin synthesis (Satoh et al., 1981). The ulcers in the small intestine were morphologically similar to those occurring in the stomach and they were distributed mainly in the mucosa on the mesenteric aspect of the bowel wall.

Recent single-dose studies with indomethacin and ibuprofen in rats by Suwa and colleagues (1987) have, however, demonstrated histopathological differences between the induced gastric and intestinal damage. Gastric damage was superficial, occurred within six hours and was fully repaired two weeks after dosing. Ulcers in the jejunum and ileum reached a maximum area at 48–72 hours after dosing, occurred on the mesenteric border, penetrated through the muscularis mucosa and were accompanied by inflammation and oedema. Ulcers were still present two weeks later.

Rainsford (1978) has shown that potent intestinal ulcerogens such as indomethacin inhibit the incorporation of [35_S]sulphate into glycoproteins of the upper intestinal mucosa as well as the stomach of rats. This may decrease the capacity of the mucus in the intestine to act as a buffer for hydrogen ions.

Indomethacin given orally to dogs in doses of 2.5 mg/kg/day for one to 23 days was also shown to produce intestinal ulceration. These ulcers were deep, punched-out lesions, many of which were lying over Peyer's patches (Stewart et al., 1980). Some ulcers involved the whole circumference of the small intestine wall. Histologically, the ulcers were associated with an intense inflammatory response principally of mononuclear cells which infiltrated the bowel wall to the serosa particularly adjacent to Peyer's patches. It was suggested that this striking distribution of ulcers was a result of an exaggerated immune response to normal intestinal antigens. These antigens may have been produced by inhibition of suppressor cells in Peyer's patches, following depression of prostaglandin synthetase by indomethacin (Stewart et al., 1980). This unrestrained immune response may have produced immune-mediated damage to adjacent intestinal mucosa.

Special dye techniques, scanning and transmission electron microscopy have also shown that non-steroidal anti-inflammatory drugs also produce adverse effects on the small intestine mucosa without overt pathological changes being evident by light microscopy (Brodie et al., 1970; Djaldetti and Fishman, 1981). Following administration of aspirin to mice for five weeks, shortening and frank erosion of microvilli and increased numbers of goblet cells were only demonstrated in the duodenum and jejunum by scanning and transmission electron microscopy (Djaldatti and Fishman, 1981). Such submicroscopic findings support the idea that non-steroidal anti-inflammatory agents may induce damage to the small intestine more commonly than supposed.

Although non-steroidal, anti-inflammatory drugs are well recognized for their effects on gastrointestinal mucosa, small intestinal inflammation and ulceration are produced by other agents through quite different pharmacological mechanisms. Agents of particular interest are cysteamine, propionitrile and their structural analogues as well as 1-methyl-4-phenyl-1,2,3,6-tetrahydropyridine (MPTP) which are capable of producing ulcers of chronic type in the duodenum of rats and mice (Szabo and Cho, 1988).

These compounds vary in their ulcerogenic capacity but they are all able to produce ulcers of chronic type with crater formation, granulation tissue and reactive changes in adjacent mucosa in the anterior and posterior wall of the proximal segment of the duodenum of rodents. Although these different agents influence gastric acid secretion in different ways, structure-activity relationships suggest that they produce duodenal dysmotility, decrease bicarbonate production and reduce its delivery from the distal to proximal duodenum. These factors decrease the neutralization of gastric acid in the first part of the duodenum and this may contribute to the development of ulceration (Szabo and Cho, 1988). Furthermore, these effects can be attenuated or prevented by dopamine agonists or their precursors whereas dopamine antagonists can potentiate their effects. This suggests that the central or peripheral dopamine-mediated actions of these agents may be involved in the pathogenesis of duodenal ulceration (Szabo, 1979; 1984).

Anticancer drugs and other therapeutic agents which affect cell proliferation, depress the bone marrow or the immune system can also produce intestinal mucosal necrosis, haemorrhage, inflammation and opportunistic gastrointestinal overgrowth when administered to dogs or rodents in high doses (Martin et al., 1985; Bregman et al., 1987). Lymphoid infiltrates without tissue damage were also reported in the small intestine of rats treated with human recombinant interleukin-2 (Anderson and Hayes, 1989).

Fatty change (lipidosis)

Using appropriate fixation and staining procedures, fine granular lipid droplets may be normally visualized in the apical parts of epithelial cells covering the upper third of small intestinal villi. Administration of drugs and chemicals may produce an excessive accumulation of lipid through specific effects on lipid metabolism or as part of general cellular toxicity.

In the preclinical toxicity studies with 2,6-di-tert-butylamino-3-acetyl-4-methylpyridine (Sa H51–055), an inhibitor of glucose transport intended for use as an anti-obesity drug, lipid accumulation occurred in the lamina propina of the small intestinal villi of Sprague-Dawley rats and guinea pigs but not in dogs or primates (Visscher et al., 1980). These findings in animals caused development of

Sa H51–055 to be suspended and it is therefore unknown whether this agent would also produce similar changes in the human small bowel.

After administration of Sa H51–055 to rats, there was histological evidence of a progressive accumulation of lipid droplets in the epithelial cells over the tips of the duodenal villi demonstrable by osmium tetroxide staining. Ultrastructural examination revealed uniform electron-luscent droplets within profiles of the smooth endoplasmic reticulum and Golgi apparatus. Lipid droplets increased with time, accumulated and coalesced to form large droplets in the lamina propria. Larger droplets were phagocytosed by macrophages in the lamina propria but there was no evidence of epithelial damage or necrosis.

The lipid was shown to accumulate with time over a period of up to 63 days and it remained even after cessation of dosing for up to 28 days. Changes were most pronounced in the duodenum but were also noted to a lesser extent in jejunum and ileum. They were not seen in colon or stomach.

Sequential studies using electron microscopy showed that lipid rapidly accumulated within several hours in the profiles of smooth endoplasmic reticulum and Golgi apparatus of the epithelial cells and formed droplets or chylomicra in the intercellular space. The absence of any other subcellular changes or evidence of derangement of protein synthesis suggested that the pathways of lipid resynthesis or transport were being altered by Sa H51–055. This was consistent with the distribution of the lipid in the upper third of the jejunal villus epithelium, a zone most active in lipid absorption, resynthesis and transport (Dobbins, 1969). It was suggested fatty change may have taken place because of alterations in the sugar moiety of chylomicra brought about by interference with glucose transport (Visscher et al., 1980).

Lipid droplets which stained with oil-Red-O in formalin-fixed frozen sections and which showed uniform electron density characteristic of neutral lipid were also observed in the epithelial cells and macrophages in the lamina propria of jejunum and duodenum and mesenteric lymph nodes in rats given a synthetic 2′-dodecyl glutaramide ester of erythromycin (Gray et al., 1974). Unlike the erythomycin base, this ester was poorly tolerated by rats. It appeared that the ester was absorbed unhydrolyzed and converted to chylomicron-like droplets which then accumulated in the macrophages of the lamina propria and local mesenteric lymph nodes, without overt damage to epithelial cells.

Accumulation of lipid in epithelial cells of intestinal villi has been observed in rats following administration of puromycin (Friedman and Cardell, 1972) and ethionine (Hyams et al., 1966), agents which have inhibitory effects on protein synthesis. Detailed morphological study of the intestinal epithelial cell in rats treated with puromycin have shown that there is concomitant accumulation of lipid with a decrease in the quantity of rough endoplasmic reticulum and Golgi membranes (Friedman and Cardell, 1972). These morphological findings were in keeping with the concept that lipid accumulates as a result of inhibition of the synthesis of membrane components of the Golgi by the rough endoplasmic reticulum which are important for the transport of lipid. Therefore, membrane-bound or matrix fat droplets accumulate in the cell.

In addition to lipid droplets forming as a result of altered lipid metabolism, they may form in the epithelial cells of the intestinal mucosal as a result of a direct toxic effect of the ingested drugs on the small intestinal mucosa. In such instances atrophy of villi and degenerative changes in the epithelial cells may also be observed (see following).

Phospholipidosis (myelin figures, myeloid bodies, myelinoid bodies)

The small intestinal mucosa is also one of the many sites at which drug-induced accumulation of polar lipids form laminated structures (myeloid bodies) or crystalloid structures within lysosomes. This form of lipid storage disorder is produced by a diverse range of amphiphilic cationic drugs in both man and laboratory animals probably as a result of drug interaction with polar lipids rendering them difficult to digest (Lüllmann-Rauch, 1979) Species differences in susceptability and tissue distribution of phospholipid are probably not only related to physiochemical characteristics of the inducing drugs which influences their ability to permeate selective biomembranes and react with different lipids, but also to tissue concentrations of drugs achieved and the ability of organs to metabolize parent drug to less amphiphilic products.

In general terms, this form of disorder is characterized by membrane-bound, acid phosphatase-positive cytoplasmic inclusions which on ultrastructural study are seen as lamellated or crystalloid structures in lysosomes. These appearances are characteristically reversible on cessation of treatment with the inciting agent.

An example of this phenomenon occurring in the small intestine is provided by the iodinated amphiphilic drug, amiodarone, which has been used clinically in Europe for the past 20 years in the treatment of angina and more recently in the control of supraventricular cardiac arrhymias. Its adverse effects in man are believed to be the result of accumulation of drug in lysosomes particularly in liver, skin and eye (D'Amico et al., 1981; Shepherd et al., 1987).

When high doses of amiodarone were administered orally to rats and beagle dogs, multilamellated lysosomal inclusion bodies first accumulated in the jejunal mucosa and mesenteric lymph nodes before becoming widely distributed in other organs particularly in the lungs (Mazué et al., 1984). In both rats and dogs the small intestinal lesions were characterized by the presence of foamy macrophages with pale finely vacuolated cytoplasm and condensed eccentric nuclei within the lamina propria of the jejunal villi (Mazué et al., 1984). Mesenteric lymph nodes were also involved early after the onset of treatment. In the dog, jejunal villi were somewhat flattened and widened or showed a variable degree of villous atrophy, most marked in the proximal and middle jejunum (Vic et al., 1985). Electron microscopy confirmed the presence of lamellated lysosomal bodies distending macrophages. The lesions were associated with increases in plasma cholesterol and perturbations in the low density and high density lipoproteins.

The early accumulation of foam cells in the jejununal macrophages was probably a reflection of the disposition of drug following oral absorption for although similar lipidosis was seen in many organs following intravenous administration in dogs, more lipidosis was seen in the jejunum after oral dosing. It is also of interest to note that there were species differences in sensitivity to these changes, baboons being relatively insensitive compared to dogs. Furthermore, Fischer 344 rats were very sensitive to these changes compared to Sprague-Dawley rats and Wistar rats were almost completely resistant to lipidosis induced by amiodarone under similar conditions (Mazué et al., 1984).

Similar cytological changes have been reported in cells of some organs in patients treated with amiodarone (D'Amico et al., 1981; Shepherd et al., 1987).

Villous atrophy, hypoplasia

Villous shortening or stunting results when the proliferative activity of the crypt epithelium is reduced or under circumstances in which crypt cell proliferation is insufficient to compensate for increased cell loss as a result of mucosal cell damage.

Decreased cell proliferation can be seen segments which are surgically bypassed, or following decreased food intake, parenteral nutrition, hypophysectomy or thyroidectomy (Williamson, 1978a; Bastie et al., 1982).

As adrenergic factors are important in the control of small intestinal epithelial cell division. Agents which alter α or β-adrenoreceptor activity may influence the proliferative capacity of the epithelium. In mice, proliferation of crypt cells is diminished by increased α1 or β-receptor stimulation by appropriate agonists (eg. phenylephrine) but it is increased by stimulation of α2-receptor activity (Kennedy et al., 1983). Yohimbine, an α2-antagonist also reduces cell proliferation in the same animal model. Some of the effects of these agents may be mediated by changes in splanchnic blood flow (Williamson, 1978b).

The detailed morphological study of the small intestinal mucosa in the rat following hypophysectomy by Bastie et al (1982) has shown a reduction in the height of the small intestinal villi associated with reduction in mitoses in the crypt epithelium. The number of goblet cells was shown to fall particularly in the jejunum and the number of Paneth cells increase in the ileum. Ultrastructural examination showed that the height of the micro-villi of absorptive cells also decreases and their intracytoplasmic organelles and ribosomes become less numerous. These authors also showed significant decreases in brush border enzyme activities of alkaline phosphatase, aminopeptidase, maltase and lactase about one week following hypophysectomy.

Substances which reduce mitotic activity and therefore lower regenerative capacity of the intestinal epithelium also produce shortening or stunting of small intestinal villi and eventually flattening of the mucosa.

A wide variety of anticancer agents and antiviral drugs with radio-mimetic properties interfere with cell division in the crypts thereby reducing the number of epithelial cells produced. Histologically, the effects of such agents are characterized by bluntening, shortening or complete atrophy of villi. Mitotic activity is reduced in the crypts and the crypts become dilated and lined by flattened cells (Fig. 62). The overlying epithelium loses its normal regular arrangement and

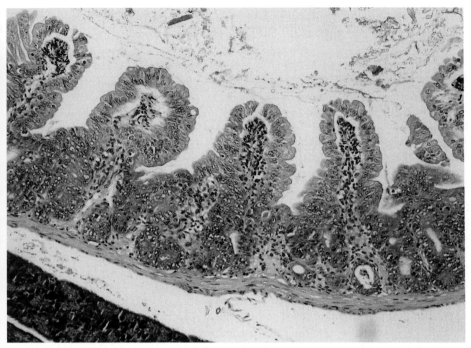

Fig. 62. Duodenum of a CD-1 mouse treated for five days with an antimitotic agent. The epithelium is intact but shows maturation arrest characterised by mild cellular degeneration and focal epithelial flattening, loss of mitotic activity in the crypts and vesiculation of nuclei. (HE, ×150.)

cells show pleomorphic nuclei with irregular chromatin patterns. Increased numbers of inflammatory cells may infiltrate the lamina propria and epithelium. Ulceration, haemorrhage and secondary infection of the gut wall ensue if there is overwhelming cell damage.

Comparison of the gastrointestinal toxicity expressed by antimitotic anti-cancer drugs of different classes in rodents, dogs, non-human primates and man have suggested that there is a higher degree of correspondence between effects in man and dog than between man and other species (Owens, 1962; Schein et al., 1970). In studies with the antiviral agent acyclovir, a radiomimetic effect was noted in the gastrointestinal tract of dogs at high doses but not rodents (Tucker et al., 1983).

Another example is the villous atrophy described in rats following treatment with an antibacterial agent ICI 17,363. This was believed to arise as a result of both interference with cell division and a direct effect on the surface epithelial cells (Murgatroyd, 1980). The effects of ICI 17,363 were characterized by atrophy of villi with dilatation of crypts and atypical features in the crypt epithelium suggestive of an effect on mitotic activity. In addition, vacuolated lipid-laden epithelial cells were observed over the tips of villi accompanied by reductions in the numbers of goblet cells and reduced activity of acid and alkaline phos-

345

phatase, esterase, adenosine triphosphatase, glucose-6-phosphatase and succinic dehydrogenase, compatable with a direct adverse effect on superficial mature epithelial cells.

Hypertrophy and hyperplasia

A variety of different factors stimulate cell proliferation in the small intestinal epithelium, including enterectomy, increased feeding, stimulation of autonomic nerves, administration of neurotransmitters, thyroxine, growth hormone, corticosteroids, testosterone, gastrin and glucagon (Williamson, 1978a). Most causes of greater cell production lead to increased villous height and mucosal hyperplasia, although intense crypt cell proliferation as a compensatory regenerative response can be associated with villous atrophy (see previous).

The compensatory response to the surgically resected or bypassed intestine has been the focus of the most detailed studies of increased cell renewal in the small intestine. Partial resection in both rats and man is accompanied by increased villous height and crypt length (Hanson et al., 1977). This is primarily the result of hyperplasia for it has been shown that the numbers of cells per unit length of villus remains unchanged (Hanson et al., 1977) but there is an overall increase in the cell population of villus and crypt (Hanson and Osborne, 1971). DNA/RNA ratios also remain largely unaltered (Williamson, 1978a). No gross changes in villous shape have been reported after resection and the total number of crypts remains constant. Although increased intestinal uptake of substances from the bowel lumen occurs in hypertrophied segments per unit length of bowel, disaccharide and dipeptidase activities are normal or even decreased after resection suggesting a comparative immaturity of cells in the residual mucosa. Functional adaptation therefore is achieved by a larger number of cells, the individual absorptive capacity of which is not increased (Williamson, 1978a).

Increased numbers of specific goblet cell populations are also seen in hyperfunctional states. Following jejunoileal bypass operations in rats, increased numbers of PAS-positive goblet cells develop in the villi and crypts of the hyperfunctional segements of the duodenum, jejunum and ileum (Olubuyide et al., 1984). Mucin histochemistry using the high-iron diamine and alcian blue techniques have shown that the goblet cells in the hyperfunctional segments contain increased sialomucins in the villi and crypts of the jejunum and ileum but not in the duodenum and increased sulphomucins in the distal ileal segment. Sialomucin production may reflect relative cellular immaturity of the more rapidly proliferating cells under these circumstances. However, as sialic acid conveys more viscoelastic properties to mucin, it has been suggested that the goblet cells change following intestinal bypass fulfills a protective function against the increased flow of gastrointestinal contents (Olubuyide et al., 1984).

Other stimuli, notably various forms of induced hyperphagia and dietary manipulation have also been shown to produce increased cell proliferation and hyperplasia of the small intestinal epithelium. In rats hypothalamic damage, hyperthroidism, tube feeding, diabetes mellitus and insulin injections have been shown to produce intestinal hyperplasia (MacKay et al., 1940; Levin and Smyth, 1963; Forrester, 1972; Jarvis and Levin, 1966).

A number of nutritional factors, particularly dietary fibre, can influence the proliferative characteristics of the small bowel mucosa. Carefully controlled studies in rats given different forms of dietary fibre have shown that the proliferative characteristics of the small intestine can be modified by both the quantity and the quality of the fibre. A decrease in the length of villi, crypt cell hyperplasia and shorter transit times were observed in rats fed pectin-supplemented diet whereas guar produced a marked increase in mucosal growth without alteration in relative differences in crypt and villous length compared with rats fed fibre-free diet. These different effects have been the result of differences in solubility, gel formation, water holding capacity, effect on transit time, ion-exchange activity or bile acid adsorption of the different fibres (Jacobs, 1983).

Administration of an inhibitor of cholesterol biosynthesis, 5α-cholest-8-(14)-en-3β-ol-15-one, to rats for up to nine days was also shown to produce enlargement of the small intestine in a way which was morphologically similar to the changes found following intestinal bypass (Smith et al., 1989). The enlargement was most marked in the proximal segment of the small intestine and progressively diminished towards the ileocaecal junction, sparing the stomach, caecum and colon. Histological examination and morphometric analysis revealed an increase in smooth muscle mass, lengthening of the villi as well as an increase in the depth and cellular proliferation in the crypts of Lieberkuhn without evidence of cell damage or fatty change. Like the changes following jejunal bypass procedures, there was also an increase in acid mucosubstances in the goblet cell population overlying he villous mucosa (Smith et al., 1989). The mechanism for this change in the rat was not clear, particularly as intestinal hyperplasia was not seen in baboons treated with this 15-ketosterol for long periods. However, it was suggested that it was an adaptive response, possibly related to inhibition of cholesterol metabolism and cholesterol absorption from the diet, particularly as the laboratory diet employed in the rat study was particularly low in cholesterol.

Local and systemic changes in hormones and various transmitter substances also influence the number of cells in the small intestinal epithelium. Morphometric studies of the small intestinal mucosa in mice following gastrin administration have shown increases in villous area associated with decreases in microvillous area, increased number of goblet cells and Paneth cells (Balas et al., 1985). Studies in which rats were treated with the prolactin-inhibitor, bromocryptine, have shown that the total number of mucous cells and the number staining with alcian blue at pH 1.0 increase in the ileal crypts, possibly as a result of increased synthesis of sulphated mucosubstances (Gona, 1981).

In this context, it is of interest that chronic treatment with the Rauwolfia neuroleptic, reserpine, causes an increase in the sulphation of goblet cell mucin in the small intestine as demonstrated by alcian blue staining at pH 1.0 and the high iron diamine technique without changes in the goblet cell numbers (Park et al., 1987).

Agents which affect activity of the sympathetic nervous system can also alter epithelial cell proliferation in the small (and large) intestine. Treatment of rats with adrenaline, isoprenaline, phenylephrine, phentolamine and yohimbine all result in decreased mitotic activity of jejunal and colonic crypt cells (Tutton and Helme, 1974; Kennedy et al., 1983). By contrast, administration of metaraminol, clonidine, propranolol, prazosin and labetolol as well as simultaneous injection of propranolol and adrenaline all resulted in an increased rate of crypt cell proliferation (Kennedy et al., 1983). These results suggest that agents which stimulate α2-adrenergic receptor activity and those which are α1-antagonists and β-adrenergic receptor antagonists increase proliferative activity in the rodent intestinal mucosa. Caffeine is also reported to produce an increase in thickness of the intestinal mucosa when administered in high doses to rats (Lachance, 1982). This raises the possibility that intestinal mucosal hyperplasia can be produced by phosphodiesterase inhibition and resultant increases in intracellular cAMP in a similar way to the hypertrophy induced in salivary tissue.

This is supported by recent findings in rats treated for periods of up to six months with the inotropic vasodilator, ICI 153,100, a phosphodiesterase inhibitor intended for treatment of congestive cardiac failure. Administration of high doses not only produced salivary gland hypertrophy but also marked thickening of the small and large intestinal mucosa. This was characterised histologically by an increase in villous length and deepening of intestinal glands, with a relatively unchanged number of epithelial cells per unit length of gland or villus (Westwood et al., 1990).

Although prostaglandin E analogues produce most of their effects in the stomach, increased thickness of the small intestine characterized by longer villi, deeper crypts and increase in cell size have been reported in rats treated with these agents (Levin, 1988).

Focal hyperplasia, focal avillous hyperplasia, focal atypical hyperplasia, duodenal plaque, polypoid hyperplasia, polyp: mouse

Irregular or atypical glandular hyperplasia may be found in the small intestinal mucosa of several strains of aged, untreated mice. The lesions may be single or multiple and are usually located in the first part of the duodenum where they form discrete, raised plaques composed of elongated, irregular or branched glands which replace the normal villous structure of the mucosa (Rowlatt and Chesterman, 1979). The glands are lined by hyperchromatic columnar cells which show marked pseudostratification and proliferative activity. Paneth cells and mucin-secreting goblet cells may also be prominant. Some glands are cystic and the stroma is fibrous and infiltrated by chronic inflammatory cells. The lesions become pedunculated or polypoid in appearance and show a fibrovascular core which is infiltrated by inflammatory cells. They resemble adenomatous polyps described in man.

The cause of these changes in the mouse small intestine is unknown but their prevalence can be altered by dietary fibre and panthothenic acid deficiency as well as by administration of drugs and chemicals (Hare and Stewart, 1956; Seronde, 1965; 1970; Ito et al., 1981).

In their study of DBA mice, Hare and Stewart (1956) considered that the lesions were not genuine neoplasms since they were composed of a mixture of cell types which normally populate the mucosa. Furthermore, they suggested that the presence of an inflammatory component in the stroma and the fact that the prevalence of these lesions was increased in mice fed a high roughage diet were consistent with the concept that they represent an inflammatory adenomatoid hyperplasia. Seronde (1965; 1970) reported these lesions in mice fed purified diets, particularly when deficient in panthothenic acid. Panthothenic acid deficiency was also associated with inflammation and deep penetrating chronic ulcers of the duodenum in affected mice, compatable with an inflammatory aetiology of the lesions.

An increase in the prevalence of these duodenal changes was recently described in CD-1 mice treated with the synthetic prostaglandin E1 analogue, misoprostol for 21 months (Port et al., 1987). These authors suggested that the findings posed no real concerns for the safety of patients treated with misoprostol on the grounds that the mouse was unique in this aspect of the response to misoprostol because the mouse had a particular liability to develop such changes in the small intestine. The proliferative lesions were found in a few control CD-1 mice in the same study. In addition, it was also argued that the lesions were neither neoplastic nor preneoplastic in nature (Port et al., 1987). They were not seen in rats treated with misoprostol for two years (Dodd et al., 1987).

Of course it is difficult to be certain that lesions characterized by such intense proliferative activity are not in themselves at increased risk for neoplastic change. Indeed chronic administration of hydrogen peroxide to C57BL/6J mice in drinking water was not only shown to potentiate the development of a similar type of duodenal hyperplasia but also to produce frankly invasive adenocarcinomas (Ito et al., 1981). Whether this phenomenon in mice has relevence for man remains uncertain.

LARGE INTESTINE

The large intestine is anatomically similar in man and laboratory animals employed in toxicology, although certain morphological differences are undoubtably of a physiological significance with potential to influence the expression of toxicity. Understanding of comparative aspects morphology and function and the interrelationships of the various colonic cells types among different species however remains incomplete. The rat colon is probably one of the best studied of the laboratory animal species because the rat is widely used for experimental work on colon carcinogenesis (Shamsuddin and Trump, 1981a). As the canine model is popular for oral dosage-form testing, differences in colonic physiology between dog and man may be better understood than between man and many other species (Dressman, 1986).

In man, as well as in the non-human primates, the large intestine can be anatomically dividied into caecum, appendix, ascending colon, transverse colon, sigmoid colon rectum and anal canal. Like the small bowel, the colon comprises mucosa, submucosa, muscularis mucosa and serosa. Mucosal plicae are only found in the rectum although plicae semilumaris, formed by folds of the entire thickness of the bowel wall, are found in the colon. The large intestine of the dog resembles that of man more than that of most other domestic species. It is a simplified tubular structure only slightly larger in diameter than the small intestine. The colon of the dog is divided anatomically into ascending, transverse and descending parts, but there is no well-defined sigmoid segment. The caecum in dog is a small diverticulum, similar to that found in other carnivorous species and it communicates directly with the colon.

The colon of the rat and mouse is shaped like an inverted V which can be divided into ascending and descending segments. There is no clearly-defined transverse colon. A characteristic feature in both rat and mouse is the presence of a curved kidney-shaped caecum. The functional significance of the caecum in rodents should not be overlooked. It is of a size which is intermediate between the large and anatomically complex caecum of herbivors such as the rabbit and the small caecum of carnivorous species. This size is perhaps a reflection of the omnivorous nature and flexibility of the rat and mouse in their dietary habits, particularly their ability to break-down cellulose (Rérat, 1978).

The caecum of the rat and mouse is a blind pouch from which the colon and ileum exit in close proximity and in which antiperistaltic movements occur. This structure and the presence of bacteria undoubtably contributes to its ability to function as a fermentation organ in which breakdown of substances can occur in a reasonably controlled milieu (Snipes, 1981).

The potential importance of intestinal microflora in the metabolism of both endogeneous and exogeneous substances has been well demonstrated in the rodent caecum (Rowland, et al., 1986; Rowland, 1988). The usual stock diets for rodents contain abundant plant fibre which provides bulk and fermentable carbohydrate for the microbial population in the caecum. Rats fed stock diets have been shown to possess high levels of reductive and hydrolytic enzyme activity (eg. azoreductase, nitroreductase, nitrate reductase, β-glucosidase and β-glucuronidase) in their caecal contents compared with rats fed purified fibre-free diets (Wise et al., 1986). Intestines of germ free animals have thinner lamina propria, lower cell turnover, enlarged caecum, altered metabolism of cholesterol, bilirubin and bile salts and larger amounts of mucin in faeces compared with animals passing gastrointestinal microflora (Midtvedt, 1987).

Species differences in microflora are also reported. Comparative studies with human and rat intestinal microflora have suggested that each population of organisms possesses a degree of autonomous self-regulation and capable of responding quite differently to dietary changes (Mallett et al., 1987).

Comparative studies in Australian laboratories have shown large differences in the numbers of faculative anaerobic gram negative bacteria in the gastro-intestinal tract of mice from three, major specific pathogen free units. It was shown that these differences could influence the immune system, susceptability to infection and experimental results (O'Rourke et al., 1988).

The caecum in the rat and mouse is the site of absorption of many substances including calcium, magnesium, water and electrolytes vitamin K and fatty acids (Snipes, 1981). Caecectomy in these species has been shown to decrease digestion of carbohydrates and protein and increase loss of faecal water (Ambuhl et al., 1979).

Histological and histochemical characteristics

The colon and caecum in man and laboratory animals is lined by a fairly uniform mucosa devoid of villi. The surface epithelium is covered by columar cells of two main types, absorptive and mucous cells similar to those found in the small intestine. Intestinal glands or crypts of Lieberkuhn extend downwards from the surface generally as simple, unbranched tubules lined principally by mucous cells with smaller populations of absorptive, endocrine and undifferentiated cells. In certain pathological conditions of the human colon the Paneth cell may also be occasionally encountered.

The mucosa in man and laboratory animals is not entirely flat but shows a slightly corrugated or uneven pattern which varies with the particular site within the colon. In histological sections of the colon in man, this corrugated pattern is seen as an anthemion-like structure of crypts reminescent of a Greek architectural feature (Filipe and Branfoot, 1974). This is also seen in larger laboratory animal species.

In rats and mice the crypts of the caecal mucosa are wider near the lumen than in the crypt base and crypts may be branched, features which may be related to the absorptive function of this zone (Snipes, 1981).

The proliferative zone in the large bowel is found in the lower part of the gland and mitotic figures are normally limited to this zone. As in the small bowel, multipotent, undifferentiated stem cells situated in the gland base give rise to the principle cell types which migrate to the cell surface with subsequent differentiation and alteration of their enzyme activities and morphological features (Chang and Leblond, 1971). In studies with mouse aggregation chimaeras in which mosaic cell populations of the intestinal epithelium were localised immunocytochemically, it was demonstrated that the entire epithelium of each adult gland descended from a single progenitor cell (Ponder et al., 1985). The single progenitor may itself give rise to several stem cells reponsible for the cell renewal in the complete crypt.

Although the control of the proliferation of the colonic mucosa is probably similar to that of the small intestinal mucosa, much is less known about the adaptive responses of the colon to different stimuli than in the jejunum and ileum (Williamson, 1978a).

Absorptive cells are found most commonly in the surface epithelium but also to a lesser extent in the glandular epithelium. They are morphologically similar to those in the small intestine each possessing apical plasma membranes with

351

uniform microvilli and a well-formed glycocalyx. Microvilli of absorptive cells have been shown by electron microscopic study to become longer and more dense with increasing distance distally in the gastro-intestinal tract. Thus, they are longer and more dense in the ileum than in the caecum and least dense and shortest in the colon, perhaps reflecting their relative absorptive capacity (Snipes, 1981). This is reflected at light microscopic level by the less conspicuous brush border in the large intestine compared with that in the small intestine.

The colon, like many other tissues also possess drug metabolising activity, although less than in the liver. However, it has been shown that the activity of cytochromes P450 involved in hydroxylation of benzo[α]pyrene in microsomes prepared from the colons of Sprague-Dawley rats retain their activity and responsiveness to inducers better than those in the liver with advancing age. (Sun and Strobel, 1986). It was therefore suggested that colonic and other extrahepatic drug metabolising enzymes may play an increasingly significant role in older animals.

There are also species and regional differences in the glycoconjugates found in the brush border of the large intestine, although they generally contain predominantly acidic mucosubstances. In the mouse and rat, sialomucins with some neutral mucins are found. In hamsters, dogs, non-human primates and man both sulpho- and sialomucins may be seen in the brush border (Sheahan and Jervis, 1976). The glycocalyx is important in the protective function of the colonic mucosa for its disruption by agents such as salicylates has been shown to increase absorption of xenobiotics from the rat rectal mucosa (Sithigorngul et al., 1983).

The morphological features of mucin-secreting cells vary. Although there has been some debate about the precise nature of the mucous cell populations based on structural studies in mice and rats (Chang, 1981; Shamsuddin and Trump, 1981c), for practical purposes two principle types of mucous cell can be defined. One of these is the typical goblet cell with cytoplasmic mucous droplets forming a goblet shape which is found both in glandular and surface epithelium. The other type, the so-called vacuolated cell or mucous cell, is found only in the crypts (Chang and Leblond, 1971; Thomopoulos et al., 1983).

These vacuolated or mucous cells show empty-appearing vacuoles in the cytoplasm which rather than being empty contain abundant sialomucins of a type different from those in goblet cells (Spicer, 1965; Wetzel et al., 1966). Detailed structural studies and cytochemistry using lectin probes have suggested that these vacuolated cells are able to differentiate into absorptive cells with the cellular apparatus to produce the cell surface glycoconjugates of the glycocalyx (Thomopoulos et al., 1983).

It is important to recognize that considerable differences exist throughout the colon among mucin-containing cells which stain uniformly with haematoxylin and eosin. Some of the most useful tools for the characterization of heterogeneity among these colonic cells are histochemical stains for mucosubstances, many of which are applicable to formalin-fixed, paraffin-embedded tissue (Tables 1 and 2).

In most species, including man, neutral mucins are present throughout the colon but acid mucins are the predominant type (Sheahan and Jervis, 1976). Sulphomucins, as demonstrated by the high-iron diamine technique, generally predominate in the distal colonic segment. In both rat and mouse, goblet cells of the proximal colonic mucosa contain largely sialomucins in the lower parts of the crypts with sulphomucins predominating in the upper parts of the crypt. The distal colon, contains largely sulphomucins. The only difference between rat and mouse appears to be the fact that the mouse caecum contains almost exclusively sulphomucins but sulphomucins and sialomucins are found in the rat caecal mucosa. In hamsters, the entire colon contains predominantly sulphomucins.

Neutral mucins and sulphomucins predominate throughout the dog colon with occasional goblet cells containing sialomucin. In non-human primates, neutral mucins, sialomucins and sulphomucins are seen throughout the colon with sialomucins generally more prominant in the proximal colon and sulphomucins in the distal segment.

In man, neutral mucins are found mostly in the caecum. In the caecum and ascending colon, sulphomucins are found in the upper crypts and sialomucins in the crypt base. The converse occurs in the distal colon where sulphomucins predominate in the lower two-thirds of the glands and sialomucins in the upper third of the glands and in the surface epithelium.

Lectin-labelling shows even greater heterogeneity of mucins in the colonic mucosal cell population, probably reflecting differentiation patterns and changes in glycosyltransferase activity as cells migrate upwards (Freeman et al., 1980; Thomopoulos et al., 1983). Lectin probes therefore also represent potentially powerful tools for use with the light and electron microscopic in defining changes in differentiation patterns in the colon mucosa.

The lamina propria of the large bowel is arranged in a similar way to that of the small bowel. By virtue of the presence of lymphocytes, plasma cells, macrophages and dendritic cells as well as scattered small lymphoid aggregates or patches, it forms an integral and important part in the mucosal immune defence system. Most of the lymphocytes in the lamina propria of the human colonic mucosa, like that of the ileum, have been shown to be T cells with helper T cells out numbering the T suppressor phenotype (Hirata et al., 1986; Pabst, 1987). This contrasts with intra-epithelial lymphocytes of the human colonic mucosa which are also T cells but more than 80% of which possess characteristics of the suppressor/cytotoxic phenotype and only 10–20% being helper T cells.

This distribution of lymphocyte subsets is seen immunocytochemically in the rat colon using the monoclonal antibodies W3/13, W3/25 and MRC OX8 (see Haemopoietic and Lymphatic Systems, Chapter III). The pan T cell marker W3/13 shows the presence of T lymphocytes in the lamina propria and most of these are labelled by W3/25 demonstrating their helper phenotype (Bland and Warren, 1985). Monoclonal antibody W3/25 also labels many non-lymphoid cells with macrophage morphology in the lamina propria. MRC OX8 demonstrates that few lymphocytes in the lamina propria are of suppressor/cytotoxic type which contrasts with the high proportion of MRC OX8 positive lymphocytes in the colonic epithelium (Bland and Warren, 1985). The monoclonal antibodies MRC OX6 and MRC OX17, specific for the rat Ia antigen, also label numerous cells with macrophage and dendritic cell morphology in the large bowel of the rat (Bland and Warren, 1985; Martin et al., 1986).

Mature, small B lymphocytes are relatively uncommon in the colonic lamina propria of man and laboratory animals. However, the lamina propria contains large numbers of plasma cells which are mainly of IgA type, followed by smaller numbers of IgM an IgG subtypes (Pabst, 1987).

A feature of the colonic mucosa is the presence of lymphoid aggregates also called lymphoid nodules, patches, lymphoid-glandular complexes or microbursa. These are similar to Peyer's patches of the small intestine as they are composed principally of lymphoid cells of the B cell series arranged in follicles with germinal centres with interfollicular and perifollicular zones composed of T cells (Pabst, 1987). They are distributed along the entire length of the colonic mucosa although they are generally smaller than Peyer's patches. In Sprague-Dawley rats, lymphoid aggregates are usually about 5 mm diameter except in the distal colon where they attain sizes of up to 10 mm in maximum diameter (Martin et al., 1986).

Immunocytochemistry using monoclonal antibodies to T cells and antisera to immunoglobins in the rat colon has confirmed that a large majority of cells in the lymphoid patches are of B cell type containing IgM and IgG and that many perifollicular cells are lymphocytes reactive with the pan T monoclonal antibody W3/13 (Martin et al., 1986). Many perifollicular cells with macrophage morphology are also stained with the W3/25 monoclonal antibody (Bland and Warren, 1985).

Unlike Peyer's patches which are characteristically not associated with crypts or villi, the colonic lymphoid aggregates frequently contain irregular atypical mucosal glands which may enter deeply in the lymphoid tissue and penetrate below the muscularis mucosa both in man and laboratory animals (Kealy, 1976a; Scott, 1982; Martin et al., 1986). In some strains of rat, cells in these glands express the Ia antigen, unlike the other parts of the colonic epithelium (Martin et al., 1986). These glandular structures, which are intimately associated with lymphoid tissue may be important in the immune protection of the colonic mucosa, perhaps by acting as a special local receptor for antigens (Kealy, 1976a). It has been proposed that these glandular structures represent sites of predilection for the spread of inflammatory disease to the submucosa by allowing micro-organisms to pass through the muscularis mucosa (Scott, 1982). It has also been suggested that they constitute physical weak points in the bowel wall and may play a part in the pathogenesis of diverticular disease of the colon in man (Kealy, 1976b). Colonic carcinomas induced by dimethylhydrazine in the rat also appear to develop more commonly in the lymphoid aggregates than in other zones (Martin et al., 1986). M cells have been described over the lymphoid aggregates in the caecum of the mouse (Owen and Nemanic, 1978) (see Small Intestine).

Although micro-organisms are important causes of inflammatory disease in the large intestine of man and animals, among laboratory animals, they are usually only evident in non-human primates and hamsters. In the strains of rats and mice and in beagle dogs commonly employed in drug safety evaluation, spontaneous disease of the colon as a result of infectious agents is uncommon. Nevertheless, even in rats, mice and dogs, the potential importance of micro-organisms should not be forgotten. Treatment with some therapeutic agents may alter the normal bacterial flora to permit overgrowth of pathogenic organisms or disturb the normal balance between antigens in the lumen or control mechanism to evoke inflammation. Inflammation induced by organisms may also confound the histological assessment of drug-induced changes in the colon.

However, ulceration and inflammation of the colon as a direct result of administration of potential therapeutic agents is not commonly reported. This is perhaps surprising when it is considered that the usual long colonic residence time is likely to prolong contact of drugs or metabolites with the colonic mucosa and in some cases permit their absorption through the colonic mucosa (Dressman, 1986). It has been suggested from studies of the effects of anticancer compounds on neoplastic colonic cells that intestinal cells may possess inherent protective properties in the form of an accelerated efflux pump which can serve to protect them from potentially damaging agents (Klohs and Steinkampf, 1986).

Ulceration and inflammation can be induced by the local application of drugs and vehicles to the rectal mucosa. Assessment of these effects in an appropriate animal model is important in the safety evaluation of preparations designed for use in man as rectal suppositories.

Although inflammatory conditions of the large bowel may possess certain morphological features typical for some inducing agents, inflammation of the large intestinal mucosa is usually characterized by a spectrum of non-specific histological features. In early or mild inflammation, the surface and glandular mucosa remains intact but shows mucin depletion. This is characterized by reduction in the mucus in goblet cells and increased cytoplasmic basophilia (Figs. 63 and 64). Scattered neutrophils may be seen in the epithelium and adjacent lamina propria. In more severe cases, crypts become filled or distended with acute inflammatory cells (crypt abscesses). The lamina propria is variably hyperaemic and congested and contains increased numbers of mononuclear cells.

Severe changes are characterized by attenuation or frank erosion of the epithelium and the formation of penetrating ulcers filled with fibrinous exudate and surrounded by intense inflammation, granulation tissue and eventually fibrosis (Fig. 65). Residual glands may be dilated and lined by flattened epithelium or show reactive changes and mitotic activity. Regenerative hyperplasia, which can become florid in chronic ulcerative conditions, is characterized by lengthening, irregularity and cystic dilatation of glands which are often lined by hyperplastic epithelial cells and goblet cells distended with mucin. Where ulcerative damage has destroyed glands and supporting stroma, regeneration of glands

355

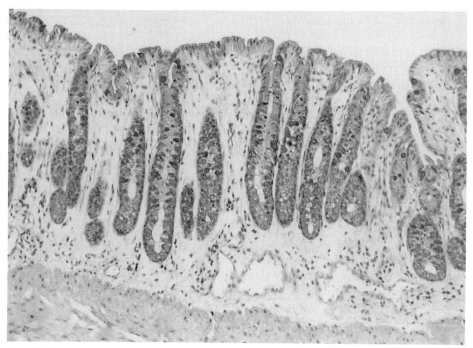

Fig. 63. Normal rectal mucosa from a New Zealand rabbit showing regular glands lined by cells replete with mucin and surrounded by a lamina propria containing abundant connective tissue. (HE, ×150.)

may not occur in the normal regular fashion and branching of crypts may be evident.

If the regenerative hyperplasia is marked and if inflammation is no longer intense, it may be difficult to distinguish it from neoplasia. The mixed population of cells, the lack of cytological atypia and absence of abnormal mitoses should help to make this distinction, although the association of chronic colonic inflammation with the development of colonic cancer in both man and laboratory animals makes this distinction more difficult than may be supposed.

Infections and infestations

Clostridium difficile may cause inflammatory changes in the colon of laboratory animals, particularly hamsters, and this may extend into the distal ileum. As in man this form of colitis, often referred to as *pseudomembranous colitis*, is usually associated with antibiotic therapy. In man it was originally associated with lincomycin and clindamycin therapy but other antibiotics have been implicated. It has been shown that both in man and the hamster experimental model that the enteritis is the result of the toxin produced by *Clostridium difficile* (Bartlett et al., 1977; 1978; Milligan and Kelly, 1979).

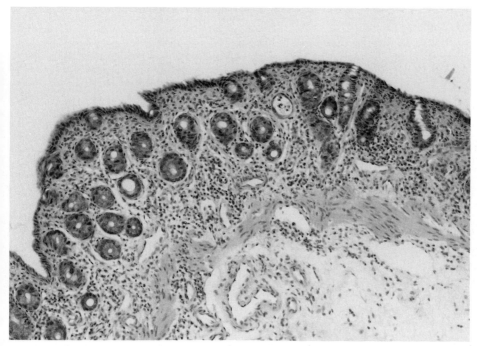

Fig. 64. Rectal mucosa taken from a New Zealand rabbit, same site as in Figure 63 but after a 21 day rectal irritancy study with a clinically employed suppository formulation. The mucosa is intact but there is reactive change and mucin depletion of the epithelium and an increase in number of chronic inflammatory cells in the lamina propria. (HE, ×150.)

In man this condition, which may be life-threatening, is histologically characterized by the presence of plaques or pseudomembranes on the colonic mucosal surface. The pseudomembrane is composed of mucus, fibrin, blood cells, inflammatory cells and cell debris, which has an appearance of streaming from the underlying mucosa. The mucosa may be partly necrotic or mucosal glands are dilated and lined by flattened or hyperplastic cells. The ileal mucosa may show similar changes (Milligan and Kelly, 1979).

Similar features are observed in the antibiotic-treated hamster although the pseudomembrane is less prominant and it may be distributed more proximally with involvement of the terminal ileum (Rehg, 1985). In the hamster, the condition is characterized histologically by erosion of the colonic epithelium and the variable presence of a pseudomembranous plaque of mucin and cell debris. Intact but affected mucosa is thickened with reactive changes accompanied by mucin loss in the epithelium and infiltration of a hyperaemic and oedematous lamina propria and submucosa by polymorphonuclear cells (Rehg, 1985).

Although most instances of this form of clostridial colitis in the hamster have been associated with antibacterial therapy, it has also been reported in untreated hamsters (Rehg and Lu, 1982) and those treated with antineoplastic drugs

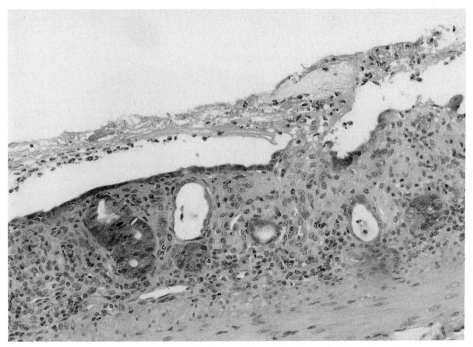

Fig. 65. Analogous section to that seen in Figure 64 but following administration of a more irritant suppository formulation. Here, erosion of the superficial epithelium has occurred, there is an inflammatory exudate and marked reactive alterations in the glandular epithelium. (HE, ×150.)

(Cudmore et al., 1980). Similar changes have been reported in antibiotic-treated guinea pigs and rabbits (Rehg and Lu, 1981; Rehg and Pakes, 1981). Guinea pigs are particularly sensitive to antibiotics especially those active against gram-positive organisms (Young et al., 1987). These drugs are believed to alter the intestinal flora, permitting overgrowth of *Clostridium difficile* as well as gram-negative organisms, resulting in a severe and frequently fatal enterocolitis. A study of the disposition of ampicillin administered parenterally to guinea pigs showed that this drug was rapidly eliminated from the systemic circulation and excreted in urine and bile, possibly favoring this effect on flora in the colon (Young et al., 1987).

Citrobacter freundii, a gram-negative, short, plump rod and member of the family of Enterobacteriaceae, is the causative agent of naturally occurring transmissible colonic hyperplasia of mice. This agent usually produces a mild or even asymtomatic enteritis in susceptable mouse populations, although it is a common cause of rectal prolapse in mice (Ediger et al., 1974). Marked strain differences have been noted in mice infected with this organism. NIH Swiss mice show the most severe histological changes and C57BL/6J mice appear the least affected (Barthold et al., 1977). Rats and hamsters seem to be unaffected by *Citrobacter freundii* (Barthold et al., 1977).

Microscopic changes are found primarily in the descending colon, although proximal segments of the colon and the caecum may also be affected. An important morphological feature is epithelial hyperplasia which occurs maximally two to three weeks after experimental inoculation with Citrobacter freundii (Barthold et al., 1977). The colonic glands are elongated and lined by cells which show mucin depletion or loss of goblet cells, considerable immaturity and mitotic activity. The surface epithelium may be covered with numerous coccobacilli which can be visualized in routine haematoxylin and eosin stained sections. An inflammatory component may also be evident with crypt abscesses and inflammatory cells in the lamina propria. Mucosal erosions and ulceration are also features (Barthold et al., 1976; 1978). In regressing lesions there is a rebound increase in goblet cells which are often distended with mucin. The colonic glands may be branched or irregular (Barthold et al., 1978).

Most laboratory animals are naturally resistant to *Shigella* infections but this is not the case for most non-human primates (Takeuchi, 1982). In infections with *Shigella*, the colon shows a superficial acute inflammatory reaction comprising oedema, congestion, haemorrhage and infiltration by acute inflammatory cells. The surface epithelium shows mucin loss and formation of microulcers where total destruction of the epithelium has occurred. Ulcers can extend into the lamina propria but in general terms the inflammatory process remains relatively superficial (Takeuchi, 1982). Organisms are also located predominantly in the superficial epithelium.

Another bacterial infection of the gastrointestinal tract which affects the colon in primates is that produced by non-tuberculosis *Mycobacterium* species (Holmberg et al., 1982b). Large intestinal lesions are characterized by massive accumulation of epitheloid macrophages in the lamina propria which may extend into the submucosa and muscular layers and along lymphatics to involve mesenteric lymph nodes. Small intestinal lesions may also occur, characterized by the presence of similar large macrophages in the lamina propria of villus tips. Superficial ulcers may occur in severely affected segments of intestine (Holmberg et al., 1982b). Acid fast bacteria are typically found within macrophages. Other organs, including spleen, liver, bone marrow and lungs, may also be involved by focal accumulations of bacteria-laden macrophages or occasionally discrete granulomas with multi-nucleated giant cells.

Protozoa and metazoal infections of the colon

Numerous protozoal and metazoal organisms have been described as inhabitants of the caecum and colon of the non-human primate (Toft, 1982). Far fewer are observed in the usual laboratory rodents and beagle dogs.

Amoebiasis caused by *Entamoeba histolytica* is a widespread disease among non-human primates characterized histologically by an ulcerative colitis. There are necrotizing ulcers which reach the muscularis mucosa to form typical flank-shaped ulcers containing or surrounded by trophozoites. Extensive hemorrhage may be seen as well as an inflammatory infiltrate composed of neutrophils and mononuclear cells (Toft, 1982).

The ciliate, *Balantidium coli*, can also cause an ulcerative process in the colon of primates, characterized by ulcers which extend down to the muscularis mucosa accompanied by lymphocytic infiltrate and *Balantidium coli* trophozoites of up to 150 μm in greatest diameter (Toft, 1982).

A variety of metazoan parasites can be observed in the primate colon and usually can be reasonably well identified in tissue sections (see review by Chitwood and Lichtenfels, 1973). The nematode of species *Strongyloides* is an important parasite which may be observed in the intestinal mucosa of primates. *Oxyurids* commonly known as pinworms are essentially innocuous parasites seen in man, non-human primates and rodents. *Enterobius vermicularis* is found in the large intestine and appendix of man and non-human primates, *Syphacia muris* and *Syphacia obvelata* in rodents.

Oesophagostomum species (nodular worms) are especially common nematode parasites of non-human primates forming characteristic nodules up to 5 mm diameter most frequently on the serosal surface of the large intestine and caecum and adjoining mesentery as well as in other sites in the peritoneal cavity. Histologically, the nodules are composed of parasite cell debris surrounded by

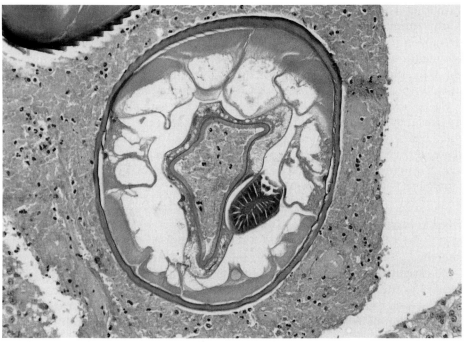

Fig. 66. Section taken through the submucosa of the small bowel wall of a cynomologus monkey showing the typical cross-sectional appearance of Oesophagostomum species. (HE, ×250.)

fibrous tissue and a variable mantle of chronic inflammatory cells and occasional foreign-body giant cells (Fig. 66). They are frequently found in close proximity to small arteries and arterioles in the submucosa and subserosa of the colon and may be associated with a local granulomatous arteritis (Lumb et al., 1985).

The inflammatory process may spread to surrounding or draining tissues, particularly if nodules rupture. Mild periportal hepatic chronic inflammation is sometimes associated with the presence of this parasite in the mesentery and this may lead to problems of interpretation if these are also drug-induced hepatic changes in the non-human primate.

Drug-induced inflammation, erosions, ulcers

Although the stomach and to a certain extent the small intestine remain the primary sites of predilection for the ulcerogenic action of non-steroidal anti-inflammatory, the colonic mucosa may become involved under certain conditions. Dogs administered 2.5 mg/kg indomethecin orally each day for periods of up to 23 days developed not only gastric and small intestinal ulceration but also scattered haemorrhagic erosions in the colon and rectum. Histologically, these lesions were characterized by loss of superficial epithelial cells, mucus-depletion of glandular epithelium, crypt abscesses, frequently with acute inflammation in adjacent lymphoid aggregates in the submucosa (Stewart et al., 1980). It was suggested that the large intestinal lesions may have been triggered by an inappropriate immune response.

An important example of chemically induced colitis of relevance to safety assessment of therapeutic agents is that induced by degraded carrageenans or synthetic sulphated dextrans. Carrageenans are a heterogeneous group of sulphated polysaccharides composed mainly of long chains of D-galactose subunits (D-galactan) derived from red seaweed species which are widely used as food emulsifiers, stabilizers, thickeners and gelling agents (Ishioka et al., 1987). When carrageenans are degraded by acid hydrolysis into smaller molecular weight fragments of about 20,000 to 40,000 and administered orally in high doses (eg. 10% of diet) to rats, mice, guinea pigs, rabbits and rhesus monkeys, colitis results (Sharratt et al., 1970; Marcus and Watt, 1971; Benitz et al., 1973; Fath et al., 1984; Kitano et al., 1986). Similarly, colitis has been induced in rats following administration of a 5% dietary admixture of dextran sulphate sodium, a sulphated polymer of glucose (a D-glucose) of molecular weight of 54,000 (Hirono et al., 1981) and a very high molecular weight D-glucan, amylopectin sulphate (Ishioka et al., 1987). A major difficulty in the safety assessment of these agents for man is the fact that long term administration of high doses to rats leads to the development of colorectal cancer despite their being devoid of any mutagenic potential.

Although histological features of this form of induced colitis varies between study, species and strain, the colitis is generally characterized mucosal ulceration mainly in the caecum but also in the distal ileum, distal colon and rectum. There is mucus-depletion with variable acute inflammatory infiltrate of the intact

361

epithelium, crypt abscesses, inflammatory infiltrate of the lamina propria with oedema, hyperaemia and even vascular thrombosis in the submucosa (Hirono et al., 1981; Fath et al., 1984). Proliferative activity of the mucosa is increased and this is confirmed by an increase in the tritiated thymidine index compared with controls (Fath et al., 1984).

In the caecum of rats, ulcers are linear but often circulating the entire circumference of the intestinal wall with subsequent scarring and stricture formation (Oohashi et al., 1981). Ulcerating lesions in the rectum and at the anal margin are associated with squamous metaplasia. Both the squamous metaplasia and the regenerative hyperplasia of the columnar epithelium have been shown to progress even after cessation of treatment (Oohashi et al., 1981). Foamy macrophages containing metachromatic material, presumably polysaccharide, are also seen in the lamina propria, submucosa, regional lymph nodes, liver and spleen (Hirono et al., 1981; Oohashi et al., 1981).

The cause of this colitis (and subsequent cancer) is unclear. Low dose levels which may be expected to mimic human exposure do not produce colitis. Dextrans, carrageenans and other polysaccharides of molecular weights outside

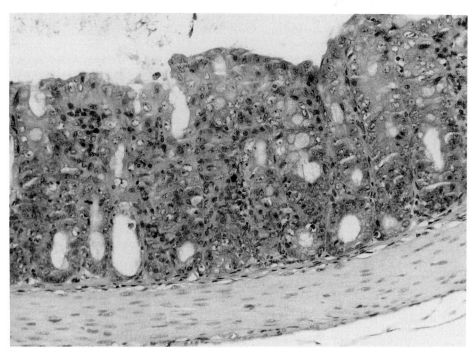

Fig. 67. Colon of a CD-1 mouse treated with a similar antimitotic regimen to that shown in Figure 62. Here again, the epithelium remains intact but its normal appearance has been lost. There is mucin depletion, focal flattening of the epithelium, loss of mitotic activity from the glands and vesiculation of nuclei. (HE, ×250.)

the range 20,000 to 60,000 tend not to incite colitis. An exception to this is the agent amylopectin sulphate which has a far higher molecular weight. However, amylopectin is composed of polysaccharide chains which can be degraded by amylase and therefore smaller molecular weight fragments may be formed in vivo (Ishioka et al., 1987).

It has been suggested that colonic disease produced by these agents is in some way linked to induced changes in intestinal microflora (Marcus and Watt, 1971) although the evidence for this is conflicting (Ishioka et al., 1987). A recent study in guinea pigs and rats using permeability markers of different molecular weights has suggested that degraded carrageenans enhance intestinal permeability in the absence of overt ulceration (Delahunty et al., 1987). It was therefore proposed that carrageenan-induced colitis could be the result of increased intestinal permeability to antigenic or inflammatory substances normally resident in the large intestine. However, the only clear feature which is common to a number of other cancer models using non-genotoxic xenobiotics is increased proliferative activity.

The rectal administration of therapeutic agents and surfactants may also induce similar ulcerative and inflammatory changes (Figs. 63, 64 and 65). Chemical colitis resembling pseudomembranous colitis has been reported in man as a result of chemical cleaning agents accidentally induced by endoscopic examination (Jonas et al., 1988). Cellular degeneration, with loss of mitotic activity and mucin depletion can also occur in the colon following treatment with antimitotic drugs (Fig. 67).

Lymphoid infiltrates without tissue damage were reported in the large bowel of rats treated with human recombinant interleukin-2 (Anderson & Hayes 1989).

Pigmentation

Melanosis coli is a well-described phenomenon in man associated with chronic ingestion of anthraquinone purgatives. It is considered to be due to the excessive accumulation of lipofuscin-like pigment in the macrophages of the colonic lamina propria (Schrodt, 1963; Ghadially and Parry, 1966; Steer and Colin-Jones, 1975). This pigment probably originates from organelles of epithelial cells or macrophages which are damaged by treatment. Similar morphological changes have been induced in laboratory animals (guinea pigs) by treatment with anthraquinones (Walker et al., 1988). As a result of these animal studies, Walker and colleagues (1988) suggested that the primary process is a treatment-induced increase in apoptotic bodies in the surface colonic epithelium which are phagocytosed by intraepithelial macrophages and transported to the lamina propria.

Lipofuscin and iron pigment is occasionally be observed in the lamina propria of untreated rodents, notably hamsters, presumably a result of aging or previous inflammatory processes and haemorrhage.

Hyperplasia, focal hyperplasia, diffuse hyperplasia, atypical hyperplasia, dysplasia and 'transitional mucosa'

As in the small intestine, cell proliferation in the large intestinal mucosa can be stimulated by a variety of different factors although these functional adaptive responses have been less well studied. Physical stimulation by distension or increased dietary bulk is sufficient to initiate hyperplasia including thickening of the muscle coats (Dowling et al., 1967; Stragand and Hagemann, 1977). One of the most clearly documented forms of compensatory hyperplasia is that which occurs as a response to surgical resection or bypass of a segment of the colon.

Following resection of a segment of colon in rats, Barkla and Tutton (1985) showed that the remaining proximal segment of the right side of the colon showed an increase in the thickness of the mucosa and the muscularis externa as well as enlargement of lymphoid aggregates. Histologically, the mucosa of the right side of the colon was uniformly thickened showing accentuated folds, elongated mucosal glands with increased height of the surface columnar cells. The changes were most marked up to 30 days following surgery but were less pronounced after 72 days. There was also a significant increase in the mitotic index in the proximal segment at seven days although at 14 days and later the mitotic index had returned to normal. The distal, down-stream segment reacted

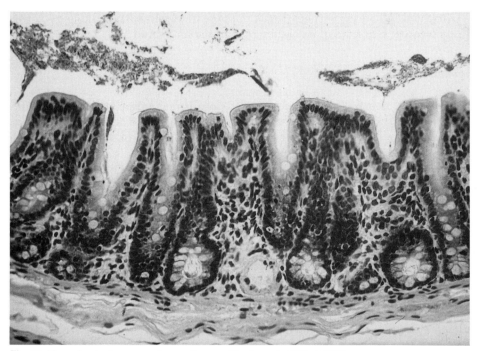

Fig. 68. Normal colonic mucosa from a Spague-Dawley rat. (HE, ×300.)

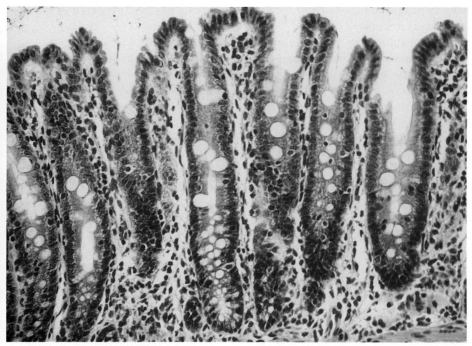

Fig. 69. Colon from a Sprague-Dawley rat, same site as in Figure 68 but following oral administration of 10% dextran sodium sulphate (molecular weight 500,000) in diet for two weeks. There is considerable thickening of the mucosa which shows elongation of colonic glands lined by slightly enlarged, but fairly normal epithelial cells with prominent vesicular nuclei. (HE, ×300.)

differently for it showed little or no morphological change but rather a long-lived increase in mitotic activity. It was suggested that these differences were related to the different embryological origin of the segments (Barkla & Tutton, 1985).

A similar form of uniform colonic hyperplasia affecting principally the caecal and right-sided colonic mucosa also occurs in rats following oral administration of sulphated dextrans of approximately 400,000 molecular weight (Figs. 68 and 69).

Similarly, oral administration of a wide range of compounds such as raw and chemically modified starches, caramels, sugar alcohols (lactitol, sorbitol, mannitol, xylilol), lactose, a synthetic polydextrose, polythylene glycol and magnesium sulphate to rats or hamsters has also been linked to an increase caecal size and colonic mucosal hyperplasia (Leegwater et al., 1974; Roe and Bar, 1985; Newberne et al., 1988). The characteristic histological appearance of the caecum following administration of these agents is lengthening of the mucosal glands which are lined by epithelium composed of increased numbers of enlarged epithelial cells (i.e. hypertrophy and hyperplasia) showing increased proliferative activity and more rapid incorporation of tritiated thymidine (Newberne et al.,

1988). In addition, mucosal and submucosal oedema has been reported in association with the administration of lactose and increased mucosal lymphoid aggregates following lactose or xylitol feeding (Newberne et al., 1988).

As the increase in caecal size and mucosal hypertrophy appears generally related to the osmotic activity of the caecal contents in rodents treated with these agents, it has been postulated that the changes represent a physiological adaptation to increased osmotic forces, irrespective of the contributing compounds (Leegwater et al., 1974).

Treatment of rodents with antibiotics also causes caecal enlargement or dilatation without significant histopathological changes, probably as a result of changes in caecal microflora. It has been suggested that the enlargement relates to accumulation of urea as a result of inhibition of bacterial ureases (Juhr and Ladeburg, 1988). However, histochemical studies of the intestinal mucosa of rats treated with neomycin have also shown treatment-related reductions in activities of NAD tetrazolium reductase, succinate dehydrogenase, esterase, alkaline and acid phosphatase in the distal ileum, suggesting that some antibiotics also posses the potential to directly influence absorption and metabolic functions of mucosal cells (Van Leeuwen et al., 1986).

Long-term administration of 16,16-dimethyl prostaglandin E2 to rats also produced thickening of the proximal colonic mucosa, although this was less marked than in the stomach and duodenum (Reinhart et al., 1983) and similar changes have been reported in rats treated with other prostaglandin E analogues (Levin, 1988).

Focal regenerative hyperplasia accompanies ulceration and other inflammatory conditions of the intestine (see above). In common with other epithelial surfaces, atypical hyperplasia is associated with the development of colonic cancer in both man and laboratory animals. The early alterations observed in rats treated with colonic carcinogens are similar to those found in the immediate vicinity of human colorectal carcinomas. The changes are characterized by lengthening, dilatation and branching of glands. The epithelium lining these glands shows mucous cell hyperplasia (goblet cell hyperplasia), goblet cells containing predominantly sialomucin instead of the normal sulphomucin (Filipe and Branfoot, 1974; Filipe, 1975; Shamsuddin and Trump, 1981b; Olubuyide et al., 1985). Despite mucin alterations, activities of glucose-6-phosphatase, glucose-6-phosphate dehydrogenase and glyceraldehyde-3-phosphate dehydrogenase were shown to be normal in this epithelium in rats treated with 1,2-dimethylhydrazine (Mayer et al., 1987). In man, this form of hyperplastic mucosa associated with cancer, has been termed 'transitional mucosa' (Filipe and Branfoot, 1974).

In rats treated with the carcinogens azoxymethane or 1,2-dimethylhydrazine, these changes are followed by the development of atypical or dysplastic histological features. Crypts show diminution of mucus secretion, increased cytoplasmic basophilia, prominant, rounded or enlarged nuclei which show variable degrees of pseudostratification and which eventually develop into frankly invasive glands (Shamsuddin and Trump, 1981b). In contrast to goblet cell hyperplasia, these atypical zones show increased activity of glucose-6-phosphate, glucose-6-phosphate dehydrogenase and glyceraldehyde-3-phosphate dehydrogenase (Mayer et al., 1987).

Note: Some compounds may induce qualitative and quantitative changes in mucin content in the colonic mucosa without marked morphological alterations. An example of this phenomenon was described in rats treated with reserpine for seven days. The colonic mucosa showed an increase in sulphomucin-(high-iron diamine positive) containing goblet cells in the surface epithelium (Park et al., 1987).

Neoplasia

Adenomas and adenocarcinomas of the small and large intestine are infrequent spontaneous neoplasms in laboratory animals compared with man where colorectal carcinoma is one of the most prevalent neoplasms in the Western world. Adenomas and adenocarcinomas probably occur spontaneously in older dogs more than in any other animal species and as in man these are located most frequently in the distal colon and rectum (Lingeman and Garner, 1972). In non-human primates glandular neoplasms of the intestine occur with increasing age in the ileum and in the colon with a predilection for the zones near the ileocaecal valve (DePaoli and McClure, 1982).

In rats and mice, spontaneous intestinal neoplasms are uncommon although adenocarcinomas are occasionally observed in the ileum or colon in mice and rats used in chronic toxicity studies and carcinogenicity bioassays (Burn et al., 1966; Wells, 1971; Greaves and Faccini, 1984; Maeda et al., 1985). Many of these neoplasms appear to originate in the distal part of the small intestine, caecum and right side of the colon. In a review of spontaneous adenocarcinomas developing over a 17 year period in Wistar rats, Vandenberghe and colleagues (1985) identified 17 adenocarcinomas, all in ascending colon. In 15 of these cases there appeared to be an intimate relationship with Campylobacter-like organisms together with diverticulae and chronic inflammation. These authors suggested that the organisms and the associated inflammation were involved in the pathogenesis of these cancers.

Certain hamster colonies, liable to develop inflammatory bowel disease (see above), also have a high incidence of small and large intestinal polyps, adenomas and adenocarcinomas (Fortner, 1957; Van Hoosier et al., 1971; personal observations). Poorly differentiated carcinomas may infiltrate local lymph nodes and it may be difficult to locate the primary neoplasm. Polyps are predominantly adenomatous in nature although inflammatory or regenerative polyps are observed (Van Hoosier et al., 1971).

Adenocarcinomas are commonly induced experimentally in the rodent intestine by the carcinogens 1,2-dimethylhydrazine and azoxymethane. The histogenesis of these induced carcinomas has been extensively studied and it is generally accepted that they resemble human colorectal cancer (Ward, 1974; Shamsuddin and Trump, 1981b; Freeman, 1983). However, there are differences between reported studies. Some have shown that these experimental carcinomas arise from pre-existing adenomas consistent with the 'adenoma-carcinoma sequence' theory (Ward, 1974; Ward et al., 1977). Others suggest that they arise 'de novo' from altered mucosa as microinvasive carcinomas (Maskens and Dujardin-Loits, 1981; Rubio et al., 1986; Sunter et al., 1978). These differences may be partly the result of different dosage schedules. Rubio and colleagues (1988) have shown that a single dose of 1,2-dimethyhydrazine produces non-polypoid, microinvasive carcinomas, particularly in the mucosa overlying lymphoid aggregates, whereas in their earlier studies using multiple doses in the same strain of rat, an adenoma-carcinoma sequence was more evident. In addition, there are undoubtably species and strain differences in the response to these agents. Teague et al (1981) demonstrated clear differences in the distribution and both macroscopic and histological types of adenomas and adenocarcinomas between three different inbred strains of rat given a similar dosage regimen of 1,2-dimethylhydrazine.

In general however, many of these carcinomas develop in the distal colonic segments similar to the distribution of human colorectal cancer, although tumours also develop in the proximal colon and in the ileum in rats treated with this agent (Ward, 1974; Shamsuddin and Trump, 1981b; Teague et al., 1981).

Neoplasms occurring in the rat colon following administration of high doses of degraded carrageenans and sulphated dextran also commonly occur in the distal colon and rectum and are commonly polypoid adenomas and adenocarcinomas (Oohashi et al., 1981; Hirono et al., 1981; Ishioka et al., 1987). However, in these models adenomas and adenocarcinomas also occur in the caecum and proximal colon and squamous carcinomas are sometimes seen in association with squamous metaplasia at the colorectal junction (Oohashi et al., 1981).

The pathogenesis of neoplasms induced by carrageenans and dextrans remains unexplained. Although they are biologically active compounds, they are non-mutagenic in the usual short-term tests (Ishioka et al., 1987). It has been suggested that carrageenans act as tumour promoters (Hirono et al., 1981), consistent with the studies that have shown that they potentiate the appearance of carcinomas in rats treated with standard intestinal carcinogens (Watanabe et al., 1978). It has also been suggested that these agents are tumour initiators based on the appearance of carcinomas in rats treated with degraded carrageenans for only two months (Oohashi et al., 1981). However, in rats which developed cancer, inflammation, regenerative changes and squamous metaplasia persisted throughout a period of 18 months after treatment was withdrawn before development of cancer.

The only consistent association of carrageenans with development of carcinoma in rats is that of chronic inflammation. Although dose levels needed to produce inflammation are far higher than any exposure likely to be achieved in man, interpretation of this inflammation-cancer sequence in rats remains a challenge in safety assessment for similar xenobiotics. This situation is perhaps also a challenge for human medicine in view of the unquestionable risk of carcinogenesis in ulcerative colitis in man which is also unexplained (Riddell et al., 1983).

A similar range of neoplasms can be defined histologically in both human and

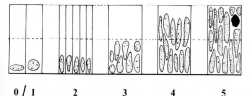

0 / 1   2   3   4   5

Fig. 70. Schematic diagram showing the concept for grading of hyperplastic and adenomatous alterations in colonic epithelium based on nuclear size, shape and pseudostratification proposed by Kozuka (1975). Grades 0/1 represent normal epithelium and grades 2 to 5 demonstrate increasing degrees of hyperplasia.

experimental pathology. It is appropriate, to use the same classification for all species including man. Lingeman and Garner (1972) who reviewed a range of tumours from domestic and laboratory animals were able to employ the classification for human gastrointestinal neoplasms. This classification can be summarized as follows:

Adenomatous polyps

These represent localized, sessile or polypoid neoplasms composed of proliferating tubular glands which show varying degrees of nuclear hyperchromatism, pseudostratification and cellular pleomorphism. A useful scheme for grading the carcinogenic potential of hyperplastic mucosa and adenomatous polyps in man based on epithelial pseudostratification has been proposed by Kozuka (1975). Although experimental neoplasms may not always show the full spectrum of these changes reported in man, this grading provides a useful baseline concept for the assessment of these non-invasive proliferative lesions (Fig. 70).

With increased nuclear pseudostratification and atypical branching of the glandular structures of these polyps becomes more prominant. If neoplastic cells or glands are seen in the stroma of the stalk or base the diagnosis of carcinoma is made.

Villous adenoma

These represent similar neoplasms in which the epithelial proliferation takes the form of elongated villi with a sparse fibrovascular stroma. They can be graded in a similar way to adenomatous polyps.

Adenocarcinoma

These are glandular neoplasms of variable differentiation, sometimes originating in adenomatous polyps or villous adenomas but which show infiltration of the intestinal wall, i.e. beyond the boundary of the muscularis mucosa.

Squamous carcinomas also occur in the anorectal zone but are similar to those which occur in squamous epithelium elsewhere. Similarly, mesenchymal neop-

369

lasms also are found in the small and large intestinal wall (see Integumentary System, Chapter I).

REFERENCES

AASE, S. and ROLAND, M. (1977): Light and electron microscopical studies of parietal cells before and one year after proximal vagotomy in duodenal ulcer patients. *Scand.J.Gastroenterol.*, 12, 417–420.

ALLEN, J.R. (1975): Response of the non-human primate to polychlorinated biphenyl exposure. *Fed.Proc.*, 34, 1675–1679.

ALTMANN, G.G. and ENESCO, M. (1967): Cell number as a measure of distribution and renewal of epithelial cells in the small intestine of growing and adult rats. *Am.J.Anat.*, 121, 319–336.

ALTMANN, H-J., WESTER, P.W., MATTHIASCHK, G., GRUNOW, W. and VAN DER HEIJ-DEN, C.A. (1985): Induction of early lesions in the forestomach of rats by 3-tert-butyl-4-hydroxy-amisole (BHA). *Food Chem.Toxicol.*, 23, 723–731.

AMBUHL, S., WILLIAMS, V.J. and SENIOR, W. (1979): Effects of caecectomy in the young adult female rat on digestibility of food offered ad libitum and in restricted amounts. *Aust.J.Biol.Sci.*, 32, 205–213.

ANDERSON, L.M., GINER-SOROLLA, A., HALLER, I.M. and BUDINGER, J.M. (1985): Effects of cimetidine, nitrite, cimetidine plus nitrite, and nitrosocimetidine on tumors in mice following transplacental chronic lifetime exposure. *Cancer Res.*, 45, 3561–3566.

ANDERSON, D.D. and HAYES, T.J. (1989): Toxicity of human recombinant interleukin-2 in rats. Pathologic changes are characterized by markedlymphocytic and eosinophilic proliferation and multisystem involvement. *Lab.Invest.*, 60, 331–346.

ANVER, M.R., COHEN, B.J., LATTUADA, C.P. and FOSTER, S.J. (1982): Age-associated lesions in barrier-reared male Sprague-Dawley rats: A comparison between Hap:(SD) and CrL:COBS[R] CD[R] (SD) stocks. *Exp.Aging Res.*, 8, 3–24.

ARSECULERATNE, S.N., PANABOKKE, R.G., NAVARATNAM, C. and WELIANGE, L.V. (1981): An epizootic of Klebsiella aerogenes infection in laboratory rats. *Lab.Anim.*, 15, 333–337.

AZUUMI, Y., OHARA, S., ISHIHARA, K., OKABE, H. and HOTTA, K. (1980): Correlation of quantitative changes of gastric mucosal glycoproteins with aspirin-induced gastric damage in rats. *Gut*, 21, 533–536.

BALAS, D., SENEGAS-BALAS, F., PRADAYROL, L., VAYSSETTE, J., BERTRAND, C. and RIBET, A. (1985): Long-term comparative effect cholecystokinin and gastrin on mouse stomach, antrum, intestine, and exocrine pancreas. *Am.J.Anat.*, 174, 27–43.

BARKA, T. (1980): Biologically active peptides in submandibular glands. *J.Histochem.Cytochem.*, 28, 836–859.

BARKA, T., CHANG, W.W.L. and VAN DER NOEN, H. (1972): The effect of 6-hydro-xydopamine on rat salivary glands and on their response to isoproterenol *Lab.Invest.*, 27, 594–599.

BARKER, I.K. and VAN DREUMEL, A.A. (1985): The alimentary system. In: K.V.F. Jubb, P.C. Kennedy and N. Palmer (Eds), *Pathology of Domestic Animals* 3rd Ed. Vol. 2, Chap. 1, pp. 1–237 Academic Press, Orlando.

BARKLA, D.H. and TUTTON, P.J.M. (1985): Proliferative and morphologic changes in rat colon following bypass surgery. *Am.J.Pathol.*, 119, 402–411.

BARTHOLD, P.M. (1987): Cyclosporin and gingival overgrowth. *J.Oral Pathol.*, 16, 463–468.

BARTHOLD, S.W. (1985)a: Mouse hepatitis virus infection, intestine, mouse. In: T.C. Jones, U. Mohr and R.D. Hunt (Eds), *Digestive System. Monographs on Pathology of Laboratory Animals*, pp. 317–321. Springer-Verlag, Berlin.

BARTHOLD, S.W. (1985)b: Murine rotavirus infection, intestine, mouse. In: T.C. Jones, U. Mohr and R.D. Hunt (Eds), *Digestive System. Monographs on Pathology of Laboratory Animals*, pp. 321–325. Springer-Verlag, Berlin.

BARTHOLD, S.W. (1985)c: Adenovirus infection, intestine, mouse. In: T.C. Jones, U. Mohr and R.D. Hunt (Eds), Digestive System. *Monographs on Pathology of Laboratory Animals*, pp.325–327. Springer-Verlag, Berlin.

BARTHOLD, S.W., COLEMAN, G.L., BHATT, P.N., OSBALDISTON, G.W. and JONAS, A.M. (1976): The etiology of transmissible murine colonic hyperplasia. *Lab.Anim.Sci.*, 26, 889–894.

BARTHOLD, S.W., COLEMAN, G.L., JACOBY, R.O., LIVSTONE, E.M. and JONAS, A.M. (1978): Transmissible murine colonic hyperplasia. *Vet.Pathol.*, 15, 223–236.

BARTHOLD, S.W., OSBALDISTON, G.W. and JONAS, A.M. (1977): Dietary, bacterial, and host genetic interactions in the pathogenesis of transmissible murine colonic hyperplasia. *Lab.Anim.Sci.*, 27, 938–945.

BARTLETT, J.G., CHANG, T.W., GURWITH, M., GORBACH, S.L. and ONDERDONK, A.B. (1978): Antibiotic-associated pseudomembranous colitis due to toxin-producing clostridia. *N.Engl.J.Med.*, 298, 531–534.

BARTLETT, J.G., ONDERDONK, A.B., CISNEROS, R.L. and KASPER, D.L. (1977): Clindamycin-associated colitis due to a toxin-producing species of Clostridium in hamsters. *J.Infect.Dis.*, 136, 701–705.

BASTIE, M.J., BALAS, D., LAVAL, J., SENEGAS-BALAS, F., BETRAND, C., FREXINOS, J. and RIBERT, A. (1982): Histological variations of jejunal and ileal mucosa on days 8 and 15 after hypophysectomy in rat: Morphometric analysis in light and electron microscopy. *Acta.Anat.*, 112, 321–337.

BASTIE, M.J., BALAS, D., LAVAL, J., BETRAND, J. and RIBET, A. (1985): Comparative study of histological and kinetic variations of the digestive mucosa and pancreatic parenchyma after hypophysectomy in the rat. *Acta.Anat.*, 124, 133–144.

BEATTIE, D. (1977): Effect of drugs on rats exposed to cold-restraint stress. *J.Pharm.Pharmacol.*, 29, 748–751.

BEGHI, E., DI MASCIO, R. and TOGNONI, G. (1986): Adverse effects of anticonvulsant drugs: a critical review. *Adv.Drug React.Ac.Pois.Rev.*, 2, 63–86.

BELLANDER, T., ÖSTERDAHL, B-G. and HAGMAR, L. (1985): Formation of N-mono-nitrosopiperazine in the stomach and its secretion in the urine after oral intake of piperazine. *Toxicol.Appl.Pharmacol.*, 80, 193–198.

BENITZ, K.F., GOLDBERG, L. and COULSTON, F. (1973): Intestinal effects of carrageenans in the rhesus monkey (Macaca mulatta). *Food Cosmet.Toxicol.*, 11, 565–575.

BENNETT, H.S. (1969): The cell surface: components and configurations. In: A. Lima-De-Faria (Ed.), *Handbook of Molecular Cytology*, pp. 1261–1293. North Holland, Amsterdam.

BERENSON, M.M., SENNELLA, J. and FRESTON, J.W. (1976): Ménétrier's disease. Serial morphological, secretory, and serological observations. *Gastroenterology*, 70, 257–263.

BERGER, E.G., BUDDECKE, E., KAMERLING, J.P., KOBATA, A., PAULSON, J.C. and VLIEGENTHART, J.F.G. (1982): Structure, biosynthesis and functions of glycoprotein glycans. *Experientia*, 38, 1129–1258.

BETTON, G.R., DORMER, C., WELLS, T., PERT, P., PRICE, C.A. and BUCKLEY, P. (1987): Fundic mucosal ECL cell hyperplasia and carcinoids in rodents following chronic administration of the histamine H2-receptor antagonist SK&F 93479 and other antisecretory agents. *Toxicol.Pathol.*, 15, 365.

BETTON, G.R., DORMER, C.S., WELLS, T., PERT, P., PRICE, C.A. and BUCKLEY, P. (1988): Gastric ECL-cell hyperplasia and carcinoids in rodents following chronic administration of the H2 antagonist SK&F 93479 and oxmetidine and omeprazole. *Toxicol.Pathol.*, 16, 288–298.

BETTON, G.R. and SALMON, G.K. (1984): Pathology of the forestomach in rats treated for 1 year with a new histamine H2-receptor antagonist, SK&F 93479 trihydrochloride. *Scand.J.Gastroenterol.*, 19, Suppl 101, 103–108.

BISHOP, A.E., ALLEN, J.M., DALY, M.J., LARSSON, H., CARLSSON, E., BLOOM, S.R. and POLAK, J.M. (1986): Gastric regulatory peptides in rats with reduced acid secretion. *Digestion*, 35, Suppl 1, 70–83.

BJARNASON, I., ZANELLI, G., SMITH, T., PROUSE, P., WILLIAMS, P., SMETHURST, P.,

DELANEY, G., GUMPEL, M.J. and LEVI, A.J. (1987): Non-steroidal anti-inflammation in humans. *Gastroenterology*, 93, 480–489.

BLAND, P.W. and WARREN, L.G. (1985): Immunohistologic analysis of the T-cell and macrophage infiltrate in 1,2-dimethylhydrazine-induced colon tumors in the rat. *J.N.C.I.*, 75, 757–764.

BLOK, J., FRANSEN, J.A.M. and GINSEL, L.A. (1984): Turnover of brush-border glycoproteins in human intestinal absorptive cells: Do lysosomes have regulatory function? *Cell Biol.Int.Rep.*, 8, 993–1014.

BLOM, H. (1986): Alterations in gastric mucosal morphology induced by long-term treatment with omeprazole in rats. *Digestion*, 35, Suppl 1, 98–105.

BOGART, B.I. (1970): The effect of aging on the rat submandibular gland. An ultrastructural, cytochemical and biochemical study. *J.Morphol.*, 130, 337–352.

BONAVINA, L., DEMEESTER, T.R., McCHESNEY, L., SCHWIZER, W., ALBERTUCCI, M., and BAILEY, R.T. (1987): Drug-induced esophageal strictures. *Ann.Surg.*, 206, 173–183.

BONKOVSKY, H.L., HAURI, H.-P., MARTI, U., GASSER, R. and MEYER, U.A. (1985): Cytochrome P450 of small intestinal epithelial cells. Immunocytochemical characterization of the increase in cytochrome P450 caused by phenobarbital. *Gastroenterology*, 88, 458–467.

BOORMAN, G.A., VAN HOOFT, J.I.M., VAN DER WAAIJ, D. and VAN NOORD, M.J. (1973): Synergistic role of intestinal flagellates and normal intestinal bacteria in a post-weaning mortality of mice. *Lab.Anim.Sci.*, 23, 187–193.

BOTT, S.J. and McCALLUM, R.W. (1986): Medication-induced oesophageal injury. Survey of the literature. *Med.Toxicol.*, 1, 449–457.

BOYD, E.M., CEHN, C.P. and MUIS, L.F. (1970): Resistance to starvation in albino rats fed from weaning on diets containing from 0 to 81% of protein as casein. *Growth*, 34, 99–112.

BOYD, W. (1970): Diseases of the kidney. In: *A Textbook of Pathology. Structure and Function in Disease*. 8th Ed. Chap. 23, pp. 613–688, Henry Kimpton, London.

BRANDTZAEG, P., VALNES, K., SCOTT, H., ROGNUM, T.O., BJERKE, K. and BAKHEN, K. (1985): The human gastrointestinal secretory immune system in health and disease. *Scand.J.Gastroenterol.*, 20, Suppl 114, 17–38.

BRECKENRIDGE, A. (1987): Enzyme induction in humans. Clinical aspects: an overview. *Pharmacol.Ther.*, 33, 95–99.

BREGMAN, C.L., COMERESKI, C.R., BUROKER, R.A., HIRTH, R.S., MADISSOO, H. and HOTTENDORF, G.H. (1987): Single-dose and multiple-dose intravenous toxicity studies of BMY-25282 in rats. *Fundam.Appl.Toxicol.*, 9, 90–109.

BRENNER, G.M. and STANTON, H.C. (1970): Adrenergic mechanisms responsible for submandibular salivary glandular hypertrophy in the rat. *J.Pharmacol.Exp.Ther.*, 173, 166–175.

BRODIE, D.A., TATE, C.L. and HOOKE, K.F. (1970): Aspirin: Intestinal damage in rats. *Science*, 170, 183–185.

BRORS, O. (1987): Gastrointestinal mucosal lesions: A drug formulation problem. *Med. Toxicol.*, 2, 105–111.

BUREK, J.D., MAJKA, J.A. and BOKELMAN, D.L. (1985): Famotidine: Summary of preclinical safety assessment. *Digestion*, 32, Suppl 1, 7–14.

BURN, J.I., SELLWOOD, R.A. and BISHOP, M. (1966): Spontaneous carcinoma of the colon of the rat. *J.Pathol.Bacteriol.*, 91, 253–254.

BURNETT, R.A., BROWN, I.L. and FINDLAY, J. (1987): Cresyl fast violet staining method for Campylobacter-like organisms. *J.Clin.Pathol.*, 40, 353.

CALE, A.E., FREEDMAN, P.D. and LUMERMAN, H. (1988): Pigmentation of the jawbone and teeth secondary to minocycline hydrochloride therapy. *J.Peridontol.*, 59, 112–114.

CARLBORG, B. and DENSERT, O. (1980): Esophageal lesions caused by orally administered drugs. An experimental study in the cat. *Eur.Surg.Res.*, 12, 270–282.

CARLBORG, B., DENSERT, O. and LINDQVIST, C. (1983): Tetracycline induced esophageal ulcers. A clinical and experimental study. *Laryngoscope*, 93, 184–187.

CARTHEW, P. and SLINGER, R.P. (1981): Diagnosis of sialodacryoadenitis virus infection of rats in a virulent enzootic outbreak. *Lab.Anim.*, 15, 339–342.

CASEMORE, D.P., SANDS, R.L. and CURRY, A. (1985): Cryptosporidium species a 'new' human pathogen. *J.Clin.Pathol.*, 38, 1321–1336.

CHABOT, J.-G., WALKER, P. and PELLETIER, G. (1987): Thyroxine accelerates the differentiation of granular convoluted tubule cells and the appearance of epidermal growth factor in the submandibular gland of the neonatal mouse. A fine structural immunocytochemical study. *Cell Tissue Res.*, 248, 351–358.

CHANG, W.W.L. (1981): Two types of mucous cells in the colon crypt. *J.N.C.I.*, 67, 746–747.

CHANG, W.W.L. and LEBLOND, C.P. (1971): Renewal of the epithelium in the descending colon of the mouse. I. Presence of three cell populations: vacuolated-columnar, mucous and argentaffin. *Am.J.Anat.*, 131, 73–100.

CHENG, H. and LEBLOND, C.P. (1974): Origin, differentiation and renewal of the four main epithelial cell types in the mouse small intestine. III Entero-endocrine cells. *Am.J.Anat.*, 141, 521–536.

CHEVILLE, N.F. (1979): Uremic gastropathy in the dog. *Vet.Pathol.*, 16, 292–309.

CHEVILLE, N.F. and OLSON, C. (1964): Cytology of the canine oral papilloma. *Am.J.Pathol.*, 45, 849–872.

CHHABRA, R.S. and EASTIN, W.C. Jr. (1984): Intestinal absorption and metabolism of xenobiotics in laboratory animals. In: C.M. Schiller (Ed.), *Intestinal Toxicology*, pp. 145–160. Raven Press, New York.

CHITWOOD, M. and LICHTENFELS, J.R. (1973): Parasitological review. Identification of parasitic metazoa in tissue section. *Exp.Parasitol.*, 32, 407–519.

CHIU, T. and CHEN, H.C. (1986): Spontaneous basophilic hypertrophic foci of the parotid glands in rats and mice. *Vet.Pathol.*, 23, 606–609.

CHVÉDOFF, M., CLARKE, M.R., IRISARRI, E., FACCINI, J.M. and MONRO, A.M. (1980): Effects of housing conditions on food intake, body weight and spontaneous lesions in mice. A review of the literature and results of an 18-month study. *Food Cosmet.Toxicol.*, 18, 517–520.

COCKRELL, B.Y., VALERIO, M.G. and GARNER, F.M. (1974): Cryptosporidiosis in the intestines of rhesus monkeys (Macaca mulatta). *Lab.Anim. Sci.*, 24, 881–887.

COHEN, S. (1962): Isolation of a mouse submaxillary gland protein accelerating incisor eruption and eyelid opening in the newborn animal. *J.Biol.Chem.*, 237, 1555–1562.

COLIN-JONES, D.G., LANGMAN, M.J.S., LAWSON, D.H. and VESSEY, M.P. (1985): Post marketing surveillance of the safety of cimetidine: Mortality during second, third, and fourth years of follow-up. *Br.Med.J.*, 291, 1084–1088.

COOK, R.W., WILLIAMS, J.F. and LICHTENBERGER, L.M. (1981): Hyperplastic gastropathy in the rat due to Taenia taeniaeformis infection: Parabiotic transfer and hypergastrinaemia. *Gastroenterology*, 80, 728–734.

CORNES, J.S. (1965): Number, size and distribution of Peyer's patches in the human small intestine. *Gut*, 6, 225–233.

CORREA, P., HAENSZEL, W., CUELLO, C., TANNENBAUM, S.R. and ARCHER, M. (1975): A model for gastric cancer epidemiology. *Lancet*, 2, 58–60.

CREAN, G.P., DANIEL, D., LESLIE, G.B. and BATES, C. (1978): The effect of prolonged administration of large doses of cimetidine on the gastric mucosa of rats. In: C. Wastell and P. Lance (Eds), *Cimetidine*. The Westminster Hospital Symposium, Chap. 18, pp. 191–206. Churchill Livingstone, Edinburgh.

CREAN, G.P., GUNN, A.A. and RUMSEY, R.D.E. (1969): The effects of vagotomy on the gastric mucosa of the rat. *Scand.J.Gastroenterol.*, 4, 675–680.

CREUTZFELDT, W., STÖCKMANN, F., CONLON, J.M., FÖLSCH, U.R., BONATZ, G. and WÜLFRATH, M. (1986): Effect of short- and long-term feeding of omeprazole on rat gastric endocrine cells. *Digestion*, 35, Suppl 1, 84–97.

CUDMORE, M., SILVA, J. and FEKETY, R. (1980): Clostridial enterocolitis produced by antineoplastic agents in hamsters and humans. In: J.D. Nelson and C. Grassi (Eds), *Current Chemotherapy and Infectious Disease*. p. 1460. Proceedings, American Society of Microbiology, Washington, DC.

CULLEN, J.M., RUEBNER, B.H., HSIEH, D.P.H. and BURKES Jr E.J. (1987): Odontogenic tumours in Fischer rats. *J.Oral Pathol.*, 16, 469–473.

CULLING, C.F.A., REID, P.E., CLAY, M.G. and DUNN, W.L. (1974): The histo-chemical demonstration of O-acylated sialic acid in gastrointestinal mucins: Their association with the potassium hydroxide-periodic acid-Schiff effect. *J.Histochem.Cytochem.*, 22, 826–831.

CULLING, C.F.A., REID, P.E. and DUNN, W.L. (1976): A new histochemical method for the identification and visualization of both side chain acylated and non-acylated sialic acids. *J.Histochem.Cytochem.*, 24, 1225–1230.

D'AMICO, D.J., KENYON, K.R. and RUSKIN, J.N. (1981): Amiodarone kerato-pathy, drug-induced lipid storage disease. *Arch.Ophthalmol.*, 99, 257–261.

DAMJANOV, I., MILDNER, B. and KNOWLES, B.B. (1986): Immunohistochemical localization of the epidermal growth factor receptor in normal human tissues. *Lab.Invest.*, 55, 588–592.

DARDICK, I., JEANS, M.T.D., SINNOTT, N.M., WITTKUHN, J.F., KAHN, H.J. and BAUMAL, R. (1985): Salivary gland components involved in the formation of squamous metaplasia. *Am.J.Pathol.*, 119, 33–43.

DAVENPORT, H.W. (1964): Gastric mucosal injury by fatty and acetylsalicylic acids. *Gastroenterology*, 46, 245–253.

DAVIS, A.J. and JENKINS, S.J. (1986): Cryptosporidosis and proliferative ileitis in a hamster. *Vet.Pathol.*, 23, 632–633.

DAWE, C.J. (1979): Tumours of the salivary and lacrymal glands, nasal fossa and maxillary sinuses. In: V.S. Turusov (Ed.), *Pathology of Tumours in Laboratory Animals. Tumours of the Mouse*, Vol. 2, pp. 91–133. IARC, Scientific Publ. No. 23, Lyon.

DEBRAY, H., DECOUT, D., STRECKER, G., SPIK, G. and MONTREUIL, J. (1981): Specificity of twelve lectins towards oligosaccharides and glyco-peptides related to N-glycosylproteins. *Eur.J.Biochem.*, 117, 41–55.

DELAHUNTY, T., RECHER, L. and HOLLANDER, D. (1987): Intestinal permeability changes in rodents. A possible mechanism for degraded carrageenan-induced colitis. *Food Chem.Toxicol.*, 25, 113–118.

DELANEY, J.P., MICHEL, H.M., BONSACK, M.E., EISENBERG, M.M. and DUNN, D.H. (1979): Adrenal corticosteroids cause gastrin cell hyperplasia. *Gastroenterology*, 76, 913–916.

DENKO, C.W. (1958): The effect of hydrocortisone and cortisone on fixation of 35S in the stomach. *J.Lab.Clin.Med.*, 51, 174–177.

DENKO, C.W. (1964): The effect of phenylbutazone and its derivatives, oxyphenbutazone and sulfinpyrazole, on 35S sulfate incorporation in cartilage and stomach. *J.Lab.Clin.Med.*, 63, 953–958.

DEPAOLI, A. and McCLURE, H.M. (1982): Gastrointestinal neoplasms in non-human primates: A review and report of new cases. *Vet.Pathol.*, 19, Suppl 7, 104–125.

DJALDETTI, M. and FISHMAN, P. (1981): The effect of aspirin on small intestinal mucosa. *Arch.Pathol.Lab.Med.*, 105, 144–147.

do'NASCIMENTO, A., BARRETO, R-de-C., BOZZO, L. and de ALMEIDA, O.P. (1985): Interaction of phenytoin and inflammation induces gingival overgrowth in rats. *J.Peridont.Res.*, 20, 386–391.

DOBBINS, W.O. III (1969): Morphologic aspects of lipid absorption. *Am.J.Clin.Nutr.*, 22, 257–265.

DODD, D.C., PORT, C.D., DESLEX, P., REGNIER, B., SANDERS, P. and INDACOCHEA-REDMOND, N. (1987): Two-year evaluation of misprostol for carcino-genicity in CD Sprague-Dawley rats. *Toxicol.Pathol.*, 15, 125–133.

DOI, K., MAEDA, N., DOI, C., ISEGAWA, N., SUGANO, S. and MITSUOKA, T. (1985): Distribution and incidence of calcified lesions in DBA/2NCrj and BALB/cAnNCrj mice. *Jpn.J.Vet.Sci.*, 47, 479–482.

DOWLING, R.H., RIECKEN, E.O., LAWS, J.W. and BOOTH, C.C. (1967): The intestinal response to high bulk feeding in the rat. *Clin.Sci.*, 32, 1–9.

DRESSMAN, J.B. (1986): Comparison of canine and human gastrointestinal physiology. *Pharm.Res.*, 3, 123–131.

DUBOIS, A. (1987): Stress ulceration-clinical relevance of animal and human studies. *Chronobiol.Int.*, 4, 69–73.

DUNN, T.B. (1967): Amyloidosis in mice. In: E. Cotchin and F.J.C. Roe (Eds), *Pathology of Laboratory Rats and Mice*, Chap. 7, pp. 181–212. Blackwell, Oxford.

EASTWOOD, G.L. and QUIMBY, G.F. (1982): Effect of chronic aspirin ingestion on epithelial proliferation in rat fundus, antrum and duodenum. *Gastroenterology*, 82, 852–856.

ECTORS, N. and DIXON, M.F. (1986): The prognostic value of sulphomucin positive intestinal metaplasia in the development of gastric cancer. *Histopathology*, 10, 1271–1277.

EDIGER, R.D., KOVATCH, R.M. and RABSTEIN, M.M. (1974): Colitis in mice with a high incidence of rectal prolapse. *Lab.Anim. Sci.*, 24, 488–494.

EDWARDS, G.S., FOX, J.G., POLICASTRO, P., GOFF, U., WOLF, M.H. and FINE, D.H. (1979). Volatile nitrosamine contamination of laboratory animal diets. *Cancer Res.*, 39, 1857–1858.

EKMAN, L., HANSSON, E., HAVU, N., CARLSSON, E. and LUNDBERG, C. (1985): Toxicological studies on omeprazole. *Scand.J.Gastroenterol.*, 20, Suppl 108, 53–69.

ELDER, J.B., GANGULI, P.C. and GILLESPIE, I. (1979): Cimetidine and gastric cancer. *Lancet*, 1, 1005–1006.

ELDER, J.B., GANGULI, P.C., KOFFMAN, C.G., WELLS, S. and WILLIAMS, G. (1982): Possible role of cimetidine and its nitrostated products in human stomach cancer. In: P.N. Magee (Ed.), Banbury Report 12. *Nitrosamines and Human Cancer*, pp. 335 349. Cold Spring Harbor Laboratory, New York.

EMMINGER, A. and MOHR, U. (1982): Tumours of the oral cavity, check pouch, salivary glands, oesophagus, stomach and intestines. In: V.S. Turusov (Ed.), *Pathology of Tumours in Laboratory Animals. Tumours of the Hamster*, Vol.3, pp. 45–68. IARC Scientific Publ. No. 34, Lyon.

ERMAK, T.H. and OWEN, R.L. (1986): Differential distribution of lymphocytes and accessory cells in mouse Peyer's patches. *Anat.Rec.*, 215, 144–152.

FATH, R.B., DESCHNER, E.E., WINAWER, S.J. and DWORKIN, B.M. (1984): Degraded carrageenan-induced colitis in CF1 mice. A clinical, histo-pathological and kinetic analysis. *Digestion*, 29, 197–203.

FELLENIUS, E., BERGLINDH, T., SACHS, G., OLBE, L., ELANDER, B., SJÖSTRAND, S.-E. and WALLMARK, B. (1981): Substituted benzimidazoles inhibit acid secretion by blocking (H + + K +) ATPase. *Nature*, 290, 159–161.

FICH, A., ARBER, N., OKON, E., ZAJICEK, G. and RACHMILEWITZ, D. (1988): Effect of chronic misoprostol ingestion on rat gastric morphology and turnover. *Arch.Toxicol.*, 61, 314–317.

FILIPE, M.I. (1975): Mucous secretion in rat colonic mucosa during carcinogenesis induced by dimethylhydrazine. A morphological and histo-chemical study. *Br.J.Cancer*, 32, 60–77.

FILIPE, M.I. (1979): Mucins in the human gastrointestinal epithelium: A review. *Invest.Cell Pathol.*, 2, 195–216.

FILIPE, M.I. and BRANFOOT, A.C. (1974): Abnormal patterns of mucous secretion in apparently normal mucosa of large intestine with carcinoma. *Cancer*, 34, 282–290.

FORRESTER, J.M. (1972): The number of villi in rat's jejunum and ileum: Effect of normal growth, partial enterectomy and tube feeding. *J.Anat.*, 3, 283–291.

FORTNER, J.G. (1957): Spontaneous tumors including gastrointestinal neoplasms and malignant melanoma, in Syrian hamster. *Cancer*, 10, 1153–1156.

FOWLER, P.D. (1987): Aspirin, paracetamol and non-steroidal anti-inflammatory drugs. A comparative review of side effects. *Med.Toxicol.*, 2, 338–366.

FOX, J.G., CLAPS, M.C., TAYLOR, N.S., MAXWELL, K.O., ACKERMAN, J.I. and HOFFMAN, S.B. (1988): Campylobacter jejuni/coli in commercially reared beagles. Prevalance and serotypes. *Lab.Anim. Sci.*, 38, 262–265.

FRANZIN, G. and NOVELLI, P. (1981): Gastritis cystica profunda. *Histo-pathology*, 5, 535–547.

FREEMAN, H.J. (1983): Lectin histochemistry of 1,2-dimethylhydrazine-induced rat colon neoplasia. *J.Histochem.Cytochem.*, 31, 1241–1245.

FREEMAN, H.J., LOTAN, R. and KIM, Y.S. (1980): Application of lectins for detection of goblet cell glycoconjugate differences in proximal and distal colon of the rat. *Lab.Invest.*, 42, 405–412.

FRIEDMAN, H.I. and CARDELL, R.R. Jr. (1972): Effects of puromycin on the structure of rat intestinal epithelial cells during fat absorption. *J.Cell Biol.*, 52, 15–40.

FUJITA, M., TAGUCHI, T., TAKAMI, M., USUGANE, M., TAKAHASHI, A. and SHIBA, S. (1974): Carcinoma and related lesions in dog stomach induced by oral administration of N-methyl-N'-nitro-N-nitrosoguanidine. *Jpn.J.Cancer Res.* (Gann), 65, 207–214.

FUJINO-KURIHARA, H., FUJITA, H., HAKURA, A., NONAKA, K. and TARUI, S. (1985): Morphological aspects on pancreatic islets of non-obese diabetic (NOD) mice. *Virchows Arch.[B]*, 49, 107–120.

FUKUSHIMA, K. and HELMAN, R.G. (1984): Cryptosporidiosis in a pup with distemper. *Vet.Pathol.*, 21, 247–248.

FUKUSHIMA, S. and ITO, N. (1985): Squamous cell carcinoma, forestomach, rat. In: T.C. Jones, U. Mohr and R.D. Hunt (Eds), *Digestive System. Mono-graphs on Pathology of Laboratory Animals*, pp. 292–295. Springer-Verlag, Berlin.

GANAWAY, J.R. (1985)a: Tyzzer's disease, intestine, mouse, rat, hamster. In: T.C. Jones, U. Mohr and R.D. Hunt (Eds), *Digestive System. Mono-graphs on Pathology of Laboratory Animals*, pp. 330- 333. Springer-Verlag, Berlin.

GANAWAY, J.R. (1985)b: Salmonellosis, intestine, mouse, rat, hamster. In: T.C. Jones, U. Mohr and R.D. Hunt (Eds), *Digestive System. Mono-graphs on Pathology of Laboratory Animals*, pp. 333–337. Springer-Verlag, Berlin.

GARTHOFF, B., HOFFMANN, K., LUCKHAUS, G. AND THURAU, K. (1982): Adequate substitution with electrolytes in toxicological testing of 'loop' diuretics in the dog. *Toxicol. Appl.Pharmacol.*, 65, 191–202.

GERARD, A. (1965): Histochemie de la muqueuse gastrique fundique du chien traité par des drogues ulcérigène. *C.R.Soc.Biol.(Paris)*, 159, 1473–1476.

GHADIALLY, F.N. and PARRY, E.W. (1966): An electron-microscope and histo-chemical study of melanosis coli. *J.Pathol.Bacteriol*, 92, 313–317.

GHADIALLY, F.N. (1982): Mitochondria. In: *Ultrastructural Pathology of the Cell and Matrix* (2nd Edition), Chap. 3, pp. 149–263. Butterworth, London.

GHOOS, Y. and VANTRAPPEN, G. (1971): The cytochemical localization of lysozyme in Paneth cell granules. *Histochem.J.*, 3, 175–178.

GILLATT, P.N., PALMER, R.C., SMITH, P.L.R., WALTERS, C.L. and REED, P.I. (1985): Susceptibilities of drug to nitrosation under simulated gastric conditions. *Food Chem.Toxicol.*, 23, 849–855.

GILLON, J., ALTHAMERY, D. and FERGUSON, A. (1982): Features of small intestinal pathology (epithelial cell kinetics, intra-epithelial lymphocytes, disaccharidases) in a primary Giardia muris infection. *Gut*, 23, 498–506.

GIMENEZ, D.F. (1964): Staining Rickettsiae in yolk sac cultures. *Stain Technol.*, 39, 135–140.

GJURLDSEN, S.T., MYREN, J. and FRETHEIM, B. (1968): Alterations of gastric mucosa following a graded partial gastrectomy. *Scand.J.Gastroenterol.*, 3, 465–470.

GLUCKSMANN, A. and CHERRY, C.P. (1973): Tumours of the salivary glands. In: V.S. Turusov (Ed.), *Pathology of Tumours in Laboratory Animals. Tumours of the Rat*, Vol. 1, Part 1, pp. 75–86. IARC Scientific Publ. No. 5, Lyon.

GOEPP, R.A. (1982): The oral cavity. In: R.H. Riddell (Ed.), *Pathology of Drug-Induced and Toxic Diseases*, Chap. 7, pp. 147–154. Churchill Livingstone, New York.

GÖGGELMANN, W., ROBISCH, G. and SCHIMMER, O. (1982): Aristolochic acid is a direct mutagen in S.typhimurium. *Mutat.Res.*, 105, 201–204.

GOLDBERG, D.M., CAMPBELL, R. and ROY, A.D. (1969): Studies of the binding of trypsin and chymotrypsin by human intestinal mucosa. *Scand.J. Gastroenterology*, 4, 217–226.

GOLDENBERG, M.M. (1973): Study of cold plus restraint stress gastric lesions in spontaneously hypertensive, Wistar and Sprague-Dawley rats. *Life Sci.*, 12, 519–527.

GOLDMAN, H. and MING, S.C. (1968): Mucins in normal and neoplastic gastro-intestinal epithelium. *Arch.Pathol.*, 85, 580–586.

GOLDSTEIN, I.J. and HAYES, C.E. (1978): The lectins: Carbohydrate-binding proteins of plants and animals. *Adv.Carbohydr.Chem.Bioch* 35, 127–340.

GONA, O. (1981): Prolactin and ergocryptine effects mucus glycoproteins of the rat ileum. *Histochem.J.*, 13, 101–107.

GRACON, S.I., MARTIN, R.A., BARSOUM, N., MITCHELL, L., STURGESS, J.M. and de la IGLESIA, F.A. (1982): Hypopigmentary changes with a platelet aggregation inhibitor. *Fed.Proc.*, 41, 402 (Abstract #2526).

GRAY, J.E., WEAVER, R.N., SINKULA, A.A., SCHURR, P.E. and MORAN, J. (1974): Drug-induced enteropathy characterized by lipid in macrophages. *Toxicol.Appl.Pharmacol.*, 27, 145–157.

GREAVES, P. and BOIZIAU, J.-L. (1984): Altered patterns of mucin secretion in gastric hyperplasia in mice. *Vet.Pathol.*, 21, 224–228.

GREAVES, P. and FACCINI, J.M. (1984): Digestive system. In: *Rat Histopathology. A Glossary for Use in Toxicity and Carcinogenicity Studies*, Vol. VI, pp. 86–143. Elsevier, Amsterdam.

GREENLEE, J.E. (1985): K virus infection, intestine, mouse. In: T.C. Jones U. Mohr and R.D. Hunt (Eds), *Digestive System. Monographs on Pathology of Laboratory Animals*, pp. 328–329. Springer-Verlag, Berlin.

GRIMELIUS, L. (1968): A silver nitrate stain for alpha-2 cells in human pancreatic islets. *Acta.Soc.Med.Upsal*, 73, 243–270.

HÅKANSON, R., BÖTTCHER, G., SUNDLER, F. and VALLGREN, S. (1986)a: Activation and hyperplasia of gastrin and enterochromaffin-like cells in the stomach. *Digestion*, 35, Suppl 1, 23–41.

HÅKANSON, R., LARSSON, L.-I., LIEDBERG, G., OSCARSON, J., SUNDLER, F. and VANG, J. (1976): Effects of antrectomy or porta-caval shunting on the histamine-storing endocrine-like cells in oxyntic mucosa of rat stomach. A fluorescence histochemical, electron microscopic and chemical study. *J.Physiol.(Lond)*, 259, 785–800.

HÅKANSON, R., OSCARSON, J. and SUNDLER, F. (1986)b: Gastrin and the trophic control of gastric mucosa. In: K.O. Borg, L. Olbe, S.J. Rune and A. Walan (Eds), Proceedings of the 1st International Symposium on *Omeprazole*, pp. 18–30. A.B. Hassle, Molndal, Sweden.

HÅKANSON, R., VALLGREN, S., EKELUND, M., REHFELD, J.F. and SUNDLER,F. (1984): The vagus exerts trophic control of the stomach in the rat. *Gastroenterology*, 86, 28–32.

HAMPERL, H. (1950): Onkocytes and so-called Hürthle cell tumor. *Arch.Pathol.*, 49, 563–567.

HANHIJÄRVI, H., KOUKKARI, T., KOSMA, V.-M., NEVALAINEN, T., COLLAN, Y. and MÄNNISTÖ, P. (1986): Dog and swine as models for testing indomethacin-induced gastrointestinal irritation. *Arch.Toxicol.*, Suppl 9, 252.

HANNA, P.E., PERCY, D.H., PATURZO, F. and BHATT, P.N. (1984): Sialodacryoadenitis in the rat: Effects of immunosuppression on the course of the disease. *Am.J.Vet.Res.*, 45, 2077–2083.

HÄNNINEN, O., LINDSTRÖM-SEPPÄ, P. and PELKONEN, K. (1987): Role of gut in xenobiotic metabolism. *Arch.Toxicol.*, 60, 34–36.

HANSON, W.R. and OSBORNE, J.W. (1971): Epithelial cell kinetics in the small intestine of the rat 60 days after resection of 70 percent of the ileum and jejunum. *Gastroenterology*, 60, 1087–1097.

HANSON, W.R., OSBORNE, J.W. and SHARP, J.G. (1977): Compensation by the residual intestine after intestinal resection in the rat. *Gastroenterology*, 73, 692–700.

HANSSON, E., HAVU, N. and CARLSSON, E. (1986): Toxicology studies with omeprazole. In: K.O. Borg, L. Oble, S.J. Rune and A. Walan (Eds), *Proceedings of the 1st International Symposiim on Omeprazole*, pp. 89–91. A.B. Hässle, Mölndal, Sweden.

HARE, W.V. and STEWART, H.L. (1956): Chronic gastritis of the glandular stomach, adenomatous polyps of the duodenum, and calcareous pericarditis in strain DBA mice. *J.N.C.I.*, 16, 889–911.

HARKNESS, J.E. and FERGUSON, F.G. (1979): Idiopathic megaoesophagus in rat. *Lab.Anim.Sci.*, 29, 495–498.

HASEGAWA, H., WATANABE, K., NAKAMURA, T. and NAGURA, H. (1987): Immunocytochemical localization of alkaline phosphatase in absorp cells of rat small intestine after colchicine treatment. *Cell Tissue Res.*, 250, 521–529.

HASSEL, T.M., PAGE, R.C., NARAYANAN, A.S. and COOPER, C.G. (1976): Diphenylhydantoin (dilantin) gingival hyperplasia: Drug-induced abnormality of connective tissue *Proc.Natl.Acad.Sci. USA*, 73, 2902.

HATTORI, T. (1974): On cell proliferation and differentiation of the fundic mucosa of the golden hamster. Fractographic study combineh microscopy and 3H-thymidine autoradiography. *Cell Tissue Res.*, 148, 213–226.

HATTORI, T. and FUJITA, S. (1976): Tritiated thymidine autoradiographic study on cellular migration in the gastric gland of the golden hamster. *Cell Tissue Res.*, 172, 171–184.

HAVU, N. (1986): Enterochromaffin-like cell carcinoids of gastric mucosa in rats after life long inhibition of gastric secretion. *Digestion*, 35, Suppl 1, 42–55.

HAWKER, R.C., MUSCROFT, T.J. and KEIGHLEY, M.R.B. (1980): Gastric cancer after cimetidine in patient with two negative pre-treatmen biopsies. *Lancet*, 1, 709–710.

HAYASHI, Y., KURASHIMA, C., UTSUYAMA, M. and HIROKAWA, K. (1988): Spontaneous development of auto-immune sialodenitis in aging BDF1 mice. *Am.J.Pathol.*, 132, 173–179.

HAYASHI, Y., SATO, M. and HIROKAWA, K. (1985): Induction of experimental allergic sialadenitis in mice. *Am.J.Pathol.*, 118, 476–483.

HERMON-TAYLOR, J., PERRIN, J., GRANT, D.A.W., APPLEYARD, A., BUBEL, M. and MAGEE, A.I. (1977): Immunofluorescent localization of enterokinase in human small intestine. *Gut*, 18, 259–265.

HIRATA, I., BERRIBI, G., AUSTIN, L.L., KEREN, D.F. and DOBBINS, W.O. III (1986): Immunohistological characterization of intra-epithelial and lamina propria lymphocytes in control ileum and colon and inflammatory bowel disease. *Dig.Dis.Sci.*, 31, 593–603.

HIRONO, I., KUHARA, K., HOSAKA, S., TOMIZAWA, S. and GOLDBERG, L. (1981): Induction of intestinal tumors in rats by dextran sulphate sulfate sodium. *J.N.C.I.*, 66, 579–583.

HIRTH, R.S., EVANS, L.D., BUROKER, R.A. and OLESON, F.B. (1988): Gastric enterochromaffin-like hyperplasia and neoplasia in the rat: An indirect effect of the histamine H2-receptor antagonist BL-6341. *Toxicol.Pathol.* 16, 273–287.

HOENSCH, H., WOO, C.H., RAFFIN, S.B. and SCHMID, R. (1976): Oxidative metabolism of foreign compounds in rats small intestine: Cellular localization and dependence on dietary iron. *Gastroenterology*, 70, 1063–1070.

HOLMBERG, C.A., LEINIGER, R., WHEELDON, E., SLATER, D., HENRICKSON, R. and ANDERSON, J. (1982)a: Clinicopathological studies of gastrointestinal disease in macaques. *Vet.Pathol.*, 19, Suppl 7, 163–170.

HOLMBERG, C.A., HENRICKSON, R.V., MALAGA, R., SCHNEIDER, R. and GRIBBLE, D. (1982)b: Non-tuberculous myobacterial disease in rhesus monkeys. *Vet. Pathol.*, 19, Suppl 7, 9–16.

HOWLEY, P.M. (1986): On human papillomaviruses. *N.Engl.J.Med.*, 315, 1089–1090.

HSU, C.-K. (1979): Parasitic diseases. In: H.J. Baker, J.R. Lindsey and S.H. Weisbroth (Eds), *The Laboratory Rat. Biology, Diseases,* Vol. 1, Chap. 12, pp. 305–331.

HYAMS, D.E., SABESIN, S.M., GREENBERGER, N.J. and ISSELBACHER, K.J. (1966): Inhibition of intestinal protein synthesis and lipid transport by ethionine. *Biochem.Biophys.Acta.*, 125, 166–173.

IMAI, K., YOSHIMURA, S., OHTAKI, T. and HASHIMOTO, K. (1981): Experimental toxicity studies with captopril, an inhibitor of angiotensin 1-converting enzymes 2. One month studies of chronic toxicity of captopril in rats. *J.Toxicol.Sci.*, 6, Supp. 2, 189–214.

IMAOKA, K., HONJO, K., DOI, K. and MITSUOKA, T. (1986): Development of spontaneous tongue calcification and polypoid lesions in DBA/2NCrj mice. *Lab.Anim.*, 20, 1–4.

IMONDI, A.R., BALIS, M.E. and LIPKIN, M. (1969): Changes in enzyme levels accompanying differentiation of intestinal epithelial cells. *Exp.Cell Res.*, 58, 323–330.

INGBAR, S.H. (1985): The thyroid gland. In: J.D. Wilson and D.W. Foster (Eds), *Textbook of Endocrinology*, Chap. 21, pp. 682–812. Saunders, Philadelphia.

INNES, J.R.M. and STANTON, M.F. (1961): Acute disease of the submaxillary and harderian glands (sialodacryoadenitis) of rats with cytomegaly and no inclusion bodies. *Am.J.Pathol.*, 38, 455–468.

INOKUCHI, H., FUJIMOTO, S. and KAWAI, K. (1983): Cellular kinetics of gastrointestinal mucosa, with special reference of gut endocrinecells. *Arch.Histol.Jpn.*, 46, 137–157.

ISHIHARA, K., OHARA, S., AZUUMI, Y., GOSO, K. and HOTTA, K. (1984): Changes of gastric mucus glycoproteins with aspirin administration inrats. *Digestion*, 29, 98–102.

ISHIOKA, T., KUWABARA, N., OOHASHI, Y. and WAKABAYASHI, K. (1987): Induction of colorectal tumors in rats by sulphated polysaccharides. CRC Crit. *Rev.Toxicol.*, 17, 215–244.

ITO, A., WATANABE, H., NAITO, M. and NAITO, Y. (1981): Induction of duodenal tumors in mice by oral administration of hydrogen peroxide. *Jpn.J.Cancer Res.* (Gann), 72, 174–175.

ITO, N., FUKUSHIMA, S., HAGIWARA, A., SHIBATA, M. and OGISO, T. (1983): Carcinogenicity of butylated hydroxyanisole in F344 rats. *J.N.C.I.* 70, 343–352.

ITO, N., HIROSE, M., FUKUSHIMA, S., TSUDA, H., TATEMATSU, M. and ASAMOTO, M. (1986): Modifying effects anti-oxidants on chemical carcinogenesis. *Toxicol.Pathol.*, 14, 315–323.

IVERSON, F., LOK, E., NERA, E., KARPINSKI, K. and CLAYSON, D.B. (1985)a: A 13-week feeding study of butylated hydroxyanisole: The subsequent regression of the induced lesions in male Fischer 344 rat forestomach epithelium. *Toxicology*, 35, 1–11.

IVERSON, F., TRUELOVE, J., NERA, E., WONG, J. and CLAYSON, D.B. (1985)b: An 85-day study of butylated hydroxyanisole in the cynomolgus monkey. *Cancer Lett.*, 26, 43–50.

JACKSON, C.D. and BLACKWELL, B.-N. (1988): Subchronic studies of doxylamine in Fischer 344 rats. *Fundam.Appl.Toxicol.*, 10, 243–253.

JACOBS, L.R. (1983): Effects of dietary fiber on mucosal growth and cell proliferation in the small intestine of the rat: A comparison of oat, bran, pectin, and guar with total fiber deprivation. *Am.J.Clin.Nutr.*, 37, 954–960.

JACOBY, R.O. (1985): Transmissible ileal hyperplasia, hamster. In: T.C. Jones, U. Mohr and R.D. Hunt (Eds), *Digestive Sysgem. Monographs of Pathology of Laboratory Animals*, pp. 346–355. Springer-Verlag, Berlin.

JARVIS, E.L. and LEVIN, R.J. (1966): Anatomic adaptation of the alimentary tract of the rat to the hyperphagia of chronic alloxan-diabetes. *Nature*, 210, 391–393.

JASS, J.R. (1980): Role of intestinal metaplasia in the histogenesis of gastric carcinoma. *J.Clin.Pathol.*, 33, 801–810.

JASS, J.R. and FILIPE, M.I. (1979): A variant of intestinal metaplasia associated with gastric carcinoma: A histochemical study. *Histopathology*, 3, 191–199.

JAYASEKARA, M.U., DEWIT, R.H., PETER, G.K. and FITZGERALD, J.E. (1986): Subchronic toxicity of C1–930, a novel cardiotonic agent in rats and dogs. *Toxicologist*, 6, 203.

JEURISSEN, S.H.M., DAVID, S., and SMIMIA, T. (1985): Uptake of particulate and soluble antigens in the small intestines of the rat. *Cell Biol.Int.Rep.*, 9, 523.

JONAS, G., MAHONEY, A., MURRAY, J. and GERTLER, S. (1988): Chemical colitis due to endoscopic cleaning solutions: A mimic of pseudomembranous colitis. *Gastroenterology*, 95, 1403–1408.

JUBB, K.V.F. and KENNEDY, P.C. (1970): *Pathology of Domestic Animals* (2nd Edition), pp. 74–81. Academic Press, New York.

JUHR, N.-C. and LADEBURG, M. (1986): Intestinal accumulation of urea in germ-free animals: a factor in caecal enlargement. *Lab.Anim.*, 20, 238–241.

JUNQUEIRA, L.C.U., TOLEDO, A.M.S. and DOINE, A.I. (1973): Digestive enzymes in the parotid and submandibular glands of mammals. *Ann.Acad.Brasil Ciênc*, 45, 629–633.

KADUK, B. and HAÜSER, H. (1980): Morphologishe Veränderungen der Magenmukosa von Ratten nach chronischer Antazidagabe. *Z.Gastroenterol.*, 18, 138–147.

KALTER, S.S. (1982): Enteric viruses of nonhuman primates. *Vet.Pathol.*, 19, Suppl 7, 33–43.

KANTOR, M.I. and HASEL, T.M. (1983): Increased accumulation of sulfated glycosaminoglycans in cultures of human fibroblasts from phenytoin-induced gingival overgrowth. *J.Dent.Res.*, 62, 383.

KATAOKA, K. (1970): Electron microscopic observations on cell proliferation and differentiation in the gastric mucosa of the mouse. *Arch.Histol. Jpn.*, 32, 251–273.

KEALY, W.F. (1976)a: Colonic lymphoid-glandular complex (microbursa): Nature and morphology. *J.Clin.Pathol.*, 29, 241–244.

KEALY, W.F. (1976)b: Lymphoid tissue and lymphoid-glandular complexes of the colon: Relation to diverticulosis. *J.Clin.Pathol.*, 29, 245–249.

KELLY, D.F., LUCKE, V.M., DENNEY, H.R. and LANE, J.G. (1979): Histology of salivary gland infarction in the dog. *Vet.Pathol.*, 16, 438–443.

KENNEDY, M.F.G., TUTTON, P.J.M. and BARKLA, D.H. (1983): Adrenergic factors involved in the control of crypt cell proliferation in jejunum and descending colon of mouse. *Clin.Exp.Pharmacol. Physiol.* 10, 577–586.

KING, T.P., PUSZTAI, A., GRANT, G. and SLATER, D. (1986): Immunogold localization of ingested kidney bean (Phaseolus vugaris) lectins in epithelial cells of the rat small intestine. *Histochem.J.*, 18, 413–420.

KITANO, A., MATSUMOTO, T., HIKI, M., HASHIMURA, H., YOSHIYASU, K., OKAWA, K., KUWAJIMA, S. and KOBAYASHI, K. (1986): Epithelial dysplasia of the rabbit colon induced by degraded carrageenan. *Cancer Res.*, 46, 1374–1376.

KLEIN-SZANTO, A.J.P., MARTIN, D. and SEGA, M. (1982): Hyperkeratinization and hyperplasia of the forestomach epithelium in vitamin A deficient rats. *Virchows Arch.[B]*, 40, 387–394.

KLOHS, W.D. and STEINKAMPF, R.W. (1986): Intrinsic resistance of colon tumors to anthrapyrazoles and antracyclines may be linked with a detoxification mechanism of intestinal cells. *Proceedings of 77th Annual Meeting of Amer. Assoc. Cancer Res.*, 27, 262 (Abstract #1040).

KOJIMA, A., TAGUCHI, O. and NISHIZUKA, Y. (1980): Experimental production of possible autoimmune gastritis followed by macrocytic anemia in athymic mice. *Lab.Invest.*, 42, 387–395.

KOPPANG, H.S. (1973): Histomorphologic investigations on the effect of cyclophosphamide on dentinogenesis of the rat incisor. *Scand.J.Dent. Res.*, 81, 383–396.

KOTSONIS, F.N., DODD, D.C., REGNIER, B. and KOHN, F.E. (1985): Preclinical toxicology profile of misoprostol. *Dig.Dis.Sci.*, 30, 1425–1465.

KOZUKA, S. (1975): Premalignancy of the mucosal polyp in the large intestine: I. Histologic gradation of the polyp on the basis of epithelial pseudostratification and glandular branching. *Dis.Colon.Rectum*, 18, 483–493.

KRAMER, A.W., DOUGHERTY, W.J., BELSON, A.R. and IATROPOULOS, M.J. (1985): Morphologic changes in the gastric mucosa of rats and dogs treated with an analog of prostaglandin E1. *Toxicol.Pathol.*, 13, 26–35.

KUHLMANN, W.D., PESCHKE, P. and WURSTER, K. (1983): Lectin-peroxidase conjugates in histopathology of gastrointestinal mucosa. *Virchows Arch.[A]*, 398, 319–328.

LACHANCE, M.P. (1982). The pharmacology and toxicology of caffeine. *J.Food Safety*, 4, 71–112.

LAMBERT, R., ANDRE, C. and MARTIN, F. (1969): Incorporation of radiosulfate in the gastric mucosa of the rat subjected to restraint. *Gastroenterology*, 56, 200–205.

LANGMAN, M.J.S. (1985): Antisecretory drugs and gastric cancer. *Br.Med.J.*, 290, 1850–1852.

LARSSON, H., CARLSSON, E., MATTSSON, H., LUNDELL, L., SUNDLER, F., SUNDELL, G., WALLMARK, B., WATANABE, T. and HÅKANSON, R. (1986): Plasma gastrin and gastric enterochromaffin-like cell activation and proliferation. Studies with omeprazole and ranitidine in intact and antrectomized rats. *Gastroenterology*, 90, 391–399.

LARSSON, L.-I. (1980): Gastrointestinal cells producing endocrine, neurocrine and paracrine messengers. *Clin.Gastroenterol.*, 9, 485–516.

LATIMER, K.S., RAKICH, P.M., PURSWELL, B.J. and KIRCHER, I.M. (1986): Effects of cyclosporin A administration in cats. *Vet.Immunol. Immunopathol.*, 11, 161–173.

LEDERMAN, D., LUMERMAN, H., REUBEN, S. and FREEDMAN, P.D. (1984): Gingival hyperplasia associated with nifedipine therapy. *Oral Surg.*, 57, 620–622.

LEEGWATER, D.C., DE GROOT, A.P. and VAN KALMTHOUT-KUPER, M. (1974). The aetiology of caecal enlargement in the rat. *Food Cosmet.Toxicol.* 12, 687–697.

LEHY, T., GRÈS, L. and BONFILS, S. (1978): Effect de l'administration prolongée d'un antisécrétoire gastrique, le pirenzepin, sur les populations cellulaires de l'estomac de rat. *Gastroenterol.Clin.Biol.*, 2, 1001–1009.

LESLIE, G.B. and WALKER, T.F. (1977): A toxicological profile of cimetidine. In. W.L. Burland and M. Alison-Simkins (Eds), *Cimetidine. Proceedings of the Second International Symposium on Histamine H2-receptor Antagonists*, pp. 24–33. Exerpta Medica, Amsterdam.

LEV, R. (1966): The mucin histochemistry of normal and neoplastic gastric mucosa. *Lab.Invest.*, 14, 2080–2100.

LEV, R. and SPICER, S.S. (1964): Specific staining of sulphate groups with alcian blue at low pH. *J.Histochem.Cytochem.*, 12, 309.

LEVIN, R.J. and SMYTH, D.H. (1963): The effect of the thyroid gland on intestinal absorption of hexoses. *J.Physiol.(Lond)*., 169, 755–769.

LEVIN, S. (1988): Structural changes of the gastrointestinal mucosa induced by prostaglandins. *Toxicol.Pathol.*, 16, 237–244.

LEVINE, M.J., REDDY, M.S., TABAK, L.A., LOOMIS, R.E., BERGEY, E.J., JONES, P.C., COHEN, R.E., STINSON, M.W. and AL-HASHIMI, I. (1987): Structural aspects of salivary glycoproteins. *J.Dent.Res.*, 66, 436–441.

LEWIN, K. (1969): Histochemical observations on Paneth cells. *J.Anat.*, 105, 171–176.

LINGEMAN, C.H. and GARNER, F.M. (1972): Comparative study of intestinal adenocarcinoma of animals and man. *J.N.C.I.*, 48, 325–346.

LIJINSKY, W. and TAYLOR, H.W. (1975): Carcinogenicity of methylated dinitro-sopiperazines in rats. *Cancer Res.*, 35, 1270–1273.

LOVE, L.A., LIJINSKY, W., KEEFER, L.K. and GARCIA, H. (1977): Chronic oral administration of l-nitrosopiperazine at high doses to MRC rats. *Z.Krebsforsch.*, 89, 69–73.

LUCAS, R.M., HOWELL, L.P. and WALL, B.A. (1985): Nifedipine-induced gingival hyperplasia : A histochemical and ultrastructural study. *J.Periodontol.*, 56, 211–215.

LÜLLMANN-RAUCH, R. (1979): Drug-induced lysosomal storage disorders. In: J.T. Dingle, P.J. Jacques and I.H. Shaw (Eds), *Lysosomes in Applied Biology and Therapeutics*, Vol. 6, Chap. 3, pp. 49–130. North Holland, Amsterdam.

LUMB, G.D., BEAMER, P.R. and RUST, J.H. (1985): Oesophagostomiasis in feral monkeys (Macaca mulatta). *Toxicol.Pathol.*, 13, 209–214.

MACKAY, E.M., CALLAWAY, J.W. and BARNES, R.H. (1940): Hyperalimentation in normal animals produced by protamine insulin. *J.Nutr.*, 20, 59–66.

MACLEOD, R.I., WELBURY, R.R. and SOAMES, J.V. (1987): Effects of cytotoxic chemotherapy on dental development. *J.R.Soc.Med.*, 80, 207–209.

MACNAB, J.C.M., WALKINSHAW, S.A., CORDINER, J.W. and CLEMENTS, J.B. (1986): Human papillomavirus in clinically and histologically normal tissue of patients with genital cancer. *N.Engl.J.Med.*, 315, 1052–1058.

MAEDA, H., GLEISER, C.A., MASORO, E.J., MURATA, I., MCMAHAN, C.A. and YU, B.P. (1985): Nutritional influences on aging of Fischer 344 rats: II. Pathology. *J.Gerontol.*, 40, 671–688.

MALLETT, A.K., BEARNE, C.A., ROWLAND, I.R., FARTHING, M.J.G., COLE, C.B. and FULLER, R. (1987): The use of rats associated with a human faecal flora as a model for studying the effects of diet on the human gut microflora. *J.Appl.Bacteriol.*, 63, 39–45.

MARCUS, R. and WATT, J. (1971): Colonic ulceration in young rats fed degraded carrageenan. *Lancet*, 2, 765–766.

MARSHALL, B.J. and WARREN, J.R. (1984): Unidentified curved bacilli in the stomach of patients with gastritis and peptic ulceration. *Lancet*, 1, 1311–1314.

MARTIN, M.S., HAMMANN, A. and MARTIN, F. (1986): Gut-associated lymphoid tissue and 1,2-dimethylhydrazine intestinal tumors in the rat: A histological and immunoenzymatic study. *Int.J.Cancer*, 38, 75–80.

MARTIN, R.A., BARSOUM, N.J., STURGESS, J.M. and DE LA IGLESIA, F.A. (1985). Leucocyte and bone marrow effects of a thiomorpholine quinazosin antihypertensive agent. *Toxicol.Appl.Pharmacol.*, 81, 166–173.

MARVOLA, M., JAJANIEMI, M., MARTTILA, E., VAHERVUO, K. and SOTHMANN, A. (1983): Effect of dosage form and formulation factors on the adherence of drugs to the esophagus. *J.Pharm.Sci.*, 72, 1034–1036.

MASCRES, C., MING-WEN, F. and JOLY, J.C. (1984): Morphologic changes of esophageal mucosa in the rat after chronic alcohol ingestion. *Exp.Pathol.*, 25, 147–153.

MASKENS, A.P. and DUJARDIN-LOITS, R.-M. (1981): Experimental adenomas and carcinomas of the large intestine behave as distinct entities: Most carcinomas arise de novo in flat mucosa. *Cancer*, 47, 81–89.

MASSON, P. (1914): La glande endocrine de l'intestin chez l'homme. *C.R.Seanc.Acad.Sci.*, 158, 59–61.

MATSUYAMA, M. and SUZUKI, H. (1970): Differentiation of immature mucous cells into parietal, argyrophil, and chief cells in stomach grafts. *Science*, 169, 385–387.

MAYER, D., TROCHERIS, V., HACKER, H.J., VIALLARD, V., MURAT, J.-C. and BANNASCH, P. (1987): Sequential histochemical and morphometric studies on preneoplastic and neoplastic lesions induced in rat colon by 1,2-dimethylhydrazine. *Carcinogenesis*, 8, 155–161.

MAZUE, G., VIC, P., GOUY, D., REMANDET, B., LACHERETZ, F., BERTHE, J., BARCHE-WITZ, G. and GAGNOL, J.P. (1984): Recovery from amiodarone-induced lipidosis in laboratory animals: A toxicological study. *Fundam.App.Toxicol.*, 4, 992–999.

MAZZACCA, G., CASCIONE, F., BUDILLON, G., D'AGOSTINO, L., CIMIMO, L. and FEMIANO, C. (1978): Parietal cell hyperplasia induced by long-term administration of antacids to rats. *Gut*, 19, 798–801.

McBRIDE, R.K., HARPER, C. and SIEGEL, I.A. (1987): Methotrexate-induced changes in rat parotid and submandibular gland function. *J.Dent.Res.*, 66, 1445–1448.

McCONNELL, E.E., HASS, J.R., ALTMAN, N. and MOORE, J.A. (1979): A spontaneous outbreak of polychlorinated biphenyl (PCB) toxicity in rhesus monkeys (Macaca mulatta): Toxicopathology. *Lab.Anim.Sci.*, 29, 666–673.

McCORMACK, K. and BRUNE, K. (1987): Classical absorption theory and the development of gastric mucosal damage associated with non-steroidal anti-inflammatory drugs. *Arch.Toxicol.*, 60, 261–269.

McDERMOTT, M.R., HORSLEY, B.A., WARNER, A.A. and BIENENSTOCK, J. (1985): Mesenteric lymphoblast localization throughout the murine small intestine: Temporal analysis relating intestinal length and lymphoblast division. *Cell Tissue Kinet.*, 18, 505–519.

McMARTIN, D.N. (1979): Morphologic lesions in aging Syrian hamsters. *J.Gerontol.*, 34, 502–511.

McMULLEN, L., WALKER, M.M., BAIN, L.A., KARIM, Q.N. and BARON, J.H. (1987): Histological identification of Campylobacter using Gimenez technique in gastric antral mucosal. *J.Clin.Pathol.*, 40, 464–465.

MENGS, U., LANG, W. and POCH, J-A. (1982): The carcinogenic action of aristolochic acid in rats. *Arch.Toxicol.*, 51, 107–119.

MICHALEK, S.M., RAHMAN, A.F.R. and McGHEE, J.R. (1975): Rat immunoglobulins in serum and secretions: Comparison of IgM, IgA and IgG in serum, colostrum, milk and saliva of protein malnourished and normal rats. *Proceedings, Society of Experimental Biology and Medicine*, 148, pp. 1114–1118.

MIDTVELD, T. (1987). Influence of ofloxacin on the faecal flora. *Drugs*, 34 (Suppl 1), 154–158.

MILLER, H.R.P. (1980): The structure, origin and function of mucosal mast cells. A brief review. *Biol.Cell*, 39, 229–232.

MILLIGAN, D.W. and KELLY, J.K. (1979): Pseudomembranous colitis in a leukaemia unit: A report of five fatal cases. *J.Clin.Pathol.*, 32, 1237–1243.

MIRVISH, S.S. (1975): Formulation of N-nitroso compounds: Chemistry kinetics, and in vivo occurrence. *Toxicol.Appl.Pharmacol.*, 31, 325–351.

MIRVISH, S.S. (1983): The etiology of gastric cancer: Intragastric nitro-samide formation and other theories. *J.N.C.I.*, 71, 629–647.

MOCH, R.W. (1988): Forestomach lesions induced by butylated hydroxyanisole and ethylene dibromide: A scientific and regulatory perspective. *Toxicol.Pathol.*, 16, 172–183.

MOOLENBECK, C. and RUITENBERG, E.J. (1981): The 'Swiss Roll': A simple technique for histological studies of the rodent intestine. *Lab.Anim.*, 15, 57–59.

MOOSKER, M.S., POLLARD, T.D. and FUJIWARA, K. (1978): Characterization and localization of myosin in the brush border of intestinal epithelial cells. *J.Cell Biol.*, 79, 444–453.

MOOSKER, M.S. and TILNEY, L.G. (1975): Organization of an actin filament-membrane attachment in the microvilli of intestinal epithelial cells. *J.Cell Biol.*, 67, 725–743.

MORGAN, R.W., WARD, J.M. and HARTMAN, P.E. (1981): Aroclor 1254-induced intestinal metaplasia and adenocarcinoma in the glandular stomach of F344 rats. *Cancer Res.*, 41, 5052–5059.

MORI, M., HAMADA, K., NAITO, R., TSUKITAN, K. and ASANO, K. (1983): Immuno-histochemical localization of epidermal growth factor in rodent submandibular glands. *Acta.Histochem.Cytochem.*, 16, 536–548.

MORSON, B.C. (1955): Intestinal metaplasia of the gastric mucosa. *Br.J.Cancer*, 9, 365–376.

MORSON, B.C., SOBIN, L.H., GRUNDMANN, E., JOHANSEN, A., NAGAYO, T. and SERCK-HANSSEN, A. (1980): Precancerous conditions and epithelial dysplasia in the stomach. *J.Clin.Pathol.*, 33, 711–721.

MOWAT, A.M. and FERGUSON, A. (1981): Hypersensitivity reactions in the small intestine. 6. Pathogenesis of the graft-versus-host reaction in the small intestinal mucosa of the mouse. *Transplantation*, 32, 238–243.

MOWRY, R.W. and MORARD, J.C. (1957): The distribution of acid mucopoly-saccharides in normal kidneys as shown by the alcian blue feulgan (AB-F) and alcian blue-periodic acid-Schiff (AB-PAS) stains. *Am.J.Pathol.*, 3, 620–621.

MÜLLER, J., KIRCHNER, T. and MÜLLER-HERMELINK, H.K. (1987): Gastric endocrine cell hyperplasia and carcinoid tumors in atrophic gastritis type A. *Am.J.Surg.Pathol.*, 11, 909–917.

MURGATROYD, L.B. (1980): A morphological and histochemical study of a drug-induced enteropathy in the Alderley Park rat. *Br.J.Exp.Pathol.*, 61, 567–578.

MUNHOZ, C.O.G. (1971): Histochemical classification of acini and ducts of parotid glands from artiodactyles, carnivores and rodents. *Acta.Histochem.*, 39, 302–317.

MURPHY, R.A., WATSON, A.Y., METZ, J. and FORSSMANN, W.G. (1980): The mouse submandibular gland: An exocrine organ for growth factors. *J.Histochem.Cytochem.*, 28, 890–902.

NAGAYO, T. (1981): Dysplasia of the gastric mucosa and its relation to the precancerous state. *Jp.J.Cancer Res.*, (Gann), 72, 813–823.

NAGAYO, T. and TANDLER, B. (1986): Ultrastructure of dog parotid gland. *J.Submicrosc.Cytol.*, 18, 67–74.

NAIR, K.V., GILLON, J. and FERGUSON, A. (1981): Corticosteroid treatment increases parasite numbers in murine giardiasis. *Gut*, 22, 475–480.

NAIR, P.N.R. and SCHROEDER, H.E. (1986): Duct-associated lymphoid tissue (DALT) of minor salivary glands and mucosal immunity. *Immunology*, 57, 171–180.

NAIR, P.N.R., ZIMMERLI, I. and SCHROEDER, H.E. (1987): Minor salivary gland duct-associated lymphoid tissue (DALT) in monkeys, changes with age. *J.Dent.Res.*, 66, 407–411.

NAKAMURA, R. (1985): Quantitative light and electron microscopic studies on the effect of vagotomy on parietal cells in rats. *Tohoku J.Exp.Med.*, 145, 269–282.

NALIN, D.R., LEVINE, M.M., RHEAD, J., BERGQUIST, E., RENNELS, M., HUGHS, T., O'DONNELL, S. and HORNICK, R.B. (1978): Cannabis, hypochlorhydria and cholera. *Lancet*, 2, 859–862.

NATIONAL TOXICOLOGY PROGRAM TECHNICAL REPORT (1987): Toxicology and carcinogenesis studies of ampicillin trihydrate in F344/N rats and B6C3F1 mice. *NIH Publication No. 87-2574*, pp. 9–10.

NEILSEN, J.A., HESSTHAYSEN, E., OLESEN, H. and NIELSEN, R. (1972): Fundal gastritis after Billroth-II-type resection in patients with duodenal ulcer. *Scand.J.Gastroenterol.*, 7, 337–343.

NELSON, L.W., KELLY, W.A. and WEIKEL, J.H. (1972): Mesovarial leiomyomas in rats in a chronic toxicity study of musuprine hydrochloride. *Toxicol.Appl.Pharmacol.*, 23, 731–737.

NEWBERNE, P.M., CONNER, M.W. and ESTES, P. (1988). The influence of food additives and related materials on lower bowel structure and function. *Toxicol.Pathol.*, 16, 184–197.

NICOLSON, G.L. (1974): The interactions of lectins with animal cell surfaces. *Int.Rev.Cytol.*, 39, 89–190.

NODA, Y., TAKI, Y., HIKOSAKA, N., MEENAGHAN, M.A. and MORI, M. (1986): Immunohistochemical localization of carbonic anhydrase in submandibular salivary glands of mice and hamsters treated with phenylephrine, testosterone or duct ligation. *Arch.Oral Biol.*, 31, 441–447.

O'ROURKE, J., LEE, A. and McNEILL, J. (1988): Differences in the gastro-intestinal microbiota of specific pathogen free mice: an often unknown variable in biomedical research. *Lab.Anim.* 22, 297–303.

ODASHIMA, S. (1979): Tumours of the oral cavity, pharynx, oesophagus and stomach. In: V.S. Turusov (Ed.), *Pathology of Tumours in Laboratory Animals. Tumours of the Mouse*, pp. 147–167. IARC Scientific Publ. No. 23, Lyon.

OGASAWARA, T., HOENSCH, H. and OHNHAUS, E.E. (1985): Distribution of glutathione and its related enzymes in small intestinal mucosa of rats. *Arch.Toxicol.*, Suppl 8, 110–113.

OLOVSON, S.G., BJÖRKMAN, J.A., Ek, L. and HAVU, N. (1983): The ulcerogenic effect on the oesophagus of three β-adrenoceptor antagonists, investigated in a new porcine oesophagus test model. *Acta.Pharmacol.Toxicol.*(Copenh), 53, 385–391.

OLUBUYIDE, I.O., WILLIAMSON, R.C.N., BRISTOL, J.B. and READ, A.E. (1984): Goblet cell hyperplasia is a feature of the adaptive response to jejunoileal bypass in rats. *Gut*, 25, 62–68.

OOHASHI, Y., ISHIOKA, T., WAKABAYASHI, K. and KUWABARA, N. (1981): A study on carcinogenesis induced by degraded carrageenan arising from squamous metaplasia of the rat colorectum. *Cancer Lett.*, 14, 267–272.

OVERVOLD, C.R., SMITH, R.B., PAIKOWSKY, S.J. and HALE, M.H. (1987): Entero-hepatic cycling in rats plays a major role in fatal NSAID intestinal ulcerogenicity. *Toxicol.Pathol.*, 15, 373.

OWEN, R.L. (1977): Sequential uptake of horseradish peroxidase by lymphoid follicle epithelium of Peyer's patches in the normal unobstructed mouse intestine: an ultrastructural study. *Gastroenterology*, 72, 440–450.

OWEN, R.L. and BHALLA, D.K. (1983): Cytochemical analysis of alkaline phosphatase and esterase activities and of lectin-binding and anionic sites in rat and mouse Peyer's patch M cells. *Am.J.Anat.*, 168, 199–212.

OWEN, R.L. and NEMANIC, P. (1978): Antigen processing structures of the mammalian intestinal tract: an SEM study of lymphoepithelial organs. In: R.P. Becker and O. Johari (Eds), *Scanning Electron Microscopy* Part II, pp. 367–378. Scanning Electron Microscopy Inc., AMF O'Hare Ill.

OWENS, A.H. Jr. (1962): Predicting anticancer drug effects in man from laboratory animal studies. *J.Chronic.Dis.*, 15, 223–228.

PABST, R. (1987): The anatomical basis for the immune function of the gut. *Anat.Embryol.*(Berl.), 176, 135–144.

PARK, C.M., REID, P.E., OWEN, D.A., SANKER, J.M. and APPLEGRATH, D.A. (1987): Morphological and histochemical changes in intestinal mucosa in the reserpine-treated rat model of cystic fibrosis. *Exp.Mol.Pathol.*, 47, 1–12.

PARKER, F.G., BARNES, E.N. and KAYE, G.I. (1974): The pericryptal fibro-blast sheath. IV. Replication, migration and differentiation of the subepithelial fibroblasts of the crypts and villus of the rabbit jejunum. *Gastroenterology*, 67, 607–621.

PEARSE, A.G.E. (1968): Histochemistry : Theoretical and Applied, Vol. 1, pp. 659–660 (3rd Edition). Churchill Livingstone, Edinburgh.

PENSTON, J. and WORMSLEY, K.G. (1986): H2-receptor antagonists and gastric cancer. *Med.Toxicol.*, 1, 163–168.

PERCY, D.H., HAYES, M.A., KOCAL, T.E. and WOJCINSKI, Z.W. (1988): Depletion of salivary gland epidermal growth factor by sialodacryoadenitis virus infection in the Wistar rat. *Vet.Pathol.*, 25, 183–192.

PERCY, D.H. and WOJCINSKI, Z.Z. (1986): Diagnostic exercise: Inter-mandibular swelling in rats. *Lab.Anim.Sci.*, 36, 665–666.

PFISTER, H. (1984): Biology and biochemistry of papillomaviruses. *Rev.Physiol.Biochem.Pharmacol.*, 99, 111–181.

PINKSTAFF, C.A. (1980): The cytology of salivary glands. *Int.Rev.Cytol.*, 63, 141–261.

PLANTEYDT, H.T. and WILLIGHAGEN, R.G.J. (1960): Enzyme histochemistry of the human stomach with special reference to intestinal metaplasia. *J.Pathol.Bacterol.*, 80, 317–322.

POCOCK, S.J. (1985): Nitrates and gastric cancer. *Hum.Toxicol.*, 4, 471–474.

PONDER, B.A.J., SCHMIDT, G.H., WILKINSON, M.M., WOOD, M.J., MONK, M. and REID, A. (1985): Derivation of mouse intestinal crypts from single progenitor cells. *Nature*, 313, 689–691.

PORT, C.D., DODD, D.C., DESLEX, P., REGNIER, B., SANDERS, P. and INDACOCHEA-REDMOND, N. (1987): Twenty-one month evaluation of misoprostol for carcinogenicity in CD-1 mice. *Toxicol.Pathol.*, 15, 134–142.

POYNTER, D., PICK, C.R., HARCOURT, R.A., SELWAY, S.A.M., AINGE, G., HARMAN, I.W.,

SPURLING, N.W., FLUCK, P.A. and COOK, J.L. (1985): Association of long lasting unsurmountable histamine H2 blockade and gastric carcinoid tumours in the rat. *Gut*, 26, 1284–1295.

POYNTER, D., SELWAY, S.A.M., PAPWORTH, S.A. and RICHES, S.R. (1986): Changes in the gastric mucosa of the mouse associated with long lasting unsurmountable histamine H2 blockade. *Gut*, 27, 1338–1346.

PRESCOTT, J.F. and MUNROE, D.L. (1982): Campylobacter jejuni enteritis in man and domestic animals. *J.Am.Vet.Med.Assoc.*, 181, 1524–1530.

PUURUNEN, J., HUTTUNEN, P. and HIRVONEN, J. (1980): Is ethanol-induced damage of the gastric mucosa a hyperosmotic effect? Comparative studies on the effects of ethanol, some other hyperosmotic solutions and acetyl-salicylic acid on rat gastric mucosa. *Acta.Pharmacol.Toxicol.(Copenh.)*, 47, 321–327.

RAINSFORD, K.D. (1975): Synergistic interaction between aspirin, or other non-steroidal anti-inflammatory drugs, and stress which produces severe gastric mucosal damage in rats and pigs. *Agents Actions*, 5, 553–558.

RAINSFORD, K.D. (1978): The effects of aspirin and other non-steroid anti-inflammatory/analgesic drugs on gastrointestinal mucus glycoprotein biosynthesis in vivo: Relationship to ulcerogenic actions. *Biochem.Pharmacol.*, 27, 877–885.

RAINSFORD, K.D., WILLIS, C.M., WALKER, S.A. and ROBINS, P.G. (1982): Electron microscopic observations comparing the gastric mucosal damage induced in rats and pigs by benoxaprofen and aspirin, reflecting their differing actions as prostaglandin-synthesis-inhibitors. *Br.J.Exp.Pathol.*, 63, 25–34.

RALL, L.B., SCOTT, J., BELL, G.I., CRAWFORD, R.J., PENSCHOW, J.D., NIALL, H.D. and COGHLAN, J.P. (1985): Mouse prepro-epidermal growth factor synthesis by kidney and other tissues. *Nature*, 313, 228–231.

RANDELIA, H.P. and LALITHA, V.S. (1988): Megaoesophagus in ICRC mice. *Lab.Anim.*,22, 23–26.

REED, K.D. and BERRIDGE, B.R. (1988): Campylobacter-like organisms in the gastric mucosa of rhesus monkeys. *Lab.Anim.Sci.*, 38, 329–333.

REED, P.I., CASSELL, P.G. and WALTERS, C.L. (1979): Gastric cancer in patients who have taken cimetidine. *Lancet*, 1, 1234–1235.

REED, P.I., SMITH, P.L.R., HAINES, K., HOUSE, F.R. and WALTERS, C.L. (1981): Effect of cimetidine on gastric juice N-nitrosamine concentration. *Lancet*, 2, 553–556.

REHG, J.E. (1985): Clostridial enteropathies, hamster. In: T.C. Jones, U. Mohr and R.D. Hunt (Eds), *Digestive System. Monographs on Pathology of Laboratory Animals*, pp. 340–346. Springer-Verlag, Berlin.

REHG, J.E., LAWTON, G.W. and PAKES, S.P. (1979): Cryptosporidium cuniculus in the rabbit (Oryctolagus cuniculus). *Lab.Anim.Sci.*, 29, 656–660.

REHG, J.E. and LU, Y.-S. (1981): Clostridium difficile colitis in a rabbit following antibiotic therapy for pasteurellosis. *J.Am.Vet.Med.Assoc.*, 179, 1296–1297.

REHG, J.E. and LU, Y.-S. (1982): Clostridium difficile typhlitis in hamsters not associated with antibiotic therapy. *J.Am.Vet.Med.Assoc.*, 181, 1422–1423.

REHG, J.E. and PAKES, S.P. (1981): Clostridium difficile antitoxin neutrali-zation of cecal toxin(s) from guinea pigs with penicillin-associated colitis. *Lab.Anim.Sci.*, 31, 156–160.

REHM, S., SOMMER, R. and DEERBERG, F. (1987): Spontaneous non-neoplastic gastric lesions in female Han: NMRI mice, and influence of food restriction throughout life. *Vet.Pathol.*, 24, 216–225.

REID, P.E., CULLING, C.F.A. and DUNN, W.L. (1973): Saponification-induced increase in the periodic-acid-Schiff reaction in the gastrointestinal tract. Mechanism and distribution of the reactive substance. *J.Histochem.Cytochem.*, 21, 473–482.

REIFEL, C.W. and TRAVILL, A.A. (1972): Structure and carbohydrate histo-chemistry of postnatal canine salivary glands. *Am.J.Anat.*, 134, 377–394.

REINHART, W.H., MÜLLER, O. and HALTER, F. (1983): Influence of long-term 16,16-dimethyl prostaglandin E2 treatment on the rat gastrointestinal mucosa. *Gastroenterology*, 85, 1003–1010.

RERAT, A. (1978): Digestion and absorption of carbohydrate and nitrogeneous matter in hindgut of the omnivorous non-reminant animal. *J.Anim.Sci.*, 46, 1808–1837.

REUTERVING, C.O., HÄGG, E., HENRIKSSON, R. and HOLM, J. (1987): Salivary glands in long-term alloxan-diabetic rats. A quantitative light and electron-microscopic study. *Acta.Pathol.Microbiol.Immunol.Scand.[A]*, 95, 131–136.

RHODIN, J.A.G. (1974): Digestive system: intestines. In: *Histology. A Text and Atlas.*, Chap. 29, pp. 554–577. Oxford University Press, New York.

RIDDELL, R.H. (1982): The gastrointestinal tract. In: *Pathology of Drug-Induced and Toxic Diseases*, Chap. 8, pp. 515–606. Churchill Livingstone, New York.

RIDDELL, R.H., GOLDMAN, H., RANSOHOFF, D.F., APPELMAN, H.D., FENOGLIO, C.M., HAGGITT, R.C., ÅHREN, C., CORREA, P., HAMILTON, S.R., MORSON, B.C., SOMMERS, S.C. and YARDLEY, J.H. (1983): Dysplasia in inflammatory bowel disease: Standardized classification with provisional clinical applications. *Hum.Pathol.*, 14, 931–968.

RIEKEN, E.O. and PEARSE, A.G.E. (1966): Histochemical study on the Paneth cell in the rat. *Gut*, 7, 86–93.

ROBINS, P.G. (1980): Ultrastructural observations on the pathogenesis of aspirin-induced gastric erosions. *Br.J.Exp.Pathol.*, 61, 497–504.

ROBINSON, M. (1985): Dietary related periodontitis and oro-nasal fistulation in rats. *J.Comp.Pathol.*, 95, 489–498.

ROBINSON, P.B., HARRIS, M. and HARVEY, W. (1983): Abnormal skeletal and dental growth in epileptic children. *Br.Dent.J.*, 154, 9–13.

ROBINSON, P.B. and HARVEY, W. (1989): Tooth root resorption induced in rats by diphenylhydantoin and parathyroidectomy. *Br.J.Exp.Pathol.*, 70, 65–72.

RODNING, C.B., ERLANSEN, S.L., WILSON, I.D. and CARPENTER, A.-M. (1983): Light microscopic morphometric analysis of rat ileal mucosa. I. Component quantitation of IgA-containing immunocytes. *Dig.Dis.Sci.*, 28, 742–750.

RODRIGUES, C., LOK, E., NERA, E., IVERSON, F., PAGE, D., KARPINSKI, K. and CLAYSON, D.B. (1986): Short-term effects of various phenols and acids on the Fischer 344 male forestomach epithelium. *Toxicology*, 38, 103–117.

ROE, F.J.C. (1984): Do detergents damage the gut? *Lancet*, 2, 525.

ROE, F.J.C. and BÄR, A. (1985): Enzootic and epizootic adrenal medullary proliferative diseases of rats: Influence of dietary factors which affect calcium absorption. *Hum.Toxicol.*, 4, 2752.

ROGERS, S., BARSOUM, N., DIFONZO, C., GRACON, S., HOUSTON, B., MARTIN, R., SMITH, G., STURGESS, J. and DE LA IGLESIA, F. (1985): Intravenous toxicology of a new cardiotonic agent. Toxicologist, 5, 111.

ROUVROY, D., BOGAERTS, J., NSENGIUMWA, O., OMAR, M., VERSAILLES, L., and HAOT, J. (1987): Campylobacter pylori, gastritis, and peptic ulcer disease in central Africa. *Br.Med.J.*, 295, 1174.

ROWLAND, I.R. (1988): Interactions of the gut microflora and the host in toxicology. *Toxicol.Pathol.*, 16, 147–153.

ROWLAND, I.R., MALLETT, A.K. and WISE, A. (1986): The effect of diet on the mammalian gut flora and its metabolic activities. *CRC Crit.Rev.Toxicol.*, 16, 31–103.

ROWLATT, C. and CHESTERMAN, F.C. (1979): Tumors of the intestines and peritoneum. In: V.S. Turusov (Ed.), *Pathology of Tumours in Laboratory Animals. Tumours of the Mouse*, Vol. 2, pp. 169–191. IARC Scientific Publ No. 23, Lyon.

ROWLATT, C., FRANKS, L.M., SHERIFF, M.U. and CHESTERMAN, F.C. (1969): Naturally occurring tumors and other lesions of the digestive tract in untreated C57BL mice. *J.N.C.I.*, 43, 1353–1368.

RUBEN, Z., ROHRBACHER, E. and MILLER, J.E. (1983): Esophageal impaction in BHE rats. *Lab.Anim.Sci.*, 33, 63–65.

RUBIO, C.A., NYLANDER, G., SVEANDER, M., DUVANDER, A. and ALUN, M.-L. (1986): Minimal invasive carcinoma of the colon in rats. *Am.J.Pathol.*, 123, 161–165.

RÜDIGER, H. (1982): Phytohemagglutinins. *Planta Medica.*, 46, 3–9.

SAGSTRÖM, S., SCARLETT, S.M., SAGULIN, G.B. and ROOMANS, G.M. (1987): Early effects of alloxan on rat submandibular gland. *J.Submicrosc.Cytol.*, 19, 555–559.

SANDOW, J.M. and WHITEHEAD, R. (1979): The Paneth cell. *Gut*, 20, 420–431.

SARNA, S.K. (1985): Cyclic motor activity; migrating motor complex: 1985. *Gastroenterology*, 89, 894–913.

SASHIMA, M. (1986): Age-related changes of rat submandibular gland: A morphometric and ultrastructural study. *J.Oral Pathol.*, 15, 507–512.

SATOH, H., INADA, I., HIRATA, T. and MAK, Y. (1981): Indomethacin produces gastric antral ulcers in the refed rat. *Gastroenterology*, 81, 719–725.

SATOH, Y., ISHIKAWA, K., TANAKA, H. and ONO, K. (1986): Immunohistochemical observations of immunoglobin A in the Paneth cells of germ-free and formerly-germ-free rats. *Histochemistry*, 85, 197–201.

SATOH, Y. and VOLLRATH, L. (1986): Quantitative electron microscopic observations on Paneth cells of germ-free and ex-germ-free Wistar rats. *Anat.Embryol.(Berl.)*, 173, 317–322.

SAVAGE, N.W., BARBER, M.T. and ADKINS, K.F. (1986): Pigmentary changes in the rat oral mucosa following antimalaria therapy. *J.Oral Pathol.*, 15, 468–471.

SAWREY, J.M. and SAWREY, W.L. (1986): Age, weight and social effects on ulceration in rats. *J.Comp.Psychol.*, 61, 464–466.

SCHEIN, P.S., DAVIS, R.D., CARTER, S., NEWMAN, J., SCHEIN, D.R. and RALL, D.P. (1970): The evaluation of anticancer drugs in dogs and monkeys for the prediction of qualitative toxicities in man. *Clin.Pharmacol.Ther.*, 11, 3–40.

SCHMEISER, H.H., POOL, B.L. and WIESSLER, M. (1986): Identification and mutagenicity of metabolites of aristolochic acid formed by rat liver. *Carcinogenesis*, 7, 59–63.

SCHRODT, G.R. (1963): Melanosis coli: A study with the electron micro-scope. *Dis.Colon Rectum*, 6, 277–283.

SCHULTE, B.A. (1987): Genetic and sex-related differences in the structure of submandibular glycoconjugates. *J.Dent.Res.*, 62, 442–450.

SCHULTE, B.A. and SPICER, S.S. (1983): Light microscopic detection of sugar residues in glycoconjugates of salivary glands and the pancreas with lectin-horseradish peroxidase conjugates. I. Mouse. *Histochem.J.*, 15, 1217–1238.

SCHULTE, B.A. and SPICER, S.S. (1984): Light microscopic detection of sugar residues in glycoconjugates of salivary glands and the pancreas with lectin-horseradish peroxidase conjugates. II. Rat. *Histochem.J.*, 16, 3–20.

SCOTT, G.B.D. (1982): Mucosal microhernias in the nonhuman primate colon: Their role in the pathogenesis of colonic disease. *Vet.Pathol.*, 19 (Suppl 7), 134–140.

SCOTT, J. (1977): Quantitative age changes in the histological structure of human submandibular salivary glands. *Arch.Oral Biol.*, 22, 221–227.

SELBY, W.S., JANOSSY, G. and JEWELL, D.P. (1981): Immunohistological characterization of intra-epithelial lymphocytes of the human gastro-intestinal tract. *Gut*, 22, 169–176.

SERONDE, J. Jr (1965): Chronic duodenal ulcers in pantothenate deficient mice. *Gastroenterology*, 48, 612–615.

SERONDE, J. Jr (1970): Focal avillous hyperplasia of the mouse duodenum. *J.Pathol.*, 100, 245–248.

SHAMSUDDIN, A.K.M. and TRUMP, B.F. (1981)a: Colon epithelium. I. Light microscopic, histochemical, and ultrastructural features of normal colon epithelium of male Fischer 344 rats. *J.N.C.I.*, 66, 375–388.

SHAMSUDDIN, A.K.M. and TRUMP, B.F. (1981)b: Colon epithelium. II. In vivo studies of colon carcinogenesis. Light microscopic, histochemical, and ultrastructural studies of histogenesis of azoxymethane-induced colon carcinomas in Fischer 344 rats. *J.N.C.I.*, 66, 389–401.

SHAMSUDDIN, A.K.M. and TRUMP, B.F. (1981)c: Two types of mucous cells in the colon crypt. *J.N.C.I.*, 67, 747.

SHARRATT, M., GRASSO, P., CARPANINI, F. and GANGOLLI, S.D. (1970): Carrageenan ulceration as a model for human ulcerative colitis. *Lancet*, 2, 932.

SHEAHAN, D.G. and JARVIS, H.R. (1976): Comparative histochemistry of gastro-intestinal mucosubstances. *Am.J.Anat.*, 146, 103–132.

SHEPHARD, S.E., SCHLATTER, C.H. and LUTZ, W.K. (1987): Assessment of risk of formulation of carcinogenic N-nitroso compounds from dietary precursors in the stomach. *Food Chem.Toxicol.*, 25, 91–108.

SHEPHERD, N.A., DAWSON, A.M., CROCKER, P.R. and LEVISON, D.A. (1987): Granular cells as a marker of early amiodarone hepatotoxicity: a patho-logical and analytical study. *J.Clin.Pathol.*, 40, 418–423.

SHIRAI, T., TAKAHASHI, M., FUKUSHIMA, S. and ITO, N. (1985): Marked epithelial hyperplasia of the rat glandular stomach induced by long-term administration of iodoacetamide. *Acta.Pathol.Jpn.*, 35, 35–43.

SHRIVER, D.A., WHITE, C.B., SANDOR, A. and ROSENTHALE, M.E. (1975): A profile of the gastrointestinal toxicity of drugs used to treat inflammatory diseases. *Toxicol.Appl.Pharmacol.*, 32, 73–83.

SIMSON, J.A.V., SPICER, S.S. and HALL, B.J. (1974): Morphology and cyto-chemistry of rat salivary gland acinar secretory granules and their alteration by isoproterenol. I. Parotid gland. *J.Ultrastr.Res.*, 48, 465–482.

SITHIGORNGUL, P., BURTON, P., NISHIHATA, T. and CALDWELL, L. (1983): Effects of sodium salicylate on epithelial cells of the rectal mucosa of the rat: A light and electron microscopic study. *Life Sci.*, 33, 1025–1032.

SMITH, B. and BUTLER, M. (1978): The effects of long-term propranolol on the salivary glands and intestinal mucosa of the mouse. *J.Pathol.*, 124, 185–187.

SMITH, G.S., BARSOUM, N.J., DIFONZO, C.J., MCEWEN, B.J., MACALLUM, G.E. and GREAVES, P. (1988): Effects of cardiotonic phosphodiesterase inhibitors on rat salivary gland. Presented at the 39th Annual ACVP meeting, Kansas.

SMITH J.H., KISIC, A., DIAZ-ARRASTIA, R., PELLY, R.P. and SCHROEPFER, G.J. (1989). Inhibitors of sterol synthesis. Morphological studies in rats after dietary administration, administration of 5 α-cholest-8(14)-en-3β-ol-15-one, a potent hypocholesterolemic compound. *Toxicol.Pathol.*, 17, 506–515.

SMITH, M.W., JAMES, P.S. and TIVEY, D.R. (1987): M cell numbers increase after transfer of SPF mice to a normal animal house environment. *Am.J.Pathol.*, 128, 385–389.

SNELL, K.C. (1967): Renal diseases of the rat. In: E. Cotchin and F.J.C. Roe (Eds), *Pathology of Laboratory Rats and Mice*, Chap. 5, pp. 105–145. Blackwell Scientific, Oxford.

SNIPES, R.L. (1981): Anatomy of the cecum of the laboratory mouse and rat. *Anat.Embryol* (Berl.), 162, 455–474.

SOLCIA, E., CAPELLA, C., SESSA, F., RINDI, G., CORNAGGIA, M., RIVA, C. and VILLANI, L. (1986): Gastric carcinoids and related endocrine growths. *Digestion*, 35, Suppl 1, 3–22.

SOLL, A.H. (1990). Pathogenesis of peptic ulcer and implications for therapy. *N.Engl.J.Med.*, 322, 909–916.

SPEECE, A.J. (1964): Histochemical distribution of lysozyme activity in organs of normal mice and radiation chimeras. *J.Histochem.Cytochem.*, 12, 384–391.

SPENCER, J., FINN, T. and ISAACSON, P.G. (1986): Human Peyer's patches: an immuno-histochemical study. *Gut*, 27, 405–410.

SPICER, S.S. (1965): Diamine methods for differentiating mucosubstances histochemically. *J.Histochem.Cytochem.*, 13, 211–234.

ST. JOHN, D.J.B., YEOMANS, N.D., BOURNE, C.A.J. and de BOER, W.G.R.M. (1977): Aspirin-induced glandular dysplasia of the stomach. Histologic and histochemical studies in rats. *Arch.Pathol.Lab Med.*, 101, 44–48.

STEER, H.W. (1984): Surface morphology of the gastroduodenal mucosa in duodenal ulceration. *Gut*, 25, 1203–1210.

STEER, H.W. and COLIN-JONES, D.G. (1975): Melanosis coli: Studies of the toxic effects of irritant purgatives. *J.Pathol.*, 115, 199–205.

STENE, T. and KOPPANG, H.S. (1976): The effect of vincristine on dentino-genesis in the rat incisor. *Scand.J.Dent.Res.*, 84, 342–344.

STENE, T. and KOPPANG, H.S. (1980): Autoradiographic investigation of dentine production in rats incisors after vincristine administration. *Scand.J.Dent.Res.*, 88, 104–112.

STEPHENS, L.C., KING, G.K., PETERS, L.J., ANG, K.K., SCHULTHEISS, T.E. and JARDINE, J.H. (1986)a: Acute and late radiation injury in rhesus monkey parotid glands. Evidence of interphase death. *Am.J.Pathol.*, 124, 469–478.

STEPHENS, L.C., KING, G.K., PETERS, L.J., ANG, K.K., SCHULTHEISS, T.E. and JARDINE, J.H. (1986)b: Unique radiosensitivity of serous cells in rhesus monkey submandibular glands. *Am.J.Pathol.*, 124, 479–487.

STEWART, H.L. and ANDERVONT, H.B. (1938): Pathologic observations on the adenomatous lesions of the stomach in mice of strain I. *Arch.Pathol.*, 26, 1009–1022.

STEWART, H.L., SNELL, K.C., MORRIS, H.P., WAGNER, B.P. and RAY, F.E. (1961): Carcinoma of the glandular stomach of rats ingesting N,N'2,7-fluorenyl-bisacetamine. *N.C.I.Monogr.*, 5, 105–139.

STEWART, T.H.M., HETENYI, C., ROWSELL, H. and ORIZAGA, M. (1980): Ulcerative enterocolitis in dogs induced by drugs. *J.Pathol.*, 131, 363–378.

STRAGAND, J.J. and HAGEMANN, R.F. (1977): Effect of lumenal contents on colonic cell replacement. *Am.J.Physiol.*, 233, E208-E211.

STREETT, C.S., CIMPRICH, R.E. and ROBERTSON, J.L. (1984): Pathologic findings in the stomach of rats treated with the H2-receptor antagonist tiotidine. *Scand.J.Gastroenterol.*, 19 (Suppl 101), 109–117.

STREETT, C.S., ROBERTSON, J.L. and CRISSMAN, R.E. (1988): Morphologic stomach findings in rats and mice treated with the H2-receptor antagonists, ICI 125211 and ICI 162846. *Toxicol.Pathol.*, 16, 299–304.

SUGANUMA, T., TSUYAMA, S., SUZUKI, S. and MURATA, F. (1984): Lectin-peroxidase reactivity in rat gastric mucosa. *Arch.Histol.Jpn.*, 47, 197–207.

SUGIMURA, T. and FUJIMURA, S. (1967): Tumour production in glandular stomach of rat by N-methyl-N'-nitro-N-nitrosoguanidine. *Nature*, 216, 943–944.

SUN, J. and STROBEL, H.W. (1986): Aging affects the drug metabolism systems of rat liver, kidney, colon and lung in a differential fashion. *Exp.Gerontol.*, 21, 523–534.

SUNDBERG, J.P. and EVERITT, J.I. (1986): Diagnostic exercise: Lingual growths in rabbits. *Lab.Anim.Sci.*, 36, 499–500.

SUNDBERG, J.P., JUNGE, R.E. and EL SHAZLY, M.O. (1985): Oral papillomatosis in New Zealand white rabbits. *Am.J.Vet.Res.*, 46, 664–668.

SUNDBERG, J.P., JUNGE, R.E. and LANCASTER, W.D. (1984): Immunoperoxidase localization of papillomaviruses in hyperplastic and neoplastic epithelial lesions of animals. *Am.J.Vet.Res.*, 45, 1441–1446.

SUNDLER, F., HÄKANSON, R., CARLSSON, E., LARSSON, H. and MATTSSON, H. (1986): Hypergastrinemia after blockade of acid secretion in the rat. Trophic effects. *Digestion*, 35, Suppl 1, 56–69.

SUNTER, J.P., APPLETON, D.R., WRIGHT, N.A. and WATSON, A.J. (1978): Patho-logical features of the colonic tumors induced in rats by the administration of 1,2-dimethylhydrazine. *Virchows Arch.[B].*, 29, 211–223.

SUWA, T., URANO, H., KOHNO, Y., SUZUKI, A. and AMANO, T. (1987): Comparative studies on the gastrointestinal lesions caused by several non-steroidal anti-inflammatory agents in the rats. *Agents Actions*, 21, 167–172.

SUZUKI, Y., TAGUCHI, O., KOJIMA, A., MATSUYAMA, M. and NISHIZUKA, Y. (1981): Fine structure of giant hypertrophic gastritis developed in thymectomized mice. *Lab.Invest.*, 45, 209–217.

SUZUKI, S., TSUYAMA, S. and MURATA, F. (1983): Cells intermediate between mucous neck cells and chief cells in rat stomach. *Cell Tissue Res.*, 233, 475–484.

SYRJAMEN, S.M. and SYRJAMEN, K.J. (1979): Hyperplastic gingivitis in a child receiving sodium valproate treatment. *Proc.Finn.Dent. Soc.*, 75, 95–98.

SZABO, S. (1979): Dopamine disorderin duodenal ulceration. *Lancet*, 11, 880–882.

SZABO, S. (1984): Biology of disease. Pathogenesis of duodenal ulcer disease. *Lab Invest.*, 51, 121–147.

SZABO, S. and CHO, C.H. (1988): From cysteamine to MPTP: Structure-activity studies with duodenal ulcerogens. *Toxicol.Pathol.*, 16, 205–212.

SZENTIRMAY, Z. and SUGAR, J. (1985): Adenocarcinoma, glandular stomach, rat. In: T.C. Jones, U. Mohr and R.D. Hunt (Eds), *Digestive System. Mono-graphs on Pathology of Laboratory Animals*, pp. 301–309. Springer-Verlag, Berlin.

TABAK, L.A., LEVINE, M.J., MANDEL, I.D. and ELLISON, S.A. (1982): Role of salivary mucins in the protection of the oral cavity. *J.Oral Pathol.*, 11, 1–17.

TABATA, K. and OKABE, S. (1980): Effects of 16,16-dimethyl prostaglandin E2-methyl ester on aspirin- and indomethacin-induced gastrointestinal lesions in dogs. *Dig.Dis.Sci.*, 25, 439–448.

TAKEDA, Y., SUZUKI, A. and ISHIKAWA, G. (1985): Nodular hyperplasia of oncocytes in mouse submandibular glands. *J.Oral Pathol.*, 14, 182–189.

TAKEUCHI, A. (1982): Early colonic lesions in experimental shigella infections in rhesus monkeys: Revisited. *Vet.Pathol.*, 19, Suppl 7, 1–8.

TEAGUE, C.A., GAVIN, J.B. and HERDSON, P.B. (1981): The response of three inbred strains of rat to the carcinogen 1,2-dimethylhydrazine. *Pathology*, 13, 473–485.

TEGLBJAERG, P.S. and NIELSON, H.O. (1978): 'Small intestinal type' and 'colonic type' intestinal metaplasia of the human stomach and their relationship to the histogenetic types of gastric adenocarcinoma. *Acta.Pathol.Microbiol.Scand.*[A], 86, 351–355.

THOMOPOULOS, G.N., SHULTE, B.A. and SPICER, S.S. (1983): Light and electron microscopic cytochemistry of glycoconjugates in the recto-sigmoid colonic epithelium of the mouse and rat. *Am.J.Anat.*, 168, 239–256.

THOMPSON, G.R., BAKER, J.R., FLEISCHMAN, R.W., ROSENKRANZ, H., SHAEPPI, U.H., COONEY, D.A. and DAVIS, R.D. (1972): Preclinical toxicologic evaluation of bleomycin (NSC 125 006), a new anti-tumor antibiotic. *Toxicol.Appl.Pharmacol.*, 22, 544–555.

TOFT, J.D. (1982): The pathoparasitology of the alimentary tract and pancreas of non-human primates: A review. *Vet.Pathol.*, 19, Suppl 7, 44–92.

TSIFTSIS, D., JASS, J.R., FILIPE, M.I. and WASTELL, C. (1980): Altered patterns of mucin secretion in the precancerous lesions induced in the glandular part of the rat stomach by the carcinogen N-methyl-N'-nitro-N-nitrosoguanidine. *Invest.Cell Pathol.*, 3, 399–408.

TSUKITANI, K. and MORI, M. (1986): Immunohistochemistry and radioimmunoassay of EGF in submandibular glands of mice treated with secretogogues. *Cell Mol.Biol.*, 32, 677–683.

TUCKER, W.E. Jr., MACKLIN, A.W., SZOT, R.J., JOHNSON, R.E., ELION, G.B., de MIRANDA, P. and SZCZECH, G.M. (1983): Preclinical toxicology studies with acyclovir: Acute and subchronic tests. *Fundam.Appl.Toxicol.*, 3, 573–578.

TUTTON, P.J.M. and HELME, R.D. (1974): The influence of adrenoreceptor activity on crypt cell proliferation in rat jejunum. *Cell Tissue Kinet.*, 7, 125–136.

TYZZER, E.E. (1907): A sporozoan found in the peptic glands of the common mouse. *Proc.Soc.Exp.Biol.Med.*, 5, 12–13.

VAN ESCH, E., DREEF-VAN DER MEULEN, H.C. and FERON, V.J. (1986): Spontaneous hyperplastic and metaplastic duct epithelium in the sublingual salivary glands of Wistar rats. *Lab.Anim.*, 20, 127–131.

VAN HOOSIER, G.L. Jr., SPJUT, H.J. and TRENTIN, J.J. (1971): Spontaneous tumors of the Syrian hamster: Observations in a closed breeding colony and a review of the literature. In: *Defining the Laboratory Animal. IVth Symposium International Committee on Laboratory Animals and Institute of Laboratory Animal Resources*. National Research Council, pp. 450–473. National Academy of Sciences, Washington.

VAN LEEUWEN, P.A.M., DRUKKER, J., VAN DER KLEYN, N.M., VAN DEN BOOGAARD, A.E.J.M. and SOETERS, P.B. (1986): Morphological effects of high dose neomycin sulphate on the small and large intestine. *Acta.Morphol.Neerl Scand.*, 24, 223–234.

VANDERBERGHE, J., VERHEYEN, A., LAUWERS, S. and GEBOES, K. (1985): Spontaneous adenocarcinoma of the ascending colon in Wistar rats: The intracytoplasmic presence of a Campylobacter-like bacterium. *J.Comp.Pathol.*, 95, 45–55.

VANE, J.R. (1971): Inhibition of prostaglandin synthesis as a mechanism of action of aspirin-like drugs. *Nature*, 231, 232–235.

390

VIC, P., GOUY, D., LACHERETZ, F., VERSCHUERE, B., CROS, M., REMANDET, J., BERTHE, J. and MAZUE, G. (1985): Intestinal pathology in the dog induced by sublethal doses of amiodarone. *Arch.Toxicol.*, Suppl 8, 104–109.

VISSCHER, G.E., ROBINSON, R.L. and HARTMAN, H.A. (1980): Chemically induced lipidosis of the small intestinal villi in the rat. *Toxicol.Appl.Pharmacol.*, 55, 535–544.

WAGGIE, K.S., THORNBURG, L.P., GROVE, K.J. and WAGNER, J.E. (1987): Lesions of experimentally induced Tyzzer's disease in Syrian hamsters, guinea pigs, mice and rats. *Lab.Anim.*, 21, 155–160.

WAGNER, J.E., DOYLE, R.E., RONALD, N.C., GARRISON, R.C. and SCHMITZ, J.A. (1974): Hexamitis in laboratory mice, hamsters, and rats. *Lab.Anim.Sci.*, 24, 349–354.

WALKER, N.I., BENNETT, R.E. and AXELSEN, R.A. (1988): Melanosis coli: A consequence of anthraquinone-induced apoptosis of colonic epithelial cells. *Am.J.Pathol.*, 131, 465–476.

WALKER, T.F., WHITEHEAD, S.M., LESLIE, G.B., CREAN, G.P. and ROE, F.J.C. (1987): Safety evaluation of cimetidine: Report at the termination of a seven-year study in dogs. *Hum.Toxicol.*, 6, 159–164.

WALSH, K.M. and GOUGH, A.W. (1989): Hypopigmentation in dogs treated with an inhibitor of platelet aggregation. *Toxicol.Pathol.*, 17, 549–554.

WANER, T., NYSKA, A., NYSKA, M., PIRAK, M., SELA, M. and GALIANO, A. (1988): Gingival hyperplasia in dogs induced by oxodipine, a calcium channel blocking agent. *Toxicol.Pathol.*, 16, 327–332.

WARD, J.M. (1974): Morphogenesis of chemically induced neoplasms of the colon and small intestine in rats. *Lab Invest.*, 30, 505–513.

WARD, J.M., RICE, J.M., ROLLER, P.P. and WENK, M.L. (1977): Natural history of intestinal neoplasms induced in rats by a single injection of methyl(acetoxymethyl) nitrosamine. *Cancer Res.*, 37, 3046–3052.

WARD, J.M. (1985): Proliferative lesions of the glandular stomach and liver in F344 rats fed diets containing aroclor 1254. *Environ. Health Perspect.*, 60, 89–95.

WARD, F.W. and COATES, M.E. (1987): Gastrointestinal pH measurement in rats: Influence of microbial flora, diet and fasting. *Lab.Anim*, 216–222.

WATANABE, H. (1978): Experimentally induced intestinal metaplasia in Wistar rats by X-ray irradition. *Gastroenterology*, 75, 796–799.

WATANABE, H., FUJII, I. and TERADA, Y. (1980): Induction of intestinal metaplasia in the rat gastric mucosa by local X-irradiation. *Pathol.Res.Pract.*, 70, 104–114.

WATANABE, H., NAITO, M. and ITO, A. (1984)a: The effect of sex difference on induction of intestinal metaplasia in rats. *Acta.Pathol.Jpn.*, 32, 305–312.

WATANABE, K., REDDY, B.S., WONG, C.Q. and WEISBURGER, J.H. (1978): Effect of dietary undegraded carrageenan on colon carcinogenesis in F344 treated with azoxymethane or methylnitrosourea. *Cancer Res.*, 38, 4427–4430.

WATANABE, T., TAGUCHI, Y., SHIOSAKA, S., TANAKA, J., KUBOTA, H., TERANO, Y., TOHYAMA, M. and WADA, H. (1984)b: Distribution of the histaminergic neuron system in the central nervous system of rats; a fluorescent immunohistochemical analysis with histidine decarboxylase as a marker. *Brain Res.*, 295, 13–25.

WATERHOUSE, J.P., CHISOLM, D.M., WINTER, R.B., PATEL, M. and YALE, R.S. (1973): Replacement of functional parenchymal cells by fat and connective tissue in human submandibular salivary glands. An age-related change. *J.Oral Pathol.*, 2, 16–27.

WATRACH, A.M., SMALL, E. and CASE, M.T. (1970): Canine papilloma: Progression of oral papilloma to carcinoma. *J.N.C.I.*, 45, 915–920.

WEISBROTH, S.H. (1979): Bacterial and mycotic disease. In: H.J. Baker, J.R. Lindsey and S.H. Weisbroth (Eds), *The Laboratory Rat, Biology and Diseases*, Vol. 1, Chap. 9, pp. 191–241. Academic Press, New York.

WELBURY, R.R., CRAFT, A.N., MURRAY, J.J. and KERNAHAN, J. (1984): Dental health of survivors of malignant disease. *Arch.Dis.Child.*, 59, 1186–1187.

WELLS, D.J. and HUMPHREYS-BEHER, M.G. (1985): Analysis of protein synthesis in rat salivary glands after chronic treatment with β-receptor agonists and phosphodiesterase inhibitors. *Biochem.Pharmacol.*, 34, 4229–4237.

WELLS, G.A.H. (1971): Mucinous carcinoma of the ileum in the rat. *J.Pathol.*, 103, 271–275.

WELLS, M., STEWART, M. and DIXON, M.F. (1982): Mucin histochemistry of gastric intestinal metaplasia. *J.Pathol.*, 137, 70–71.

WESTWOOD, F.R., ISWARAN, T.J. and GREAVES, P. (1990): Long-term effects of an inotropic phosphodiesterase inhibitor (ICI 153,110) on the rat salivary gland and intestinal mucosa. (In preparation).

WETZEL, M.G., WETZEL, B.K. and SPICER, S.S. (1966): Ultrastructural localization of acid mucosubstances in the mouse colon with iron-containing stains. *J.Cell Biol.*, 30, 299–315.

WHITTLE, B.J.R. (1981): Temporal relationship between cyclooxygenase inhibition, as measured by prostacyclin biosynthesis, and the gastro-intestinal damage induced by indomethacin in the rat. *Gastroenterology*, 80, 94–98.

WHITTLE, B.J.R., HIGGS, G.A., EAKINS, K.E., MONCADA, S. and VANE, J.R. (1980): Selective inhibition of prostaglandin production in inflammatory exudates and gastric mucosa. *Nature*, 284, 271–273.

WHITTLE, B.J.R. and VANE, J.R. (1984): A biochemical basis for the gastro-intestinal toxicity of non-steroid antirheumatoid drugs. *Arch.Toxicol.*, Suppl 7, 315–322.

WILLEMS, G. and LEHY, T. (1975): Radioautographic and quantitative studies on parietal and peptic cell kinetics in the mouse: A selective effect of gastrin on parietal cell proliferation. *Gastroenterology*, 69, 416–426.

WILLIAMSON, R.C.N. (1978)a: Intestinal adaptation. Structural, functional and cytokinetic changes. *N.Engl.J.Med.*, 298, 1393–1402.

WILLIAMSON, R.C.N. (1978)b: Intestinal adaptation. Mechanisms of control. *N.Engl.J.Med.*, 298, 1444–1450.

WINGREN, U. and ENERBÄCK, L. (1983): Mucosal mast cells of the rat intestine: a re-evaluation of fixation and staining properties, with special reference to protein blocking and solubility of the granular glycosaminoglycan. *Histochem.J.*, 15, 571–582.

WISE, A., MALLETT, A.K. and ROWLAND, I.R. (1986): Effect of mixtures of dietary fibres on the enzyme activity of the rat caecal microflora. *Toxicology*, 38, 241–248.

WITZEL, L., HALTER, F., OLAH, A.J. and HÄCKI, W.H. (1977): Effect of prolonged metiamide medication on the fundic mucosa. *Gastroenterology*, 73, 797–803.

WOLF, J.L. and BYE, W.A. (1984): The membraneous epithelial (M) cell and the mucosal immune system. *Annu.Rev.Med.*, 35, 95–112.

WORLD HEALTH ORGANIZATION (1978): Nitrosatable drugs: an assessment of the risks. *Drug Information Report*, PD/Dl/78.2, pp. 4–8.

WORMSLEY, K.G. (1984): Assessing the safety of drugs for the long-term treatment of peptic ulcers. *Gut*, 25, 1416–1423.

WYLLIE, E., WYLLIE, R., CRUSE, R.P., ROTHNER, A.D. and ERENBERG, G. (1986): The mechanism of mitrazepam-induced drooling and aspiration. *N.Engl.J.Med.*, 314, 35–38.

YAMAGUCHI, K. and SCHOEFL, G.I. (1983): Blood vessels of the Peyer's patch in the mouse. III High endothelial venules. *Anat.Rec.*, 206, 419–438.

YAMAMOTO, T. (1982): Ultrastructural basis of intestinal absorption. *Arch.Histol.Jpn.*, 45, 1–22.

YASHIRO, K., KAMEYAMA, Y., MIZUNO, M. and YOKOTA, Y. (1987): Alteration of membrane phospholipids in hypertrophied rat salivary glands induced by chronic administration of isoproterenol. *Arch.Oral Biol.*, 32, 799–805.

YOSHITOMI, K., MARONPOT, R.R., SOLLEVELD, H.A., BOORMAN, G.A. and EUSTIS, S.L. (1986): Forestomach ulcers in Crj:B6C3 (C57BL/6NCrj x C3H/HeNCrj) F1 mice. *Lab.Anim.Sci.*, 36, 501–503.

YOUNG, J.D., HURST, W.J., WHITE, W.J. and LANG, C.M. (1987): An evaluation of ampicillin pharmacokinetics and toxicity in guinea pigs. *Lab.Anim.Sci.*, 37, 652–656.

ZENTLER-MONRO, P.L. and NORTHFIELD, T.C. (1979): Drug-induced gastro-intestinal disease. *Br.Med.J.*, 1, 1263–1265.

VIII. Digestive System 2

LIVER

As the principle site of drug metabolism and detoxification, the liver is a frequent site of drug-induced injury in man and commonly undergoes changes in preclinical toxicity studies.

Drug-induced hepatic injury in man includes virtually all known types of both acute and chronic hepatic injury and it may be difficult, if not impossible to distinguish histologically between drug induced and spontaneous hepatic disease (Scheuer, 1981). Although some drugs produce hepatic injury in man but apparently not in experimental animals, a number of factors need to be considered in the extrapolation of hepatic findings in experimental animals to man. Some reactions recorded in man are considered predictable (Type I), as they are dose and time dependent, they occur in most or all subjects exposed to appropriate doses and are reproducible in laboratory animals. Other reactions are regarded as non-predictable (Type II), being dose and time independent, occurring sporadically in man and not reproducible in laboratory animals.

This simple division into predictable and non-predictable has been criticised as an oversimplification. Zimmerman (1981), has suggested that non-predictable reactions may be of at least two types. Drug reactions occurring after one to five weeks of commencing drug therapy seem to involve hypersensitivity reactions. Those occurring after weeks to months of starting a drug appear to be the result of metabolic idiosyncrasy. Furthermore, Zimmerman, (1981) has suggested that models for these idiosyncratic reactions can be developed in experimental animals, if account is taken of metabolism and disposition of the drug in question.

There have been relatively few studies which have tried to correlate adverse hepatic findings occurring with therapeutic agents in man with those which can be produced in laboratory animals. Making this comparison is not straightforward because much of the preclinical data for many agents remains unpublished. It is not only necessary to critically compare histopathological findings in both man and animal, but also evaluate differences in drug metabolism and tissue distribution. Nevertheless, a comprehensive literature review of substances causing liver damage in man and laboratory animals suggested that evidence of drug-induced hepatic toxicity in rodents or non-rodent species should be taken as suggestive that an agent possesses potential to cause hepatic toxicity in man, (Hayes et al., 1982).

Most diagnostic work with human liver biopsies takes place using light microscopy and paraffin-embedded tissue sections, with correlation of clinical data and blood chemistry findings. The same is true of hepatic tissue in preclinical toxicity studies. However, it has become clear that electron microscopy and a wide variety of other techniques including cytochemistry and immunocytochemistry which have increasingly helped our understanding of human hepatic disease (Goldblatt and Gunning, 1984), are assuming increasing importance in the explanation of hepatic changes observed with novel pharmaceutical agents in preclinical safety studies. Scanning electron microscopy has been particularly instructive in providing a deeper insight into the three-dimensional structure of the liver and the pathophysiology of liver disease (see reviews by Motta, 1984; Goldblatt and Gunning, 1984) and these newer structural considerations are worth briefly reviewing here.

Hepatocytes compose about 60% of the liver (Weibel et al., 1969) and are arranged into interconnecting plates or laminae of a single cell thickness giving rise to a continuous labyrinth of spaces or lacunae in which blood vessels are suspended. Lobules and acini are the smallest units in this structure as Malpighi (1666) first described. There are three concepts of liver structure, that of the *classical lobule* (Kiernan, 1833), the *portal lobule* (Mall, 1906) and the *liver acinus of Rappaport* (1954). However, the complex, dynamic metabolism gradients within the hepatic laminae suggests that these concepts have limited use and should be used with caution (Teutsch, 1984).

Hepatocytes are polyhedral, usually possessing six facets, all covered with microvilli. Half of the facets are attached to adjacent hepatocytes and form complementary walls of bile canuliculi (bile facets or bile poles). In central areas of the lobule (Rappaport zone III), bile canaliculi are approximately 0.5 μm wide but they become wider (1–2.5 μm) in peripheral zones (Rappaport zone I) where they may be bounded by three hepatocytes. The bile canaliculi are visualized by certain cytochemical techniques at light microscopic level (McMillan et al., 1984; Masson et al., 1986).

The remaining liver cell facets are particularly well-endowed with microvilli. They are adjacent to the sinusoidal walls but separated from them by a perisinusoidal space, the space of Disse. As a consequence, the spaces of Disse form a continuous labyrinth of microlacunae within the liver and contain variable amounts of tissue fluid. The space of Disse is notable for the absence of basal lamina and infrequent numbers of collagen fibres (Goldblatt and Gunning, 1984). Lipocytes or fat storing cells of Ito (1951) [1] are also located in the space of

---

[1] The 'fat storing cells' are identical to the stellate cells (Sternzellen) first observed by von Kupffer (1876) which react with gold chloride, while the phagocytic cells in the sinusoids are designated Kupffer cells (Wake, 1974). For a detailed historical review see Aterman (1986).

Disse. These cells are occasionally prominant in paraffin-embedded sections from normal rodent livers. The precise function of these cells remains unknown although they appear to be the main storage site for vitamin A in the liver (Yamamoto and Ogawa, 1983) and may be responsible for intraparenchymal collagen formation under certain circumstances (Okanoue et al., 1983). In vitamin A-deficient rats, lipid droplets in Ito cells become particularly sparse whilst the converse is true when vitamin A is administered in excess (Yamamoto and Ogawa, 1983).

Hepatic sinusoids represent small capillaries which connect perilobular and portal vessels with the central veins, forming a rich vascular network within the lobule. The sinusoids are lined by cells of two distinct types, endothelial cells and Kupffer cells, the latter distinguishable by their phagocytic activity and ultrastructural characteristics of macrophages (Goldblatt and Gunning, 1984)

The endothelial cells lining the sinusoids appear to be functionally different to those lining larger vessels such as the central or interlobular veins, at least in the rat, as shown by their difference endocytic activities (Yokota, 1985). The endothelial cells contain, fenestrations arranged in groups or 'sieve plates'. In vivo, an open communication exists between the sinusoidal lumen and the space of Disse so that solutes and particles up to a certain size can exchange freely between blood and lymph in these two compartments (Bradfield, 1984). Another sinusoidal cell described in the rat is the *pit cell* (Wisse, 1976). These cells are characterized by dense cytoplasmic granules and rod-cored vesicles, but their function remain unknown (Bradfield, 1984).

Arterial and venous components in the portal zones are surrounded by connective tissue fibres and wide spaces (spaces of Mall) containing tissue fluid. Bile duct cells commence in the transitional ductal epithelium that lines the terminal portion of the bile canaliculi as they join the finest radicals of the bile duct system at the canals of Herring (canicular-ductular junctions).

Functional hepatocellular heterogeneity

Although hepatocytes have a fairly uniform structure, histochemical study as well as the newer biochemical sampling methods, in conjunction with microfluorometric assays of high sensitivity, have revealed considerable functional heterogeneity of hepatocytes within the hepatic lobule (Teutsch, 1984, 1985). This is perhaps not surprising in view of the way the liver plates are perfused with blood in the sinusoids. Since the quality of blood changes during its passage from the portal tracts, functional demands on hepatocytes must be different in different parts of the hepatic lobule (Jungerman and Katz, 1982).

Knowledge of functional heterogeneity is clearly of importance in assessment of the histopathological changes found in preclinical toxicity studies. In general terms, most experiments suggest that oxidative energy metabolism, β-oxidation, aminoacid catabolism, ureagenesis from aminoacids, gluconeogenesis, bile acid and bilirubin secretion are preferentially located in the periportal zone, whereas glycolysis, liponeogenesis and ureagenesis from ammonia appear predominantly situated in the perivenous or centrilobular zones (Jungerman and Katz, 1982; Matsumura and Thurman, 1984; Lawrence et al., 1986).

Periportal hepatocytes are well-endowed with protective properties against toxic oxygen reduction products such as superoxide anion radicals, hydrogen peroxide and hydroxyl radicals (Jungerman and Katz, 1982). This is shown by the presence of abundant glutathione and glutathione peroxidase in the periportal zones (Smith et al., 1979; Yoshimura et al, 1980).

Conversely, biotransformation of foreign substances, whether by oxidation, reduction, hydrolysis or conjugation appear to be preferentially located in perivenous zones (Jungerman and Katz, 1982; Conway et al., 1984). For example, the NADPH-generating enzyme, glucose-6-phosphate dehydrogenase and the NADPH utilising enzyme NADPH-cytochrome c reductase (Baron et al., 1978), cytochrome P450 and cytochrome b5 (Gooding et al., 1978) have a centrilobular, perivenous distribution.

In the rat liver, similar regional variations have been observed in the activity of a number of other enzymes using quantitative cytochemical techniques (James et al., 1986; Frederiks et al., 1987; Mompon et al., 1987). Immunocytochemical approaches to the zones of cytochromes P450 have shown a variable regional distribution, usually with most immune-reactive enzyme being found in perivenous zones (Moody et al., 1985). However, immunocytochemical distribution of immune-reactive cytochrome P450 is dependent on the particular antibody or technique employed, for under some conditions a diffuse pattern has been reported (Moody et al., 1985; Foster et al., 1986).

These differences are undoubtably partly due to the immunological cross-reactivity of the multiple forms of cytochrome P450 enzymes present in hepatocytes as a result of varying degrees of aminoacid sequence homology (Thomas et al., 1987). It is believed that phenobarbitone-inducible cytochromes P450 (P450b and P450e of rat) are present in higher concentrations in centrilobular regions whereas the P448 family of cytochromes (P450c and P450d of rat or polycyclic hydrocarbon-inducible forms) are found in greater concentrations in perivenous zones (Ioannides and Parke, 1987).

Furthermore, there is heterogeneity of total cytochrome P450 content between the different lobes of the rat liver, with highest levels being reported in the right lobe (Sumner and Lodola, 1987). These differences may influence the susceptability of the various lobes to the effects of xenobiotics.

Xenobiotic metabolizing enzymes have also been demonstrated in the non-parenchymal cells of the rat liver (Lafranconi et al., 1986). Although the total level of metabolizing enzyme activity is lower in these cells than in hepatocytes, they can be induced by administration of xenobiotics. As non-parenchymal cells are located mainly along sinusoids, they are the first cells in the liver to be exposed to blood borne substances and may therefore have considerable impact on hepatic disposition and toxicity of administered xenobiotics (Lafranconi et al., 1986).

Other zonal differences also exist because there are undoubtedly hormone gradients and hormone receptor differences within the hepatic lobule (Jungerman and Katz, 1982).

It is important to stress however, that much of the knowledge related to zonal heterogeneity is based on data from the rat liver and not only are there species, strain or sex differences but also zonal heterogeneity is not an absolute or static phenomenon but rather a dynamic process which responds to demands imposed by changes in environmental conditions as well as to physiological and pathological states.

For example, species differences have been noted for the aldehyde dehydrogenase, which are found in greatest concentrations in the liver and appear important in the metabolism of acetylaldehyde, the proximate metabolite of ethanol (Dietrich, 1966; Marjanen, 1972; Smolen et al., 1981, 1982). These enzymes are components of the cytosol, mitochondria and microsomes but the proportion in each subcellular fraction is species-dependent. For instance, 60% of total hepatic activity in the rat is mitochondrial whereas most activity is cytosolic in the mouse. (Dietrich, 1966; Marjanen, 1972; Smolen et al., 1981). Furthermore, quite marked differences in the activity of this enzyme have been found between inbred mouse strains (Smolen et al., 1982). Pentobarbitone sleeping time, believed to reflect microsomal enzyme activity in the liver, has also shown marked differences between inbred mouse strains (Lovell, 1986).

Note. Over the last twenty years a variety of different names have been used for the increasing number of different forms of cytochromes P450 which have been isolated in various laboratories. Although the original P448 name is employed in this text, a new nomenclature for the P450 gene superfamily has been recently proposed in which P448 refers to the haemoproteins of the P450I gene family which comprises at least two P448 isoenzymes (Nebert et al., 1987).

Studies on isolated hepatocytes from rat and dog have shown considerable species differences in surface receptors for insulin, glucogen and pancreatic polypeptide, which suggests that hormone-target cell interactions in the liver may also be different between species (Bonnevie-Nielsen et al., 1982).

Variations with age

Clinical study in man have established that aging is accompanied by a significant decline in disposition rates of a variety of drugs. Although this decline can be attributed to a number of different factors including reduced intestinal absorption or hepatic blood flow and lowered renal clearance of metabolites, there is considerable evidence for an age-related decrease in the capacity of the liver to metabolise drugs, (Schmucker, 1979, 1985).

Such findings in man have been generally corroborated in both in vivo and in vitro experimental studies with rats and mice, although there remain differences between man and rodent (Schmucker and Wang, 1983). It has also been shown that aging influences the susceptability of rats to hepatotoxic injury (Rikans,

1984). The aging process has also been shown to influence the inducability of component enzymes of the hepatic drug metabolising system in rats (Sun and Strobel, 1986). Studies in rats have shown that decreases in hepatic blood flow occur over the first 12 months of life which are capable of diminishing the biotransformation capacity of the liver (VanBezooijen, 1984).

Ploidy, the state of the cell nucleus which relates to the number of genomes present, also changes with increasing age. There is an increase in ploidy with advancing age which is marked in mice and strain-dependent in rats (Shima and Sugahara, 1976; Grice and Burek, 1984). It has been shown in rats that because ploidy and binucleation increase with advancing age, nuclear/cytoplamic ratios also alter as a function of age (Englemann et al., 1981). It has been suggested that age-related changes in hepatic drug metabolism are partly due to these age-related changes in ploidy status of hepatocytes (Grice and Burek, 1984).

Morphometric studies at electron microscopic level using male Fischer rats have also shown that the volume occupied by smooth endoplastic reticulum decreases in the liver with age (Schmucker et al., 1977) although the converse has been reported in female Wistar rats (Pieri et al., 1975). A variety of experiments in rodents designed to study the activity of the hepatic mixed function oxidase system and hepatic microsomal drug metabolising enzymes have also shown declining activity with age (van Bezooijen, 1984).

The studies with microsomal NADPH cytochrome c (P450) reductase from the male rat liver have demonstrated several marked, age-dependent changes including a decline in specific activity, reduced inducability and enhanced thermolability (Schmucker and Wang, 1983). It is also pertinant to note that hepatic microsomal drug metabolising enzyme activity is strongly sex-dependent in rats being generally higher in males. However, our understanding of the role of sex hormones on liver function in man remains fairly poor (Johnson, 1984). Studies of hepatic microsomal mono-oxygenase activities in liver tissue of aging male and female Wistar rats have shown that this sex-related difference tends to disappear with age due mainly to a decline in enzyme activity in the males (Kitagawa et al., 1985).

Phase II metabolism or conjugation activities in rodents also appear to decline with advancing age (Stohs et al., 1982; Fujita et al., 1985), although van Bezooijen (1984) has suggested that changes in the capacity of rodents to conjugate foreign substanceswith glutathione in advancing age are probably small.

Age-related changes in other hepatic activities have been described in the rodent. Key enzymes involved in liver energy metabolism change with age. Enzymes such as pyruvate kinase involved in glycolysis and enzymes involved in lipogenesis appear to decrease in activity with age in the rat, whereas those involved in gluconeogenesis are maintained or even increase with age (Vitorica et al., 1981). Lysosomal enzyme activity is higher in periportal zones in young rats but in old rats the hepatocytes around the central vein possess greater lysosomal activity (van Manen et al., 1983).

Although the contribution of sinusoidal cells to drug metabolizing capacity of the liver with age has not been studied in great detail, age-related decline in the capacity for antigen handling by Kupffer and endothelial cells have been reported in Fischer rats (Caperna and Garvey, 1982).

Environmental factors

Among the environmental factors which influence hepatic function, diet is considered one of the most important. Morphometric evaluation of rat hepatocytes has shown marked differences in nuclear and cytoplasmic volume, changes in the amounts of glycogen, lipid and rough endoplasmic reticulum in response to diets of varying carbohydrate, protein and fat content (Berlin et al., 1982). Dietary protein levels can have a profound effect on liver metabolism. A high protein diet given to rats is associated with active gluconeogenesis and ureagenesis accompanied by marked increases in the number of mitochondria and increases in mitochondrial cytochrome oxidase activity in the liver (Didier et al., 1985).

Activity of the drug metabolising mixed function oxidase system in the rat liver is also influenced by diet for it has been shown to be more active in rats given a cereal-based diet than those given an equivalent purified diet (Proia et al., 1984).

Fasting is of particular interest in toxicology, for animals are often fasted prior to blood sampling or autopsy. Yet this procedure can markedly influence the rodent liver over a fairly short period of time. A quantitative cytochemical study of glycogen and glutathione in the liver of mice over a 12 hour period of fasting under conditions usual in toxicity studies, showed age-dependent losses in glycogen and glutathione of up to about 50% (Irisarri and Mompon, 1983). The glycogen distribution pattern also altered over the period. These findings carry implications for protocol design in toxicology and for the timing of final sacrifice, for both glycogen metabolism and glutathione may influence the capacity of the liver to metabolise drugs. By immunocytochemical study, calmodulin, a key protein in the calcium messenger system, important in the regulation of glycogenolysis (Rasmussen, 1986), was also shown to disappear from glycogen particles in the rat hepatocyte during fasting (Harper et al., 1980). Routine overnight starvation also reduces the hepatic albumin content in rats, notably in periportal and midzonal regions (Le Bouton, 1982).

Other environmental factors also influence liver function. Altered light-dark cycles may affect liver glycogen and enzymatic activities (Bhattacharya, 1983). Diurnal variation in 5'-nucleotidase activity has also been shown using quantitative histochemical study (Frederiks et al., 1987). Although it has been suggested that certain spontaneous liver lesions affect drug metabolising capacity (van Bezooijen, 1984), there is little evidence for this being a major factor. However, the presence of the gastrointestinal parasite, Syphacia muris, in mice has been shown to influence the hepatic microsomal monooxygenase system (Mohn and Philipp, 1981). Cage bedding has also been shown to influence microsomal cytochrome P450-dependent drug metabolising activity in rats, cedar chip bedding enhancing and pinewood bedding decreasing enzyme activity (Weichbrod et al., 1988).

Tissue sampling

As with most tissues from toxicity studies, immersion fixation of the liver at autopsy is usually sufficient to provide good morphological detail for light microscopy in routine paraffin embedded sections, although there appears to be considerable interlaboratory variation in the quantity of liver from each animal which is examined histologically. For rats, this may vary from between one to over four sections of liver for pivotal regulatory studies, (personal observations). In two-year rat carcinogenicity studies the National Toxicology Program practice is to take two liver samples representing cross sections of the widest parts of the left lobe and right median lobe (Maronpot et al., 1989).

It becomes more complex, if in order to keep numbers of animals used low by avoiding use of satellite groups or performing additional studies, liver tissue is sampled from toxicity studies for histological, biochemical, cytochemical and ultrastructural study. Conflicts arise between the necessity to randomize the autopsies and the need to assure that livers for cytochemical or biochemical study have all been harvested over a short period of time to avoid the effects of prolonged fasting. Although perfusion fixation is ideal for electron microscopy, this may not always be feasible in routine toxicity studies. A compromise for rodent livers has been transparenchymal perfusion, in which a lobe is removed at the time of autopsy and perfused directly through the hepatic substance (Roberts et al., 1990).

Zbinden (1981) has suggested that hepatic biopsies are useful for monitoring liver tissue in a small number of rodents. This may be useful in the rat under some circumstances, although tissue samples are very small and only effective for monitoring widespread or diffuse hepatic changes. Nevertheless, neoplastic alterations may be detected in the rodent liver by this method (Giampaolo et al., 1989).

Liver weight changes

Dose-related increases in liver weight are commonly observed in repeat-dose toxicity studies performed in rodents, although in dog or other large animal studies, the individual variations and the small numbers of animals used makes assessment of liver weight changes less certain. The cause for the liver weight changes may be evident in tissue sections when caused by accumulation of lipid, glycogen or other substances, cell damage, congestion, hepatocellular hypertrophy or hyperplasia. Liver weight is also greatly influenced by circulatory factors, although these are difficult to assess (Barka and Popper, 1967). Biochemical or ultrastructural study may be necessary to define the cause of the liver weight changes, particularly if initial morphological studies do not provide a clear explanation for the weight changes. It is important to carefully characterise

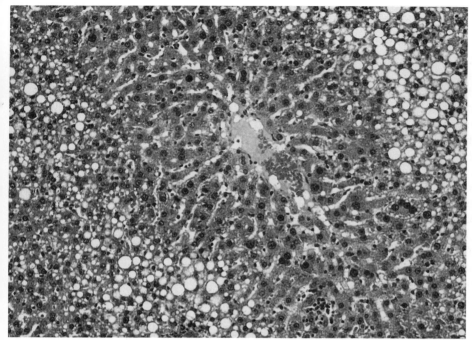

Fig. 71. Liver from a 24-month-old Sprague-Dawley rat showing a periportal, fatty change of macrovesicular type. (HE, ×200.)

the nature of the liver weight changes to be able to critically assess any potential risk for man.

Fatty changes (steatosis)

Zimmerman (1978a) has listed a large number of agents which can produce fatty change in rat hepatocytes and a variety of drugs have also produced hepatic fatty change in mouse, dog, primate and man (Hayes et al., 1982). The fatty change may be of fine, lipid-containing cytoplasmic vacuoles (microvesicular type) or large, single vacuoles within each cell (Fig. 71) (macrovesicular type). Fat may be distributed in a diffuse or regional manner. The different types and distribution of fatty change are seen sporadically in control animals, presumably as a result of nutritional, metabolic or hormonal derangements (Greaves and Faccini, 1984).

Although hepatic steatosis can be a manifestation of cell damage and be associated with hepatic necrosis in animals treated with medicinal agents, steatosis may result from quite different mechanisms. It has been suggested that most agents which lead to the development of steatosis do so by interference with the process of removal of lipid from the cell rather than increase entry of lipid into the cell (Zimmerman, 1978b).

Usually, the pathologist assessing preclinical toxicity studies is faced with increased hepatic lipid without necrosis or other cellular changes, particularly as special stains for lipid are often routinely performed on frozen sections of liver. Cytochemical and ultrastructural study can be helpful in the interpretation of such drug-induced findings. Mori (1983) has shown that a number of chemical agents each affecting different parts of the lipoprotein transport process produced fatty change in the rat liver, associated with fairly specific ultrastructural and cytochemical changes of help in the understanding of the processes involved. For instance, cycloheximide, believed to inhibit protein synthesis, produced immunohistochemical evidence of depletion of the apoprotein B component of lipoprotein in hepatocytes. At ultrastructural level loss of lipoprotein particles from the rough endoplasmic reticulum was observed. Ethionine, which decreases hepatic ATP biosynthesis, produced an accumulation of lipoprotein particles in the terminal parts of the rough endoplasmic reticulum and the smooth endoplasmic reticulum but not in the Golgi apparatus, suggesting a hiatus in the ATP-dependent transport processes. Colchicine, known to depolymerize cytoplasmic microtubules, caused fatty change with a marked decrease in cytoplasmic microtubules of the liver when examined ultrastructurally, in keeping with the concept that microtubules are important in the transport of lipoproteins from the Golgi to the plasma membrane.

Lipid also accumulates in the Ito cell (see above) and this can occur in livers from quite normal rodents, where it is characterized by a scattering of small clear cells closely related to the sinusoids. Long-term administration of vitamin A and β-carotene, a food colorant, may accentuate lipid accumulation in sinusoidal cells of the liver in dogs and rodents (Heywood et al., 1985; Wake, 1974).

Clear cell change

This is characterised by hepatocytes with clear cytoplasm, a well defined eosinophilic cytoplasmic membrane and centrally placed nuclei. Special stains usually reveal the presence of glycogen after appropriate fixation procedures. It may be quite commonly observed in well-fed, untreated rodents, particularly if fasting of the rodents is not practiced before autopsy. In certain inbred strains of rat a specific deficiency of hepatic phosphorylase kinase also leads to an accumulation of glycogen in the liver (Clark et al., 1980; Haynes et al., 1983). In larger animals such as dog and primate this type of clear cell is variably prominent in the normal state.

Certain pharmaceutical agents cause glycogen accumulation in the rat liver. Clavulanate, an agent used to potentiate antibiotic activity, produced increases in hepatic glycogen in toxicity studies in rats but not in dogs (Jackson et al., 1985). It was argued that the rat findings were an adaptive response to the extensive hepatic metabolism of the compound in this species. As the dog metabolised clavulanate in a manner more like man than the rat, it was suggested that this finding represented little risk for man at therapeutic doses. Similar glycogen accumulation has been reported in the rat following administration of tetracycline and it was postulated to result from an inhibiting effect on glycogen utilisation. (Proksová 1973).

Dogs may show marked accumulation of hepatocellular glycogen and clear cell change predominantly in midzonal distribution following administration of prednisone (Fittschen and Bellamy, 1984). Although the exact mechanism for this particular accumulation of glycogen is uncertain, glucocorticoid treatment probably alters the balance between glycogenesis and glycogenolysis in the dog leading to hepatomegaly through intracellular glycogen accumulation (Fittschen and Bellamy, 1984).

A marked variation in the degree of hepatic clear cell change as a result of cytoplasmic glycogen accumulation has been reported in New Zealand white rabbits used as controls in 28 and 90 day percutaneous toxicity studies (Wells et al., 1988) Not only were variations in severity reported between individual studies and within the same study, the vacuolation was more marked in females and in animals with greater body weight and relative liver weight. Animals evaluated in this study, were however fed ad libitum up until the time of death.

Hepatocellular hypertrophy and hyperplasia

A large number of medicinal agents with different chemical structures and therapeutic activities produce liver enlargement when given in high doses to species used in toxicity studies. In many instances, this enlargement is accompanied by an increase in activity of the hepatic microsomal drug metabolising enzymes in the absence of any morphological evidence of hepatocellular damage (Schulte-Hermann, 1974). Hepatic enlargement may be accompanied by evidence of hepatocyte hypertrophy, hepatocyte hyperplasia or both. Conventionally, hypertrophy is considered to be an increase in cell volume and hyperplasia an increase in cell number. Whereas hypertrophy may be relatively easy to assess if it is distributed in a zonal manner, diffuse hypertrophy or hyperplasia is not so evident. The occurrence of mitotic figures can be misleading if single cell necrosis is present, although hyperplasia can be reflected by the presence of liver plates comprising two cell layers (Barka and Popper, 1967). However, it should be noted that certain authors use the functional definition proposed by Barka and Popper (1967) in which hyperplasia refers to the state in which there is an increase in genetic material whether derived from cell division, increase in ploidy or binuclearity, assessed by measurement of DNA content of the liver.

In hypertrophy, electron microscopic examination typically reveals proliferation of the smooth endoplasmic reticulum which manifest at light microscopic level as a 'ground glass' eosinophilic, or granular cytoplasm and increased size of hepatocytes (Fig. 72). Biochemical studies show evidence of increased activity of enzymes of the drug metabolising system as well as increases in microsomal protein. Cytochemical studies of equivalent enzyme systems also show increased activity, particularly in centrilobular zones with little or no disturbance of the normal pericanalicular distribution of lysosomal enzyme activity. The changes are typically reversible on cessation of treatment, although this may take more

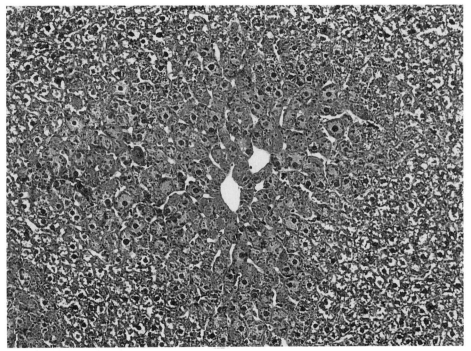

Fig. 72. Liver from a Sprague-Dawley rat treated for one month with phenobarbitone showing the typical centrilobular hypertrophy. Affected hepatocytes are characterised by an eosinophilic, 'ground glass' cytoplasm. (HE, ×200.)

than one month in rodent species. Studies in the rat after up to seven days following cessation of treatment with phenobarbitone have shown that much of the excess smooth endoplasmic reticulum is removed by being sequestered into autophagic vacuoles to be digested by lysosomal enzymes (Feldman et al., 1980).

Findings of this nature are in favour of an adaptive response (Crampton et al., 1977a) and this reasoning has been recently applied to the liver changes occurring in rodent toxicity studies with a number of novel pharmaceutical agents such as imidazole antifungals (Marriott et al., 1983), LY171883, an anti-asthmatic agent (Eacho et al., 1985, 1986) and tilidine fumarate, a synthetic analgesic (McGuire et al., 1986) as well as numerous others, data from which remain unpublished.

However, this apparently simple situation of liver enlargement or hypertrophy accompanied by induction of drug metabolising enzymes being an adaptive response is complicated by a variety of factors which need to be considered when an assessment of this type is made. Indeed, it is not entirely certain that this simple adaptive response is entirely without risk for man because the enhanced metabolism which serves to prevent the accumulation of the administered drug may also serve to accelerate the metabolism of other drugs or the generation of toxic metabolites of other chemicals (Schulte-Hermann, 1979). For this reason, drug regulatory authorities are wary of licencing enzyme inducing agents unless the potential therapeutic benefit is great (Breckenridge, 1987). Thus, dose levels at which enzyme induction occurs are quite clearly of importance in the assessment of potential risk.

Experience from long-term studies in rodents with some enzyme inducers has also shown certain adverse effects, notably nodular lesions, the precise nature and relevance of which remain disputed (see below). Based on long-term rat studies of a number of agents which produced hepatic enlargement accompanied by increases in drug metabolising activity in the absence of overt cell damage, Crampton and his colleagues (1977 a,b) distinguished different types of effect in the rat. Certain agents such as phenobarbitone produced the classical changes outlined above with increased drug-metabolising activity which was sustained over long periods. Other agents, exemplified by safrole and Ponceau MX, produced increases in metabolising activity without evidence of cell damage but this was not sustained. Following long term treatment with safrole and Ponceau MX, a decline in metabolising enzyme activities occurred, accompanied by increases in lysosome number, lysosomal enzyme activity, autophagocytic vacuoles and dilatation of rough endoplasmic reticulum. Eventually, light microscopic evidence of individual hepatocyte necrosis, fatty change occurred and finally hepatic nodules appeared. It was this latter spectrum of changes that Crampton and colleagues (1977b) suggested provided early evidence of long-term toxicity.

It has been suggested that such differences may be related to the activity and induction of the different cytochromes. Thus, cytochromes of the P448 type (P450c and P450d of rat), generally appear to convert xenobiotics to reactive electrophiles giving rise to cellular toxicity or carcinogenicity whereas the phenobarbitone-inducible form of P450, i.e. P4540b and P450e of rat, usually direct metabolism to the formation of inactive metabolites and detoxification processes (Ioannides and Parke, 1987). Cytochromes P448 are induced by a variety of xenobiotics although in the rat the levels of P450c and P450d may be increased to different extents. For example 3-methylcholanthrene and β-naphthoflavone induce primarily P450c whereas safrole and 3,4,5,3′,4′5′-hexochlorophenyl induce mainly P450d. (Thomas et al., 1983).

This association of P448 type induction with toxicity and carcinogenicity poses questions for the development of novel therapeutic agents with P448-inducing properties in experimental animals. A number of drugs being developed have been shown to have P448 inducing potential, although none appears to have yet successfully completed a full development programme or been in extensive clinical use. (McKillop and Case, 1990).

However, these concepts are based on studies of enzyme-inducing properties of xenobiotics in the rat liver and far less is known about the roles of the various human P450 proteins in the metabolism of such agents (Guengerich, 1988). There are species and strain differences in the induction of the mixed function oxidase system by some xenobiotics and selective patterns occur suggesting involvement of different forms of cytochrome P450 in different species (Dent et al., 1980; Smith et al., 1986).

Considerable strain differences in the inducibility of cytochromes of the P448 type in hepatic and other tissues also have been demonstrated in inbred mice, with C57 BL/6 strains showing high and DBA/2 strains characterised by low inducibility (Nebert, 1979). Guinea pigs also are more resistant to the induction of cytochrome P448 by 3-methylcholanthrene than rats (Abe and Watanabe, 1983). It has been suggested that there is a correlation between resistance to cytochrome P448-induction and low susceptibility to cancer among laboratory animal populations (Ioannides and Parke, 1987).

By contrast to effects in laboratory animals, the number of drugs exhibiting significant enzyme-inducing properties in man is quite small and largely limited to anticonvulsant drugs and rifampicin. Although this low number may be related to species differences in sensitivity to enzyme induction, it may also relate to the lower doses employed in clinical practice compared with experimental studies (Breckenridge, 1987). In addition to drugs, environmental factors, diet and smoking may also induce the synthesis of specific cytochrome P450 isoenzymes in man, although there is considerable inter-individual viability (Conney, 1986).

Many compounds which modify drug metabolising activity have also been shown to exhibit a biphasic effect, inhibition followed by induction (Conney, 1967). For example, studies with various novel imidazol antimycotics, some of which produce hepatic enlargement in preclinical toxicity studies as well as hepatic toxicity in man (Lewis et al., 1984), have been shown to produce time and dose-dependent, biphasic effects in rat liver which vary considerably between different agents (Niemegeers et al., 1981). Clearly, it is important to measure drug metabolising activity at the dose levels and according to the dose schedules actually used in the toxicity studies in order to assess such hepatic changes correctly and to provide some idea of potential for enzyme induction in man.

Peroxisomal proliferation

Clofibrate, a hypolipidaemic agent indicated for the treatment of certain types of hyperlipidaemia, produces liver enlargement accompanied by proliferation of smooth endoplasmic reticulum and increases in hepatic cytochrome P450 and cytochrome c reductase levels (Orton and Higgins, 1979). However, clofibrate and other hypolipidemic agents also produce proliferation of peroxisomes in the rodent liver (Figs. 73, 74, 75 and 76). Although it is questioned whether this particular effect represents an adaptive response or is evidence of injury (Jezequel & Orlandi, 1972), agents which produce peroxisomail proliferation in the rodent liver are associated with the development of hepatic neoplasia when administered for long periods to these species. This association has given rise to the concept that peroxisomal proliferators represent a special class of 'non-genotoxic' carcinogens capable of giving rise to excess hydrogen peroxide, oxidative injury

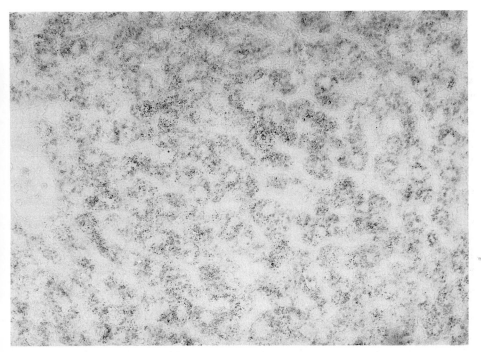

Fig. 73. Liver from a Sprague-Dawley rat showing the usual level of peroxisomal activity in an untreated animal. (Frozen section, catalase reaction, ×300.)

to DNA or other macromolecules and ultimately a carcinogenic response (Reddy et al., 1980; Reddy and Lalwani, 1983).

The causal link between peroxisomal proliferation and cancer still remains to be established, although it is probable that this type of carcinogenic effect is not directly attributable to the chemical but to the adaptive response of the host to its effects (Reddy and Rao, 1987). Peroxisomal proliferation does not show a quantitative correlation with tumour development (Marsman et al., 1988) nor has DNA injury by peroxisomal proliferations been identified.

These agents have also been shown to possess promoting activity (Conway et al., 1989). In contrast to the lack of correlation between degree of peroxisomal proliferation and tumorigenesis, a recent study has shown a correlation between the sustained hepatocyte DNA synthesis produced by di(2-ethylhexyl)phthalate and WY 14,643 in rats and the degree of tumour response (Marsman et al., 1988).

A more recent study which compared the effects of phenobarbitone with clofibrate and the potent hypolipidaemic agent ICI 53072 on the rat liver confirm that phenobarbitone increases liver size mainly by hepatocyte enlargement, whereas hepatomegaly produced by hypolipidaemic agents was a result of both proliferation and hepatocyte enlargement (Berman et al., 1983). These authors also showed by using radioactive microspheres that the hypolipidaemic

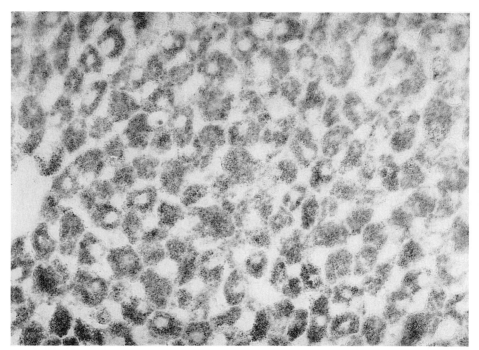

Fig. 74. Similar reaction to that seen in Figure 73 but performed on a section of liver taken from a Sprague-Dawley rat treated for four weeks with 400 mg/kg/day of clofibrate. It shows a striking increase in the number of peroxisomes. (Catalase reaction, ×300.)

agents also had a significant effect on hepatic blood flow, possibly a factor in the development of hepatic nodules in the rat.

Note. Microbodies, including peroxisomes of vertebrate cells, protozoa and fungi and glycosomes of plants and fungi probably belong to the same family of single membrane-bound bodies involved in different metabolic pathways but sharing some role in respiration based on peroxide metabolism and fatty acid oxidation (Borst, 1986). All the available evidence suggested that peroxisomes arise from pre-existing ones by a process of budding or fission (Lazarow and Fujiki, 1985; Borst, 1986).

Cohen and Grasso (1981) suggested that peroxisomal proliferation is a phenomenon which occurs in rodents but not man. More recent findings suggest that other species such as dog and monkey can also show peroxisomal proliferation when treated with some hypolipidaemic agents (Lake and Gray, 1985; Fitzgerald et al., 1986). In this respect, it appears that species differences in disposition and metabolism of particular compounds are especially important. However, quantitative sterological studies in animals treated with the lipid regulating agent, gemfibrozil, have shown considerable interspecies differences in the susceptabil-

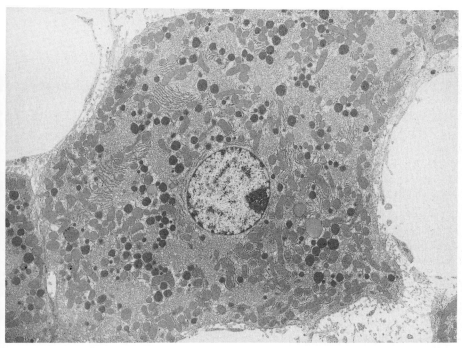

Fig. 75. Transmission electron micrograph of the liver from a Wistar rat treated with 400 mg/kg/day of clofibrate for 14 days showing characteristic hepatocyte enlargement with proliferation of smooth endoplasmic reticulum and a slight increase in peroxisomes. Illustration by courtesy of Dr. N.G. Read. (EM, ×4500.)

ity of laboratory animals to hepatic peroxisomal proliferation, with dog and primate being less sensitive than the rat or hamster (Gray and de la Iglesia, 1984). In addition, quantitative microscopy of liver biopsies from eight patients treated with gemfibrozil for periods of up to 27 months failed to demonstrate an increase in number of hepatic peroxisomes. (de la Iglesia et al., 1981).

Comparative studies on nafenopin-induced peroxisomal proliferation has also shown marked species differences. Following 21 days oral administration, rats and to a lesser extent, hamsters, showed dose-related increases in liver size, peroxisomal numbers, peroxisomal and microsomal fatty acid oxidizing enzyme activities (Lake et al., 1989). By contrast, no effects on liver size and only small changes in these enzyme activities were found in guinea pigs and marmosets treated similarly with nafenopin although increases in microsomal cytochrome P450 and mixed function oxidase activities were observed in these species.

Other evidence which suggests lack of peroxisomal proliferation in man is the paucity of response in cultured human hepatocytes under conditions in which rodent hepatocytes show marked proliferation of peroxisomes (Elcombe and Mitchell, 1987; Butterworth et al., 1989).

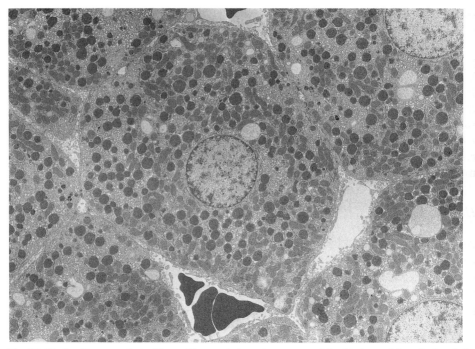

Fig. 76. Similar liver sample to Figure 75 except the rat was treated for 21 days with a similar daily dose of clofibrate. Peroxisomal proliferation is more pronounced. Illustration by courtesy of Dr. N.G. Read. (EM, ×3500.)

Drugs of totally different therapeutic classes and chemical structures also produce peroxisomal proliferation in toxicity studies. The anti-asthmatic agent, LY171883, produced proliferation of hepatic peroxisomes in rats but not dogs or rhesus monkeys (Eacho et al., 1985, 1986; Hoover et al., 1990) Methaphenilene, an analogue of antihistamine methapyrilene, has been shown to produce a similar effect. (Reznik-Schüller and Lijinsky, 1983). Thromboxane synthetase inhibitors, dehydroepiandosterone and structural analogues as well as non-steroidal antioestrogens have also been shown to produce peroxisomal proliferation in rodents (Watanabe et al., 1986; Schwartz et al., 1988; Ahotupa and Hirsimäki, 1989). It is probable that drugs of other classes are capable of producing peroxisomal proliferation, although this effect is not always searched for by enzyme histochemistry or ultrastructural study.

The hepatic peroxisomal proliferation observed in rats treated with LY171883, a tetrazole-substituted alkoxyacetophenone, occurred at high doses and was associated with reversible hepatomegaly which DNA analysis showed was a combination of hypertrophy and hyperplasia (Eacho et al., 1985). There were no histological changes of hepatocyte damage (Eacho et al., 1985). Although similar changes occurred in mice given LY171883, the fact that these changes only

410

occurred at high doses and not at all in dog or rhesus monkeys, Eacho and coworkers (1986) argued that this effect was unlikely to occur in man.

Although man and higher species in general appear less susceptible to the production of an increase in hepatic peroxisomes than rodents, each agent must be assessed individually with respect to dose at which changes occur in the rodent, the degree of proliferation, paying attention to species differences in drug disposition. Indeed, the variety of these features including peroxisomal proliferation which may be associated with hepatic enlargement in toxicity studies, serves to underline the need to assess morphological and functional aspects of the changes with some care to enable a reasonable risk assessment for man to be made.

Hepatic necrosis

Although both zonal and massive hepatic necrosis occasionally occurs in man treated with quite a variety of drugs (Sherlock, 1982; Ludwig and Axelsen, 1983), it is doubtful today whether novel pharmaceutical agents which are found to cause significant hepatic necrosis at modest dose levels by a direct mechanism in preclinical toxicity studies will usually be developed for use in man. Neverthe-

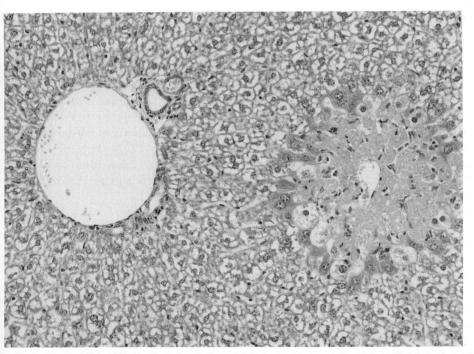

Fig. 77. Liver from a CD-1 mouse showing centrilobular necrosis produced by administration of paracetamol. (HE, ×250.)

less, drugs in current clinical use can produce significant hepatic necrosis in animals (Fig. 77) (Hayes et al., 1982; Falzon et al., 1985). Hepatic necrosis can be found in preclinical toxicity studies without this necessarily ruling out further development of a drug. Hepatic necrosis occurs spontaneously in laboratory animals and can develop following treatment with high doses of therapeutic agents as a result of an indirect mechanism such as tissue anoxia from circulatory derangements. In such cases, it is clearly necessary to precisely define the nature and distribution of the hepatic necrosis and assess any accompanying histological changes such as fatty change, congestion, inflammation, bile stasis and presence of Mallory bodies. Ultrastructural study may also give clues to pathogenesis.

Necrosis may be *zonal*, i.e. centrilobular, mid-zonal or periportal, *confluent or massive* or affect individual hepatocytes (*single cell necrosis*). It may also occur focally in an irregular distribution. '*Piecemeal necrosis*' is a component of chronic hepatitis.

Focal necrosis

In rodents one of the most prevalent forms of necrosis is the sporadic occurrence of well-defined foci of necrotic hepatocytes with or without inflammation (necrotizing inflammation) or repair. These lesions may be the results of infective processes in the gastrointestinal tract, notably Tyzzer's disease (Bacillus piliformis) and salmonellosis. Clues to the pathogenesis are obtained by special stains for the causative agent, but care is needed for drugs produce similar morphological changes, particularly in mice. Focal areas of parenchymal necrosis also occur following bile duct obstruction in the rat (Kountouras et al., 1984).

Similar foci are also seen in otherwise healthy beagle dogs, presumably the result of subclinical infection. This is perhaps not surprising in view of the fact that even young beagle dogs from well-run colonies occasionally develop fairly marked hepatic inflammatory disease including development of abscesses as a result of bacterial infection (Hargis and Thomassen, 1980). Foci of hepatic inflammation composed predominantly of macrophages have been associated with Ebola virus infection in cynomolgus monkeys (Jahrling et al., 1990).

Centrilobular necrosis

Centrilobular necrosis is particularly liable to occur following the administration of drugs and chemicals. The centrilobular zone is particularly vulnerable to ischaemic damage by virtue of the vascular supply of the liver and the resultant oxygen gradient. Centrilobular hepatocytes are also well-endowed with drug-metabolising enzymes and reactive metabolites are especially liable to be formed in the centrilobular zone and damage tissue by covalent binding directly with vital organelles or indirectly by promotion of lipid peroxidation of membrane unsaturated fatty acids (Comporti, 1985). It may not be possible to distinguish between the two mechanisms on histological evidence. Both mechanisms may also operate in the development of centrilobular necrosis. It has been suggested from studies conducted in the mouse, that paracetamol (acetaminophen) initially produces cytotoxic damage to centrilobular hepatocytes by the generation of reactive metabolites but that the necrosis extends with time as a result of the anoxia which results from the severe congestion accompanying the initial tissue damage (Walker et al., 1985).

However, as a variety of aldehydes including several 4-hydroxyalkenals are produced following peroxidation of cellular membrane lipids, histochemical detection of bound aldehydes represents a powerful tool in the study of lipid peroxidation. It has been shown that a modified, direct Schiff's reaction performed on frozen sections is capable of demonstrating the results of lipid peroxidation produced in rat liver by carbon tetrachloride or choline deficient diet (Rushmore et al., 1987; Taper at al., 1988).

Histologically, centrilobular necrosis is characterized by hepatocytes which show marked eosinophilia, accompanied by variable congestion and inflammation which is dependent on the actual time of observation following the insult (Fig. 77).

Periportal necrosis

Focal hepatic necrosis is seen in periportal zones following treatment with agents such as α-naphthylisothiocyanate which damage the bile ducts or following bile duct ligation and subsequent increase in intrahepatic bile levels.

Single cell necrosis (single cell degeneration, apoptosis)

Single, degenerate hepatocytes may be seen in the rodent, dog and primate livers following treatment with drugs and chemicals and under certain other circumstances such as ischaemia (Kerr, 1971) as well as occasionally in normal liver tissue. Histologically, they are seen as isolated extracellular, dense eosinophilic bodies sometimes possessing pyknotic nuclear fragments and unaccompanied by any inflammatory change. They also undergo apparent phagocytosis by viable hepatocytes and represent the so-called *Councilman body* described in a variety of pathological conditions in human liver.

One hypothesis advanced for the presence of these bodies is that they represent evidence of shrinkage necrosis or necrobiosis of individual hepatocytes which is the expression of programmed or controlled cell death in response to physiological or pathological changes (Kerr, 1971; Kerr and Searle, 1977; Wyllie, 1980). Careful quantitative histological and histochemical study of these bodies in the liver of rats treated with the synthetic progestin, cyproterone acetate, has tended to support this hypothesis (Bursch et al., 1985). This synthetic progestin produces liver weight increases in the rat, liver largely as a result of hyperplasia (Schulte-Herman et al., 1980). Following withdrawal of treatment these eosinophilic bodies or apoptopic bodies increase markedly and rapidly in number (in matter of hours) after withdrawal of treatment. The process was shown to be inhibited by growth stimuli and it was therefore argued to be a controlled event serving to eliminate excess cells rather than a manifestation of toxic hepatocellular damage (Bursch et al., 1985).

However, there may be no sharp separation between apoptosis which is a controlled adaptive change from apoptosis which is a manifestation of toxic damage. For instance, it has been recently shown that the centrilobular, acute haemorrhagic hepatic necrosis produced in rats by a single dose of dimethylnitrosamine is preceded by a period during which centrilobular hepatocytes become apoptotic (Pritchard and Butler, 1989). It was suggested that apoptosis may be a mode of cell injury distinct from that associated with hepatotoxins such as carbon tetrachloride which produce hydropic degeneration and coagulative necrosis of hepatocytes.

Apoptotic bodies are seen occasionally in the liver in control rats, other rodents, dogs and primates. They may be common in animals in preclinical studies suffering from general ill-health or non-specific toxic or ischaemic phenomena, not directly related to the liver (personal observations, Kerr, 1971).

Inflammation

One of the most prevalent forms of hepatic inflammation in preclinical toxicity studies is mild focal inflammation characterised by small aggregates of acute or chronic inflammatory cells grouped around small zones of necrotic or degenerate eosinophilic hepatocytes In general, these lesions are unrelated to treatment with drugs and chemicals under study for they are observed in untreated rodents, dogs and primates. Small granulomatous foci may also occasionally be seen in control animal livers (Fig. 78).

These foci may become more prevalent in rodents, primates and dogs in treatment groups in toxicity studies. Although it is not always clear exactly why this occurs, these foci can often be regarded as non-specific changes in animals subject to exaggerated effects of potent pharmaceutical agents given at high doses.

Focal inflammation may also localise in and around portal tracts in untreated laboratory animals and this inflammation may be associated with bile duct changes. The cause of spontaneous portal tract inflammation is often unclear but it can be associated with inflammatory changes in the gastrointestinal tract. This is particularly obvious in primates infested with the strongoloid nematode larva, Oesophagostomum which localise in mesenteric tissues and excite an inflammatory response in the peritoneal cavity. Portal inflammation may also accompany certain stages of the life cycle of Taenia taeniaeformis in the rat (Cook et al., 1981).

A more diffuse inflammatory process or hepatitis is uncommonly observed in laboratory animals used in toxicology, although hepatitis can result from viral inflammation in both dogs and rodents. Canine hepatitis virus is a well-known cause of hepatitis in young dogs. It is characterized by scattered foci of hepato-

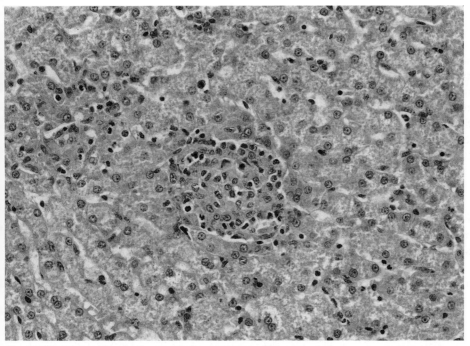

Fig. 78. Liver from a beagle dog containing typical granulomatous lesions or macrophage aggregates sometimes found spontaneously in this species. (HE, ×400.)

cellular necrosis, vascular dilatation, haemorrhage and characteristic, intranuclear inclusions (Jones and Hunt, 1983).

Furthermore, certain viruses such as rat parvovirus which usually only provoke hepatitis with focal cell lysis and intranuclear inclusions in mitotically active neonatal liver, can be reactivated in adult animals by immunosuppression, partial hepatectomy or administration of hepatotoxins (Jacoby et al., 1979).

Although drug-induced hepatic necrosis may be accompanied by an inflammatory response and agents which provoke cholestatic injury also excite inflammation of the portal zones, primary drug-induced inflammation is more unusual (Zimmerman, 1978a).

Complex therapeutic agents such as Corynebacterium parvum and some liposome preparations produce *focal granulomatous inflammation* in the rodent or primate liver following parenteral administration (Roumiantzeff et al., 1975; Allen and Smuckler, 1985).

Allen and Smuckler (1985) have demonstrated the formation of small randomly distributed granulomas composed of rounded histiocytic cells in the livers of mice following repeated intravenous injection of liposomes of certain types. Furthermore, granulomas disappeared on cessation of treatment with most but not all types of liposomes. These differences appeared to relate to changes in phagocytic function accompanying injection of these liposomes, perhaps as a

415

result of the metabolism of the different phospholipid components or the rigidity of the liposome particles (Allen and Smuckler, 1985).

Similar changes occur with the immune modulating agent, Corynebacterium parvum which causes liver weight increase, diffuse histiocytic infiltration and discrete granuloma formation on repeated injection into laboratory animals. In addition, increase of serum hepatic enzymes and slight jaundice have been detected in its clinical use in man (Milas and Scott, 1978), suggesting that similar changes occur in man. Granulomatous hepatitis has been reported in man following treatment with another bacterial immune modulator, bacillus Calmette-Guérin (BCG)(Lamm et al, 1986).

Chronic active hepatitis

This chronic inflammatory condition is characterized histologically by the presence of an inflammatory infiltrate composed mainly of lymphocytes and plasma cells with variable numbers of neutrophils and eosinophils which expands the portal areas and extends into the liver lobule to erode the limiting plate. Individual or small groups of necrotic liver cells may be found in this expanding inflammatory process accompanied by collapse of reticulin and extending fibrous strands (Scheuer, 1980). This may ultimately progress to cirrhosis.

In man, chronic active hepatitis is commonly precipitated by an acute infection with the hepatitis B virus, the outcome of which may be determined by lymphocyte function. When lymphocyte function is defective, viral replication continues and a carrier state with or without chronic hepatitis results. Such lymphocyte failure may occur as a result of increased suppressor-T-cell function, a defect in cytotoxic (K) lymphocytes, blocking antibodies on the cell membrane, or to lack of recognition of genetic HLA markers on the hepatocyte membrane (Sherlock, 1982).

Drugs are also a well described cause of chronic active hepatitis in man, notably the extensively used drugs methyldopa and nitrofurantoin (Goldstein et al., 1973; Maddrey, 1981), the formerly widely employed laxative oxyphenisatin (Reynolds et al., 1971), as well as sulphonamides (Tönder et al., 1974) and isoniazid (Black et al., 1975). Although clinical experience with this type of drug-induced injury indicates that there is gradual improvement following withdrawal of the offending agent (Maddrey, 1981), it may be a progressive condition after cessation of treatment. It has been suggested that parent drug or metabolite can act as a hapten by combining with liver macromolecules rendering them antigenic with resultant lymphocyte sensitisation and hepatocyte damage on subsequent or repeated exposure to the drug (Sherlock, 1982).

This type of chronic active hepatitis found in man is less well described in animals used in toxicology. However, a form of chronic active hepatitis has been described in dogs which may follow infection with canine hepatitis virus and may be accompanied by cholestasis and jaundice (Strombeck and Gribble, 1978; Meyer et al., 1980) and it may occasionally be seen in untreated beagles. However, this type of hepatitis in dogs is quite distinctive possessing certain

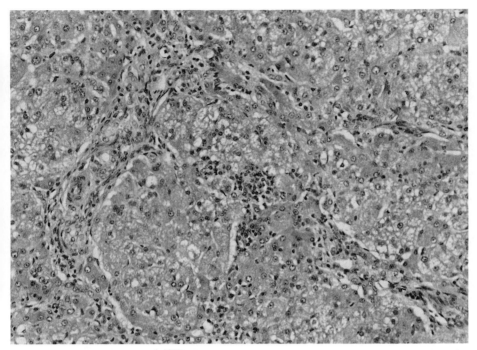

Fig. 79. Liver from a beagle dog showing the histological appearances of chronic dissecting hepatitis. There is some disruption of lobular architecture by fine collagenous bands giving rise to a suggestion of nodularity, mild chronic inflammatory infiltration and slight ballooning of a few hepatocytes. (HE, ×400.)

histological features not normally found in chronic active hepatitis in man and for this reason the term *lobular dissecting hepatitis* has been proposed for the condition (Bennett et al., 1983). This process is characterized histologically by disruption of the hepatic parenchyma by fine collagen and reticulin fibres with formation of small or medium sized regenerative nodules (Figs. 79 and 80). Disruption of limiting plates is quite prominant, hepatocytes show ballooning, granular or eosinophilic cytoplasmic changes and focal piecemeal necrosis. There is bile duct proliferation but relatively sparse portal tract inflammation. Vascular changes are prominant with characteristic dilatation of portal venous sinuses, and pooling of blood, but there is no evidence of primary vascular damage or thrombosis (Bennett et al., 1983).

This histopathological picture can also be observed in the beagle dog following treatment with therapeutic agents which produce hepatic damage (personal observations).

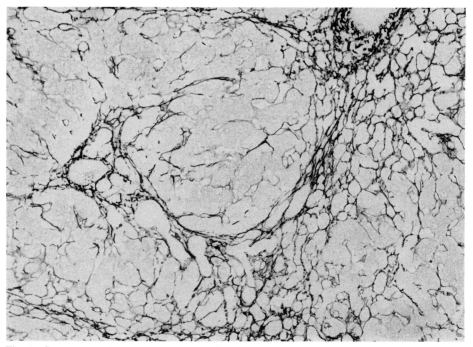

Fig. 80. Same case as in Figure 79 but stained for reticulin. The distinct regenerative nodularity is more evident. (Reticulin, ×250.)

Mallory bodies

These cytoplasmic inclusions were first described by Mallory (1911) in the human liver in alcoholic cirrhosis but they have also been observed in the human liver in a variety of other circumstances including bile duct obstruction (Phillips et al., 1986) hepatocellular carcinoma and following treatment with drugs such as glucocorticoids (Itoh et al., 1977), the cardiovascular agents perhexiline maleate (Paliard et al., 1978) diethylaminoethoxyhexestrol (Itoh and Tsukada, 1973) and amiodarone (Simon et al., 1984; Poucell et al., 1984; Tordjman et al., 1985; Babany and Dhumeaux, 1985; Rinder et al., 1986).

Similar inclusions have been reported in primates given choline-deficient diets or after chronic administration of alcohol (Wilgram and Taylor, 1959; Rubin and Lieber, 1974), in mice given the antifungal agent, griseofulvin (Denk et al., 1979), in aged mice fed a vitamin A deficient-diet for long periods (Akeda et al., 1986), in hepatic nodules in mice given dieldrin (Meierhenry et al., 1981) and in the cells of diethylnitrosamine-induced hepatocellular carcinomas in rats (Borenfreund et al., 1980a). Mallory body formation is also associated with bile duct obstruction in laboratory rats (Kountouras et al., 1984).

Histologically, Mallory bodies are characterized by homogeneous, dense eosinophilic material in the hepatocyte cytoplasm arranged either as small

418

spherical or irregular aggregates or as fairly homogeneous dense intracytoplasmic bodies. Their light microscopic staining characteristics vary with time but in general they appear similar in man and rodent. Immunocytochemical study has shown Mallory bodies contain cytokeratins (Hazen et al., 1986). Human and mouse Mallory bodies possess common antigenic determinants which cross-react with antibodies to prekeratin (Denk et al., 1979), although rat hepatocellular carcinoma Mallory bodies bind to both antiprekeratin and anti-vimentin antibodies (Borenfreund et al., 1980b; French, 1981).

At ultrastructural level they contain filaments which are orientated randomly or in parallel and which vary in diameter from four to over 20 nm (Denk et al, 1979). This suggests that they form as a result of condensation or collapse of intermediate filaments (French, 1981; Okanoue et al., 1985).

French (1981) has reviewed the various theories related to the pathogenesis of Mallory bodies. It has been proposed that they occur as a result of microtubular failure, based on the observation that when microtubules are caused to disassemble by agents such as alcohol and griseofulvin, intermediate filaments accumulate in the cell. Another theory proposed by Denk et al., (1979) is that Mallory bodies are a pathological expression of a hepatocyte-specific form of keratinization, analogous to squamous metaplasia which occurs in various epithelia in vitamin A deficiency. The occurrence of Mallory bodies in neoplastic hepatocytes of both man and rodents and their close association with γ-glutamyl transpeptidase activity and α-foetoprotein expression, have led to the suggestion that Mallory bodies may represent a genetically controlled characteristic of neoplastic or preneoplastic hepatocytes (French, 1981; Tazawa et al., 1983; Nakanuma and Ohta 1985, 1986).

Myelin figures (myeloid bodies, myelinoid bodies, myelinosomes)

Various names have been given to single membrane-bound, lysosomal bodies containing electron-dense smooth membranes arranged in a reticular manner, in stacks or as concentric whorls (Ghadially, 1982). They are seen at light microscopic level as small dense or dark particles within the cell cytoplasm. Although they are found in normal cells, a large variety of amphiphilic drugs can produce these bodies in the liver of experimental animals usually as part of generalised phospholididosis. (Hruban et al., 1972; Hruban, 1984). The preferential involvement of the liver depends on drug disposition, dosage and duration of treatment as well as the potency of amphiphilic drug (Hruban, 1984). The study by Hruban and colleagues (1972) suggested that these bodies are modified secondary lysosomes which persist as a result of protracted degradation of membranous material. Drugs or their metabolites may be responsible for this change through several mechanisms. They may bind to membranes and inhibit their digestion, they may inhibit cholesterol synthesis, thereby allowing precursors of cholesterol to accumulate, they may selectively inhibit lysosomal enzymes concerned with membrane digestion or prevent fusion of primary lysosomes with heterogenesis dense bodies (Hruban et al., 1972).

Although most of the 50 or so drugs which cause phospholididosis in laboratory animals have not shown similar effects in man, a small number are associated with hepatic phospholididosis and hepatic damage in humans (reviewed by Hruban, 1984).

Mitochondrial crystalloid inclusions

Filamentous or crystalline inclusions have been observed in hepatic mitochondria in man in a variety of conditions including viral hepatitis, cholestasis and biliary lithiasis, hyperlipoproteinaemia. Dubin-Johnson syndrome, Wilson's disease, obesity, diabetes and alcoholic liver disease (Theman and von Bassewitz 1969; Bhagwat and Ross, 1971; Kovacs et al., 1972; Burns et al., 1972; Friedman et al., 1977). They have also been found in man following oral contraceptive administration, methotrexate, and lidoflazine therapy and after environmental exposure to organochlorine pesticides (Lundbergh and Westman, 1970; Verheyen et al., 1975; Guzelian et al., 1980; Horvath et al., 1978). Identical inclusions have also been observed in biopsies taken from apparently quite normal human livers (Verheyen et al., 1975).

Similar mitochondrial crystalloid are also found in the dog liver (Ghadially, 1982). They are very occasionally seen in apparently normal dogs (Verheyen and Borgers, 1976; personal observations) and they have also been described in the liver of the normal rhesus monkey (Kennedy, 1979). Their development can be potentiated by administration of pharmaceutical agents of different classes, in the absence of evidence of structural cell damage (Simpson et al., 1974).

Although large mitochondria containing needle-like inclusions can be seen in epon-embedded sections by light microscopy (Friedman et al., 1977), the crystalline inclusions are only clearly visualized at ultrastructural level. They are characterized both in man and dog by bundles of parallel arranged filaments of somewhat variable thickness, but usually 5–10 nm and separated by a space of 4–6 nm orientated longitudinally in the mitochondrial matrix (Simpson et al., 1974; Friedman et al., 1977).

Electron microscopic study suggests that these filaments originate from mitochondrial cristae (Friedman et al., 1977). Optical diffraction methods have shown that these inclusions originate from mitochondrial proteins and phospholipids (Kiechle, 1979). Histochemical techniques have demonstrated high cytochrome oxidase activities in these inclusions (Theman and von Bassewitz, 1969).

When seen in the absence of adverse cellular or subcellular changes, the presence of crystalloid does not appear to be indicative of hepatotoxicity. The careful study of liver biopsies of obese patients undergoing intestinal bypass surgery showed that the number of inclusions were related to the degree of hepatic steatosis and they tended to disappear as steatosis cleared. This finding supports the concept that the presence of intramitochondrial inclusions represents ultrastructural evidence of an adaptation to an altered metabolic environment which is reversible when the inciting stimulus is removed (Friedman et al.,

1977). However, the finding of hepatic mitochondrial inclusions in toxicity studies needs to be evaluated in the context of any other hepatic changes which may be found.

Note. Crystalloid inclusions are also seen in abnormally large mitochondria (giant mitochondria, megamitochondria). These are found in hepatocytes from man, dog, rat and mouse in a variety of circumstances including after administration of alcohol, drugs, hormones, in various nutritional states as well as in apparently normal livers (Ghadially, 1982). They may also be the result of exaggerated demands on fatty acid metabolism (Kovacs et al., 1972) or associated with a decrease in number of mitochondria by fusion of pre-existing ones as a result of defects in the respiratory system (Kimberg and Loeb, 1972). In haematoxylin and eosin-stained sections of liver they can be seen as rounded homogeneous pink structures 3–10 m diameter in hepatocyte cytoplasm where they need to be distinguished from Mallory bodies (Chedid et al., 1986).

Drug crystals

Whilst crystallization of certain poorly soluble drugs is a well-recognised phenomen in the distal part of the nephron, drug crystals may form in hepatocytes or bile caniliculi where they need to be distinguished from endogeneous crystalloid substances.

An example of this phenomenon has been reported in cynomolgus monkeys treated with an investigative benzopyran-4-one, cerebral dopamine autoreceptor agonist, PD 119819 (Macallum et al., 1988, 1989).

Needle-like drug crystals were demonstrated in bile canaliculi and hepatocytes (as well as kidney), associated with granulomatous inflammation and biochemical evidence of hepatic damage (Fig. 81). It was postulated that this form of crystallization was primarily the result of the insolubility of PD 119189 at alkaline pH. Although the phenomenon did not occur in rodents, it occurred at sufficiently low doses in the primate model, to preclude its administration to man (Macallum et al., 1989a).

Other cytoplasmic inclusions

A variety of less-well characterised eosinophilic cytoplasmic inclusions also develop in the hepatocytes of laboratory animals both spontaneously and following treatment with xenobiotics. Homogeneous, globular eosinophilic inclusions may be found in the hepatic cytoplasm of untreated laboratory beagle dogs (Harleman et al., 1987). These are PAS positive, stain with Sudan black for bound lipids and are characterised by electron microscopy as membrane-bound homegeneous, moderately electron dense bodies. Their significance is unclear.

Eosinophilic cytoplasmic inclusions are also sometimes visible in hepatocytes in laboratory animals treated with agents which increase smooth endoplasmic reticulum formation and induce mixed function oxidase activity in the liver.

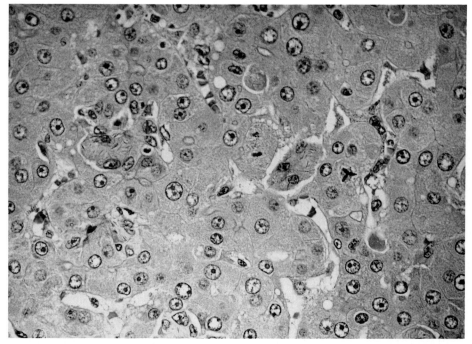

Fig. 81. Liver from cynomolgus monkey treated with a novel dopamine autoreceptor agonist, PD 119819, as reported by Macallum et al., (1989). This field shows the presence of fine needle-like crystals of drug in some hepatocytes. (HE, ×550.)

These inclusions correlate with the presence of concentric arrays of smooth membranes continuous with smooth endoplasmic reticulum which form following administration of these agents (Walker et al., 1988).

The presence of rounded, eosinophilic cytoplasmic inclusions composed of condensed electron dense material within the dilated cisternae of rough endo- plasmic reticulum in mouse hepatocellular carcinoma cells has been associated with low thymidine labelling indices (Kakizoe et al., 1989).

Pigmentation

Various ceroids or lipofuscin are seen in the livers of untreated rodents non-hu- man primates and dogs, particularly in older animals and the accumulation of these pigments can be accelerated by treatment with drugs and chemicals, trauma, circulatory disturbances and dietary abnormalities. The outstanding feature of these pigments is their insolubility in alcohols and xylene and other solvents used to prepare tissue sections. They are characterized by pale yellow to deep brown colour, sudanophilia and typically show autofluorescence under ultraviolet light (Hartroft and Porta, 1972).

Ceroid granules are heterogeneous in nature when viewed under the electron microscope. They may be translucent, compact rounded bodies of variable density or laminated in nature (Hartroft and Porta, 1972; Ikeda et al., 1985). They are usually bounded by a discrete limiting membrane consistent with a lysosomal location. They appear to be formed from unsaturated fats by reactions which begin with lipid peroxidation and subsequent polymerization to an insoluble substance.

Whereas ceroid may accumulate following tissue necrosis produced by administration of xenobiotics, a number of therapeutic agents increase the amount of ceroid observed in the liver in the absence of overt necrosis. Hypolipidaemic agents which produce peroxisomal proliferation in the rodent liver, increase the amount of lipofuscin in rodent liver cells after prolonged treatment probably by a process of increased lipid peroxidation (Goel et al., 1986).

Indeed, the presence of lipofucsin in the liver following long-term treatment of rodents with peroxisomal proliferators has been interpreted as evidence of lipid peroxidation and supporting the concept of free radical production by these agents (Reddy and Lalwani, 1983). Lipofuscin deposition accompanied by

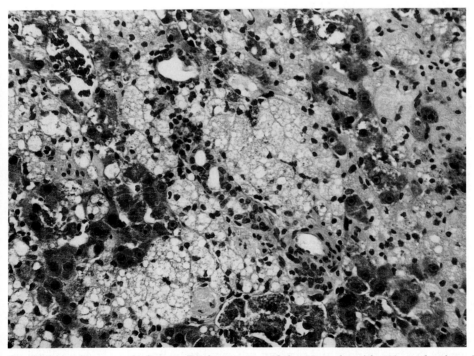

Fig. 82. Liver from a male Sprague-Dawley rat treated for 86 weeks with 400 mg/kg/day of clofibrate and killed 17 weeks after withdrawal of treatment. There is massive accumulation of lipofuscin pigment between residual hepatocytes. (HE, ×300.)

hepatocyte vacuolation has also been reported in rats treated for six months with an imidazole antifungal drug (Nishikawa et al., 1984).

Increased lipochrome has also been observed in the Kupffer cells of dogs treated with the synthetic ergot derivative, bromocriptine, apparently as a non-specific effect accompanying general adverse changes such as shown by body weight loss and diminished food intake at exaggerated dose levels (Richardson et al., 1984). During the preclinical toxicity testing of the novel histamine H1 receptor antagonist, temelastine, increased hepatocellular lipofuscin pigment was also found in both treated dogs and rats. Although in neither species was there histological evidence of hepatocellular necrosis, the associated increases in plasma alanine aminotransferase, glutamine dehydrogenase and alkaline phosphatase in treated dogs led to the suggestion that temelastine could be inducing mild hepatocellular membrane damage which led to accumulation of lipofuscin (Poole et al., 1990). Ceroid deposition may also be found in areas of fibrosis in the liver or around hepatic nodules in rodents (Fig. 82). Ceroid pigment together with lipogranulomas have been found in increased amounts in the hepatic parenchyma and portal tracts in dogs which develop hyperplastic nodules of the liver (Berman, 1983).

Other pigments may be found, particularly iron, which accumulates in hepatocytes and Kupffer cells after injection of iron-containing compounds or following breakdown of red blood cells.

For instance, a slight increase in haemosiderin was reported in hepatocytes and Kuffer cells as well as in the spleen in rats treated for 12 months with high doses of the angiotensin converting enzyme inhibitor, captopril. (Hashimoto et al., 1981). This was associated with slight reductions in haemoglobin and increased erythropoiesis and was probably the result of increase breakdown of red blood cells.

Porphyrin pigments can also be deposited in the liver of rats, mice or dogs following aministration of a number of different xenobiotics including griseofulvin, 3,5-diethoxycarbonyl-1,4-dihydrocollidine (DDC), hexachlorobenzene and an antiarthritic agent 3-[2-(2,4,6-trimethylphenyl)-thiothyl]-4 methylsydnone (TTMS) (Tschudy and Bonkowsky, 1972; Stejskal et al., 1975; Poh-Fitzpatrick et al., 1983; De Matteis et al., 1987).

Typically, these agents produce a similar histological picture, characterised by the presence of red-brown pigment globules in bile ductules and bile canaliculi and small granules in hepatocytes, Kupfer cells and portal macophages. This is accompanied by a variable acute and chronic portal tract inflammation and bile duct proliferation. The pigment is characterised by birefringent properties and red autofluorescence in ultraviolet light and is believed to be protoporphyrin. (De Matteis et al., 1987).

Administration of TTMS to rat, mouse and dog produced hepatic porphyria in all three species although periportal focal hepatocyte necrosis was found in mice but not rats or dogs and pigment appeared to be limited to bile canaliculi in dogs (Stejskal et al., 1975).

Based on studies with griseofulvin and DDC in rodents, it has been postulated that this type of drug-induced porphyria is a result of inhibition of ferrochelatase which leads to accumulation of its substrate protoporphyrin and compensatory stimulation of the first enzyme in this pathway, 5-aminolevulinate synthase (De Matteis et al., 1987).

Whereas accumulation of protoporphyrin can produce hepatocellular damage in these experimental animals, there is little or no clinical evidence of drug-induced protoporphyria in humans (Bloomer, 1988).

Amyloid

In amyloid-prone species, particularly the hamster, amyloid may be deposited in the liver with advancing age. It may appear in the walls of blood vessels or accumulate to a major extent in the portal tracts, giving rise to dilatation or degeneration of bile ducts and blood vessels. Amyloid may also extend from the portal tracts into the hepatic parenchyma to produce a cirrhosis-like appearance.

Vascular changes

The liver vasculature may develop pathology seen in other parts of the cardiovascular system including vasculitis, thrombosis and deposition of amyloid (see Cardiovascular System, Chapter VI). Vascular changes specific to the liver are described below.

Peliosis hepatis

In man, this condition is characterized by the presence of blood-filled cystic spaces or lacunae of variable size usually devoid of an endothelial lining. Their presence has been associated with chronic wasting diseases as well as administration of anabolic steroids and oral contraceptives (Yanoff and Rawson, 1964; Naeim et al., 1973; Bagheri and Boyer, 1974). The association of peliosis with oral contraceptive agents is somewhat controversial, as adequate human liver biopsy material is scanty (Portman et al., 1981). The pathogenesis of hepatic peliosis is uncertain. Recent ultrastructural study has suggested that the lesion results from weakening of the sinusoidal supporting structure, possibly by impairment of the ability of endothelial cells to maintain collageneous reticulum (Zafrani et al., 1984). This study showed no definite evidence that hepatocellular necrosis or blockage of liver blood flow at the junction of sinusoids and centrilobular veins were primary events in the development of peliosis hepatitis in man.

A similar histological pattern is found in untreated aged rats of various strains (Boorman and Hollander, 1973; Lee, 1983). Ultrastructural study has suggested this also arises from disruption of the sinusoidal epithelium (Lee, 1983).

The lesion can be induced in mice and rats by exposure to viruses (Bergs and Scotti, 1967) or administration of various compounds including the pyrrolizidine alkaloid, lasiocarpine (Ruebner et al., 1970), sodium lithocholate (Bagheri et al, 1973) and phalloidin, a cyclic peptide isolated from the mushroom, Amanita phalloides, (Tuchweber et al., 1973). It has also been induced in rats with an anti-rat glomerular basement membrane antibody in rats pre-sensitised with a rare earth metal complex, neodymium pyrocatechin disulphonate, which is known to depress reticulo-endothelial activity (Husztik et al., 1984).

Since all these experimental procedures produce damage to endothelium and cell membranes, they are consistent with the concept that peliosis is associated with damage or weakening of the sinusoidal walls.

Sinusoidal dilatation

Sinusoidal dilatation in centrilobular zones (Rappaport zone III) with a variable degree of atrophy of hepatocyte plates is reported in man in a variety of conditions associated with hypoxia or hypoperfusion such as right sided heart failure, compression or thrombosis of hepatic veins, amyloid infiltration and the presence of neoplastic or granulomatous disease (Bruguera et al., 1978). Similar histological appearances are found in aged rodents suffering from various sponta-neous disease but particularly the aged hamster which is especially prone to develop cardiac and vascular thrombosis and amyloid infiltration of the liver. Sinusoidal dilatation also occurs both in and around hepatic nodules in the rodent liver.

By contrast, periportal sinusoidal dilatation (Rappaport zone I) in man appears to be almost exclusively associated with the long-term effect of con-traceptive steroids (Winkler and Poulsen, 1975; Ishak, 1981; Camilleri et al., 1981). The cause of this change is not clear. It appears not to be associated with haemodynamic changes, although it may represent a direct effect of contracep-tive steroids or metabolites on hepatocytes. (Winkler and Poulsen, 1975). Certain authors have noted a similarity between this type of sinusoidal dilatation in man and changes preceding the development of angiosarcoma produced by vinyl chloride, thorotrast or arsenic (Thung and Gerber, 1981) although there is no convincing evidence that such lesions are related in any way.

A similar histological picture has been observed in rats, mice and guinea pigs treated with glucocorticoids or in mice bearing hormone-secreting testicular intesti-nal neoplasms, presumably also a result of locally altered haemodynamics (Wolstenholme and Gardner, 1950; Bhagwat and Deodar, 1968).

Foci of cellular alteration, hepatic nodules and hepatic carcinoma

Focal and nodular proliferation of hepatocytes occurs spontaneously or in associ-ated with the administration of drugs and chemicals both in man and laboratory animals. Unlike in the rodent, the largest proportion of hepatocellular neoplasms in man throughout the world are associated with cirrhosis which influences the range of focal or nodular histopathological changes seen in clinical practice. However, hepatic nodules of various types and hepatocellular neoplasms occur in the human liver without cirrhosis and in association with pharmaceutical agents such as oral contraceptives and anabolic steroids (Baum et al., 1973; Bernstein et

TABLE 1   *Classification of focal hepatocellular lesions and neoplasia*

Characteristics	Man (Edmondson, 1958) Rodents (Newberne, 1982) Hamster (Greenblatt, 1982) Dog (Fabry et al., 1982)	Rat (Squire and Levitt, 1975; Stewart et al., 1980)	Mouse, rat and hamster (Hayashi, 1985)
No compression	Foci of cellular alteration	Foci of cellular alteration	Foci of cellular alteration
With compression but no invasion	Focal nodular hyperplasia Adenoma	Neoplastic nodule	Hyperplastic nodule
With invasion and/or metastases	Hepatocellular carcinoma	Hepatocellular carcinoma	Hepatocellular carcinoma

Characteristics	Mouse (Ward and Vlahakis, 1978; Turusov and Takayama,	Mouse (Walker et al., 1972)	Mouse (Gellatly, 1975)	Mouse (Becker, 1982)
No compression	Foci of cellular alteration		Type 1 nodule *	MLT 1
		Type a hepatoma		
With compression but no invasion	Adenoma		Type 2 nodule	MLT II
With invasion and/or metastases	Hepatocellular carcinoma	Type b hepatoma	Type 3 nodule	MLT III
				MLT IV

Note: Type I nodule defined as not compressing surrounding liver tissue

al., 1971; Sherlock, 1978; Ishak, 1981). Indeed, the proliferation of case reports of nodules associated with sex hormone administration in man has led to quite a debate concerning their terminology (Portman et al., 1981), somewhat analogous to the differences of opinion about the classification of rodent liver nodules. However, more recent critical evaluation of these nodular lesions in human liver has served to reaffirm the basic histological criteria outlined nearly 30 years ago by Edmundson (1958).

A number of different histopathological classifications have been proposed for rodent liver nodules and neoplasia (Table 1), none entirely satisfactory in all situations. A major difficulty in the experimental situation is obtaining a clear indication of biological behaviour of the different lesions which are only usually observed at one point in time: at autopsy. By the use of syngeneic animals, transplantation procedures are sometimes used to assess biological behaviour, but results from this technique do not always give rise to a convincing assessment of biological behaviour (Stewart et al., 1980). This contrasts with the clinical situation in man where modern imaging techniques can now closely monitor the progression of hepatic nodules. Here the problem is more often the converse: lack of sufficient biopsy material to assure a realistic histological evaluation of large, often heterogenous nodular lesions (Portman et al., 1981).

Apart from the difficulties in classification of hepatic nodules in rodents, a variety of other factors need to be considered in their evaluation when they are found in carcinogenicity bioassays conducted with medicinal agents.

The rodent liver model has been used extensively for the study of the initiation and promotion sequence of neoplasia. The basic characteristics of this system, using powerful genotoxic carcinogens, appear similar to the mouse skin model from which much of our understanding of the initiation and promotion sequence has evolved (Pitot, 1983). The sequence has been particularly well studied in the rat liver, where initiation with a powerful carcinogen is followed by rapid development of foci of cellular alteration with distinct morphological characteristics which appear to represent the clonal progeny of initiated cells (Williams, 1980; Bannasch et al., 1982; Farber, 1982; Rabes et al., 1982). After further exposure to carcinogens or promoting agents, various nodules and hepatocellular carcinomas are found. A similar sequence also appears to occur both in mice (Becker and Sell, 1979) and hamsters (Stenbäck et al., 1986), when similar carcinogens and dose schedules are employed, although in mice the effects of hepatocarcinogens has been shown to be strain dependent (Kakizoe et al., 1989).

Unfortunately, this straightforward situation is complicated by the occurence of similar hepatic foci, nodules and hepatocellular carcinomas spontaneously in certain strains of rat, mouse and hamster with advancing age. They also occur in association with administration of chemical agents which are neither considered powerful carcinogens nor are mutagenic in the various short-term tests. (Tennant et al., 1987). Schulte-Hermann and colleagues (1983, 1985) have questioned whether it is in fact possible to distinguish promoting agents from initiators in the rodent liver if foci of cellular alteration, which are generally believed to represent the progeny of initiated cells, occur in untreated rats. This is obviously of importance because initiation is considered irreversible and without a threshhold dose level, whereas promotion, at least in the mouse skin and rat liver, is a dose-dependent phenomenon (Pitot, 1983). A further complicating factor is the influence of diet on the development of enzyme altered foci in the rat liver occurring after initiation and promotion sequences (Hei and Sudilovsky, 1985). Rats fed diets devoid of choline and low in methionine in the absence of any known or added carcinogen also develop hepatic neoplasms (Mikol et al., 1983; Ghoshal and Farber, 1984; Yokayama et al., 1985).

Unfortunately, our understanding of the development and progression of liver cancer in rodents following administration of non-genotoxic agents such as the peroxisomal proliferators or after dietary manipulation remains poor (Farber and Sarma, 1987). Consequently, when a totally novel pharmaceutical agent showing no genotoxic activity in conventional short term tests induces increased numbers of hepatic foci, nodules and neoplasia in rodent carcinogenicity bioassays, elucidation of the mechanism and evaluation of human risk remains a major challenge.

Nevertheless, it is becoming apparent that foci and nodules produced by genotoxic agents are not necessarily identical to those occurring spontaneously in the rodent liver or following long-term treatment with high doses of therapeutic agents (see Figs. 83 and 84). Ward (1981) has suggested that some types of hepatocarcinogen produce specific morphological types of hepatic tumours in the rat. Different metabolic characteristics, rate of onset and reversibility patterns have also been noted between foci of cellular alteration and nodules in rats treated with genotoxic carcinogens such as diethylnitrosamine and the hypo-lipidaemic agent, clofibrate (Rao et al., 1982a; Greaves et al., 1986).

The eosinophilic nodules which were induced in C3H/the mice by chronic administration of phenobarbitone were also shown to be different from the distinctly basophilic nodules arising spontaneously in this strain and unlike basophilic nodules produced by administration of N-nitrosodiethylamine (Gangolli et al., 1987). Retrospective characterisation of morphological character-istics of altered hepatocellular foci in six conventional two year carcinogenicity studies conducted in Fischer 344 rats by the National Toxicology Program (NTP) has also shown morphological variability of foci induced by different agents (Harada et al., 1989a,b).

Markers and metabolic patterns in foci and nodules

Nodules produced in the various rat hepatic cancer liver models which employ agents such as 2-acetylaminofluorene, diethylnitrosamine or dimethylhydrazine are characterised by common metabolic patterns of activity. The particular nodules found in these models generally show low activity of enzymes such as microsomal cytochrome P450, cytochrome b_5 and aminopyrine demethylase which are associated with phase I reactions. By contrast, they contain elevated components of conjugation or detoxification reactions (phase II) such as is demonstrated by the presence of increased amounts of glutathione and height-ened activity of glutathione-S-transferases and gamma glutamyl transpeptidase (Fig. 85) (Farber, 1984; Roomi et al., 1985). Although these changes do not represent an unique tumour enzyme pattern, it has been suggested that they indicate an adaptive process, hepatocytes in nodular lesions being better equipped to survive the adverse effects of repeated administration of carcinogens or promoting agents (Farber, 1984; Farber and Sarma, 1987).

This hypothesis also embraces the putative pre-neoplastic cell marker, gamma-glutamyl transpeptidase. Studies of this enzyme, particularly in the kidney, have suggested that hydrolysis of glutathione and its thiol derivatives at the cell membrane is the major significant reaction catalysed by gamma-gluta-myl transpeptidase (Curthoys and Hughey, 1979). Many compounds, including carcinogens, are conjugated with glutathione in the liver and excreted in the bile, and it has been suggested by Hanigan and Pitot (1985) that this may be partly why gamma-glutamyl transpeptidase activity is so heavily concentrated on the luminal surface of intrahepatic bile ducts, thereby allowing reabsorption of

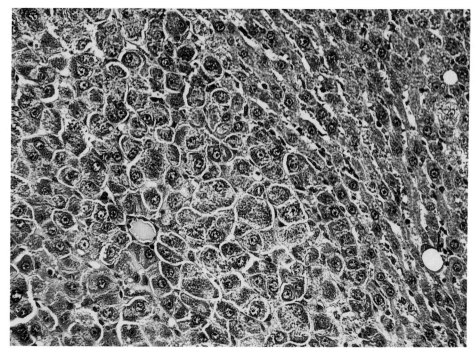

Fig. 83. Hyperplastic nodule developing spontaneously in a two-year-old Sprague-Dawley rat. It is composed or large hepatocytes and there is early displacement of the surrounding normal parenchyma. (HE, ×300.)

glutathione in the form of its constituent amino acids from fluids which are being excreted.

Whereas these enzyme patterns, including that of elevated gamma-glutamyl transpeptidase activity seem to correlate with the evolution of hepatic neoplasia in other systems or species including man (Gerber and Thung, 1980), they cannot simply be regarded as diagnostic of pre-neoplastic or neoplastic change. Enzymatic changes in foci of cellular alteration and nodules in the rat and mouse after initiation with powerful carcinogens seems to depend in part on the nature of the subsequent promoting agent (Ohmori et al., 1981; Ward et al. 1983; Schulte-Hermann et al., 1984; Numoto et al., 1985). Although similar enzymatic patterns have been produced by carcinogenic chemicals in the mouse (Stout and Becker, 1986), it appears that enzymatic changes occurring in the mouse hepatic neoplasia models are generally less consistent to those occurring in the rat (Butler and Hempsall, 1978; Essigman and Newberne, 1981; Ruebner et al., 1982).

In the hamster, gamma-glutamyl transpeptidase activity is notable by its absence in hepatocellular lesions produced by dimethylnitrosamine followed by phenobarbitone (Stenbäck et al., 1986) Similarly, foci and nodules occurring in the rat liver following administration of hypolipidaemic agents are also characterised by lack of gamma-glutamyl transpeptidase activity (Rao et al., 1982a).

Typical foci positive for gamma-glutamyl transpeptidase are not found in the rat liver after portocaval anastomosis (Evarts et al., 1986), despite the fact that this procedure can produce nodules in the rat liver (Weinbren and Washington, 1976; Weinbren, 1978). Although a relationship between protooncogene expression and neoplasia in the rat liver has also been described (Hayashi et al., 1984; Corcos et al., 1984), the expression of such protooncogenes does not correlate very well with gamma-glutamyl transpeptidase activity in the rat liver (Beer et al., 1986).

Immunohistochemical demonstration of a placental form of glutathione S-transferase has also been shown to be a useful marker of foci in the rat liver although it fails to show foci induced by peroxisomal proliferators (Popp and Goldsworthy, 1989). The enzyme glucose-6-phosphate dehydrogenase, an important rate limiting enzyme in the pentose phosphate shunt which provides ribose for synthesis of nucleic acids and NADPH for biosynthetic processes, is also of interest. When neotetrazolium chloride is used as a cytochemical indicator of activity of this enzyme, oxygen competes with neotetrazolium and eliminates the reaction in normal cells but not those in a range of human of human malignant cell types and hepatocellular carcinomas developing in the rat

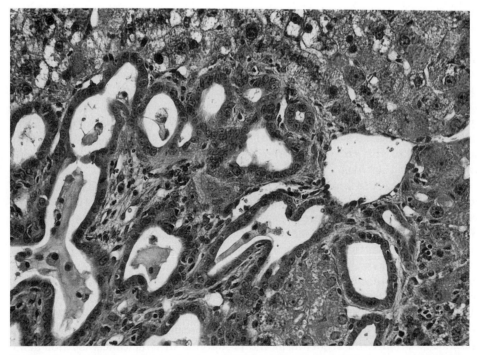

Fig. 84. Hepatocellular carcinoma showing glandular differentiation. This tumour developed in a Sprague-Dawley rat treated with diethynitrosamine followed by phenobarbitone promotion. (HE, ×300.)

after the administration of diethylnitrosamine followed by promotion with phenobarbitone (Fig. 86) (Greaves et al., 1986).

Correlative histochemical studies of foci, nodules and hepatocellular carcinomas occurring in the rat following administration of N-nitrosomorpholine have also shown that although glycogen storage occurs initially in many foci (clear cell foci), there is a progressive shift away from glycogen metabolism with time in foci and subsequent nodules and carcinomas (Hacker et al., 1982).

This shift, during which focal lesions become mixed or more basophilic in character, is accompanied by a parallel shift to the pentose phosphate pathway and glycolysis as shown by the increase in activity of glucose-6-phosphate dehydrogenase (Fig. 86) and glyceraldehyde-3-phosphate dehydrogenase (Hacker et al., 1982).

In addition to these enzymatic changes a variety of other phenomena have been studied in experimental liver cancer models such as resistance to iron storage (Williams, 1980), expression of α-foetoprotein (Becker and Sell, 1979) and a number of other cell markers and enzymes which can be demonstrated in tissue sections by immunocytochemical and lectin histochemical techniques (Holmes et al., 1984; Schulte-Hermann et al., 1984; Enomoto et al., 1981; Pritchard and Butler, 1986; Villanove and Greaves, 1983; Ogino et al., 1982).

Another approach to distinguishing between agents which induce neoplasms by genotoxic mechanisms from those which may potentiate the growth of background tumours has been the study of activated cellular oncogenes (c-oncs) in hepatic tissue from treated rodents. Using hybridisation techniques and transfection assays, it has been shown that hepatic neoplasms induced in rodents by xenobiotics show enhanced expression of certain oncogenes and that the patterns of expression may be different from those found in spontaneously developing hepatic tumours. (Corcos et al., 1984; Reynolds et al., 1987). The polymerase chain reaction (PCR) which is able to detect any short chain DNA sequence in tissue sections (Goudie, 1989) represents another powerful technique which may be able to detect differences in oncogene expression using paraffin wax-embedded sections.

Although these techniques and findings are of considerable interest in experimental tumour pathology, they possess less immediate application in the safety assessment of novel therapeutic agents. Nevertheless, many of these methods have potential in safety assessment by aiding the characterization of foci and nodules developing in carcinogenicity bioassays. This is especially true of enzymes and markers such as cytochrome P450, gamma-glutamyl transpeptidase and α-foetoprotein, the presence of which can be demonstrated immunocytochemically in formalin fixed or paraffin embedded material (Kuhlmann, 1981; Woods, 1983; Schulte-Hermann et al., 1984). However, the sheer diversity of these characteristics and our general lack of understanding of the initiation-promotion-progression sequence in the production of liver cancer by non-genotoxic agents serves to underline that the assessment of focal and nodular hepatic lesions found in bioassays should be based on a thorough histopathological assessment of liver sections. This should be conducted in the context of a thorough knowledge of the precise morphological characteristics of lesions occurring spontaneously in the test species, metabolic changes occurring in the nodular and non-nodular liver of treated animals, coupled with a good understanding of the pharmacology, genetic activity, metabolism and disposition of the test agent.

Histopathology of foci of cellular alteration

It is convenient for comparative purposes to consider focal or nodular lesions of the liver as three main groups, foci and areas of cellular alteration, hepatic nodules and hepatocellular carcinomas (see Table 1).

1) *Foci and areas of cellular alteration* are characterised by small groups of hepatocytes with cytological features distinctive from adjacent liver cells but with little or no alteration in architectural pattern and no evidence of compression of surrounding tissue.

They have been most clearly characterized in the rat liver, where they may show cytoplasmic basophilia (*basophilic focus*), eosinophilic or ground glass change (*eosinophilic focus*), clear cell change (*clear cell focus*), vacuolation (*vacuolated focus*) or mixed appearances (*mixed cell focus*) (Squire and Levitt, 1975; Stewart et al., 1980; Greaves and Faccini, 1984).

More recently, Harada and collegues (1989a) have defined a number of other morphological subtypes of hepatic foci in control Fischer 344 rats, although their biological significance is unclear. Basophilic foci can be composed of cells showing homogeneous cytoplasmic basophilia (*homogenous basophilic foci*) or bands of basophilia located in the peripheral cytoplasm, the so-called '*tigroid foci*'. Five variations of eosinophilic foci have also been described each with different functional characteristics (Harada et al., 1989a).

A further point made recently by Squire (1989) is that there has been an evolution in the diagnostic criteria applied by some pathologists to foci since the NCI workshop in 1974. This change is the acceptance of a greater degree of displacement or compression of the surrounding liver tissue by hepatocellular foci. Thus, the presence of some compression alone is considered by some workers not sufficient evidence to clarify a focal lesion as neoplastic (Squire, 1989).

Rats usually develop foci of cellular alteration spontaneously with age but their prevalence and cytological type vary markedly between strain of rat (Burek, 1978). In the Fisher-344 rat, basophilic foci, generally devoid of gammaglutamyl transpeptidase activity, are particularly common (Ward, 1981). In other strains, basophilic foci may also be prominent (Schulte-Hermann et al., 1983) but variations in the cytological nature of foci have been recorded in the same strain of rat with time even in the same laboratory using standard housing and diet (Greaves et al., 1986).

Similar foci occur in the various rat models for rapid production of liver neoplasms using powerful genotoxic carcinogens, and they are believed to represent the clonal progeny of initiated cells (see above). As they appear prior to the development of frank neoplasms in these models, foci occurring in carcinogenic-

433

ity bioassays of pharmaceutical agents need to be carefully evaluated (Bannasch, 1986).

The fact that foci occur spontaneously in the rat with increasing age suggests that treatment-related increase in the prevalence of foci in rat carcinogenicity assays do not necessarily represent carcinogenic risk for man. Foci in the various models for hepatic neoplasia occur rapidly at a time when spontaneous foci do not generally occur (Greaves et al., 1986). Those which occur following treatment with pharmaceutical agents in widespread clinical use, notably clofibrate and phenobarbitone, occur much later in the life of rats and tend to be predominantly eosinophilic in type (Ward et al., 1983; Rao et al., 1984; Greaves et al., 1986).

More recently, high doses of lovastatin, a HMG CoA reductase inhibitor and cholesterol lowering agent, were reported to produce an increase in the prevalence of both eosinophilic and basophilic foci but not hepatocellular neoplasms in a rat carcinogenicity study (MacDonald et al., 1988). As coadministration of mevalonic acid, the immediate product of HMG CoA reductase, prevented the development of foci, it was argued that their development was related to the exaggerated biochemical mechanism of action of lovastatin, of little or no relevance to the appropriate therapeutic use of the drug in man.

Similar foci of cellular alteration have been produced in the mouse after administration of carcinogens (Vesselinovitch et al., 1985). They also occur spontaneously in the hamster liver (McMartin, 1979) and are occasionally seen in man (Altmann, 1978). They appear to be a less common finding in species other than the rat. The precise reason for this species difference is not certain, but the variety of other changes seen in the livers of mice and hamsters with advancing age are perhaps of greater importance.

Quite clearly, it is important to record the type of foci occurring spontaneously in the test strain, the type occurring in treatment groups and their rate of onset in carcinogenicity bioassays with pharmaceutical agents.

Other types of foci

Metaplastic foci (foci of pancreatic tissue) Discrete foci of pancreatic acinar tissue have been found in the livers of rats fed with polychlorinated biphenyls such as Arochlor 1254 (Kimbrough, 1973). These foci resemble pancreatic tissue at ultrastructural level and immunocytochemical study has shown the presence of both amylase and typsinogen, confirming that these foci are both morphologically and functionally similar to pancreatic acinar tissue (Rao et al., 1986). This phenomenon is another example of *metaplasia* illustrative of the multipotent nature of some cells in mature animals. Similar phenomena are illustrated by the intestinal metaplasia of intrahepatic bile ductular epithelium, conversion of pancreatic acinar cells to hepatocytes and epidermal metaplasia of bronchial epithelium (Scarpelli and Rao 1981; Reddy et al., 1984; Scarpelli, 1985).

This histogenesis of pancreatic foci in the liver remains uncertain. The most probable pathway is the conversion of a parent cell to an intermediate one which then fully differentiates to a metaplastic cell (Scarpelli, 1985). It is likely that the experimental conditions allow derepression of genes with subsequent morphological and functional differentiation of a different nature. Whether pancreatic foci develop from hepatocytes, oval cells or bile duct cells remains uncertain (Rao et al., 1986).

Spongiosis hepatis (focal cystic change) Foci or zones of multilocular cavities separated by thin walls composed of connective tissue and containing pale granular or flocculent pink acid mucopolysaccharide are found in the untreated rat liver, as well as in the livers of rats treated with nitrosomorpholine (Bannasch et al., 1981). Unlike peliosis hepatis the cavities are generally devoid of blood.

Electron microscopic examination reveals that the foci comprise connective tissue cells, resembling fibroblasts and fat storing cells with extremely elongated cytoplasmic processes closely associated with a thick, basement membrane-like material.

Bannasch and his colleagues (1981) from their study of spongiosis hepatis induced by N-nitrosomorpholine, suggested that the lesions result from carcinogen-induced metabolic disturbance of perisinusoidal cells which gives rise to excessive accumulation of acid mucopolysaccharide and collageneous material. However, there is no evidence that spongiosis hepatis is in itself a pre-neoplastic lesion.

2) *Focal nodular lesions showing compression but not infiltration of the surrounding parenchyma*

The classification of these lesions remains one of the most controversial in human, experimental and veterinary hepatic pathology. For comparative purposes these lesions can be considered *focal hyperplasias, benign neoplasms* or *adenomas*, although in rodents, large animals and in man the distinction between hyperplasia and benign neoplasia remains difficult.

In man, these nodular lesions have been fairly well characterized into focal nodular hyperplasia and adenoma (Edmondson, 1958), although the precise nature of the lesions is still disputed. Indeed, focal nodular hyperplasia is regarded as a multinodular adenoma by some workers (Altmann, 1980).

Histologically, *focal nodular hyperplasia* in man is a circumscribed lesion composed of normal-looking hepatic cells subdivided into pseudolobules by fibrous tracts and bands which often coalesce at the centre of the lesion. The connective tissue stroma usually contains many small proliferating bile ducts. Lymphocytic infiltration is common but central veins are not seen.

Although probably not causally related to oral contraceptive therapy growth of nodular hyplasia may be enhanced or modified by contraceptive steroids (Portmann et al., 1981). They tend to be found incidentally.

A *liver cell adenoma* is a benign neoplasm, usually solitary in nature, characterized by fairly normal to somewhat atypical cells arranged in cords which may occasionally form bile. These lesions are *devoid of portal tracts, bile ducts and central veins*, but in man they are nearly always encapsulated by fibrous tissue.

Adenomas found in association with anabolic steroid administration may regress or persist on withdrawal of treatment. (Westaby and Williams, 1981).

Bile duct adenoma (cholangioma) is an uncommon tumour in all species. It is characterised as a well-demarcated nodule composed of tubules lined by cuboidal epithelium with clear cytoplasm and small, moderately chromatic nuclei. There is no infiltration of the surrounding tissue.

In rodents and larger animals, nodular non-infiltrative lesions of the liver do not fall so easily into well-defined clinicopathological groups, due in part to the great variety of models employed by different pathologists. This situation has given rise to diverse terminology for nodular non-infiltrative lesions found in the livers of experimental animals (see Table 1).

Newberne (1982) has suggested that in rodents both *adenomas* and focal hyperplasias (*hyperplastic nodules*) can be delineated in a manner analogous to the division of hepatic nodules in man. This grouping has also been employed by Greenblatt (1982) for nodules in the hamster liver. Thus, a *hyperplastic nodule* is characterized as a rounded or irregular lesion compressing surrounding hepatic parenchyma but retaining vasculature and bile ducts and showing a fairly uniform controlled proliferation of cells with little cellular pleomorphism and mitotic activity (Fig. 83). An *adenoma* in the rodent liver, also characterized by an expanding non-infiltrative growth pattern, is composed of enlarged eosinophilic cells, but showing complete loss of lobular architecture, including a complete absence of portal triads and central veins (Newberne, 1982; Greenblatt, 1982).

Although it seems reasonable to try and make the distinction between adenoma and hyperplastic nodule on histopathological grounds, this may pose some difficulty in some species, particularly as data relating to their biological nature may not be available. A common approach therefore is to avoid this division and regard all such non-invasive nodular lesions found in rodent bioassays of pharmaceutical agents as hyperplastic nodules. This system has some merit for although nodules in the rodent liver may be one of the sites of development of hepatocellular carcinoma, it remains uncertain whether they are themselves autonomous neoplastic lesions. Indeed, it has been shown that many of these nodules produced in the rat by clofibrate administration actually regress following withdrawal of treatment (Greaves et al., 1986). The term hyperplastic nodule has also been recently employed in this way by a group of Japanese pathologists (Hayashi, 1985).

For non-infiltrative hepatic nodules found in the rat, the term *neoplastic nodule* has also been proposed on the basis that these nodules are proliferative lesions which can be induced by carcinogens and thus represent a manifestation of an early stage in carcinogenesis. (Squire and Levitt, 1975; Stewart et al., 1980). This group of pathologists believed that the term *adenoma* for these lesions is best avoided because such non-infiltrative nodules produced by carcinogens are

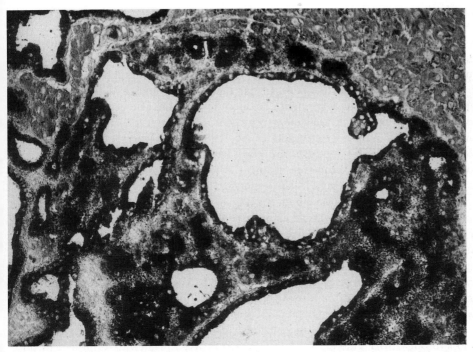

Fig. 85. Same neoplasm as shown in Figure 84 but showing gamma glutamyl transpeptidase activity using method of Albert et al. (1961). (Frozen section, ×300.)

progressive and do not represent an end-stage benign hepatic neoplasm (Stewart et al., 1980).

In contrast, Ward and Vlahakis (1978) in their review of hepatic tumours in male C3H-A^vyfB mice propose that small, non-invasive nodules should be regarded at least as adenomas as they appeared to possess progressive growth potential. Similarly, non-invasive nodular lesions of the mouse liver are considered adenomas in the IARC classification (Turusov and Takayama, 1979).

Although it is widely believed that hepatocellular carcinomas induced by genotoxic agents in the rodent liver develop from hepatic nodules which are often considered to be preneoplastic, this may not be the case. Studies of phenotypic markers in developing hepatic carcinomas in the rat have suggested that carcinomas may arise from pluripotential primitive stem cells and that altered foci and nodules are adaptive, non-oncogenic responses to the toxic effects of these xenobiotics. (Sell and Dunsford, 1989).

Similar difficulties of classification are also encountered in the assessment of nodular hepatocellular lesions occuring in the dog, although those usually occur only after the age of five years (Patnaik et al., 1980; Trigo et al., 1982; Bergman, 1985) and are only rarely encountered in routine toxicity studies. However, focal hepatic nodular hyperplasia was reported to occur in a dose-related manner in

437

beagle dogs treated for seven years with oral contraceptive steroids. (Johnson, 1989).

The deficiences in our understanding of non-infiltrative hepatic nodules and difficulties in classification, naturally give rise to problems in the safety assessment of pharmaceutical agents when nodules occur in greater prevalence in treated animals than in controls in carcinogenicity bioassays. Although there appears to be a general agreement that nodules and hepatic neoplasms occurring in the rat as a results of treatment represent a higher risk to man than nodules induced in the mouse (Bannasch et al., 1982), perception of risk is greatly dependent on whether nodules are considered simply reactive hyperplasias or exaggeration of a spontaneous change, whether nodules represent end-stage benign neoplasms or a stage in the evolution of hepatocellular carcinoma.

Despite these considerations, a variety of quite different therapeutic agents have produced benign proliferative hepatocellular lesions in rodents when administered in high doses for long periods without substantial risk for man or any apparant adverse impact on the overall clinical benefits for appropriate therapeutic indications. Examples not only include sex steroids in rats and dogs. (Schardein et al., 1970; Schuppler et al., 1982; Machnik et al., 1983; Johnson, 1989) but also cyproterone acetate in rats (Schuppler and Günzel, 1979) phenobarbitone in rats and mice (Butler, 1978; Gangolli et al., 1987) the antidepressant bupropion and the minor tranquillizers ripazepam and oxazepam in rats (Fox and Lahcen, 1974; Tucker, 1983; Fitzgerald et al., 1984) and rifampicin in mice (Della Porta et al., 1978).

For these reasons, the assessment of nodules and extrapolation of findings in experimental animals to man must include an evaluation of changes likely to occur in untreated animals, the distribution of nodules in treated groups, the presence or absence of foci of cellular alteration and malignant neoplasms, the nature of the effect of the test compound on the hepatocyte itself (e.g. enzyme inhibition, enzyme induction, peroxisomal proliferation, cell damage) as well as a detailed comparison of drug disposition in the various test species at the doses employed compared with drug kinetics and metabolism in man at therapeutic doses.

Multifocal nodular hyperplasia / cirrhosis Multifocal nodular hyperplasia is the term employed for the regenerative hyperplasia which occurs in cirrhosis as a result of the proliferation of normal liver cells to form pseudolobules (Edmondson, 1958). Nodules in cirrhosis are variable in size but they show an intimate relationship with bile ducts and pseudobile ducts which can be found deep within their parenchyma. This feature serves to aid in the distinction of these nodules from adenomas, which are devoid of such structures and show more striking cellular pleomorphism.

The World Health Organisation (WHO) definition of cirrhosis, 'a diffuse process characterised by fibrosis and the conversion of normal liver architecture into structurally abnormal nodules' (Anthony et al., 1977) has been criticized on the basis that no consideration was given to the profound vascular derangements which have a key role in the development of this condition (Rappaport et al., 1983). Tridimensional studies of Rappaport and colleagues (1983) have suggested that zonal scarring of the liver produced by a variety of insults results in profound changes in microcirculatory dynamics. These alter oxygenation and the normal regional functional heterogeneity of the liver which may be important in the development of nodules in cirrhosis.

Administration of a number of xenobiotics to laboratory animals can give rise to cirrhosis. Some of these chemicals have been used to develop models for the human disease (Nuber et al., 1980). Dietary manipulation can also produce a cirrhotic picture in rodents (Rogers and Newberne, 1973) and primates (Wilgram and Taylor, 1959) although the non-human primate appears to be much more like man because it is sensitive to the cirrhosis-inducing effects of alcohol even when given a nutritionally adequate diet (Rubin and Lieber, 1974).

Cirrhosis occurs spontaneously in certain strains of Syrian hamsters although the cause for this is uncertain (Chesterman and Pomerance, 1965). A cirrhotic-like nodular hyperplasia may occasionally be found in untreated rats.

Liver cell carcinoma, hepatocellular carcinoma

These are a heterogeneous group of malignant tumours generally bearing a close resemblance to hepatic parenchymal cells. In man, liver cell carcinomas are graded histologically according to quantity and character of the cytoplasm, size and degree of hyperchromatism of nuclei, nuclear-cytoplasmic ratio, cohesive nature of the tumour cells and general histological architecture. Histologically, they vary from easily recognizable adult cell types to highly anaplastic neoplasms (Edmondson, 1958). In man the clinical progression of liver cell carcinoma associated with cirrhosis is very rapid, being a matter of a few months. Survival of patients with circumscribed hepatic cancers in non-cirrhotic livers such as those associated with oral contraceptive or anabolic steroid use may be better (Neuberger et al., 1981; Westaby and Williams, 1981).

In rodents and other species, similar histological criteria are employed in the diagnosis of hepatocellular carcinoma. Thus, the presence of abnormal tubeculae, cellular pleomorphism, prominent or abnormal mitoses, anaplastic zones, and infiltration of individual or small group of tumour cells into connective tissue stroma or adjacent liver tissue are important diagnostic features (Fig. 84). Metastatic deposits also develop in other organs.

In laboratory animals the biological behaviour of hepatocellular carcinoma is less easily followed clinically and the assessment of tumour behaviour in drug safety evaluation usually rests simply on two functional characteristics which can be observed in fixed tissue sections, that of ability to produce metastases in distant sites and invasion of blood vessels and surrounding tissues.

Questions concerning histogenesis of hepatic neoplasia also influence diagnostic criteria and terminology. Some workers believe that glandular hepatic carcinomas, characterized by mucin secretion and abundant connective tissue

439

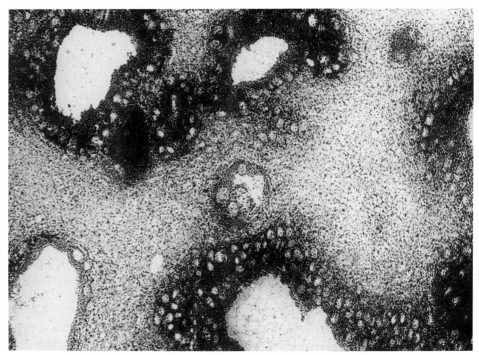

Fig. 86. Same tumour as in Figure 84 showing the reaction for glucose-6-phosphate dehydrogenase when the reaction is performed in an atmosphere of oxygen. This type of activity appears to correlate with malignant cell types as shown in the rat liver by Greaves and colleagues in 1986. (Frozen section, ×300.)

stroma, arise from bile duct cells (i.e. bile duct carcinomas *cholangiocarcinomas*), although this is disputed by others(Stewart et al., 1980).

Recent studies of morphological, autoradiographic and phenotypic expression of cellular attentions in developing liver cancer in rats have suggested that both hepatocellular and ductular carcinomas arise from pluripotential liver stem cells located in the periportal zone which are capable of undergoing differentiation in various directions to produce different histological patterns (Sell and Dunsford, 1989).

Hepatocellular carcinomas occur spontaneously in small numbers of treated rats (Ward, 1981; Greaves and Faccini, 1984), mice (Ward and Vlahakis, 1978), hamsters (Fortner, 1957; Van Hoosier and Trentin, 1979) and beagle dogs (Patnaik et al., 1980) with advancing age. Although genotoxic agents which produce hepatocellular carcinomas rapidly in rodents are regarded as potential carcinogens, there is dispute about the relevance of such findings for drugs such as clofibrate which produce carcinomas only after extremely long periods of treatment in rodents at high doses (Cohen and Grasso, 1981).

Hepatocellular carcinomas have also been reported to develop in the rat or mouse liver following administration of other therapeutic agents of different classes including certain tranquillizers (Fitzgerald et al., 1984), some oral contraceptive steroids at high multiples of the human contraceptive dose (Schuppler and Günzel, 1979), non-steroidal antioestrogens (Ahotupa and Hirsimäki, 1989), rifampicin (Della Porta et al., 1978) and cisplatin (Ewen et al., 1987).

BILE DUCTS, BILIARY SYSTEM

Structure

Liver structure has been briefly outlined above but it is worth noting the anatomical division in the intrahepatic biliary system:

Bile ducts are biliary channels found in the large and small portal tracts and which are accompanied by branches of the hepatic artery and lined by cuboidal or columnar biliary epithelial cells.

Bile ductules are smaller, lined by biliary cuboidal or flattened epithelial cells which are found in portal areas but not accompanied by hepatic arterial branches.

Ducts of Hering / cholangioles are thin connecting channels situated between the bile duct system and bile canaliculi, formed partly by biliary cells and partly by hepatocytes.

Canaliculi are the smallest channels bounded by hepatocytes.

Bile Secretion

Knowledge about normal bile flow is incomplete and this has hampered our understanding of cholestasis (Phillips et al., 1986). Our understanding of the process has been reviewed in detail by Boyer (1980, 1981). Normal bile secretion is highly polarized within the hepatocyte, bile secretion being directed over a small part of the cell surface, the canalicular membrane. The canaliculus is delimited by tight junctions which represent the only anatomical barrier between blood and bile.

The actin-containing microfilaments of the cytoskeleton are important in the maintainance of the integrity and orientation of the surface membrane and junctional complexes of the canaliculus. Transport of bile acids represents one of the important factors in biliary secretion. They enter the hepatocyte by a process linked to the sodium gradient which is dependent on the activity of Na, K-ATPase located in the sinusoidal and lateral parts of the hepatocyte plasma membrane (Latham and Kashgarian, 1979). By contrast, alkaline phosphatase and Mg^{++}-ATPase are localized mainly around the canalicular membrane. This regional distribution of transport enzymes suggests that the transport system for bile acids by the liver cell is analogous to the sodium linked anion transport of many secretory epithelia and compounds which inhibit Na, K-ATPase or alter liver plasma membrane may be expected to impair this energy dependent process for bile acid transport (Boyer, 1981). A point here is that bile acids stimulate bile secretion to a variable degree in different animals (Boyer, 1981).

Several other factors are also important. A lobular gradient exists in which periportal hepatocytes normally remove the majority of bile acid anions from sinusoidal blood so that centrilobular hepatocytes are exposed to lower concentrations of bile acids. This may partly be reponsible for the centrilobular intracanalicular cholestasis which follows drug-induced injury (Boyer, 1981). Other negatively charged solutes also accumulate in the canalicular lumen and their osmotic effects influence bile secretion and bile flow. Studies in dogs have shown that the diuretics chlorothiazide and ethacrynic acid, increase bile flow probably as a direct result of their cellular actions, producing fluid shifts in the biliary tract as well as in the kidney (Maxwell et al., 1974).

The rat, which does not possess a gall bladder, has a complex bile ductular periportal plexus not found in other species which may also influence bile flow (Yamamoto and Phillips, 1984). Although the precise function of this plexus is not known, it may modify canalicular bile by sequestration and reabsorption of water and electrolytes, it may store and concentrate bile or act as a collecting system (Yamamoto and Philips, 1984). Comparative studies have shown that man and rhesus monkeys but not dog, rabbit and guinea pig, possess less complex, irregular biliary periportal side branches or pouches which arise from intrahepatic bile ducts and which may also store or modify bile (Yamamoto et al., 1985).

Cholestasis

Cholestasis represents an impairment in the excretion of bile which results in the retention of biliary constituents both in the liver and in the blood. The various types of cholestasis occurring in man have been well delineated (Phillips et al., 1986). Spontaneous disease in aged laboratory rodents, notably space occupying lesions, hepatic amyloidosis and inflammatory disease similarly result in intrahepatic or extrahepatic biliary obstruction. Certain experimental procedures such as ligation of bile ducts produce a cholestatic picture of bile stasis, bile infarcts, bile duct proliferation, fibrosis and cirrhosis, change which mirrors that seen in biliary obstructive disease in man (Kountouras et al., 1984).

Drugs from nearly all of the major therapeutic classes have been reported to produce cholestatic reactions in man (Zimmerman and Lewis, 1987). These compounds can be grouped into those such as anabolic or contraceptive steroids which produce a bland or pure cholestasis characterized by the presence of bile plugs, limited initially to centrilobular zones, without overt evidence of hepatocellular damage, and those producing the more variegated response of cholestasis with hepatocellular or cholangiocellular injury (Ishak, 1982). It is the latter group of compounds which are associated with the bulk of cholestatic drug reactions in man (Plaa and Priestly, 1977; Ishak, 1982; Ludwig and Axelsen, 1983).

Putative mechanisms involved in the development of drug-induced cholestasis at therapeutic doses in man have been reviewed by Zimmerman and Lewis (1987). They can be grouped into those caused by the compound itself or a normal metabolite (intrinsic), a relatively rare metabolite (metabolic idiosyncrasy) or an immunological reaction (hypersensitivity). Cholestasis may follow disturbance to the anatomical structures involved in bile formation and flow as a reult of damage to the canalicular membrane itself, the microfibrillar network, microtubules and microvesicles, tight junctions around canaliculi, bile ducts or bile ductules. However, functional alterations may also be important and have particular relevance to high-dose toxicity studies. Impaired formation of canicular bile can result from decreased uptake of bile acids and other key constituents from sinusoidal blood, deficient transport into the canaliculus and impaired propulsive action of the canalicular network. Other factors such as electrolyte balance and bile viscosity also influence bile flow independent of bile acids (Zimmerman and Lewis, 1987).

Despite extensive study, many cholestatic drug reactions in the human liver have been difficult to reproduce in experimental animals and this may be one of the major reasons for the lack of predictability of the cholestatic potential of drugs from experimental studies (Plaa and Priestly 1977; Plaa and Hewitt, 1982). Even the well-studied drug, chlorpromazine which is associated with a modest incidence of cholestatic drug reactions in man, seems not to produce a typical cholestatic picture in rats even in the presence of additional immunological manipulation (Mullock et al., 1983).

Although the cholestatic reaction associated with steroids can be reproduced in mice, there is considerable inter-strain and inter-animal differences in sensitivity and Sprague-Dawley rats appear totally resistant to these effects (Imai and Hayashi, 1970).

These authors showed that administration of norethisterone to DS mice for five days produced a dose-related increase in bile plugs in canaliculi and interlobular bile ducts. At high doses this was associated with swollen hepatocytes sometimes containing cytoplasmic pigment granules, single cell necrosis and periportal round cell infiltration. Electron microscopy showed dilation of bile canaliculi and distortion or loss of canalicular microvilli. Dose-related increases in plasma bilirubin, alkaline phosphatase and amino-transferases were also found. CS and C57B mice were shown to be most sensitive, ICR mice least sensitive and Sprague-Dawley rats completely resistant to these effects even at the highest doses. Other C17 α-substituted steroids produced similar effects but testosterone propionate, progesterone and oestradiol were devoid of this activity in this model (Imai and Hayashi, 1970). These results are of interest because anabolic steroids which cause jaundice in man all have an alkyl group in the C-17 position (Zimmerman and Lewis, 1987).

It is perhaps because cholestastis has been difficult to reproduce in the rat, that the experimental agent α-napthylisothiocyanate (ANIT) has been so extremely well studied in the rat as a model for cholestatic disease in man. It also provides a useful comparative agent in toxicology when trying new methods for hepatotoxicity assessment.

Despite the difficulties in reproducing cholestatic reactions experimentally, certain agents which do not produce a cholestatic reaction in rodents have done

443

so in dogs. Unfortunately, studies have not been conducted to establish the mechanism of such changes and the reasons for species differences. For example, intrahepatic cholestasis, exemplified by the presence of bile plugs in canaliculi but little overt hepatocellular damage apart from 'feathery' and single cell degeneration has been observed in dogs treated with the hypnotic agent 2-ethyl-2 phenyl butyramide (Keysser et al., 1963). The flavour-suspending agent, sucrose acetate isobutyrate, used in the manufacture of soft drinks produced mild reversible cholestasis in beagle dogs, but not rats or squirrel monkeys (Procter et al., 1973). This was shown by impaired bromsulphophthalein clearance from plasma, increased serum alkaline phosphatase and microscopic evidence of dilatation of bile canaliculi and increased bile pigment accumulation in the beagle dog liver. It is possible therefore, that dogs are more sensitive to cholestasic agents than rodent species.

However, as Plaa and Priestly (1977) have aptly pointed out, the idea that there is a single mechanism for cholestasis is undoubtedly far too simplistic and probably a variety of different mechanisms lead to a cholestatic response, each of which may represent a different hazard to man.

Bile duct changes

Dilatation of intrahepatic bile ducts and a range of cystic and proliferative intrahepatic lesions of biliary epithelium are observed in untreated laboratory rats (Burek, 1978; Greaves and Faccini, 1984), mice (Lewis, 1984), hamsters (McMartin, 1979) and beagle dogs (Anderson, 1970). Both degenerative and proliferative lesions of the biliary epithelium are produced by agents which are directly cytotoxic to bile duct epithelium or mediate damage indirectly by interference with bile flow (Zimmerman and Lewis, 1978).

In the rat, solitary or multiple thin-walled, multiloculated cysts containing clear or amber fluid and lined by cuboidal or flattened epithelium are found with increasing frequency with increasing age (Burek, 1978). These may derive from bile duct epithelium (Stewart et al., 1980). Cystic change of a similar nature may also be closely related to portal tracts where walls of the cysts may be thicker and more fibrous in nature (Greaves and Faccini, 1984). Identical thin-walled cysts occur in the aged hamster (McMartin, 1979). In addition, multiloculated cystic dilation of bile ducts also occur in portal zones in the hamster liver but this change appears to relate to deposition of amyloid.

Non-neoplastic proliferation of the bile ducts and ductules is also found spontaneously in both rat and hamster (Stewart et al., 1980; Greenblatt, 1982). Microscopically, these changes are characterised by varying degrees of proliferation and hyperplasia of the biliary epithelium which may be associated with fibrosis, sclerosis or mild inflammatory change. Glandular or intestinal metaplasia may also be occasionally observed.

Lewis (1984) has documented the spontaneously occurring adenomatoid, tumour-like lesions of the intrahepatic biliary system in aged CD-1 mice. Other strains of mice also show this change (Rabstein et al., 1973; Turusov and

Takayama, 1979; Enomoto et al., 1974). These striking morphological changes are uncommon but they occur spontaneously in small numbers and more frequently in females. Histologically, these lesions are characterised by focal or nodular proliferation of intrahepatic bile ducts surrounded by inflammation and fibrosis. The cells lining the proliferating ducts may be hyperplastic with acidophilic or basophilic cytoplasm or show glandular metaplasia including the presence of goblet cells. These changes are associated with intracytoplasmic and intraluminal angular, rhomboid or needle-like acidophilic crystalloid material. These changes may be associated glandular hyperplasia of the gall bladder epithelium and frank cholecystitis. Similar changes are also sometimes seen in pancreatic ducts. The precise cause of these changes is unknown but the ubiquitous presence of biliary crystalloid material in bile ducts in the mice studied by Lewis (1984) suggested that these biliary lesions were a response to bile stasis, cholelithiasis and inflammation. Despite the florid nature of the changes they should not be regarded as neoplastic.

The expression of these spontaneous cystic and proliferative lesions of the liver in rats, mice and hamsters can be modulated in each species by dietary factors (Tepperman et al., 1964; Chesterman and Pomerance, 1965; Enomoto et al., 1974; Yu et al., 1982).

Intrahepatic bile ducts may be dilated and contain intrahepatic bile pigment in aged beagles and these changes is also associated with cystic hyperplasia in the gall bladder mucosa (Anderson, 1970). Occasionally, young beagle dogs used in toxicity studies show these changes. Congenital unilocular or multilocular cysts lined by a single layer of cuboidal, columnar or flattened epithelial cells have also been reported in dogs (Van den Ingh and Rothuizen, 1985).

In rodents as well as in larger animals used in toxicology, a variety of different chemical agents produce proliferative, hyperplastic and cystic changes in the bile duct epithelium. Bile duct proliferation (adenofibrosis, cholangiofibrosis), associated with oval cell proliferation and intestinal metaplasia of duct cells, is associated with administration of powerful carcinogens and non-carcinogenic hepatotoxins (Farber, 1963, 1976; Kimbrough et al., 1973; Stewart et al., 1980; Greenblatt, 1982; Dunsford et al., 1985; Tryphonas et al., 1986) as well as some therapeutic agents (Gregory et al., 1983; McGuire et al., 1986). Whereas bile duct proliferation occurs in rodents following treatment with carcinogens, of more direct relevance to drug safety evaluation are the changes produced by non-carcinogenic agents such as α-naphthylisothiocyanate (ANIT).

Following a single dose of ANIT, the rat liver shows mild hepatocellular changes only, comprising loss of glycogen and possibly fatty change. By contrast, bile ducts show marked cell damage, desquamation of epithelium, associated with oedema and inflammatory infiltrate of portal tracts which subsides over a number of days to be followed by bile duct proliferation.

Dilatation and tortuosity of biliary canaliculi are seen both ultrastructurally and at light microscopical level using histochemical techniques (Steiner et al., 1963); Leonard et al., 1981; Masson et al., 1986). Although there is evidence of increased bilirubin in the circulation of rats treated with ANIT, biliary stasis as shown by the presence of bile plugs in histological sections of liver does not seem to be a prominant feature.

Following repeated dosing with ANIT, the proliferation of bile ducts may be more marked (Steiner and Carruthers, 1963) and associated with elevations in gamma-glutamyl transpsptidase and α-foetoprotein expression. Unlike the increases following administration of powerful carcinogens, the elevations of gamma glutamyl transpeptidase and α-foetoprotein are reversible on cessation of treatment with ANIT (Richards et al., 1982).

Similar morphological changes have been described with potential therapeutic agents. In the preclinical toxicity studies on the synthetic analgesic agent, tilidine fumarate, proliferative and cystic changes were observed in rats treated with high doses of this agent, but this was not associated with neoplastic change even after two years treatment (McGuire et al., 1986). The schistosomicide, oxamniquine, produced bile duct proliferation in rats but not in mice, rabbits or dogs after a single oral dose (Gregory et al., 1983). Female rats were more sensitive to this effect and although species and sex differences in metabolism of oxamniquine could not entirely explain this effect in the rat, oxamniquine did not produce this change even after prolonged treatment of dogs, mice and hamsters and has been successfully used in man for a number of years for the treatment of Schistosoma mansoni (Chvédoff et al., 1984).

Note. Oval cells represent small bile duct-like cells with scanty, basophilic cytoplasm and pale blue oval nuclei showing a fine chromatin pattern. They become prominent in and around portal areas in rodent hepatocarcinogenesis models using different carcinogens as well as following treatment with some non-carcinogenic hepatotoxins (Farber, 1976; Richards et al., 1982; Tatematsu et al., 1984, 1985; Dunsford et al., 1985). The histogenesis and fate of oval cells remains poorly understood, although they appear to derive predominantly from bile ductular epithelium rather than hepatocytes or hepatocyte stem cells (Tatematsu et al., 1984). They show at least three biological options, disappearance, presumably by cell death, differentiation to hepatocytes or rearrangement to form ducts and cholangiofibrosis (Ogawa et al., 1974; Tatematsu et al., 1985). Cytochemical study shows that oval cells induced by 2-acetylaminofluorene, contain prekeratin and possess gamma glutamyl transpeptidase activity, similar to bile duct epithelium. However, unlike hepatocytes, they are devoid of epoxide hydrolase or leucine aminopeptidase activity (Tatematsu et al., 1984, 1985). By contrast, Dunsford and colleagues (1985) have shown that the proliferating oval cells in rats fed 2-acetylaminofluorene contain α-foetoprotein, a marker for proliferating hepatocytes, suggesting oval cells possess a relationship to immature hepatocytes. Similar conclusions have been reached with differential cytokeratin and α-foetoprotein expression of epithelial cells in the rat liver emerging following treatment with 4-dimethylaminoazobenzene (Germain et al., 1985).

446

Gall bladder

As much preclinical safety evaluation is performed in the rat which does not possess a gall bladder, this organ seldom features prominantly in toxicity studies. Nevertheless, spontaneous pathology of the gall bladder is sporadically observed in the other species and the gall bladder can affected by drugs and chemicals. Much experimentalwork has concerned the mouse gall bladder.

In the young beagle dog, cystic change or cystic hyperplasia of the gall bladder mucosa is occasionally found. This lesion, seen commonly in aged beagles, is characterised by the presence of papillary and cystic formations lined or covered by simple cuboidal or columnar epithelium which may show copious mucin production (Anderson, 1970). Although the pathogenesis of this condition is uncertain, it appears to be of little pathological significance.

The aged mouse and hamster more frequently show lesions of the gall bladder. In general, these lesions are characterised by inflammation, erosion, hyperplasia or mucous metaplasia of the gall bladder mucosa, often seen in the presence of fragments of crystalline biliary debris (Rabstein et al., 1973; Lewis, 1984). Adenomatous polyps form in the gall bladder of the aged hamster (Pour et al., 1976).

Studies in the mouse have shown that drugs and chemicals can affect mucus secretion from gall bladder mucosa as well as the discharge of bile. The secretory behaviour of the gall bladder is affected not only by fasting and refeeding,but also cholecystokinin/pancreozymin (Wahlin et al., 1976), adrenergic and cholinergic drugs (Axelsson et al., 1979). Colchicine which interferes with microtubules and can interfere with glandular secretion in a number of tissues also produces cholestasis with marked dilatation of the gall bladder when administered to the mouse (Hopwood et al., 1986).

EXOCRINE PANCREAS

The bulk of the pancreas, embryonically derived from dorsal and ventral pancreatic buds of entodermal epithelium, is concerned with exocrine secretion. The islets of Langerhans, situated throughout the pancreatic parenchyma are discussed in detail below.

Among laboratory animals the pancreas is more variable macroscopically than in its microscopic appearances. Two basic anatomical patterns have been recognised. The mesenteric type, as is found in the rabbit, is diffusely distributed in the mesentery of the small bowel. The more compact type is seen in hamster, dog, primate and man (Doerr and Becker, 1958). The pancreas of the rat and mouse is of mesenteric type, although fairly close-packed in form. The drainage of the pancreatic ducts into the small bowel is also different between species. The pancreatic ducts of rat and mouse often open directly into the common bile duct, those in the rabbit into the lower duodenum whereas in the dog, the pancreatic duct or ducts open into the duodenum at or near the papilla of Vater as in man.

Pancreatic exocrine secretions are stored and secreted in an inactive form and their activation usually occurs in the lumen of the gastrointestinal tract. The initial step is the activation of trypsinogen to trypsin in the presence of calcium by the glycoprotein enzyme, enterokinase.

In man, this is produced only at the brush border of absorptive cells at the apical parts of the villi in the duodenum and in the proximal 15 cms of proximal jejunum (Hermon-Taylor, 1977). Similar enzyme patterns have been observed in the rat (Nordström, 1971, 1972; Schneider et al., 1975). Trypsin then activates the other pancreatic zymogens. This system, therefore, prevents the pancreas from destroying itself by enzymatic digestion. Profiles of pancreatic zymogens and lysosomal enzymes secreted in response to secretin and cholecystokinin may also vary between species (Rinderknecht et al., 1983).

Significant species differences exist in the extent of direct arterial blood supply to the exocrine pancreas. In the dog and primate most of the exocrine tissue is supplied by efferent vessels from the islets of Langerhans whereas in the rat, acinar arterioles which supply the acini directly are more abundant (Bonner-Weir and Orchi, 1982; Fujita and Murakami, 1973; Williams and Goldfine, 1985). The subsequent perfusion of the acini by blood from the islets of Langerhans (the insulo-acinar portal system) plays an important part in the regulation of the exocrine pancreas.

Drug metabolising enzymes are also present in exocrine pancreatic tissue and are inducible by the administration of certain chemicals (Scarpelli et al., 1980). Immunocytochemical techniques have clearly demonstrated the these drug-metabolising enzymes in both pancreatic acinar (especially apical regions) and ductular cellsin the rat and hamster (Kawabata et al., 1984). The pancreas, like the liver, may sometimes contain very high concentrations of an administered drug (Vollmer at al., 1986).

Acute inflammation, acute pancreatitis, pancreatic necrosis

A variety of derangements are known to predispose to the development of acute pancreatitis in man, including diseases of biliary and pancreatic ducts, abdominal trauma, ischaemia, viral and other systemic infective diseases, hyperlipidaemia, hypercalcaemia and excessive alcohol consumption. Although some of the clinical reports of pancreatitis following administration of therapeutic agents are difficult to evaluate, acute pancreatitis has been associated with the administration of a wide range of drugs including oestrogens, corticosteroids, thiazide diuretics, antibiotics, some antimitotics, notably azathiaprine and analgesic or anti-inflammatory agents such as paracetamol, indomethacin and salicylates (Riddell and Straus, 1982; Bannerjeee et al., 1989). The pathogenesis of pancreatitis in man is poorly understood but the final common pathway in its development is related to release of the inactive enzymes from exocrine tissue, their activation and action both in the pancreatic tissues and systemically.

Postulated mechanisms include pancreatic duct obstruction of stasis, direct cytoxicity, immune suppression, osmotic or pressure effects, ionic changes or arteriolar thrombosis (Bannerjee et al., 1989).

Acute pancreatitis is occasionally observed in untreated, aged laboratory rats (Greaves and Faccini, 1984), mice (Seamer, 1967) and hamsters (Takahashi and Pour, 1978). It is also associated with arteritis occurring spontaneously in the pancreatic vasculature in these species. In the rat, this inflammatory process has a tendency to develop in association with arteritis of the pancreatoduodenal artery (Coleman et al., 1977). Acute and chronic pancreatitis occurs more commonly in diabetic BB Wistar rats than their non-diabetic counterparts (Wright et al., 1985). It can occur in dogs and is seen in primates (McClure and Chandler, 1982).

Factors associated with the development of pancreatitis in man have been explored in a wide variety of experimental models, particularly using the rat, mouse and dog. Most of these methods produce stasis or damage in the pancreatic ducts by procedures such as ligation of the duodenum to form a closed loop, or by the intraductal injection of blood, bacteria, bile, detergent and trypsin or other enzymes (Rao et al., 1981; Aho and Nevalainen, 1982).

Pancreatitis has been induced in mice by feeding a choline-deficient diet containing 0.5% DL-ethionine (Virji and Rao, 1985). It is believed that this form of pancreatitis results from the potentiation of ethionine toxicity by the choline deficient diet. The effect is greater in female than in male mice and can be potentiated in males by administration of oestrogen (Rao et al., 1982b).

Pancreatitis has been induced in rats by infusion of the cholecystokinin-pancreazymin analogue, caerulein, at a dose in excess of that which stimulates maximal pancreatic secretion (Steer and Meldolesi, 1987). The precise mechanisms involved in these models are not clear but it is believed that derangement of intracellular transport of secretory proteins in acinar cells may be a common factor (Steer and Meldolesi, 1987). Pancreatic necrosis with little or no inflammation develops in rats fed a copper deficient diet (Rao et al., 1987).

Pancreatitis also follows experimental infection with Reo and Coxsackie viruses (Papadimitriou and Walters, 1986; Seamer, 1967). Drug-induced acute pancreatitis in experimental animals is less commonly described. In rabbits, adrenocorticoid administration may produce focal necrotizing pancreatitis associated with proliferating duct epithelium, probably as a result of ductal obstruction which follows changes in viscosity of secreted material or cortisone-induced ductular changes (Bencosme and Lazarus, 1956).

Pancreatic acinar necrosis and inflammation have also been reported in dogs treated with a novel anxiolytic agent C1–918, (Smith et al., 1985) and an adenosine agonist C1–936, [N-(2,2-diphenylethyl) adenosine] with antipsychotic activity (Macallum et al., 1989b). From the same laboratory, a novel neuroleptic drug was also reported to produce pancreatic acinar cell degeneration associated with mild periductal inflammation and fibrosis in rats following administration for thirteen weeks (Smith et al., 1984). The mechanisms involved remained unclear.

Histologically, the early phase of acute pancreatitis in rats or in the other experimental models is characterised by varying degrees of focal necrosis, diffuse parenchymal acute inflammation, haemorrhage, oedema and inflammation in and around ducts. Proliferature changes may also be found in duct epithelium. Fat necrosis and granulomatous inflammation may also be present (Greaves and Faccini, 1984; Rao et al., 1981; Aho and Nevalainen, 1982; Virji and Rao, 1985; Bencosme and Lazarus, 1956). Vasculitis and fibrinoid necrosis of small vessels and marked haemorrhage into the pancreatic parenchyma and surrounding tissues can occur (haemorrhagic pancreatitis). In some models the inflammatory component may be sparse, notably in mice given choline deficient diets and in copper deficient rats (Rao et al., 1987).

Chronic inflammation and atrophy of the exocrine pancreas

Focal and diffuse chronic inflammation with or without fibrosis and atrophy or atrophy without inflammation appears to be a fairly common finding in the exocrine pancreas in untreated aged rats (Kendry and Roe, 1969). It is also found sporadically in mice (Ward et al., 1979; Chvédoff et al., 1982), hamsters (Takahashi and Pour, 1978) and in young beagle dogs (Prentice et al., 1980). These changes may be associated with changes in the pancreatic duct system and endocrine cells.

Kendry and Roe (1969) have described the chronic inflammatory and atrophic changes seen in the rat exocrine in considerable detail using the term *chronic relapsing pancreatitis*. The prevalence and severity of this condition is strain dependent (Anver and Cohen, 1979) but it becomes more marked with advancing age. Chronic pancreatitis also occurs more commonly in diabetic (BB)Wistar rats than the corresponding non-diabetic Wistar rat (Wright et al., 1985). Early changes are characterised histologically by infiltration of the tromal tissue by mononuclear cells with varying degrees of mild parenchymal damage. In more advanced cases, there is progressive loss acinar tissue which is replaced by simplified, microcystic glandular tissue lined by flattened cells. Single lobules or the entire gland may be affected. Eventually there is almost complete replacement of the gland by adipose tissue (fatty atrophy). There is usually fairly prominant chronic inflammation associated with the pancreatic duct system and this suggests a ductal origin for the condition (Kendry and Roe, 1969). Proliferative changes in the duct epithelium are not usually prominent.

Although islets of Langerhans remain relatively unaffected by this process, they become disrupted in later stages of the disease and single endocrine cells or isolated proliferating groups of insulin-containing cells may be observed (Spencer et al., 1986).

It is surprising that such a striking condition occurs in the rat but not generally in the mouse. This is perhaps a result of the anatomy of the pancreatic ducts which open directly into the common bile duct (Greaves and Faccini, 1984). However, chronic inflammation of the pancreatic parenchyma is seen sporadically in aged mice of various strains (Ward et al., 1979; Chvédoff et al., 1982).

Chronic inflammation and marked exocrine atrophy also occurs after acute pancreatitis induced by reovirus infection in the mouse, and this may be associated with proliferative changes of pancreatic duct cells (Walters, 1966). Electron microscopy of the pancreas in this experimental model has shown that virus replication is limited to the epithelial cells of the main pancreatic duct, suggesting that most of the damage to pancreatic parenchyma is a direct result of obstruction rather than a direct effect of the virus on these cells (Papadimitriou and Walters, 1967).

In hamsters, a similar spectrum of changes in the exocrine pancreas may be seen, although its prevalence is variable between various strains and seems to be sex-dependent. As in the rat, the changes are characterised by chronic inflammation, focal atrophy and replacement by fibrous and adipose tissue but there appears to be a more prominant proliferative component involving the pancreatic duct system and endocrine tissue (Takahashi and Pour, 1978).

In the young Beagle dog used in toxicity studies, focal inflammation is also sporadically seen. Non-inflammatory atrophy with loss of acinar lobules and replacement by fatty tissue is a well-described change (Prentice et al., 1980).

In primates, lobular atrophy with fibrosis, replacement by fatty tissue and infiltration with chronic inflammatory cells also occur usually without clear cause. Sometimes atrophy is found in association with cryptosporidosis or other parasites (McClure et al., 1978). Perivascular granulomas associated with birefringent fragments of Oesophogostomum are occasionally seen in feral monkeys (Lumb et al., 1985).

Some experimental procedures and administration of xenobiotics also induce or potentiate the development of chronic inflammation and atrophy of the pancreas in experimental animals. In rats, chronic protein deficiency or hypophysectomy have been reported to result in the loss of pancreatic weight associated with loss of zymogen granules, degeneration of rough endoplasmic reticulum and increased autophagocytic activity (Svoboda et al., 1966; Murata et al., 1985; Kitagawa and Ono, 1986). High doses of glucagon have been also shown to produce loss of zymogen granules and pancreatic atrophy in the rat (see islets of Langerhans). As noted previously, copper deficiency in rats produces pancreatic necrosis with little or no inflammation which ultimately leads to pancreatic atrophy (Rao et al., 1987).

Degenerative alterations and atrophy of acinar cells of uncertain histogenesis have also been reported in beagle dogs treated for thirteen weeks with the novel anxiolytic agent, 4-(2-chlorophenyl)-1,6-dihydro-1,3,9-trimethylimidazo-(1,2-a)pyrazolo-(4,3-f)diazepine (CI-918). Islet cells were unaffected. Similar changes were seen neither in dogs treated for two weeks nor in rats treated for thirteen weeks with CI-918 (Smith et al., 1985).

Pancreatic hypertrophy and hyperplasia

Although the pancreas is less widely weighed in toxicity studies than other organs such as liver and kidney, a number of dietary and tropic factors have been

451

shown to be capable of increasing the size and weight of the pancreas in experimental animals.

Feeding rats with raw but not heated soya flour for long periods has been shown to increase pancreatic growth (Crass and Morgan, 1982). Initially, during the first week of feeding, this increase in size appears to be a result of simple acinar cell hypertrophy but by the second week of feeding there is a marked increase in total DNA, indicative of hyperplasia (Oates and Morgan, 1982). As heated soya flour has the composition as raw flour except for the absence of active trypsin inhibitors, it has been suggested that this is the key factor involved in the increase in pancreatic size (Oates and Morgan, 1982). Pancreatic growth is believed to be regulated by cholecystokinin, which is in turn controlled by a negative feedback mechanism involving intestinal trypsin. The removal of trypsin by binding to a trypsin inhibitor such as is presentin raw soya flour is believed to be sufficient to stimulate the release of cholecystokinin from the small intestine with resultant increase pancreatic size and enzyme content. Not only can raw soya flour feeding increase pancreatic weight but it also potentiates the action of pancreatic carcinogens (Morgan et al., 1977; Levison et al., 1979).

Administration of cholecystokinin or synthetic peptides containing a similar C-terminal tetrapeptide-amide sequence (e.g. pentagastrin) have also been shown to increase pancreatic size and enzyme secretion (Rothman and Wells, 1967; Mayston and Barrowman, 1971; Johnson, 1976; Howatson and Carter, 1985). The increase in pancreatic size as a result of administration of pentagastrin for short periods appears principally a result of acinar cell hypertrophy (Mayston and Barrowman, 1971). Studies with cholecystokinin given to hamsters have shown that the treatment schedule may influence the nature of the hypertrophy or hyperplasia (Howatson and Carter, 1985). Cholecystokinin can also act as a co-carcinogen or promotor of pancreatic carcinoma development in hamsters treated with carcinogenic nitosamines (Howatson and Carter, 1985). Other hormones may also increase pancreatic weight. Hyperprolactinaemia in mice produced by pituitary grafting can also increase pancreatic size mainly as a result of hyperplasia of acinar cells (Mori et al., 1986). It may also increase the prevalence of benign pancreatic neoplasms (see below).

Daily injections of 10 mg or 25 mg of isoprenaline for twelve day in rats has also been shown to increase pancreatic weight (Sturgess and Reid, 1973). Microscopic examination revealed hypertrophy of the acinar cell with an increase in secretory granules and a more strongly basophilic cell base. These changes were accompanied by alterations in salivary gland (See Digestive System, Part 2, Chapter VII)

Duct proliferation

Proliferative changes are seen sporadically in the epithelium of the pancreatic duct in association with inflammation of exocrine tissue or as a response to duct obstruction, the presence of calculi or parasites in the duct lumen. Such changes are prominant in the aged untreated Syrian hamster where they are associated with inflammatory and proliferative changes in the pancreatic parenchyma and biliary tree (Pour et al., 1976, 1979). These changes are characterised by proliferation of the duct epithelium, which may be polypoid in nature and show mucous or squamous metaplasia. There may be associated proliferation of endocrine cells.

These changes are of note because treatment of the hamster with pancreatic carcinogens produces exaggerated but similar morphological changes, whereas other species appear resistant to the pancreatic effects of the same agents (Takahashi and Pour, 1978). On this basis, Takahashi and Pour (1978) suggested that genetically linked susceptibility of the hamster pancreas might be a determinant in the neoplastic response.

Duct proliferation has also been described in mice experimentally infected with reo-virus 3 which proliferates in the cells of the main pancreatic duct (Walters, 1966; Papadimitriou and Walters, 1967) and in rabbits treated with corticosteroids (Bencosme and Lazarus, 1956).

Eosinophilic change of the exocrine pancreas

Zones of exocrine cells exhibiting increased eosinophilic staining of the cell cytoplasm, usually observed close to or around islets of Langerhans should be distinguished from true foci of cellular alteration. In these peri-insular areas, acinar cells appear larger and possess more prominent nuclei than surrounding cells. Their cell cytoplasm contains abundant zymogen granules which gives rise to the increased eosinophilic appearances. These peri-insular zones or peri-insular 'halos' have been recognised for many years (Jarotzky, 1899). Their presence is believed to reflect the intimate functional links between the endocrine and exocrine cells of the pancreas. Not only do these peri-insular islets contain more zymogen granules but the pattern of enzymatic content is different from the surrounding acinar cells (Malaisse-Lagae et al., 1975; Bendyan and Ito, 1979; Henderson et al., 1981). It has been suggested that these zonal differences are the result of high levels of insulin reaching the peri-insular acini through the insulo-acinar portal system because the peri-insular halos are more prominent in hyperinsulinaemic mice and disappear after treatment with alloxan (Hellman et al., 1962). However, this relationship is undoubtedly complex because these peri-insular zones are also prominent in rats made diabetic with streptozotocin, implying that other secretory products are involved in this process (Malaisse-Lagae et al., 1975).

Focal lesions of the exocrine pancreas including neoplasia

In the assessment of focal lesions and neoplasia of the exocrine pancreas, the pathologist is faced with conflicting or controversial terminology, somewhat analogous to the situation which occurs in the interpretation of hepatic nodules in rodents (see review by Chiu, 1985). Questions concerning the significance of foci of cellular alteration or whether nodular growths represent hyperplastic or

453

neoplastic lesions also apply to acinar pancreatic tissue. This is perhaps not surprising, for in the attempt to design experimental models for pancreatic carcinogenesis in laboratory animals, chemicals have been specifically selected for their rapid effects on the pancreas (reviewed by Rao and Reddy, 1985). Therefore, conclusions drawn from the occurrence of certain foci and nodules following administration of these selected chemicals may not be equally applicable to all types of xenobiotics. Particular caution is merited when focal lesions of the exocrine pancreas are found following long-term administration of potent therapeutic agents which cause marked physiological changes. Focal proliferative lesions of the exocrine pancreas also occur spontaneously in small numbers of untreated rats, mice and hamsters with advancing age and also develop in increasing numbers following dietary or hormonal manipulation.

Despite these uncertainties, it is probably most convenient to adhere to the customary histopathological classification of focal lesions of the pancreas which distinguishes foci of *cellular alteration, focal hyperplasia, adenoma* and *adenocarcinoma*. This grouping is widely used in the assessment of focal lesions in the rat pancreas (Boorman and Eustis, 1984; Greaves and Faccini, 1984). To aid interspecies comparison in toxicity studies, it is reasonable to adopt a similar pragmatic approach in other experimental species.

Foci of cellular alteration (focal cellular change, hypertrophic foci)

These are analogous to foci which occur in the rat liver for they show tinctoral characteristics which are different from the surrounding parenchyma but exhibit no compression or displacement of adjacent tissue. In the rat, foci observed either spontaneously or following administration of chemicals, are usually basophilic in their staining characteristics (basophilic foci) (Chiu, 1985). The cytoplasm of these cells appear basophilic because of less than their usual complement of eosinophilic zymogen granules.

Ultrastructural examination reveals the presence of abundant rough endoplasmic reticulum in the cell cytoplasm. The altered cells also possess enlarged parabasal nuclei with prominant nucleoli. The nuclei may also be mildly pleomorphic and exhibit some mitotic activity (Boorman and Eustis, 1984). The use of the term basophilic focus has been criticised by Chiu (1985) on the basis that not all foci have basophilic features and he suggested the term *hypertrophic focus*. However, the more descriptive term 'basophilic focus' possesses the merit of retaining a clear distinction from lesions of eosinophilic character which are believed to possess different proliferative characteristics. The *eosinophilic (acidophilic)* focus is the other focal lesion found in the rat pancreas which does not compress surrounding parenchyma. These foci tend to be larger than basophilic foci and are composed of cells containing abundant zymogen granules with enlarged basal nuclei with prominent nucleoli. Although by definition, acidophilic foci show no compression of the surrounding pancreatic tissue, they possess cytological proliferative characteristics which are similar to the larger eosinophilic nodular lesions which show compression and this has given rise to the suggestion that all such eosinophilic lesions should be grouped in the same category and called *focal hyperplasia* (Chiu, 1985). It is important to distinguish this type of focus from those zones of acinar cell parenchyma around islets of Langerhans which show increased eosinophilic staining (see above).

Both basophilic and eosinophilic foci are occasionally observed in untreated rats but they also occur in the pancreas of rats treated with 4-hydroxy-aminoquinoline-l-oxide, the proximate carcinogen of 4-nitroquinoline-l-oxide (Hayashi et al., 1972) and azaserine (Roebuck et al., 1984). In untreated rats, the prevalence of these lesions rises with age but they tend to be small and few in each pancreas, whereas in carcinogen-treated rats they develop rapidly in numbers over 100 in each pancreas (Longnecker et al., 1981).

It is important to note that the proliferative characteristics of basophilic and eosinophilic foci appear quite different from each other under the conditions where this has been investigated. Basophilic foci appear to have proliferative features similar to normal pancreatic tissue whereas acidophilic foci have greater proliferative characteristics as shown by mitotic activity and autoradiography using tritiated thymidine (Rao et al., 1982c). Eustis and Boorman (1985) showed that although nodular lesions in the rat pancreas (focal hyperplasia and adenoma) were increased in rats treated with corn oil for long periods (see below), an increase in the prevalence of basophilic foci was not seen. They therefore suggested that basophilic foci do not represent part of the same biological process as nodules and frank neoplasia of the pancreas. Thus, it appears that an increase in the prevalence of basophilic foci is not necessarily a harbinger of neoplasia in the rat pancreas and should not be considered a preneoplastic change.

Although not so extensively studied, similar foci of cellular alteration also occur in mice (Roebuck et al., 1980). In hamsters, foci of cellular alteration also occur spontaneously with advancing age, although these are characterised by intense eosinophilic staining of the cell cytoplasm without prominant nuclear changes (Takahashi and Pour, 1978; McMartin, 1979). Such lesions are often associated with inflammatory change in the hamster pancreas. Focal acinar lesions also occur in the human pancreas, although their significance is quite unknown. These lesions also composed of acinar cells which show variable tinctoral changes including reduced basophilia, reduced zymogen content or cytoplasmic vacuolization and mild nuclear changes (Longnecker et al., 1980). They are occasionally found in the pancreatic tissue of children but their prevalence seems not to increase markedly during adulthood. There is no evidence that they are associated with neoplasia (Longnecker et al., 1980).

Metaplastic foci

Foci of eosinophilic cells with morphological and functional characteristics of hepatocytes develop under certain circumstances in both the rat and hamster pancreas (Fig. 87).

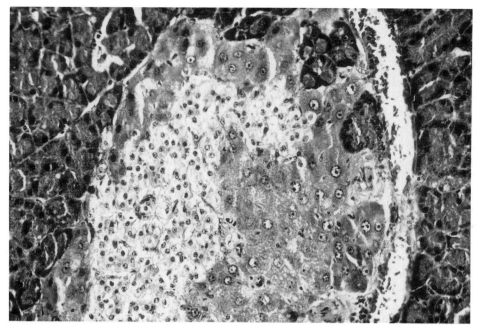

Fig. 87. Pancreas from a Wistar rat showing the appearances of hepatic metaplasia in the exocrine cells around an islet. (HE, ×300.)

Administration of a single dose of the carcinogen N-nitrosobis(2-oxopropyl)amine to hamsters at the peak of regenerative activity induced in the pancreatic exocrine tissue following pancreatic injury, leads eventually to moderate pancreatic exocrine atrophy and the appearance of foci of polyhedral eosinophilic cells resembling hepatocytes (Scarpelli and Rao, 1981). These cells contain glycogen, possess catalase activity and show the ultrastructural characteristics of hepatocytes. Unlike pancreatic exocrine cells, immunocytochemical staining shows them to be devoid of amylase and carboxypeptidase A. Administration of ciprofibrate, a peroxisomal proliferator in doses of 10 mg/kg/day for F344 rats for 60–72 weeks was also shown to produce clusters of polyhedral hepatocyte-like cells distributed adjacent to islets of Langerhans (Reddy et al., 1984). Reddy and his colleagues (1984) showed that these cells were ultrastructurally identical to rat hepatocytes. In addition, the cells contained numerous peroxisomes characterised by uricase-containing crystalloid nucleoids, typical of rat hepatocyte peroxisomes.

Such metaplastic cells, like pancreatic foci developing in the liver, probably indicate differentiation of a stem cell or intermediate cell to a metaplastic state in which pancreas specific genes are repressed while liver specific ones are simultaneously expressed (Reddy et al., 1984; Scarpelli, 1985).

Focal hyperplasia, hyperplastic nodule and adenoma

Nodular proliferative lesions of the exocrine pancreas occur spontaneously and can be induced by dietary or hormonal manipulation and by the administration of various chemicals in rats, mice, hamsters (Hayashi et al., 1972; Love et al., 1977; McGuinness et al., 1980; Abdo et al., 1985; Takahashi and Pour, 1978; Roebuck et al., 1980; Eustis and Boorman, 1985; Mori et al., 1986). Although nodular lesions of the exocrine pancreas occur in dogs and primates (McClure et al., 1978; McClure and Chandler 1982), they are extremely uncommon in the usual toxicity studies performed with young adults of these species.

Although it may be difficult on purely morphological grounds to make a valid distinction between hyperplasia and benign neoplasia in the rodent pancreas, it is usual to attempt this separation. Criteria for this have been schematized for the rat by Boorman and Eustis (1984) and are also applicable to both mouse and hamster. Thus, *focal hyperplasia* (acinar hyperplasia, hyperplastic nodule) is a focal lesion with tinctorial features distinct from the rest of the pancreas. Although usually contiguous with unaffected parenchyma and devoid of a capsule, focal hyperplasias nevertheless show mild compression or displacement

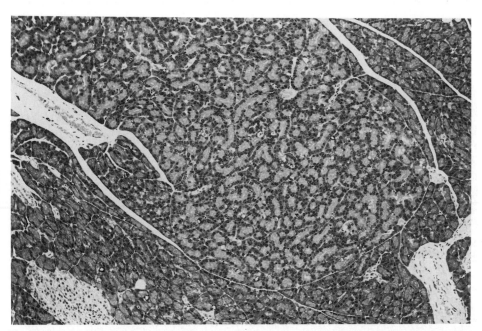

Fig. 88. Pancreas from a two-year-old Wistar rat showing a fairly well-delineated but unencapsulated, nodule composed of well-differentiated exocrine cells. Although this nodule measured less than three centimeters diameter at autopsy, it shows early compression of adjacent tissue and its cytology is distinct from that of the surrounding normal parenchyma. This would be called an adenoma by many pathologists although it is represents a borderline lesion of somewhat uncertain biological nature. (HE, ×100.)

of surrounding acinar tissue. They exhibit mild or moderate nuclear pleomorphism with variable mitotic activity.

Acinar adenomas are usually single, and sharply demarcated from the surrounding parenchyma by different cytological appearances, which is compressed or displaced. A fibrous capsule may be present and the altered cells show variable nuclear pleomorphism and mitotic activity. There is by definition no evidence of tissue or vascular invasion. Size of the lesion is not an absolute criterion but the larger the mass, the more likely it is to have compressed adjacent tissue and the more likely it is to be an autonomous growth (Rowlatt, 1967). More recently, pathologists in the National Toxicology Program have used size (greater than 3 mm diameter) as a major criterion for the diagnosis of adenoma in the rat (Boorman and Eustis, 1984). Although this has the merit of providing consistency between pathologists, such rigid criteria do not necessarily possess biological significance and particular care is needed in the interpretation of treatment-related increase in prevalence of lesions defined in this way (Figs. 88 and 89).

Treatment-related increases in benign nodular lesions of the rodent pancreas have been recorded in quite diverse situations. Adenomas were found in the pancreas of male F344/N rats but not females following two-year administration of the widely used flavouring agent, benzyl acetate, which is also found naturally

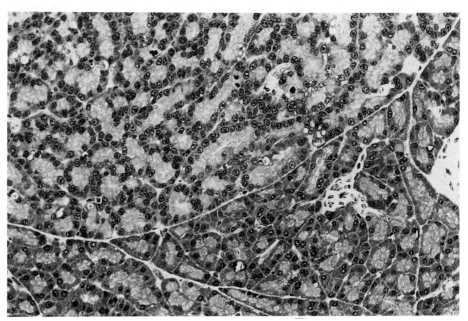

Fig. 89. Higher power view of nodule seen in Figure 88 showing cytological appearances of the nodule which in this field are distinct from those of the surrounding exocrine tissue. (HE, ×250.)

in a number of plants (Abdo et al., 1985). Focal acinar hyperplasia and acinar adenomas were found five times more frequently in male F344/N rats in carcinogenicity bioassays in which corn oil was administered by gavage than males not given corn oil and the incidence of these lesions was related to maximum mean body weights attained in the study groups (Eustis and Boorman, 1985). Hyperprolactinaemia produced in mice by ectopic pituitary grafting has also been shown to produce focal acinar hyperplasia or adenomas, indicating that prolactin may also be important in pancreatic tumorigenesis (Mori et al., 1986).

Carcinoma of the exocrine pancreas

Adenocarcinomas of the exocrine pancreas have been described in laboratory rodents, domestic animals particularly old dogs and cats, non-human primates and in man (Levison, 1979; Cotchin, 1984; McClure and Chandler, 1982). Histologically, they vary from well-differentiated neoplasms with acinar, duct like or papillary structures to quite pleomorphic or anaplastic tumours composed of small rounded cells, spindle cells or varying proportions of bizarre giant cells and multinucleated giant cells of Langhan's or Touton type (Priester, 1974a,b; Cubilla and Fitzgerald, 1975, 1979; Levison, 1979; Benitz and Roth, 1980; Madewell, 1981; Trepeta et al., 1981; Roebuck et al., 1981; McClure and Chandler 1982; Pour, 1985; Berendt et al., 1987).

Although perhaps of academic interest in drug safety evaluation, it is of note that the histological pattern of pancreatic carcinoma in man and rodents has given rise to considerable discussion concerning histogenesis. The histological appearances commonly observed in human pancreatic cancer are suggestive of mucin secreting cells of duct type and this has given rise to the traditional view that the majority of these cancers in man arise from duct or ductular epithelial cells (Cubilla and Fitzgerald, 1975; Longnecker, 1983). Similarly, pancreatic carcinomas induced in the hamster also appear to be morphologically similar to those occurring in man. (Pour et al., 1987). Immunocytochemical study has shown that these neoplasms contain a blood group A-like antigen which is normally produced by pancreatic ductal or ductular cells and this supports the concept that hamster pancreatic carcinoma is also derived from these duct cells (Pour, 1985).

This view has been challenged. Acinar differentiation is occasionally seen in human pancreatic carcinoma and even undifferentiated human pancreatic cancers may possess antigenic components of acinar cells (Parsa, 1982). Although in the rat, histological appearances of induced pancreatic carcinoma occasionally resemble those occurring in man, acinar differentiation is much more common (Levison, 1979; Roebuck et al., 1981; Eustis and Boorman, 1985). Using three-dimensional reconstruction and retrograde injection, it has been shown that the formation of ductule-like structures is a common and non-specific phenomenon in the pancreas and that duct or ductular differentiation dose not exclude the acinar cell as a cell of origin for pancreatic carcinoma (Bockman, 1981). Thus, it has been suggested that acinar cells may give rise to more human pancreatic carcinoma that has previously been thought (Levison, 1979; Longnecker, 1983).

Whether these findings represent variability in expression of a single neoplastic population or selection of a subpopulation exhibiting particular differentiation is part of a wider debate about the histogenesis and differentiation of neoplasms (Gould, 1986). However, pancreatic exocrine neoplasms, like other tumours, are capable of multidirectional differentiation, regardless of their postulated histogenesis.

Although a treatment-related increase in prevalence of pancreatic exocrine carcinomas in a rodent carcinogenicity bioassay is cause for concern, the assessment of their significance in terms of risk for man requires a critical assessment of many different factors. The prevalence of pancreatic carcinomas can be greatly influenced by dietary and hormonal factors (Roebuck et al., 1981; Howatson and Carter 1985). Somewhat surprising is the fact that invasive and metastazing carcinomas can be produced in the rat pancreas simply by feeding with raw soya flour for long periods (McGuinness et al., 1980).

The development of pancreatic acinar carcinoma in the F344 rat has also been ascribed to the administration of clofibrate and other compounds which produce peroxisomal proliferation in the liver (Reddy and Rao, 1977; Reddy and Qureshi, 1979). The precise significance of these observations for human safety of hypolipidaemic agents is uncertain, although it appears that the response of human tissues to these compounds may be different to rodent tissues and these findings do not necessarily indicate a cancer hazard to man.

These uncertainties underline the need in such instances for a general assessment of toxicity profile, comparative disposition and metabolism as well as mutagenic potential. It has been recently suggested that the cellular toxicity of certain pancreatic carcinogens correlates to a certain extent with their tumorigenic effect (Zucker et al., 1986).

Islets of Langerhans

In mammalian species, islets of Langerhans are scattered throughout the exocrine pancreatic tissue, forming 1–2% of pancreatic volume in adults and a somewhat greater percentage in foetal animals (Williams and Goldfine, 1985). Careful morphometric analysis is needed to accurately quantitate islet cell volume and number even in small rodents because islets are not randomly distributed and their size may be greater in some regions. (Bonnevie-Nielsen, 1986). It has been shown in the mouse that total islet cell mass correlates well with total pancreatic insulin content in a variety of physiological and pathological states (Bonnevie-Nielsen, 1986). Islets probably undergo some postnatal growth. Morphometric study of islets in rats has shown that islet volume increases from birth to about twelve weeks of age principally as a result in the increase in volume of B cells (Michels et al., 1986).

Classical histological techniques and immunocytochemistry have shown that the islets contain four main types of cells which synthesise and secrete insulin (beta or B cells), glucagon (alpha or A-cells), somatostatin (delta or D-cells) or pancreatic polypeptide (pp-cells).

Insulin-containing B-cells account for 80–85% of islets cells. In the rat, mouse and rabbit they occupy mainly the core of each islet (Doerr and Becker, 1985; Like et al., 1978; Smith, 1983). In the islets of guinea pigs, dogs and man, B cells are generally distributed in smaller core-like clusters mixed with other types of endocrine cells (Doerr and Becker, 1958; Smith, 1983; Anderson et al., 1986). In rhesus monkeys, B cells occupy the periphery of islets of Langerhans (Fujita and Murakami, 1973). Glucagon-containing A-cells comprise only about 10% of normal islet cells and in common with somatostatin-secreting D cells are generally located in the periphery of islets in man and animals (Smith, 1983; Fenoglio and King, 1983).

Pancreatic polypeptide containing pp-cells are located in the islet periphery but pp-cell containing islets tend to be found in the lower dorsal part of the head of the human and rat pancreas (Orci et al., 1976; Falkmer, 1979; Fiocca et al., 1983). In man, various ultrastructural types of pp-cells are apparently segregated into different parts of the pancreas (Fiocca et al., 1983). Extra-islet endocrine cells also occur in the human and animal pancreas. These appear as scattered single or small clusters of endocrine cells which most commonly immunostain for insulin (Kaitoh et al., 1986, Spencer et al., 1986, Anderson et al., 1986). Morphometric examination of endocrine tissue in the human pancreas has suggested that these single cells or small groups of endocrine cells only form a small percentage of overall endocrine cell volume in the pancreas (Kaitoh et al., 1986).

Another important feature of pancreatic islets in mammals is their distinctive blood supply because much of the blood which perfuses the exocrine pancreatic tissue passes through the islets. Pancreatic interlobular arteries give rise to islet branches which divide to form a network of capillaries in each islet. It is the vessels emerging from this network, referred to as insulo-acinar portal vessels which perfuse much of the exocrine pancreas (Williams and Goldfine, 1985).

Species differences exist in the extent to which there is a direct arterial supply to the exocrine pancreas, through vessels not passing from the islets. In the dog, primate and horse, most arterial branches to acinar cells pass via the islets whereas in the rat, part of the acinar blood supply passes directly from the pancreatic interlobular arteries into the acinar capillary network (Fujita and Murakami, 1973; Bonner-Weir and Orci, 1982). Mouse islets appear to be particularly well vascularised compared with the rat (Doerr and Becker, 1958).

This portal system has been emphasised by a number of investigators over the past few years for it is believed that the flow of blood from islets to exocrine cells plays a significant part in the metabolic activity of the exocrine pancreas. Insulin increases uptake and incorporation of glucose and amino acids into metabolically active tissues and this is important in the exocrine pancreas which has a particularly high rate of protein synthesis. It has been suggested that the synthesis of protein in the pancreas is controlled by the levels of insulin being

461

released from islet cells into the insulo-portal blood system (Henderson et al., 1981). It is of note that the exocrine pancreas in insulin-dependent diabetics is smaller than normal subjects (Maclean and Ogilvie, 1955). Conversely, administration of high doses of glucagon to rats and guinea pigs has been shown to produce degranulation and atrophy of pancreatic acinar cells (Salter et al., 1957; Cameron and Melrose, 1962; Jarrett and Lacy, 1962).

Inflammation, degeneration and atrophy of Islets of Langerhans

Inflammation (insulitis) with subsequent degeneration and atrophy of islet cells is associated with juvenile onset diabetes mellitus in man and similar changes occur in certain strains of animals which develop diabetes mellitus spontaneously. Both insulitis and a variety of degenerative changes can also be produced in laboratory animals by the administration of chemicals. The syndrome of insulin-dependent diabetes mellitus occurs in man or in laboratory animals, when more than 90% of insulin-containing Bcells are destroyed (Pipeleers and Van de Winkel, 1986). The structural changes occurring in islets of Langerhans in diabetes have been well reviewed by Wellman and Volk (1980).

Insulitis, characterized by an infiltration of islets by small lymphocytes, with smaller numbers of plasma cells, macrophages, eosinophils and neutrophils, is frequently observed in patients who die within one year of the clinical onset of juvenile-onset (type I) diabetics (Gepts and De May, 1978). It has been suggested that insulitis occurring as a result of abnormal immune mechanisms is important in the pathogenesis of human type I diabetes. This view is supported by the clinical association of diabetes type I with autoimmune diseases of the adrenal and thyroid glands and gastric parietal cells, the presence of islet cell cytoplasmic surface antibodies in the serum of recently diagnosed diabetics and evidence of T cell defects (Like and Rossini, 1984). The BB Wistar rat also develops a distinctive insulitis which resembles the juvenile diabetes occuring in man. Typically, fully developed lesions are found shortly after the development of detectable glycosuria and hyperglycaemia although the inflammatory process is initiated well in advance of the appearance of diabetes (Seemayer et al., 1982a). The affected pancreas is characterised by the presence of a monuclear infiltrate composed of small lymphocytes and monocytes both within the islets and in immediately adjacent exocrine parenchyma (Nakhooda et al., 1976; Seemayer et al., 1982a; Wright et al., 1985). Studies using monoclonal antibodies against rat lymphocytes have shown that the islet cell infiltrate is composed prodominantly of Ia$^+$ macrophages as well as helper/inducer (W3/25) and cytotoxic suppressor (OX 8) cells but few B lymphocytes (Like et al., 1983b). B islet cells in affected islets develop cytoplasmic swelling, vacuolisation, intense eosinoplilic change and pyknotic nuclei. Ultrastructural study reveals B-cell degranulation, cytoplasmic rarefaction, vesiculation, frank degeneration and cell death. (Seemayer et al., 1982a; Laupacis et al., 1983; Wright et al., 1985). Subsequently, well after the onset of overt diabetes, the lymphoid infiltrate diminishes in intensity but islet cells show residual cellular degeneration and eventually atrophy. Additionally, some irregular hyperplastic islets may develop (Wright et al., 1985).

These findings, particularly the presence of the lymphocytic insulitis at the time of the development of hyperglycaemia support the idea that the diabetes in the BB rat is also a result of cell-mediated autoimmune destruction of pancreatic cells. This concept is supported by the fact that manipulation of the immune system by neonatal thymectomy, administration of antilymphocyte serum, glucocorticoids or cyclosporin can reduce or eliminate the development of diabetes (Like et al., 1979, 1982, 1983a; Laupacis et al., 1983).

In addition, quantitation of circulating lymphocyte subsets using the monoclonal antibodies W3/13 and W3/25 (see Haemopoietic and Lymphatic Systems, Chapter III) demonstrates that the diabetic BB Wistar rat possesses fewer circulating T lymphocytes, particularly helper T (W 3/25 positive) cells compared with its non-diabetic Wister counterpart (Jackson et al., 1981). B-lymphocytic proliferative disorders, including plasma cell sarcomas, lymphomas and immunoblastic sarcomas also develop in the abdominal lymphoid tissue of diabetic BB Wistar rats maintained on insulin for their natural lifespan of about 12 months, presumably a result of immunoregulatory defects (Seemayer et al., 1982b).

Another model of juvenile onset diabetic mellitus is the non-obese diabetic mouse, a subline derived from the Jcl-ICR mouse (Makino et al., 1980). Jcl-ICR mice develop insulitis after about four weeks of age. This is followed by overt diabetes after a further period of 12 weeks. Cells infiltrating the islets of Langerhans comprise large numbers of small and medium-sized lymphocytes, some large lymphocytes, plasma cells, macrophages and a few polymorphonuclear cells. The B-islet cells show degenerative changes at about five or six weeks of age and ultrastructural examination demonstrates characteristic changes in the secretory granules (Fujino-Kurihara et al., 1985; Makino et al., 1980). Inflammation diminishes with time and when overt diabetes appears, this active inflammatory process may have ceased. Islets eventually become small and atrophic.

Mononuclear cells also appear in the periductular connective tissue of the submandibular glands of affected animals at about four or five weeks of age (see Salivary Gland, Chapter VII) (Fujino-Kurihara et al., 1985).

It has been suggested that this condition in non-obese diabetic mice is immunologically mediated, but it is of special interest that retrovirus-like (type C) particles have been observed in the cisternal of the rough endoplasmic reticulum in B islet cells of affected mice (Fujino-Kurihara et al., 1985). Immunohistochemical study using an antiserum to Kirsten murine sarcoma virus also showed strong immunoreaction localized to islet cells in non-obese diabeticmice older than four weeks but not in islet cells of their non-diabetic Jcl-ICR counterparts. The precise role of retroviruses in the non-obese diabetic mice is unclear, although they may damage islet cells directly, or induce an autoimmune reaction. Studies of type C retrovirus expression in B-islet cells of

C3H-db/db diabetic mice have suggested that type C retrovirus induction is pathogenetically linked to accelerated B-islet cell destruction (Leiter, 1985).

These spontaneous diabetic syndromes in mice and rats possess morphological features in common with diabetes which can be produced by viral infection. Mice infection with a variant of encephalomyocarditis virus (M-strain) develop degranulation, necrosis, loss of B-islet cells and hypoglycaemia (Craighead and McLane, 1986; Stefan et al., 1978). The immune system, particularly T-lymphocytes appear to be involved in the induction of diabetes by this virus for athymic (nude) mice are resistant to the effect (Buschard et al., 1976). Seemayer and colleagues (1982a) have shown that the syndrome produced by the encephalomyocarditis virus in mice is mild and transient, with characteristic ultrastructuralchanges in the endothelium of capillaries of the islets, unlike the findings in the BB rat. A similar phenomenon has been reported in non-human primates infected with coxsackie virus group B-4. Infection with this virus produces a transient diabetes mellitus in patas but not cynomolgus, rhesus or Cebus monkeys (Yoon et al., 1986).

Altered islet cell function can be produced by viral infection without evidence of cell damage. The replication of choriomeningitis virus can take place in the islet cells, particularly B cells of various strains of mice, to produce hyperglycaemia and abnormal glucose tolerance without obvious morphological change either at light or ultrastructural level (Oldstone et al., 1984; Southern and Oldstone, 1986). This is a similar phenomon to the virus induced changes in pituitary function without morphological alterations which have also been reported in mice (see Pituitary Gland, Chapter XII). Viral infections such as mumps, coxsackie virus group B-4 and rubella have also been considered responsible for the onset of diabetes in children (Like et al., 1978).

Diabetes mellitus occurs occasionally in dogs and non-human primates also the result of degeneration, atrophy or hypoplasia or pancreatic endocrine tissue (Anderson et al., 1986; Stokes, 1986).

A number of chemicals and medicinal agents can also cause direct damage on degenerative alterations in the islet cells which can also be associated under certain circumstances with insulitis and increased type C viral expression.

Streptozotocin, originally developed as an antibiotic, but with oncogenic and diabetogenic properties, exerts a direct effect on pancreatic B cells causing a loss of secretory granules several hours after a single large dose is administered to rats, mice and dogs. This early change is followed by evidence of necrosis and rapid removal of B cells with little or no evidence of cell debris or inflammation, three days after injection (Rakieten et al., 1963; Junod et al., 1967; Whiting et al., 1982). Although the same basic changes are seen in other species, some cytological differences are apparent between species when streptozotocin is administered in a similar dose schedule under similar conditions (Richter et al., 1971).

The precise way in which streptozotocin intiates damage to the islet B-cell remains unclear. A cytotoxic moiety may bind to a glucose receptor, enter the cell to alkylate DNA or interfere with respiratory enzyme activity (Le Doux et al., 1986).

The effects of streptozotocin in mice demonstrate some important factors of potential importance in safety assessment of therapeutic agents and therefore worth detailing here. CD-1 mice given a single large (200 mg/kg) injection of streptozotocin rapidly develop hypoglycaemia associated with complete destruction of B pancreatic cells, similar to that occurring in other species. In contrast, CD-mice given five daily injections of a subdiabetogenic dose (40 mg/kg) develop hypoglycaemia only after a period of five days in association with a insulitis. This is characterised by infiltration of islets with large numbers of lymphocytes and macrophages, features highly suggestive of a cell-mediated immune reaction similar to the spontaneous juvenile diabetes-like syndromes described above (Like and Rossini, 1976).

In addition, electron microscopic examination reveals increased expressions of C-type virus particles and occasional clusters of intra-cisternal type A viruses in B pancreatic cells of the affected CD-1 mice (Like and Rossini, 1976). Immunocytochemical study using antiserum to type C virus specific antigens (anti-Moloney leukaemia virus antibody) has also demonstrated the localization of viral material in affected islet cells (Appel et al., 1978). Although the significance of this finding remains uncertain, it has been suggested that because the type C virus envelope protein (gp 70) and the precursor polyprotein of the viral core are constituents of leukaemia cell membranes and are capable of serving as target hosts for the immune response, a similar phenomenon may occur in streptozotocin induced insulitis, i.e. streptozotocin-induced C-type virus expression results in structural changes of B islet cell membranes which initiate a cell-mediated immune response (Appel et al., 1978).

However, the induction of diabetes in mice by streptozotocin is undoubtedly very complex. Strain differences exist. Neither a single (200 mg/kg) nor multiple (40 mg/kg injections induced hyperglycaemia in AKR/J or Jackson BALB/c mice although the same dose under the same conditions produces changes in CD-1 mice and C57 BL/6J mice (Kim and Steinberg, 1984). LAF1 mice became hyperglycaemic after a single dose of 200 mg/kg but not after five daily doses of 40 mg/kg of streptozotocin.

In C57 BL/KSJ mice, insulitis and diabetes is also produced by streptozotocin but unlike CD-1 mice there is no increase in type C virus expression although type A virus induction occurs (Like et al., 1978). Nude mice appear resistant to the development of this insulitis, diabetes syndrome, implying that intact thymic function is necessary for development of insulitis (Paik et al., 1980). The immunological studies of Kim and Steinberg (1984) have confirmed that the T-lymphocyte system possesses a crucial role in the development of insulitis by multiple low doses of streptozotocin. They have suggested that an immunological reaction, specific to streptozotocin modified B-islet cells occurs in streptotozocin-mediated insulitis in mice.

Alloxan, a derivative of urea which structurally resembles D-glucose also has the intriguing, but well-known property of producing a profound and selective

465

effect on pancreatic B cells, causing cytoplasmic vesiculation, nuclear pyknosis and finally frank necrosis with little or no evidence of inflammation except for phagocyosis of the cellular debris. Pancreatic A-cells are spared and even appear more prominant in histological sections (Dunn et al., 1943; Bunnag et al., 1967; Patent and Alfert, 1967). Species differences in the sensitivity of pancreatic B-cells to the toxic effects of alloxan occur, human pancreatic B-cells being more resistant than those in either dog or rodent (Gorus et al., 1986). Despite considerable research, the precise mechanism for the toxic effects of alloxan on pancreatic B-cells and the reason for species specificity remains uncertain. It has been postulated that the toxic effect results from a high rate of alloxan uptake and poor enzymatic handling, perhaps allowing the generation of toxic oxygen-containing radicals (Gorus et al., 1982). There appears to be a complex relationship between cellular glucose metabolism and alloxan cytotoxicity, for glucose protects the B-cell probably by its metabolic effects and generation of reducing equivalents (Gorus et al., 1982).

Glucose and other sugars such as mannose which exert this protective effect are structurally similar to alloxan and it has also been suggested that this protective effect is a result of the prevention of inactivation of the glucose sensor of the pancreatic B-cell, glucokinase (Meglasson et al., 1986). Various *in vitro* studies and studies using spermatozoa as a source of cells have suggested that species differences in sensitivity are not related to differences in cellular uptake of alloxan or sensitivity to organic peroxides but rather differences in cellular scavenging of super-oxides anion radicals or species differences in ascorbic acid handling (Gorus et al., 1986).

Although both streptozotocin and alloxan are generally considered experimental agents, they provide well-studied models for the assessment of diabetogenic effects and degenerative changes in pancreatic B-cells produced by a number of more widely employed therapeutic agents.

For instance pentamidine, an antiprotozoal drug effective in the treatment of immunosuppressed patients with Pneumocystis carinii infection, has been reported to cause hypoglycaemia severe enough to require glucose administration as well as overt diabetes mellitus (Bouchard et al., 1982; Jha and Sharma 1984; Boillot et al., 1985). In vitro studies using rat islets have suggested that pentamidine is selectively toxic to B-islet cells causing degranulation, dilatation of the rough endoplasmic reticulum and necrosis of B-cells (Boillot et al., 1985). The damage to islet cells seems to be similar but occurs more slowly than either streptozotocin and alloxan following uptake by islet cells. Its mechanism of action remains unclear, but pentamidine is a lipophilic molecule, highly cationic and appears to be selectively taken up by islet cells. As the breakdown products include xanthine and uric acid, chemically closely related to alloxan, its mechanism of action may be similar, although this is far from clear as it may not be well metabolised in vivo (Boillot et al., 1985 for review).

A number of drugs of diverse pharmacological properties, some in current clinical use, cause cytoplasmic vacuolation and degranulation of B-islet cells in rats, associated with abnormal glucose tolerance. Cyproheptadine, an antihistamine employed as an appetite stimulant, cyclizine, a widely used antihistamine, and structurally related analogues possessing a piperidine or piperazine ring substituted at the 4 position with another group containing a ring, have been reported to produce reversible vacuolation and degranulation of pancreatic B-cells in rats and mice, sparing other species (Longnecker et al., 1972; Fisher et al., 1973; Fischer and Rickert, 1975; Klöppel et al., 1978). The changes in B-cells are characterized at light microscopic level by the loss of paraldehyde-fuchsin stained granules and the presence of clear cytoplasmic vacuoles. Ultrastructural examination shows a progressive loss of B-cell granules after the onset of treatment associated with dilatation of the cisternae of the rough endoplasmic reticulum, detachment of ribosomes, vesiculation and formation of vacuoles containing amorphous proteinaceous material. There is no morphological evidence of cell necrosis or inflammation and the changes appear entirely reversible on cessation of treatment. The changes are associated with an abnormal but reversible glucose tolerance.

The mechanism remains uncertain. Although these agents do not deplete insulin by stimulating its secretion, they may act through interference with the formation and maturation of insulin secretory granules (Fischer and Rickert, 1975). Another important factor is that all the available evidence suggests that these changes are species restricted, occurring mainly in the rat, although whether this is a result of metabolism idiosyncracy or differences in tissue sensitivity is unclear (Fischer and Rickert, 1975).

More recently, similar morphological changes have been reported to occur in the pancreatic B-cells of the Sprague-Dawley rat following administration of a novel anti-thrombotic agent SH966BS, an isoquinoline derivative with some structural features in common with cyproheptidine (Kast and Ueberberg, 1986). Cyclosporin has also been shown to inhibit insulin secretion in mice and rat islets and produce islet cell degranulation and vacuolation. (Wilson and Le Doux, 1989). Other therapeutic agents which exert effects on the pancreatic B-cell include the oral hypoglycaemic agent, tolbutamide, which causes increased insulin secretion and B-cell degranulation, diazoxide, a benzothiadiazine antihypertensive, which inhibits insulin release and produces mild ultrastructural changes in B cell granules and high doses of glucocorticoids which stimulate insulin release and B-cell degranulation in laboratory animals (see review by Fischer and Rickert, 1975; Wilson and Le Doux 1989). An increase in pancreatic islet vacuolation has also been reported in beagle dogs treated with contraceptive steroids for periods of up to seven years, probably as a consequence of overstimulation in response to decreased glucose tolerance (Johnson, 1989).

The cytotoxic drug, busulphan has also been shown to produce marked vascular congestion or haemorrhage of islets followed by fibrosis, an almost complete loss of A cells and a reduction in number of B cells when administered to rats for periods of up to twelve weeks (Kaduk et al., 1987). The mechanism for this effect is also unclear although local vascular damage favouring islet cell blood vessels may be involved.

Amyloid

Amyloid is deposited in islets of Langerhans in amyloid-prone laboratory species. In primates, this can be accompanied by total B-cell obliteration and development of frank diabetes mellitus (Palotay and Howard, 1982; Stokes, 1986). Amyloid is also found in pancreatic islets in mice with advanced amyloidosis (Williams, 1964).

Islet cell hyperplasia

Various types or degrees of islet cell hyperplasia occur in laboratory animals both spontaneously with advancing age or following the administration of chemicals. Similar changes have also been recorded in man.

Aging rats, especially males, commonly develop large hyperplastic islets of Langerhans under the usual laboratory conditions which includes ad libitum feeding (Hajdu and Rona, 1967; Greaves and Faccini, 1984). Large islets are also particularly common in genetically obese strains (Shino et al., 1973) and strains which develop late onset insulin-independent diabetes mellitus (Type II) (Michaelis et al., 1986).

Islet cell hyperplasia in the aged rat is characterized by a spectrum of appearances varying from large rounded or multilobulated islets to those showing an irregular appearance due to the presence of intra- or extra-islet fibrosis and interspersed exocrine tissue. These enlarged islets are occasionally associated with pigment-(iron) laden macrophages and chronic inflammation (Hajdu and Rona, 1967). The hyperplastic islets cells generally retain an arrangement and cytology very much like that found in normal islets. Immunocytochemical study has shown that such enlarged islets are composed mainly of insulin-containing cells but there is usually a preserved rim of glucagon-staining cells, reminiscent of normal rat islets. This distribution pattern can be helpful in the distinction of hyperplastic islets from adenomas in which the A and B cells are distributed in a more random manner (Spencer et al., 1986). In rats which develop atrophy of the exocrine tissue, the endocrine cells may become much more disorganised. Islet cells become scattered in irregular, insulin-containing masses, small clusters or even as single cells in a manner similar to that reported in destructive lesions of the human exocrine pancreas (Bartow et al., 1981).

In genetically obese rats, hyperplasia is also marked, but it occurs at an early age associated with degranulation of B-islet cells, and ultrastructural evidence of loss of secretory granules, vesicularisation of rough endoplasmic reticulum and prominance of Golgi apparatus (Shino et al., 1973). In the rat model for insulin-independent diabetes mellitus, the spontaneous hypertensive/NIH-corpulent rat, development of diabetes is associated with hyperplasia of islets involving insulin-containing B-cells which may form irregular masses enveloping islands of exocrine glands (Michaelis et al., 1986).

Reavon and Reavon (1981) showed that in normal Sprague-Dawley rats, islet cell function declines with advancing age but that hyperplasia of the islets can be prevented by increased physical activity and/or weight control. They therefore postulated that overnutrition increases insulin demand or insulin resistance such that in the face of declining islet cell function some B-cells cannot keep up increased production of insulin and consequently degenerate or die. In compensation, new cells are formed resulting in enlarged, multilobulated or hyperplastic islets. Similarly, in genetic obese rats, it has been suggested that increased demand of insulin by peripheral tissues associated with advancing obesity gives rise to a compensatory adaptation of islets with resultant hyperplasia. Hyperplasia of islet cells also occurs but far less commonly in the usual mice strains (Frith and Sheldon, 1983) and occasionally in untreated Syrian hamsters (personal observations).

As these forms of spontaneous hyperplasia are partly a response to increased insulin demand, it is not surprising that certain chemicals which increase the demand for insulin or stimulate its release from B pancreatic cells also stimulate the development of islet cell hyperplasia. Administration of synthetic corticosteroids in high doses to rats for up to six months produced rounded and enlarged hyperplastic islets as well as irregular proliferative changes in islet cells associated with fibrosis in a manner quite similar to that occurring spontaneously in aged rats (Kast et al., 1970). Morphometric study showed that both the number and the percentage volume of islets were increased in a dose-related fashion and that the changes were reversable on cessation of treatment. Islet cell enlargement, characterised by an increase in islet cell numbers has also been reported in hamsters given adrenocorticosteroids for periods of one month (Frenkel, 1983). The mechanisms for corticosteroid-induced islet cell changes are uncertain. However, B cells are those mainly affected and this is presumably related to corticosteroid-induced alterations in hepatic gluconeogenesis. Similar changes have been reported in rabbits given glucagon for long periods (Lazarus and Volk, 1958).

Neoplasia of pancreatic islets

Most laboratory animal species develop islet cell tumours spontaneously with advancing age. Islet cell neoplasms have been fairly well characterized in laboratory rodents where their morphological appearances and functional characteristics bear a close resemblance to pancreatic islet cell neoplasms in man. The difficulties in the distinction between hyperplasia and neoplasia in islets and the assessment of true malignant potential of islet tumours is common to all the species which have been studied in detail.

Typically, islet cell adenomas in rats (Rowlatt, 1967), hamsters (Pour et al., 1979), mice (Cardesa et al., 1979; Frith and Sheldon, 1983), guinea pigs (Yoshida et al., 1979), beagle dogs (Priester, 1974b), and man (Frantz, 1959) are single and characterised by rounded contours, with variable compression and condensation of surrounding tissue and inconstant capsule formation. Cytologically, the adenoma cells resemble normal islet cells but they may possess enlarged vesicular nuclei which show increased mitotic activity (Fig. 90). Adenoma cells may be

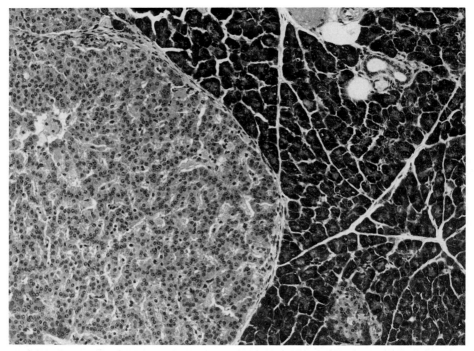

Fig. 90. Pancreas from a Sprague-Dawley rat showing a well-differentiated islet cell adenoma. (HE, ×200.)

arranged in ribbons or in glandular structures and vascularity may be prominant. Groups of tumour cells commonly penetrate surounding connective tissue, giving an impression of tissue invasion but such features do not appear to represent malignant biological behaviour, either in man where clinical follow-up is complete (Franz, 1959) or in laboratory species (Rowlatt, 1967; Mohr and Reznik, 1982; Frith and Sheldon, 1983).

The only unequivocal criterion for the diagnosis of islet cell carcinoma is the presence of metastatic growth (Rowlatt, 1967; Lewis et al., 1982). Therefore, careful study of local tissues, particularly regional lymph nodes and liver is warranted.

Immunohistochemical studies of islet cell tumours in man and those occurring spontaneously in Fischer (Stromberg et al., 1983), Sprague-Dawley, and Long-Evans rats (Spencer et al., 1986) and dogs (Hawkins et al., 1987; O'Brien et al., 1987) have all tended to confirm previous work using classical histological stains and ultra-structural examination, that islet cell neoplasms are composed mainly of insulin-producing B-cells. Although composed prodominantly of insulin-containing cells, they are not uncommonly multihormonal, containing a scattering of cells possessing immunoreactivity for glucagon, somatostatin and/or pancreatic polypeptide (Heitz et al., 1982; Liu et al., 1985; Spencer et al., 1986; Hawkins et al., 1987; O'Brien et al., 1987). The random distribution of these various pancreatic hormones within the islet-cell neoplasms can be helpful in the distinction between neoplasia and hyperplasia. In hyperplasia the distribution of cell types retains the more ordered distribution found in normal islets of Langerhans (Spencer et al., 1986).

Similar pancreatic islet cell neoplasms can be produced experimentally in rats by the administration of certain chemicals, notably single injections of streptozotocin or alloxan with or without nicotinamide or picolinamide (Rakieten et al., 1971; Kazumi et al., 1978; Michels et al., 1986; Yamagami et al., 1985).

The mechanism for the potentiation of the pancreatic tumorigenic activity by nicotinamide or picolinamide is not clear but it has been suggested that both streptozotocin and alloxan cause DNA strand breaks in islet B-cells which is associated with activation of poly (ADP-ribose) synthetase. This causes NAD^+ depletion which in turn leads to impairment of B-cell functions including pro-insulin synthesis (Yamamoto et al., 1981). As this enzyme is inhibited by aromatic acid amides such as nicotinamide and picolinamide it has been suggested that cellular NAD + levels are maintained when these substances are administered with streptozotocin or alloxan, allowing islet B-cells to survive, although in a state in which DNA remains fragmented. This may be one of the reasons for enhanced tumorigenesis (Yamagani et al., 1985). Furthermore as poly (ADP-ribose) synthetase inhibitors retard the joining of DNA strand breaks, this repair inhibition may increase the frequency of alteration in gene structure which may result in abnormal expression of genes involved in tumorigenesis. Recently, a novel gene which is expressed in rat insulinomas has been described and designated the rat insulinoma gene (Takasawa et al., 1986).

These induced rat tumours are principally of insulin-containing cells with additional glucagon, somatostatin and pancreatic polypeptide-positive cells as demonstrated by immunocytochemistry (Morohoshi et al., 1984), similar to those occurring spontaneously the rat.

REFERENCES

ABE, T. and WATANABE, M. (1983): Purification and characterization of three forms of microsomal }ytochrome P-450 in liver from 3-methycholanthrene-treated guinea pigs. *Mol.Pharmacol.*, 23, 258, 264.

ABDO, K.M., HUFF, J.E., HASEMAN, J.K., BOORMAN, G.A., EUSTIS, S.L., MATTHEWS, H.B., BURKA, L.T., PREJEAN, J.D. and THOMPSON, R.B. (1985): Benzyl acetate carcinogenicity, metabolism, and disposition in Fischer 344 rats and B6C3F1 mice. *Toxicology*, 37, 159–170.

AHO, H.J. AND NEVALAINEN, T.J. (1982): Experimental pancreatitis in the rat. Light and microscopical observations on early pancreatic lesions induced by intraduct injection of trypsin, phospholipase A2, lysolecithin and non-ionic detergent. *Virchows Arch.*[B], 40, 347–356.

AHOTUPA, M. and HIRSIMÄKI, P. (1989): The effect of tamoxifen citrate and tomerifene citrate on lipid peroxidation, antioxidation enzymes and xenobiotic metabolizing enzymes in rat liver. Presented at Vth International Congress of Toxicology, 16–21 July 1989, Brighton, England.

AKEDA, S., FUJITA, K., KOSAKA, Y. and FRENCH, S.W. (1986): Mallory body formation and amyloid deposition in the liver of aged mice fed a vitamin A deficient diet for a prolonged period. *Lab.Invest.*, 54, 228–233.

ALBERT, Z., ORLOWSKI, M. and SZEWCZUK, A. (1961): Histochemical demonstration of gamma-glutamyl transpeptidase. *Nature*, 191, 767–768.

ALLEN, T.M. and SMUCKLER, E.A. (1985): Liver pathology accompanying chronic liposome administration in the mouse. *Res.Commun.Chem.Pathol.Pharmacol.*, 50, 281–290.

ALTMANN, H.W. (1978): Pathology of human liver tumours. In: H. Remmer, H.M. Bolt, P. Bannasch and H. Popper (Eds), *Primary Liver Tumours*, Chap. 4, pp. 53–71. M.R.P.Press Ltd., Lancaster, England.

ALTMANN, H.W. (1980): Drug-induced liver reactions : A morphological approach. In: E. Grundmann (Ed.), *Drug Induced Pathology*. Current Topics in Pathology, 69, pp. 69–142. Springer-Verlag, Berlin.

ANDERSON, A.C. (1970): General pathology. In: A.C. Anderson and L.S Good (Eds), *The Beagle as an Experimental Dog*. Chap.23A, pp. 520–546. Iowa State University Press, Ames, Iowa.

ANDERSON, P.G., BRAUND, K.G., DILLON, A.R. and SARTIN, J.L. (1986): Polyneuropathy and hormone profiles in a chow puppy with hypoplasia of the islets of Langerhans. *Vet.Pathol.*, 23,528–531.

ANVER, M.R. and COHEN, B.J. (1979): Lesions associated with aging. In: Baker, H.J., Lindsey, J.R. and Weisbroth, S.H. (Eds), *The Laboratory Rat, Vol.1, Biology & Diseases*, Chap. 14, p. 377. Academic Press, New York.

ANTHONY, P.P., ISHAK, K.G., NAYAK, N.C., PULSEN, H.E., SCHEUER, P.J. and SOBIN, L.H. (1970): The morphology of cirrhosis : Definition, nomenclature, and classification. *Bull.WHO*, 540, 521–540.

APPEL, M.C., ROSSINI, A.A., WILLIAMS, R.M. and LIKE, A.A. (1978): Viral studies in streptozotocin-induced pancreatic insulitis. *Diabetologica*, 15, 327–336.

ATERMAN, K. (1986): The parasinusoidal cells of the liver : a historical account. *Histochem.J.* 18, 279–305.

AXELSSON, H., DANIELSSON, A., HENRIKSSON, R. and WAHLIN, T. (1979): Secretory behaviour and ultrastructural changes in mouse gall bladder principle cells after stimulation with cholinergic and adrenergic drugs. *Gastroenterology*, 76, 335–340.

BABANY, G. and DHUMEAUX, D. (1985): L'amidarone hépatotoxique? *Gastroenterol.Clin.Biol.*, 9, 505–507.

BAGHERI, S.A. and BOYER, J.L. (1974): Peliosis hepatitis associated with androgenic-anabolic steroid therapy. *Ann.Intern.Med.*, 81, 610–618.

BAGHERI, S.A., PALMER, R.H., BOYER, J.L. and HUNTER, R.L. (1973): Production of peliosis hepatitis in mice by oral administration of sodium lithocholate (abstract). *Gastroenterology, 64*, 879.

BANNERJEE, A.K., PATEL, K.J. and GRAINGER, S.L. (1989): Drug-induced acute pancreatitis. A critical review. *Med.Toxicol.*, 4, 186–198.

BANNASCH, P. (1986): Preneoplastic lesions as end points in carcinogenicity testing. I. Hepatic preneoplasia. *Carcinogenesis*, 7, 689–695.

BANNASCH, P., BLOCH, M. and ZERBAN, H. (1981): Spongiosis hepatis. Specific changes of the perisinusoidal liver cells induced in rats by N-nitrosomorpholine. *Lab.Invest.*, 44, 252–264.

BANNASCH, P., MOORE, M.A., KLIMEK, F. and ZERBAN, H. (1982): Biological markers of preneoplastic foci and neoplastic nodules in rodent liver. *Toxicol.Pathol.*, 10, 19–34.

BARKA, T. and POPPER, H. (1967): Liver enlargement and drug toxicity. *Medicine*, 46, 103–117.

BARON, J., REDICK, J.A., GREENSPAN, P. and TAIRA, Y. (1978): Immunohistochemical localisation of NADPH-cytochrome c reductase in rat liver. *Life Sci.*, 22, 1097–1102.

BARTOW, S.A., MUKAI, K. and ROSAI, J. (1981): Pseudoneoplastic proliferation of endocrine cells in pancreatic fibrosis. *Cancer*, 47, 2627–2633.

BAUM, J.K., HOLTZ, F., BOOKSTEIN, J.J. and KLEIN, E.W. (1973): Possible association between benign hepatomas and oral contraceptives. *Lancet*, 2, 926–929.

BECKER, F.F. (1982): Morphological classification of mouse liver tumors based on biological characteritics. *Cancer Res.*, 42, 3918–3923.

BECKER, F.F. and SELL, S. (1979): α-Fetoprotein levels and hepatic alterations during chemical carcinogenesis in C57BL/6N mice. *Cancer Res.*, 39, 3491–3494.

BEER, D.G., SCHWARTZ, M., SAWADA, N. and PITOT, H.C. (1986): Expression of H-ras and c-myc protooncogenes in isolated gamma-glutamyl transpeptidase-positive rat hepatocytes and in hepatocellular carcinomas induced by diethylnitrosamine. *Cancer Res.*, 46, 2435–2441.

BENCOSME, S.A. and LAZARUS, S.S. (1956): The pancreas of cortisone-treated rabbits : a pathogenic study *Arch.Pathol.*, 62, 285–295.

BENDYAN, M. and ITO, S. (1979): Immunohistochemical localization of exocrine enzymes in normal rat pancreas. *J.Histochem.Cytochem.*, 27, 1029–1034.

BENITZ, K.F. and ROTH, R.N. (1980): A spontaneous metastasizing exocrine adenocarcinoma of the pancreas in the rat. *Lab.Anim.Sci.*, 30, 64–66.

BENNETT, A.M. DAVIES, J.D., GASKELL, C.J. and LUCKE, V.M. (1983): Lobular dissecting hepatitis in the dog. *Vet.Pathol.*, 20, 179–188.

BERENDT, R.C., SHNITKA, T.K., WIENS, E. MANICKAVEL, V. and JEWELL, L.D. (1987): The osteoclast-type giant cell tumor of the pancreas. *Arch.Pathol.Lab.Med.*, 111, 43–48.

BERGMAN, J.R. (1985): Nodular hyperplasia in the liver of the dog : An association withchanges in the Ito cell population. *Vet.Pathol.*, 212, 427–438.

BERGS, V.V. and SCOTTI, T.M. (1967): Virus-induced peliosis hepatitis in rats. *Science*, 158, 377–378.

BERLIN, J., CASTRO, C.E., BAILEY, F. and SEVALL, J.S. (1982): Adaptation of rat parenchymal hepatocyte to nutritional variation: Quantitation by stereology. *Nutr.Res.*, 2, 51–63.

BERMAN, J.S., HILLEY, C.R. and WILSON, A.C. (1983):Comparison of the effects of the hypolipidaemic agents ICI 53072and clofibrate with those of phenobarbitone on liver size, blood flow and DNA content in the rat. *Br.J.Pharmacol.*, 78, 533–541.

BERNSTEIN, M.S. HUNTER, R.L. and YACHNIN, S. (1971): Hepatoma and peliosos hepatis developing in a patient with Fanconi's anaemia. *N.Engl.J.Med.*, 284, 1135–1136.

BHAGWAT, A.G. and ROSS, R.C. (1971): Hepatic intramitrochondrial crystalloids. *Arch.Pathol.*, 91, 70–77.

BHAGWAT, A.G. and DEODAR, S.D. (1968): Experimental hepatic injury produced in the rabbit by glucocorticoids. *Arch.Pathol.*, 85, 346–356.

BHATTACHARYA, R.D. (1983): Heterogeneity in circadian phase shifting of some liver variables in altered light-dark cycle. *Cell.Mol.Biol.*, 29, 483–487.

BLACK, M., MITCHELL, J.R., ZIMMERMAN, H.J., ISHAK, K.G. and EPLER, G.R. (1975): Isoniazid-associated hepatitis in 114 patients. *Gastroenterology*, 69, 289–302.

BLOOMER, J.R. (1988): The liver in protoporphyria. *Hepatology*, 8, 402–407.

BONNEVIE-NIELSEN, V. (1986): The endocrine pancreas. Aspects of β-cell function in relation to morphology, insulin secretion and insulin content. *Scand.J.Clin.Lab.Invest.*, 46, Suppl. 183, 1–47.

BONNEVIE-NEILSEN, V., POLONSKY, K.S., JASPAN, J.J., RUBENSTEIN, A.H., SCHWARTZ, T.W. and TAGER, H.S. (1982): Surface receptors for pancreatic hormones in dog and rat hepatocytes. Qualitative and quantitative differences in hormone-target cell interaction. *Proc.Natl.Acad.Sci.*, USA, 79, 2167–2171.

BOCKMAN, D.E. (1981): Cell of origin of pancreatic cancer : Experimental animal tumors related to human pancreas *Cancer*, 47, 1528–1534.

BOILLOT, D., in't VELD, P., SAI, P., FEUTREN, G., GEPTS, W. and ASSAN, R. (1985): Functional and morphological modifications induced in rat islets by pentamidine and other diamidines in vitro. *Diabetologia*, 28, 359–364.

BONNER-WEIR, S. and ORCI, L. (1982):New perspectives on the microvasculature of the islets of Langerhans in the rat. *Diabetes*, 31, 883–889.

BOORMAN, G.A. and HOLLANDER, C.F. (1973): Spontaneous lesions in the female WAG/Rij (Wistar) rat. *J.Gerontol.*, 28, 152–159.

BOORMAN, G.A. and EUSTIS, S.L. (1984): Proliferative lesions of the exocrine pancreas in male F344/N rats. *Environ.Health Perspect.*, 56, 213–217.

BORENFREUND, E., HIGGENS, P.J., and PETERSON, E. (1980)a: Intermediate-sized filaments in cultured rat liver tumour cells with Mallory body-like cytoplasm abnormalities. *J.N.C.I.*, 64, 323–33.

BORENFREUND, E., SCHMID, E., BENDICH, A. and FRANKE, W.W. (1980)b: Constitutive aggregates of intermediate-sized filaments of the vimentin and cytokeratin type in cultured hepatoma cells and their dispersal by butyrate. *Exp.Cell.Res.*, 127, 215–235.

BORST, P. (1986): How proteins get into microbodies (peroxisomes, glyoxisomes, glycosomes). *Biochim.Biophys.Acta*, 866, 176–203.

BOUCHARD, Ph., SAI, P., REACH, G., CAUBARRERE, I., GANEVAL, D. and ASSAN, R. (1982): Diabetes mellitis following pentamidine-induced hypoglycemia in humans. *Diabetes*, 31, 40–45.

BOYER, J.L. (1980): New concepts of mechanisms of hepatocyte bile formation. *Physiol.Rev.*, 60, 303–326.

BOYER, J.L. (1981): Membrane events in mechanisms of bile formation and drug-induced cholestasis. In: M. Davis, J.M. Tredger and R. Williams (Eds), *Drug Reactions and the Liver*, pp. 64–71. Pitman Medical, London.

BRADFIELD, J.W.B., (1984): Liver sinusoidal cells. *J.Pathol.*, 142, 5–6.

BRECKENRIDGE, A. (1987): Enzyme induction in humans. Clinical aspects: an overview. *Pharmaco.Ther.*, 33, 95–99.

BRUGUERA,M., ARANGUIBEL,F., ROS, E and RODES, J. (1978): Incidence and clinical significance of sinusoidal dilatation in liver biopsies. *Gastroenterology*, 75, 474–478.

BUNNAG, S.C., WARNER, N.E. and BUNNAG, S. (1967): Microcirculation of islets of Langerhans in alloxan diabetes of mice. *Bibl.Anat.*, 9, 169–175.

BUREK, J.D. (1978): Age-associated pathology. In: *Pathology of Aging Rats*. Chap. 4, pp. 29–168. CRC Press Inc., Boca Raton, Florida.

BURNS, W., WEIDE, G.V. and CHAN, C. (1972): Laminated mitochondrial inclusions in hepatocytes of liver biopsies. *Arch.Pathol.*, 94, 75–80.

BURSCH, W., TAPER, H.S., LAUER, B. and SCHULTE-HERMANN, R. (1985): Quantitative histological and histochemical studies on the occurrence and stages of controlled cell death (apoptosis) during regression of rat liver hyperplasia. *Virchows.Arch.[B]*, 50, 153–166.

BUSCHARD, K., RYGAARD, J. and LUND, E. (1976) The inability of a diabetogenic virus to induce diabetes mellitis in athymic (nude) mice. *Acta.Pathol.Microbiol.Scand [C].*, 84, 299–303.

BUTLER, W.H. (1978): Long-term efforts of phenobarbitone-Na on male Fischer rats. *Br.J.Cancer*, 37, 418–423.

BUTLER, W.H. and HEMPSALL, V. (1978): Histochemical observations on nodules induced in the mouse liver by phenobarbitone. *J.Pathol.*, 125, 155–161.

BUTTERWORTH, B.E., SMITH-OLIVER, T., EARLE, L., LOURY, D.J., WHITE, R.D., DOOLITTLE, D.J., WORKING, P.K., CATTLEY, R.C., JIRTLE, R., MICHALOPOULOS, G. and STROM, S. (1989): Use of primary cultures of human hepatocytes in toxicology studies. *Cancer Res.*, 49, 1075–1084.

CAMERON, J.M. and MELROSE, A.G. (1962): Changes in liver, pancreatic and stomach morphology following chronic glucagon administration in guinea pigs. *Br.J.Exp.Pathol.*, 43, 384–386.

CAMILLERI, M., SCHAFLER, K., CHADWICK, V.S., HODGSON, H.J. and WEINBREN, K. (1981): Periportal sinusoidal dilatation, inflammatory bowel disease, and the contraceptive pill. *Gastroenterology*, 80, 810–815.

CAPERNA, T.J. and GARVEY, J.S. (1982): Antigen handling in aging II. The role of Kupffer and endothelial cells in antigen processing in Fischer 344 rats. *Mech.Ageing Dev.*, 20, 205–221.

CARDESA, A., BULLON-RAMIREZ, A. and LEVITT, M.H. (1979): Tumours of the pancreas. In: V.S. Turusov (Ed.),*Pathology of Tumours in Laboratory Animals, Vol.2, Tumours of the Mouse.* pp. 235–241. IARC Scientific Publ. No.23, Lyon.

CHEDID, A., MENDENHALL, C.L., TOSCH, T., CHEN, T., RABIN, L., GARCIA-PONT, P., GOLDBERG, S.J., KIERNAN, T., SEEFF, L.B., SORRELL, M., TAMBURRO, C., WEESNER, R.E. and ZETTERMANN, R. (1986): Significance of mega mitochondria in alcoholic liver disease. *Gastroenterology*, 90, 1858–1864.

CHESTERMAN, F.C. and POMERANCE, A. (1965): Cirrhosis and liver tumours in a closed colony of golden hamsters. *Br.J.Cancer*, 19, 802–811.

CHIU, T. (1985): Hypertrophic foci of pancreatic acinar cells in rats. *CRC Crit. Rev.Toxicol.*, 14, 133–157.

CHVEDOFF, M., CHIGNARD,G., DANCLA, J.L., FACCINI, J.M., LOYEAU, F., PERRAUD, J. and TARADACH, C. (1982): Le rongeur agé : observations recueillies an cours d'essais de carcinogenicité. *Sci.Tech.Anim.Lab.*, 7, 87–97.

CHVEDOFF, M., FACCINI, J.M., GREGORY, M.H., HULL, R.M., MONRO, A.M., PERRAUD, J., QUINTON, R.M. and REINERT, H.H. (1984): The toxicology of the schistosomicidal agent oxamnaquine. *Drug Dev.Res.*, 4, 229–235.

CLARKE, D.G., TOPPING, D.L., ILLMAN, R.J., TRIMBLE, R.P. and MALTHUS, R.S. (1980): A glycogen storage disease (gsd/gsd) rat : Studies on lipid metabolism, lipogenesis, plasma metabolites and bile acid secretion. *Metabolism*, 29, 415–420.

COHEN, A.J. and GRASSO, P. (1981): Review of the hepatic response to hypolipidaemic drugs in rodents and assessment of its toxicological significance to man. *Food Cosmet.Toxicol.*, 19, 585–605.

COLEMAN, G.L., BARTHOLD, S.W., OSBALDISTON, G.W., FOSTER, S.J. and JONAS, A.M. (1977): Pathological changes during aging in barrier-reared Fischer 344 male rats. *J.Gerontol.*, 32, 258–278.

COMPORTI, M. (1985): Biology of disease. Lipid peroxidation and cellular damage in toxic liver injury. *Lab.Invest.*, 53, 599–623.

CONNEY, A.H. (1967): Pharmacological implications of microsomal enzyme induction. *Pharmacol.Rev.*, 19, 317–366.

CONNEY, A.H. (1986): Induction of microsomal cytochrome P-450 enzymes: The first Bernard B. Brodie Lecture at Pennsylvania State University. *Life Sci.*, 39, 2493–2518.

CONWAY, J.G., KAUFFMAN, F.C., TSUKADA, T. and THURMAN, R.G. (1984): Glucuronidation of 7-hydroxycoumarin in periportal and pericentral regions of the liver lobule. *Mol.Pharmacol.*, 25, 487–493.

CONWAY, J.G., CATTLEY, R.C., POPP, J.A. and BUTTERWORTH, B.E. (1989): Possible mechanisms in hepatocarcinogenesis by the peroxisomal proliferator di(2-elthylhexyl)phthalate. *Drug Metab.Rev.*, 21, 65–102.

COOK, R.W., TRAPP, A.L. and WILLIAMS, J.F. (1981): Pathology of Taenia taeniaeformis in the rat : Hepatic, lymph node and thymic changes. *J.Comp.Pathol.*, 91, 219–226.

CORCOS, D., DEFER, N., RAYMONDJEAN, M., PARIS, B., CORRAL, M., TICHONICKY, L., KRUH, J., GLAISE, D., SAULNIER, A. and GUGUEN-GUILLOUZO, C. (1984): Correlated increase of the expression of the c-ras genes in chemically induced hepatocarcinomas. *Biochem.Biophys.Res.Commun.*, 122, 259–264.

COTCHIN, E. (1984): Veterinary oncology : A survey *J.Pathol.*, 142, 101–127.

CRAIGHEAD, J.E. and MCLANE, M.F. (1968): Diabetes mellitus : Induction in mice by encephalomyocarditis virus. *Science*, 162, 913–914.

CRAMPTON, R.F., GRAY, T.J.B., GRASSO, P. and PARKE, D.V. (1977)a: Long-term studies on chemically induced liver enlargement in the rat. I. Sustained induction of microsomal enzymes with absence of liver damage on feeding phenobarbitone or butylated hydroxytoluene. *Toxicology*, 7, 289–306.

CRAMPTON, R.F., GRAY, T.J.B., GRASSO, P. and PARKE, D.V. (1977)b: Long-term studies on chemically induced liver enlargement in the rat. II. Transient induction of microsomal enzymes leading to liver damage and nodular hyperplasia produced by safrole and Ponceau MX. *Toxicology*, 7, 307–326.

CRASS, R.A. and MORGAN, R.G.H. (1982): The effects of long-term feeding of soya-bean flour diets on pancreatic growth in the rat. *Br.J.Nutr.*, 47, 119–129.

CUBILLA, A.L. and FITZGERALD, P.J. (1975): Morphological patterns of primarily nonendocrine human pancreas carcinoma. *Cancer Res.*, 35, 2234–2246.

CUBILLA, A.L. and FITZGERALD, P.J. (1979): Cancer of the pancreas (nonendocrine) : A suggested morphological classification. *Semin.Oncol.*, 6, 285–297.

CURTHOYS, N.P. and HUGHEY, R.P. (1979): Characterisation and physiological function of rat renal gamma-glutagamyltranspeptidase. *Enzyme*, 24, 383–403.

DE LA IGLESIA, F.A., PINN, S.M., LUCAS, J. and MCGUIRE, E.J. (1981): Quantitative sterology of peroxisomes in hepatocytes from hyperlipoproteinemic patients receiving gemfibrozil. *Micron.*, 12, 97–98.

DE MATTEIS F., GIBBS, A.H. and HOLLEY, A.E. (1987): Occurrence and biological properties of N-methyl protoporphyrin. *Ann.N.Y.Acad.Sci.*, 514, 30–40.

DELLA PORTA G., CABRAL, J.R. and ROSSI, L. (1978): Carcinogenicity study of rifampicin in mice and rats. *Toxicol.Appl.Pharmacol.*, 43, 293–302.

DENK, H., FRANKE, W.W., KERJASCHKI, D. and ECKERSTORFER, R. (1979): Mallory bodies in experimental animals and man. *Int.Rev.Exp.Pathol.*, 20, 77–121.

DENT, J.G., GRAICHEN, M.E., SCHNELL, S. and LASKER, J. (1980): Constitutive and induced hepatic microsomal cytochrome P-450 monooxygenase activities in male Fischer-344 and CD rats. A comparative study. *Toxicol.Appl.Pharmacol.*, 52, 45–53.

DIDIER, R., REMESY, C., DEMIGNE, C. and FAFOURNOUX, P. (1985): Hepatic proliferation of mitochondria in response to a high protein diet. *Nutr.Res.*, 5, 1093–1102.

DIETRICH, R.A. (1966): Tissue and subcellular distribution of mammalian aldehyde oxidizing capacity. *Biochem.Pharmacol.*, 15, 1911–1922.

DOERR, W. and BECKER, V. (1958): Bauchspeicheldrüse. In: P. Cohrs, R. Jaffe and H. Meeson (Eds), *Pathologie der Laboratoriumstiere. Vol.1*, pp. 130–155. Springer-Verlag, Berlin.

DUNN, J.S., SHEENAN, H.L. and MCLETCHIE, N.G.B. (1943): Necrosis of islets of Langerhans produced experimentally. *Lancet*, 1, 484–487.

DUNSFORD, H.A., MASET, R., SALMAN, J. and SELL, S. (1985): Connection of duct-like structures induced by a chemical hepatocarcinogen to portal bile ducts in the rat liver detected by injection of bile ducts with a pigmented barium gelatin medium. *Am.J.Pathol.*, 118, 218–224.

EACHO, P.I., FOXWORTHY, P.S., JOHNSON, W.D. and VAN LIER, R.B.L. (1985): Characterisation of liver enlargement induced by compound LY171883 in rats. *Fundam.Appl.Toxicol.*, 5, 7943–803.

EACHO, P.I., FOXWORTHY, P.S., JOHNSON, W.D., HOOVER, D.M. and WHITE, S.L. (1986): Hepatic peroxisomal changes induced by a tetrazole-substituted alkodyacetophenone in rats and comparison with other species. *Toxicol.Appl.Pharmacol.*, 83, 430–437.

EDMONDSON, H.A. (1958): Tumors of the liver and intrahepatic bile ducts. *Atlas of Tumor Pathology*, Section VII, Fascicle 25. Armed Forces Institute of Pathology, Washington D.C.

ELCOMBE, C.R. and MITCHELL, A.M. (1987): Peroxisome proliferation due to di(2-elthylhexyl)phthalate (DEHP): Species differences and possible mechanisms. *Environ.Health Perspect.*, 70, 211–219.

ENGELMANN, G.L., RICHARDSON, A., KATZ, A. and FIERER, J.A, (1981): Age-related changes in isolated rat hepatocytes. Comparison of size, morphology, binucleation, and protein content. *Mech.Ageing Dev.*, 16, 385–395.

ENOMOTO, K., YING, T.S., GRIFFIN, M.J. and FARBER, E. (1981): Immunohistochemical study of epoxide hydrolase during experimental liver carcinogenesis. *Cancer Res.* 41, 3281–3287.

ENOMOTO, M., NAOE, S., HARADA, M., MIYATA, K., SAITO, M. and NOGUCHI, Y. (1974): Carcinogenesis in extrahepatic bile duct and gall bladder: carcinogenic effects of N-hydroxy-2-acetamidofluorene in mice fed a 'gallstone-inducing' diet. *Jpn.J.Exp.Med.*, 44, 37–54.

ESSIGMAN, E.M. and NEWBERNE, P.M. (1981): Enzymatic alterations in mouse hepatic nodules induced by a chlorinated hydrocarbon pesticide. *Cancer Res.* 41, 2823–2839.

EUSTIS, S.L. and BOORMAN, G.A. (1985): Proliferative lesions of the exocrine pancreas : Relationship to corn oil gavage in the National Toxicology Program. *J.N.C.I.*, 75, 1067–1073.

EVARTS, R.P., RAAB, M., MARSDEN, E. and THORGEIRSSON, S.S. (1986): Histochemical changes in livers from portacaval-shunted rats. *J.N.C.I.*, 76, 731–738.

EWEN, C., MOORE, J.V. and HARRIS, M. (1987): Proliferative lesions in the livers of mice treated 18 months previously with ciplatin. *Br.J.Cancer*, 55, 109–110.

FABRY, A., BENJAMIN, S.A. and ANGLETON, G.M. (1982): Nodular hyperplasia of the liver in the beagle dog. *Vet.Pathol.*, 19, 109–119.

FALKMER, S. (1979): Immunocytochemical studies on the evolution of islet hormones. *J.Histochem.Cytochem.*, 27, 1281–1282.

FALZON, M., WHITING, P.H., EWEN, S.W.B., MILTON, A.S. and BURKE, M.D. (1985): Comparative effects of indomethacin on hepatic enzymes and histology and on serum indices of liver and kidney function in the rat. *Br.J.Exp.Pathol.*, 66, 527–534.

FARBER, E. (1963): Ethionine carcinogenesis. *Adv.Cancer Res.*, 7, 383–474.

FARBER, E. (1976): The pathology of experimental liver cell cancer. In: H.M. Cameron, D.A. Linsell and G.P. Warwick (Eds), *Liver Cell Cancer*, pp. 243–277. Elsevier, Amsterdam.

FARBER, E. (1982): Chemical carcinogenesis. A biological perspective. *Am.J.Pathol.*, 106, 271–296.

FARBER, E. (1984): The biochemistry of preneoplastic liver : a common metabolite pattern in hepatocyte nodules. *Can.J.Biochem.Cell.Biol.*, 62, 486–494.

FARBER, E. and SARMA, D.S.R. (1987): Hepatocarcinogenesis: A dynamic cellular perspective. *Lab.Invest.* 56, 4–22.

FELDMAN, D., SWARM, R.L. and BECKER, J. (1980): Elimination of excess smooth endoplasmic reticulum after phenobarbital administration. *J.Histochem.Cytochem.*, 28, 997–1006.

FENOGLIO, C.M. and KING, D.W. (1983): Somatostatin : An update. *Hum.Pathol.*, 14, 475–479.

FIOCCA, R., SESSA, F., TENTI, P., USELLINI, L., CAPELL, A.C., O'HARE, M.M.T. and SOLCIA, E. (1983): Pancreatic polypeptide (PP) cells in the PP-rich lobe of the human pancreas are identified ultrastructurally and immunocytochemically as F cells. *Histochemistry*, 77, 511–523.

FISCHER, L.J., WOLD, J.S. and RICKERT, D.E. (1973): Structure-activity relationships in drug-induced pancreatic islet cell toxicity. *Toxicol.Appl.Pharmacol.*, 26, 288–298.

FISCHER, L.J. and RICKERT, D.E. (1975): Pancreatic islet-cell toxicity. *CRC Crit.Rev.Toxicol.*, 3, 231–263.

FITTSCHEN, C. and BELLAMY, J.E.C. (1984): Predisone-induced morphologic and chemical changes in the liver of dogs. *Vet.Pathol.*, 21, 399–406.

FITZGERALD, J.E., DE LA IGLESIA, F.A. and McGUIRE, E.J. (1984): Carcinogenicity studies in rodents with ripazepam, a minor tranquilizing agent. *Fundam.Appl.Toxicol.*, 4, 178–190.

FITZGERALD, J.E., PETRERE, J.A., MCGUJIRE, E.J. and DE LA IGLESIA, F.A. (1986): Preclinical toxicology studies with the lipid-regulating agent gemcadiol. *Fundam.Appl.Toxicol.*, 6, 520–531.

FORTNER, J.G. (1957): Spontaneous tumors including gastrointestinal neoplasms and malignant malanomas in the Syrian hamster. *Cancer*, 10, 1153–1156.

FOX, K.A. and LAHCEN, R.B. (1974): Liver cell adenomas and peliosis hepatis in mice associated with oxazepam. *Res.Commun.Chem.Pathol.Pharmacol.*, 8, 481–488.

FOSTER, J.R., ELCOMBE, C.R., BOOBIS, A.R., DAVIES, D.S., SESARDIC, D., McQUADE, J., ROBSON, R.T., HAYWARD, C. and LOCK, E.A. (1986): Immunocytochemical localisation of cytochrome P-450 in hepatic and extrahepatic tissues of the rat with a monoclonal antibody against cytochrome P-450c. *Biochem.Pharmacol.*, 35, 4543–4554.

FRANTZ, V.K. (1959): Islet cell tumors. In: Tumors of the Pancreas. *Atlas of Tumor Pathology*, Section VII, Fascicle 27, pp. 79–141. Armed Forces Institute of Pathology, Washington D.C.

FREDERIKS, W.M., MARX, F., BOSCH, K.S. and VAN NOORDEN, C.J.F. (1987): Diurnal variation in 5'-nucleotidase activity in the rat liver. *Histochemistry*, 87, 439–443.

FRENCH, S.W. (1981): The Mallory body : Structure, composition and pathogenesis. *Hepatology*, 1, 76–83.

FRENKEL, J.K. (1983): Pancreatic islet-cell hyperplasia, golden hamster. In: T.C.Jones, U.Mohr and R.D.Hunt (Eds), *Endocrine System*, pp. 304–307. Springer Verlag, Berlin.

FRIEDMAN, H.I., CHANDLER, J.G. and NEMETH, T.J. (1977): Hepatic intramitochondrial filaments in morbidly obese patients undergoing intestinal bypass. *Gastroenterology*, 73, 1353–1361.

FRITH, C.H. and SHELDON, W.D. (1983): Hyperplasia, adenoma and carcinoma of pancreatic islets, mouse. In: T.C.Jones, U.Mohr and R.D.Hunt (Eds), *Endocrine System*, pp. 297–303. Springer Verlag, Berlin.

FUJINO-KURIHARA, H., FUJITAS, H., HAKURA, A., NONAKA, K. and TARUI, S. (1985): Morphological aspects on pancreatic islets of non-obese diabetic (NOD) mice. *Virchows Arch.[B]*, 49, 107–120.

FUJITA, T. and MURAKAMI, T. (1973): Microcirculation of monkey pancreas with special reference to the insulo-acinar portal system. A scanning electron microscopic study of vascular casts. *Arch.Histol.Jpn.*, 35, 255–263.

FUJITA, S., KITAGAWA, H., ISHIZAWA, H., SUZUKI, T. and KITANI, K., (1985): Age-associated alterations in hepatic glutathione-s-transferase activities. *Biochem.Pharmacol.*, 34, 3891–3894.

GANGOLLI, S.D., LAKE, B.G. and EVANS, J.G. (1987): The histopathology and biochemistry of phenobarbitone-induced liver nodules in C3H mice. *Arch.Toxicol.Suppl.*, 10, 95–107.

GELLATLY, J.B.M. (1975): The natural history of hepatic parenchymal nodule formation in acolony of C57BL mice with reference to the effect of diet. In:W.H. Butler and P.M. Newberne (Eds), *Mouse Hepatic Neoplasia*. Chap. 5, pp. 77–109, Elsevier, Amsterdam.

GEPTS, W. and DE MAY, J. (1978): Islet cell survival determined by morphology : An immunocytochemical study of the islets of Langerhans in juvenile diabetes mellitus. *Diabetes*, 27 (Suppl.1), 251–261.

GERBER, W.A. and THUNG, S.N. (1980): Enzyme patterns in human hepatocellular carcinomas. *Am.J.Pathol.*, 98, 395–400.

GERMAIN, L., GOYETTE, R. and MARCEAU, N. (1985): Differential cytokeratin and alpha-fetoprotein expression inmorphologically distinct epithelial cells emerging at the earlystage of rat hepatocarcinogenesis. *Cancer Res.*, 45, 673–681.

GHADIALLY, F.N. (1982): Mitochondria. In: *Ultrastructural Pathology of the Cell and Matrix*, 2nd Ed., Chap. 3, pp. 149–263. Butterworths, London.

GHADIALLY, F.N. (1982): Lysosomes: In: *Ultrastructural Pathology of the Cell and Matrix*,2nd Ed., Chap. 7, pp. 435–579.

GHOSHAL, A.K. and FARBER, E. (1984): The induction of liver cancer by dietary deficiency of choline and methionine without added carcinogens. *Carcinogenesis*, 5, 1367–1370.

GIAMPAOLO, C., BRAY, K., KOWALSKI, B. and ROGERS, A.E. (1989): Cytologic characteristics of neoplastic and regenerating hepatocytes in fine needle aspirates of rat liver. *Toxicol.Pathol.*, 17, 743–753.

GOEL, S.K., LALWANI, N.D. and REDDY, J.K. (1986): Peroxisomal proliferation and lipid peroxidation in rat liver. *Cancer Res.* 46, 1324–1330.

GOLDBLATT, P.J. and GUNNING, W.T. (1984): Ultrastructure of the liver and biliary tract in health and disease. *Ann.Clin.Lab.Sci.*, 14, 159–167.

GOLDSTEIN, G.B., LAM, K.C. and MISTILIS, S.P. (1973): Drug-induced active chronic hepatitis. *Am.J.Dig.Dis.*, 18, 177–184.

GOODING, P.E., CHAYEN, J., SAWYER, B. and SLATER, T.F. (1978): Cytochrome P_{450} distribution in rat liver and the effect of sodium phenobarbitone administration. *Chem.Biol.Interact.* 20, 299–310.

GORUS, F.K., MALAISSE, W.J. and PIPELEERS, D.G. (1982): Selective uptake of alloxan by pancreatic B-cells. *Biochem.J.*, 208, 513–515.

GORUS, F.K., FINSY, R. and PIPELEERS, D.G. (1986): Alloxan toxicity in human and canine spermatozoa. Possible biochemical basis for a species difference in sensitivity. *Biochem.Pharmacol.*, 35, 1725–1729.

GOUDIE, R.B. (1989): The polymerase chain reaction and histopathology. *J.Pathol.*, 158, 183–184.

GOULD, V.E. (1986): Histogenesis and differentiation: A re-evaluation of these concepts as criteria for the classification of tumours. *Hum.Pathol.* 17, 212–215.

GRAY, R.H. and DE LA IGLESIA, F.A. (1984): Quantitative microscopy comparison of peroxisomal proliferation by the lipid-regulating agent gemfibrozil in several species. *Hepatology*, 4, 520–530.

GREAVES, P. and FACCINI, J.M. (1984): Digestive system. In: *Rat Histopathology*. A glossary for use in toxicity and carcinogenicity studies. Chap. 6, pp. 86–125. Elsevier, Amsterdam.

GREAVES, P., IRISARRI, E. and MONRO, A.M. (1986): Hepatic foci of cellular and enzymatic alteration and nodules in rats treated with clofibrate or diethnylnitrosamine followed by phenobarbital : Their rate of onset and their reversibility. *J.N.C.I.*, 76, 475–484.

GREENBLATT, M. (1982): Tumours of the liver. In: V.S. Turusov, (Ed.), *Pathology of Tumours in Laboratory Animals*, Vol. 3, Tumours of the Hamster, pp. 69–101. I.A.R.C. Sci.Publ., Lyon.

GREGORY, M., MONRO, A., QUINTON, M. and WOOLHOUSE, N. (1983): The acute toxicity of oxamniquine in rats; sex-dependent hepatotoxicity. *Arch.Toxicol.*, 54, 247–255.

GRICE, H.C. and BUREK, J.D. (1984): Age-associated (geriatric) pathology: In: *Current Issues in Toxicology*, pp. 57–107. Springer-Verlag, Berlin.

GUENGERICH, F.P. (1988): Roles of cytochrome P-450 enzymes in chemical carcinogenesis and cancer chemotheraphy. *Cancer Res.*, 48, 2946–2954.

GUZELIAN, P.S., VRANIAN, G., BOYLAN, J.J., COHN, W.J. and BLANKE, R.V. (1980): Liver structure and function in patients poisoned in the chlordecone (Kepone). *Gastroenterology*, 78, 206–213.

HACKER, H.J., MOORE, M.A., MAYER, D. and BANNASCH, P. (1982): Correlative histochemistry of some enzymes of carbohydrate metabolism in preneoplastic and neoplastic lesions in the rat liver. *Carcinogenesis*, 3, 1265–1272.

HAJDU, A. and RONA, G. (1967): Morphological observations on spontaneous pancreatic islet changes in rats. *Diabetes*, 16, 108–110.

HANIGAN, M.H. and PITOT, H.C. (1985): Gamma-glutamyl transpeptidase: its role in hepatocarcinogenesis. *Carcinogenesis*, 6, 165–172.

HARADA, R.T., MARONPOT, R.R., MORRIS, R.W., STITZEL, K.A. and BOORMAN, G.A. (1989)a: Morphological and stereological characterisation of hepatic foci of cellular alteration in control Fischer 344 rats. *Toxicol.Pathol.* 17, 579–593.

HARADA, T., MARANPOT, R.R., MORRIS, R.W. and BOORMAN, G.A. (1989)b: Observations on altered hepatocellular foci in National Toxicology Program two-year carcinogenicity studies in rats. *Toxicol.Pathol.*, 17, 690–708.

HARLEMAN, J.H., SUTER, J. and FISCHER, M. (1987): Intracytoplasmic eosinophilic inclusion bodies in the liver of beagle dogs. *Lab.Anim.Sci.*, 37, 229–231.

HARTROFT, W.S. and PORTA, E.A. (1972): Observation and interpretation of lipid pigments (lipofuscins) in the pathology of laboratory animals. *CRC Crit.Rev.Toxicol.*, 1, 379–411.

HARGIS, A.M. and THOMASSEN, R.W. (1980): Hepatic abscesses in beagle puppies. *Lab.Anim.Sci.*, 30, 689–693.

HARPER, J.F., CHEUNG, W.Y., WALLACE, R.W., HUANG, H-L., LEVINES, S.N. and STEINER, A.L. (1980): Localisation of calmodiulin in rat tissues. *Proc.Natl.Acad.Sci.*, USA, 77, 366–370.

HASHIMOTO, K., IMAI, K., YOSHIMURA, S. and OHTAKI, T. (1981): Experimental toxicity studies with captopril, an inhibitor of angiotensin 1-converting enzyme. 3. 12 month studies of chronic toxicity of captopril in rats. *J.Toxicol.Sci.*, 6, Suppl.2, 215–246.

HAYASHI, Y., FURUKAWA, H. and HASEGAWA, T. (1972): Pancreatic tumors in rats induced by 4-nitroquinoline l-oxide derivatives. In W.Nakahara, S.Takayama, T.Sugimura and S.Odashima (Eds), *Topics In Chemical Carcinogenesis.*, pp. 53–61. University Park Press, Baltimore, MD.

HAYASHI, K., MAKINO, R. and SUGIMURA, T. (1984): Amplification aznd over-expression of the c-myc gene in Morris hepatomas. *Jp.J.Cancer Res.* (Gann), 75, 475–478.

HAYASHI, Y. (1985): Histologic typing of liver tumours in rats, mice and hamsters: a workshop report. *Exp.Pathol.*, 28, 140–141.

HAWKINS, K.L., SUMMERS, B.A., KUHAJDA, F.P. and SMITH, C.A. (1987): Immunocytochemistry of normal pancreatic islets and spontaneous islet cell tumors in dogs. *Vet.Pathol.*, 24, 170–179.

HAYES, A.W., FEDOROWSKI, T., BALAZS, T., CARLTON, W.W., FOWLER, B.A., GILMAN, M.R., HEYMAN, I., JACKSON, B.A., KENNEDY, G.L., SHAPIRO, R.E., SMITH, C.C., TARDIFF, R.G. and WEIL, C.S. (1982): Correlation of human hepatotoxicants with hepatic damage in animals. *Fundam.Appl.Toxicol.*, 2, 55–66.

HAYNES, D., HALL, P. and CLARK, D. (1983): A glycogen storage disease in rats. Morphological and biochemical investigations. *Virchows.Arch.*[B], 42, 289–301.

HAZAN, R., DENK, H., FRANKE, W.W., LACKINGER, E. and SCHILLER, D.L. (1988): Change of cytokeratin organisation during development of Mallory bodies as revealed by a monoclonal antibody. *Lab.Invest*, 54, 543–553.

HEI, T.K. and SUDILOVSKY, O. (1985): Effects of a high sucrose diet on the development of enzyme-altered foci in chemical hepatocarcinogenesis in rats. *Cancer Res.*, 45, 2700–2705.

HEITZ, P.U., KASPER, M., POLAK, J.M. and KLOPPEL, G. (1982): Pancreatic endocrine tumors : Immunocytochemical analysis of 125 tumors. *Hum.Pathol.*, 13, 263–271.

HELLMAN, B., WALLGREN, A. and PETERSSON, B. (1962): Cytological characterstics of the exocrine pancreatic cells with regard to their positions in relation to the islets of Langerhans. A study in normal and obese-hyperglycaemic mice. *Acta.Endocrinol.*(Copenh), 93, 465–473.

HENDERSON, J.R., DANIEL, P.M. and FRASER, P.A. (1981): The pancreas as a single organ : the influence of the endocrine upon the exocrine part of the gland. *Gut*, 22, 158–167.

HERMON-TAYLOR, J., PERRIN, J., GRANT, D.A.W., APPLEYARD, A., BUBEL, M. and MAGEE, A.I. (1977): Immunofluorescent localization of enterokinase in human small intestine. *Gut*, 18, 259–265.

HEYWOOD, R., PALMER, A.K., GREGSON, R.L. and BUMMLER, H. (1985): The toxocity of beta-carotone. *Toxcicology*, 36, 91–100.

HOLMES, C.H., AUSTIN, E.B., FISK, A., GUNN, and BALDWIN, R.W.(1984): Monoclonal antibodies reacting with normal rat liver cells as probes in hepatocarcinogenesis. *Cancer Res.*, 44, 1611–1624.

HOOVER, D.M., BENDELE, A.M., HOFFMAN, W.P., FOXWORTHY, P.S. and EACHO, P.I. (1990): Effects of chronic treatment with the leukotriene D_4 antagonist compound LY 171883 on Fischer 344 rats and rhesus monkeys. *Fundam.Appl.Toxicol.*, 14, 123–130.

HOPWOOD, D., MILNE, G., ROSS, P.E., CLARK, A. and WOOD, R.A.B. (1986): Effects of colchicine on the gall bladder of the mouse. *Histochem.J.*, 18, 80–89.

HORVATH, E., SAIBEIL., F.G., KOVACS, K., KERENYI, N.A. and ROSS, R.C. (1978): Fine structural changes in the liver of methtrexate-treated psoriatics. *Digestion.* 17, 488–502.

HOWATSON, A.G. and CARTER, D.C. (1985): Pancreatic carcinogenesis: enhancement by cholecystokinin in the hamster-nitrosamine model. *Br.J.Cancer*, 51, 107–114.

HRUBAN, Z., (1984): Pulmonary and generalised lyosomal storage induced by amphiphilic drugs. *Environ.Health Perspect.*, 55, 53–76.

HRUBAN, Z., SLESERS, A. and HOPKINS, E. (1972): Drug-induced and naturally occurring myeloid bodies. *Lab.Invest.*, 27, 62–70.

HUSZTIK, E., LAZAR, G. and SZABO, E. (1984): Immunologically induced peliosis hepatis in rats. *Br.J.Exp.Pathol.*, 65, 313–318.

IKEDA, H., TAUCHI, H. and SATO, T. (1985): Fine structural analysis of lipofuscin in various tissues of rats of different ages. *Mech.Ageing Dev.*, 33, 77–93.

IMAI, K. and HAYASHI, Y. (1970): Steroid-induced intrahepatic cholestasis in mice. *Jnp.J.Pharmacol.*, 20, 473–481.

IOANNIDES, C. and PARKE, D.V. (1987): The cytochromes P-488: a unique family of enzymes involved in chemical toxicity and carcinogenesis. *Biochem.Pharmacol.*, 36, 4197–4207.

IRISARRI, E. and MOMPON, P. (1983): Hepatic effects of fasting on 6 and 12 week old mice: A quantitive histochemical study. *J.Pathol.*, 140, 176.

ISHAK, K.G. (1981): Hepatic lesions caused by anabolic and contraceptive steroids. *Semin.Liver Dis.*, 1, 6–128.

ISHAK, K.G. (1982): The Liver. In: R.H.Riddell (Ed.), *Pathology of Drug-Induced and Toxic Diseases.* Chap. 17, pp. 457–513. Churchill Livingstone, New York.

ITO, T. (1951): Cytological studies on stellate cells of Kupffer fat storing cells in the capillary wall of the human liver. *Acta.Anat.Nippon*, 26, 42–74.

ITOH, S., IGARASHI, M., TSUKADA, Y. and ICHINOE, A. (1977): Non-alcoholic fatty liver with alcoholic hyalin after long term glucocorticoid therapy. *Acta.Hepato.Gastroenterol.*, 24, 415–418.

ITOH, S. and TSUKADA, Y. (1973): Clinico-pathological and electron microscopic studies on a coronary dilating agent: 4-4′ diethyl-aminoethoxyhexestrol-induced liver injuries. *Acta.Hepato.Gastroenterol.*, 20, 204–215.

JACKSON, D., COCKBURN, A., COOPER, D.L., LANGLEY, P.F., TASKER, T.C.G, and WHITE, D.J. (1985): Clinical Pharmacology and safety evaluation of Timentin. *Am.J.Med.*, 73, Suppl. 5B, 44–55.

JACKSON, R., RASSI, N., CRUMP, T., HAYNES, B. and EISENBARTH, G.S. (1981): The BB diabetic rat. Profound T-cell lymphocytopenia. *Diabetes*, 30, 887–889.

480

JACOBY, R.O., BHATT, P.N. and JONAS, A.M. (1979): Viral diseases. In: H.J.Baker, J.R. Lindsey and S.H Weisbroth (Eds), *The Laboratory Rat. Vol. 1, Biology and Diseases*, Chap 11, pp. 271–306. Academic Press, New York.

JAHRLING, P.B., GEISBERT, T.W., DALGARD, D.W., JOHNSON, E.D., KSIAZEK, T.G., HALL, W.C. and PETERS, C.J. (1990): Preliminary report: isolation of Ebola virus from monkeys imported to USA. *Lancet*, 335, 502–505.

JAMES, J., FREDERIKS, W.M., VAN NOORDEN, C.J.F. and TAS, J. (1986): Detection of metabolic changes in hepatocytes by quantitive cytochemistry. *Histochemistry*, 84, 308–316.

JARRETT, L. and LACY, P.E. (1962): Effect of glucagon on the acinar portion of the pancreas. *Endocrinology*, 70, 867–873.

JAROTZKY, A.J. (1899): Uber die Veränderungen in der Grösse und im Bau der Pankreaszellen mit einigen Arten der Inanition. *Virchows Arch. [A]*, 156, 409–429.

JEZEQUEL, A.M. and ORLANDI, F. (1972): Fine morphology of the human liver as a tool in clinical pharmacology. In: F. Orlandi and A.M. Jezequel (Eds), *Liver and Drugs*, Chap. 6, pp. 176–178. Academic Press, New York.

JHA, T.K. and SHARMA, V.K. (1984): Pentamidine-induced diabetes mellitus. *Trans.R.Soc.Trop.Med.Hyg.*, 78, 252–253.

JOHNSON, P.J. (1984): Sex hormones and the liver. *Clin.Sci.*, 66, 369–376.

JOHNSON, A.N. (1989): Comparative aspects of contraceptive steroids: effects observed in beagle dogs. *Toxicol.Pathol.* 17, 389–395.

JOHNSON, L.R. (1976): The trophic action of gastrointestinal hormones. *Gastroenterology*, 70, 278–288.

JONES, T.C. and HUNT, R.D. (1983): Diseases caused by viruses. In: *Veterinary Pathology*, Chap. 9, pp. 286–510. Lea & Febiger, Philadelphia.

JUNGERMAN, K. and KATZ, N. (1982): Functional hepatocellular heterogeneity. *Hepatology*, 2, 385–395.

JUNOD, A., LAMBERT, A.E., ORCHI, L., PICTET, R., GONET, A.E. and RENOLD, A.E. (1967): Studies of the diabetogenic action of streptozotocin. *Proc.Soc.Exp.Biol.Med.*, 126, 201–205.

KADUK, B., HUSSLEIN, E-M. and SIEGFRIED, A. (1987): Morphology of the chronic toxicity of busulfan on the islets of Langerhans. *Hepatogastroenterology*, 34, 108–112.

KAITOH, T., MASUDA, T., SASANO, N. and TAKAHASHI, T. (1986): The size and number of Langerhans islets correlated with their endocrine function : A morphometry on immunostained serial sections of adult human pancreases. *Tohoku J.Exp.Med.*, 149, 1–10.

KAKIZOE, S., GOLDFARB, S. and PUGH, T.D. (1989): Focal impairment of growth in hepatocellular neoplasms of C57BL/6 mice: A possible explanation for the strain's resistance to hepatocarcinogenesis. *Cancer Res.*, 49, 3985–3989

KAST, A., HAMATAKE, H., HIGASHI, T. and NISHIMURA, T. (1970): Gewebemessungen am Inselorgan mit Corticoid behandelter Ratten. *Arzneimittelforschung*, 20, 1259–1265.

KAST, A. and UEBERBERG, H. (1986): Cytoplasmic vacuolation of pancreatic beta cells of rats after oral administration of a derivative of isoquinoline. *Toxicol.Appl.Pharmacol.*, 85, 274–285.

KAWABATA, T.T., WILK, D.G., GUENGERICH, F.P. and BARON, J. (1984): Immunohistochemical localization of carcinogen metabolizing enzymes within the rat and hamster exocrine pancrease. *Cancer Res.*, 44, 215–223.

KAZUMI, T., YOSHINO, G., FUJII, S. and BABA, S. (1978): Tumorigenic action of streptozotocin on the pancreas and kidney in male Wistar rat. *Cancer Res.*, 38, 2144–2147.

KENDRY, G. and ROE, F.J.C. (1969): Histopathological changes in the pancreas of laboratory rats. *Lab.Anim.*, 3, 207–220.

KENNEDY, S.J.(1979): Ultrastructure of normal monkey liver. *Lab.Anim.*, 13, 125–129.

KERR, J.F. (1971): Shrinkage necrosis disticnt mode of cellular death. *J.Pathol.*, 105, 13–19.

KERR, J.F.R. and SEARLE, J. (1973): Depletion of cells by apoptosis during castration induced involution of rat prostate. *Virchows Arch.[B]*, 13, 87–102.

KEYSSER, C.H., WILLIAMS, J.A., VAN PETTEN, L.E. and COY, N. (1963): Experimental production by 2-ethyl-2-phenyl butyramide of intrahepatic cholestasis with bile plugs in dogs. *Nature*, 199, 498–499.

481

KIECHLE, F.L. (1979): Optical diffraction studies of paracrystalline mitochondrial inclusions in hepatocytes of liver biopsies. *Lab.Invest.*, 40, 264.

KIERNAN, F. (1833): The anatomy and physiology of the liver. *Philos.Trans.R.Soc.Lond.*[Biol], 123, 711–770.

KIM, Y.T. and STEINBERG, C. (1984): Immunologic studies on the induction of diabetes in experimental animals. Cellular basis for the induction of diabetes by streptozotocin. *Diabetes*, 33, 771–777.

KIMBERG, D.V. and LOEB, H.N. (1972): Effects of cortisone administrationon rat liver mitochondria : Support for the concept of mitochondrial fusion. *J.Cell.Biol.*, 55, 635–643.

KIMBROUGH, R.D. (1973). Pancreatic-type tissue in livers of rats fed polychlorinated biphenyls. *J.N.C.I.*, 52, 679–681.

KIMBROUGH, R.D., LINDER, R.E., BURSE, V.W. and JENNINGS, R.W. (1973): Adenofibrosis in the rat liver with persistence of polychlorinated biphenyls in adipose tissue. *Arch.Environ.Health*, 27, 390–395.

KITAWAGA, H., FUJUTA, S., SUZUKI, T. and KITANI, K. (1985): Disappearance of sex differences in rat liver drug metabolism in old age. *Biochem.Pharmacol.*, 34, 579–581.

KITAGAWA, T. and ONO, K. (1986): Ultrastructure of pancratic exocrine cells of the rat during starvation. *Histol.Histopathol.*, 1, 49–57.

KLÖPPEL, G., BOMMER, G., RUTTMANN, E. and SCHAFER, H-J (1978): Qualitative and semi-quantitative calcium cytochemistry in B cells of mice treated with cyproheptidine and mannoheptulose. *Acta.Endocrinol.*, 87, 786–798.

KOUNTOURAS, J., BILLING, B.H. and SCHEUER, P.J. (1984): Prolonged bile duct obstruction : a new experimental model for cirrhosis in the rat. *B.J.Exp.Pathol.*, 65, 305–311.

KOVACS, K., LEE, R. and LITTLE, J.A. (1972): Ultrastructural changes of hepatocytes in hyperlipo-proteinaemia. *Lancet 1*, 752–753.

KUHLMANN, W.D. (1981): Alpha-fetoprotein : cellular origin of a biological marker in rat liver under various experimental conditions. *Virchows Arch* [A], 393, 9–26.

LAFRANCONI, W.M., GLATT, H. and OESCH, F. (1986): Xenobiotic metabolizing enxymes of rat liver nonparenchymal cells. *Toxicol.Appl.Pharmacol.*, 84, 500–511.

LAKE, B.G. and GRAY, T.J.B. (1985): Species differences in hepatic peroxisomal proliferation. *Biochem.Soc.Trans.*, 13, 859–861.

LAKE, B.G., EVANS, J.G., GRAY, T.J.B., KÖRÖSI S.A. and NORTH, C.J. (1989): Comparative studies on nafenopin-induced hepatic peroxisome proliferation in the rat, Syrian hamster, guinea pig and marmoset. *Toxicol.Appl.Pharmacol.*, 99, 148–160.

LAMM, D.L., STOGDILL, V.D., STODGILL, B.J. and CRISPEN, R.G. (1986): Complications of ballicus Calmette-Guérin immunotherapy in 1,278 patients with bladder cancer. *J.Urol.*, 135, 272–274.

LATHAM, P.S. and KASHGARIAN, M. (1979): The ultrastructural localization of transport ATPase in the rat liver at non-bile canalicular plasma membranes.*Gastroenterology*, 76, 988–996.

LAUPACIS, A., STILLER, C.R., GARDELL, C., KEOWN, P., DUPRE, J., WALLACE, A.C. and THIBERT, P. (1983): Cyclosporin prevents diabetes in BB Wistar rats. *Lancet*, 1, 10–12.

LAWRENCE, G.M., JEPSON, M.A., TRAYER, I.P. and WALKER, D.G. (1986): The compartmentation of glycolytic and gluconeogenic enzymes in rat kidney and liver and its significance to renal and hepatic metabolism. *Histochem.J.*, 18, 45–53.

LAZARUS, S.S. and VOLK, B.W. (1958): The effect of protracted glucagon administration on blood glucose and on pancreatic morphology. *Endocrinology*, 63, 359–371.

LAZAROW, P.B. and FUJIKI, Y. (1985): Biogenesis of peroxisomes. *Annu.Rev.Cell Biol.*, 1, 489–530.

LE BOUTON, A.V. (1982): Routine overnight starvation and immunocytochemistry of hepatocyte alubumin content. *Cell Tissue Res.*, 227, 423–427.

LE DOUX, S.P., WOODLEY, S.E., PATTON, N.J. and WILSON, G.L. (1986): Mechanisms of nitrosourea-induced beta-cell damage. *Diabetes*, 35, 866–872.

LEE, K.P. (1983): Peliosis hepatis-like lesion in aging rats. *Vet Pathol.*, 20, 410–423.

LEITER, E.H. (1985): Type C retrovirus production by pancreatic beta cells. Association with accelerated pathogenesis in C3H-db/db ('diabetes') mice. *Am.J.Pathol.*, 119, 22–32.

LEONARD, T.B., POPP, J.A., GRAICHEN, M.E. and DENT, J.G. (1981): Alpha-naphthylisothiocyanate induced alterations in hepatic drug metabolizing enzymes and liver morphology : implications concerning anticarcinogenesis. *Carcinogenesis*, 2, 473–482.

LEVISON, D.A. (1979): Carcinoma of the pancreas. *J.Pathol.* 129, 203–223.

LEVISON, D.A., MORGAN, R.G.H., BRIMACOMBE, J.S., HOPWOOD, D., COGHILL, G. and WORMSLEY, K.G. (1979): Carcinogenic effects of di-(2-hydroxypropyl) nitrosamine (DHPN) in male Wistar rats : promotion of pancreatic cancer by raw soya flour diet. *Scand.J.Gastroenterol.*, 14, 217–224.

LEWIS, D.J. (1984): Spontaneous lesions of the mouse biliary tract. *J.Comp.Pathol.*, 94, 263–271.

LEWIS, D.J., OFFER, J.M. and PRENTICE, D.E. (1982): Metastasizing pancreatic islet cell tumours in the rat. *J.Comp.Pathol.*, 92, 139–147.

LEWIS, J.H., ZIMMERMAN, H.J., BENSON, G.D. and ISHAK, K.G. (1984): Hepatic injury associated with ketoronazole therapy. Analysis of 33 cases. *Gastroenterology*, 86, 503–513.

LIKE, A.A., APPEL, M.C., WILLIAMS, R.M. and ROSSINI, A.A. (1978): Streptozotocin-induced pancreatic insulitis in mice. Morphologic and physiologic studies. *Lab.Invest.*, 38, 470–486.

LIKE, A.A., ROSSINI, A.A., GUBERSKI, D.L. and WILLIAMS, R.M. (1979): Spontaneous diabetes mellitus : Reversal and prevention in the BB/W rat with antiserum to rat lymphocytes. *Science*, 206, 1421–1423.

LIKE, A.A., KISLAUSKIS, E., WILLIAMS, R.M and ROSSINI, A.A. (1982): Neonatal thymectomy pevents spontaneous diabetes in the BB/W rat. *Science*, 216, 644–646.

LIKE, A.A. and ROSSINI, A.A. (1976): Streptozotocin-induced pancreatic insulitis : New model of diabetes mellitus. *Science*, 193, 415–417.

LIKE, A.A. and ROSSINI, A.A. (1984): Spontaneous autoimmune diabetes mellitus in the Bio Breeding/Worcester rat. *Surv.Synth.Pathol.Res.*, 3, 131–138.

LIKE, A.A., ANTHONY, M., GUBERSKI, D.L. and ROSSINI, A.A. (1983)a: Spontaneous diabetis mellitus in the BB/W rat. Effects of glucocorticoids, cyclosporin A and antiserum to rat lymphocytes. *Diabetes*, 32, 326–330.

LIKE, A.A., FORSTER, R.M., WODA, B.A. and ROSSINI, A.A. (1983)b: T-cell subsets in islets and lymph nodes of Bio Breeding/Worcester (BB/W) rats. *Diabetes*, 32, 51A.

LIU, T-H., TSENG, H-C., ZHU, Y., ZHONG, S-X, CHEN, J. and CUI, Q-C. (1985): Insulinoma. An immunocytochemical and morphologic analysis of 95 cases. *Cancer*, 56, 14020–1429.

LONGNECKER, D.S. (1983): Carcinogenesis in the pancreas. *Arch.Pathol.Lab.Med.*, 107, 51–58.

LONGNECKER, D.S., HASHIDA, Y. and SHINOZUKA, H. (1980): Relationship of age to prevalence of focal acinar cell dysplasia in the human pancreas. *J.N.C.I.*, 65, 63–66.

LONGNECKER, D.S., ROEBUCK, B.D., YAGER, J.D., LILJA, H.S. and SIEGMUND, B. (1981): Pancreatic carcinoma in azaserine-treated rats : Induction, classification, and dietary modulation of incidence. *Cancer*, 47, 1562–1572.

LONGNECKER, D.S., WOLD, J.S. and FISCHER, L.J. (1972): Ultrastructural study of alterations in beta cells of pancreatic islets from cyproheptidine-treated rats. *Diabetes*, 21, 71–79.

LOVE, L., PELFRENE, A. and GARCIA, H. (1977): Acinar adenomas of the pancreas in MRC-Wistar rats. *J.Comp.Pathol.*, 87, 307–310.

LOVELL, D.P. (1986): Variation in pentobarbitone sleeping time in mice. 1. Strain and sex differences. *Lab.Anim.*, 20, 85–90.

LUDWIG, J. and AXELSEN, R. (1983): Drug effects on the liver. An updated tabular compilation of drugs and drug-related hepatic diseases. *Dig.Dis.Sci.*, 28, 651–666.

LUMB, G.D., BEAMER, P.R. and RUST, J.H. (1985): Oesophagostomiasis in feral monkeys (Macaca mulatta). *Toxicol.Pathol.*, 13, 209–214.

LUNDBERGH, P. and WESTMAN, J. (1970): Hepatic filamentous mitochondrial inclusions associated with oral contraceptives. *Scand.J.Infect.Dis.*, 2, 105–109.

MACALLUM, G.E., SMITH, G.S., BARSOUM, N.J., WALKER, R.M., and GREAVES, P. (1988): Renal and hepatic toxicity of a benzopyran-4-one in the cynomolgus monkey. *Toxicologist*, 8, 220.

MACALLUM, G.E. SMITH, G.S., BARSOUM, N.J., WALKER, R.M., and GREAVES, P.(1989)a: Renal and hepatic toxicity of a benzopyran-4-one in the cytomologus monkey. *Toxicology*, 59, 97–108.

MACALLUM, G.E., WALKER, R.M., BARSOUM, N.J., SMITH, G.S. and GREAVES, P. (1989)b: Preclinical toxicity studies of an adenosine agonist CI-936. *Toxicologist*, 9, 178.

MACHNIK, G., CHEMNITIUS, K-H. and NIEKRENZ, H. (1983): Liver neoplasms after long-term steroid application in rats. *Exp.Pathol.*, 24, 183–187.

MACDONALD, J.S., GERSON, R.J., KORNBRUST, D.J., KLOSS, M.W., PRAHALADA, S., BERRY, P.H., ALBERTS, A.W. and BOKELMAN, D.C. (1988): Preclinical evaluation of lovastatin. *Am.J.Cardiol.*, 62, 16J-27J.

MACLEAN, N. and OGILVIE, R.F. (1955): Quantitative estimation of pancreatic islet tissue in diabetic subjects. *Diabetes*, 4, 367–376.

McCLURE, H.M. and CHANDLER, F.W. (1982): A survey of pancreatic lesions in non-human primates. *Vet.Pathol.*, 19 (Suppl.7), 193–209.

McCLURE, H.M., CHAPMAN, W.L. Jr., HOOPER, B.E., SMITH, F.G. and FLETCHER, O.J. (1978): The digestive system. In: K.Benirschke, F.M. Garner and T.C.Jones (Eds), *Pathology of Laboratory Animals*, Vol.1, Chap. 4, pp. 175–317. Springer-Verlag, New York.

McGUINNESS, E.E., MORGAN, R.G.H., LEVISON, D.A., FRAPE, D.L., HOPWOOD, D. and WORMSLEY, K.G. (1980): The effects of long-term feeding of soya flour on the rat pancreas. *Scand.J.Gastroenterol.*, 15, 497–502.

McGUIRE, E.J., DIFONZO, C.J., MARTIN, R.A. and DE LA IGLESIA, F.A. (1986): Evaluation of chronic toxicity and carcinogenesis in rodents with the synthetic anagesic, tilidine fumarate. *Toxicology*, 39, 149–163.

McKILLOP, D. and CASE, D.E. (1990): A summary of the mutagenicity, carcinogenicity and toxicity data on the potent P448 inducer, beta-naphthoflavone. *Biochem.Phamacol.*, In Press.

McMARTIN, D.N. (1979): Morphological lesions in aging Syrian hamsters. *J.Gerontol*, 34, 502–511.

McMILLAN, P.N., FERAYORNI, L.S., GERHARDT, C.O. and JAUREGUI, H.O., (1984): Light and electron microscope analysis of lectin binding to adult rat liver in situ. *Lab.Invest.*, 50, 408–420.

MADDREY, W.C. (1981): Drug-induced chronic active hepatitis. In: M. Davis, J.M. Tredger and R. Williams (Eds), *Drug Reactions and the Liver*, pp. 58–63. Pitman Medical, London.

MADEWELL, B.R. (1981): Neoplasms in domestic animals : A review of experimental and spontaneous carcinogenesis. *Yale J.Biol.Med.*, 54, 111–125.

MAKINO, S., KUNIMOTO, K., MURAOKA, Y., MIZUSHIMA, Y., KATAGIRI, K. and TOCHINO, Y. (1980): Breeding of a non-obese, diabetic strain of mice. *Exp. Anim.*, 29, 1–13.

MALAISSE-LAGAE, F., RAVAZZOLA, M., ROBBSTRECHT, P., VANDERMEERS, A., MALAISSE, W.J. and ORCI, L. (1975): Exocrine pancreas : Evidence for topographic partition of secretory function. *Science*, 190, 795–797.

MALL, F.P. (1906): A study of the structural unit of the liver. *Am.J.Anat.*, 5, 227–308.

MALLORY, F.B. (1911): Cirrhosis of the liver. Five different types of lesions from which it may arise. *Bull.John Hopkins Hosp.*, 22, 69–74.

MALPIGHI, M. (1966): De hapate. Bologna.

MARJANEN, L. (1972): Intracellular localization of aldehyde dehydrogenases in rat liver. *Biochem.J.*, 127, 633–639.

MARRIOTT, M.S., BRAMMER, K.W., FACCINI, J., FAULKNER, J.K, JEVONS, S., MONRO, A.M., NACHBAUR, J., PERRAUD, J. and TARBIT, M.H. (1983): Tioconazole, a new broad-spectrum antifungal agent : Preclinical studies related to vaginal candidiasis. *Gynacol.Rundsch.*, 23, 1–11.

MARONPOT, R.R., HARADA, T., MURTHY, A.S.K. and BOORMAN, G.A. (1989): Documenting foci of hepatocellular alteration in two-year carcinogenicity studies: Current practices of the National Toxicology Program. *Toxicol.Pathol.* 17, 675–684.

MARSMAN, D.S., CATTLEY, R.C., CONWAY, J.G. and POPP, J.A. (1988): Relationship of hepatic peroxisome proliferation and replicative DNA synthesis to the hepatocarcinogencity of the peroxisomal proliferators, di(2-ethylhexyl)phthalate and [4-chloro-6-(2,3,xylidino)-2 pyrimidiny (thio)acetic acid (Wy 14, 643)] in rats. *Cancer Res.*, 48, 6739–6744.

MASSON, M.T., VILLANOVE, F. and GREAVES, P. (1986): Histological demonstration of wheat germ lectin binding sites in the liver of normal and ANIT treated rats. *Arch.Toxicol.*, 59, 121–123.

MATSUMURA, T. and THURMAN, R.G. (1984): Predominance of glycosis in pericentral regions of the liver lobule. *Eur.J.Biochem.*, 140, 229–234.

MAXWELL, D.R., SZWED, J.J., HAMBERGER, R.J., YU, P-L and KLEIT, S.A. (1974): Influence of diuretics on simultaneous thoracic duct lymph, bile and urine flows in the dog. *Am.J.Physiol.*, 226, 540–543.

MAYSTON, P.D. and BARROWMAN, J.A. (1971): The influence of chronic administration of pentagastrin on the rat pancreas. *Q.J.Exp.Physiol.*, 56, 113–122.

MEGLASSON, M.D., BURCH, P.T., BERNER, D.K., NAJAFI, H. and MATSCHINSKY, F.M. (1986): Identification of glucokinase as an alloxan-sensitive glucose sensor of the pancreatic beta-cell. *Diabetes*, 35, 1163–1173.

MEIERHENRY, E.F., RHEBNER, B.H., GERSHWIN, M.E., HSIEH, L.S. and FRENCH, S.W. (1981): Mallory body formation in hepatic nodules of mice ingesting dieldren. *Lab.Invest.*, 44, 392–396.

MEYER, D.J., IVERSON, W.O. and TERRELL, T.G. (1980): Obstructive jaundice associated with chronic active hepatitis in a dog. *J.Am.Vet.Med.Assoc.*, 176, 41–44.

MICHAELIS, O.E., PATRICK, D.H., HANSEN, C.T., CANARY, J.J., WERNER, R.M. and CARSWELL, N. (1986): Insulin-independent diabetes mellitis (type II). Spontaneous hypertensive/NIH-corpulent rat. *Am.J.Pathol.*, 123, 398–400.

MICHELS, J.E., BAUER, G.E., JOHNSON, D. and DIXIT, P.K. (1986): Morphometric analysis of the endocrine cell composition of rat pancreas following treatment with streptozotocin and nicotinamide. *Exp.Mol.Pathol.*, 44, 247–258.

MIKOL, Y.B., HOOVER, K.L., CREASIA, D. and POIRER, L.A. (1983): Hepatocarcinogenesis in rats fed methyl-deficient, amino acid defined diets. *Carcinogenesis*, 4, 1619–1629.

MILAS, L. and SCOTT, M.T. (1978): Antitumour activity of Corynebacterium parvum. In: G. Klein, and S. Weinhouse. *Advances in Cancer Research*, Vol. 26, pp. 257–306.

MITCHELL, J.R., NELSON, S.D., THORGEIRSSON, S.S., MCMURPHY, R.J. and DYBING, D.E. (1976): Metabolic activation : biochemical basis for many drug-induced injuries. *Prog.Liver Dis.*, 5, 259–279.

MOHN, G and PHILLIP, E-M. (1981): Effects of Syphacia muris and the antihelmintic fenbendazole on the microsomal mono-oxygenase system in mouse liver. *Lab.Anim.*, 15, 89–95.

MOHR, U. and REZNIK, G. (1982): Tumours of the pancreas. In: V.S. Turusov (Ed.), *Pathology of Tumours in Laboratory Animals*. Vol. 3, Tumours of the Hamster. pp. 103–114, IARC Scientific Publ. No. 34, Lyon.

MOMPON, P., GREAVES, P., IRISARRI, E., MONRO, A.M. and BRIDGES, J.W. (1987): A cytochemical study of the livers of rats treated with diethylnitrosamine/phenobarbital, with benzidine/phenobarbital, or with clofilorate. *Toxicology*, 46, 217–236.

MOODY, D.E., TAYLOR, L.A. and SMUCKLER, E.A. (1985): Immunofluorescent determination of the lobular distribution of a constitutive form of microsomal cytochrome P_{450}. *Hepatology*, 5, 440–451.

MORGAN, R.G.H., LEVISON, D.A., HOPWOOD, D., SAUNDERS, J.H.B. and WORMSLEY, K.G. (1977): Potentiation of the action of azaserine on the rat pancreas by raw soya bean flour. *Cancer Lett.*, 3, 87–90.

MORI, M. (1983): Ultrastructural changes of hepatocyte organelles induced by chemicals and their relationship to fat accumulation in the liver. *Acta.Pathol.Jpn.*, 33, 911–922.

MORI, T., NAGASAWA, H., NAMIKI, H. and NIKI, K. (1986): Development of pancreatic hyperplasia in female SHN mice receiving ectopic pituitary isographs. *J.N.C.I.*, 76, 1193–1198.

MOROHOSHI, T., KANDA, M. and KLOPPEL, G. (1984): On the histiogenesis of experimental pancreatic endocrine tumours. An immunocytochemical and electron microscopical study. *Acta.Pathol.Jpn.*, 34, 271–281.

MOTTA, P.M. (1984): The three-dimensional microanatomy of the liver. *Arch.Histol.Jpn.*, 47, 1–30.

MULLOCK, B.M., HALL, D.E., SHAW, L.J and HINTON, R.H. (1983): Immune responses to chlorpromazine in rats. Detection and relation to hepatotoxicity. *Biochem.Pharmacol.*, 32, 2733–2738.

MURATA, Y., YOKOSE, Y. and KONISHI, Y. (1985): Exocrine pancreas of hypophysectionized rats. In: T.C. Jones, U. Mohr and R.D. Hunt (Eds), *Digestive System. Monographs on Pathology of Laboratory Animals*, pp. 245–248, Springer-Verlag, Berlin.

NAEIM, F., COPPER, P.H. and SEMION, A.A. (1973): Peliosis hepatis. possible etiologic role of anabolic steroids. *Arch.Pathol.*, 95, 284–285.

NAKANUMA, Y. and OHTA, G. (1986): Expression of Mallory bodies in hepatocellular carcinoma in man and its significance. *Cancer*, 56, 81–86.

NAKANUMA, Y. and OHTA, G. (1985): Is Mallory body formation a preneoplastic change? A study of 181 cases of liver bearing hepatocellular carcinoma and 82 cases of cirrhosis. *Cancer*, 56, 2400–2404.

NAKHOODA, A.F., LIKE, A.A., CHAPPEL, C.I., MURRAY, F.T. and MARLISS, E.B. (1976): The spontaneously diabetic Wistar rat. Metabolic and morphologic studies. *Diabetes*, 26, 100–112.

NEBERT, D.W. (1979): Genetic differences in the induction of monooxygenase activities by polycyclic aromatic compounds. *Pharmacol. Ther.*, 6, 395–417.

NEBERT, D.W., ADESNIK, M., COON, M.J., ESTABROOK, R.W., GONZALEZ, F.J., GUENGERICH, F.P., GUNSALUS, I.C., JOHNSON, E.F., KEMPER, B., LEVIN, W., PHILLIPS, I.R., SATO, R. and WATERMAN, M.R. (1987): The P450 gene superfamily: Recommended nomenclature. *DNA*, 6, 1–11.

NEUBERGER, J.M., DAVIS, M. and WILLIAMS, R. (1981): Clinical aspects of oral contraceptive-associated liver tumours. In: M.Davis, J.M. Tredger and R. Williams, (Eds), *Drug Reactions and the Liver*, pp. 271–283. Pittman Medical, London.

NEWBERNE, P.M. (1982): Assessment of the hepatocarcinogenic potential of chemicals : Response of the liver. In: G. Plaa and W.R. Hewitt (eds) *Toxicology of the Liver*, pp. 243–290. Raven Press, New York.

NIEMEGEERS, C.J.E., LEVRON, J. Cl., AWOUTERS, F and JANSSEN, P.A.J. (1981): Inhibition and induction of microsomal enzymes in the rat. A comparative study of four antimycotics: Miconazole, econazole, clotrimazole and ketoconazole. *Arch.Int.Pharmacodyn.Ther.*

NISHIKAWA, S., HARA, T., MIYAZAKI, E. and OHKURO, T. (1984): Studies on the safety of KW-1414: Acute toxicity in mice and rats, and oral subacute and chronic toixicity studies in rats. *The Clinical Report*, 18, 281–305.

NORDSTRÖM, C. (1971): Enzymatic release of enteropeptidase from isolated rat duodenal brush borders. *Biochim.Biophys.Acta.*, 268, 711–718.

NORDSTRÖM, C. (1972): Release of enteropeptidase and other brush border enzymes from the small intestine wall in the rat. *Biochim.Biophys.Acta.*, 289, 367–377.

NUBER, R., TEUTSCH, H.F. and SASSE, D. (1980): Metabolic zonation in thioacetamide-induced liver cirrhosis. *Histochemistry*, 69, 277–288.

NUMOTO, S., TANAKA, T. and WILLIAMS, G.M. (1985): Morphologic and cytochemical properties of mouse liver neoplasms induced by diethylnitrosamine and promoted by 4,4'-dichlorodiphenyl-trichloroethane, chlordane, or hepatachlor.*Toxicol.Pathol.*, 13, 325–334.

O'BRIEN, T.D., HAYDEN, D.W., O'LEARY, T.P., CAYWOOD, D.D. and JOHNSON, K.H. (1987): Canine pancreatic endocrine tumors: Immunohistochemical analysis of hormone content and amyloid. *Vet.Pathol.*, 24, 308–314.

OATES, P.S. and MORGAN, R.G.H. (1982): Pancreatic growth and cell tumour in the rat fed soya flour. *Am.J.Pathol.*, 108, 217–224.

OGAWA, K., MINASE, T. and ONOE, T. (1974): Demonstration of glucose-6-phosphatase activity in the oval cells of rat liver and the significance of the oval cells in azodye carcinogenesis. *Cancer Res.*, 34, 3379–3386.

OGINO, M., OKITA, K., TSUBOTA, W., NUMA, Y., KODAMA, T. and TAKEMOTO, T. (1982): Some biochemical properties of the preneoplastic antigen in rat liver hyperplasic nodules. *Jpn.J.Cancer Res.*, (Gann) 73, 349–353.

OHMORI, T., RICE, J.M. and WILLIAMS, G.M. (1981): Histochemical characteristics of spontaneous and chemically induced hepatocellular neoplasms in mice and the development of neoplasms with gamma glutamyltranspeptidase activity during phenobarbital exposure. *Histochem.J.*, 13, 85–99

OKANOUE, T., BURBIGE, E.J. and FRENCH, S.W. (1983): The role of the Ito cell in perivenular and intralobular fibrosis in alcoholic hepatitis. *Arch.Pathol.Lab.Med.*, 107, 459–463.

OKANOUE, T., OHKA, M., OU, O., KACHI, K., KAGAWA, K., YUKI, T., OKUNO, T., TAKINO, T. and FRENCH, S.W., (1985): Relationship of Mallory bodies to intermediate filaments in hepatocytes, A scanning electron microscopy study. *Lab.Invest.*, 53, 534–540.

OLDSTONE, M.B.A., SOUTHERN, P., RODRIGUEZ, M. and LAMPERT, P. (1984): Virus persists in beta cells of islets of Langerhans and is associated with chemical manifestations of diabetes. *Science*, 224, 1440–1443.

ORCI, L., BAETENS, D., RAVAZZOLA, M., STEFAN, Y. and MAILAISSE-LAGAE, F. (1976): Ilots a polypeptide pancreatique (PP) et ilots a glucagon : Distribution topographique distincte dans le pancreas du rat. *C R Acad.Sci.*, 283, 1213–1216.

ORTON, T.C. and HIGGINS, J., (1979): The effects of hypolipidaemic agents on liver drug metabolizing enzymes. *Toxicol.Appl.Pharmacol.*, 48, A126.

PALIARD, P., VITREX, D., FOURNIER, G., BELHADJALI, L. and BERGER, F. (1978): Perhexiline maleate-induced hepatitis. *Digestion*, 17, 419–427.

PAIK, S-G., FLEISHER, N. and SHIN, S-I. (1980): Insulin-dependent diabetes mellitus induced by subdiabetogenic doses of streptozotocin : Obligatory role of cell-mediated autoimmune processes. *Proc.Natl.Acad.Sci.*, U.S.A., 77, 6129–6133.

PALOTAY, J.L. and HOWARD, C.F. Jr. (1982): Insular amyloidosis in spontaneously diabetic non-human primates. *Vet.Pathol.*, 19, Suppl.7, 181–192.

PAPADIMITRIOU, J.M. and WALTERS, M.N-I. (1967): Studies on the exocrine pancreas. II. Ultrastructural investigation of reovirus pancreatitis. *Am.J.Pathol.*, 51, 387–403.

PARSA, I. (1982): Identification of human acinar cell carcinoma by monoclonal antibody and in vitro differentiation. *Cancer Lett.*, 15, 115–121.

PATENT, G.J. and ALFERT, M. (1967): Histological changes in the pancreatic islets of alloxan-treated mice, with comments on beta-cell regeneration. *Acta.Anat.*, 66, 504–519.

PATNAIK, A.K., HURVITZ, A.I. and LIEBERMAN, P.H. (1980): Canine hepatic neoplasms : A clinicopathological study. *Vet.Pathol.*, 17, 553–564.

PHILLIPS, M.J. and POUCELL, S., ODA, M. (1986): Mechanisms of cholestasis. *Lab.Invest.*, 54, 593–608.

PIPELEERS, D. and VAN DE WINKEL, M. (1986): Pancreatic B cells possess defense mechanisms against cell-specific toxicity. *Proc.Natl.Acad.Sci.*, U.S.A., 83, 5267–5271.

PIERI, C., NAGY, I.Zs., MAZZUFFERI, G. and GUILLI, C. (1975): The aging of rat liver as revealed by electron microscopic morphometry. I. Basic parameters. *Exp.Gerontol.*, 10, 291–304.

PITOT, H.C. (1983): Contributions to our understanding of the natural history of neoplastic development in lower animals to the cause and control of human cancer. *Cancer Surv.*, 2, 519–537.

PLAA, G.L and HEWITT, W.R. (1982): Quantitative evaluation of indices of hepatotoxicity. In: G.L. Plaa and W.R. Hewitt (Eds), *Toxicology of the Liver*, pp. 103–120. Raven Press, New York.

PLAA, G.L. and PRIESTLY, B.G. (1977): Intrahepatic cholestasis induced by drugs and chemicals. *Pharmacol.Rev.*, 28, 207–273.

POH-FITZPATRICK, M.B., SKLAR, J.A., GOLDSMAN, C. and LEFKOWITCH, J.H. (1983): Protoporphyrin hepatopathy. Effects of cholic acid ingestion in murine griseofulvin-induced protoporphyria. *J.Clin.Invest.*, 72, 1449–1458.

POOLE, A., BETTON, G.R., SALMON, G., SUTTON, T. and ATTERWILL, C.K. (1990): Comparative toxicology of temelastine, novel H_1 antagonist in dog, rat and monkey. *Fundam.Appl.Toxicol.*, 14, 71–83.

POPP, J.A. and GOLDSWORTHY, T.L., (1989): Defining foci of cellular alteration in short-term and medium-term rat liver tumor models. *Toxicol.Pathol.*, 17, 561–568.

PORTMAN, B., CEVIKBAS, U., MELIA, W.M. and WILLIAMS, R. (1981): Pathology of oral contraceptive and androgenic steroid-associated liver tumours. In: M. Davis, J.M. Tredger and R. Williams (eds). *Drug Reactions and the Liver*, pp. 290–303. Pittman Medical, London.

POUCELL, S., IRETON, J., VALENCIA-MAYORAL, P. DOWNAR, E., LARRATT, L., PATTERSON, J., BLENDIS, L. and PHILLIPS, M.J. (1984): Amiodarone-associated phospholipidosis and fibrosis of the liver: light immunohistochemical and electron microscopic studies. *Gastroenterology*, 86, 926–936.

POUR, P.M. (1985): Induction of unusual pancreatic neoplasms, with morphologic simuilarity to human tumors, and evidence for their ductal/ductular cell origin. *Cancer*, 55, 2411–2416.

POUR, P.M., MOHR, U., CARDESA, A., ALTHOFF, J. and KMOCH, N. (1976): Spontaneous tumors and common diseases in two colonies of Syrian hamsters. II Respiratory tract and digestive system. *J.N.C.I.*, 56, 937–948.

POUR, P.M., ALTHOFF, J., SALMASI, S.Z. and STEPAN, K. (1979): Spontaneous tumors and common diseases in three types of hamsters. *J.N.C.I.*, 63, 797–811.

POUR, P.M., PARSA, I. and HAUSER, R. (1987): Evidence of partial exocrine acinar differentiation in experimentally induced pancreatic ductal/ductular cell tumours. *Int.J.Pancreatol.*, 1, 47–58.

PRENTICE, D.E., JAMES, R.W. and WADSWORTH, P.F. (1980): Pancreatic atrophy in young beagle dogs. *Vet.Pathol.*, 17, 575–580.

PRIESTER, W.A. (1974)a: Data from eleven United States and Canadian Colleges of veterinary medicine on pancreatic carcinoma in domestic animals. *Cancer Res.*, 34, 1372–1375.

PRIESTER, W.A. (1974)b: Pancreatic islet cell tumors in domestic animals. Data from 11 colleges of veterinary medicine in the United States and Canada. *J.N.C.I.*, 53, 227–229.

PRITCHARD, D.J. and BUTLER, W.H. (1986): The lectin histochemistry of aflatoxin B_1 induced hepatic nodules and hepatocellular carcinoma. *Histochem.J.*, 18, 57.

PRITCHARD, D.J. and BUTLER, W.H. (1989): Apoptosis: the mechanism of cell death in dimethylnitrosamine-induced hepatotoxicity. J.Pathol., 158, 253–260.

PROCTER, B.G., DUSSAULT, P. and CHAPPEL, C.I. (1973): Biochemical effects of sucrose acetate isobutyrate (SAIB) on the liver. *Proc.Soc.Exp.Biol.Med.*, 142, 595–599.

PROIA, A.D., EDWARDS, D.G., McNAMARA, D.J. and ANDERSON, K.E. (1984): Dietary influences of the hepatic mixed function oxidase system in the rat after portacaval. *Gastroenterology*, 86, 618–626.

PROKSOVA, E.G. (1973): Quantitative glycogenveränderungen in der Rattenleber nach Tetracyklin. *Anat.Anz.*, 143, 87–93.

RABES, H.M., BÜCHER, Th., HARTMANN, A., LINKE, I. and DÜNNWALD M. (1982): Clonal growth of carcinogen-induced enzyme-deficient preneoplastic cell populations in mouse liver. *Cancer Res.*, 42, 3220–3227.

RABSTEIN, L.S., PETERS, R.L. and SPAHN, G.J. (1973): Spontaneous tumors and pathologic lesions in SWR/J mice. *J.N.C.I.*, 50, 751–758.

RAKIETEN, N., GORDON, B.S., BEATY, A., COONEY, D.A. and DAVIS, R.D., SCHEIN, P.S. (1971): Pancreatic islet cell tumors produced by the combined action of streptozotocin and nicotinamide. *Proc.Soc.Exp.Biol.Med.*, 137, 280–283.

RAO, M.S., LALWANI, N.D. and SCARPELLI, D.G. (1982)a: The absence of gamma glutamyl transpeptide activity in putative preneoplastic lesions and hepatocellular carcinomas induced in rats by the hypolipidemic peroxisomal proliferator Wy-14, 643. *Carcinogenesis*, 3, 1231–1233.

RAO, K.N., EAGON, P.K., OKAMURA, K., VAN THIEL, D.H., GAVALER, J.S., KELLY, R.H. and LOMBARDI, B. (1982)b: Acute haemorrhagic pancreatic necrosis in mice. Induction in male mice treated with estradiol. *Am.J.Pathol.*, 109, 8–14.

RAO, M.S., UPTON, M.P., SUBBARAO, D.G. and SCARPELLI, D.G. (1982)c: Two populations of cells with differing proliferation capacites in atypical acinar cell foci induced by 4-hydroxyaminoquinoline-l-oxide in the rat pancreas.*Lab.Invest.*, 46, 527–534.

RAO, M.S., LALWANI, N.D. and REDDY, J.K. (1984): Sequential histologic studies of rat liver during peroxisomal proliferator [4-chloro-6(2,3-xylidino)-2-pyrimidinylthio]-acetic acid (Wy-14,643)-induced carcinogenesis. *J.N.C.I.*, 73, 983–990.

RAO, M.S. and REDDY, J.K. (1985): Induction and differentiation of exocrine pancreatic tumours in the rat. *Exp.Pathol.*, 28, 67–87.

RAO, M.S., SUBBARAO, V., YELDANDI, A.V. and REDDY, J.K. (1987): Pancreatic acinar cell regeneration following copper deficiency: induced pancreatic necrosis. *Int.J.Pancreatol.*, 2, 71–85.

RAO, S.S., WEATT, I.A., DONALDSON, L.A., CROCKET, A. and JOFFE, S.N. (1981): A serial histologic study of the development and progression of acute pancreatitis in the rat. *Am.J.Pathol.*, 103, 39–46.

RAO, M.S. BRENDAYAN, M., KIMBROUGH, R.D. and REDDY, J.K. (1986): Characterization of pancreatic-type tissue in the liver of rat induced by polychlorinated biphenyls. *J.Histochem.Cytochem.*, 34, 197–201.

RAPPAPORT, A.M., BOROWY, Z.J., LOUGHEED, W.M. and LOTTO, W.N. (1954): Subdivision of hexagonal liver lobules into a stuctural and functional unit. Role in hepatic physiology and pathology. *Anat.Rec.*, 119, 11–34.

RAPPAPORT, A.M., MACPHEE, P.J., FISHER, M.M and PHILLIPS, M.J. (1983): The scarring of the liver acini (cirrhosis). Tridimensional and microcirculatory considerations. *Virchows Arch.*[A], 402, 107–137.

RASMUSSEN, H. (1986): The calcium messenger system. *N.Engl.J.Med.*, 314, 1094–1101.

REAVON, E.P. and REAVON, G.M. (1981): Structure and function changes in the endocrine pancreas of aging rats with reference to the modulating effects of exercise and caloric restruction. *J.Clin.Invest.*, 68, 75–84.

REDDY, J.K. and QURESHI, S.A. (1979): Tumorigenicity of the hypolipidaemic peroxisome proliferator ethyl-alpha-p-chlorphenoxyisobutyrate (clofibrate) in rats. *Br.J.Cancer* 40, 476–482.

REDDY, J.K., RAO, M.S., QURESHI, S.A., REDDY, M.K., SCARPELLI, D.G. and LALWANI, N.D. (1984): Induction and origin of hepatocytes in rat pancreas. *J.Cell.Biol.*, 98, 2082–2090.

REDDY, J.K. and RAO, M.S. (1977): Malignant tumors in rats fed nafenopin, a hepatic peroxisomal proliferation. *J.N.C.I.*, 59, 1645–1650.

REDDY, J.K., RAO, M.S., QURESHI, S.A., REDDY, M.K., SCARPELLI, D.G. and LALWANI, N.D. (1984): Induction and origin of hepatocytes in rat pancreas. *J.Cell Biol.*, 98, 2082–2090.

REDDY, J.K. and RAO, M.S. (1987): Xenobiotic-induced peroxisomal proliferation: Role of tissue specificity and species differences in response in the evaluation of the implications for human health. *Arch.Toxicol.Suppl.*, 10, 43–53.

REDDY, J.K., AZARNOFF, D.L. and HIGNITE, C.E. (1980): Hypolipidaemic hepatic peroxisome proliferation form a novel class of chemical carcinogens. *Nature*, 283, 398–398.

REDDY, J.K. and LALWANI, N.D. (1983): Carcinogenesis by hepatic peroxisomal proliferators: Evaluation of the risk of hypolipidemic drugs and industrial plasticizers to humans. *CRC Crit.Rev.Toxicol.*, 12, 1–58.

REYNOLDS, T.B., PETER, P.L. and YAMADA, S. (1971): Chronic active and lupoid hepatitis caused by a laxative, oxyphenisatin. *N.Engl.J.Med.*, 285, 813–820.

REYNOLDS, S.H., STOWERS, S.J., PATTERSON, R.M., MARONPOT, R.R., AARONSON, S.A. and ANDERSON, M.W. (1987): Activated oncogenes in B6C3F1 mouse liver tumours: Implications for risk assessment. *Science,* 237, 1309–1316.

REZNIK-SCHULLER, H.M. and LIJINSKY, W. (1983): Methaphenilene, an analogue of the anti-histaminic methapyriline, is a 'peroxisomal proliferator'. *Arch.Toxicol.*, 52, 165–166.

RICHARDS, W.L, TSUKADA, Y and POTTER, V.R. (1982): Gamma-glutamyl transpeptidase and alpha-tetoprotein expression during alpha-naphthylisothiocyanate-induced hepatoxicity in rats. *Cancer Res.*, 42, 5133–5138.

RICHARDSON, B.P., TURKALJ, I., FLUCKIGER, E. (1984): Bromocriptine. In: D.R.Laurence, A.E.M.Mclean and M.Weatherall (Eds), *Safety Testing of New Drugs. Laboratory Predictions and Clinical Performance.* Chap. 3, pp. 19–63.

RICHTER, K-D, LOGE, O. and LOSERT, W. (1971): Vergleichende morphologische Untersuchungen über die diabetogene Wirkung von Streptozotocin bei Ratten, chinesischen Streifenhamstern, Meerschweinchen und Kaninchen. *Arzneimittelforschung*, 21, 1654–1656.

RIDDELL, R.H. and STRAUS, F.H. (1982): The pancreas. In: R.H. Riddell (Ed.), *Pathology of Drug-Induced and Toxic Diseases.* Chap. 19, pp 607–629. Churchill Livingston, New York.

RIKANS, L.E. (1984): Influence of aging on the susceptibility of rats to hepatotoxic injury. *Toxicol.Appl.Pharmacol.*, 73, 243–249.

RINDER, H.M., LOVE, J.C. and WEXLER, R. (1986): Amiodarone hepatotoxicity. *N.Engl.J.Med.*,314, 318–319.

RINDERKNECHT, H., MASET, R., COLLIAS, K. and CARMACK, C. (1983): Pancreatic secretory profiles of protein, digestive, and lysosomal enzymes in the Syrian golden hamster. *Diagn.Dis.Sci.*, 28, 518–525.

ROBERTS, J.C., MCROSSAN, M.V. and JONES, H.B. (1990): The case for perfusion fixation of large tissue samples for ultrastructural pathology. *Ultrastruct.Pathol.*, 14, 177–191.

ROEBUCK, B.D., BAUMGARTNER, K.J. and THRON, C.D. (1984): Characterization of two populations of pancreatic atypical acinar cell foci induced by azaserine in the rat. *Lab.Invest.*, 50, 141–146.

ROEBUCK, B.D., LILJA, H.S., CURPHY, T.J. and LONGNECKER, D.S. (1980): Pathologic and biochemical effects of azaserine in inbred Wistar/Lewis rats and non-inbred CD[R]-1 mice. *J.N.C.I.*, 65, 383.

ROEBUCK, B.D., YAGER, J.D. and LONGNECKER, D.S. (1981): Dietary modulation of azaserine-induced pancreatic carcinogenesis in the rat. *Cancer Res.*, 41, 888–893.

ROGERS, A.E. and NEWBERNE, P.M. (1973): Fatty liver and cirrhosis in lipotrope-deficient male rats. *Am.J.Pathol.*, 73, 817–820.

ROOMI, M.W., HO, R.K., SARMA, D.S.R and FARBER, E. (1985): A common biochemical pattern in preneoplastic hepatocyte nodules generated in four different models in the rat. *Cancer Res.*, 45, 564–571.

ROSAI, J. (1968): Carcinoma of the pancreas simulating giant cell tumor of bone. *Cancer*, 22, 333–344.

ROTHMAN, S.S. and WELLS, H. (1967): Enhancement of pancreatic enzyme synthesis by pancreozymin. *Am.J.Physiol.*, 213, 215–218.

ROUMIANTZEFF, M., MYNARD, M.C., COQUET, B., GOLDMAN, C. and AYME, G. (1975): Acute and chronic toxicities in mammal and subhuman primates with inactivated Corynebacterium suspension. In B. Halpern, (Ed.), *Corynebacterium parvum. Applications in Experimental and Clinical Oncology*, Chap. 2, pp. 11–27.

ROWLATT, U.F. (1967): Pancreatic neoplasms of rats and mice. In: E.Cotchin and F.J.C. Roe (Eds), *Pathology of Laboratory Rats and Mice*. Chap. 4, pp. 85–101, Blackwell Scientific, Oxford.

RUBIN, E. and LIEBER, C.S. (1974): Fatty liver, alcoholic hepatitis and cirrhosis produced by alcohol in primates. *N.Engl.J.Med.*, 290, 128–135.

RUEBNER, B.H, GERSHWIN, M.E., MEIERHENRY, E.F. and DUNN, P. (1982): Enzyme histochemical characteristics of spontaneous and induced hepatocellular neoplasms in mice. *Carcinogenesis*, 3, 899–903.

RUEBNER, B.H., WATANABE, K. and WAND, J.S. (1970): Lytic necrosis resembling peliosos hepatis produced by lasiocarpine in the mouse liver. A light and electron microscopic study. *Am.J.Pathol.*, 60, 247–269.

RUEBNER, B.H., GERSHWIN, M.E., MEIERHENRY, E.F., HSIEH, L.S. and DUNN, P.L. (1984): Irreversibility of liver tumours in C3H mice. *J.N.C.I.*, 73, 493–498.

RUSHMORE, T.H., GHAZARIAN, D.M., SUBRAHMANYAN, V., FARBER, E. and GOSHAL, A.K. (1987): Probable free radical effects on rat liver nuclei during early hepatocarcinogenesis with a choline-alevoid low methionine diet. *Cancer Res.*, 47, 6731–6740.

SALTER, J.M., DAVIDSON, I.W.F. and BEST, C.H. (1957): The pathologic effects of large amounts of glucagon. *Diabetes*, 6, 248–255.

SCARPELLI, D.G. (1985): Multipotent developmental capacity of cells in the adult animal. *Lab.Invest.*, 52, 331–332.

SCARPELLI, D.G. and RAO, M.S. (1981): Differentiation of regenerating pancreatic cells into hepatocyte-like cells. *Proc.Natl.Acad.Sci.*, USA, 78, 2577–2581.

SCARPELLI, D.G., RAO, M.S., SUBBARAO, V., BEVERSLUIS, M., GURKA, D.P. and HOLLENBERG, P.F. (1980): Activation of nitrosamines to mutagens by postmitochondrial fraction of hamster pancreas. *Cancer Res.*, 40, 67–74.

SCHARDEIN, J.L., KAUMP, D.H., WOOSLEY, E.T. and JELLEMA, M.M. (1970): Long-term toxicologic and tumorigenesis studies on an oral contraceptive agent in albino rats. *Toxicol.Appl.Pharmacol.*, 16 10–23.

SCHEUER, P.J. (1980): In: Liver Biopsy Interpretation, 3rd edition. Balliere Tindall, London.

SCHEUER, P.J. (1981): Drug hepatoxicity : Range of pathological lesions. In: M.Davis., J.M.Tredger. and R.Williams. (eds). Drug Reactions and the Liver, pp. 54–63. Pitman Medical, London.

SCHMUCKER, D.L., (1979): Age-related changes in drug deposition. *Pharmacol.Rev.*, 37, 133–148.

SCHMUCKER, D.L. (1985): Aging and drug disposition : An update. *Pharmacol.Rev.*, 37, 133–148.

SCHMUCKER, D.L., MOONEY, J.S. and JONES, A.L. (1977): Age-related changes in hepatic endoplasmic reticulum : A quantitative analysis. *Science*, 197–1007.

SCHMUCKER, D.L. and WANG, R.K. (1983): Age-dependent changes in rat liver microsomal NADPH cytochrome c (P-450) reductase : A kinetic analysis. *Exp.Gerontol.*, 18, 313–321.

SCHNEIDER, R., TROESCH, V. and HADORN, B. (1975): On the cellular distribution of sucrase and enterokinase in different populations of rat intestinal epithelial cells isolated by a vibration method. *Biol.Gastroenterol.* (Paris), 8, 11–20.

SCHULTE-HERMANN, R. (1974): Induction of liver growth by xenobiotic compounds and other stimuli. *CRC Crit.Rev.Tocicol.*, 3, 97–158.

SCHULTE-HERMANN, R. (1979); Reactions of the liver to injury. Adaption. In E. Farber. and M.M. Fisher. (Eds), *Toxic Injury of the Liver*, Chap. 9, pp. 385–444. Marcel Dekker, New York.

SCHULTE-HERMANN, R. (1985): Tumor promotion in the liver. *Arch.Toxicol.*, 57, 147–158.

SCHULTE-HERMANN, R., HOFFMAN, V. and LANDGRAF, H. (1980): Adaptive responses of rat liver to the gestagen and anti-androgen cyproterone acetate and other inducers. III Cytological changes. *Chem.Biol.Interact.*, 31, 301–311.

SCHULTE-HERMANN, R., TIMMERMAN-TROSIENER, I. and SCHUPPLER, J. (1983): Promotion of spontaneous preneoplastic cells in rat liver as a possible explanation of tumor production by non-mutagenic compounds. *Cancer Res.*, 43, 839–844.

SCHULTE-HERMANN, R., ROOME, N., TIMMERMAN-TROSIENER, I. and SCHUPPLER, J. (1984): Immunocytochemical demonstration of a phenobarbitol-inducible cytochrome P450 in putative preneoplastic foci of rat liver. *Carcinogenesis*, 5, 149–153.

SCHUPPLER, J. and GÜNZEL, P. (1979): Liver tumours and steroid hormones in rats and mice. *Arch.Toxicol.Suppl.*, 2, 181–195.

SCHUPPLER, J., SCHULTE-HERMANN, R., TIMMERMANN-TROSIENER, I. and GÜNZEL, P. (1982): Proliferative liver lesions and sex steroids in rats. *Toxicol.Pathol.*, 10, 132–143.

SCHWARTZ, A.G., LEWBART, M.L. and PASHKO, L.L. (1988): Novel dehydroepiandrosterone analogues with enhanced biological activity and reduced side effects in mice and rats. *Cancer Res*, 48, 4817–4822.

SEAMER, J.H. (1967): Some virus infections of mice. In: E. Cotchin and F.J.C. Roe (Eds), *Pathology of Laboratory Animals*. Chap. 17, pp. 537–567, Blackwell, Oxford.

SEEMAYER, T.A., TANNENBAUM, G.S., GOLDMAN, H.Y. and COLLE, E. (1982)a: Dynamic time course studies of the spontaneously diabetic BB Wistar rat. III Light-microscopic and ultrastructural observations of pancreatic islets of Langerhans. *Am.J.Pathol.*, 106, 237–249.

SEEMAYER, T.A., SCHURCH, W. and KALANT, N. (1982)b: B cell lymphoproliferation in spontaneously diabetic BB Wistar rats. *Diabetologia*, 23, 261–265.

SELL, S. and DUNSFORD, H.A., (1989): Evidence for the stem cell origin of hepatocellular carcinoma and cholangiocarcinoma. *Am.J.Pathol.*, 134, 1347–1363.

SHERLOCK, S. (1978): Hepatic tumors and sex hormones. In: H. Remmer, H.M. Bolt, P. Bannasch and H. Popper (Eds), *Primary Liver Tumours*. Chap. 16, pp. 201–212. MTP Press Ltd, Lancaster, England.

SHERLOCK, S. (1982): Patterns of hepatocyte injury in man. *Lancet*, 1, 782–786.

SHIMA, A. and SUGAHARA, T. (1976): Age-dependent ploidy class changes in mouse hepatocyte nuclei as revealed by Feulgen-DNA cytofluoremetry. *Exp.Gerentol.*, 11, 193–203.

SHINO, A., MATSUO, T., IWATSUKA, H. and SUZUOKI, Z. (1973): Structural changes of pancreatic islets in genetically obese rats. *Diabetologia*, 9, 413–421.

SIMON, J.B., MANLEY, P.N., BRIEN, J.F. and ARMSTRONG, P.W. (1984): Amiodarone hepatotoxicity stimulating alcoholic liver disease. *N.Engl.J.Med.*, 311, 167–172.

SIMPSON, C.F., BRADLEY, R.E. and JACKSON, R.F. (1974): Crystalloid inclusions in hepatocyte mitochondria of dogs treated with levamisol. *Vet.Pathol.*, 11, 129–137.

SMITH, G.S., BARSOUM, N.J., GOUGH, A.W., STURGESS, J.M. and DE LA IGLESIA, F.A. (1984): Pathologic changes in rats following subchronic oral administration of a novel neuroleptic agent. *Fed.Proc.*, 43, 575.

SMITH, G., BARSOUM, N.J., DIFONZO, C., GRACON, S., MARTIN, R., STURGESS, J.M. and DE LA IGLESIA, F.A.(1985): Subacute oral toxic of an anxiolytic agent. *Toxicologist*, 5, 227.

SMITH, J.H., RUSH, G.F. and HOOK, J.B. (1986): Induction of renal and hepatic mixed funxtion oxidases in the hamster and guinea pig. *Toxicology*, 38, 209–218.

SMITH, M.T., LOVERIDGE, N., WILLIS, E.D. and CHAYEN, J. (1979): The distribution of glutathione in the rat liver lobule. *Biochem.J.*, 182, 103–108.

SMITH, P.H. (1983): Immunocytochemical localization of glucagon-like and gastric inhibitory polypeptide-like peptides in the pancreatic islets and gastrointestinal tract. *Am.J.Anat.*, 168, 109–118.

SMOLEN, A., WAXMAN, A.L., SMOLEN, T.N., PETERSEN, D.R. and COLLINS, A.C. (1981): Subcellular distribution of hepatic aldehyde dehydrogenase activity in four inbred mouse strains. *Comp.Biochem.Physiol.*[C], 69, 199–204.

SMOLEN, A., SMOLEN, T.N. and COLLINS, A.C. (1982): The influence of age, sex and genotype on the subcellular distribution of hepatic aldehyde dehydrogenase activity in the mouse. *Comp.Biochem.Physiol.*[B], 73, 815–822.

SOUTHERN, P. and OLDSTONE, M.B.A. (1986): Medical consequences of persistent viral infection. *N.Engl.J.Med.*, 314, 359–367.

SPENCER, A.J., ANDREU, M. and GREAVES, P. (1986): Neoplasia and hyperplasia of pancreatic endocrine tissue in the rat : An immunocytochemical study. *Vet.Pathol.*, 23, 11–15.

SQUIRE, R.A. and LEVITT, M.H. (1975): Report of a workshop on classification of specific hepatocellular lesions in rats. *Cancer Res.*, 35, 3214–3223.

SQUIRE, R.A. (1989): Evaluation and grading of rat liver foci in carcinogenicity tests. *Toxicol.Pathol.*, 17, 685–689.

STEER, M.L. and MELDOLESI, J. (1987): The cell biology of experimental pancreatitis. *N.Engl.J.Med.*, 316, 144–150.

STEFAN, Y., MALAISSE-LAGAE, F., YOON, J.W., NOTKINS, A.L. and ORCI, L. (1978): Virus-induced diabetes in mice : A quantitative evaluation of islet cell population by immunofluorescent technique. *Diabetologica*, 15, 395–401.

STEINER, J.W. and CARRUTHERS, J.S. (1963): Electron microscopy of hyperplastic ductular cells in alpha-naphthyl isothiocyanate-induced cirrhosis. *Lab.Invest.*, 12, 471–498.

STEINER, J.W., PHILLIPS, M.J. and BAGLIO, C.M. (1963): Electron microscopy of the excretory pathways in the liver in alpha-naphthyl isothiocyanate intoxication. *Am.J.Pathol.*, 43, 677–696.

STEJSKAL, R., ITABASHI, M., STANEK, J. and HRUBAN, Z. (1975): Experimental porphyria induced by 3-[2-(2,4,6-trimethylphenyl)-thioethyl]-4-methylsydnone. *Virchows Arch.*[B], 18, 83–100.

STENBÄCK, F., MORI, H., FURUYA, K. and WILLIAMS, G.M. (1986): Pathogenesis of dimethylnitrosamine-induced hepatocellular cancer in hamster liver and lack of enhancement by phenobarbital. *J.N.C.I.*, 76, 327–333.

STEWART, H.L., WILLIAMS, G., KEYSSER, C.H., LOMBARD, L.S. and MONTALI, R.J. (1980): Histologic typing of liver tumors of the rat. *J.N.C.I.*, 64, 178–106.

STOHS, S.J., AL-TURK, W.A. and ANGLE, C.R. (1982): Glutathione S-transferase and glutathione reductase activities in hepatic and extrahepatic tissues of female mice as a function of age. *Biochem.Pharmacol.*, 31, 2113–2116.

STOKES, W.S. (1986): Spontaneous diabetes mellitus in a baboon (Papio cynocephalus anubis). *Lab.Anim.Sci.*, 36, 529–533.

STOUT, D.L. and BECKER F.F. (1986): Xenobiotic metabolizing enzymes in genetically and chemically initiated mouse liver tumors. *Cancer Res.*, 46, 2693–2696.

STROMBECK, D.R. and GRIBBLE, D. (1978): Chronic active hepatitis in the dog. *J.Am.Vet. Med.Assoc.*, 173, 380–386.

STROMBERG, P.C., WILSON, F. and CAPEN, C.C. (1983): Immunocytochemical demonstration of insulin in spontaneous pancreatic islet cell tumors of Fischer rats. *Vet.Pathol.*, 20, 291–297.

STURGESS, J. and REID, L. (1973): The effect of isoprenaline and pilocarpine on (a) brochial mucus-secreting tissue and (b) pancreas, salivary glands, heart, thymus, liver and spleen. *Br.J.Exp.Pathol.*, 54, 388–403.

SUMNER, I.G. and LODOLA, A. (1987): Total cytochrome P-450, but not the major phenobarbitone or 3-methylcholanthrene induced isoenzyme, is differentially induced in the lobes of the rat liver. *Biochem.Pharmacol.*, 36, 391–393.

SUN, J. and STROBEL, H.W. (1986): Aging affects the drug metabolism systems of rt liver, kidney, colon and lung in a differential fashion. *Exp.Gerontol.*, 21, 523–534.

SVOBODA, D., GRADY, H. and HIGGINSON, J. (1966): The effects of chronic protein deficiency in rats. II. Biochemical and ultrastructural changes. *Lab.Invest.*, 15, 731–749.

TAKAHASHI, M. and POUR, P. (1978): Spontaneous alterations in the pancreas of the aging Syrian golden hamster. *J.N.C.I.*, 60, 355–364.

TAKASAWA, S., YAMAMOTO, H., TERAZONO, K. and OKAMOTO, H. (1986): Novel gene activated in rat insulinomas. *Diabetes*, 35, 1178–1180.

TAPER, H.S., SOMER, M.P., LANS, M., DE GERLACHE, J. and ROBERFROID, M. (1988): Histochemical detection of the in vivo produced cellular aldehydes by means of direct Schiff's reaction in CCL₄ intoxicated rat liver. *Arch.Toxicol.*, 61, 406–410.

TATEMATSU, M., HO, R.H., KAKU, T., EKEM, J.K. and FARBER, E. (1984): Studies on the proliferation and fate of oval cells in the liver of rats treated with 2-acetylaminofluorene and partial hepatectomy. *Am.J.Pathol.*, 114, 418–430.

TATEMATSU, M., KAKU, T., MEDLINE, A. and FARBER, E. (1985): Intestinal metaplasia as a common option of oval cells in relation to cholangiofibrosis in liver of rats exposed to 2 acetyl-aminofluorene. *Lab.Invest.*, 52, 354–362.

TAVASSOLI, M., OZOLS, J., SUGIMOTO, G., COX, K.H. and MULLER-EBERHARD, U. (1976): Localization of cytochrome b₅ in rat organs and tissues by immunocytochemistry. *Biochem.Biophys.Res.Commun.*, 72, 281–287.

TAZAWA, J., IRIE, T. and FRENCH, S.W. (1983): Mallory body formation runs paralell to gamma-glutamyl transferase induction in hepatocytes of griseofulvin-fed mice. *Hepatology.*, 3, 989–1001.

TENNANT, R.W., MARGOLIN, B.H., SHELBY, M.D., ZEIGER, E., HASEMAN, J.K., SPALDING, J., CASPARY, W., RESNICK, M., STASIEWICZ, S., ANDERSON, B and MINOR R. (1987): Prediction of chemical carcinogenicity in rodents from in vitro genetic toxicity assays. *Science*, 236, 933–941.

TEPPERMAN, J., CALDWELL, F.T. and TEPPERMAN, H.M. (1964): Induction of gallstones in mice by feeding a cholesterol-cholic acid containing diet. *Am.J.Physiol.*, 206, 628–634.

TEUTSCH, H.F. (1984): Functional liver cell heterogeneity. *Acta.Histochem.Cytochem.*, 17, 687.

TEUTSCH, H.F. (1985): Quantitative histochemical assessment of regional differences in hepatic glucose uptake and release. *Histochemistry*, 82, 159–164.

THEMAN, H. and VON BASSEWITZ, D.B. (1969): Parakristalline Einschlusskörper der Mitochondrien des menschlichen Leberparenchyms. Elektronenmikroskopische und histologische Untersuchungen. *Cytobiol.*, 1, 135–151.

THOMAS, P.E., REIK, L.M., RYAN, D.E. and LEVIN, W. (1983): Induction of two immunochemically related rat liver cytochrome P-450 isozymes cytochromes, P-450c and P450d, by structurally diverse xenobiotics. *J.Biol.Chem.*, 258, 4590–4598.

THOMAS, P.E., BANDIERA, S., REIK, L.M., MAINES, S.L., RYAN, D.E. and LEVIN, W. (1987): Polyclonal and monoclonal antibodies as probes of rat hepatic cytochrome P-450 isozymes. *Fed.Proc.*, 46, 2563–2566.

THUNG, S.N. and GERBER, M.A. (1981): Percusor stage of hepatocellular neoplasm following long exposure to orally administered contraceptives. *Hum.Pathol.*, 12, 472–474.

TÖNDER, M., NORDAY, A. and ELGIO, K. (1974): Sulfonamide-induced chronic liver disease. *Scand.J.Gastroenterol.*, 9, 93–96.

TORDJMAN, K., KATZ, I., BURSZTYN, M. and ROSENTHAL, T. (1985): Amiodarone and the liver. *Ann.Intern.Med.*, 102, 411–412.

TREPETA, R.W., MATHUR, B., LAGINS, S. and LIVOLSI, V.A. (1981): Giant cell tumor ('osteoclastoma') of the pancreas : A tumor of epithelial cell origin. *Cancer*, 48, 2022–2028.

TRIGO, F.J., THOMPSON, H., BREEZE, R.G. and NASH, A.S. (1982): The pathology of liver tumours in the dog. *J.Comp.Pathol.*, 92, 21–39.

TRYPHONAS, L., ARNOLD, D.L., ZAWIDZKA, Z., MES, J., CHARBONNEAU, S. and WONG, J. (1986): A pilot study in adult rhesus monkeys (M.mulatta) treated with Aroclor 1254 for two years. *Toxicol.Pathol.*, 14, 1–10.

TSCHUDY, D.P., ROSE, J., HELLMAN, E., COLLINS, A. and RECHCIGL, M. (1962): Biochemical studies of experimental porphyria. *Metabolism*, 11, 1287–1301.

TUCHWEBER, B., KOVACS, K., KHANDEHAR, J.D. and GORG, B.D. (1973): Peliosis-like changes induced by phalloidin in the rat liver. A light and electron microscopic study. *J.Med.*, (Basel), 4, 327.

TUCKER, W.E. (1983): Preclinical toxicity of bupropion: An overview. *J.Clin.Psychiatry*, 44, 60–62.

TURUSOV, V.S. and TAKAYAMA, S. (1979): Tumours of the liver. In: V.S. Turusov (Ed.), Pathology of Tumours in Laboratory Animals Vol.12, Tumours of the Mouse, pp. 193–233. IARC Lyon.

VAN BEZOOIJEN, C.F.A. (1984): Influence of age-related changes in rodent liver morphology and physiology on drug metabolism. A review. *Mech.Aging Dev.*, 25, 1–22.

VAN DER INGH, T.S.G.A.M. and ROTHUIZEN, J. (1985): Congenital cystic disease of the liver in seven dogs. *J.Comp.Pathol.*, 95, 405–414.

VAN HOOSIER, G.L. and TRENTIN, J.J. (1979): Naturally occurring tumors in the Syrian hamster. *Prog.Exp.Tumor Res.*, 23, 1–12.

VAN MANEN, R., DE PRIESTER, W. and KNOOK, D.L. (1983): Lysosomal activity in aging rat liver. I. Variation in enzyme activity within the liver lobule. *Mech.Aging Dev.*, 22, 159–165.

VERHEYEN, A. and BORGERS, M. (1976): Effects of levamisole on the ultrastructure of mitochondria in the liver of beagle dogs. *Vet.Pathol.*, 13, 131–137.

VERHEYAN, A., BORGERS, M., BLATON, H. and SOWA, H. (1975): The ultrastructure of human livers after prolonged lidoflazine therapy. *Toxicol.Appl.Pharmacol.*, 34, 224–232.

VESSELINOVITCH, S.D., HACKER, H.J. and BANNASCH, P. (1985): Histochemical characterisation of focal hepatic lesions induced by single diethyl-nitrosamine treatment of infant mice. *Cancer Res.*, 45, 2774–2780.

VILLANOVE, F. and GREAVES, P. (1983): Sialoconjugates in normal and neoplastic rat liver : A histochemical study. *Pathol.Res.Prac.*, 178, 171.

VIRJI, M.A. and RAO, K.N. (1985): Acute hemorrhagic pancreatitis in mice. A study of glucoregulatory hormones and glucose metabolism. *Am.J.Pathol.*, 118, 162–167.

VITORICA, J., SATRUSTEGUI, J. and MACHADO, A. (1981): Metabolic implications of aging : Changes in activities of key lipogenic and gluconeogenic enzymes in the aged rat liver. *Enzyme*, 21, 144–152.

VOLLMER, K-O., VON HODENBERG, A. and KÖLLE, E.U. (1986): Pharmacokinetics and metabolism of gabapentin in rat, dog and man. *Arzneimittelforschung*, 36, 830–839.

VON PROKSOVCI, E.G. (1973): Quantitative Glykogenveranderugen in der Rattenleber nach Teracyklin: *Anat.Anz.*, 134, 87–93.

WAKE, K. (1974): Development of vitamin A rich lipid droplets in multivesicular bodies of rat liver stellate cells. *J.Cell.Biol.*, 63, 683–691.

WALKER, R.M., DIFONZO, C.J., BARSOUM, N.J., SMITH, G.S. and MACALLUM, G.E. (1988): Chronic toxicity of the anticonvulsant zonisamide in beagle dogs. *Fundam.Appl.Toxicol.*, 11, 333–342.

WALKER, A.I.T., THORPE, E. and STEVENSON, D.E. (1972): The toxicology of dieldrin (HEOD). I: Long-term oral toxicity studies in mice. *Food Cosmet Toxicol.*, 11, 415–432.

WALKER, R.M., RACZ, W.J., and McELLIGOTT, T.F. (1985): Acetaminophen-induced hepatoxic congestion in mice. *Hepatology*, 5, 233–240.

WALTERS, M.N. (1966): Adipose atrophy of the exocrine pancreas. *J.Pathol.Bacteriol.*, 92, 547–557.

WARD, J.M., GOODMAN, D.G., SQUIRE, R.A., CHU, K.C. and LINHART, M.S. (1979): Neoplastic and non-neoplastic lesions in aging (C57BL/6N × C3H/HeN)F1 (B6C3F1) mice. *J.N.C.I.*, 63, 849–854.

WARD, J.M. (1981): Morphology of foci of altered hepatcoytes and naturally-occurring hepatocellular tumors in F344 rats. *Virchows Arch.*[A]., 390, 339–345.

WARD, J.M., RICE, J.M., CREASIA, D., LYNCH, P and RIGGS, C. (1983): Dissimilar patterns of promotion by di(2-ethylhexyl)phthalate and phenobarbital of hepatocellular neoplasia initiated by diethylnitrosamine in B6C3F1 mice. *Carcinogenesis*, 4, 1021–1029.

WARD, J.M. and VLAHAKIS, G. (1978): Evaluation of hepatocellular neoplasms in mice. *J.N.C.I.*, 61, 807–811.

WATANABE, T., UTSUGLI, M., MITSUKAWA, M., SUGAT. and FUJITANI, H. (1986): Hypolipidemic effect and enhancement of peroxisome β-oxidation in the liver of rats by sodium-(E)-3-[4-(3-pyridylmethyl)phenyl]-2-methyl propenoate(OKY-1581), a potent inhibitor of TXA$_2$ synthetase. *J.Pharmacobiodyn.*, 9, 1023–1031.

WEIBEL, E.R., STAUBLI, W., GNAGI, H.R. and HESS, F.A. (1969): Correlation morphometric and biometric studies on the liver cell. I. Morphometric model, stereologic methods, and normal morphometric data for rat liver. *J.Cell Biol.*, 42, 68–91.

WEICHBROD, R.H., CISAR, C.F., MILLER, J.G., SIMMONDS, R.C., ALVARES, A.P. and UENG T-H (1988): Effects of cage beddings on microsomal oxidative enzymes in rat liver. *Lab.Anim.Sci.*, 38, 296–298.

WEINBREN, K. (1978): Induction of liver nodules after portacaval anastomasis in rats. In: H. Remmer, H.M. Bolt, P. Bannasch, H. Popper (Eds), *Primary Liver Tumours*. Chap. 32, pp. 395–399. MTP Press Ltd., Lancaster, England.

WEINBREN, K. and WASHINGTON, S.L.A. (1976): Hyperplastic nodules after portacaval anastomosis in rats. *Nature*, 264, 440–442.

WELLMAN, K.F. and VOLK, B.W. (1980): Islets of Langerhans : Structure and function in diabetes. *Pathobiol.Annu.*, 10, 105–133.

WELLS, M.Y., WEISBRODE, S.E., MAURER, J.K., CAPEN, C.C. and BRUCE, R.D. (1988): Variable hepatocellular vacuolation associated with glycogen in rabbit. *Toxicol.Pathol.*, 16, 360–365.

WESTABY, D. and WILLIAMS, R. (1981): Androgen and anabolic steroid-related liver tumours. In: M. Davis, J.M. Tredger and R. Williams (Eds), *Drug Reactions and the Liver*, pp. 284–289.

WHALIN, T., BLOOM, G.D. and DANIELSSON, A. (1976): Effect of cholecystokinin-pancreozymin epithelium. *Cell Tissue Res.*, 171, 425–435.

WHALIN, T., BLOOM, G.D. and DANIELSSSON, A. (1976): Effects of fasting and refeeding on secretory granules of the mouse gall bladder epithelium. *Gastroenterology*, 70, 353–358.

WHITING, P.H., MIDDLETON, B., THOMAS, N. and HAWTHORNE, J. (1982): Studies on a stable, mild diabetes induced by streptozotocin in rats. *Br.J.Exp.Pathol.*, 63, 408–413.

WILGRAM, G.F., and TAYLOR, W.J. (1959): Experimental cirrhosis of the liver in primates. *Lancet*, 1, 26–27.

WILLIAMS, G. (1964): Amyloidosis in parabiotic mice. *J.Pathol.Bacteriol.*, 88, 35–41.

WILLIAMS, G.M. (1980): The pathogenesis of rat liver cancer caused by chemical carcinogens. *Biochem.Biophys.Acta.*, 605, 165–189.

WILLIAMS, J.A. and GOLDFINE, I.D. (1985): The insulin-pancreatic acinar axis. *Diabetes*, 34, 980–986.

WILSON, G.L. and LeDOUX, S.P. (1989): The role of chemicals in the etiology of diabetes mellitus. *Toxicol.Pathol.*, 17, 357–363.

WINKLER, K. and POULSEN, H. (1975): Liver disease with periportal sinusoidal dilation. A possible complication to contraceptive steroids. *Scand.J.Gastroenterol.*, 10, 699–704.

WISSE, E., VAN'T NOORDENDE, J.M., VAN DER MEULEN, J. and DAENS, W.Th. (1976): The pit cell : description of a new type of cell occurring in rat liver sinusoids and peripheral blood. *Cell Tissue Res.*, 173, 423–435.

WOLSTENHOLME, J.T. and GARDNER, W.U. (1950): Sinusoidal dilation occurring in livers of mice with a transplanted testicular tumor. *Proc.Soc.Exp.Biol.Med.*, 74, 659–661.

WOODS, J.A. (1983): Cellular immunlocalization of alpha-fetoprotein in rat liver. *Histochem.J.*, 15, 1021–1028.

WRIGHT, J., YATES, A., SHARMA, H. and THIBERT, P. (1985): Histopathological lesions in the pancreas of the BB Wistar rat as a function of age and duration of diabetes. *J.Comp.Pathol.*, 95, 7–14.

WYLLIE, A.H., KERR, J.F.R. and CURRIE, A.R. (1980): Cell death : the significance of apoptosis. *Int.Rev.Cytol.*, 68, 251–306.

YAMAGAMI, T., MIWA, A., TAKASAWA, S., YAMAMOTO, H. and OKAMOTO, H. (1985): Induction of rat pancreatic B-cell tumors by the combined administration of streptozotocin or alloxan and poly (adenosine diphosphate ribose) synthetase inhibitors. *Cancer Res.*, 45, 1845–1849.

YAMAMOTO, K., FISHER, M.M. and PHILLIPS, M.J. (1985): Hilar biliary plexus in human liver. A comparative study of the intrahepatic bile ducts in man and animals. *Lab.Invest.*, 52, 103–106.

YAMAMOTO, K and OGAWA, K. (1983): Fine structure and cytochemistry of lysosomes in the Ito cells of the rat liver. *Cell Tissue Res.*, 233, 45–57.

YAMAMOTO, K. and PHILLIPS, M.J. (1984): A hitherto unrecognised bile ductular plexus in normal rat liver. *Hepatology*, 4, 381–385.

YAMAMOTO, H., UCHIGATA, Y. and OKAMOTO, H. (1981): Streptozotocin and alloxan induce DNA strand breaks and poly (ADP-ribose) synthetase inpancreatic islets. *Nature* (London), 294, 284–286.

YANOFF, M. and RAWSON, A.J. (1964): Peliosis hepatis. An anatomic study with demonstration of two varieties. *Arch.Pathol.*, 77, 159–165.

YOKOTA, S. (1985): Functional differences between sinusoidal endothelial cells and interlobular or central vein endothelium in rat liver. *Anat.Rec.*, 212, 74–80.

YOKAYAMA, S., SELLS, M.A., REDDY, T.V. and LOMBARDI, B. (1985): Hepatocarcinogenesis and promoting action of a choline-devoid diet in the rat. *Cancer Res.*, 45, 2834–2842.

YOON, J-W., LONDON, W.T., CURFMAN, B.L., BROWN, R.L. and NOTKINS, A.L. (1986): Coxsackie virus B4 produces transient diabetes in non-human primates. *Diabetes*, 35, 712–716.

YOSHIDA, A., IQBAL, Z.M. and EPSTEIN, S.S. (1979): Spontaneous pancreatic islet cell tumours in guinea pigs. *J.Comp.Pathol.*, 89, 471–480.

YOSHIMURA, S., KOMATSU, N. and WATANABE, K. (1980): Purification and immuno-histochemical localization of rat liver glutathione peroxidase. *Biochem.Biophys.Acta.*, 621, 130–137.

YU, B.P., MASORO, E.J., MURATA, I., BERTRAND, H.A. and LYND, F.T. (1982): Life span study of SPF Fischer 344 male rats fed ad libitum or restricted diets : Longevity, growth, lean body mass and disease. *J.Gerontol.*, 37, 130–141.

ZAFRANI, E.S., CAZIER, A., BAUDELOT, A-M. and FELDMAN, G. (1984): Ultrastructural lesions of the liver in human peliosis. *Am.J.Pathol.*, 114, 349–359.

ZBINDEN, G. (1981): New methods of screening for hepatotoxicity. In M.Davis, J.M.Tredger and R.Williams (Eds), *Drug Reactions and the Liver*, pp. 337–343. Pittman Medical, London.

ZIMMERMAN, H.M. (1978)a: The expressions of hepatoxicity. In: *Hepatotoxicity. The Adverse Effects of Drugs and other Chemicals on the Liver*. Chap. 4, pp. 47–90, Appleton Century Crofts, New York.

ZIMMERMAN, H.J. (1978)b: Classification of hepatoxins and mechanisms of toxicity. In: *Hepatotoxicity. The Adverse Effects of Drugs and other Chemicals on the Liver*. Chap. 5, pp. 91–121.

ZIMMERMAN, H.J. (1978)c: Drugs used in cardiovascular disease. In: *Hepatoxicity. The Adverse Effects of Drugs and Other Chemicals on the Liver*. Chap. 22, pp. 510–522. Appletone Century Crofts. New York.

ZIMMERMAN, H.J. (1981): Drug hepatoxicity: Spectrum of clinical lesions. In: M. Davis., J.M. Tredger and R. Williams (Eds), *Drug Reactions and the Liver*, pp. 35–53. Pitman Medical, London.

ZIMMERMAN, H.J. and LEWIS, J.H. (1987): Drug-induced cholestasis. *Med.Toxicol.*, 2, 112–160.

ZUCKER, P.F., CHAN, A.M. and ARCHER, M.C. (1986): Cellular toxicity of pancreatic carcinogens. *J.N.C.I.*, 76, 1123–1127.

IX. Urinary Tract

KIDNEY

Many therapeutic and diagnostic agents used in man can damage the kidney, although incrimination of a particular drug may be difficult because some disease processes for which drugs are used also adversely affect the kidney. Hypertension, dehydration, or fluid and electrolyte loss by vomiting also potentiate the nephrotoxic effect of drugs (Schreiner and Maher, 1965).

A paucity of renal tissue diagnoses of drug-induced changes in man leads to difficulties in the understanding of the pathological processes involved in renal toxicity in clinical practice. Although experimental studies in animals have provided understanding of direct toxic effects, they have been less helpful in our understanding of indirect mechanisms (Heptinstall, 1983a).

Renal changes are particularly liable to be observed in preclinical toxicity studies which employ excessive doses of highly active and novel therapeutic agents, in view of the fact that many drugs and chemicals or their metabolites are eliminated primarily by the kidneys.

The kidneys possess drug-metabolising activity. Mixed-function oxidases are present in the proximal renal tubules and can be selectively induced or inhibited by xenobiotics (Rush et al., 1983, 1986). Although the activity of these enzymes are generally less than in the liver and concerned more with phase II metabolism, they may be important in extrahepatic metabolism of drugs and play a part in the local generation of reactive metabolites responsible for renal toxicity (Litterst et al., 1975, 1977; Fry et al., 1978).

In addition, the kidney is rendered susceptible to toxic damage by virtue of its high blood flow and its potential to be exposed quickly to peak concentrations of chemicals, even those only present transiently in the circulation. Its high oxygen consumption makes it also sensitive to ischaemia and volume depletion. Its ability to concentrate toxic solutes in parenchymal cells and in tubular luminal fluid is a further risk factor (Schreiner and Maher, 1965). It has been aptly pointed out by Mudge (1984) that skeletal muscle, which is fairly resistant to the adverse effects of chemicals, also has a high blood flow but it is the unique

497

functional organization of the kidney which is of critical importance in its sensitivity to the damaging effect of xenobiotics.

In view of the sensitivity of the kidney in both man and animals to damage by therapeutic agents, a high degree of judgement is called for in the assessment of renal pathology or weight changes occurring in one or more of the test species in the preclinical evaluation of a potential new drug. It is essential to carefully evaluate the nature of the renal changes, if necessary using biochemical, cytochemical, ultrastructural or functional techniques. An assessment of the dose levels at which changes occur in the light of comparative pharmacokinetics and metabolism as well as intended use of the agent in man is also important.

Strain differences in sensitivity of renal tissue to drugs should also be considered and even difference between individual animals can be important. Within the same strain of Sprague-Dawley rats subgroups have been found which are more highly sensitive than others to the renal effects of drugs (Frazier et al. 1986a; Riviere et al., 1986). Animals with mild subclinical renal dysfunction are also more sensitive to renal effects of drugs than normal animals even when similar blood drug levels are maintained (Frazier et al., 1986a). Whereas a degree of nephrotoxicity at high doses in an animal model does not rule out administration to man in the relevant clinical situation at appropriate dose levels under carefully controlled conditions, a potential for renal toxicity may not be desirable in some therapeutic areas and raise sufficient additional hurdles to preclude effective development of a drug candidate. Studies which have attempted to address the predictive potential of animal studies for man have shown that renal changes in the rat often correctly predict clinical effects on the urinary system with a modest degree of overprediction (Lumley and Walker, 1986a, b).

The potential for non-renal factors to influence renal function should also not be forgotten. So called, pre-renal azotaemia, may be caused by disorders which decrease renal blood flow such as depletion of salt and water or severe depression of cardiac output. Post-renal causes include obstruction to urinary outflow or reduction in venous drainage.

Anatomy and physiology

A number of specific anatomical and physiological factors need to be considered in the histopathological evaluation of renal changes in preclinical studies and extrapolation of the results to man and it is worthwhile briefly reviewing them. A standard nomenclature for the complex structures of the kidney has been recently proposed, see Fig. 91 (Kriz et al., 1988).

In rat, mouse, hamster, rabbit and dog, the kidneys are unilobar (unipyramidal) whereas in man each kidney is composed of 10–14 lobes, the prominence of which are most marked in the foetus. The monkey kidney is generally like that of man, although it is unilobular in type (Horacek et al., 1984). Renal weight, as a correlate of body weight, varies greatly between species. Studies of renal weight among inbred strains of rats and mice housed under identical conditions have, however, demonstrated a close correlation between renal and body weight within a particular species (Hackbarth et al., 1981; Hackbarth and Hackbarth, 1981).

In the rodent, rabbit and dog the cortex forms a cap over the medulla. The medulla has the shape of a pyramid, the tip of which, the papilla, projects into the renal sinus. The cut surface of the pyramid appears striated and the striations extend into the cortex as medullary rays.

Blood supply

Each kidney is supplied by a main renal artery. On the right the main renal artery usually arises from the aorta more caudally than on the left side in rat, mouse, dog and man, although there is considerable individual variation.

In man, each renal artery divides into *segmental arteries* which give way to so called *interlobar arteries*, which then lead to *arcuate arteries*. For the unilobar kidneys of species used in toxicology, the term 'interlobar' is ambiguous and difficult to define, although interlobar arteries may be considered to be continua-

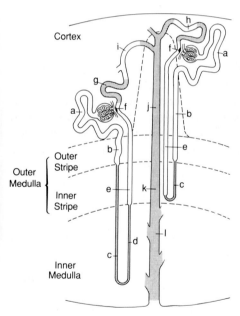

Fig. 91. Schematic diagram redrawn from Kriz et al. (1988) showing the standard nomenclature for the nephron as defined by the Renal Commission of the International Union of Physiological Sciences: (a) Proximal Convoluted tubule. (b) Proximal straight tubule. (c) Descending thin limb. (d) Ascending thin limb. (e) Distal straight tubule (thick ascending limb). (f) Macular densa located within the final portion of the thick ascending limb. (g) Distal convoluted tubule. (h) Connecting tubule. (i) Connecting tubule of the juxtamedullary nephron that forms an arcade. (j) Cortical collecting duct. (k) Outer medullary collecting duct. (l) Inner medullary collecting duct.

tion of the segmental arteries which give rise to arcuate arteries. The arcuate arteries traverse the renal parenchyma at the level of the cortico-medullary junction and give rise to *interlobar arteries*. The term '*cortical radial artery*' has been proposed in the standard nomenclature as more appropriate than 'interlobular artery' for describing these vessels (Kriz et al., 1988). These extend outwards to become *afferent arteries, glomerular capillaries*, and *efferent arteries*. Efferent arteries, which arise from glomeruli near the medulla, give rise to *arterial vasa recta* (spuria) through which the medulla receives most of its relatively poor blood supply. Arterial vasa recta turn back into *venous vasa recta* which drain into *arcuate veins* at the cortico-medullary junction. The efferent arteries arising from glomeruli near the cortex break up into rich interconnected peritubular network in the cortex. This network drains into the *interlobular veins* which also enter into arcuate veins.

The main structural and functional unit of the kidney is of course the *nephron*, composed of the glomerulus and the *renal tubule*. Its distal end is at the point it enters the *common collecting system* (Fig. 91).

Glomerulus

The glomerulus consists of a coil of specialized capillaries projecting into a capsular space (Bowman's capsule) which opens into the proximal convoluted tubule. Glomeruli show interspecies and strain variation in total number, distribution, size and microanatomy.

In adults of several laboratory species the number and size of glomeruli is a relatively constant function of body and kidney weight, although glomerular size relative to kidney weight may be smaller in the mouse than other laboratory species (Randerath and Hieronymi, 1958). Morphometric studies in two strains of Wistar rats have shown that the size of Bowman's capsule and the capillary tuft can vary between strain and generally increases in size with advancing age (Hackbarth et al., 1983). The study by Hackbarth and his colleagues (1983) confirmed that, in common with other species including man, the distribution of glomeruli in the renal cortex is not homogeneous but that there is a continuous decrease in glomerular density from the outer to inner zones. A higher number of glomeruli are located near the surface in young rats and certain strains such as the Munich Wistar strain (Hackbarth et al., 1983).

Electron microscopic examination of the glomerulus in a number of species has shown that there is a single basement membrane in the capillary tuft composed of a central lamina densa with less dense zones on either side, referred to as the lamina rara externa and lamina rara interna. Fine fibrils of variable width have been described in all layers of the basement membrane in several species as well as man, although they are arranged more compactly in the lamina densa than in the lamina rara. The relative prominence of these zones varies according to species. The basement membrane is thicker in human adults than either in children or laboratory animals (Karnovsky and Ainsworth, 1972). The basement membrane is also negatively charged because of anionic sites of glycosaminoglycans principally heparan sulphate in the lamina rara (Rennke et al., 1975; Farquhar and Kamwar, 1980; Kanwar and Farquhar, 1979).

A point of distinction between the basement membrane in man and laboratory species is the fact that C3 receptors are present in human glomeruli but scarcely, if at all, in animals. These receptors may affect immune complex deposition within the glomerulus (Shin et al., 1977).

Urine formation begins in the glomerulus with the elaboration of an ultrafiltrate across the walls of the glomerular capillaries. The glomerular filtration rate depends on the balance of hydrostatic and oncotic pressures acting across the capillary, the rate of plasma flow through the glomeruli and the permeability and the total area of the filtering capillaries (Brenner et al., 1976). It is, therefore, not surprising that there are considerable interspecies and strain differences in glomerular filtration rate. In various strains of rats and mice it has been shown that there are greater correlations between glomerular filtration rate and body weight than glomerular filtration rate and renal weight (Hackbarth et al., 1981; Hackbarth and Hackbarth, 1981). Proteins and other macromolecules are hindered at the glomerulus in proportion to their molecular size, shape and net charge. Molecules smaller than 25,000 daltons usually cross the glomerular barrier and attain concentrations in the glomerular filtrate of more than 50% of their concentration in plasma (Maack et al., 1979).

Renal tubule

The various parts of the renal tubule can usually be identified in routine haematoxylin and eosin stained sections although special stains such as PAS, lectin histochemistry, plastic embedded sections and ultrastructural examination allow greater precision (see Maunsbach, 1966; Rhodin, 1974; Schulte and Spicer, 1983). Cross sections of the proximal convoluted tubule are observed in routine sections around the glomeruli, cells being columnar and cuboidal with a brush border and granular eosinophilic cytoplasm. There is a wide variation in morphology of the proximal tubule between species, so care is needed in cross species generalisations (Bulger, 1986). However, ultrastructural study has defined three segments of the proximal tubule most clearly in the rat, S1, S2 and S3 or P1, P2 or P3 (Maunsbach, 1966; Jacobsen and Jorgensen, 1973). The S1 segment represents the first part of the convoluted tubule, possessing a thick well-developed brush border (2–3 μm in rats, 1 μm man and mouse), prominent endocytic vacuoles, a well-developed phagosomal system, numerous, elongated mitochondria and complex basolateral interdigitations. The S2 segment represents the remaining part of the convoluted tubule and the first part of the straight segment. In this segment, the brush border is shorter, lysosomal bodies are more prominent, mitochondria are fewer and there are fewer and shallower basolateral interdigitations than in the S1 segment.

The transition from S2 to S3 is abrupt in some species (rat and dog), but gradual in others such as the rabbit (Kriz et al., 1988). The S3 segment comprises the remaining proximal straight tubule in the medullary ray and outer stripe of the outer medulla. In the rat it shows an increase in brush border height but a less well-developed endophagocytic system. Basolateral interdigitations are sparse. For comparison between man, rat and mouse, see review by Trump et al., (1984a). The structure of these segments correlates with function. The S1 and S2 segments are primarily involved in solute and fluid reabsorption, coupled to sodium reabsorption mediated by sodium/potassium ATPase located in the highly developed basolateral membrane. The distal segment of the proximal tubule (S3) is particularly well endowed with enzymes of the mixed/function oxidase system, although less than in the liver, making it particularly sensitive to compounds which are toxic after metabolic activation (Dees et al., 1980).

The highly convoluted segment of the tubule ends before entering the medullary ray as the straight descending limb or pars recta before abruptly becoming the thin descending and ascending part of the loop of Henle in the medulla. The actual level at which the thin segment commences depends on the location of the nephron in the cortex. Juxtamedullary nephrons have long thin segments, with the turn located near the papilla, whereas nephrons located more superficially in the cortex have short thin segments located at varying levels within the outer medulla. The thin ascending limb becomes the thick ascending limb which returns to the cortex via the medullary ray. Traditionally, the thick ascending limb of Henle's loop is considered to end at the macula densa. However, ultrastructural evidence and the distribution of the specialized Tamm-Horsfall protein suggests that the transition between the ascending limb and the distal convoluted tubules is a little beyond the macula densa (Kriz and Kaissling., 1985; Kaissling et al., 1977). The distal tubules drain into the collecting duct system (Fig. 91).

Fluid reabsorption across the proximal tubule is isosmotic and accounts for about two-thirds of the glomerular ultrafiltrate. Under normal conditions one-third of the glomerular filtrate enters the descending limb of the tubule. The thin descending limb is highly permeable to water but not to sodium ions, so passive absorption of water occurs. Conversely, the ascending thick limb is impermeable to water but a large proportion of sodium chloride is reabsorbed in this segment by active transport of chloride ions (Burg and Green, 1973; Rocha and Kokko, 1973). In consequence, intratubular fluid entering the distal tubule is always dilute and the surrounding medullary interstitium hypertonic. The distal tubule and collecting ducts also reabsorb water under the influence of antidiuretic hormone in plasma. Salt reabsorption in this segment is enhanced by aldosterone.

The distal tubule which includes the thick ascending link of Henle's loop, the distal convoluted tubule and the collecting duct also shows both structural and functional heterogenicity. As the thick ascending limb extends from the medulla to cortex, the surface area of its apical plasma membrane increases whilst that of the basolateral membrane and its interdigitations decreases (Madsen and Tischer, 1986). The interdigitating cell processes contain numerous mitochondria that are closely associated with the basolateral plasma membrane.

The main function of both the ascending limb and the distal convoluted tubule is the absorption of sodium, potassium, chloride and divalent ions, a process which is dependent on the Na-K-ATPase that has been located in the basolateral membrane of the distal tubule (Madsen and Tischer, 1986). The collecting duct epithelium is composed of two distinct cell types: the principal cell and the intercalated cell.

The juxtaglomerular apparatus and the renin-angiotensin system

The functional anatomy of the renin-angiotensin system has been reviewed for pathologists by Lindop and Lever (1986) but see also Kritz and Kaissling (1985). Classically, the juxtaglomerular apparatus comprises afferent and efferent arterioles, complete with granular, renin-secreting cells, the macula densa, a specialized group of distal tubular cells and lacis cells (Goormaghtigh cells, polar cushion, extraglomerular mesangium cells). Lacis cells form a pyramid of small cells situated between the afferent and efferent arterioles, with its base on the macula densa and apex continuous with the glomerular mesangium.

Other epithelial cells situated between the visceral and parietal epithelial cells at the vascular pole of the glomerulus have also been described. These cells contain secretory granules devoid of immunoreactive renin (Ryan et al., 1979). Renal sympathetic fibres innervate the juxtaglomerular apparatus.

The juxtaglomerular apparatus can be considered as an anatomical unit which is important in tubuloglomerular feedback control of renal blood flow, glomerular filtration rate and possibly also tubular control of renin secretion (Barajas and Salido, 1986).

The most specific reaction in the renin-angiotensin cascade as well as the rate limiting factor in the generation of angiotensin II is the release of renin (Tree et al., 1985). Immunocytochemical study has confirmed that much of the renin in the kidney is localized in the outer media of the afferent arterioles but normally to a greater extent in superficial cortex than in juxtamedullary regions. It appears that renin release occurs outwards into the extravascular space and into renal capillaries (Lindop and Lever, 1986). Immunocytochemical demonstration of renin is a greatly superior method for the demonstration and localization of renin-containing cells than the previously used variations of Bowie's stain (Faraggiana et al., 1982).

Renin-secreting cells are also found in more proximal parts of the afferent arterioles and in interlobular arteries as well as in efferent arterioles (Taugner et al., 1982a, 1982b, 1983). Immunoactivity to renin is also found in tubular cells but this latter finding is a result of reabsorption of renin which filters through the glomerulus (Taugner et al., 1982a).

Immunocytochemical study of the distribution of angiotensin II in the mouse kidney has shown the distribution pattern similar to that of renin, suggesting that both renin and angiotensin II co-exist in the same cells (Taugner et al., 1983).

Interstitium

The interstitium forms a small proportion of total renal volume but it may be altered by many pathological states (Kriz and Napiwotzky, 1979; Bohle et al., 1979). It has been suggested that the increase in kidney weight during aging is largely due to an increased volume of the interstitium (Christensen and Madsen, 1978). It is composed of a matrix and a number of interstitial cells, which have been shown to be abundant in the rat renal medulla (Bohman, 1974).

Ultrastructural study of the rat kidney has delineated three type of interstitial cells in the medulla (Bohman, 1974). The first (Type I) is an irregular cell with long cytoplastic processes closely related to loops of Henle and capillaries. The cytoplasm of this cell contains variable numbers of lipid droplets and abundant rough endoplasmic reticulum. Type I cells, containing lipid droplets, have been associated with prostaglandin production although significant prostaglandin synthetase activity is also present in the collecting duct cells (Bohman, 1977). The second type of cell (Type 2) is rounded with a large nucleus, scanty cytoplasm which is devoid of long processes and lipid droplets but contains abundant free ribosomes and sparse endoplasmic reticulum.

The final type (Type 3), a flattened cell with thin cytoplasmic processes, is a pericyte related mainly to the vasa recta.

Renal pelvis

In species used in toxicology, the renal pelvis is an elaborately shaped chamber with folds which extend deep into the medulla to form specialised fornices and ridges of the medullary outer zone, termed secondary pyramids. It is believed that this anatomical arrangement is related to the ability to increase the osmotic ceiling of urine because higher papillary urea concentrations are found in mammals with specialised fornices than in those without them (Pfeiffer, 1968). The epithelium lining the renal pelvis appears to be important in the function of the renal pelvis. In the rat, in common with the hamster and mouse, transitional epithelium extends from the ureters to the insertion of the pelvis onto the renal parenchyma. It is fairly typical transition epithelium except for fewer cell layers, fewer apical fusiform vesicles, less pronounced deep invaginations and a less scalloped surface than in the bladder. Functionally, this epithelium appears to be relatively impermeable, similar to the transitional epithelium in ureter or bladder.

From the point of insertion of the pelvis, the thickness of the epithelium diminishes and cells become covered with short microvilli as shown by scanning electron microscopy (Verani and Bulger, 1982). Over the secondary pyramids some transitional cells remain but from the base of the true pyramid to the tip of the papilla there is only a single layer of cuboidal cells covered by microvilli similar to the relatively permeable papillary collecting ducts. This is consistent with a recycling function of this zone (Verani and Bulger, 1982).

Enzyme distribution in the nephron

Enzyme activity varies markedly in the different segments of the nephron. As the variations have considerable functional significance, knowledge of their distribution can be of considerable help in the study of drug-induced renal changes. Much of the precise information concerning enzyme distribution has been obtained by microdissection techniques (Schmidt and Guder, 1976; Guder and Ross, 1984), although enzyme cytochemistry is of help in the correlation of morphological changes with alterations in enzyme activities in toxicity studies (Faccini, 1982; Wachsmuth, 1984). Enzymes from the nephron may spill over into the urine where their activities may be monitored as non-invasive indicators of renal integrity both in animals and in man (Kluwe, 1981; Halman et al., 1985; Price, 1982). The study of urinary enzymes has proved of help in the assessment of the precise site and nature of cellular damage with different nephrotoxins (Josepovitz et al., 1985). Quantitative urine analysis including enzyme analysis in rats has been shown to be particularly sensitive in the screening of chemicals for nephrotoxic effects (Fent et al., 1988, Zbinden et al., 1988). Enzymuria in patients has been used to define a rank order of nephrotoxic potential of aminoglycoside antibiotics (Palla et al., 1985). The location of enzymes along the nephron has been reviewed in detail by Schmidt and Guder (1976) and more recently by Guder and Ross (1984).

It is established that fatty acids and acetoacetate are the main exogeneous fuels of respiration in the rat kidney cortex when available in physiological concentrations (Weidmann and Krebs, 1969). In contrast, the renal medulla possesses a rapid rate of aerobic and anaerobic glucose metabolism and probably depends mainly on glucose as a respiratory fuel (Lee and Peter. 1969; Abodeely and Lee, 1971). This glycolytic capacity, highest in the distal part of the nephron, is reflected by high levels of enzymes such as hexokinase and pyruvate kinase which catalyze reactions of glucose metabolism in this segment. By contrast, enzymes which characterize gluconeogenesis such as glucose-6-phosphatase are generally restricted to the proximal tubular cells. Enzymes involved in fructose and glycerol metabolism of the pentose phosphate shunt such as glucose-6-phosphate dehydrogenase are fairly well distributed throughout the nephron.

Mitochondria are unevenly distributed along the nephron. Mitochondrial density appears greatest in the thick ascending limb of the loop of Henle and the proximal convoluted tubule in the rat (Pfaller, 1982). Mitochondrial enzyme activity seems in general to parallel this distribution.

Not surprisingly, lysosomal enzyme activity is particularly high in the proximal tubular cells, reflecting the role of this segment in degradation of reabsorbed macromolecules. It is also of note that peroxisomes and peroxisomal enzyme activities are also prominent in the proximal renal tubular cell (Guder and Ross, 1984).

Of particular interest to the pathologist as cytochemical markers are the brush border enzymes, although their precise function is not well understood.

Alkaline phosphatase, 5'-nucleotidase and gamma-glutamyl transpeptidase activity increases towards the end of the the proximal tubule. In the rat, renal brush border enzyme activity decreases with advancing age (Nakano et al., 1985).

The proximal tubule contains the highest activities of enzymes involved in glutathione synthesis and degradation, as well as high microsomal mixed function oxidase activity and cytochrome P450, suggesting that the proximal renal tubule can be site of renal drug metabolism (Fry et al., 1978; Endou et al., 1982).

Study of renal mixed function oxidases in rats, mice and rabbits have shown that these enzymes vary in response to different inducers depending on the species and that induction of these renal enzymes may develop in different segments of the proximal tubules (Rush et al., 1983, 1986).

Immunocytochemistry

A variety of antisera to various antigens present in the kidney can be used to study renal changes in both laboratory animals and man.

Cell surface markers for the lymphocyte and monocyte populations have been used in the study of conditions such as experimental graft-host reactions in which lymphocytes infiltrate renal parenchyma (see Claesson et al., 1965). The theta or Thy-1 antigen has been shown to present on the surface of mesangial cells in the rat glomerulus and monoclonal antibodies to this antigen (e.g. 0X7) are useful markers for mesangial cells (Paul et al., 1984). In mouse kidney, Thy-1 antigen appears to be absent (Morris and Ritter 1980), whereas in the dog, Thy-1 has been localized in medullary tubular basement membrane (McKenzie and Fabre, 1981).

In the normal rat glomerulus, 35 to 70% of the mesangial population of mononuclear leukocytes express class II major histocompatability complex antigens. These can be demonstrated immunocytochemically by monoclonal antibodies to rat common leukocyte antigen (MRC 0X1) and rat Ia antigen (MRC 0X3 and 0X4) (Schreiner and Unanue, 1984; Gurner et al., 1986). Monoclonal antibodies to rat T cells and T cell subsets are also useful for identifying lymphocytic cells in the rat glomerulus (Eddy et al., 1986). In general, these surface antigens do not resist routine formalin fixation and paraffin embedding and, therefore, frozen sections must be used (see Haemopoietic and Lymphatic Systems, Chapter III).

A variety of other antigens resist formalin or other routine fixation and paraffin embedding and can be used as markers in renal tissue sections. Many of these antisera are readily available, particularly as many antisera, designed for use against human antigens, cross react with those in rat, mouse and dog. Examples of these include polypeptides such as atrial natriuretic factor (ANF) located in the renal collecting duct cells (McKenzie et al., 1985a), calmodulin, a calcium binding protein in the podocytes and/or mesangial cells as well as collecting duct cells (Seto-Ohshima et al, 1985), renin, present in the juxtaglomerular apparatus, myoepithelial cells of the renal arteries and afferent arterioles (Taugner et al., 1983; Lindop and Lever, 1986).

The unique Tamm-Horsfall proteins, localized at the surface membrane of the thick ascending limb of Henle's loop, have also been localized by immuno-cytochemical techniques (Bach and Bridges, 1982; Holthöfer et al., 1983). They appear to form a gel or aggregate in response to increasing concentrations of electrolytes and influence the permeability characteristics of the thick segment (Hoyer and Seiler, 1979). Antibodies to the various intermediate filaments such as the cytokeratins, desmin and vimentin, are also used to selectively stain nephron segments and mesenchymal cells (Holthöfer et al., 1983; Bachman et al., 1983).

Although renal excretory function cannot usually be determined with preci-sion using histological examination, there is some evidence to suggest that a functional and morphological correlate can be achieved using immunocytochemi-cal characterisation of renal tubular segments. Using point counting of tubules in human kidneys stained immunocytochemically for proximal brush border anti-gen and Tamm-Horsefall protein, Howie and colleagues (1990) demonstrated a correlation between the reciprocal of plasma creatinine concentration and ratios of tubules staining positively and negatively to these antigens. This suggests that more precise and sensitive localisation of tubular changes using immunocy-tochemistry has potential for characterization of functional renal alterations.

Immunocytochemical techniques can also be used to selectively stain for the presence of enzyme antigenic sites. In this way the presence of cytochrome P450 has been demonstrated in the proximal renal tubule in rats and other animals (Dees et al., 1980, 1982). Gamma-glutamyl transpeptidase has also been demon-strated in the brush border of proximal convoluted tubules by the use of monoclonal antibodies to this enzyme (Yasuda and Yamashita, 1985).

Lectin histochemistry

Over recent years peroxidase and fluorescence-labelled lectins have been used as histochemical probes for the localization of specific sugar groups or sequences in the kidney of various species including man and these probes represent useful tools in the study of renal changes in experimental studies (Schulte and Spicer, 1983; Murata et al., 1983).

It has been shown by a number of workers that there are consistent lectin staining patterns of the various segments of the nephron, although only some structures stain similarly in several species (Holthöfer, 1983; Schulte and Spicer, 1983). Also of considerable practical value is the fact that staining with labelled lectins can often be performed after paraffin wax embedding.

For instance, Arachis hypogaea (peanut) and Ricinus comminis (castor bean) labelled lectins, specific for β-galactose or N-acetyl galactosamine groups stain the S1 and S3 segments of the proximal tubule of the rat intensely whereas the S2 segment remains only poorly stained (Schulte and Spicer, 1983). Cortical collecting tubules of the rat also show intense but focal staining with these two lectins. By contrast, these lectins show only poor staining of the mouse proximal tubule. However, heavy staining of the brush border of the mouse proximal renal tubule occurs with another labelled lectin, Lotus tetragonolobus, which has α-L-fucose specificity. This lectin does not mark the rat proximal tubule (Schulte and Spicer, 1983).

In both rat and mouse, the glomerular endothelium as well as endothelial cells of other vessels, stain heavily with the labelled-lectin, Bandeiraea simplicifolia (BSA lB4) which has binding specificity for α-D-galactose. This is in contrast to the human endothelial cells which are labelled with Ulex europeus (UEA1), specific for α-L-fucose (Schulte and Spicer 1983; Holthöfer et al., 1983).

Prior sialidase digestion which removes terminal sialic acid groups reveals β-galactose residues in the glomeruli of both rats and mice which can then be stained with labelled-lectin specific for this group, peanut lectin (Arachis hypogaea) (Schulte and Spicer, 1983).

Labelled wheat germ lectin (Triticum vulgare), which possesses a nominal sugar specificity for sialic acid and N-acetylglucosamine, also binds to the capillary walls in the glomerulus of the rat as well as in the mouse, dog and man (Holthöfer, 1983). This staining pattern of the glomerular capillary loop probably reflects the presence of the major sialoprotein, podocalyxin on the renal glomerular cell. This protein possesses a molecular weight of 140,000, has a high affinity for wheat germ lectin, and binds peanut lectin after neuraminidase treatment (Kerjaschki et al., 1984). The N-acetylgalactosamine-specific lectin, Dolichos biflorus, also binds a common structure, the distal tubule, in many species including man (Holthöfer, 1983).

Although greater understanding of the functional significance of the cell membranes may result from the use of these techniques, they have empirical value for the pathologist in defining structural components in fixed tissue sections (Spicer and Schulte, 1982).

Renal weight changes

Little dispute exists concerning the importance of weighing the kidneys in preclinical safety studies, for it has been shown that this measurement compares favourably with various functional tests for renal toxicity (Kluwe, 1981). Increase in renal weight, associated with macroscopic evidence of swelling and pallor have been accepted as signs of renal toxicity for many years. However, histopathological examination is essential in the assessment of renal weight changes for increases in renal weight have not only been associated with renal tubular necrosis, but a wide variety of other renal changes such as the vacuolation following sucrose administration (Monserrat and Chandler, 1975), partial or total blockage of the nephron by drug crystal deposition or ligation of a ureter (Taylor et al., 1968).

It is common in toxicity studies for mild dose-related changes in renal weight to occur, unassociated with histopathological evidence of cell damage. These weight changes may be simply adaptive responses to the major physiological changes which can occur following administration of large doses of highly active pharmaceutical agents. These changes are perhaps analogous to those occurring following nephrectomy or administration of high protein diet in which increase in renal tissue mass occurs as a result of hypertrophy of the nephron (Fine and Bradley, 1985). Renal tubular hypertrophy has been linked to the elevation of the glomerular filtration rate and the altered tubular fluid flow which occurs in these circumstances (Finn, 1982; Fine and Bradley, 1985). Spontaneous diseases in laboratory animals such as amyloid deposition in the mouse and hamster and nephrosis in the rat, also produce renal weight changes.

Glomerular vacuolation

Various types of vacuoles can be seen in the glomerulus in toxicity studies. Occasional glomeruli in the normal Beagle dog may contain foam cells (Fig. 92). These cells contain lipid and are considered a normal variation of no pathological significance, although deposits may be more frequent in older obese dogs.

Vacuoles appear in the glomerulus after administration of drugs (Fig. 93). One example is doxorubicin (adriamycin). In the rat treated with doxorubicin, these vacuoles consist of variably sized, round, empty vacuoles in glomerular epithelial cells or podocytes, mainly in juxtamedullary zones (Bertani et al., 1982; Fajardo et al., 1980). The vacuoles are limited to the visceral epithelial cells but may

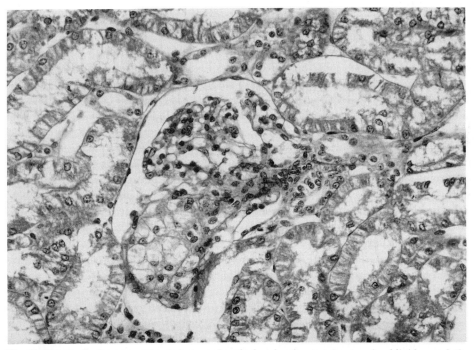

Fig. 92. Glomerulus from an untreated, young beagle dog showing spontaneous focal lipid vacuolation within the glomerular tuft. (PAS, ×400.)

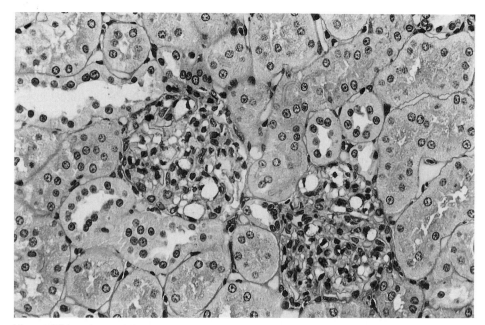

Fig. 93. Kidney from a Wistar rat showing a drug-induced form of glomerular vacuolation without evidence of tubular damage. (HE, ×400.)

affect cells lining Bowman's membrane (Giroux et al., 1984). Their precise pathogenesis remains uncertain, although it has been suggested that the formation of vacuoles may relate to changes in the plasma membrane of epithelial cells (Giroux et al., 1984). In the rat, the onset of renal lesions and cardiomyopathy is simultaneous, suggesting that the phenomena are independent of each other (van Hoesel et al., 1986).

The vacuolar glomerular changes in doxorubicin toxicity may be associated with tubular degeneration and interstitial inflammation. In the rat, a nephrotic syndrome may develop following anthracycline administration, which is associated with complex changes in plasma lipoproteins (Calandra et al., 1983). Structural alterations induced in the kidneys by anthracyclines were first noted in the Sprague-Dawley rat by Sternberg and Philips (1967) but have since been observed in other strains of rats and rabbits (Herman et al., 1985). Chronic glomerulonephritis, characterised by glomerular fibrinoid necrosis and fibrosis has also been reported in rats treated with anthracyclines (Sternberg et al., 1972). There are no clear descriptions of such changes occurring in man (Fajardo et al., 1980), where it appears that anthracyline-induced renal toxicity is uncommon (Herman et al., 1985). Studies in the LOU/M/WS1 rat have suggested that the nephrotoxicity produced by doxorubicin is quite independent of the cardiomyopathy produced by this agent (van Hoesel et al., 1986) (see Cardiovascular System, Chapter VI).

This is the most important spontaneous renal disease in laboratory rats although its prevalence and its age of onset varies considerably between strains (Gray et al., 1982, Solleveld and Boorman 1986) and it is usually more severe in males (Gray, 1977). Unfortunately, this disease process possesses a number of histological features which have the potential to confound results in toxicity and carcinogenicity studies. It can also reduce survival of rats in carcinogenicity studies to below acceptable limits.

In its established form, the disease is easy to recognize, being characterised macroscopically by enlarged pale kidneys, with a microcystic cut surface, visible to the naked eye. Microscopically, glomeruli show segmental sclerosis which can extend to involve the entire tuft (global sclerosis). There is usually little evidence of marked hypercellularity although mesangial thickening may be evident and epithelial cells can contain PAS-positive granules (Magro and Rudofsky, 1982). Bowman's capsule can also be focally thickened and accompanied by periglomerular sclerosis and fibrosis, but epithelial crescents are not seen.

Electron microscopic examination of the glomerulus shows considerable thickening of the capillary basement membrane. Swollen epithelial cells contain dense cytoplasmic droplets and exhibit partial fusion of foot processes but little or no change in mesangial or endothelial cells (Gray et al., 1974).

Histopathological changes extend to the renal tubules where casts are observed, tubular basement membrane is thickened and tubules are focally sclerotic with variable degeneration, basophilia, atrophy and dilatation. In advanced cases, the tubular cells show a variety of cytological changes including the accumulation of intracytoplasmic protein droplets, pigmentation, as well as hypertrophy and hyperplasia. The interstitium may also contain an inflammatory infiltrate. A mild fibroblastic reaction may be seen and wedge-shaped cortical scars have also been described (Gray et al., 1982).

Although these florid changes are easy to recognize, it is important to be aware of the features of mild disease for the focal tubular alterations in mild glomerulosclerosis may complicate the assessment of potential nephrotoxic agents. Mild changes can be seen in surprisingly young rats from some strains and can affect interpretation of short toxicity studies. Early sclerotic changes are found in scattered glomeruli, with mild focal tubular basophilia in areas near affected glomeruli, tubular basement membrane thickening and cast formation at the cortico-medullary junction (Gray et al., 1982).

The morphological features of focal glomerular sclerosis are associated with functional changes, notably increased glomerular basement membrane permeability and loss selectivity as shown by proteinuria. The degree of proteinuria increases with advancing age as the severity of the condition increases. Protein electrophoresis shows that albumin is the major urinary component but later a full spectrum of serum proteins can be demonstrated in the urine (Bolton et al., 1976).

The pathogenesis of this condition remains uncertain, despite the fact that it has been studied in some detail since the suggestion that it represents an appropriate model for focal and segmental glomerular hyalinosis and sclerosis which occurs in man in a variety of progressive kidney diseases (Couser and Stilment, 1975; Elema and Arends, 1975; Kreisberg and Karnovsky, 1978; Grond et al., 1986). Notwithstanding our incomplete knowledge of this condition, it appears to be primarily an age-related basement membrane dysfunction (Couser and Stilment, 1975) associated with changes in its amino acid composition and increased degrees of hydroxylation and glycosylation (Taylor and Price, 1982). Its onset can be accelerated and its severity increased by a variety of different factors including administration of high calorie or high protein diets (Newburgh and Curtis, 1928; Tucker et al., 1976; Everitt et al., 1982) salt loading (Elema and Arends, 1971; Koletsky, 1959; Jaffe et al., 1970) and hormonal factors, notably prolactin (Addis et al., 1950, Richardson and Luginbühl, 1976).

Large rats within the same study also appear to be at greater risk of developing nephropathy (Turnbull et al., 1985), whereas food or protein restriction retards or prevents its development (Everitt et al., 1982).

Its development has also been associated with changes in activity of the renin-angiotensin system and it has been suggested that spontaneous or induced changes in the chromaffin cells of the juxtaglomerular apparatus can initiate or exacerbate this condition (Magro and Rudofsky, 1982).

Over recent years a number of studies have shown that partial nephrectomy in rats also accelerates the appearance of glomerulosclerosis (Shimamura and Morrison, 1975; Grond et al., 1986). Studies have shown that early changes in partially nephrectomized rats consist of rounded or crescent like accumulations of homogeneous, hyaline-like, PAS-positive material under the endothelial cells, principally near the hilus of the capillar tuft and sometimes associated with foamy macrophages, lipid droplets and fibrin strands (Olson et al., 1985). Structural and functional studies in this model have tended to confirm previous suggestions that subendothelial deposition and mesangial overloading by macromolecular substances such as proteins, lipids and immunoglobulins is important in the development of this renal lesion by causing increased production of mesangial matrix and sclerosis (Grond et al., 1986). Local haemodynamic factors are particularly important. It has been suggested that ad libitum feeding or protein-rich diets contribute to the development of this nephropathy by their ability to produce sustained elevations in renal perfusion and glomerular filtration, a change which perhaps facilitates excretion of metabolic end products (Brenner, 1985; Goldstein et al., 1988).

A variety of pharmaceutical agents have also been shown to influence the prevalence and severity of glomerulosclerosis in rat toxicity and carcinogenicity studies.

For instance, the angiotensin inhibitor, captopril has been shown to inhibit the development of glomerulosclerosis at pharmacological doses (Hall et al., 1985). Interestingly enough, however, captopril has no ameliorating effect on renal damage induced by adriamycin treatment (Hall et al., 1986). There is also some evidence that it may improve renal function in certain forms of nephrotic

512

syndrome in man (Taguma et al., 1985), although conversely, high doses of captopril have been associated with the development of nephrotic syndrome and membranous glomerulonephritis (Case et al., 1980). A dramatic treatment-induced reduction in glomerulosclerosis was reported in the two year rat toxicity and carcinogenicity studies conducted with bromocriptine, a drug which selectively inhibits pituitary prolactin secretion (Richardson et al., 1984). This finding supports the concept that prolactin is involved in the development of glomerulosclerosis in rats (Richardson and Luginbühl, 1976). Dehydroepiandrosterone, an adrenal steroid, has also been shown to inhibit proteinuria development in aging Sprague-Dawley rats (Pashko et al., 1986).

A variety of drugs of widely differing types accelerate or advance the progression of glomerulosclerosis in the rat. For instance, this effect has been reported in the preclinical toxicity studies with the novel gastric antisecretory drug, omeprazole (Ekman et al., 1985), dazoxiben, a thromboxane synthetase inhibitor (Irisarri et al., 1985), ibopamine, a dopamine analogue (Casagrande et al., 1985) and cyclosporin A (Ryffel et al., 1983). The distinction between agents that produce this effect by exaggerated pharmacological alterations or physiological mechanisms from those which exacerbate rat renal disease by a direct toxic effect and renal tubular cell damage, calls for an extremely critical assessment of the preclinical findings. Whilst it is important to avoid falling into the trap of assuming that agents which exacerbate rat glomerulosclerosis in long term toxicity studies are completely devoid of nephrotoxic potential, it is probable that many drugs which exacerbate this condition at high doses, possess little or no nephrotoxicity in normal clinical practice.

Immune complex deposition and glomerulonephritis

Although immune complex deposition in the glomerulus and glomerulonephritis is not a common problem in the toxicity testing of conventional pharmaceutical agents, in certain situations treatment-induced glomerulonephritis is observed. It has become increasingly common in preclinical toxicity experiments to undertake the repeated intravenous injection or continuous infusion of complex macromolecules such as polypeptides, proteins and glycoproteins and these substances may be immunogenic and immune complexes may form in the circulation (Wilson et al., 1985). As the kidney is important in the filtration of macromolecules in view of its large surface area of endothelial cells relative to its weight (Schreiner and Maher, 1965), they may accumulate in the glomerulus and lead to glomerular injury.

Certain substances modulate the immune response and permit immune complex formation. Other chemicals modifying the antigenic determinants of endogenous macromolecules can also lead to autoimmune damage.

Damage to the glomerulus may result from subsequent activation of complement system either by the classical or alternative pathways with formation of membrane attack complex or production of potent neutrophil chemotactic factors (Couser et al., 1985).

513

Recent advances in immunology have brought about the realization that failure of mechanisms involved in tolerance to self-antigens, notably those involving T lymphocytes, can lead to excessive immune complex formation and autoimmune disease (Oliviera and Peters, 1989). The strong major histocompatibility linkage (MHC) of many autoimmune diseases is believed to stem from the way in which T lymphocytes interact with cell surface antigen, in particular the specific molecular interaction with MHC products. It is now realised that generation of immune complexes is a frequent occurrence in normal individuals and that abnormalities in the clearance of such complexes is also important in disease such as systemic lupus erythematosus (Oliviera and Peters, 1989).

A number of different factors have been shown to stimulate glomerular (mesangial) cell proliferation including interleukin 1, platelet derived growth factor, epidermal growth factor, insulin-like growth factor, as well as platelets which themselves contain many growth factors (Johnson et al., 1990).

The precipitating cause in individual cases of glomerulonephritis remains usually unknown. Its development in man has been associated with streptococcal, staphylococcal and pneumococcal infections, bacterial endocarditis, secondary syphilis, hepatitis B, malaria and neoplasia (Germuth and Rodiguez, 1973; Morrison and Wright, 1977; McCluskey, 1983).

Various types of glomerulonephritis have been reported after drug therapy in man (Curtis, 1979) although the membranous type appears most common (Hill, 1986). A syndrome resembling systemic lupus erythematosus with antinuclear antibodies may be triggered by drugs such as hydralazine, procainamide and a variety of anticonvulsants (Alarcon-Segovia, 1976; Hill, 1986). Clinical features of drug-induced lupus are similar to those of the natural disease. It is also an immune complex-type glomerulonephritis. The mechanism for the initiation of the condition by drugs is not clear, although it probably resides in the antigenicity of the drugs or their capacity to act as haptens (Alarcon-Segovia, 1976).

Evidence of drug-induced immune complex glomerulonephritis has also appeared in man during treatment with levamisole (Hansen et al., 1978; Hoorntje et al., 1980), gold salts (Törnroth and Skrifvars, 1974) mercurial agents, certain anticonvulsants, captopril (Hill, 1986) immune stimulants and adjuvants, Corynebacterium parvum (Dosik et al., 1978), mycobacteria (Krutchik et al., 1980; Davies, 1986) and penicillamine (Gartner, 1980). The pathology of penicillamine-induced nephropathy has been particularly well studied and it illustrates a drug which can induce both main types of glomerulonephritis. In one type, cellular proliferation is slight or absent but the glomerular basement membrane may show spikes and electron microscopic examination reveals subepithelial electron dense deposits. Immunofluorescence shows a granular pattern of IgG and C3. The features are similar to idiopathic membranous glomerulonephritis, although the mechanism for the production of immune-complexes remains unclear (Gartner, 1980; Heptinstall, 1983a). A second form of glomerulonephritis with crescents with many of the features of Goodpastures syndrome (antibasement membrane disease) has also been reported following treatment with penicillamine (Gibson et al., 1976). Captopril, in common with penicillamine, contains a sulphydryl group which may be a factor in the induction of glomerulonephritis by these agents.

Interferon A has also been implicated in the development of nephrotic syndrome in man, associated with minimal change nephropathy although the precise pathogenesis also remains obscure (Averbuch et al., 1984; Selby et al., 1984).

Susceptibility to these drug-induced immune complex disorders in man is influenced by the major histocompatibility complex and this has undoubtedly implications for the prediction of these effects occurring following treatment with novel drugs. Associations have been reported between systemic lupus erythematosus induced by hydralazine and HLA-DR4 antigens as well as pro-teinuria produced by gold salts in rheumatoid arthritis patients and HLA-DRW3 or HLA-B8 antigens (Batchelor et al., 1980; Wooley et al., 1980). However, other interrelationships are important. For instance, the development of systemic lupus erythematosus is also more common in female patients and the poor acetylator phenotype (Batchelor et al., 1980).

Some compounds are also believed to produce glomerular damage in man by direct injury, although the evidence for this is largely based on animal experiments.

Glomerulonephritis in animals

Virtually all species of animals develop glomerulonephritis. It can be primary or secondary to a variety of disease processes including bacterial, parasitic and viral infections (Casey and Splitter, 1975; Morrison and Wright, 1977), neoplasia (Müller-Peddinghaus and Trautwein, 1977a), derangements in the immune system (Theofilopoulos and Dixon 1981) and administration of therapeutic agents. In parallel with the influence of genetic factors and the MHC complex in autoimmune disorders in man, development of glomerulonephritis in animals, including that induced by xenobiotics, is highly species and strain dependent.

Glomerulonephritis: dog In the dog, primary glomerular disease represents one important disease responsible for persistent proteinuria, another being amyloidosis, which is generally limited to older dogs (Slausen and Lewis, 1979). Glomerulonephritis can affect fairly young dogs, even beagle dogs under one year of age (Guttman and Anderson, 1968; Robertson 1986). Its prevalence is uncertain for subtle changes, detectable in semithin plastic embedded sections, may be overlooked in haematoxylin and eosin stained, paraffin embedded sections (Müller-Peddinghaus and Trautwein, 1977 a,b). Several morphological types of glomerulonephritis occur in dogs, although it is not certain whether they have distinct causes.

A pure membranous form exists in which there is little or no proliferation in the mesangium but the glomerular basement membrane is thickened and may show subepithelial spike formation. Immunofluorescence studies have shown focal or granular deposits of IgG and C3 in both types (Müller-Peddinghaus and Trautwein, 1977a).

The membrano-proliferative type is characterized by mesangial proliferation or sclerosis with a thickened but split glomerular basement membrane, also with deposits of IgG and C3. Finally, a mesangial-proliferative form has been described in which the glomerular basement membrane is essentially unaltered but there is proliferation of mesangial cells and mesangial deposition of IgG and C3. It is this latter type which occurs more commonly in young dogs and it has been suggested that the mesangial proliferative glomerulonephritis represents an early form of other types of glomerulonephritis (Müller-Peddinghaus and Trautwein, 1977a). This is perhaps not surprising in view of the importance of mesangial cells in the processing of macromolecules. For this reason the mesangial cells may represent the first site of damage following deposition of immune complexes (Kashgarian, 1985).

There appears to be no direct correlation between canine glomerulonephritis and interstitial nephritis which is also common in the dog (see below). The cause of glomerulonephritis in the dog is uncertain but it has been associated with extra-renal lesions, including heart worm infestation (Dirofilaria immitis) (Casey and Splitter, 1975), neoplasia, hepatic disease, pyometria and endometriosis. Its prevalence increases with age (see reviews by Müller-Peddinghaus and Trautwein, 1977b; Slausen and Lewis, 1979). Many breeds of dogs may also be affected by a syndrome resembling systemic lupus erythematosus in man and mouse (see below), including glomerulonephritis associated with basement membrane thickening and electron dense deposits composed of IgG and complement (Lewis, 1977). Although antinuclear antibodies have been produced in pure bred beagle dogs by treatment with hydralazine or procainamide for periods of many months, drug-induced disease did not develop and the dogs remained healthy (Balazs et al., 1981; Balazs and Robinson, 1983).

Subclinical glomerulonephritis has also been described in dogs treated with high doses of ampicillin. The lesions were characterised by focal mesangial hypercellularity, granular glomerular deposits of IgG, C3 and some IgM as well as electron-dense deposits both in the mesangium and subendothelial locations (Wright and Nash, 1984). These changes are believed to be immunologically mediated due to the presence of high molecular weight, immunogenic molecules associated β-aminopenicillanic acid nucleus. These are common to many penicillins and may occur as a result of reaction of degradation products or polymers of the penicillin molecule with autologous proteins making them immunogenic (Shaltiel et al., 1971). Immunologically mediated renal damage as a result of penicillin or penicillin derivatives have also been reported in man, although this is typically a nephritis of interstitial type (Linton et al., 1980; Appel et al., 1981).

Glomerulonephritis: mouse A number of mouse strains, the most familiar of which is the inbred New Zealand Black (NZB) mouse, spontaneously develop a disease which possesses many of the manifestations of systemic lupus erythematosus (SLE) in man. These models have been extensively studied and the

516

results have helped in the understanding of the human syndrome (Schwartz, 1981). The expression of the syndrome is variable among the different predisposed strains of mice. It may not only comprise glomerulonephritis but also haemolytic anaemia, necrotizing polyarteritis of renal and coronary arteries and arthritis. Arthritis presents with swollen joints and there is degeneration of articular cartilage, pannus formation and proliferation of synovium. There may also be thymic atrophy, especially marked in the cortex associated with cystic medullary hyperplasia. Hyperplasia of lymph nodes, circulating anti-DNA and antilymphocyte antibodies and immune complexes including those of retroviral origin are also found (Andrews et al., 1978).

The glomerular changes vary with the age and stage of development of the lesions as well as with the strain of mouse. The changes can be acute with an active proliferative glomerulonephritis and accompanying infiltration by polymorphonuclear leukocytes. A subacute proliferative form may develop with proliferation of endothelial and mesangial cells, occasional crescents and basement membrane thickening. There also may be a more classical obliterative lesion in the NZB/W female mouse, comprising heavy mesangial proteinaceous deposition and generalized cellular proliferation (Andrews et al., 1978). Immunofluorescent study shows granular deposits of IgG and C3 in glomerular capillary walls, mesangium and tubulo-interstitial zones. Murine retrovirus has also been found in the glomerular deposits, although the precise role of viruses in its pathogenesis remain uncertain (Andrews et al., 1978).

Murine lupus erythematosus as well as that in man appears to represent not a single disease but rather a syndrome brought about by a complex interaction of genetic and environmental factors on the immune system (Steinberg et al., 1981; Theofilopoulos and Dixon 1981; Schwartz, 1981).

The progression of this disease process in NZB mice can be accelerated by certain therapeutic regimens, notably treatment with interferon (Heremans et al., 1978). The mechanism for such acceleration remains unknown although it has been suggested that impurities such as foreign proteins or residual viral components in the injected substances may be responsible (Heremans et al., 1978). However, NZB/NZW mice treated with the synthetic interferon inducer, tilorone, also showed accelerated development of glomerulonephritis (Walker, 1977), suggesting a direct effect of interferons.

Glomerulonephritis has also been induced by interferon in young laboratory mice of other strains. This is characterized by mesangial thickening and proliferation, thickening of capillary loops and accumulation of focal and segmental granular deposits of IgG, IgM and C3 within the mesangium and along the basement membrane (Gresser et al., 1976). In advanced disease marked hyalinization, large subendothelial deposits and epithelial crescents were described (Gresser et al., 1976, 1981). In more formal toxicity studies with interferon, electron-dense glomerular deposits without inflammation have also been observed. These changes are presumably also the result of immune complex deposition or formation in the renal glomerulus.

The relevance of these experimental findings in safety assessment of the

517

interferons remains uncertain. Although several different interferons are being used in man and have a variety of side-effects, glomerulonephritis seems to be of relatively little clinical importance for both interferons produced by purification or recombinant DNA technology (Priestman, 1980; Scott et al., 1981; Spiegel et al., 1986; Talpaz et al., 1986).

Other agents, used in man, have also produced glomerulonephritis in the mouse. Corynebacterium parvum has been used in patients with malignant disease because of its stimulatory effects on the immune system, increasing antibody production, activating complement and stimulating interferon (Milas and Scott, 1978). However, its use in man was associated with nephrotoxicity, probably due to immune complex glomerulonephritis (Dosik et al., 1978). When Corynebacterium parvum is injected into mice, a mesangio-proliferative glomerulonephritis occurs, characterized by mesangial proliferation, thickening of capillary loops, small foci of necrosis, polymorphonuclear accumulation and occasional crescents (Uff et al., 1981). There was ultrastructural evidence of mesangial and subendothelial dense deposits with deposition of basement membrane-like material between deposits and endothelial cells and immunocytochemical evidence of complement deposition. A segmental necrotizing arteritis was also described. The glomerulonephritis induced in the mouse by this agent appeared to be of immune complex type. Although the antigen responsible was not identified, it may have been a component of the bacteria injected or the powerful adjuvant activity of the agent may have stimulated a response to other antigens (Uff et al., 1981).

Studies examining the effects of mercuric choride, gold sodium thiomalate and D-penicillamine in mice have shown that development of antinuclear antibodies and glomerulonephritis is highly strain dependent (Robinson et al., 1983, 1984; Joseph et al., 1986). Experiments in a series of 10 inbred strains of mice showed that only one strain, the ASw/SnJ bearing the specific $H-2^s$ (murine major histocompatibility complex) haplotype, was capable of developing autoimmune responses following chronic administration of mercuric chloride, gold sodium thiomalate and D-penicillamine, although even this strain appeared resistant to the induction of similar responses by hydralazine or procainamide (Joseph et al., 1986). Affected mice developed autoantibodies against nuclear components. Microscopic examination of the kidneys revealed dilation of the glomerular capillary loops with accumulation of eosinophilic material, proliferation of the mesangium and glomerular capsular cells with immunofluorescent evidence of immunoglobulin deposition in the tuft.

These studies emphasized that the strain-sensitivity to the autoantibody-inducing effects of drugs is selective for certain chemical structures. Joseph and colleagues (1986) suggested that their results in mice were analogous to findings in man where autoimmune effects of gold salts and D-penicillamine are linked to HLA haplotypes which are different from those associated with hydralazines and procainamide where the slow acetylator phenotype is an important risk factor (Batchelor et al., 1980). Recent experiments with mercury-induced immune complex disease in the sensitive BALB/c strain have shown that T-function is important in the strain sensitivity to development of renal immune complex deposition and that immunocomplex disease can be prevented by prior administration of a cyclophosphamide (Hultman and Eneström, 1989).

Finally, it is of note that mouse strains which do not normally develop overt glomerulonephritis, may show immune complex deposition in the glomeruli. These deposits may be granular or smooth and linear in nature distributed along the capillary wall or in the mesangium and most commonly IgM, but also IgG and IgA with complement. Their incidence increases in age, and they may be associated with mild proteinuria (Markham et al., 1973). They develop less commonly in germ free mice. The actual antigens involved remain uncertain but it has been suggested they are the result of an immune response to natural viral antigens nuclear or other endogenous tissue antigens (Markham et al., 1973).

Glomerulonenephritis: rat   The most common spontaneous glomerular condition in the rat is of course glomerulosclerosis (see above). Although immunofluorescence studies have demonstrated deposits of complement and immunoglobulins, particularly IgM in the glomerular capillaries in this condition (Bolton et al., 1976), there is little evidence that they represent evidence of immune complex disease but rather incidental findings (Elema and Arends, 1975).

Much more rarely, frank necrotizing glomerulonephritis is reported in aged untreated rats (Kroes et al., 1981), although this condition has not been described in detail.

Despite the relative rarity of spontaneous glomerulonephritis in the rat, the rat has been extensively used for the experimental induction of glomerulonephritis as a model for the human disease. Two main types of glomerular disease have been produced experimentally in rats, one following the deposition of antigen-antibody complexes from the circulation (immune complex disease), the other a result of antibodies directed against antigenic determinants within glomerular basement membranes (antiglomerular basement membrane antibody disease).

Immune complex disease: rat

The classic form of immune complex disease is serum sickness, which may result from the injection of a single large amount of foreign protein such as bovine serum albumin (acute serum sickness) or repeated injections of foreign protein or serum (chronic serum sickness). Much work with serum sickness has also been performed in the rabbit. Although chronic serum sickness is less easily produced in the rat by simple intravenous injection of foreign protein, it can be produced by prior subcutaneous immunization with bovine serum albumin in incomplete Freund's adjuvant followed by repeated injections of the antigen (Arisz et al., 1979). In the early phase, glomerular changes are characterized by mild mesangial hypercellularity and mesangial deposits of IgG, C3 and bovine serum albumin or other injected antigens. After the onset of proteinuria, there is diffuse proliferation of endocapillary cells, accumulation of polymorphonuclear leukocytes, focal thickening of glomerular capillary walls and segmental fibrinoid necrosis, in the absence of crescents. Fine and coarse granular deposits of IgG, C3 and bovine serum albumin (or other foreign protein) may be seen by fluorescence microscopy. Electron microscopic examination shows subepithelial, subendothelial and occasional intramembranous and mesangial electron dense deposits, and loss of epithelial foot processes (Arisz et al., 1979).

The second form of immune complex disease is characterized by glomerular deposits which contain complexes composed of auto-antibody and autologous antigens (autologous immune complex disease, Heymann Nephritis) which was originally produced by intraperitoneal injection of rats with homologous kidney homogenates in Freund's adjuvant (Heymann et al., 1959). This model has been extensively studied and it has been shown that it can be induced by minute quantities of renal tubular antigen preparations given in Freund's adjuvant (Edgington et al., 1968). It therefore appears that the immunizing preparation does not provide a source of antigen which forms glomerular deposits but that immunization stimulates the production of auto-antibodies and these react with autologous antigens. There has been some debate whether circulating complexes form or whether auto-antibodies are directed against constituents of the glomerular basement membrane but it now appears that the latter is more likely (McCluskey, 1983). The antigen is probably a 300 kd brush border protein, also expressed by the glomerular epithelial cell, located on the subepithelial side of the glomerular basement membrane and epithelia of several other organs (Assmann et al., 1985, 1986).

Histologically, Heymann nephritis is very similar to human membranous glomerulonephritis being characterized by thickening of the glomerular capillary loops, spikes on the epithelial side of the basement membrane in silver methenamine stained sections, and granular, electron dense deposits of IgG (Alousi et al., 1969). The development of immune complex nephritis can be influenced by immunization schedule, type of adjuvant, the nature of the antigen and the strain of rat used. Lewis rats are very sensitive to its development, Fischer rats less so and Sprague-Dawley rats are more resistant (Watson and Dixon, 1966).

An immune complex model of mesangioproliferative glomerulonephritis can be induced in Lewis rats by injection of a Thy-1 antibody (Johnson et al., 1990). This antibody binds Thy-1 antigen on mesangial cells resulting in a complement-mediated mesangiolysis followed by mesangial hypercellularity.

Administration of the simple chemical, mercuric chloride, to some strains of rat can also produce glomerulonephritis and immune derangements which are believed to be comparable to drug-induced autoimmune disorders in man (Weening et al., 1981).

Antinuclear antibodies, with granular immune complex deposition along the glomerular basement membrane have been demonstrated in PVG/C rats (Weening et al., 1978, 1981). By contrast, a biphasic autoimmune glomerulonephritis characterized initially by antiglomerular antibasement membrane antibodies and linear IgG deposition along the glomerular capillary walls followed by granular

IgG deposits of an immune complex glomerulonephritis has been demonstrated in Brown Norway rats (Pelletier et al., 1988). Lewis rats appear resistant to this type of mercury-induced effect (Pelletier et al., 1984).

The precise pathogenesis is uncertain, but mercury has high affinity for the kidney, is able to form covalent bonds with sulphur groups and has been shown to produce a T-lymphocyte-dependent polyclonal activation of B-cells in Brown Norway rats (Pelletier et al., 1988).

Anti-glomerular basement membrane antibody disease: rat (Masugi nephritis)

This is an experimental glomerular disease produced by intravenous injection of heterologous antibodies against glomerular basement membrane, usually in rats and rabbits (McCluskey, 1983). The condition possesses two phases, one which begins shortly after injection and results in the fixation of the antibodies to the glomerular basement membrane (heterologous phase), and the second which begins several days later when host antibodies combine with the heterologous gamma-globulin in the basement membrane (autologous phase). Both types of immunoglobulin can be demonstrated in a continuous linear pattern, characteristic of anti-basement membrane disease. This contrasts with the granular deposits found in immune complex disease.

Histologically, glomerular changes are dependent on the type and source of antigen and the test animal strain or species. Early changes are characterized by accumulation of mononuclear cells in glomerular capillaries, swelling and focal detachment of endothelial cells, followed by neutrophil infiltration (Kreisberg et al., 1979). This is associated with loss in negative charge from the lamina rara interna and fenestrated endothelium as demonstrated by staining with colloidal iron (Kreisberg et al., 1979). Later changes include hypercellularity of the tufts as a result of mononuclear cell infiltration, deposition of fibrin in Bowman's space, breaks in the glomerular basement membrane, capsular adhesions and crescent formation, although the latter is easier to produce in the rabbit than in other species (Shigematsu and Kobayashi, 1971, 1973; Thomson et al., 1979; Kondo and Akikusa, 1982). The dose of antibody, however, may be critical in the development of crescents which are composed of proliferating epithelial cells associated with macrophages (Morley and Wheeler, 1985).

Many of these models, especially those in the rat, employ adjuvants, particularly Freund's complete and incomplete adjuvant. When these substances are injected alone into the rat, glomerulonephritis may result. Freund's complete adjuvant is composed of a mineral oil, an emulsifier and Mycobacterium tuberculosis or butyricum. When the mycobacteria are omitted the mixture is referred to as an incomplete Freund's adjuvant.

This glomerulonephritis is characterized by proliferation of endothelial and mesangial cells, and neutrophil infiltration (Heymann et al., 1959; Cuppage 1965; McCluskey and Vassalli, 1969).

Finally, it is of note that normal rats develop mesangial deposits of immunoglobulins which can be detected using immunofluorescence techniques as early as at five days of age (Goode et al., 1988). In young rats, these deposits are unaccompanied by complement, supporting the concept that they represent filtration residues of circulating macromolecules which constantly perfuse the normal kidney (Goode et al., 1988).

Bowman's capsule: high cuboidal epithelium (metaplasia, hyperplasia, adenomatoid transformation)

The parietal layer of Bowman's capsule is usually lined by a layer of simple squamous epithelium but high cuboidal epithelium, similar to the proximal tubular epithelium is reported in man, mouse and rat.

In the mature male mouse this cuboidal epithelium is commonly seen and its prevalence seems to be influenced by age and circulating levels of testosterone (Crabtree, 1941). Long-Evans rats also seem more predisposed to develop this type of Bowman's capsule (Jakowski, 1982). It appears to be more prevalent in spontaneously hypertensive rats than in their normotensive counterparts, but in both strains its prevalence increases with advancing age (Haensly et al., 1982). It is not clear whether this predisposition in the hypertensive rat is a result of hypertension (Haensly et al., 1982). In man, tubular-type epithelium lining Bowman's capsule has been reported in association with malignant disease but it has also been described in normal subjects (Ward, 1970; Chappell and Phillips, 1950; Eisen, 1946; Eulderlink, 1964; Reibord, 1968). The parietal epithelium may also show hypertrophy and hyperplasia in advanced glomerulonephrosis of rats (Peter et al., 1986). This structural change within Bowman's capsule should be distinguished from artefactual herniation of proximal tubular cytoplasm into the glomerular capsular space which can occur under certain fixation conditions (Murray, 1979).

Amyloidosis

Amyloidosis of considerable severity occurs in the kidneys of the hamster and the mouse, although the rat remains generally unaffected by this disease (see Haemopoietic and Lymphatic Systems, Chapter III). In both mouse and hamster, the glomeruli are frequently involved. In severe cases, particularly in the hamster, renal tubules and collecting ducts may be surrounded by amyloid or massive interstitial formation of amyloid can develop in the renal papilla. Extensive secondary degenerative changes occur in the tubules which become dilated and develop casts. The histological picture may superficially resemble glomerulosclerosis in the rat. Ultrastructural study of the kidney reveals extensive involvement of mesangial cells and the capillary basement membrane by amyloid fibrils.

Although rhesus monkeys are also liable to develop amyloidosis, the kidneys are not frequently involved (Blanchard et al., 1986).

Drugs and chemicals influence the development of amyloid (see Haemopoietic and Lymphatic Systems, Chapter III). For instance, it has been reported that colchicine can prevent the development of renal amyloid in both man and experimental animals, although the precise mechanism remains uncertain (Shirahama and Cohen, 1974; Zemer et al., 1986).

Severe amyloidosis, in the hamster, may be associated with hyperplasia of the epithelium in the renal pelvis (Pour et al., 1979).

Tubular necrosis

Acute renal failure associated with tubular necrosis occurs in man following a variety of different insults including hypotension, blood loss, shock, dehydration, crush injury, infections, transfusion incompatability, as well as following administration of therapeutic and diagnostic agents, notably aminoglycoside antibiotics and radiographic contrast media (Solez et al., 1979). Two groups of tubular lesions have been defined, those in which there is a direct adverse effect by chemical agents on the tubule, principally the proximal convoluted tubule and those which are associated with renal ischaemia (Solez, 1983).

Although a lesion which results from a direct chemical insult on the tubular cell is of obvious concern to the toxicological pathologist, ischaemia-related injury has nevertheless important implications in the interpretation of renal tubular damage. It is this second type of lesion which has generated the most conflicting ideas about pathogenesis, reflected by the variety of different names applied to the tubular lesions: traumatic necrosis, lower nephron nephrosis, vasomotor nephropathy, post ischaemic acute renal failure and ischaemic nephropathy. This latter type has generally been considered to be a patchy focal necrosis not limited to the proximal tubule (Oliver et al., 1951). More recent work on renal oxygen deprivation has helped understanding of the pathophysiology of this anoxia-related tubular damage (see review by Brezis et al., 1984a). It has been shown in perfusion experiments that the medullary thick ascending limb of Henle's loop is particularly at risk from ischaemic damage, particularly because this part of the nephron normally operates on the verge of anoxia (Brezis et al., 1984a). Ischaemic lesions are prominent in the thick ascending limbs which are most removed from vascular bundles, situated in parts of the outer medulla close to the junction with the inner medulla. Furthermore, as in other organs, it has also been shown that oxygen deficiency in this region is related to demand as well as supply, a principle which has important implications in the understanding of certain drug-induced damage of the kidney.

The thick ascending segment is impermeable to water and involved in active transport of chloride ions. Inhibition to this cell transport activity with agents such as furosemide or ouabain can protect against ischaemic damage in the perfused kidney (Brezis et al., 1984b). By contrast, agents such as the polyene antibiotics, amphoteracin or nystatin which increase membrane permeability and stimulate the sodium pump, reproduce extensive anoxic-like lesions in the medullary thick ascending limb of Henle's loop (Brezis et al., 1984c).

Hypoxia also causes damage to proximal tubules although the S3 segment is particularly sensitive to ischaemia and reflow injury (Shanley et al., 1986). As the straight segment of the proximal tubule of the rat nephron is sensitive to the toxic effects of the immunosuppressive agent cyclosporin A, it has been suggested that this may be due, in part to tissue anoxia as a result of reduction in glomerular filtration rate, mediated by the renin-angiotensin system or other mechanism affecting renal blood flow (McKenzie et al., 1985; Whiting et al., 1985). A similar phenomenon may be responsible for tubular changes found after high doses of angiotensin-converting enzyme (ACE) inhibitors (MacDonald, 1984).

Further complicating factors can alter the final expression of cell damage. For instance, Tamm-Horsfall protein normally localized in the thick ascending limb may be released by damaged tubular cells and obstruct distal tubules (Hoyer and Seiler, 1979). Defective solute reabsorption in the thick ascending limb activates tubuloglomerular feedback mechanism. Tubular necrosis allows backleak of toxic substances (Brezis et al, 1984a). Regional impairment to blood supply as a result of endothelial damage, derangements in viscosity and coagulation, tubular swelling, release of humoral mediators or activation neural reflexes (Frega et al., 1976; Mason and Thiel, 1982; Solez et al., 1980a).

These considerations are important in the evaluation of tubular necrosis. Although necrosis may be confined to the proximal segment, the changes may extend to or be found exclusively in other nephron segments or in the collecting ducts. In addition to the intrinsic toxicity of an agent, toxicity depends on a variety of other influences notably pharmacokinetic factors such as the maximum concentrations achieved and the duration of high drug levels in the tissues. Careful assessment of the nature and distribution of the renal tubular changes is necessary, using, where appropriate, special stains, plastic sections, electron microscopic examination, enzyme cytochemistry and immunocytochemistry, quantitative and semi-quantitative analysis, in the context of the type of agent and dosage schedule. Assessment of mitotic activity in the tubules is also helpful (Charuel et al., 1984).

Although use of more sensitive techniques may make the delineation of a clear no-effect dose level more difficult, they allow a more complete picture of the changes to be built up and a firmer basis from which to extrapolate such findings of importance to man (Faccini, 1982).

Affected tubules show a variety of histological changes which are not only dependent on the nature of the insult but also on severity and the time at which the tissues are taken for study. Damaged tubules are frequently dilated and lined by flattened cells with basophilic cytoplasm, hyperchromatic irregular nuclei or nuclei in mitosis. Amorphous eosinophilic material or cellular debris may be present in the tubular lumens. Casts also accumulate in the distal segments and collecting tubules. Oedema and inflammation may be seen in the interstitium. Although glomeruli are usually spared, cells lining Bowman's capsule can show microscopic changes similar to those occurring in the tubules. Tubular necrosis may be accompanied by other cytoplasmic changes, such as vacuolation or hyaline droplet formation (see below).

Gentamycin and other aminoglycoside antibiotics have been widely used as experimental agents for producing tubular necrosis particularly in the rat. It is generally believed that the effects of gentamycin in the rat closely resemble those occurring in man, particularly because the pharmacokinetics of gentamycin is similar in the two species (Hottendorf and Williams, 1986). Rats treated with gentamycin develop fairly typical tubular necrosis involving the proximal tubule. This is characterized histologically by cytoplasmic degeneration and necrosis with formation of protein casts, tubular regeneration with a variable degree of interstitial round cell infiltration and fibrosis. Hyaline droplets may also be numerous in affected proximal tubular segments (Frazier et al., 1986a,b). Indeed, the earliest ultrastructural change is an increase in the size and number of *secondary lysosomes* (*myeloid bodies, myelinoid bodies, myelinosomes*) in the proximal tubular cell cytoplasm in both experimental animals and in man (Kosek et al., 1974; Haughton et al., 1976; Spangler et al., 1980; Ghadially, 1982; Jao et al., 1983). These myeloid bodies are characteristically composed of membrane-bound, osmiophilic structures containing concentrically arranged smooth membranes, believed to be lysosomal in nature (Ghadially, 1982; Jao et al., 1983). It has now become clear that there is preferential uptake of aminoglycoside antibiotics in the renal cortex followed by slow, inconstant release (Silverblatt and Kuehn, 1979; Kaloyanides and Pastoriza-Munoz, 1980; Morin et al., 1980; Charuel et al., 1984). The primary route of uptake into the cortex is reabsoption from the proximal tubular lumen through the brush border by endocytosis and incorporation into lysosomes. As the aminoglycoside accumulates in the lysosomes, myeloid bodies appear, probably as a result of the impairment of biodegradation of complex polar lipids (Kaloyanides and Pastoriza-Munoz, 1980; Aubert-Tulkens et al., 1979). As dosing continues, lysosomes continue to take up aminoglycoside, enlarge and finally appear to rupture with release of myeloid bodies into the tubular lumen and concomitant tubular cell damage. It has not been clearly established whether lysosomal disruption is an essential part of the process of tubular cell damage (Whelton and Solez, 1982).

Gentamycin produces similar morphological changes in the kidneys of dogs. It has been shown that changes induced by gentamycin in dogs can be increased, if renal function is impaired by subtotal surgical nephrectomy (Frazier et al., 1986b).

Tubular dilation, cystic change

In histological sections of kidneys from repeated dose toxicity studies in which there has been an adverse effect on renal tubules, necrotic cells may not be evident, but tubules may appear dilated and lined by flattened epithelial cells. Under these circumstances the term 'tubular necrosis' can be avoided and the changes described as tubular dilatation or tubular cystic change. Frequently, these changes are the expression of a milder but chronic adverse effect on renal tubular cells causing tubular cell degeneration and loss with ongoing repair. They need to be distinguished from simple tubular dilatation without cell degeneration.

Cystic changes have been striking in rats following chronic treatment with lithium (Christensen and Ottosen, 1986), and in rats, hamsters and dogs treated with agents such as modified starches, sugar alcohols, lactose and synthetic polydextrose, which modify calcium absorption and calcium renal excretion (Newberne et al., 1988). Tubular dilatation has also been reported in the kidneys of rats following a temporary period of ischaemia produced by vascular manipulation or administration of a single dose of serotonin (Koletsky, 1954; Sheehan and Davis, 1960; Murray, 1979).

In rats, chronic hypokalaemia has been associated with renal tubular dilatation due to luminal obstruction by hyperplastic and hypertrophic changes of the epithelium in the collecting ducts (Oliver et al., 1957). Potassium depletion induced in young rabbits by certain long-acting adrenal corticosteroids has also been linked to the development of progressive cystic changes in the cortical nephrons (Perey et al., 1967). It has been suggested that similar phenomena may be the cause of the association between hypokalaemia, aldosteronism and renal cysts in human patients (Torres et al., 1990).

In chronic toxicity studies performed in dogs and rats with angiotensin-converting enzyme (ACE) inhibitors, tubular dilatation is also reported (Goodman et

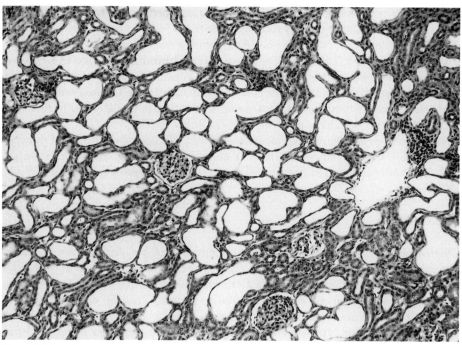

Fig. 94. Kidney from a beagle dog treated with an excessive dose of an angiotensin converting enzyme (ACE) inhibitor showing marked but characteristic tubular dilatation described with this type of agent. (HE, ×150.)

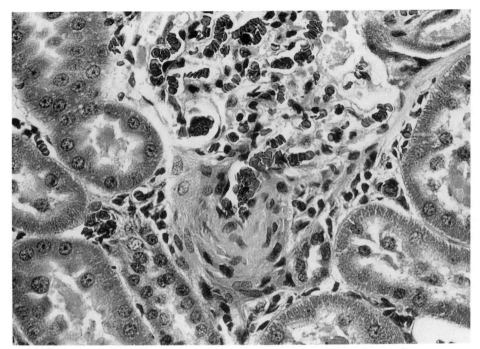

Fig. 95. Kidney from a Wistar rat treated with a high dose of an ACE inhibitor showing marked hyperplasia of the juxtaglomerular apparatus. (HE, ×550.)

al., 1985; Bagdon et al., 1985). High doses of ACE inhibitors produce this type of cystic dilatation of renal tubules, particularly in juxtaglomerular nephrons in both dogs (Fig. 94) and rats. This has been associated with histological evidence of renal tubular cell degeneration or necrosis, interstitial oedema and increased blood urea as well as juxtaglomerular hyperplasia (Fig. 95) (Bagdon et al., 1985; Goodman et al., 1985; MacDonald et al., 1987). As these effects can be potentiated by concomitant administration of hydrochlorthiazine and alleviated by saline supplementation and as their distribution within the kidney shares characteristics of ischaemic damage, it has been postulated that they result from excessive renal haemodynamic changes rather than a direct nephrotoxic effect (MacDonald, 1984; MacDonald et al., 1987). The beagle dog seems more sensitive to this type of effect than the rat.

High doses of some diuretics alone elicit similar renal changes. These are also more pronounced in the dog than in the rat and can also be alleviated by electrolyte replacement. Studies in which dogs were given high doses of the diuretics, furosemide or muzolimine, for periods of 13 or 52 weeks, dose-dependent increases in blood urea and creatinine as well as cystic dilatation of distal tubules were observed. Affected tubules were lined by flattened epithelial cells and contained occasional desquamated cells (Garthoff et al., 1982).

In addition, mild interstitial round cell infiltration, focal fibrosis and subcapsular cyst formation were observed after chronic treatment with these diuretics, although addition of electrolytes in the drinking water reduced these effects. Kief and Westen (1980) noted that these changes can occur in the dog kidney following doses of furosemide which are considered to be within the therapeutic range.

The fact that electrolyte and consequent fluid volume replacement alleviates the renal changes is fully compatible with the concept that they are secondary to excessive electrolyte and water loss, rather than the result of primary, drug-induced tubular damage.

Tubular vacuolation

Tubular vacuolation is seen under a variety of circumstances in preclinical toxicity studies and may indicate the presence of increased water (hydropic change), fat (fatty change), glycogen or other substances. Hydropic change, characterized histologically by swollen tubular cell cytoplasm which is pale staining and sometimes granular in appearance may be seen sporadically in the proximal renal tubules in aged rats dying from spontaneous disease. A similar histological picture has been described in an autopsy series in man, associated with conditions such as congestive cardiac failure, abdominal complications of peritonitis, ileus and fistulae as well as cirrhosis, which were often complicated by hyponatremia, hypochloremia and uraemia (Brewer, 1961). The vacuolation of proximal renal tubular cells, which occurs in potassium deficient humans, does not appear to occur in hypokalaemic rats (Alpern and Toto, 1990).

Tubular cell vacuolation is also seen in both patients and laboratory animals following administration of hypertonic sugar solutions and dextrans (Maunsbach et al., 1962; Monserrat and Chandler, 1975; Trump and Janigan, 1962). Ultra-structural study has shown that the vacuoles occurring after administration of sucrose solutions are large and pale bounded by a simple membrane and show acid phosphatase activity, features suggestive of lysosomes (Maunsbach et al., 1962; Trump and Janigan, 1962).

Although the precise pathogenesis of the hydropic changes following administration of hypertonic solution remains uncertain, the early appearance of droplets under the brush border of the renal tubular cell, has led to the suggestion that they result from pinocytosis of the injected carbohydrates (Maunsbach, 1966). More recently, a study injecting tritium labelled dextran into the rat and using a dextran-retaining fixative for renal ultrastructural study has confirmed lysosomal accumulation of dextran, although lysosomal functions such as protein catabolism do not appear to be altered. The changes appear to be fully reversible (Monserrat and Chandler, 1975).

An important point here is that despite this mild morphological renal changes, acute, reversible renal failure may result from infusion of dextrans in man or laboratory animals, particularly when there is compromise of the circulatory system. It has been shown in man that infusion of dextran 40 (average molecular weight 40,000, range 10,000 to 80,000) can induce acute renal failure in the presence of atherosclerotic vascular disease which is rapidly reversible by removal of dextran by plasmapheresis (Moran and Kapsner, 1987). A similar phenomenon has also been reported following dextran infusion in laboratory animals when there is constriction of the renal arteries (Mailloux et al., 1967). It has been postulated that administration of dextrans produces a hyperoncotic state in the cirulation leading to an increase in negative oncotic forces within the glomerular capillaries, which retard fluid movement into Bowman's space (Moran and Kapsner, 1987). If the positive hydraulic forces promoting fluid movement into Bowman's space are also reduced by vascular disease on narrowing of renal arteries, glomerular filtration may cease and acute renal failure becomes clinically evident.

Clear vacuoles as a result of abnormal accumulation of glycogen, the so-called 'Armanni-Ebstein' lesion are found in the renal tubular epithelium of diabetic patients and rats. Their prevalence and severity correlate with blood glucose levels. In diabetic rats, these vacuolated cells are located mainly in the distal convoluted and cortical collecting tubules and appear as swollen, clear cells with prominent cell boundaries and condensed nuclei (Tsuchitani et al., 1990). Cells stain with PAS and electron microscopy reveals abundant cytoplasmic glycogen granules.

Tubular vacuolation has been reported following the administration of nitrilotriacetate, a chelating agent, although the mechanism for the formation of the vacuoles may not be the same as the sucrose and dextran type of vacuolation (Merski and Meyers, 1985).

Tubular vacuoles may also represent lipid which is lost in the routine preparation of histological sections. The normal kidney contains appreciable amounts of lipid although there is considerably interspecies variation. In toxicity studies, fatty droplets (fatty change) are most commonly observed as a normal variation in the beagle dog where both proximal and distal tubular cells may be laden with fine vacuoles of fat.

Vacuolation of the renal tubules is also observed in association with frank tubular necrosis. A good illustration of this phenomenon occurs in the rat given cyclosporin A. Tubular vacuolation is observed at light microscopic level in the straight segment of the proximal tubule. This appears to be the result of dilatation of both smooth and rough endoplasmic reticulum (Blair et al., 1982; Whiting et al., 1982; Ryffel et al., 1983; Ryffel and Mihatsch, 1986). Vacuoles are also seen in the proximal-tubular cells in rats treated with the nephrotoxic agent cisplatin (Bulger and Dobyan, 1984). This serves to underline that in the assessment of any tubular vacuolation, a careful search for tubular damage should be undertaken.

Crystal deposition, crystalluria

Compounds or metabolites of low solubility may precipitate in the concentrated filtration fluid in the nephron, particularly in the context of high-dose toxicity studies. As urine concentrates mainly in the distal nephron, crystals are most likely to be found distally (Figs. 96 and 97). This is a point of distinction between

529

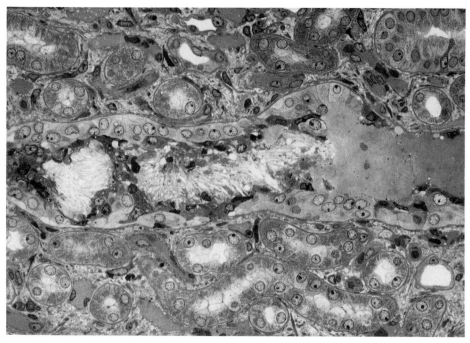

Fig. 96. This and the following figure demonstrate the clarity of cytological detail achieved with semithin plastic embedded sections. This represents the renal papilla of a cynomolgus monkey from a 28-day toxicity study in which administered drug or its metabolite was deposited as crystals within the collecting tubules. The crystals dissolved from the tissues during processing leaving these clefts in the section. By courtesy of Dr N.G. Read. (Methylene blue, ×500.)

crystals of drug or metabolite and crystalloid structures in lysosomes which are found in proximal tubular cells. Crystal deposition has been reported for a number of drugs notably the sulphonamides and severe obstructive nephropathy with cell damage can result both in laboratory animals and in man (Appel and Neu, 1977; Zbinden, 1969). Quinolone antibiotics may also produce crystalleria and crystal deposition when high doses are administered to rats and dogs (Corrado et al., 1987; Mayer, 1987; Schlüter, 1987). Deposits of metabolites of low solubility also occur after administration of purine analogues (Zbinden, 1969) and adenine (Farebrother, 1984).

More recently, an acyclic purine nucleoside analogue, acyclovir, produced dose-related crystal deposition in the distal part of the nephron in rat intravenous toxicity studies (Tucker et al., 1983). Birefringent crystals were seen in fresh frozen tissue sections, although in routine formalin fixed section, only crystal clefts were observed. These crystals were deposited principally in collecting tubules and ductules in the papillae and were accompanied by focal tubular dilatation, tubular cell hyperplasia with a variable interstitial inflammatory response and foreign body giant cell formation. Overlying transitional epithelium was hyperplastic. Although the cortex and outer medullary did not contain

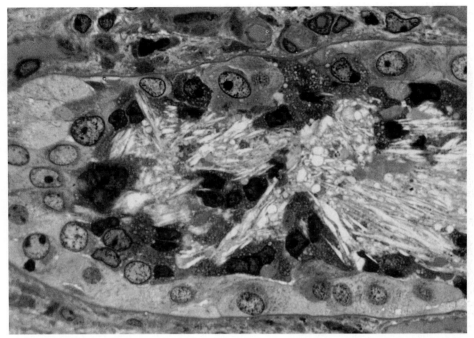

Fig. 97. Higher power view of section seen in Fig. 96. By courtesy of Dr N.G. Read. (Methylene blue, ×1200.)

crystal deposits, tubules were focally dilated and showed focal atrophy. Glomeruli were also be focally shrunken within distended and thickened Bowman's capsules. Ultrastructural study revealed increased numbers of lysosomal bodies in both proximal and distal tubules.

Although it was suggested by Tucker et al. (1983) that the rat was particularly susceptible to deposition of acyclovir crystals because it normally produces concentrated urine, similar changes were also observed in the dog treated with intravenous acyclovir. Furthermore, high intravenous bolus doses of acyclovir in patients with severe Herpes simplex infections have produced adverse effects on renal function, probably due to a similar mechanism (Brigden et al., 1982).

Crystalluria which is pH-dependent and obstructive nephropathy is reported in rats, dogs and primates treated with high doses of the quinolone antibiotics, although renal toxicity appears to be uncommonly associated with their therapeutic use in man (Corrado et al., 1987; Mayer 1987; Schlüter, 1987).

Another example was reported in cynomolgus monkeys but not rodents treated with an investigative benzopyran-4-one, a brain dopamine autoreceptor agonist, PD 119819. The kidneys of treated animals contained highly birefringent drug crystals which were primarily located in the proximal renal tubules (Macallum et al., 1988, 1987). The nephrons also showed extensive tubular degeneration and associated acute and chronic inflammation (Figs. 98 and 99).

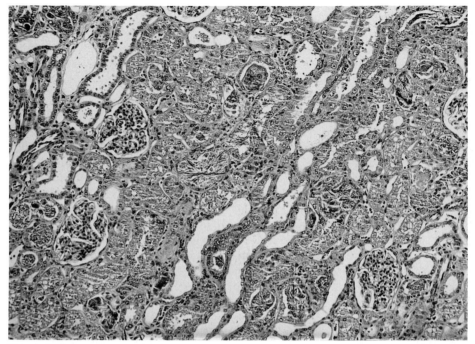

Fig. 98. Kidney of a cynomolgus monkey treated with PD 119819, a novel dopamine autoreceptor agonist as described by Macallum et al., (1989). In this field crystalline deposits of drug have formed within the renal tubules and have provoked disruption and damage to tubular epithelium. (HE, ×150.)

There was also a dose-related rise in blood urena nitrogen and creatinine. Although PD 119819 possessed good aqueous solubility, it was practically insoluble at alkaline pH. It was postulated that sufficient concentrations of drug were achieved in the alkaline milieu of the proximal tubule for crystallization to occur in this way (Macallum et al., 1989).

Hyaline droplets

Dense eosinophilic, 'hyaline droplets' of variable size are seen in the cytoplasm of the cells of the proximal tubule both in man and experimental animals under a number of circumstances. They may be particularly prominent in untreated male rats (Logothetopoulos and Weinbren, 1955). They also form in male rats following the injection of a variety of proteins, immunoglobulin light chains and after systemic administration of drugs and chemicals. Examples include volatile hydrocarbons (Oliver, 1954; Sumpio and Hayslett, 1985; Fajardo et al., 1980; Phillips and Cockerell, 1984; Alden et al., 1984), the established anthelmintic and immunomodulator, levamisol, a pyrazoline antiflammatory, BW 540c and a naphthoquinone antimalarial, BW 58c (Evans et al., 1988; Read et al., 1988).

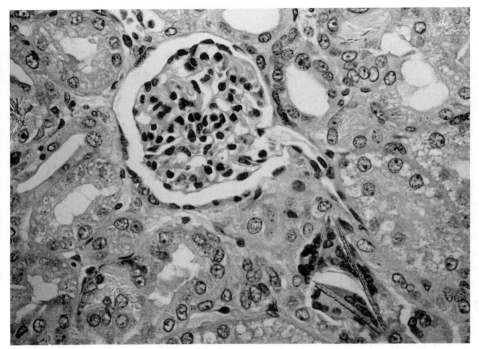

Fig. 99. Higher power view of the same case seen in Figure 98 showing the presence of needle-like drug crystals and a foreign-body giant cell reaction. (HE, ×550.)

They have also been described in the rat following administration of a cellulose used as a food additive (Hjortkjaer et al., 1986) and in rabbit kidneys with obstructed renal veins (Sheehan and Davis, 1960).

Much of our understanding about hyaline droplets and their relationship to renal protein handling extends from the work of Oliver, Straus and colleagues who studied the excretion of protein in the rat, a species in which this process is marked (Oliver et al., 1954, 1955; Straus, 1954, 1956, 1964; Sumpio and Hayslett, 1985). The kidney is an important site of uptake and catabolism of low molecular weight proteins such as albumin, immunoglobulin light chains, complement protein D, lysozyme, insulin, growth hormone, parathyroid hormone and glucagon (Maack et al., 1979; Rabkin and Kitaji, 1983; Sanders et al., 1987).

The main pathway for the extraction of proteins from the circulation is by glomerular filtration and the amount of protein reaching the urinary space is dependent on glomerular filtration rate, plasma concentration and the physicochemical characteristics of the protein (Sumpio and Hayslett, 1985). The degree of renal uptake is inversely related to molecular size of the protein (Maack et al., 1979). The majority of protein within the tubular fluid is taken up into the proximal renal tubular cell by endocytosis. Absorbed proteins within endocytotic vacuoles are transported to regions of the cell rich in lysosomes where fusion takes place and hydrolysis to aminoacids occurs. Aminoacids are

533

then returned to the circulation. It appears that it is the disturbance of this balance, either by increased filtered loads of proteins or their decreased catabolism, which results in accumulation of protein as ('hyaline') droplets in lysosomes (Maack et al., 1979). Thus, the mere presence of increased numbers of hyaline droplets in renal tubules does not in itself indicate cell damage but rather proof of functional and structural integrity; at least until a point is reached at which the adaptive responses of the cell is exceeded and cell damage results.

Although hyaline droplets are seen in the proximal tubules in both sexes of all species including man, the male rat appears particularly liable to show these changes, both spontaneously and after treatment with drugs and chemicals. This appears to be principally due to the presence of a specific protein, α_{2U} globulin which is the major normal male rat urinary protein, synthesized by the liver under synergistic control of testosterone and endogenous corticosterone (Irwin et al., 1971; Alden et al., 1984). Although humans excrete proteins of a similar nature to α_{2U} globulin, they are only in trace amounts (Olson et al., 1990). This protein, possessing a molecular weight of 18 to 20,000 daltons, is filtered freely by the glomerulus and reabsorbed by the proximal tubular cell in adult but not immature male rats (Irwin et al., 1971). Immunocytochemical study has shown that α_{2U} globulin is localized mainly in the S2 segment of the male rat proximal tubule (Stonard et al., 1986). Protein tracer studies using ovalbumin have also shown that in the proximal tubule of the rat kidney, the rates of reabsorption and catabolism of ultrafiltrate protein are higher in females than in males, demonstrating a lower capacity for renal protein handling in male rats (Asan et al., 1986).

In rats, hyaline droplets appear of variable size, rounded and densely eosinophilic in haematoxylin and eosin stained sections. In plastic embedded sections stained with toluidine blue they are particularly easy to identify by their dense blue staining (Fig. 100). Ultrastructural examination shows the droplets to be membrane-bound and to contain crystalloid structures composed of arrays of an ordered electron-dense lattice with distinct periodicity (Fig. 101), features suggestive of crystalline protein or other macromolecular substances (Maunsbach, 1966). These hyaline bodies also possess high levels of lysosomal enzyme activity (Fig. 102), supporting the concept that they are intimately associated with lysosomes (Oliver et al., 1955; Straus, 1956; Maunsbach, 1966; Read et al., 1988). Their presence in rats also correlates with renal cortical patterns of low molecular weight proteins determined by two dimensional gel electrophoresis (Kanerva et al., 1987).

Hyaline droplets which form in the male rat or ovariectomized female rats treated with testosterone after administration of volatile hydrocarbons or other xenobiotics, attain much larger sizes and contain prominent angular crystalloid structures visible in haematoxylin and eosin stained sections and prominent with Mallory-Heidenhain stain or toluidine blue stained resin-embedded sections (Fig. 100) (Phillips and Cockerell, 1984; Alden et al., 1984; Dodd et al., 1987; Kanerva et al., 1987; Bomhard et al., 1988; Swenberg et al., 1989). With high doses of these agents the tubular cell cytoplasm becomes overloaded with droplets and

534

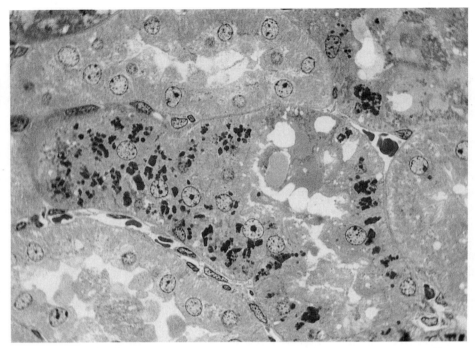

Fig. 100. Proximal renal tubule from a male Wistar rat showing the typical angular appearance of xenobiotic-induced hyaline droplet accumulation. Although hyaline droplets are not easily visible in routinely embedded, haematoxylin-stained sections, they are prominent in this toluidine blue-stained section. Some early tubular degeneration is also evident. Similar, but smaller droplets may be seen in untreated rats. (Resin-embedded, toluidine blue, ×550.)

crystalloid structures with consequent loss of cytoplasmic integrity, cell death and repair which is manifest in histological sections by small regenerative basophilic foci in the tubular epithelium. Granular cellular debris may also accumulate as casts and dilate tubules at the junction of the inner and outer bands of the outer medullary zone. Studies with tritiated thymidine have shown a marked increase in the labelling index in proximal tubular cells, although other segments show increased cell turnover (Short et al., 1986).

The precise cause of the massive accumulation of hyaline droplets after administration of hydrocarbons has not been elucidated, although biochemical study shows that they contain α_{2U} globulin (Alden et al., 1984). Immuno-cytochemical study of treated male rats has also confirmed an increase in α_{2U} globulin in the S2 segment of renal tubular cells and its extension into S1 and S3 segments which normally do not contain α_{2U} globulin (Stonard et al., 1986). For this reason, the term 'α_{2U} globulin nephropathy' has been employed to describe these changes (Swenberg et al., 1989).

Although it has been suggested that the presence of these droplets may represent increased production of α_{2U} globulin by the liver, it seems more

535

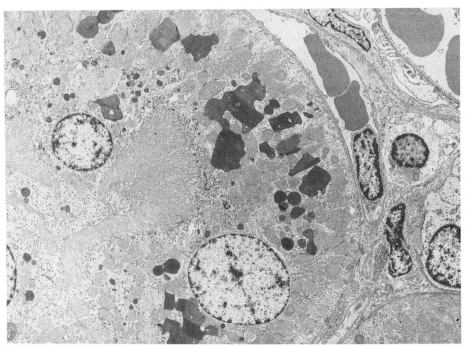

Fig. 101. Transmission electron micrograph of a renal tubule from a Wistar rat treated with levamisole, 75 mg/kg/day for 14 days. Typical, moderately electron-dense globular and angular crystalloid inclusions similar to those seen in Figure 100 are seen. Illustration by courtesy of Dr N.G. Read. (EM, ×4500.)

probable that the mechanism is related to binding of hydrocarbon and α_{2U} globulin within tubular cell lysosomes and their accumulation because the complex is poorly catabolized (Alden, 1986; Swenberg et al., 1989). This concept is supported by the presence of entirely normal hepatic levels of α_{2U} globulin in treated male rats (Viau et al., 1986).

Treatment of male rats for long periods with hydrocarbons which produce massive accumulation of these droplets with subsequent increased proximal tubular cell death and cell turnover may potentiate rat renal disease (glomerulosclerosis), development of proliferative lesions of tubular cells, primary renal adenomas and adenocarcinomas (MacFarland 1984). The significance of these longer term effects in the rat for man remains uncertain (Trump et al., 1984b). It has been suggested that increased human risk would probably only occur if exposure to these agents were sufficient to produce increased tubular cell proliferation (Swenberg et al., 1989).

Urinary enzyme measurements in male rats after oral administration of decalin, a prototype volatile hydrocarbon have shown increases in lactate dehydrogenase associated with increased excretion of aspartate aminotransferase and N-acetylglucosamidase as the cytoplasmic droplet accumulation becomes marked

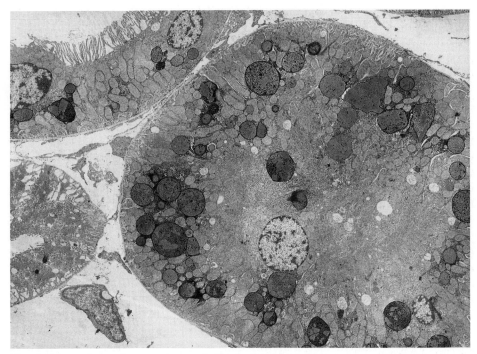

Fig. 102. Transmission electron micrograph illustrating the localisation of acid phosphatase in a rat proximal renal tubular cell containing hyaline droplets. The reaction product is distributed around the matrices of the inclusions, confirming their lysosomal nature. Illustration by courtesy of Dr N.G. Read. (EM, ×3500.)

and associated with single cell degeneration in the tubular epithelium (Evans and Morgan, 1986). These results are compatible with the concept outlined above, that renal tubular cell damage occurs only when droplet accumulation becomes excessive.

Hyaline droplets which form in rat tubules following injection or perfusion of proteins may be more numerous than those found spontaneously, but they possess identical morphological and cytochemical characteristics. However, different proteins may possess different nephrotoxic potentials. For instance, perfusion of rat kidneys with human immunoglobulin kappa light chains of molecular weights between 20 and 50,000 daltons was associated with acute tubular injury, as well as droplet formation, whereas albumin was devoid of this effect (Sanders et al., 1987). The reason for this difference was unclear, although their individual physicochemical properties are probably important in this respect. Kappa immunoglobulin light chains may also produce acute tubular injury in man (Case records of Massachusetts General Hospital, 1984).

Similar morphological changes may also be observed in the male rat following administration of pharmaceutical agents (Figs. 100, 101 and 102). These changes may also be a result of binding of drug with lysosomal constituents in the proximal tubule which impairs their catabolism (Peter et al., 1986).

Male but not female Wistar rats developed hyaline droplets in the proximal renal tubules following administration of three unrelated pharmaceutical agents, levamisole an anthelmintic, BW 58c a naphthoquinone antimalarial and BW 540c a pyrazoline antiflammatory drug (Read et al., 1988). Droplets were similar to those observed in hydrocarbon treated rats, developing in males, mainly in S1 and S2 tubular segments and only in severe cases in the S3 region. Ultrastructural cytochemical study showed that the droplets possessed lysosomal enzyme activity and immunocytochemical examination revealed the presence of α_{2U} globulin (Read et al., 1988). Rats treated with levamisole also showed increased urinary excretion of asparate aminotransferase and N-acetylglucosamidase similar to that found in rats treated with the volatile hydrocarbon, decalin (Evans et al., 1988).

The precise cause for the hyaline droplet accumulation with these three agents was not identified although interference of drug with lysosomal breakdown of protein was suggested. However, tissue distribution studies with BW 58c and BW 540c showed no evidence for renal accumulation of parent drug or metabolite. In terms of human experience, there is little evidence to suggest that levamisole is nephrotoxic in man (Symöens et al., 1979). Hyaline droplets of lysosomal nature have also been found in the proximal tubular ureas of rats treated with gentamycin (see above) and cyclosporin (Ryffel and Mihatsch, 1986).

Although hyaline droplets have been best characterized in the laboratory rat, some strains of mice such as the inbred T70, 'beige', (C3H × 101)F_1, hybrid show PAS-positive, lysosomal inclusions in the straight part of the proximal tubule (Morley and Wheeler, 1985). The mouse kidney also exhibits a testosterone-mediated sexual dimorphism, characterized by the accumulation of cytoplasmic droplets in the apical cytoplasm of proximal tubules. Studies in A/JAX mice have shown that males and testosterone-treated females develop these droplets in proximal tubular cells. These droplets are characterized by acid phosphatase and β-glucuronidase activity and appear ultrastructurally as membrane-bound, membranous or myeloid lysosomal bodies (Koenig et al., 1978, 1980). Mitochondria were also shown to be larger and characterized by greater enzyme activity in male mice. It was suggested that testosterone not only stimulates RNA and protein synthesis, but also modulates mitochondrial size and function and enhances lysosomal activity in proximal tubular cells, increasing autophagy (Koenig et al., 1980).

Pigment droplets

Pigments are found in the kidneys of most laboratory animals, particularly rodents. The renal pigments have been most fully documented in the rat, where they occur in most strains (Coleman et al., 1977; Anver et al., 1982).

Most commonly, yellowish-brown droplets, which are essentially Perl's negative and weak by PAS positive seen in the proximal renal tubular cell cytoplasm in general represent lipofucsin (lipochrome) granules (Ward and Reznik-Schüller, 1980). These granules are autofluorescent and increase in number with advancing age (Ikeda et al., 1985). These droplets represent accumulation of pigment in lysosomes which are numerous in the proximal tubules (see above).

Certain drugs potentiate the appearance of lipofucsin granules in the renal tubular cell. This has been described in male rats treated with high doses of benzodiazepines (Owen et al., 1970). Lipochrome droplets were found in renal tubules in the dog but not rat toxicity studies performed with bromocriptine, an inhibitor of pituitary prolactin, although this finding has not been of any significance in the clinical utilization of this agent (Richardson et al., 1984). Lipochrome pigment may also develop spontaneously in the tubular cells of untreated primates.

Other pigments may also be seen in the kidney. At the site of spontaneous or drug-induced renal tubular damage, iron pigment may accumulate. Iron pigment also accumulates in the Fischer 344 rats with mononuclear cell leukaemia (Solleveld and Boorman, 1986). Bile pigment is also occasionally seen in the renal tubules of laboratory animals, particularly when there is liver damage and bilirubinaemia.

Tubular hypertrophy

Although tubular hyperplasia is not always sharply separable from hypertrophy, hypertrophy of the renal tubules or collecting ducts occurs in response to the increased renal demand which is associated with partial nephrectromy, high protein diet, dietary excess of sodium chloride or administration of high doses of xenobiotics which increase kidney demand.

Studies in rats, mice or rabbits with reduced cell mass or fed high protein diets, have indicated that hypertrophy involves the entire nephron, but augmentation in the size of the proximal tubule accounts for most of the increase in renal cell mass (Fine and Bradley, 1985). In partial nephrectomy models, it has been shown that an increase in tubular cell size (hypertrophy) predominates over an increase in cell number (hyperplasia) (Johnson and Roman, 1966; Skraastad, 1987). Although tubular cell proliferation also occurs, this response is age-dependent, being most prominent in juvenile animals (Celsi et al., 1988). Compensatory growth has also been shown to be greater in rats partially nephrectomized at five days than at 55 days (Celsi et al., 1986).

Physiological studies have demonstrated a close link between hypertrophy of the proximal tubular cells and elevation of glomerular filtration rate, although the precise ultrafiltration dynamics involved and the nature of the primary trigger for hypertrophy are uncertain (Finn, 1982; Fine and Bradley, 1985).

Accurate structural characterization of proximal tubular cell hypertrophy under these circumstances requires careful morphometric analysis following appropriate fixation. Studies using these techniques have shown that proximal

539

tubular cell hypertrophy following partial nephrectomy is asymmetric with increase in tubular diameter and cell volume being accompanied by greater increases in the area of basolateral membranes than luminal membrane area per cross section of tubule, morphological features consistent with adaptive increases in active transcellular transport capacity of tubular cells (Fine and Bradley, 1985).

Analogous studies in rats and rabbits have also shown that a high dietary intake of sodium chloride or chronic administration of the diuretic furosemide leads to hypertrophy of the *distal* convoluted tubule (Kaissling and Le Hir, 1982; Kaissling et al., 1985; Ellison et al., 1989).

In rats given furosemide by continuous infusion for six days using osmotic pumps and provided free access to water and saline, it was shown that distal convoluted tubules were more prominent than in controls and were characterized by increase in epithelial height, large nuclei and ultrastructural evidence of increased basolateral cell membrane area (Kaissling et al., 1985).

Based on such studies, it has been postulated that high rates of ion delivery to the distal nephron cause distal tubular hypertrophy which is in turn associated with an adaptive increase in ion transport capacity (Ellison et al., 1989).

Hypertrophy of the distal tubular epithelial cells has also been observed in toxicity studies performed in rats, dogs and monkeys with the novel isouricaemic diuretic agent, indacrinone (MK-196). It was argued that this also represented an adaptive response of the distal nephron to the increased demand for ion transport (Abrams et al., 1985).

Although lithium, used extensively in psychiatric diseases, is associated with renal tubular degeneration and interstitial fibrosis in man and experimental animals (Ottosen et al., 1986; Hetmar et al., 1987), studies in rats at doses equivalent to those used in clinical practice have shown that hypertrophy of the collecting ducts occurs (Jacobsen et al., 1982; Ottosen et al., 1987). Histologically, both principle and intercalated cells of collecting ducts were shown to be enlarged, bulging into the duct lumen creating a 'hob-nail' appearance. Nuclear enlargement and an increase in the number of nuclear profiles suggested that hyperplasia also occurred (Jacobsen et al., 1982). Whereas changes in more proximal segments of the nephron have indicated that cellular damage occurs, the alterations to the collecting ducts suggest an adaptive effect, possibly a consequence of the effects of lithium on distal nephron potassium and hydrogen ion transport (Ottosen et al., 1987).

Swelling of the collecting tubular cells is also reported in potassium deficient rats, although this appears to be associated with degeneration and hyperplasia of the tubular epithelium (Oliver et al., 1957).

Tubular hyperplasia

Chronic renal damage may lead to hyperplastic changes in the tubular epithelium. This is commonly seen in rat carcinogenicity studies in association with advanced spontaneous glomerulosclerosis (Peter et al., 1986). Administration of drugs which produce chronic renal injury also produce proliferative or hyperplastic lesions of renal tubules, in common with a number of other chemicals. A single dose of the antineoplastic agent, cisplatin, has been shown to produce tubular necrosis, with subsequent development of cystic lesions and areas of tubular hyperplasia in the rat (Bulger and Dobyan, 1984; Dobyan, 1985). These hyperplastic lesions are characterized by a variety of different appearances ranging from nodules of enlarged tubular cells to proliferation of cords of hyperchromatic tubular cells in a thickened or fibrous matrix. These changes may be associated with renal functional derangements. Tubular damage accompanied by atypical hyperplasia characterized by nuclear pleomorphism and polypoid proliferation has also been described in the kidneys of patients treated with cisplatin (Tanaka et al., 1986).

Sequential morphological studies of the kidneys of rats treated with streptozotocin have shown that proximal tubular injury induced by this agent is followed by distal tubular degeneration and regeneration, which is associated with a form of focal hyperplasia of the cells lining the collecting ducts in the inner medulla (Dees and Kramer, 1986). This hyperplasia is characterized histologically by the presence of numerous large collecting duct cells containing large bizarre pleomorphic nuclei. These cells are also seen in the epithelium overlying the papilla. In view of the oncogenic potential of streptozotocin, it was suggested such hyperplastic renal changes may possess potential to progress to neoplasia (Dees and Kramer, 1986).

Interstitial nephritis

The term interstitial nephritis is used to describe conditions in which the renal interstitium is infiltrated by lymphocytes, plasma cells, polymorphonuclear cells accompanied by oedema (acute interstitial nephritis) or fibrosis with sparse numbers of chronic inflammatory cells with tubular loss (chronic interstitial nephritis, chronic interstitial fibrosis). Although, interstitial inflammation may accompany a variety of primary renal conditions such as glomerulonephritis, pyelonephritis and papillary necrosis, the term 'interstitial nephritis' is reserved for primary inflammatory diseases of the interstitium.

Interstitial nephritis in man has been increasingly recognized as a complication of drug treatment of which methicillin is the best studied example (Linton et al., 1980; Appel et al., 1981). Drug-induced interstitial nephritis consists of a moderate to severe interstitial infiltrate composed of lymphocytes, plasma cells and eosinophils with interstitial oedema and variable tubular damage (Linton et al., 1980). It appears that some of these cases are immunologically mediated with formation of anti-tubular basement membrane antibody. Acute interstitial nephritis has also been reported following therapy with recombinant leukocyte interferon therapy (Averbuch et al., 1984). Focal interstitial fibrosis is also described in man and rats following administration of lithium (Ottosen et al., 1986; Hetmar et al., 1987) and in chronic potassium deficiency (Alpern and Toto, 1990).

Interstitial nephritis may accompany infections such as leptospirosis which has been described in the dog (Krohn et al., 1971). Diseases in which anti-basement membrane antibodies form or immune complex deposition takes place may involve the tubular basement membranes with an interstitial inflammatory reaction (see review by Heptinstall, 1983b). Interstitial nephritis can be induced in the Brown-Norway or Lewis-Brown Norway F1 rats and in some mouse strains, by the production of anti-tubular basement antibodies in a manner analogous to experimental glomerulonephritis (Lehman et al., 1974; Sugisaki et al., 1973; Ueda et al., 1988). Studies immunizing different strains of mice with purified murine tubular basement membrane antigen have shown that the induction of interstitial nephritis and the immune response to this antigen are controlled by one or a few dominant genes whose loci are within or closely linked to the H-2 complex (Ueda et al., 1988). By far the most common interstitial inflammation observed in usual toxicity studies is the spontaneous focal inflammatory infiltrate, composed of mononuclear cells which occurs in control rats, hamsters, mice and occasionally beagle dogs.

Vascular changes

The kidney is a common site for vascular pathology in rodents and dogs in toxicity studies and is an organ of predilection for drug-induced vascular disease. Histopathological features of the various vascular changes are described under Cardiovascular System (Chapter VI).

Infarction

Wedge-shaped infarcts are sporadically observed in aged rodents in toxicity studies, usually associated with renal disease such as glomerulosclerosis or amyloidosis of severity sufficient to produce focal renal ischaemia. Infarcts may also be produced by primary vascular disease, thrombosis or embolization of the renal vasculature.

Similar wedge-shaped zones of infarction may follow administration of drugs which produce focal renal ischaemia by potentiation of thrombosis or arterial vasoconstriction. An example of this is the administration of serotonin to rats (Murray, 1979).

Histologically, recent renal infarcts are characterized by a zone of clearly necrotic parenchyma surrounded by a zone of inflammatory tissue. Older lesions show scarring of varying degrees with collapses of renal tubules, basement membrane thickening, fibrosis and even mineralization (dystrophic calcification).

To a certain extent, the renal infarcts can be dated on their histological appearances, congestion and necrosis appearing quite early with polymorphonuclear cells appearing at about 12 hours. Subsequently, there is a loss of staining of the infarcted zone increased numbers of polymorphonuclear cells which begin to undergo karyorrhexis about four days. Subsequently, repair occurs with appearance of fibroblasts and capillaries (Solez, 1983).

Hypertrophy and hyperplasia of the juxtaglomerular apparatus

Hypertrophy, hyperplasia, increased granularity or an extension of immunostaining for renin has been demonstrated in the kidneys of laboratory animals under circumstances in which there is increased stimulation of the renin-angiotensin system and increased demand for renin. This has been reported following adrenalectomy, sodium depletion, experimental renal ischaemia, hypertension and following administration of ACE inhibitor (Taugner et al., 1983). Similar changes have been found in the kidneys of human patients (Lindop and Lever, 1986).

As noted above, the bulk of renal renin is localized in the media of afferent arterioles. Under conditions of increased demand, immunocytochemical study has shown that the distribution of renin extends to involve more proximal segments of the afferent arterioles, the efferent arterioles and the interlobular arteries (Taugner et al., 1982b, 1983; Lindop and Lever, 1986). Increased immunostaining for renin has been associated with morphological changes variably described as increased granularity, hypertrophy or hyperplasia of juxtaglomerular cells, or hypertrophy and hyperplasia of afferent arterioles and interlobular arteries (Fig. 95). Although increased numbers of renin-containing cells develop under these circumstances, it has also been suggested, based on study of the rat renal hypertension model, that this arises by a process of *metaplasia* of pre-existing medial smooth muscle cells (Cantin et al., 1977).

Sodium depletion has also been shown to increase the percentage of renin containing cells in the efferent arterioles in the superficial cortex of the kidney. It is believed that this represents an adaptive response under circumstances of decreased renal blood flow in an attempt to maintain glomerular filtration by efferent arteriolar constriction (Taugner et al., 1982b). Renin-secreting cells may also increase in ischaemic renal lesions or at the edges of renal infarcts in man (Camilleri et al., 1980).

Of importance to the toxicologic pathologist are the changes following the administration of angiotensin-converting enzyme (ACE) inhibitors such as captopril, enalapril, ramipril, quinapril and SCH 31846. These agents also produce hypertrophy of juxtaglomerular cells in rats, mice, dogs and monkeys (La Rocca et al., 1986; Baum et al., 1985; Ohtaki et al., 1981; Hashimoto et al., 1981; Zaki et al., 1982; Donaubauer and Mayer, 1988; Dominick et al., 1989). This hypertrophy is accompanied by a distinct increase in granularity of the juxtaglomerular cells which can be demonstrated by special techniques for renin-containing granules such as the Bowie and Hartroft stains (Bowie, 1935; Hartroft and Hartroft, 1953).

These granules are also well visualized in toluidine blue-stained plastic embedded sections. Immunocytochemical study using antisera to renin has shown increased staining reactions in the afferent arterioles of rats, mice and primates treated with captopril (Zaki et al., 1982). These changes are generally considered to be an exaggerated pharmacological effect caused by stimulation of the renin-secreting cells due to loss of feedback inhibition by angiotensin II (La Rocca et al., 1986).

A further finding under these circumstances relates to the immunostaining for angiotensin II. The distribution of immunoactive angiotensin II has been shown to parallel that of renin in mice subjected to adrenalectomy or unilateral renal ischaemia. However, following prolonged administration of captopril, a disassociation between renin and angiotensin II is observed. Immunostaining for renin increases whilst that of angiotensin II decreases (Taugner et al. , 1983).

Papillary necrosis

Since Spühler and Zollinger (1953) noted an association between chronic interstitial nephritis, papillary necrosis and chronic analgesic consumption, the association of papillary necrosis with non-steroidal anti-inflammatory agents and analgesics has been subject to an enormous amount of epidemiological and experimental study reviewed in detail by Bach and Bridges (1985a,b).

Most experimental work has been conducted in the rat, although papillary necrosis can be produced experimentally in the mouse (Macklin and Szot, 1980) the rabbit (Mandel and Popper, 1951; Davies, 1968, 1970; Clausen, 1964) and dog (Mandel and Popper, 1951; Ellis et al., 1973). Although it has been suggested that the rat kidney is unduly sensitive to the adverse effects of non-steroidal inflammatory agents compared with man (Faccini, 1982), experimental variables in reported studies as well as strain and sex differences, render the extrapolation of findings in the rodent to man difficult (Bach and Bridges, 1985b). The use of a known positive control is a prudent measure in the assessment of papillary necrosis produced by a novel pharmaceutical agent.

The study of Bokelman et al. (1971) of a novel non-steroidal anti-inflammatory agent in the rat is particularly interesting in this respect. These workers showed that not only were two strains of rat quantitatively different in their sensitivity to the adverse renal effects of this agent but also gave rise to qualitatively different renal pathology. A further point was that the male rat was particularly affected by this agent whereas, with another anti-inflammatory agent, sudoxicam, the female rat was more affected (Wiseman and Reinert, 1975). In the latter case, there was a sex-related difference in plasma concentrations of sudoxicam, which were higher in the female rat. Other workers have also noted rat strain differences in sensitivity to non-steroid anti-inflammation drugs (Owen and Heywood, 1986) and strain differences in the metabolism of these agents have also been reported (Bach and Bridges, 1985b).

Although histological appearances vary with the agent, dose, length of study and other variables, the fully developed lesion is characterized by frank necrosis of the tip of the renal papilla, which may be completely lost. Usually an inflammatory reaction is sparse or completely lacking although there may be a band of polymorphonuclear cells at the junction with viable renal tissue. There may be haemorrhage, casts and cell debris in the remaining tubules and mineralization can occur. Ulceration and reactive changes appear in the transitional epithelium of the papilla and renal pelvis (see below). Proximal tubules within the non-necrotic cortex also show dilatation, casts and degenerative change. Early or mild changes are characterized by mild interstitial oedema or 'mucoid' change in the renal papillary matrix.

In general, papillary necrosis occurring in toxicity studies increases in prevalence and sensitivity with increasing length of toxicity study (see Wiseman and Reinert, 1975). In the study of a novel anti-inflammatory agent by Bokelman et al. (1971), the Sprague-Dawley rat developed lesions as described above. By contrast, in another strain (Manor Farms SPF) the focal polypoid hyperplasia of the renal papillary epithelium was far more prominent and was associated with small foci of necrosis and fibrosis in the immediately underlying renal papilla rather than lesions being limited to the interior of the papilla.

Pathogenesis of the primary lesion remains controversial. Clausen (1964) suggested changes were the direct result of a toxic effect on the tubular epithelium, principally at the corticomedullary junction. It has also been proposed that both precipitation of analgesic breakdown products and ischaemia may contribute to the development of this lesion (Kincaid-Smith, 1967; Kincaid-Smith et al., 1968).

The detailed morphological study of Molland (1978) has also suggested that early papillary changes are the result of ischaemia, possibly as a result of inhibition of prostaglandin synthesis with subsequent reduction of medullary blood flow. It has also been suggested that drug-induced changes in the glycosaminoglycan content of the medullary matrix may also play a part in the development of renal papillary necrosis (Bach et al., 1983).

Mineralization (calcification, nephrocalcinosis)

Calcium deposition in the organs and tissues of man has been studied for over a century since the early description by Virchow (1855) and its classification into two principal types, *metastatic* and *dystrophic* (Jaccottet, 1959). Detailed clinicopathological study in man has shown that metastatic renal calcification is essentially a tubular process but with a highly variable distribution within the nephron which appears dependent on the underlying clinical condition or precipitating cause (Jaccottet, 1959).

By contrast, dystrophic calcification is usually closely associated with damaged renal tissue, although dystrophic and metastatic calcification cannot always be clearly separated from each other on morphological grounds.

Different forms of calcium deposition develop spontaneously in laboratory rats, mice, hamsters and dogs and different types of mineralization can be induced by the administration of drugs and chemicals. Renal calcium deposition in laboratory animals may follow the administration of calcium and vitamin D (Duffy et al., 1971; Ganote et al., 1975; Scarpelli, 1965), oxalates (Khan et al., 1982), phosphate loading (Craig, 1959), parathyroid hormone (Caulfield and Schrag, 1964), certain drugs such as acetazolamide (Harrison and Harrison 1955) as well as chloride depletion (Sarkar et al., 1973), magnesium deficiency (Schneeberger and Morrison, 1965) and pyridoxine B6 deficiency (Lilian et al., 1981). Assessment and interpretation therefore of drug-induced nephrocalcinosis found in toxicity studies may be difficult in view of its development under such a wide range of conditions.

Intratubular lithiasis (calcinosis, mineralization)

A characteristic form of intratubular mineralization occurs in the female rat. These are rounded concretions of variable size situated mainly with the tubular lumen at the corticomedullary junction. They stain with variable intensity with haematoxylin, some staining intensely blue others quite pale in colour suggesting an inconstant mineral content. It has been shown that these concretions are composed of calcium, phosphorus and a glycoprotein matrix and appear to form as a result of shedding of vesiculated microvilli and microvesicles from the S1 segment of the proximal renal tubule. These vesicles increase in size as they descend the nephron and tend to accumulate in the straight segment (S3) of the proximal tubule at the corticomedullary junction (Nguyen and Woodard, 1980). The prevalence of these concretions varies considerably between rat strains different laboratories and even in the same rat strain housed in the same laboratory over a period of time.

Severe forms of this type of nephrolithiasis occur in very young female rats as well as older animals (Silverman and Riverson, 1980). Clapp and colleagues (1982) have demonstrated that the prevalence and severity of this nephrolithiasis in the rat is highly dependent on the calcium-phosphorus ratio in the diet, those with high calcium-phosphate ratios (high calcium-low phosphate) being protective. They also showed that diets which produced these lesions in the rat did not do so in the mouse, underlining the fact that the mouse is relatively resistant to such nephrocalcinosis. Precise pathogenesis is uncertain. Nguyen and Woodard (1980) have suggested that there is a disequilibrium in the handling of calcium and phosphate in the proximal tubule which is more marked in the female. It has been shown from micropuncture techniques that resorption of phosphate in the proximal tubule is less avid in the female than in the male (Harris et al., 1974). In a detailed disposition study of calcium and phosphorus in female rats during the period in which nephrocalcinosis developed, no gross changes in calcium or phosphorus metabolism were detected (Phillips et al., 1986). This also suggests that there is no simple relationship between mineral utilization and nephrocalcinosis. The female sex predominance of mineralization at the corticomedullary junction of the rat is reflected by the fact that it can be prevented by ovariectomy and induced in castrated male and female rats by administration of oestrogen (Cousins and Geary, 1966).

A similar distribution of nephrocalcinosis has been reported after administration of carbonic anhydrase inhibitors such as acetazolamide (Harrison and Harrison, 1955; Greaves and Faccini, 1984) and it has been suggested this occurs because these agents lower urinary citrate and pH with consequent precipitation of calcium as found in renal tubular acidosis in man (Harrison and Harrison,

1955). However, it is of importance to note that these authors also reported that when rats on low phosphate, high calcium diets were treated with acetazolamide, calcified plaques were formed at the tips of the papillary ducts with formation of calculi in the pelvis (see below), indicating that dietary factors can influence in the way drug-induced mineralization is expressed.

Corticomedullary nephrocalcinosis also develops in an accentuated form in rats, particularly in females, following the administration of modified starches, sugar alcohols and lactose. When these agents are given in large quantities they are capable of increasing calcium absorption and urinary excretion (Roe and Bär, 1985; Newberne et al., 1988; Roe, 1989). Renal tubular mineralization associated with tubular dilation and scarring has also been reported in dogs given a synthetic polydextrose (Newberne et al., 1988). As identical lesions were produced in the dogs following infusion of 84 mg/kg body weight of calcium, but not sodium lactate over a seven hour period, it has been postulated that the renal tubular damage was a consequence of excessive calcium retention and excretion. Roe (1989) has argued that this type of change in the rodent kidney, which follows administration of high doses of these agents, has little relevance for the human use of these agents under normal circumstances.

Another form of intratubular mineral deposition is found commonly in the normal beagle dog, characterized by small flocculent haematoxylin staining deposits in the collecting ducts of the renal papilla. They have no pathological significance.

Renal pelvic mineralization

Most severe nephrocalcinosis and formation of calculi occurs in or adjacent to the renal pelvis in aged rodents. These occur both in rats and mice but the aged hamster seems particularly disposed to develop this form of mineral deposition. Free-lying deposits may be seen in the pelvis itself, located in the fornix or at the base of the renal papilla. Very occasionally, massive calculi are found in the renal pelvis in young rats, accompanied by hydronephrotic changes in the renal parenchyma and hyperplasia of the urothelium. There is usually advanced degeneration and sclerosis of renal tubules in affected kidneys, with relative sparing of the glomeruli.

Deposits are liable to form under the surface epithelium of the renal papilla, especially in the rat. These deposits are often associated with local tissue changes which include oedema, fibrosis, cystic degeneration, telangiectasis, ulceration or hyperplasia of the adjacent surface epithelium (Fig. 103). Certain drugs such as carbonic anhydrase inhibitors may also accentuate mineral deposition at this particular site in the renal papilla and form striking linear deposits along the basement membrane of the epithelium covering the papilla.

Renal pelvic mineralization has also been reported in rats following the administration of the sweetening agent aspartame which was associated with a high urinary calcium (Ishii et al., 1981). It can also be found accompanying the

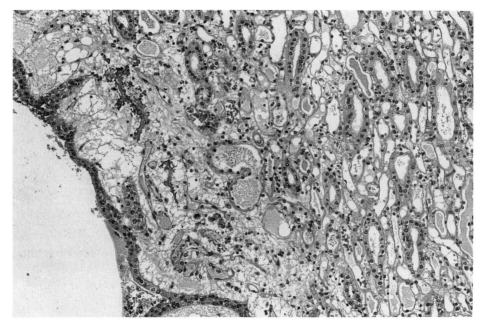

Fig. 103. Renal papilla in an aged, female Sprague-Dawley rat exhibiting the accumulation of mineral and associated degenerative changes just below the surface of the papilla. (HE, ×200.)

renal tubular lithiasis which occurs following administration of modified starches and related materials (Newberne et al., 1988).

Mineralization in the papilla may also accompany the renal papillary necrosis which follows the administration of drugs and chemicals (see above).

Dystrophic calcification

Mineralization which is dystrophic may accompany other forms of renal damage, including the spontaneous forms of glomerulonephritis and tubular damage occurring in aged rodents. Even this form of renal calcification may be accentuated in long-term toxicity studies in the rat as has been described with the novel inhibitor of thromboxane synthesis, dazoxiben (Irisarri et al., 1985).

Epithelial hyperplasia, renal pelvis

Hyperplasia of the epithelium lining of the renal pelvis and covering the renal papilla may be a spontaneous change or induced directly or indirectly by treatment with drugs and chemicals. It may be focal or diffuse in distribution.

It is seen most commonly in a sporadic manner and clearly related to focal damage to the pelvic or peri-pelvic tissues as a result of spontaneous disease in aged rodents. Epithelial hyperplasia may be associated with pyelonephritis, glomerulosclerosis in the rat and spontaneous renal mineralization and calculi. There is usually focal thickening of the epithelium, closely associated with eroded epithelium. Likewise hyperplasia of the pelvic epithelium is associated with drug-induced damage to the papilla such as renal papillary necrosis, drug-induced mineralization, and deposition of drug crystals. Focal polypoid urothelial hyperplasia has been reported on the papillary epithelium in rats treated with cisplatin (Bulger and Dobyan, 1984).

Drug administration may also produce a more diffuse or widespread hyperplasia of the urothelium which can involve the pelvic epithelium without light microscopic evidence of cell damage. Such changes, characterized by increased numbers of cells in the urothelium are most commonly found in the bladder (see below), presumably as urine, drug or metabolites remain for extended periods in bladder rather than the renal pelvis. However, a number of factors can explain the presence of such changes in the pelvic epithelium. Urine may stagnate in the renal pelvis, due to the presence of casts and stones or administration of drugs and chemicals with pharmacological effects on smooth muscle and subsequent effects on ureter peristalsis. Metabolic activation of endogenous and exogenous compounds within the surrounding medulla and the pelvis may also be important (Bach and Bridges, 1985b).

A problem in the interpretation of diffuse urothelial hyperplasia is assessment of risk for man, particularly as hyperplasia of the pelvic epithelium is sometimes associated with the development of transitional cell papillomas and carcinoma in laboratory rodents. However, urothelial hyperplasia can occur in preclinical toxicity studies with pharmaceutical agents associated with neither increase in urothelial neoplasia in carcinogenicity studies nor risk for man when used in therapeutic doses. This is perhaps not surprising when hyperplasia has been shown to occur following the administration of agents which produce pH changes in the urine or after diets supplemented with sodium chloride (Lalich et al., 1974). Therefore, to a large extent urethelial hyperplasia must be considered an adaptive response to urinary alterations.

Hydronephrosis, pelvic dilatation

Dilatation of the renal pelvis or hydronephrosis is a recurring finding in rats, mice and hamsters in toxicity studies, although its pathogenesis remains uncertain. In the rat, it usually affects the right side, possibly as a result of the anatomic arrangement of the overlying spermatic or ovarian artery compressing the ureter (Burton et al., 1979). This change is not usually a toxicological problem, unless accompanied by other pathological changes.

Modest dilatation of the renal pelvis without pathological changes in the renal parenchyma should be distinguished from hydronephrosis in which there is histological evidence of renal parenchymal damage as a result of outflow obstruction. In such cases there is usually more marked dilatation of the renal pelvis, which may contain calculi or drug crystals and show transitional cell hyperplasia. There is evidence of tubular damage and sclerosis, with variable amounts of interstitial inflammation and fibrosis, but with relative sparing of renal glomeruli.

Renal neoplasia

Primary renal tumours are found sporadically in untreated rats of most strains and they appear histologically similar to those occurring in man (Greaves and Faccini, 1984). Identical neoplasms are reported in mice and hamsters. Although beagle dogs used in toxicity studies do not normally develop these tumours, the range of renal neoplasms reported in aging dogs is similar to those in rodents and man (Baskin and De Paoli, 1977; Diters and Wells, 1986). Most types of renal neoplasms reported in man can be induced in laboratory animals by administration of xenobiotics and a number of experimental renal tumour models have been created (reviewed by Hard, 1986).

Renal neoplasms are categorized histological into epithelial, mesenchymal, embryonal and mixed or composite types.

Adenomas and adenocarcinomas form the largest group in older animals and present a wide range of cytological appearances in all species, notably eosinophilic or oncocytic, basophilic or clear cell features and solid, tubular or papillary growth patterns. Each tumour must be assessed on its individual appearances in order to distinguish between adenoma and adenocarcinoma because clinical behaviour of these neoplasms is less well known in dogs and rodents than in man.

In laboratory rodents, the distinction between focal hyperplasia, adenoma and carcinoma of the renal parenchyma, remains somewhat arbitrary. Focal hyperplasia is usually considered a proliferation of tubular epithelial cells which remains within the confines of an intact renal tubule. Extension of the proliferation beyond the confines of a tubule is considered to be evidence of autonomous growth, i.e. adenoma. Typically, adenomas exhibit relatively little cellular pleomorphism and mitotic activity. By contrast, carcinomas are usually larger growths characterized by increased cellular pleomorphism, mitotic activity, and vascularization with infiltration of tumour cells into the surrounding parenchyma. There may be considerable necrosis and haemorrhage in large neoplasms and ultimately blood borne metastatic deposits develop.

Adenomas and carcinomas have been induced in rats by administration of several different chemicals including N-(4′-fluoro-4-biphenylyl) acetamide (Dees et al., 1980; Hinton et al., 1984), N-nitrosomorpholine (Bannasch, 1984; Bannasch et al., 1986), N-ethyl-N-hydroxy-ethylnitrosamine (Hiasa et al., 1979) and streptozotoxin (Rakieten et al., 1968). Aristolochic acid, used previously in pharmaceutical preparations but with mutagenic activity, is also capable of inducing cortical adenomas and adenocarcinomas as well as urothelial neoplasms in rats (Mengs et al., 1982).

Hydrocarbons which produce hyaline droplet nephropathy in the male rat also induce a low incidence of renal epithelial tumours in male rats after long latent periods, although they appear not to develop in female rats or other species treated with these agents (Macfarland, 1984; Kitchen, 1984).

Chemicals associated with tubular cell tumour development in mice include dimethylnitrosamine, N-nitrosomethylurea, cyclasin, basic lead acetate, tris(2,3-dibromopropyl) phosphate, 2-acetylaminofluorene and the diabetogenic agent, streptozotoxin (Shinohara and Frith, 1980; Hard, 1985). A single dose of streptozotoxin administered to six week old CBA/H/TBJ mice resulted in a high incidence of renal cell carcinomas (Hard, 1985). A single dose of this agent was also shown to induce well-differentiated neoplasms of renal tubular cell type, up to 2 cm diameter in the renal cortex and medulla of Sherman and Holtzman rats (Rakieten et al., 1968). Bucetin (3-hydroxy-p-butyrophenetidide), which structurally resembles phenacetin and also used as an analgesic and antipyretic, produced renal cell adenomas and carcinomas as well as dysplastic tubular changes in male but not female B6C3F1, mice when administered at high doses for 76 weeks (Togei et al., 1987).

Renal cell carcinomas have been induced in male, female and castrated male Syrian hamsters by continuous treatment with synthetic or natural oestrogens (Kirkman and Robbins, 1959; Li et al., 1983). These neoplasms are typically, well-demarcated, unencapsulated nodules or masses composed of branching and anastomosing cords and plates of cuboidal or columnar cells, characteristic of renal cell carcinomas (Kirkman and Robbins, 1959; Liehr et al., 1988). Some tumour cells have been shown to possess cilia and in larger tumours, foci showing spindle cell differentiation have been described. Whereas many of these spindle cell foci probably arise by metaplasia from cells of epithelial derivation, spindle cells showing smooth muscle differentiation or containing cytoplasmic vimentin and desmin filaments, but no cytokeratins, have also been found in these tumours (Kirkman and Robbins, 1959; Hacker et al., 1988). It has therefore been suggested that cells of mesenchymal origin in the kidney may also be capable of participating in the tumorigenic response of the hamster kidney to oestrogens (Hacker et al., 1988).

Tumour cell nuclei are usually only moderately hyperchromatic and mitotic activity is not striking. However, growth through the renal capsule with peritoneal spread to other intra-abdominal organs is quite common and occasionally metastases are found in lungs and lymph nodes (Kirkman and Robbins, 1959).

It has been suggested that although there is a close relationship between hormonal and renal tumorigenic activity in the hamster, neoplasms do not result from a direct hormonal action, but by the effects of oestrogen-induced growth factors (Liehr et al., 1988).

Nephroblastoma occurs more commonly in young rodents (Figs. 104 and 105) and dogs. A similar, age-related trend is found in human cases. This neoplasm comprises variable proliferating populations of blastematous, epithelial and stromal cells, as well as glomerular bodies or primitive glomeruli of varying maturation (Greaves and Faccini, 1984; Baskin and De Paoli, 1977; Bennington and Beckwith, 1975).

Although a number of unconventional laboratory animal models have been used for the study of nephroblastoma, transplacental administration of N-ethyl-nitrosourea (ENU) is an effective method for inducing nephroblastoma in the

551

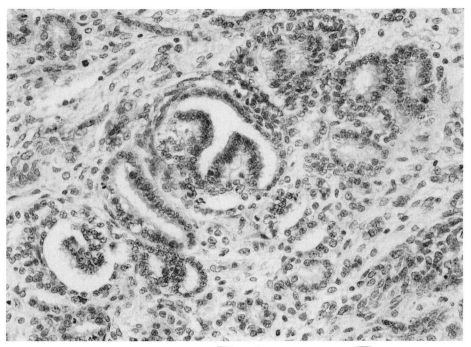

Fig. 104. Nephroblastoma 2.0 cm maximum diameter found in the kidney of a young Wistar rat. It shows the typical primitive tubular and glomerular structures. (HE, ×550.)

rat, notably in the inbred Nb hooded rat, which has a natural deposition to develop this tumour spontaneously (Hard, 1986). Nephroblastomas were also induced at an early age in cynomolgus monkeys exposed in the prenatal period to 1,2-dimethylhydrazine (Beniashvili, 1989).

Various neoplasma of *mesenchymal* origin are also found in rodents and dogs. Typical neoplasms of connective tissue are described, including spindle cell tumours of fibroblastic type (see Integumentary System, Chapter I) (Baskin and De Paoli, 1977; Diters and Wells, 1986).

The so-called *mesenchymal tumour* of the rat kidney is a highly characteristic neoplasm which rarely, if ever, develops spontaneously in most rat populations, but it can be induced by injection of dimethylnitrosamine, particularly if rats are fed a protein-free, high carbohydrate diet (Swan et al., 1980). This neoplasm is believed to be a neoplasm of mesenchymal cells, characterized histologically by a heterologous mixture of fibroblast-like spindle or stellate cells, elements of smooth or skeletal muscle, vascular, cartilageneous or osteoid differentiation.

Although tubular profiles are found deeply embedded within these neoplasms, it has been suggested that they simply represent remnants of pre-existing non-neoplastic tubular epithelium (Hard, 1986). Unlike nephroblastoma, the mesenchymal tumour of the rat possesses an irregular outline and spreads diffusely into the surrounding parenchyma.

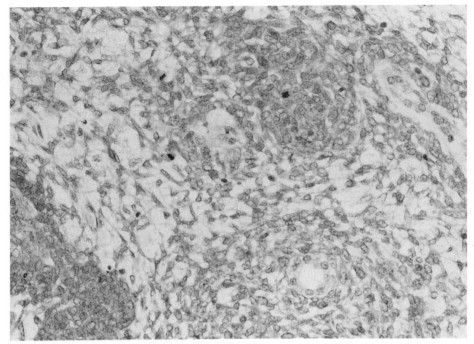

Fig. 105. Another field of the same neoplasm seen in Figure 104 but showing the primitive spindle cell pattern. (HE, ×550.)

Sequential studies have suggested that these neoplasms develop from primitive stem cells of connective or vascular tissue within the renal interstitium (Hard, 1986).

These mesenchymal features are not commonly reported in renal tumours in other species.

Benign neoplasm composed of fat and smooth muscle are common mesenchymal renal tumours in older human populations (Bennington and Beckwith, 1975). Similar tumours are found spontaneously in small numbers in old rats. Histologically, these tumours replace segments of the renal parenchyma and are composed of a variable population of mature fat cells, lipoblasts, prominant blood vessels and spindle cells. They may show haemorrhage and necrosis and considerable mitotic activity. Most are slow growing, benign neoplasms, but undoubtedly a small proportion show marked cellular and nuclear pleomorphism, extend widely in the kidney and produce distant metastatic deposits (Goodman et al., 1980; Gordon, 1986). Their histogenesis remains unclear. This is reflected in a variety of different terms employed for these tumours, including lipoma, liposarcoma, lipomatous hamartoma, angiolipoma, myolipoma, angiomyolipoma and mixed tumours (Greaves and Faccini, 1984).

Transitional cell tumours develop in the renal pelvis, but for full description see below. Some strains of rats such as DA/Han rats with a high spontaneous incidence of transitional cell neoplasms of the bladder also develop renal pelvic carcinomas more commonly (Deerberg and Rehm, 1985). Very occasionally, transitional cell carcinoma are reported in the upper outflow tract of laboratory beagles (Hanika and Rebar, 1980).

Urothelial carcinomas of the renal pelvis have been associated with administration of non-steroidal anti-inflammatory drugs and analgesics in both human populations and experimental animals. The molecular mechanisms involved are unclear, although a variety of associated factors, such as bacterial infection, calculi, alterations to the mucoid layer covering the mucosa, necrosis and repair may be involved in the process (Bach and Bridges, 1985 a,b). Without a full understanding of the mechanisms, it is difficult to develop predictive tests for the assessment of the risks of the development of papillary urothelial neoplasms in man following therapy. However, as with the assessment urothelial neoplasms in the bladder in experimental studies, a thorough study of any associated non-neoplastic changes including calculi is essential.

URINARY BLADDER

Inflammation, cystitis

Inflammation of the bladder is not a common spontaneous finding amongst most laboratory animal populations, but it is found sporadically in isolated cases.

It is seen more frequently in some colonies of aged rats, mice and hamsters in association with other urinary tract pathology, such as urolithiasis, pyelonephritis, prostatitis, urethral stasis or infestations such as Trichosomoides crassicauda in the rat (Tuffery, 1966; Pour et al., 1976; Burek, 1978; Zubaidy and Majeed, 1981).

Some drugs or their urinary metabolites are also associated with erosion, haemorrhage and inflammation of the bladder mucosa. A notable example is the anticancer agent, cyclophosphamide, which is activated by hepatic microsomal enzymes to potent alkylating cytotoxic metabolites. Administration of this agent is associated with the development of haemorrhagic cystitis in cancer patients and this effect can be reproduced in laboratory animals (Fig. 106) (Koss and Lavin, 1970).

Urothelial damage, characterized histologically by cytoplasmic exfoliation, vacuolation and ballooning, microabscess formation and the accumulation of PAS positive, diastase resistant cytoplasmic bodies, was also reported in rats treated for two weeks with a novel non-dopaminergic antipschyotic agent (Barsoum et al., 1985).

The crystalluria produced by administration of high doses of poorly insoluble drugs in toxicity studies can induce haematuria, with haemorrhage, ulceration and inflammation of the urothelium. There is also evidence for nephrotoxicity of drug crystals in human patients, provided crystals are formed in vivo (Lehmann, 1987). However, in drawing the conclusion that drug crystals are the cause of

554

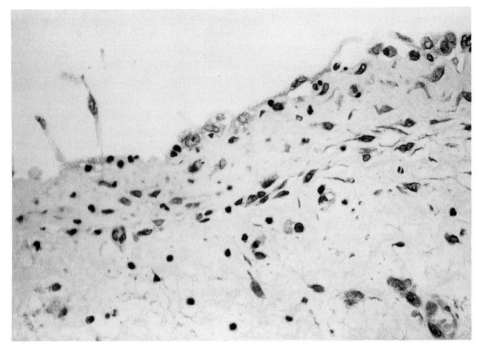

Fig. 106. Bladder mucosa from a Wistar rat treated for two days with cyclophosphamide. This shows almost complete denudation of the transitional epithelium. (HE, ×350.)

urothelial damage, it is necessary to demonstrate in vivo presence of drug crystals either by evidence of their presence in tissues in histological sections or in the urine immediately after voiding or sampling before cooling of the specimen occurs.

Mineralization, calcification, calculi, stones

Mineralization in the bladder can take the form of a single large calculus or multiple bladder stones, characteristically with facetted surfaces. They are found sporadically in most colonies of rats, mice and hamsters, but only very occasionally in laboratory beagles and non-human primates. The cause of the spontaneous development of bladder calculi is not always clear, although as in renal mineralization, diet and hormone balance are important.

It has been postulated that bladder surface glycosaminoglycans are important antiadherence factors which prevent calcium, which is often supersaturated in the urine, from depositing on the bladder surface to form a nidus for stone formation (Parsons et al., 1980).

Other factors which influence the development of urolithiasis include urinary tract infections, presence of foreign bodies, drug crystals and abnormalities in the anatomy of the urinary outflow tract.

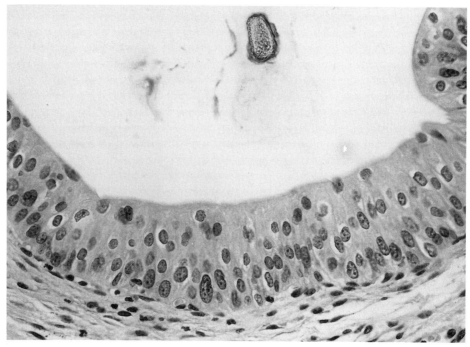

Fig. 107. Diffuse hyperplasia of the bladder epithelium of a Wistar rat treated orally with an anti-inflammatory drug for a period of one month. The transitional epithelium contains increased layers of enlarged, pseudostratified nuclei but there is no cytological atypia. (HE, ×350.)

Genetic pre-disposition is important because certain strains of rats appear to have a higher prevalence of urinary stones even when husbandry conditions are identical (Kunstyr et al., 1982). The spontaneously hypertensive rat (SHR) is also prone to develop bladder stones which appear to form from microscopic foci of renal papillary mineralization which become detatched, and lodged in the bladder to form the nidus for the development of bladder calculi (Wexler and McMurtry 1981). These authors suggested that this pre-disposition of SHR rats is also genetically programmed.

In some laboratories, rats of a few weeks of age have been shown to develop multiple bladder stones spontaneously (Paterson, 1979). This suggests that calculi can develop within a few weeks under appropriate conditions.

The rapidity of calculi development has been shown in a rat model of urolithiasis in which calculi of heterogeneous composition were induced in Fischer 344 rats in less than two weeks by exposure to terephthalic acid or dimethyl terephthalate, both of which were associated with aciduria and hyper-calciuria (Chin et al., 1981; Wolkowski-Tyl et al., 1982).

Composition of urinary tract calculi in the rat is variable, but they are usually mixed, comprising proteins, calcium carbonates, calcium or ammonium magnesium phosphates (Paterson, 1979; Kunstyr et al., 1982).

Bladder calculi of uncertain aetiology are occasionally reported in laboratory cynomolgus monkeys (Renlund et al., 1986). Bladder uroliths are commonly seen in certain strains of dogs, presumably as a result of their particular metabolic characteristics (Robertson, 1986). Beagles appear less pre-disposed to develop bladder calculi than a number of other breeds.

The presence of bladder stones or calculi is typically associated with transitional cell hyperplasia. This may be marked and accompanied by submucosal inflammation and fibrosis (see below).

Urothelial hyperplasia

Hyperplasia of transitional bladder epithelium occurs in response to a variety of adverse stimuli including chronic inflammation, urinary stasis, presence of calculi, crystals, parasites or other foreign bodies as well as following administration of xenobiotics. An issue in the histological assessment of urothelial hyperplasia in drug safety assessment is that a number of studies have shown that the progression to neoplasia in the rodent bladder following administration of carcinogens such as N-[4-(5.nitro-Z-furyl)-2-thiazolyl formamide (FANFT) or N-(4-hydroxybutyl) nitrosamine passes through a stage of simple hyperplasia which is indistinguishable on light and electron microscopic examination from a simple reactive hyperplasia (Ito et al., 1969; Fukushima et al., 1981). A further complication is that prolonged episodes of bladder mucosal hyperplasia produced by stones and other foreign bodies in rodents are also associated with the development of bladder neoplasia (Clayson 1974; Grasso, 1987).

Histologically, uncomplicated focal or diffuse hyperplasia is characterized by an increase in the number of epithelial cell layers compared with unaffected or control animals (Fig. 107). In making comparisons of epithelial thickness between control and treated groups, it is important to employ a uniform sampling and fixation procedure. This is ideally performed after inflation of the bladder with fixative for fixation of the collapsed bladder may increase the apparent thickness of the mucosa in histological sections.

Marked hyperplasia is associated with the development of infolding, cystic downgrowth of the epithelium into the bladder wall or the formation of small papillary mucosal structures. The florid nature of marked hyperplasia has led to the use of terms such as *nodular* or *papillary hyperplasia* in these circumstances (Hicks et al., 1976). Morphological studies of the rat urinary bladder following single episodes of surgical trauma, freezing damage or intravesicular instillation of formalin have shown that florid changes of this type are fully reversible within three or four weeks and lead to no long-term hyperplasic or neoplastic sequelae (Fukushima et al., 1981).

Scanning electron microscopy has been shown to be a very sensitive technique for the detection of mucosal bladder lesions and characteristic surface charges have also been described in urothelial hyperplasia (Murasaki and Cohen, 1981). In the normal rat bladder, the large superficial polygonal cells exfoliate to reveal underlying round intermediate cells with uniform short microvilli (Fig. 108). As

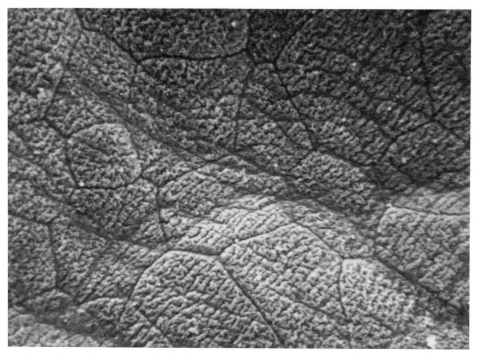

Fig. 108. Scanning electron micrograph of the surface of the bladder mucosa from a normal Wistar rat. The superficial epithelium is composed of an intact pavement of homogeneous cells showing a highly scalloped surface. Illustration by courtesy of Dr N.G. Read. (SEM, ×575.)

these intermediate cells mature, their microvilli merge and develop into so-called ropy microridges. Thus, the rate of exfoliation and replacement of urothelium can be estimated from the extent of the surface with ropy microridges and uniform microvilli. In rats, reactive hyperplasia in the urinary bladders produced by local trauma, formalin instillation or following dosing with saccharin, increased numbers of zones showing ropy microridges and uniform short microvilli are found (Fig. 109) (Fukushima et al., 1981; Murasaki and Cohen, 1981). Epithelial cells in marked or prolonged reactive hyperplastic states also develop pleomorphic surface microvilli, which have been associated with early lesions of experimental bladder cancer (Jacobs et al., 1976). However, they do not appear to be specific for malignant transformation (Fukushima et al., 1981).

Whereas reactive hyperplasia is usually observed in association with some clear evidence of bladder pathology, uncomplicated reactive hyperplasia can occur following the administration of high doses of pharmaceutical agents without evidence of lithiasis or crystal formation. For instance, the β-adreno-receptor antagonist, practalol, produced diffuse hyperplasia of the bladder mucosa of rats in the high dose group of a 13 week oral toxicity study by gavage (Cruickshank et al., 1984). Histologically, the affected bladders were lined by mucosa of up to six cells thick instead of the normal three cells in control rats.

558

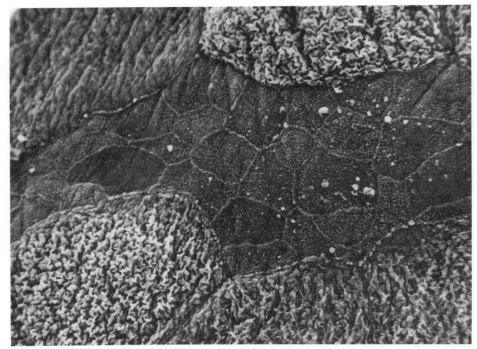

Fig. 109. Similar micrograph to that in Figure 108 but taken from a rat treated with a drug which produced light microscopic alterations in the epithelium. Treatment has produced shedding of some superficial cells to reveal intermediate cells with short stubby microvilli. The residual epithelial cells show prominent surface ridges. Illustration by courtesy of Dr N.G. Read. (SEM, ×1250.)

The changes were found to be fully reversible after cessation of treatment. The findings were attributed to the local irritant effects as a result of transient peak urinary concentrations of drug associated with administration of practalol by gavage, because hyperplasia was not seen in later studies in which practalol was administered in higher doses in the diet. Bladder neoplasms were not found in carcinogenicity bioassays performed with practalol and, although there were major clinical problems with this agent, adverse urinary effects were not reported in man (Cruickshank et al., 1984).

An important part of the evaluation of bladder hyperplasia in drug safety studies in the characterization of any atypical or dysplastic cytological features for such features have traditionally been associated with the progression of urothelial hyperplasia to bladder neoplasia in a number of experimental rodent models and in man. Experimental models only include rodents treated with agents such as nitrosamines, a FANFT (Ito et al., 1969; Cohen et al., 1976; Cohen and Friedell, 1979; Rowland et al., 1980), but also rats treated with alkylating anti-cancer drug, cyclophosphamide, which produces atypical and persistent hyperplasia even after a single dose and bladder cancer following continued treatment (Philips et al., 1961; Koss and Lavin, 1970; Schmähl and Habs, 1979).

Persistence of urothelial hyperplasia following withdrawal of treatment has also been correlated with the development bladder neoplasia in BALB/C female mice treated with 2-acetylaminofluorine (Littlefield et al., 1979).

A large body of data obtained from biopsies and cytological preparations from human bladders has also demonstrated a close relationship between cytological atypia and the development of bladder cancer. Cytological abnormalities of the urinary bladder epithelium have also been reported in patients treated with cyclophosphamide (Forni et al., 1964).

Atypia of bladder epithelium is characterised by a disturbance of the normal regular cell polarity and maturation, nuclear hyperchromasia and pleomorphism, giant cells, prominent nucleoli, chromatin clumping and the presence of mitoses, particularly in upper parts of the epithelium.

Neoplasia

Tumours of the urinary bladder are uncommon in most untreated laboratory rodents, dogs and primates although they are found sporadically in aged rodents in carcinogenicity bioassays. Some strains of rats develop bladder neoplasms more frequently. Histologically, experimental bladder neoplasms resemble those found in man and a similar classification is applicable.

Most are of epithelial nature, although the bladder wall is occasionally also the site of development of mesenchymal tumours.

Transitional cell papilloma

Transitional cell papillomas are single or multiple, pedunculated growths composed of arborescent, delicate branching villi with a fibromuscular stroma. They are covered by transitional epithelium which possesses the uniform appearance of normal bladder epithelium, devoid of cellular atypia or anaplasia. These tumours can ulcerate or develop squamous metaplasia. The stroma may be oedematous and contain inflammatory cells. Invasion of the stalk is not seen.

The so-called 'inverted papilloma' described in man has also been described in DA/Han rats (Deerberg et al., 1985). This consists of transitional epithelium characterized by an endophytic or inverted growth pattern with some cells forming gland-like, cystic structures.

Transitional cell carcinoma

These take the form of papillomatous or sessile growths, distinguished from the papilloma by a greater degree of epithelial atypia including hyperchromasia, nuclear pleomorphism and mitotic activity as well as the variable presence of spindle shaped, rounded or columnar cells and evidence of stromal invasion. Squamous metaplasia may be seen, although metastatic deposits are infrequent in most series reported in laboratory animals.

Other tumour types

Other tumour types reported in smaller numbers include squamous cell carinoma, adenocarcinoma, undifferentiated and carcinomas showing mixed patterns of differentiation.

Extrapolation to man

Although administration of alkylating agents for the treatment of malignant disease increases the risk of development of further cancers, only the use of cyclophosphamide has been linked to an increased frequency of bladder neoplasia in man (Hoover and Fraumeni, 1981). This effect has been demonstrated in laboratory animals treated with this drug. A dose-related increase in transitional cell carcinomas was demonstrated in Sprague-Dawley rats treated with cyclophosphamide (Schmähl and Habs, 1979). In this study, males were shown to be more sensitive to the development of bladder neoplasms than females. The doses employed were quite low and comparable to those used in the treatment of human cancer and perhaps for this reason induction periods were quite long, ranging from about 18 months to two years (Schmähl and Habs, 1979).

Whereas cyclophosphamide appears to be a clear case of drug-induced bladder neoplasia occurring in both man and laboratory animals, in many instances where transitional cell tumours have been induced in laboratory animals, the relevance of the findings for man are less clear.

One of the main difficulties relates to the development of transitional cell neoplasms following the prolonged hyperplasia associated with the presence of bladder calculi or other extraneous materials in the bladder lumen. A close association between the presence of calculi and prolonged hyperplasia with development of bladder neoplasia has been established in a number of rodent models. For instance, strains of rats, notably BN/Bi Rij and DA/Han rats with a high spontaneous incidence of bladder neoplasms develop them only after prolonged periods in association with a high prevalence of bladder stones (Burek, 1978; Deerberg et al., 1985).

Weil and colleagues (1965) showed that urothelial neoplasms which developed in rats treated with diethylene glycol were closely associated with bladder stones and that if the stones were removed, washed and re-implanted into the bladders of young rats, transitional tumours also resulted. Other workers have also demonstrated analogous effects in mice with bladders implanted with foreign bodies of various types, including cholesterol and paraffin wax (Clayson, 1974; Grasso, 1987). Although rats treated with 4-ethylsulphonynaphthalene-1-sulphonamide developed a high incidence of bladder tumours, this was also shown to be linked to an alkaline urine, crystalluria and stone formation. Crystals, stones and the tumorigenic response disappeared when acidification of the urine was produced using ammonium chloride (Flaks et al., 1973).

Another example of the difficulties in the extrapolation of the finding of xenobiotic-induced bladder cancer in rats to man is illustrated by the controversy surrounding the sweetening agent saccharin. Sodium saccharin produces bladder mucosa hyperplasia in rats in a dose-related manner (Murasaki and Cohen, 1981). Under certain conditions following long-term administration, transitional cell neoplasms also develop (Choweniec and Hicks, 1979).

Its role in the production of carcinomas of the bladder of the rat remain unclear. However, it is poorly metabolized and there is little or no evidence of a genetic interaction. As it can only enhance the prevalence of neoplasms after administration of high doses for long periods it has been considered to be a weak carcinogen, co-carcinogen or promoting agent (Hicks, 1984). Clayson (1984) has suggested that it may act by its ability to inhibit proteases or enzymes concerned with DNA synthesis only when high cellular concentrations are achieved through damage to the integrity of the permeability barrier of the urothelium. He has suggested that the fact that the administration of known carcinogens, freeze ulceration, presence of Trichosomoides crassicauda which can potentiate the appearance of saccharin-induced neoplasia are factors which provide optimal conditions for saccharin to reach effective concentrations in the urothelium. Despite the experimental findings however, many epidemiological studies have failed to demonstrate a significant risk from artificial sweetner consumption in man (Clayson, 1984).

In view of the association between urinary tract lithiasis and the presence of foreign bodies with the development of urothelial neoplasia, a thorough examination for bladder calculi is essential in preclinical safety studies where bladder neoplasm are found.

Transitional cell neoplasms and focal transitional cell hyperplasia have also been described in the neck or trigone area of the bladder in dogs treated with oral contraceptives (Johnson, 1989). The mechanism for this effect is unknown, but oral contraceptive agents do not produce these effects in rodents or in monkeys, nor are they reported in humans. It has been postulated that the different embryonic development of the trigone and bladder neck area may render it more responsive to endocrine influences (Johnson, 1989).

REFERENCES

ALPERN, R.J. and TOTO, R.D. (1990): Hypokalemic nephropathy: a clue cystogenesis. N.Engl.J.Med., 322, 398–399.

ABODEELY, D.A. and LEE, J.B. (1971): Fuel of respiration of outer renal medulla. Am.J.Physiol., 220, 1693–1700.

ABRAMS, W.B., IRVIN, J.D., TORBERT, J.A., FERGUSON, R.K. and VLASSES, P.H. (1985): Enantiomers of indacrinone. In: A. Scriabine (Ed.), New Drugs Annual: Cardiovascular Drugs, Vol. 3, pp. 1–20. Raven Press, New York.

ADDIS, T., MARMORSTON, J., GOODMAN, H.C., SELLERS, A.L. and SMITH, M. (1950): Effect of adrenalectomy on spontaneous and induced proteinuria in the rat. Proc.Soc.Exp.Biol.Med., 74, 43–46.

ALARCON-SEGOVIA, D. (1976): Drug-induced antinuclear antibodies and lupus syndromes. Drugs, 12, 69–77.

ALDEN, C.L. (1986): A review of unique male rat hydrocarbon nephropathy. *Toxicol.Pathol.*, 14, 109–111.

ALDEN, C.L., KANERVA, R.L., RIDDER, G. and STONE, L.C. (1984): The pathogenesis of the nephrotoxicity of volatile hydrocarbons in the male rat. *Adv.Modern Environ.Toxicol.*, 7, 107–120.

ALOUSI, M.A., POST, R.A. and HEYMANN, W. (1969): Experimental autoimmune nephrosis in rats. Morphogenesis of the glomerular lesion: Immuno-histochemical and electron microscopic studies. *Am.J.Pathol.*, 54, 47–71.

ANDREWS, B.S., EISENBERG, R.A, THEOFILOPOULOS, A.N., IZUI, S., WILSON, C.B., Mc-CONAHEY, P.J., MURPHY, E.D., ROTHS, J.B. and DIXON, F.J. (1978): Spontaneous murine lupus-like syndromes. Clinical and immunopathological manifestations in several strains. *J.Exp.Med.*, 148, 1198–1215.

ANVER, M.R., COHEN, B.J., LATTUADA, C.P. and FOSTER, S.J. (1982): Age-associated lesions in barrier-reared male Sprague-Dawley rats: A comparison between Hap: (SD) and Crl:COBS-CD(SD) stocks. *Exp.Aging.Res.*, 8, 3–24.

APPEL, G.B., GARVEY, G., SILVA, F., FRANKE, E., NEU, H.C. and WEISSMAN, J. (1981): Acute interstitial nephritis due to amoxycillin therapy. *Nephron*, 27, 313–315.

APPEL, G.B. and NEU, H.C. (1977): The nephotoxic of antimicrobial agents. *N.Engl.J.Med.*, 296, 784–787.

ARISZ, L., NOBLE, B., MILGROM, M., BRENTJENS, J.R. and ANDRES, G.A. (1979): Experimental chronic serum sickness in rats. A model of immune complex glomerulonephritis and systemic immune complex deposition. *Int.Arch.Allergy Appl.Immunol.*, 60, 80–88.

ASAN, E., KUGLER, P. and SHIEBLER, T,H, (1986): Sex-related differences in the handling of florescent ovalbumin by the proximal tubule of the rat kidney. *Histochemistry*, 84, 408–417.

ASSMANN, K.J.M., LANGE, W.P.H, TANGLEDER, M.M. and KOENE, R.A.P. (1986): The organ distribution of gp-300 (Heymann antigen) and gp-90 in the mouse and the rat. *Virchows Arch.[A]*, 408, 541–553.

ASSMANN, K.J.M., RONCO, P., TENGELDER, M.M. LANGEM W.P.H., VERROUST, P. and KOENE, R.A.P. (1985): Comparison of antigenic targets involved in antibody-mediated membranous glomerulonephritis in the mouse and rat. *Am.J.Pathol.*, 121, 112–122.

AUBERT-TULKENS, G., VAN HOOF, F. and TULKENS, P. (1979): Gentamycin-induced lyosmal phospholipidosis in cultured rat fibroblasts: Quantitative ultrastructural and biochemical study. *Lab.Invest.*, 40, 481–491.

AVERBUCH, S.D., AUSTIN, H.A., SHERWIN, S.A., ANTONOVYCH, T., BUNN, P.A. amd LONGO, D.L. (1984): Acute interstitial nephritis with the nephrotic syndrome following recombibant leucocyte A interferon therapy for mycosis fungoides. *N.Engl.J.Med.*, 310–2–35.

BACH, P.H. and BRIDGES, J.W. (1982): Chemical associated renal papillary necrosis. In: P.H. Bach, F.W. Bonner, J.W. Bridges, E.A. Lock (Eds), *Nephrotoxicity, Assessment and Pathogenesis*, pp. 437–459. John Wiley & Sons, Chichester.

BACH, P.H. and BRIDGES, J.W. (1985)a: Chemically induced renal papillary necrosis and upper urothelial carcinoma I. *CRC Crit. Rev.Toxicol.*, 15, 217–329.

BACH, P.H. and BRIDGES, J.W. (1985)b: Chemically induced renal papillary necrosis and upper urothelial carcinoma II. *CRC Crit.Rev.Toxicol.*, 15, 331–437.

BACH, P.H., GRASSO, P., MOLLAND, E.A. and BRIDGES, J.W. (1983): Changes in medullary glycosaminoglycan histochemistry and microvascular filling during the development of 2-bromethanamine hydrobromide-induced renal papillary necrosis. *Toxicol.Appl.Pharmacol.*, 69, 333–344.

BACHMAN, S., KRIZ, W., KUHN, C. and FRANKE, W.W. (1983): Differentiation of cell types in the mammalian kidney by immunofluorescence microscopy using anitbodies to intermediate filament proteins and desmoplakins. *Histochemistry*, 77, 365–394.

BAGDON, W.J., BOKELMAN, D.L., STONE, C.A. and USUI, T. (1985): Toxicity study of MK-421 (enalapril meleate) III. Subacute and one-year chronic studies in Beagle dogs. *Jpn.Pharmacol.Ther.*, 13, 467–518.

BALAZS, T. and ROBINSON, C.J.G. (1983): Procainamide-induced antinuclear antibodies in beagle dogs. *Toxicol.Pharmacol.*, 71, 299–302.

563

BALAZS, T., ROBINSON, C.J.G. and BALTER, N. (1981): Hydralazine-induced antinuclear antibodies in beagle dogs. *Toxicol.Appl. Pharmacol.*, 57, 452–456.

BANNASCH, P. (1984): Sequential cellular changes during chemical carcinogenesis. *J.Cancer Res.Clin.Oncol.*, 108, 11–22.

BANNASCH, P., HACKER, H.J. and ZERBAN, H. (1986): Aberrant regulation of carbohydrate metabolism and metamorphosis during renal carcinogenesis. *Adv.Enzyme Regul.*, 25, 279–296.

BARAJAS, L. and SALIDO, E. (1986): Juxtaglomerular apparatus and the renin-angiotensin system. *Lab.Invest.*, 54, 361–364.

BARSOUM, N., GRACON, S., MCGILL, G., MOORE, J and STURGESS, J. (1985): Early urothelial toxicity induced by a novel antipsychotic agent. *Fed.Proc.*, 44, 1545.

BASKIN, G.B. and DE PAOLI, A. (1977): Primary renal neoplasms of the dog. *Vet.Pathol.*, 14, 591–605.

BATCHELOR, J.R., WELSH, K.I., TINOCO, R.M., DOLLERY, C.T., HUGHES, G.R.V., BERNSTEIN, R., RYAN, P., NAISH, P.F., ABER, G.M., BING.R.F., and RUSSELL, G.I. (1980): Hydralazine-induced systemic lupus erythematosus: Influence of HLA-DR and Sex on susceptibility. *Lancet*, 1, 1107–1109.

BAUM, T., SYBERTZ, E.J., AHNS, H.S., WATKINS, R.W., POWELL, M.L. and LA ROCCA, P.T. (1985): SCH31846. In: A. Scriabine (Ed.), *New Drugs Annual: Cardiovascular Drugs*, Vol. 3, pp. 43–55. Raven Press.

BENIASHVILI, D. Sh. (1989): Induction of renal tumors in cynomolgus monkeys (Macaca fascicularis) by prenatal exposure to 1,2-dimethylhydrazine. *J.N.C.I.*, 81, 1325–1327.

BENNINGTON, J.L. and BECKWITH, J.B., (1975): Mesenchymal tumors of kidney. In: *Tumors of the Kidney, Renal Pelvis and Ureter. Atlas of Tumor Pathology*, Second Series, Fascicle 12, p. 202, AFIP Washington, D.C.

BERTANI, T., POGGI, A., POZZONI, R., DELAINI, F., SACCHI, G., MECCA, G. and DONATI, M.B. (1982): Adriamycin-induced nephrotic syndrome in rats: sequence of pathological events. *Lab.Invest.*, 46, 16–23.

BLAIR, J.T., THOMSON, A.W., WHITING, P.H., DAVIDSON, R.J.L. and SIMPSON, J.G. (1982): Toxicity of the immune suppressant cyclosporin A in the rat. *J.Pathol.*, 138, 163–178.

BLANCHARD, J.L. BASKIN, G.B. and WATSON, E.A. (1986): Generalized amyloidosis in rhesus monkeys. *Vet. Pathol.*, 23, 625–430.

BOHLE, A., CHRIST, H., GRUND, K.E. and MACKENSEN, S. (1979): The role of the interstitium of the renal cortex in renal disease. *Contrib.Nephrol.*, 16, 109–114.

BOHMAN, S.O. (1974): The ultrastructure of the rat medulla as observed after improved fixation methods. *J.Ultrastruct.Res.*, 47, 329–360.

BOHMAN, S.O. (1977): Demonstration of prostaglandin synthesis in collecting duct cells amd other cell types of the rabbit renal medulla. *Prostaglandins*, 14, 729–744.

BOKELMAN, D.L., BAGDON, W.J., MATTIS, P.A. and STONIER, P.F. (1971): Strain-dependent renal toxicology of a non-steroidal anti-flammatory agent. *Toxicol.Appl.Pharmacol.*, 19, 111–124.

BOLTON, W.K., BENTON, F.R., MACLAY, J.G. and STURGILL, B.C. (1976): Spontaneous glomerulosclerosis in aging Spague-Dawley rats. I. Lesions associated with mesangial IgM deposits. *Am.J.Pathol.*, 85, 277–302.

BOMHARD, E., LUCKHAUS, G, VOIGT, W-H and LOESER, E. (1988): Induction of light hydrocarbon nephropathy by p-dichlorobenzene. *Arch. Toxicol.*, 61, 433–439.

BOWIE, D.J. (1935): Method for staining pepsinogen granules in gastric glands. *Anat.Rec.*, 64, 357–367.

BRENNER, B.M., DEEN, W.M. and ROBERTSON, C.R. (1976): Glomerular filtration. In: B.M. Brenner, F.C. Rector Jr (Eds). *The Kidney*. pp. 251–271. W.B. Saunders, Philadelphia.

BRENNER, B.M. (1985): Nephron adaptation to renal injury or ablation. *Am.J.Physiol.*, 249, F324-F337.

BREWER, D.B. (1961): Hydropic change of the proximal convoluted tubules of the kidney. *J.Pathol.Bacteriol.*, 81, 355–363.

BREZIS, M., ROSEN, S., SILVA, P. and EPSTEIN, F.H. (1984)a: Renal ischemia: A new perspective. *Kidney Int.*, 26, 375–383.

BREZIS, M., ROSEN, S., SILVA, P. and EPSTEIN, F.H. (1984)b: Transport dependent anoxic cell injury in the isolated perfused rat kidney. *Am.J.Pathol.*, 116, 327–341.

BREZIS, M., ROSEN, S., SILVA, P. and EPSTEIN, F.H. (1984)c: Polyene toxicity in renal medulla: Injury mediated by transport activity. *Science*, 224, 66–68.

BRIGDEN, R.E., ROSLING, A.E. and WOODS, N.C. (1982): Renal function after acyclovir intravenous injection. *Am.J.Med.*, 73, 182–185.

BULGER, R.E. and DOBYAN, D.C. (1984): Proliferative lesions found in rat kidneys after a single dose of cisplatin. *J.N.C.I.*, 73, 1235–1242.

BULGER, R.E. (1986): Kidney morphology: Update 1985. *Toxicol, Pathol.*, 14, 13–25.

BUREK, J.D. (1978): Age-associated pathology. In: *Pathology of Aging Rats*, Chap. 4, pp 29–167. CRC Press, West Palm Beach, FL.

BURG, M.B. and GREEN, N. (1973: Function of the thick ascending limb of Henle's loop. *Am.J.Physiol.*, 224, 659–668.

BURTON, D.S., MARONPOT, R.R. and HOWARD, F.L. (1979): Frequency of hydronephrosis in Wister rats. *Lab.Anim.*, 29, 642–644.

CALANDRA, S., TARUGI, P., CHISELLINI, M. and GHERADI, E. (1983): Plasma and urine lipoproteins during the development of nephrotic syndrome induced in the rat by adriamycin. *Exp.Mol.Pathol.*, 39, 282–299.

CAMILLERI, J.P., PHAT, V.N., BARIETY, J., CORVOL, P. and MENARD, J. 1980: Use of a specific antiserum for renin detection in human kidney. *J.Histochem.Cytochem.*, 28, 1343–1346.

CANTIN, M., ARAUJO-NASCIMENTO, M de F., BENCHIMOL, S. and DESORMEAUX, Y. (1977): Metaplasia of smooth muscle cells into juxtaglomerular cells in the juxtagomerular appartus, arteries, and arterioles of the ischemic (endocrine) kidney. An ultrastrutural-cytochemical and autoradiographic study. *Am.J.Pathol.*, 87, 581–602.

CASAGRANDE, C., GHIRARDI, P. and MARCHETTI, G. (1985): Ibopamine. In: A. Scriabine (Ed.), *New Drugs Annual: Cardiovascular Drugs* pp. 173–196. Raven Press, New York.

CASE RECORDS OF THE MASSACHUSETTS GENERAL HOSPITAL (1984): Case 45-1984. *N.Engl.J.Med.*, 311, 1239–1247.

CASE, D.B., ATLAS, S.A. MOURADIAN, J.A. FISHMAN, R.A. SHERMAN, R.L. and LARAGH, J.H. (1980): Proteinuria during long-term captopril therapy, *J.A.M.A.*, 244, 346–349.

CASEY, H.W., and SPLITTER, G.A. (1975): Membranous glomerulonephritis in dogs infected with Dirofilaria immitis. *Vet.Pathol.*, 12, 111–117.

CAULFIELD, J.B. and SCHRAG, P.E. (1964): Electron microscopic study of renal calcification. *Am.J.Pathol.*, 44, 365–381.

CELSI, G., JAKOBSSON, B and APERIA, A. (1986): Influence of age on compensatory renal growth in rats. *Pediatr. Res.*, 20, 347–350.

CHAPPELL, R.H. AND PHILLIPS, J.R. (1950): Adenomatoid changes of renal glomerular capsular epithelium associated with adrenal tumor. *Arch.Pathol.*, 49, 70–72.

CHARUEL, C., FACCINI, J., MONRO, A. and NACHBAUR, J. (1984): A second peak in uptake of gentamicin by rat kidney after cessation of treatment. *Biopharm.Drug Dispos.*, 5, 21–24.

CHIN, T.Y., TYL, R.W., POPP, J.A. and HECK, H. d'A. (1981): Chemical urolithiasis:1. Characteristics of bladder stone induction by terephthalic acid and dimethyl terephthalate in weanling Fischer-344 rats. *Toxicol.Appl.Pharmacol.*, 58, 307–321.

CHOWANIEC, J. and HICKS, R.M. (1979): Response of the rat to saccharin with particular influence to the urinary bladder. *Br.J.Cancer.*, 39, 355–375.

CHRISTENSEN, E.I., and MADSEN, K.M. (1978): Renal age changes. Observations on the rat kidney cortex with special reference to structure and function of the lysosomal system in the proximal tubule. *Lab.Invest.*, 39, 289–297.

CHRISTENSEN, E.I. and MAUNSBACH, A.B. (1979): Effects of dextran on lysomal ultrastructure and protein digestion in renal proximal tubule. *Kidney Int.*, 16, 301–311.

CHRISTENSEN, S. and OTTOSEN, P.D. (1986): Lithium-induced uremia in rats; Survival and renal function and morphology after one year. *Acta Pharmacol.Toxicol.(Copenh).*, 58, 339–347.

CLAESSON, K., FORSUM, U., KLARESKOG, L., ANDREEN, T., LARSSON, E., FRÖDIN, L.

Tissue distribution of T-lymphocytes and Ia-expressing cells in rat kidney grafts. *Scand.J.Immunol.*, 22, 273–278.

CLAPP, M.J.L., WADE, J.D. and SAMUELS, D.M. (1982): Control of nephrocalcinosis by manipulating the calcium: phosphorus ratio in commercial rodent diets. *Lab.Anim.*, 16, 130–132.

CLAUSEN, E. (1964): Histological changes in rabbit kidneys induced by phenacetin and acetylsalicyclic acid. *Lancet*, 2, 123–124.

CLAYSON, D.B. (1974): Bladder carcinogenesis in rats and mice. Possibility of artefact. *J.N.C.I.*, 52, 1685–1689.

CLAYSON, D.B. (1984): The mode of carcinogenic action of saccharin. *Cancer Lett.*, 22, 119–123.

COLEMAN, G.L., BARTHOLD, S.W., OSBALDISTON, G.W., FOSTER, S.J., JONAS, A.M. (1977): Pathological changes during aging in barrier-reared Fischer 344 male rats. *J.Gerontol.*, 32, 258–278.

COHEN, S.M. and FRIEDELL, G.H. (1979):Animal Model: Carcinoma of th urinary bladder induced in Fischer rats by N-[4-(5-nitro-2-furyl)-2-thiazolyl]formamide. *Am.J.Pathol.*, 95, 849–852.

COHEN, S.M., JACOBS, J.B., ARAI, M., JOHANSSON, S. and FRIEDELL, G.H. (1976): Early lesions in experimental bladder cancer: Experimental design and light microscopic findings. *Cancer Res.*, 36, 2508–2511.

CORRADO, M.L. STRUBLE, W.E., PETER, C., HOAGLAND, V. and SABBAJ, J. (1987): Norfloxacin: Review of safety studies. *Am.J.Med.*, 82, Suppl 6B, 22–26.

COUSER, W.G., BAKER, P.J. and ADLER, S. (1985): Complement mediation of immune glomerular injury: A new perspective. *Kidney Int.*, 28, 879–890.

COUSER, W.G. and STILMENT, M.M. (1975): Mesangial lesions and focal glomerular sclerosis in the aging rat. *Lab.Invest.*, 33, 491–501.

COUSINS, F.B. and GEARY, C.P.M. (1966): A sex determined renal calcification in rats. *Nature*, 211, 980–981.

CRABTREE, C. (1941): The structure of Bowman's capsule in castrate and testosterone treated mice as an index of hormonal effect on the renal cortex. *Endocrinology*, 29, 197–203.

CRAIG, J.M. (1959): Observations on the kidney after phosphate loading in the rat. *Arch.Pathol.*, 6, 306–315.

CRUIKSHANK, J.M. FITZGERALD, J.D. and TUCKER, M. (1984): Beta-adrenoceptor blocking drugs: pronethalol and practalol. In: D.R. Laurence, A.E.M. McLean and M. Weatherall, (Eds), Safety Testing of New Drugs. *Laboratory Predictions and Clinical Performance*, Chap. 5, pp 93–123. Academic Press, London.

CUPPAGE, F.E. (1965): Renal changes in the rat following intravenous injection of complete Freund's adjuvant. *Lab.Invest.*, 14, 514–528.

CURTIS, J.R. (1979): Drug-induced renal disease. *Drugs*, 18, 377–391.

DAVIES, D.J. (1968): Changes in the renal cortex following experimental medullary necrosis. *Arch. Pathol.*, 86, 377–382.

DAVIES, D.J. (1970): The early changes produced in the rabbit renal medulla by ethyleneimide: Electron-microscope and circulatory studies. *J.Pathol.*, 101, 329–332.

DAVIES, I., (1986): Immunological adjuvants of natural origin and their adverse effects. *Adv.Drug React.Act.Pois.Rev.*, 1. 1–21.

DEERBERG, F. and REHM, S. (1985): Spontaneous renal pelvic carcinoma in DA/HAN rats. *Z. Versuchstierkd.*, 27, 33–38.

DEERBERG, F. REHM, S. and JOSTMEYER, H.H. (1985): Spontaneous urinary bladder tumors in DA/HAN rsts: A feasible model of human bladder cancer. *J.N.C.I.*, 75, 1113–1121.

DEES, J.H., HEATFIELD, B.M., REUBER, M.D. and TRUMP, B.F. (1980): Adenocarcinomaof the kidney. III. Histogenesis of renal adenocarcinomas induced by N-(4'fluoro-4-biphenylyl)acetamide. *J.N.C.I.*, 64, 1537–1545.

DEES, J.H. and KRAMER, R.A. (1986): Sequential morphologic analysis of the nephrotoxicity produced in rats by single doses of chlorozotocin. *Toxicol.Pathol.*, 14, 213–231.

DEES, J.H., COE, L.D., YASUKOCHI, Y. and MASTERS, B.S. (1980): Immuno-fluorescence of

NADPH cytochrone C (P-450) resductase in rat and minipig tissues injected with phenobarbital. *Science*, 208, 1473–1475.

DEES, J.H., PARKHILL, L.K., OKITA, R.T., YASUKOCHI, Y. and MASTERSM B.S. (1982): Localization of NADPH-cytochrome P-450 reductase and cytochrome P-450 in animal kidneys. In: P.H. Bach, F.W. Bonner, J.W. Bridgesand E.A. Lock (Ed.), *Nephrotoxicity, Assessment and Pathogenesis*, pp. 246–249.

DITERS, R.W. and WELLS, M. (1986): Renal interstitial cell tumors in the dog. *Vet.Pathol.*, 23, 74–76.

DOBYAN, D.C. (1985): Long-term consequences of cisplatinum-induced renal injury: A structural and functional study. *Anat.Rec.*, 212, 239–245.

DODD, D.E., LOSCO, P.E., TROUP, C.M., PRITTS, I.M. and TYLER, T.R. (1987): Hyaline droplet nephrosis in male Fischer-344 rats following inhalation of diisobutyl ketone. *Toxicol.Ind.Health.* 3, 443–457.

DOMINICK, M.A., SUSICK, R.L. and MACDONALD, J.R. (1989): effects of the angiotensin converting enzyme inhibitor quinapril on renal structure and function. *Toxicologist*, 9, 175.

DONAUBAUER, H.H. and MAYER, D. (1988): Acute, sub-chronic and chronic toxicity of the new angiotensin converting enzyme inhibitor ramipril. *Arzneimittelforschung*, 38, 14–20.

DOSIK, G.M., GUTTERMAN, J.U., HERSH, E.M., AKHTAR, M., SONODA, T. and HORN, R.G. (1978): Nephrotoxicity from cancer immunotherapy. *Ann.Intern.Med.*, 89, 41–46.

DUFFY, J.L., YASHNOSUKE, S. and CHUNG, J. (1971): Acute calcium nephropathy: Early proximal tubular changes in the rat kidney. *Arch.Pathol.*, 91, 340–350.

EDDY, A.A.. CRARY, G.S. and MICHAEL, A.F. (1986): Identification of lympho-hemopoietic cells in the kidneys of normal rats. *Am.J.Pathol.*, 124, 335–342.

EDGINGTON, T.S., GLASSOCK, R.J. and DIXON, F.J. (1968): Autologous immune complex nephritis induced with renal tubular antigen: I. Identification and isolation of the pathogenetic antigen. *J.Exp.Med.*, 127, 555–572.

EISEN, H.N. (1946): Adenomatoid transformation of the glomerular capsular epithelium. *Am.J.Pathol.*, 22, 597–601.

EKMAN, L., HANSSON, E., HAVU, N., CARLSSON, E. and LUNBERG, C. (1985): Toxicological studies on omeprazole. *Scand.J.Gastroenterol.*, 20, Suppl. 108, 53–69.

ELEMA, J.D. and ARENDS, A. (1971): Functional overload as a possible cause for non-immune glomerular damage. Effect of nephrectomy and irradiation of the contralateral kidney. *J.Pathol.*, 103, 21–28.

ELEMA, J.D. and ARENDS, A (1975): Focal and segmental glomerular hyalinosis and sclerosis in the rat. *Lab.Invest.*, 33, 554–561.

ELLIS, B.G., PRICE, R.G. and TOPHAM, J.C. (1973): The effect of papillary damage by ethylene-imide on kidney function and some urinary enzymes in the dog. *Chem.Biol.Interact.*, 7, 131–142.

ELLISON, D.H., VELAZQUEZ, H. and WRIGHT, F.S. (1989): Adaptation of the distal convoluted tubule of the rat. Structural and functional effects of dietary salt intake and chronic diuretic infusion. *J.Clin.Invest.*, 83, 113–126.

ENDOU, H., KOSEKI, C., HASAMURA, S., KAKUNO, K., HOJO, K. and SAKAI, F. (1982): Renal cytochrome P-450: its localization along a single nephron and its induction. In: F. Morel (Ed.), *Biochemistry of Kidney Function*, pp. 319–327. Elsevier, Amsterdam.

EULDERLINK, F. (1964): Adenomatoid changes in Bowman's capsule in primary carcinoma of the liver. *J.Pathol.Bacteriol.*, 87, 251–254.

EVANS, G.O. and MORGAN, R.J.I. (1986): Urinary enzyme measurements in male rats after oral administration of decalin. *Hum.Toxicol.*, 5, 120.

EVANS, G.O., GOODWIN, D.A., PARSONS, C.E. and READ, N.G. (1988): The effects of levamisole on urinary enzyme measurements and proximal tubule cell incusions in male rats. *Br.J.Exp.Pathol.*, 69, 301–308.

EVERITT, A.V., PORTER, B.D. and WYNDHAM, J.R. (1982): Effects of caloric intake and dietary composition on the development of proteinuria, age-associated renal disease and longevity in the male rat. *Gerontology*, 28, 168–175.

567

FACCINI, J.M. (1982): A perspective on the pathology and cytochemistry of renal lesions. In: P.H. Bach, F.W. Bonner, J.W. Bridges and E.D. Lock (Eds), *Nephrotoxicity Assessment and Pathogenesis*, pp. 82–97. John Wiley & Sons, Chichester.

FAJARDO, L.F., ELTRINGHAM, J.R., STEWARD,J.R. and KLAUBER, M.R. (1980): Adriamycinnephrotixicity. *Lab.Invest.*, 43, 242–253.

FARAGGIANA, T., GRESIK,E., TANAKA, T., INAGAMI, T. and LUPO, A. (1982): Immunohistochemical localization of renin in the human kidney. *J.Histochem.Cytochem.*, 30, 459–465.

FAREBROTHER, D.A. (1984): Histopathological changes found in the renal medulla of rats in adenine toxicity. In: P.H. Bach and E.A. Lock (Eds), *Renal Heterogeneity and Target Cell Toxicity*, pp. 223–226. John Wiley & Sons, Chichester.

FARQUHAR, M.G. and KANWAR, Y.S. (1980): Characterization of anionic sites in the glomerular basement membranes of normal and nephrotic rats. In: A. Leaf, G. Giebisch, L. Bolis, S. Gorini (Eds), *Renal Pathophysiology: Recent Advances*, p. 57. Raven Press, New York.

FENT, K., MAYER, E. and ZBINDEN, G. (1988): Nephrotoxicity screening in rats: a validation study. *Arch. Toxicol.*, 61, 349–358.

FINE, L.G. and BRADLEY, T. (1985): Adaption of proximal tubular structure and function: insights into compensatory renal hypertrophy. *Fed.Proc.*, 44, 2723–2727.

FINN, W.F. (1982): Compensatory renal hypertrophy in Sprague-Dawley rats. Glomerular ultrafiltration dynamics. *Renal Physiol.*, 5, 222–234.

FLAKS, A., HAMILTON, J.M. and CLAYSON, D.B. (1973): Effect of ammonium chloride on indicence of bladder tumors by 4-ethylsulphonylnaphthalene-1-sulphonamide. *J.N.C.I.*, 51, 2007–2008.

FORNI, A.M., KOSS, L.G. and GELLER, W. (1964): Cytological study of the effect of cyclophosphamide on the bladder epithelium of the urinary bladder in man. *Cancer.* 17, 1348–1355.

FRAZIER, D.L., CARVER, M.P. DIX, L.P., THOMPSON, C.A. and RIVIERE, J.E. (1986)a: Exaggerated response to gentamycin-induced nephrotoxicity in Sprague Dawley rats: Identification of a highly sensitive outlier population. *Toxicol.Pathol.*, 14, 204–209.

FRAZIER, D.L., DIX, L.P., BOWMAN, K.F., THOMPSON, C. and RIVIERE, J.E. (1986)b: Increased gentamicin nephrotoxicity in normal and diseased dogs administered identical serum drug concentration profiles: Increased sensitivity in subclinical renal dysfuntion. *J.Pharmacol.Exp.Ther.*, 239, 946–951.

FREGA, N.S., DIBONA, D.R., GUERTLER, B. and LEAF, A. (1976): Ischemia renal injury. *Kidney Int.*, 10 (Suppl 1), S17–S25.

FRY, J.R., WEIBKIN, P., KAO, J., JONES, C.A., GWYNN, J. and BRIDGES, J.W. (1978): A comparison of drug-metabolizing capability is isolated viable rat hepatocytes and renal tubule fragments. *Xenobiotica*, 8, 113–120.

FUKUSHIMA, S., COHEN, S.M. ARAI, M., JACOBS, J.B. and FRIEDELL, G.H. (1981): Scanning electron microscopic examination of reversible hyperplasia of the rat urinary bladder. *Am.J.Pathol.*, 102, 373–380.

GANOTE, C.E., PHILIPSBORN, D.S., CHEN, E. and CARONE, F.A. (1975): Acute calcium nephrotoxicity. *Arch.Pathol.*, 99, 650–657.

GARTHOFF, B., HOFFMANN, K., LUCKHAUS, G. and THURAU, K. (1982): Adequate substitution with electrolytes in toxicological testing of 'loop' diuretics in the dogs *Toxicol.Appl.Pharmacol.*, 65, 191–202.

GARTNER, H.V. (1980): Membranous (peri-epi-extramembranous) glomerulonephritis-prototype of an immune complex glomerulonephritis. A clinical morphological study. *Veroff.Pathol.*, 113, 1–136.

GERMUTH, F.G. and RODRIGUEZ.E. (1973): Spontaneous animal diseases. In: Immunopathology of the Renal Glomerulus. *Immune Complex Deposit and Antibasement Membrane Disease*, Chap. 3, pp, 45–56. Little, Brown and Co., Boston.

GHADIALLY, F.N. (1982): Lysosomes. In: *Ultrastructural Pathology of Cell and Matrix* (2nd Edition), Chap. 7, pp. 435–579, Butterworths, London.

GIBSON, T., BURRY, H.C. and OGG, C. (1976): Goodpasture syndrome and D-penicillamine. *Ann.Intern.Med.*, 84, 100.

GIROUX, L., SMEESTERS, C., BOURY, F., FAURE, M.P. and JEAN, G. (1984): Adriamycin and adriamycin-DNA nephrotoxicity in rats. *Lab.Invest.*, 50, 190–196.

GOLDSTEIN, R.S., TARLOFF, J.B. and HOOK, J.B. (1988): Age-related nephropathy in laboratory rats. *FASEB,J.*, 2, 2241–2251.

GOODE, N.P., DAVISON, A.M. GOWLAND, G., and SHIRES, M. (1988): Spontaneous glomerular immunoglobulin deposition in young Sprague-Dawley rats. *Lab. Anim.*, 22, 287–292.

GOODMAN, F.R., WEISS, G.B. and HURLEY, M.E. (1985): Pentopril. In: A. Scriabine (Ed.), *New Drugs Annual: Cardiovascular Drugs*, Vol. 3, pp. 57–69. Raven Press, New York.

GOODMAN, D.G., WARD, J.M., SQUIRE, R.A., PAXTON, M.B., REICHARDT, W.D., CHU, K.C. and LINHARD, M.S. (1980): Neoplastic and non-neoplastic lesions in aging Osborne-Mendel rats. *Toxicol.Appl.Pharmacol.*, 55, 433–447.

GORDON, L.R. (1986): Spontaneous lipomatous tumors in the kidney of the Crl:CD (SD) BR rat. *Toxicol. Pathol.*, 14, 175–182.

GRASSO, P. (1987): Persistent organ damage and cancer production in rats and mice. *Arch. Toxicol.*, Suppl. 11, 75–83.

GRAY, J.E. (1977): Chronic progressive nephrosis in the albino rat. *CRC Crit.Rev.Toxicol.*, 5, 115–144.

GRAY, J.E., VAN ZWIETEN, M.J. and HOLLANDER, C.F. (1982): Early light microscopic changes of chronic progressive nephrosis in several strains of aging laboratory rats. *J.Gerontol.*, 37, 142–150.

GRAY, J.E., WEAVER, R.N. and PURMALIS, A. (1974): Ultrastructural observations of chronic progressive nephrosis in the Sprague-Dawley rat. *Vet.Pathol.*, 11, 153–164.

GREAVES, P. and FACCINI, J.M. (1984): Urinary tract. In: *Rat Histo-pathology*, Chap 7, pp. 144–160. Elsevier, Amsterdam.

GRESSER, I., AGUET, M., MOREL-MAROGER, L., WOODROW, D., PAVION-DUTILLEUL, F., GUILLON, J-C. and MAURY, C. (1981): Electrophoretically pure mouse interferon inhibits growth, induces liver and kidney lesions and kills suckling mice. *Am.J.Pathol.*, 102, 396–402.

GRESSER, I., MAURY, C., TOVEY, M.G.,MOREL-MAROGER, L. and PONTILLON, F. (1976): Progressive glomerulonephritis in mice treated with interferon preparations at birth. *Nature*, 263, 420–422.

GREND, J., SCHILTHUIS, M.S., KOUDSTALL, J. and ELEMA, J.D. (1982): Mesangial function and glomerular sclerosis in rats after unilateral nephrectomy. *Kidney Int.*, 22, 338–343.

GROND, J., BEUKERS, J.Y.B., SCHILTHUIS, M.S., WEENING, J.J. and ELEMA, J.D. (1986): Analysis of renal structural and functional features in two rat strains with a different susceptibility to glomerular sclerosis. *Lab.Invest.*, 54, 77–83.

GUDER, W.G. and ROSS, B.D. (1984): Enzyme distribution along the nephron. *Kidney Int.*, 26, 101–111.

GURNER, N., SMITH, J. and CATELL, V. (1986): In vivo induction of Ia antigen in resident leucocytes in normal rat renal glomerulus. *Lab.Invest.*, 55, 546–550.

GUTTMAN, P.H. and ANDERSON, A.C. (1968): Progressive intercapillary glomerulosclerosis in aging and irradiated beagles. *Radiat.Res.*, 35, 45–60.

HACKBARTH, H., BAUNACK, E. and WINN, M. (1981): Strain differences in kidney function of inbred rats: In: Glomerular filtration rate and renal plasma flow. *Lab.Anim.*, 15, 125–128.

HACKBARTH, H., BUTTNER, D., JARCK, D., POTHMANN, MESSOW, C. and GARTNER, K. (1983): Distribution of glomeruli in the renal cortex of Munich Wistar Frömter (MWF) rats. *Renal Physiol.*, 6, 63–71.

HACKBARTH, H. and HACKBARTH, D. (1981): Genetic analysis of renal function in mice: I. Glomerular filtration rate and its correlation with body and kidney weight. *Lab.Anim.*, 15, 267–272.

HACKER, H.J. BANNASCH, P. and LIEHR, J.G. (1988): Histochemical analysis of the development of estradiol-induced kidney tumors in male Syrian hamsters. *Cancer Res.*, 48, 971–976.

HAENSLY, W.E., GRANGER, H.J., MORRIS, A.C. and CIOFFE, C. (1982): Proximal tubule-like epithelium in Bowman's capsule in spontaneously hypertensive rats. Changes with age. *Am.J.Pathol.*, 107, 92–97.

569

HALL, R.L., WILKE, W.L. and FETTMAN, M.J. (1985): Captopril slows the progression of chronic renal disease in partially nephrectomized rats. *Toxicol.Appl.Pharmacol.*, 80, 517–526.

HALL, R.L., WILKE, W.L. and FETTMAN, M.J. (1986): The progression of adriamycin-induced nephrotic syndrome in rats and the effect of captopril. *Toxicol.Appl.Pharmacol.*, 82, 164–174.

HALMAN, J., FOWLER, J.S.L. and PRICE, R.G. (1985): Urinary enzymes proteinuria and renal function tests in the assessment of nephrotoxicity in the rat. In: P.H. Bach and E.A. Lock (Eds), *Renal Heterogeneity and Target Cell Toxicity. Monographs in Applied Toxicity*, 2, 295–298. Wiley & Sons, Chichester.

HANIKA, C. and REBAR, A.H. (1980): Urethral transitional cell carcinoma in the dog. *Vet.Pathol.*, 17, 643–646.

HANSEN, T.M., PETERSEN, J., HALBERG, P., PERMIN, H., ULLMA, S., BRON, C. and LARSEN, S. (1978): Levamisole-induced nephropathy. *Lancet*, 2, 737.

HARD, G.C. (1985): Identification of a high frequency model for renal carcinoma by the induction of renal tumors in the mouse with a single dose of streptozotocin. *Cancer Res.*, 45, 703–708.

HARD, G.G. (1986): Experimental models for the sequential analysis of chemically-induced renal carcinogenesis. *Toxicol.Pathol.*, 14, 112–122.

HARRIS, C.A., BAER, P.G., CHIRITO, E. and DIRKS, J.H. (1974): Composition of mammalian glomerular filtrate. *Am.J.Physiol.*, 227, 972–976.

HARRISON, H.E. and HARRISON, H.C. (1955): Inhibition of urine citrate excretion and the production of renal calcinosis in the rat by acetazolamine (Diamox) administration. *J.Clin.Invest.*, 34, 1662–1670.

HARTROFT, P.M. and HARTROFT, W.S. (1953): Studies on renal juxtaglomerular cells. *J.Exp.Med.*, 97, 415–427.

HASHIMOTO, K., YOSHIMURA, S., OHTAKI, T. and IMAI, K. (1981): Toxicological studies of captopril, an inhibitor of angiotensin converting enzyme. III: Twelve month studies on the chronic toxicity of captopril in beagle dogs. *J.Toxicol.Sci.*, 6 (Suppl. 2), 215–246.

HAUGHTON, D.G., HARTNETT, M., CAMPBELL-BOSWELL, M., PORTER, G. and BENNET, W.A. (1976): A light and electron microscopic analysis of gentamycin nephrotoxicity in rats. *Am.J.Pathol.*, 82, 589–612.

HEPTINSTALL, R.H. (1983)a: Renal complications of therapeutic and diagnostic agents, analgesic abuse and addition to narcotics. In: *Pathology of the Kidney, Vol. 3*, Chap. 23, pp. 1195–1255. Little, Brown and Company, Boston.

HEPTINSTALL, R.H (1983)b: Interstitial nephritis. In: *Pathology of the Kidney, Vol. 3*, Chap. 22, pp. 1149–1193. Little, Brown and Company, Boston.

HEREMANS.H., BILLIAU, A., COLOMBATTI, A., HILGERS, J. and DE SOMER, P. (1978): Interferon treatment of NZB mice: Accelerated progression of autoimmune disease. *Infect.Immun.*, 21, 925–930.

HERMAN, E.H., EL-HAGE, A.V., FERRANS, V.J. and ARDALAN, B. (1985): Comparison of the severity of the chronic cardiotoxicity produced by doxorubicin in normotensive and hypertensive rats. *Toxicol. Appl.Pharmacol.*, 78, 202–214.

HETMAR, O., BRUN, C., CLEMMESEN, L., LADEFOGED, J., LARSEN, S. and RAFAELSEN, O.J. (1987): Lithium: Long term effects on the kidney - II. Structural changes. *J. Psychiatr. Res.*, 21, 279–288.

HEYMANN, W., HACKEL, D.B., HARWOOD, S., WILSON, S.G.F. and HUNTER, J.L.P. (1959): Production of nephrotic syndrome in rats by Freund's adjuvants and rat kidney suspensions. *Proc.Soc.Exp.Biol.Med.*, 100, 660–664.

HIASA, Y, OHSHIMA, M., IWATA, C. and TANIKATE, T (1979): Histopathological studies on renal tubular cell tumors in rats treated with N-ethyl-N-hydroxyethylnitrosamine. *Jpn.J.Cancer Res.*, (Gann) 70, 817–820.

HICKS, R.M. (1984): Promotion: Is saccharin a promotor in the urinary bladder. *Food Chem.Toxicol.*, 22, 755–760.

HICKS, R.M. WAKEFIELD, J. St. J., VLASOV, N.N. and PLISS, G.B. (1976): Tumours of the bladder. In: V.S. Turusov (Ed.), *Pathology of Tumours in Laboratory Animals, Vol. 1, Tumours* of the Rat, Part 2, pp. 103–134. IARC Scientific Publ No. 6, Lyon. HILL, G.S. (1986): Drug-associated glomerulopathies. Toxicol. Pathol., 14, 37–44.

HINTON, D.E., HEATFIELD, B.M., LIPSKY, M.M. and TRUMP, B.F. (1980): Animal models. Chemically induced renal tubular carcinoma in rats. Am.J.Pathol., 100, 317–320.

HJORTKJAER, R.K., BILLE-HANSEN, V., HAZELDEN, K.P., McCONVILLE, M., McGREGOR, D.B., CUTHBERT, J.A. and GREENOUGH, R.J. (1986): Safety evaluation of celluclast, an acid cellulase derived from Triichoderma reesi. Food Chem.Toxicol., 24, 55–63.

HOLTHÖFER, H. (1983): Lectin binding sites in kidney. A comparative study of 14 animal species. J.Histochem.Cytochem., 31, 531–537.

HOLTHÖFER, H., MIETTINEN, A., PAASIVUO, R., LEHTO,.P., LINDER, E., ALFTHAN, O. AND VIRTANEN, I. (1983): Cellular origin and differentiation of renal carcinomas. A fluorescence microscopic study with kidney specific antibodies, anti-intermediate filament antibodies and lectins. Lab.Invest., 49, 317–326.

HOORNTJE, S.J. WEENING, J.J., THE, T.H., KALLENBERG, C.C.M., DONKER, A.J.M. and HOEDEMAEKER, P.J. (1980): Immune complex glomerulopathy in patients treated with captopril. Lancet, 1, 1212–1215.

HOOVER, R. and FRAUMENI, J.F. (1981): Drug-induced cancer. Cancer, 47, 1071–1080.

HORACEK, M.J., EARLE, A.M. and GILMORE, P. (1987): The renal vascular system of the monkey: a gross anatomical description. J. Anat., 153, 123–137.

HOTTENDORF, G.H. and WILLIAMS, P.D. (1986): Aminoglycoside nephrotoxicity. Toxicol.Pathol., 14, 66–72.

HOWIE, A.J., GUNSON, B.K. and SPARKE, J. (1990): Morphometric correlates of renal excretory function. J.Pathol., 160, 245–253.

HOYER, J.R. and SEILMER, M.W. (1979): Pathophysiology of Tamm-Horsfall protein. Kidney Int., 16, 279–289.

HULTMAN, P. and ENESTRÖM, S. (1989): Murine mercury-induced immune-complex disease: effect of cyclophosphamide treatment and importance of T-cells. Br.J.Exp.Pathol., 70, 227–236.

IKEDA, H., TAUCHI, H., SHIMASAKI, H., UETA, N. and SATO, T. (1985): Age and organ differences in amount and distribution of autofluorescent granules in rats. Mech.Ageing Dev., 31, 139–146.

IRISARRI, E., KESSEDJIAN, M.J., CHARUEL, C., FACCINI, J.M., GREAVES, P., MONRO, A.M., NACHBAUR, J. and RABEMAMPIANINA, Y. (1985): Dazoxiben, a prototype inhibitoe of thromboxane synthesis, has little toxicity in laboratory animals. Hum.Toxicol., 4, 311–315.

IRWIN, J.F., LANE, S.E. and NEUHAUS, O.W. (1971): Synergistic effect of glucocortoids and androgens on the biosynthesis of sex-dependent protein in the male rat. Biochem.Biophys.Acta., 252, 328–334.

ISHII, H., KOSHIMIZU, T., USAMA, S. and FUJIMOTO, T. (1981): Toxicity of aspartame and its diketopiperaine for Wistar rats by dietary administration for 104 weeks. Toxicology, 21, 91–94.

ITO, N., HIASA, Y., TAMAI, OKAJIMA, E. and KITAMURA, H., (1969): Histogenesis of urinary bladder tumors induced by N-butyl-N-(4-hydroxybutyl)nitrosamine in rats. Jpn.J.Cancer Res., (Gann) 60, 401–410.

JACCOTTET, M-A. (1959): Zur Histologie and Pathogenase der Nierenverkalung. (Nephrocalcinose und dystrophische Kalknephrose). Virchows Arch.[A], 332, 245–263.

JACOBS, J.B., ARAI, M., COHEN, S.M. and FRIEDELL, G.H. (1976): Early lesions in bladdercancer: Scanning electron microscopy of cell surface markers. Cancer Res., 36, 2512–2517.

JACOBSEN, N.O., OLESSEN, O.V. THOMSEN, K., OTTOSEN, P.D. and OLSEN, S. (1982): Early changes in renal distal convoluted tubules and convoluted ducts of lithium treated rats. Light microscopy, enzyme histochemistry and ^{3}H-thymidine autoradiography. Lab. Invest., 46, 298–305.

JACOBSEN, N.O. and JORGENSEN, F. (1973): Ultrastructural observations of the proximal tubule in the kidney of the male rat. Z.Zellforsch.Microsk.Anat., 136, 479–499.

JAFFE, D., SUTHERLAND, L.E. and BARKER, D.M. (1970): Effects of chronic excess salt ingestion: morphological findings in kidneys of rats with differing genetic susceptibilities to hypertension. Arch.Pathol., 90, 1–16.

JAKOWSKI, R.M. (1982): Renal tubular epithelium lining parietal layer of Bowman's capsule in adult Long-Evans rats. *Vet.Pathol.*, 19, 212–215.

JAO.W., MANALIGOD, J.R., GERADO, L.T. and CASTILLO, M.M. (1983): Myeloid bodies in drug-induced acute tubular necrosis. *J.Pathol.*, 139, 33–40.

JOHNSON, A.N. (1989): Comparative aspects of contraceptive steroids. Effects observed in beagle dogs. *Toxicol.Pathol.*, 17, 389–395.

JOHNSON, H.A. and ROMAN, J.M.V. (1968): Compensatory renal enlargement. Hypertrophy versus hyperplasia. *Am.J.Pathol.*, 49, 1–13.

JOHNSON, R.J., GARCIA, R.L. PRITZL, P. and ALPERS, C.E. (1990): Platelets mediate glomerular cell proliferation in immune complex nephritis induced by antimesangial cell antibodies in the rat. *Am.J.Pathol.*, 136, 369–374.

JOSEPH, X., ROBINSON, C.J.G., ABRAHAM, A.A. and BALAZS, T. (1986): Differences in the induction of autoimmune responses in A.SW/SnJ mice by various agents. *Arch.Toxicol.*, Suppl. 9, 272–274.

JOSEPOVITZ, C., LEVINE, R., LANE, B. and KALOYANIDES, G.J. (1985): Contrasting effects of gentamycin and mercuric chloride on urinary excretion of enzymes and phospholipids in the rat. *Lab.Invest.*, 52, 375–386.

KAISSLING, B.S., BACHMAN, S. and KRIZ, W. (1985): Structural adaptation of the distal convoluted tubule to prolonged furosemide treatment. *Am.J.Physiol.*, 248, F374–381.

KAISSLING, B. and LE HIR, M (1982): Distal tubular segments of the kidney after adaptation to altered Na and K intake. *Cell Tissue Res.*, 224, 469,492.

KAISSLING, B., PETER, S. and KRIZ, W. (1977): Transition of the thick ascending limb of Henle's loop into distal convoluted tubule in the nephron of the rat kidney. *Cell Tissue Res.*, 182, 111–118.

KALOYANIDES, G.J. and PASTORIZA-MUNOZ, E. (1980): Aminoglycoside nephrotoxicity. *Kidney Int.*, 18, 571–582.

KANERVA, R.L., RIDDER, G.M., STONE, L.C. and ALDEN, C.L. (1987): Characterisation of spontaneous and decalin-induced hyaline droplets in kidneys of adult male rats. *Food Chem. Toxicol.*, 25, 63–83.

KANWAR, Y.S. and FARQUAR, M.G. (1979): Isolation of glycosaminoglycans (heparan sulfate) from glomerular basement membranes. *Proc.Natl.Acad.Sci.*, USA 76, 4493–4497.

KARNOVSKY, M.J. and AINSWORTH, S.D. (1972): The structural basis of glomerular filtration. In: J. Hamburger, J. Crisnier and M.H. Maxwell (Eds), *Advances in Nephrology*. Year Book, Vol. 2, Chap. 3, pp. 35–60.

KASHIGARIAN, M. (1985): Mesangium and glomerular disease. *Lab.Invest.*, 52, 569–571.

KERJASCHKI, D., SHARKEY, S.J. and FARQUAR, M.G. (1984): Identification and characterization of podocalyxin: the major sialoprotein of the renal glomerular epithelial cell. *J.Cell.Biol.*, 98, 1591–1596.

KHAN.S.R., FINLAYSON, B. and HACKETT, R.L. (1982): Experimental calcium oxalate nephrolithiasis in the rat. Role of the renal papilla. *Am.J.Pathol.*, 107, 59–69.

KIEF, H. and WESTEN, H. (1980): Besonderheiten bei der Prüfung von Diuretika. In B. Schnieders and P. Grosdanoff (Eds), Zur Problematik von Chronischen Toxizitätsprufung, AMI-Bericht 1/1980, pp. 131–135. Dietrich Reimer Verlag, Berlin.

KINCAID-SMITH, P.M. (1967): Pathogenesis of the renal lesion associated with the abuse of analgesics. *Lancet*, 1, 859–862.

KINCAID-SMITH, P.M., SAKER, B.M., McKENSIE, I.F.C. and MURIDEN, K.D. (1968): Lesions in the blood supply of the papilla in experimental analgesic nephropathy. *Med.J.Aust.*, 1, 203–206.

KIRKMAN, H. and ROBBINS, M. (1959): Estrogen-induced tumors of the kidney. V. Histology and histogenesis in the Syrian hamster. *N.C.I. Monogr.*, 1, 93–139.

KITCHEN, D.N. (1984): Neoplastic renal effects of unleaded gasoline in Fischer-344 rats. In: M.A. Mehlman (Ed.), *Renal effects of Petroleum Hydrocarbons*, pp. 65–71. Princeton Scientific Publishers, Princeton.

KLUWE, W. (1981): Renal function tests as indicators of kidney injury in the subacute toxicity studies. *Toxicol.Appl.Pharmacol.*, 57, 414–424.

KOENIG, H. GOLDSTONE, A., BLUME, G. and LU, C.Y. (1980). Testosterone-mediated sexual dimorphism of mitochondria and lysosomes in mouse kidney proximal tubules. *Science*, 209, 1023–1026.

KOENIG, H, GOLDSTONE, A. and HUGHES, C. (1978). Lysosomal enzymuria in the testosterone-treated mouse. A manifestation of cell defecation of residual bodies. *Lab.Invest.*, 39, 329–341.

KOLETSKY, S. (1954). Effects of temporary interruption of renal circulation in rats. *Arch.Pathol.*, 58, 592–603.

KOLETSKY, S. (1959): Role of salt in renal mass in experimental hypertension. *Arch.Pathol.*, 68, 21–32.

KONDO, Y. (1982): Experimental glomerulonephritis. *Acta.Pathol.Jpn.*, 32 (Suppl. 1), 197–209.

KONDO, Y. and AKIKUSA, B. (1982): Chronic Masugi nephritis in the rat. An electron microscopic study on evolution and consequences of glomerular capsular adhesions. *Acta.Pathol.Jpn.*, 32, 231–242.

KOSEK, J.C., MAZZE, R.I. and COUSINS, M.J. (1974): Nephrotoxicity of gentamycin. *Lab.Invest.*, 30, 48–57.

KOSS, L.G. and LAVIN, P. (1970). Effect of a single dose of cyclophosphamide on various organs in the rat: II. Response of urinary bladder epithelium according to strain and sex. *J.N.C.I.*, 44, 1195–1200.

KREISBERG, J.I. and KARNOVSKY, M.J. (1978): Focal glomerular sclerosis in the Fawn-Hooded rat. *Am.J.Pathol.* 92, 637–645.

KREISBERG, J.I., WAYNE, D.B. and KARNOVSKY, M.J. (1979): Rapid and focal loss of negative change associated with mononuclear cell infiltration early in nephrotoxic serum nephritis. *Kidney Int.*, 16, 290–300.

KRIZ, W., BANKIR, L., BULGER, R.E., BURG, M.B., GONCHAREVSKAYA, O.A., IMAI, M., KAISSLING, B., MAUNSBACH, A.B. MOFFAT, D.B. MOREL, F., MORGAN, T.O., NATOCHIN, Y.V. TISCHER, C.C., VENKATACHALAM, M.A. WHITTEMBURY, G. and WRIGHT, F.S. (1988): A standard nomenclature for structures of the kidney. *Kidney Int.*, 33, 1–7.

KRIZ, W. and NAPIWOTZKY, P. (1979): Structural and functional aspects of the renal interstitium. *Contrib. Nephrol.*, 16, 104–108.

KRIZ, W., and KAISSLING, B. (1985): Structural organization of the mammalian kidney. In: D.W. Seldin and G. Giebisch (Eds), *The Kidney: Physiology and Pathophysiology*, Chap. 14, pp. 265–306, Raven Press, New York.

KROES, R., GARBIS-BERKVENS, J.M., De VRIES, T. and VAN NESSELROOY, J.H.J. (1981): Histopathological profile of a Wistar rat stick including a survey of the literature. *J.Gerontol.*, 36, 259–279.

KROHN, K., MERO, M., OKSANEN, A. and SANDHOLM, M. (1971): Immunologic observations in canine interstitial nephritis. *Am.J.Pathol.*, 65, 157–172.

KRUTCHIK, A.N., BUZDAR, A.U., AKHTAR, M. and BLUMENSCHEIN, G.R. (1980): Immune-complex glomerulonephritis secondary to non-specific immunotherapy. *Cancer*, 45, 495–497.

KUBES, L. (1977): Experimental immune complex glomerulonephritis in the mouse with two types of immune complex. *Virchows Arch.[B]*, 24, 343–354.

KUNSTYR, I., NAUMANN, S. and WERNER, J. (1982): Urolithiasis in female inbred SPF rats. Possible predisposition of DA and ACI strains. *Z. Versuchstierkd.*, 24, 214–218.

LA ROCCA, P.T., SQUIBB, R.E., POWELL, M.L., SZOT, R.J., BLACK, H.E. and SCHWARTZ, E. (1986): Acute and subchronic toxicity of a non-sulfhydryl angiotensin coverting enzyme inhibitor. *Toxicol.Appl.Pharmacol.*, 82, 104–111.

LALICH, J.J., PAIK, W.C.W. and PARDHAN, B. (1974): Epithelial hyperplasia in the renal papilla of rats. Induction in animals fed excess sodium chloride. *Arch.Pathol.*, 97, 29–32.

LEE, J.B. and PETER, H.M. (1969): Effect of oxygen tension in glucose metabolism in rabbit kidney cortex and medulla. *Am.J.Physiol.*, 217, 1464–1471.

LEHMAN, D.H., WILSON, C.B. and DIXON, F.J. (1974): Interstitial ephritis in rats immunized with heterologous tubular basement membrane. *Kidney Int.* 5, 185–195.

LEHMANN, D.F. (1987): Primadone crystalluria following overdose. A report of a case and an analysis of the literature. *Med.Toxicol.*, 2, 383–387.

LEWIS, R.M. (1977): Evidence for a virus in canine lupus erythematosis. L.E. Glynn and H.D. Schlumberger (Eds), *Bayer-Symposium VI Experimental Models of Chronic Inflammatory Diseases*, pp. 71–76, Springer-Verlag, Berlin.

LI, J.J., LI, S.A., KLICKA, J.K., PARSONS, J.A. and LAM, L.K.T. (1983): Relative carcinogenic activity of various synthetic and natural estrogens in the Syrian hamster kidney. *Cancer Res.*, 43, 5200–5204.

LIEHR, J.G., SIRBASKU, D.A., JURKA, E., RANDERATH, K. and RANDERATH, E. (1988): Inhibition of estrogen-induced renal carcinogenesis in male Syrian hamsters by tamoxifen without decrease in DNA adduct levels. *Cancer Res.*, 48, 779–783.

LILIAN, O.M., HAMMOND, W.S., KRAUSS, D.J., ELBADAWI, A. and SCHOONMAKER, J.E. (1981): The microgenesis of some renal calculi. *Invest.Urol.*, 81, 451–456.

LINDOP, G.M.B. and LEVER, A.F. (1986): Anatomy of the renin-angiotensin system in the normal and pathological kidney. *Histopathology*, 10, 335–362.

LINTON, A.L. CLARK, W.F. DRIEDGER, A.A., TURNBULL, D.I. and LINDSAY, R.M. (1980): Acute intestinal nephritis due to drugs. *Ann.Intern.Med.*, 93, 735–741.

LITTERST, C.L., MINAUGH, E.G. and GRAM, T.E. (1977): Comparative alterations in extrahepatic drug metabolism by factors known to affect hepatic activity. *Biochem.Pharmacol.*, 26, 749–755.

LITTERST, C.L. MINNAUGH, E.G., REAGAN, R.L. and GRAM, T.E. (1975): Comparison of in vitro drug metabolism by lung, liver and kidney of several common laboratory species. *Drug Metab.Dispos.*, 3, 259–265.

LITTLEFIELD, N.A., GREENMAN, D.L. FARMER, J.H. and SHELDON, W.G. (1979): Effects of continuous and discontinued exposure to 2-AAF on urinary bladder hyperplasia or neoplasia. *J. Environ.Pathol. Toxicol.*, 3, 35–54.

LOGOTHETOPOULOS, J.H. and WEINBREN, K. (1955): Naturally occurring droplets in the proximal tubule of the rat's kidney. *B.J.Exp.Pathol.*, 36, 402–406.

LUMLEY, C.E. and WALKER, S.R. (1986)a: Predicting the safety of medicines from animal toxicity tests. I. Rodent alone. *Arch.Toxicol.(Suppl)*, 11, 295–299.

LUMLEY, C.E. and WALKER, S.R. (1986)b: Predicting the safety of medicines from animal toxicity tests. II. Rodent and non-reodent. *Arch.Toxicol.(Suppl)*, 91, 300–304.

MAACK, T., JOHNSON, V., KAU, S.T., FIGUEIREDO, J. and SIGULEM, D. (1979): Renal filtration, transport and metabolism of low molecular weight proteins: a review. *Kidney Int.* 16, 251–270.

MACALLUM, G.E., SMITH, G.S., BARSOUM, N.J., WALKER, R.M. and GREAVES, P. (1988): Renal and hepatic toxicity of a benzopyran-4-one in the cynomolgus monkey. *Toxicologist*, 8, 220.

MACALLUM, G.E., SMITH, G.S., BARSOUM, N.H., WALKER, R.M. and GREAVES, P. (1989): Renal and hepatic toxicity of a benzopyran-4-one in the cynomolgus monkey. *Toxicology*, 59, 97–108.

MACDONALD, J. (1984): Food and Drug Administration Committee Review of Enalapril, June 20, 1984, Washington, D.C.

MACDONALD, J.S. BAGDON, W.J., PETER, C.P. SINA, J.F., ROBERTSON, R.T., ULM, E.H. and BOKELMAN, D.L. (1987): Renal effects of enalapril in dogs. *Kidney Inst.*, 31, Suppl 20, S148-S153.

MACFARLAND, H.N. (1984): Xenobiotic induced kidney lesions: Hydrocarbons. The 90-day and 2-year gasoline studies. In: M.A. Mehlman (Ed.), *Renal Effects of Petroleum Hydrocarbons*, pp. 51–56. Princeton Scientific Publishers Inc. Princeton.

MACFARLAND, H.N. (1984): Xenobiotic induced kidney lesions: Hydrocarbons. The 90 day and 2 year gasoline studies. *Adv.Modern Environ.Toxicol.*, 7, 51–56.

MACKLIN, A.W. and SZOT, R.J. (1980): Eighteen month oral study of aspirin, phenacetin and caffeine in C57NL/6 mice. *Drug Chem.Toxicol.*, 3, 135–163.

MADSEN, K.M. and TISHER, C.C. (1986): Structural-functional relationships along the distal nephron. *Am.J.Physiol.*, 250, F1-F15.

MAGRO, A.M. and RUDOFSKY, U.H. (1982): Plasma renin activity decrease preceded spontaneous focal glomerular sclerosis in aging rats. *Nephron*, 31, 245–253.

MAILLOUX, L., SWARTZ, C.D., CAPIZZI, R., KIM, K.E., ONESTI, G., RAMIREZ, O. and BREST, A.N. (1967): Acute renal failure after administration of low-molecular-weight dextran. *N.Engl.J.Med.*, 227, 1113–1118.

MANDEL, E.E and POPPER, H. (1951): Experimental medullary necrosis of the kidney: Morphologic and functional study. *Arch.Pathol.*, 52, 1–17.

MARKHAM, R.J. Jr., SUTHERLAND, J.C. and MARDINEY, M.R. Jr. (1973): The ubiquitous occurrence of immune complex localization in the renal glomeruli of normal mice. *Lab.Invest.*, 29, 111–120.

MASON, J. and THIEL, G. (1982): Workshop on the role of medullary circulation in the pathogenesis of acute renal failure. *Nephron*, 31, 289–323.

MAUNSBACH, A.B. (1966): The influence of different fixatives and fixation methods on the ultrastructure of rat kidney proximal tubules. I. Comparison of different perfusion fixation methods and of glutaraldehyde, formaldehyde and osmium tetroxide fixatives. *J.Ultrastruct.Res.*, 15, 242–282.

MAUNSBACH, A.B., MADDEN, S.C. and LATTA, H. (1962): Light and electronmicroscopic changes in proximal tubules of rats after administration of glucose, mannitol, sucrose or dextran. *Lab.Invest.*, 11, 421–432.

MAYER, D.G. (1987): The safety profile of ofloxacin in drug interaction studies. Overview of toxicological studies. *Drugs*, 34, Suppl. 1, 150–153.

MENGS, U., LANG, W. and POCH, J-A. (1982): The carcinogenic action of aristolochic acid in rats. *Arch.Toxicol.*, 51, 107–119.

MERSKI, J.A. and MEYERS, M.C. (1985): Light and electron microscopic evaluation of renal tubular cell vacuolation induced by administration of nitrilotriacetate or sucrose. *Food Chem.Toxicol.*, 23, 923–930.

McCLUSKY, R.T. (1983): Immunological mechanisms in glomerular disease. In: R.H. Heptinsall (Ed.), *Pathology of the Kidney*, Vol. 1, Chap. 7, pp. 301–385, Brown and Company, Boston.

McCLUSKEY, R.T. and VASSALLI, P. (1969): Experimental glomerular diseases. In: C.Rouiller and A.F. Muller (Eds), *The Kidney, Morphology, Biochemistry, Phyiology,Vol. 2*, Chap. 2, pp. 83–198, Academic Press, New York.

McKENZIE, J.C., TANAKA, I., MISONO, K.S. and INAGAMA, T. (1985)a: Immunocytochemical localization of atrial natriuretic factor in the kidney, adrenal medulla, pituitary and atrium of rat. *J.Histochem.Cytochem.*, 33, 828–832.

McKENZIE, J.L. and FABRE, J.W. (1981): Studies with a monclonal antibody on the distribution of Thy-1 in the lymphoid and extracellular connective tissues of the dog. *Transplantation*, 31, 275–282.

McKENZIE, N., DIVINENI, R., VIZINA, W., KEOWN, P. and STILLER, C. (1985)b: The effect of cyclosporin on organ blood flow. *Transplant.Proc.*, 17, 1973–1975.

MILAS, L. and SCOTT, M.T. (1978): Anti-tumor activity of Corynebacterium parvum. *Adv.Cancer res.*, 26, 257–306.

MOLLAND, E.A. (1978): Experimental renal papillary necrosis. *Kidney Int.*, 13, 5–14.

MONSERRAT, A.J. and CHANDLER, A.E. (1975): Effects of repeated injections of sucrose in the kidney: Histologic, cytochemical and functional studies in an animal model. *Virchows Arch.[B]*, 19, 77–91.

MORAN, M. and KAPSNER, C. (1987): Acute renal failure associated with elevated plasma oncotic pressure. *N.Engl.J.Med.*, 317, 150–153.

MORIN, J.P., VIOTTE, G., VANDEWALLE, A., VAN HOOF, F., TULKENS, P. and FILLASTRE, J.P. (1980): Gentamycin-induced nephrotoxicity: a cell biology approach. *Kidney Int.*, 18, 583–590.

MORLEY, A.R. and WHEELER, J. (1985): Cell proliferation within Bowman's capsule in mice. *J.Pathol.*, 145, 315–327.

MORRIS, R.J., and RITTER, M.A. (1980): Association of Thy-1 cell surface differentiation antigen with certain connective tissues in vivo. *Cell Tissue Res.*, 206, 459–475.

MORRISON, W.I. and WRIGHT, N.G. (1977): Viruses associated with renal disease of man and animals. *Prog.Med.Virol.*, 23, 22–50.

MUDGE, G.H. (1984): Pathogenesis of nephrotoxicity: Pharmacological principles. In: P.H. Bach and E.A. Lock (Eds), *Renal Heterogeneity and Target Cell Toxicity*, pp. 1–12, John Wiley and Sons, Chichester.

MÜLLER-PEDDINGHAUS, R. and TRAUTWEIN, G. (1977)a: Spontaneous glomerulonephritis in dogs. I. Classification and Immunopathology. *Vet.Pathol.*, 14, 1–13.

MÜLLER-PEDDINGHAUS, R. and TRAUTWEIN, G. (1977)b: Spontaneous glomerulonephritis in dogs. II. Correlation of glomerulonephritis with age, chronic interstitial nephritis and extra-renal lesions. *Vet.Pathol.*, 14, 121–127.

MURASAKI, G. and COHEN, S.M. (1981): Effect of dose of sodium saccharin on the induction of rat urinary bladder proliferation.*Cancer Res.*, 41, 942–944.

MURATA, F., TSUYAMA, S., SUZUKI, S., HAMADA, H., OZAWA, M. and MURAMATSU, T. (1983): Distribution of glyconjugates in the kidney studies by me of labelled lectins. *J.Histochem.Cytochem.*, 31, 139–144.

MURRAY, S.M. (1979): The morphology of serotonin-induced renal lesions in the rat. *J.Pathol.*, 128, 203–211.

NAKANO, M., ITO, Y., KOHTANI, K., MIZUNO, T. and TAUCHI, H. (1985): Age-related change in brush borders of rat kidney cortex. *Mech.Ageing Dev.*, 33, 95–102.

NEWBERNE, P.M., CONNER, M.W. and ESTES, P. (1988): The influence of food additives and related materials on lower bowel structure and formation. *Toxicol.Pathol.*, 16, 184–197.

NEWBURGH, L.H. and CURTIS, A.C. (1928): Production of renal injury in the white rat by the protein of the diet. *Arch.Intern.Med.*, 42, 801–821.

NGUYEN, H.T. and WOODARD, J.C. (1980): Intranephron calcinlosis in rat. *Am.J.Pathol.*, 100, 39–56.

OHTAKI, T., IMAI, K., YOSHIMURA, S. and HASHIMOTO, K. (1981): Toxicological studies of captopril, an inhibitor of angiotensin converting enzyme. IV. Three month subacute toxicity of captopril in beagle dogs. *J.Toxicol.Sci.*, 6 (Suppl. 2), 247–270.

OLIVEIRA, D.B.G. and PETERS, D.K. (1989): Antoimmunity and the kidney. *Kidney Int.*, 35, 923–928.

OLIVER, J., MACDOWELL, M. and LEE, Y.C. (1954): Cellular mechanisms of protein metabolism in the nephron. I. The structural aspects of proteinuria; tubular absorption, droplet formation, and the disposal of proteins. *J.Exp.Med.*, 99, 589–605.

OLIVER, J., MACDOWELL, M. and TRACY, A. (1951): The pathogenesis of acute renal failure associated with traumatic and toxic injury. Renal ischemia, nephrotoxic damage and the ischemuric episode. *J.Clin.Invest.*, 30, 1307–1351.

OLIVER, J., MACDOWELL, M., WELT, L.G. HOLLIDAY, M.A., HOLLANDER, W., WINTERS, R.W., WILLIAMS, T.F. and SEGAR, W.E. (1957): The renal lesions of electrolyte inbalance. The structural alterations in potassium-depleted rats. *J.Exp.Med.*, 106, 563–573.

OLIVER, J. STRAUS, W., KRETCHMER, N., LEE, Y.C., DICKERMAN, H.W. and CHEROT, F. (1955): The histochemical characteristics of absorption droplets in the nephron. *J.Histochem.Cytochem.*, 3, 277–283.

OLSON, J.L., DE URDANETA, A.G. and HEPTINATALL, R.H. (1985): Glomerular hyalinosis and its relation to hyperfiltration. *Lab.Invest.*, 52, 387–398.

OLSON, M.J., JOHNSON, J.T. and REIDY, C.A. (1990): A comparison of male rat and human urinary proteins: Implications for human resistence to hyaline droplet nephropathy. *Toxicol.Appl. Pharmacol.*, 102, 524–536.

OTTOSEN, P.D., NYENGÅRD, J.R., JACOBSEN, N.O. and CHRISTENSEN, S. (1987): A morphometric and ultrastructural study of lithium-induced changes in the medullary collecting ducts of the rat kidney. *Cell Tissue Res.*, 249, 311–315.

OTTOSEN, P.D., NYENGÅRD, J.R. OLSEN, T.S. and CHRISTENSEN. S. (1986): Interstitial focal fibrosis and induction in proximal tubular length in adult rats after lithium treatment. *Acta.Pathol.Microbiol.Immunol.Scand.*, A94, 401–403.

OWEN, G.S., SMITH, T.H.F. and AGERSBORG, H.P.K. Jr. (1970): Toxicity of some benzodiazepine compounds with CNS activity. *Toxicol.Appl.Pharmacol.*, 16, 556–570.

OWEN, R.A. and HEYWOOD, R. (1986): Strain-related susceptibility of nephrotoxicity induced by aspirin and phenylbutazone in rats. *Toxicol.Pathol.*, 14, 242–246.

PALLA, R., MARCHITIELLO, M., TUONI, M., CIRAMI, C., GIOVANNINI, L., BERTELLI, A.A.E., BERTELLI, A. (1985): Enzymuria in aminoglycoside-induced kidney damage. Comparative study of gentamycin, mikacin, sisomicin, and netilmicin. *Int.J.Clin.Pharmacol.Res.*, 5, 351–355.

PARSONS, C.L., STAUFFER, C. and SCHMIDT, J.D. (1980): Bladder surface glycosaminoglycans: An efficient mechanism of environmental adaptation. *Science*, 605–607.

PASHKO, L.L., FAIRMAN, D.K. and SCHWARTZ, A.G. (1986): Inhibition of proteinuria development in aging Sprague-Dawley rats and C57BL/6 mice by long-term treatment with dehydroepiandrosterone. *J.Gerontol.*, 41, 433–438.

PATERSON, M. (1979): Urolithiasis in the Sprague-Dawley rat. *Lab. Anim.*, 13, 17–20.

PAUL, L.C., RENNKE, H.G., MILFORD, E.L. and CARPENTER, C.B. (1984): Thy-1.1 in glomeruli of rat kidneys. *Kidney Int.*, 25, 771–777.

PELLETIER, L., PASQUIER, R., HIRSCH, F., SAPIN, C. AND DRUET, P. (1984): B cell proliferation induced by modified syngenic monoculear cells: Relevance to drug-induced autoimmune glomerulonephritis. In: P.H. Bach and E.A. Lock (Eds), *Renal Heterogeneity and Target Cell Toxicity*, pp. 249–252, John Wiley & Sons, Chichester.

PELLETIER, L., PASQUIER, R., GUETTIER, C., VIAL, M-C., MANDET, C., NOCHY, D., BAZIN, H. and DRUET, P. (1988): HgCl$_2$ induces T and B cells to proliferate and differentiate in BN rats. *Clin. Exp. Immunol.*, 71, 336–342.

PEREY, D.Y., HERDMAN, R.C. and GOOD, R.A. (1967): Polycystic renal disease: a new experimental model. *Science*, 158, 494–496.

PETER, C.P. BUREK, J.D. and VAN ZWIETEN, M.J. (1986): Spontaneous nephropathies in rats. *Toxicol.Pathol.*, 14, 91–100.

PFALLER, W. (1982): Structure function correlation on rat kidney. *Adv.Anat.Embryol.Cell.Biol.*, 70, 1–106.

PFEIFFER, E.W. (1968): Comparative anatomical observations of the mammalian renal pelvis and medulla. *J. Anat.*, 102, 321–331.

PHILLIPS, R.D. AND COCKERELL, B.Y. (1984): Kidney structural changes rats following inhalation exposure to C10-C11 isoparaffinic solvent. *Toxicology.*, 33, 261–273.

PHILLIPS, F.S., STERNBERG, S.S., CRONIN, A.P. and VIDAL, P.M. (1961): Cyclophosphamide and urinary bladder toxicity. *Cancer Res.*, 21, 1577–1589.

POUR, P., ALTHOFF, J., SALMASI, S.Z. and SEPAN, K. (1979): Spontaneous tumours and common diseases in three types of hamsters. *J.N.C.I.*, 63, 797–811.

POUR, P., MOHR, U., ALTHOFF, J., CARDESA, A. and KMOCH, N. (1976): Spontaneous tumors and common diseases in two colonies of Syrian hamsters. III Urogenital system and endocrine glands. *J.N.C.I.*, 56, 949–961.

PRICE, R.G. (1982): Urinary enzymes, nephrotoxicity and renal disease.*Toxicology.*, 23, 99–134.

PRIESTMAN, T.J. (1980): Initial evaluation of human lymphoblastoid interferon in patients with advanced malignant disease. *Lancet*, 2, 113–118.

RABKIN, R. and KITAJI, J. (1983): Renal metabolism of peptide hormones. *Miner. Electrolyte Metab.*, 9, 212–226.

RAKIETEN, N., GORDON, B.S., COONEY, D.A., DAVIS, R.D. and SCHEEN, P.S. (1968): Renal tumorigenic action of streptozotocin (NSC-55998) in rats. *Cancer Chemother.Rep.*, 52, 563–567.

RANDERATH, E. and HIERONYMI, G. (1958): Urogenital system. Erkrankungen der Harnorgane. In: P. Cohrs, R. Jaffe and H. Meeson (Eds), *Pathologie der Laboratoriumstiere*, Vol. 1, pp. 357–381, Spinger-Verlag, Berlin.

READ, N.G., ASTBURY, P.J., MORGAN, R.J.I., PARSONS, D.N. and PORT, C.J. (1988): Induction and exacerbation of hyaline droplet formation in the proximal rats receiving a variety of pharmacological agents. *Toxicology*, 52, 81–101.

REIBORD, H.E. (1968): Metaplasia of the parietal layer of Bowman's capsule. *Am.J.Clin.Pathol.*, 50, 240–242.

RENLUND, R.C., MCGILL, G.E. and CHENG, P.T. (1986): Calcite urolith in a cynomolgus monkey. *Lab. Anim. Sci.*, 36, 536–537.

RENNKE, H.G., COTRAN, R.S. and VENKATACHALAN, M.A. (1975): Role of molecular change in glomerular permeability. Tracer studies with cationized ferritins. *J.Cell.Biol.*, 67, 638–646.

RHODIN, J.A.G. (1974): The Urinary System. In: *Histology, A Text and Atlas.*, Chap. 32, pp. 647–674, Oxford University Press, New York.

RICHARDSON, B.T. and LUGINBÜHL, H-R. (1976): The role of prolactin in the development of chronic progressive nephropathy in the rat. *Virchows Arch.[A]* 370, 13–16.

RICHARDSON, B.P., TURKALJ, I. and FLÜCKIGER, E. (1984): Bromocriptine. In: D.R. Laurence, A.E.M. McLean and M. Weatherall (Eds), *Safety Testing of New Drugs. Laboratory Predicitions and Clinical Performance*, Chap.3, pp. 19–63, Academic Press, London.

RIVERE, J.E., DIX, L.P., CARVER, M.P. and FRAZIER, D.L. (1986): Identification of a subgroup of Sprague-Dawley rats highly sensitive to drug-induced renal toxicity. *Fundam.Appl.Toxicol.*, 7, 126–131.

ROBERTSON, J.L. (1986). Spontaneous renal disease in dogs. *Toxicol.Pathol.*, 14, 101–108.

ROBINSON, C.J.G., ABRAHAM, A.A. and BALAZS, T. (1984): Induction of antinuclear antibodies by mercuric chloride in mice. *Clin.Exp.Immunol.*, 58, 300–306.

ROBINSON, C.J.G., EGOROV, I. and BALAZS, T. (1983): Strain differences in the induction of antinuclear antibodies by mercuric chloride, gold sodium thiomalate and D-penicillamine in inbred mice. *Fed.Proc.*, 42, 1213.

ROCHA, A.S. and KOKKA, J.P. (1973): Sodium chloride and water transport in the medullary thick ascending limb of Henle: Evidence for active chloride transport. *J.Clin.Invest.*, 52, 612–613.

ROE, F.J.C. (1989): Relevance for man of the effects of lactose, polyols and other carbohydrates on calcium metabolism seen in rats. A review. *Hum.Toxicol.*, 8, 87–98.

ROE, F.J.C. and BÄR, A. (1985): Enzootic and epizootic adrenal medullary proliferative disease of rats: Influence of dietary factors which affect calcium absorption. *Hum.Toxicol.*, 4, 27–52.

ROWLAND, R.G., HENNEBERRY, M.O., OYASU, R. and GRAYHACK, J.T. (1980): Effects of urine and continued exposure to carcinogens on progression of early neoplastic urinary bladder lesions. *Cancer Res.*, 40, 4524–4527.

RUSH, G.F., PRATT, I.S., LOCK, E.A. and HOOK, J.B. (1986): Induction of renal mixed function oxidases in the rat and mouse. Correlation with ultra-structural changes in the proximal tubule. *Fundam.Appl.Toxicol.*, 6, 307–317.

RUSH, G.F., WILSON, D.M. and HOOK, J.B. (1983): Selective induction and inhibition of renal mixed function oxidases in the rat and rabbit. *Fundam.Appl.Toxicol.*, 3, 161–168.

RYAN, G.B., GOGHLAN, J.P. and SCOGGINS, B.A. (1979): The granulated peripolar cell: a potential secretory component of the renal juxtaglomerular complex. *Nature*, 277, 655–656.

RYFFEL, B., DONATSCH, P., MADORIN, M., MATTER, B.E., RUTTIMANN, G., SCHON, H., STOLL, R. and WILSON, J. (1983): Toxicological evaluation of cyclosporin A. *Arch.Toxicol.*, 53, 107–141.

RYFFEL, B. and MIHATSCH, M.J. (1986): Cyclosporin nephrotoxicity. *Toxicol.Pathol.*, 14, 73–82.

RYFFEL, B., SIEGL, H., MUELLER, A-M., HAUSER, R. and MIHATSCH, M.J. (1985): Nephrotoxicity of cyclosporin in spontaneously hypertensive rats. *Transplant.Proc.*, 17, 1430–1431.

SANDERS, P.W., HERRERA, G.A. and GALLA, J.H. (1987): Human Bence Jones protein toxicity in rat proximal tubule epithelium in vivo. *Kidney Int.*, 32, 851–861.

SARKAR, K., TOLNAI, G. and LEVINE, D.Z. (1973): Nephrocalcinosis in chloride depleted rats. An ultrastructural study. *Calcif.Tissue Res.*, 12, 2–7.

SCARPELLI, D.G. (1965): Experimental nephrocalcinosis: A biochemical and morphological study. *Lab.Invest.*, 114, 123–141.

SCHLÜTER, G. (1987): Ciprofloxacin: review of potential toxicologic effects. *Am.J.Med.*, 82, Suppl. 4A, 91–93.

SCHMÄHL, D. and HABS, M. (1979): Carcinogenic actions of low-dose cyclophosphamide given orally to Sprague-Dawley rats in a lifetime experiment. *Int.J.Cancer*, 23, 706–712.

SCHMIDT, U. and GUDER, W.G. (1976): Sites of enzyme activity along the nephron. *Kidney Int.*, 9, 233–242.

SCHNEEBERGER, E.E. and MORRISON, A.B. (1965): The nephropathy of experimental magnesium deficiency. *Lab.Invest.*, 14, 674–686.

SCHREINER, G.E. and MAHER, J.F. (1965): Toxic nephropathy. *Am.J.Med.*, 38, 409–449

SCHREINER, G.F. and UNANUE, E.R. (1984): Origin of the rat mesangial phagocyte and its expression of the leukocyte common antigen. *Lab.Invest.*, 51, 515–523.

SCHULTE, B.A. and SPICER, S.S (1983): Histochemical evaluation of mouse and rat kidneys with lectin-horseradish peroxidase conjugates. *Am.J.Anat.*, 168, 345–362.

SCHWARTZ, R.S. (1981): Immunologic and genetic aspects of systemic lupus erythematous. *Kidney Int.*, 19, 474–484.

SCOTT, G.M., SECHER, D.S., FLOWERS, D., BATE, J., CANTELL, K. and TYRRELL, D.A.J. (1981): Toxicity of interferon. *Br.Med.J.*, 282, 1345–1348.

SELBY, P., KOHN, J., RAYMOND, J., JUDSON, I. and McELWAIN, T. (1984): Nephrotoxic syndrome following interferon therapy. In: P.H. Bach and E.A. Lock (Eds), *Renal Heterogeneity and Target Cell Toxicity*, pp. 265–266. John Wiley & Sons, Chichester.

SETO-OHSHIMA, A., SANO, M. and MIZUTANI, A. (1985): Characteristic localization of calmodulin in human tissues: Immunohistochemical study in the paraffin sections. *Acta.Histochem.Cytochem.*, 18, 275–282.

SHALTIEL, S., MIZRAHI, R. and SELA, M. (1971): On the immunological properties of penicillins. *Proc.R.Soc.Lond.[Biol]*, 179, 411–432.

SHANLEY, P.F., ROSEN, M.D., BREZIS, M., SILVER, P., EPSTEIN, F.A., and ROSEN, S. (1986): Topography of focal proximal tubular necrosis after ischaemia with reflow in the rat kidney. *Am.J.Pathol.*, 122, 462–468.

SHEEHAN, H.L. and DAVIS, J.C. (1960): Experimental obstruction of renal veins. *J.Pathol.Bacteriol.*, 79, 347–359.

SHIGEMATSU, H. and KOBAYASHI, Y. (1971): The development and fate of the immune deposits in the glomerulus during the secondary phase of rat Masugi nephritis. *Virchows Arch.[B]*. 8, 83–95.

SHIGEMATSU, H. and KOBAYASHI, Y. (1973): The distortion and disorganization of the glomerulus in progressive Masugi nephritis in the rat. *Virchows Arch.[B]*, 14, 313–328.

SHIMAMURA, T. and MORRISON, A.B. (1975): A progressive glomerulosclerosisoccurring in partial five-sixths nephrectomised rats. *Am.J.Pathol.*, 79, 95–106.

SHIN, M.L., GELFAND, M.C., NAGLE, R.B. CARLO, J.R., GREEN, I. and FRANK, M.M. (1977): Localization of receptors for activated complement on visceral epithelial cells of the human renal glomerulus. *J.Immunol.*, 188, 869–873.

SHIRAHAMA, T. and COHEN, A.S. (1974): Blockage of amyloid induction by colchicine in an animal model. *J.Exp.Med.*, 140, 1102–1107.

SHINOHARA, Y. and FRITH, C.H. (1980): Morphologic characteristics of benign and malignant renal cell tumours in control and 2-acetylaminofluorene-treated BALB/C female mice. *Am.J.Pathol.*, 100, 455–468.

SILVERBLATT, F.J. and KUEHN, C. (1979): Autoradiography of gentamycin uptake by the rat proximal tubule cell. *Kidney Int.*, 15, 335–345.

SILVERMAN, J. and RIVERSON, A. (1980): Nephrocalcinomas in 2 young rats. *Lab.Anim.*, 14, 241–242.

SHORT, B.G., BURNETT, V.L. and SWENBERG J.A. (1986): Histopathology and cell proliferation induced by 2,2,4-trimethylpentane in the male rat kidneys. *Toxicol.Pathol.*, 14, 194–203.

SKRAASTAD, O. (1987): Compensatory cell proliferation in the kidney after unilateral nephrectomy in mice. *Virchows Arch. [B]*.53, 97–101.

SLAUSEN, D.O., and LEWIS, R.M. (1979): Comparative pathology of glomerulonephritis in animals. *Vet.Pathol.*, 16, 135–164.

579

SOLEZ, K. (1983): Acute renal failure ('Acute tubular necrosis, infarction and corticol necrosis'). In: R.H. Hepinstall (Ed.), *Pathology of the Kidney*, Vol. 2, Chap. 21, pp. 1069-1148, Little, Brown and Company, Boston.

SOLEZ, K. IDEURA, T. and SAITO, H. (1980)a: Role of thromboxane and outer medullary microvasucilature injury in post-ischemic acute renal failure (abstract). *Clin.Res.*, 28, 461A.

SOLEZ, K., IDEURA, T., SILVIA, C.B., HAMILTON, B. and SAITON, H. (1980)b: Clonidine after renal ischemia to lessen acute renal failure and microvascular damage. *Kidney Int.*, 18, 309-322.

SOLEZ, K., MOREL-MAROGER, L. and SRAER, J-D (1979): The morphology of 'acute tubular necrosis' in man. Analysis of 57 renal biopsies and a comparison with the glycerol model. *Medicine*, 58, 362-376.

SOLLEVELD, H.A. and BOORMAN, G.A. (1986): Spontaneous renal lesions in five rat strains. *Toxicol.Pathol.*, 14, 168-174.

SOLLEVELD, H.A. and BOORMAN, G.A. (1986): Spontaneous renal lesions in five rat strains. *Toxicol.Pathol.*, 14, 168-174.

SPANGLER, W.L. ADELMAN, R.D., CONZELMAN, G.M. and ISHIZAKI, G. (1980): Gentamycin nephrotoxicity in the dog: Sequential light and electron microscopy. *Vet.Pathol.*, 17, 206-217.

SPICER, S.S. and SCHULTE, B.A. (1982): Identification of cell surface consituents. *Lab.Invest.*, 47, 2-4.

SPIEGEL, R.J., SPICEHANDLER, J.R., JACOBS, S.L. and ODEN, E.M. (1986): Low incidence of serum neutralizing factors in patients receiving recombinant alfa-2b interferon (Intron A). *Am.J.Med.*, 80, 223-228.

SPÜHLER, O. and ZOLLINGER, H.U. (1953): Die chronische-interstitielle Nephritis. *Z.Klin.Med.*, 151, 1-50.

STEINBERG, A.D., HUSTON, D.P., TAUROG, J.D., COWDERY, J.S. and RAVENCHE, E.S. (1981): The cellular and genetic basis of murine lupus. *Immuno.Rev.*, 55, 121-154.

STERNBURG, S.S. and PHILIPS, F.S. (1967): Biphasic intoxication and nephrotic syndrome in rats given daunomycin. *Proc.Am.Assoc. Cancer Res.*, 8, 64.

STERNBURG, S.S., PHILLIPS, F.S. and CRONIN, A.P. (1972): Renal tumors and other lesions in rats following a single intravenous injection of daunomycin. *Cancer Res.*, 32, 1029-1036.

STONARD, M.D., PHILLIPS, P.G.N., FOSTER, J.R., SIMPSON, M.G. and LOCK, E.A. (1986): Alpha$_{2u}$-globulin: Measurement in rat kidney following administration of 2,2,4-trimethylpentane. *Toxicology*, 41, 161-168.

STRAUS, W. (1954): Isolation and biochemical properties of droplets from the cells of rat kidney. *J.Biol.Chem.*, 207, 745-755.

STRAUS, W. (1956): Concentration of acid phosphatase, ribonuclease deoxyribonuclease, beta-glucuronidase and cathepsin in 'droplets' isolated from the kidney cells of normal rats. *J.Biophys.Biochem.Cytol.*, 2, 515-521.

STRAUS, W. (1964): Cytochemical observations on the relationship between lysosomes and phagosomes in kidney and liver by combined staining for acid phosphatase and intravenously injected horseradish peroxidase. *J.Cell.Biol.*, 20, 497-507.

STUART, B.P., PREMISTER, R.D. and THOMASSEN, R.W. (1975): Glomerular lesions associated with proteinuria in clinically healthy dogs. *Vet.Pathol.*, 12, 125-144.

SUGISAKI, T., KLASSEN, J., MILGROM, F., ANDRES, G. and McCLUSKEY, R.T. (1973): Immunopathologic study of an autoimmune tubular and interstitial renal disease in Brown Norway rats. *Lab.Invest.*, 28, 658-671.

SUMPIO, B.E. and HAYSLETT, J.P. (1985): Renal handling of proteins in normal and disease states. *Q.J.Med.*, 57, 611-635.

SWAN, P.F., KAUFMAN, D.G., MAGEE, P.N. and MACE, R. (1980): Induction of kidney tumours by a single dose of dimethylnitrosamine: Dose response and influence of diet and benzo(α)pyrene treatment. *Br. J.Cancer.*, 41, 285-294.

SWENBERG, J.A., SHORT, B., BORGHOFF, S., STRASSER, J. AND CHARBONNEAU, M. (1989): The comparative pathobiology of α_{2u}-globulin nephropathy. *Toxicol.Appl.Pharmacol.*, 97, 35-46.

SYMÖENS, J., DE CREE, J., VAN BEVER, W.F.M. and JANSSEN, P.A.J. (1979):Levamisole. In: M.E. Goldberg (Ed.), *Pharmacological and Biochemical Properties of Drug Substances*, pp. 407–418. American Pharmaceutical Association, Academy of Pharmaceutical Sciences, Washington, DC.

TAGUMA, Y., KITAMOTO, Y., FUTAKI, G., UEDA, H., MONMA, H., ISHIZAKI, M., TAKA-HASHI, H., SEKINO, H. and SASAKI, Y. (1985): Effect of captopril on heavy proteinuria in azotemic diabetics. *N.Engl.J.Med.*, 313, 1617–1620.

TALPAZ, M., KANTARJIAN, H., McCREDIE, K., TURJILLO, J.M., KEATING, M.J. and GUTTERMAN, J.U. (1986): Hematologic remission and cytogenetic improvement induced by recombinant human interferon alpha A in chronic myelogenous leukaemia. *N.Engl.J.Med.*, 314, 1065–1069.

TANAKA, H., ISHIKAWA, E., TESHIMA, S. and SHIMIZU, E. (1986): Histopathological study of human cisplatin nephropathy. *Toxicol.Pathol.*, 14, 247–257.

TAUGNER, R. BURHLE, Ch,Ph., GANTEN, D., HACKENTHAL, E., INAGAMI, T., NOBILING, R. (1983): Immunohistochemistry of the renin-angiotensin-system in the kidney. *Clin.Exp.Hypertens.[A]*, 5, 1163–1177.

TAUGNER, R., HACKENTHAL, E., INAGAMI, T., NOBILING, R. and POULSEN, K. (1982)a: Vascular and tubular renin in the kidneys of mice. *Histochemistry*, 75, 473–484.

TAUGNER, R., HACKENTHAL, E., RIX, E., NOBILING, R. and POULSEN, K. (1982)b: Immunocytochemistry of the renin angiotensin system: Renin, angiotensinogen, angiotensin I, angiotensin II, and converting enzyme in the kidneys of mice and rats, and tree shrews. *Kidney Int.*, 22, Suppl. 12, 33–43.

TAYLOR, D.M., THRELFALL, G. and BUCK, A.T. (1968): Chemically-induced renal hypertrophy in the rat. *Biochem.Pharmacol.*, 17, 1567–1574.

TAYLOR S.A. and PRICE, R.G. (1982): Age-related changes in rat glomerular basement. *Int.J.Biochem.*, 14, 201–206.

THEOFILOPOULOS, A.N. and DIXON, F.J. (1981): Etiopathogenesis of murine SLE. *Immunol.Rev.*, 55, 179–216.

THOMSON, N.M., HOLDSWORTH, S.R., GLASGOW, E.F. and ATKINS, R.C. (1979):The macrophages in the development of experimental crescentric glomerulonephritis. *Am.J.Pathol.*, 94, 223–240.

TOGEI, K., SANO, N., MAEDA, T., SHIBATA, M. and OTSUKA, H. (1987): Carcinogenicity of bucetin in (C57BL/6×C3H) F1 mice. *J.N.C.I.*, 79, 1151–1158.

TÖRNROTH, T. and SKRIFVARS, B., (1974): Gold nephropathy: Prototype of membranous glomerulonephritis. *Am.J.Pathol.*, 75, 573–590.

TORRES, V.E., YOUNG, W.F., OFFORD, K.P. and HATTERY, R.R. (1990): Association of hypokalemia, aldosteronism, and renal cysts. *N.Engl.J.Med.*, 322, 345–351.

TREE, M., BROWN, J.J., LECKIE, B.J., LEVER, A.F., MANHEIM, P., MORTON, J.J., ROBERTSON, J.I.S., SZELKE, M. and WEBB, D. (1985): Renin and blood pressure. *Biochem.Soc.Trans.*, 12, 948–951.

TRUMP, B.F. and JANIGAN, D.T. (1962): The pathogenesis of cytologic vacuolization in sucrose nephrosis. An electron microscopic and histochemical study. *Lab.Invest.*, 11, 395–411.

TRUMP, B.F., JONES, T.W. and HEATHFIELD, B.M. (1984)a: The biology of the kidney. *Adv.Mod.Environ.Toxicol.*, 7, 27–49.

TRUMP, B.F., LIPSKY, M.M, JONES, T.W., HEATFIELD, B.M., HIGGINSON, J., ENDICOTT, K. and HESS, H.B. (1984)b: An evaluation of the significance of experimental hydrocarbon toxicity to man. *Adv.Mod.Environ.Toxicol.*, 7, 273–288.

TSUCHITANI, M., KURODA, J., NAGATANI, M., MIURA, K., KATOH, T., SAEGUSA, T., NARAMA, I. and ITAKURA, C. (1990): Glycogen accumulation in the renal tubular cells of spontaneously occurring diabetic WBN/Kob rats. *J.Comp.Pathol.*, 102, 179–190.

TUCKER, S.M., MASON, R.L. and BEAUCHENE, R.E. (1976): Influence of diet and feed restriction on kidney function of aging male rats. *J.Gerontol.*, 31, 264–270.

TUCKER, W.E. Jr, MACKLIN, A.W., SZOT, R.J., JOHNSTON, R.E., ELION, G.B.,de MIRANDA,

P. and SZCZECH, G.M. (1983): Preclinical toxicity studies with acyclovir: Acute and subchronic tests. *Fundam.Appl.Toxicol.*, 3, 573–578.

TUFFERY, A.A. (1966): Urogenital lesions in laboratory mice. *J.Pathol.Bacteriol.*, 91, 301–309.

TURNBULL, G.J., LEE, P.N. and ROE, F.J.C. (1985): Relationships of body-weight gain to longevity and to risk of development of nephropathy and neoplasia in Sprague-Dawley rats. *Food Chem. Toxicol.*, 23, 355–361.

UEDA, S., WAKASHIN, M., WAKASHIN, Y., YOSHIDA, H., AZEMOTO, R., IESATO, K., MORI, T., MORI, Y., OGAWA, M. and OKUDA, K. (1988): Autoimmune interstitial nephritis induced in inbred mice. Analysis of mouse tubular basement membrane antigen and genetic control of immune response to it. *Am.J.Pathol.*, 132, 304–318.

UFF, J.S., MITCHESON, H.D., PUSSELL, B.A. BRILL, M. and CASTRO, J.E. (1981): Proliferative glomerulonephritis in mice given intravenous corynebacterium parvum. *J.Pathol.*, 133, 89–105.

VAN HOESEL, Q.G.C.M., STEERENBERG, P.A., DORMANS, J.A.M.A., DE JONG, W.H., DE WILDT, D.J. and VOS,J.G. (1986): Time-course study on doxorubicin-induced nephropathy and cardiomyopathy in male and female LOU/M/WSL rats: Lack of evidence for a causal relationship. *J.N.C.I.*, 76, 299–307.

VAN HOESEL, Q.C.C.M., STEERENBERG, P.A., DORMANS, J.A.M.A., DE JONG, W.H., DE WILDT, D.J. and VOS J.G. (1988): Time course study on doxorubicin-induced nephropathy and cardiomyopathy in male and female LOU/M/WsL rats: Lack of evidence for a causal relationship *J.N.C.I.*, 76, 299–307.

VERANI, R. and BULGER, R.E. (1982): The pelvic epithelium of the rat kidney: A scanning and transmission electron microscopic study. *Am.J.Anat.*, 163, 223–233.

VIAU, C., BERNARD, A., GUERET, F., MALDAGUE, P., GENGOUX, P. and LAUWERYS, R. (1986): Isoparaffinic solvent induced nephrotoxicity in the rat. *Toxicology*, 38, 227–230.

VIRCHOW, R. (1855): Kalkemetastasen. *Virchows Arch.Pathol.Anat.*, 8, 103–113.

WACHSMUTH, E.D. (1984): Renal cell heterogeneity at a light microscopic level. In: P.A. Bach and E.A. Lock (Eds), *Renal Heterogeneity and Target Cell Toxicity*, pp. 13–30, John Wiley & Sons, Chichester.

WALKER, S.E. (1977): Accelerated mortality in young NZB/NZW mice treated with the interferon inducer tilorone. *Clin.Immunol.Immunopathol.*, 8, 204–212.

WARD, J.M. and REZNIK-SCHÜLLER, H. (1980): Morphological and histochemical characteristics of pigments in aging F344 rats. *Vet.Pathol.*, 17, 678–685.

WARD, M. (1970): Tubular metaplasia in Bowman's capsule. *J.Clin.Pathol.*, 23, 472–474.

WATSON, J.I. and DIXON, F.J. (1966): Experimental glomerulonephritis. IX. Factors influencing the development of kidney in adjuvant nephritis in rats. *Proc.Soc.Exp.Biol.Med.*, 121, 216–223.

WEENING, J.J., FLEUREN, G.J. and HOEDEMAEKER, Ph. J. (1978): Demonstration of antinuclear antibodies in mercuric chloride-induced glomerulopathy in the rat. *Lab.Invest.*, 39, 405–411.

WEENING, J.J., HOEDEMAEKER, Ph. J. and BAKKER, W.W. (1981): Immunoregulation and antinuclear antibodies in mercury-induced glomerulopathy in the rat. *Clin.Exp.Immunol.*, 45, 64–74.

WEIDMANN, M.J. and KREBS, H.A. (1969): The fuel of respiration of rat kidney cortex. *Biochem.J.*, 112, 149–166.

WEIL, C.S., CARPENTER, C.P. and SMYTH, H.F. (1965): Urinary bladder response to diethylene glycol. Calculi and tumours following repeated feeding and implants. *Arch.Environ.Health*, 11, 569–581.

WEXLER, B.C. and McMURTRY, J.P. (1981): Kidney and bladder calculi in spontaneously hypertensive rats. *Br.J.Exp.Pathol.*, 62, 369–374.

WHELTON, A. and SOLEZ, K. (1982): Aminoglycoside nephrotoxicity: a tale of two transports. *J.Lab.Clin.Med.*, 99, 148–155.

WHITING, P.H. THOMSON, A.W., BLAIR, J.T. and SIMPSON, J.G. (1982): Experimental cyclosporin A nephrotoxicity. *Br.J.Exp.Pathol.*, 63, 88–94.

WHITING, P.H., THOMSON, A.W. and SIMPSON, J.G. (1985): Cyclosporin: Toxicity, metabolsim, and drug interactions: implications from animal studies. *Transplant.Proc*, 17 (Suppl.), 134–144.

WILSON, R.M., DOUGLAS, C.A., TATTERSALL, R.B. and REEVES, W.G. (1985): Immunogenicity of highly purified bovine insulin: a comparison with conventional bovine and high purified human insulins. *Diabetologia*, 28, 667–670.

WISEMAN, E.H. and REINERT, H. (1975): Anti-inflammatory drugs and renal papillary necrosis. *Agents Actions*, 5, 322–325.

WOLKOWSKI-TYL, R., CHIN, T.Y., POPP, J.A. and HECK, Hd'A. (1982): Urolithiasis. Chemically induced urolithiasis in weanling rats. *Am.J.Pathol.*, 107, 419–421.

WOOLEY, P.H., GRIFFIN, J., PANAYI, G.S., BATCHELOR, J.R., WELSH, K.I. and GIBSON, T.J. (1980): HLA-DR antigens and toxic reaction to sodium aurothiomalate and D-penicillamine in patients with rheumatoid arthritis. *N.Engl.J.Med.*, 303, 300–203.

WRIGHT, N.G. and NASH, A.S. (1984): Experimental ampicillin glomerulonephropathy. *J.Comp.Pathol.*, 94, 357–361.

YASUDA, K and YAMASHITA, S. (1985): Immunohistochemical study on gamma-glutamyl-transpeptidase in rat kidney with monoclonal antibodies. *J.Histochem.Cytochem.*, 34, 111.

ZAKI, F.G., KEIM, G.R., TAKII, Y. and INAGAMI, T. (1982): Hyperplasia of the juxtaglomerular cells and renin localization in kidneys of normotensive animals given captopril. *Ann.Clin.Lab.Sci.*, 12, 200–215.

ZBINDEN, G. (1969): Experimental renal toxicity. In: C. Rouiller and A.F. Muller (Eds), *The Kidney. Morphology, Biochemistry, Physiology*, Vol. 2, Chap. 6, pp. 401–475.

ZBINDEN, G., FENT, K. and THOUIN, M.H. (1988): Nephrotoxicity screening in rats; general approach and establishment of test criteria. *Arch.Toxicol.*, 61, 344–348.

ZEMER, D., PRAS, M., SOHAR, E., MODAN, M., CAPBILL, S. and GAFNI, J. (1986): Colchicine in the prevention and treatment of the amyloidosis of familial Mediterranean fever. *N.Engl.J.Med.*, 314, 1001–1005.

ZUBAIDY, A.J. and MAJEED, S.K. (1981): Pathology of the nematode Trichosomoides crassicauda in the urinary bladder of laboratory rats. *Lab. Anim.*, 15, 381–384.

X. Male Genital Tract

During the course of drug development, the effects of novel compounds on the reproductive system are examined in the three segment reproductive test. This comprises Segment I, a general reproduction and fertility screen, Segment II, teratology studies, and Segment III, peri- and post-natal experiment in which there is also lactational exposure to drug. The Segment I screen is the only study which specifically evaluates the effects on male reproductive function but it is infrequently performed at an early stage of drug development. It is, therefore, important for the pathologist to realize that frequently the only assessment of the male reproductive organs performed prior to the first administration of a novel therapeutic agent to man is morphological examination of the male sex organs in conventional toxicity studies in rodent and non-rodent species. For this reason, this assessment should be performed carefully using meticulous techniques.

In mammals the male sex organs comprise the paired testes and the accessory reproductive organs. (See Eckstein and Zuckerman 1960 for review). Accessory organs are classified as follows:

1) ampullary and vesicular glands including seminal vesicles which connect with the vas deferens;

2) prostate gland and urethral glands such as bulbo-urethral or Cooper's glands which connect with or arise from the urogenital sinus;

3) glands of ectodermal origin such as preputial and anal glands which are associated with external genitalia.

PROSTATE GLAND

The prostate gland represents one of the accessory glands of the male reproductive system together with the seminal vesicles, coagulating glands, ampullary glands and epididymis. The prostate gland is both testosterone-dependent and influenced by hypothalamic control mechanisms (Grayhack, 1963). However, cell proliferation and differentiation of the prostate epithelium is primarily directed by androgens. Testosterone is converted to the active dihydrotestosterone in the prostate gland and this serves as a mediator for prostatic growth.

As prostatic epithelial cells possess androgen receptors and since androgens stimulate DNA synthesis in vivo, it has been postulated that proliferation of prostatic epithelium is regulated through these receptors. However, a series of studies in the mouse prostate gland and in chimeric prostates composed of rat mesenchyme and mouse epithelium has suggested that mesenchyme is also important in prostatic development, differentiation and functional activity and that the proliferative effects of androgens may not be the result of a direct effect on epithelium but mediated through androgen receptors on stromal cells (Cunha et al., 1980; Sugimura et al., 1986a). Furthermore, studies of the mouse prostate using autoradiography for DNA synthetic activity and androgen receptors using tritiated dihydrotestosterone have also demonstrated considerable regional heterogeneity in the distribution of androgen receptors and DNA synthetic activity (Sugimura et al., 1986a,b,c).

The prostate gland has potential for multidirectional differentiation in response to different hormonal environments and differentiation patterns serve as useful guides to the actual sex-hormone milieu present in laboratory animals or man. Therefore, histological examination of the prostate, as well as the seminal vesicles and epididymus forms a useful component of the assessment of the effects of xenobiotics on the male reproductive system.

Unfortunately, there is greater species variation in the anatomy of the prostate gland than most other internal organs and a number of basic aspects of comparative structure and function of the prostate are still quite poorly understood. This has in turn created a number of divergent views on structure and function of the mammalian prostate (McNeal, 1980). Despite interspecies differences, the prostate glands of rodents, dogs, or non-human primates have all been successfully employed as models for the common human prostatic disorders, prostatitis, nodular hyperplasia and prostatic carcinoma.

The *human prostate gland* envelopes the urethra and the neck of the bladder forming a single, firm tissue mass surrounded by a thin fibrous capsule. Traditionally, the prostate gland is considered to be formed by several lobes usually defined as an anterior, middle, posterior and two lateral lobes. However, these lobes are not anatomically distinct structures and their terminology open to some debate (see review by McNeal, 1980). Despite disagreement over these aspects of prostatic anatomy, it is clear that there is considerable histological heterogeneity within the parenchyma of the human prostate gland. McNeal (1980) has defined two principal zones, an outer zone composed of long branched glands and an inner part containing submucosal glands which open directly into the urethra. Histologically, the outer zone can be recognized by the presence of acini lined by uniform columnar cells with clear cytoplasm, distinct cytoplasmic borders and small dark basal nuclei. By contrast, the central zone contains acini lined by columnar cells which appear more crowded or densely packed with darker staining cytoplasm and larger paler nuclei (McNeal, 1980). Furthermore, the part of the prostate situated over the anterior aspect of the urethra is composed almost entirely of fibromuscular stroma, devoid of glandular tissue.

The importance of these microscopic differences is that they have been shown to be related to the development of human prostatic disease. The largest and most numerous nodules of hyperplasia almost always arise from the central zone near the urethra, whereas carcinomas develop from glands in the outer zone of the prostate (McNeal, 1980).

Acid phosphatase is the major secretory protein with enzymatic activity in human seminal fluid and its secretion from the prostate is both androgen- and age-dependent (Aumüller et al., 1983).

Unlike the human gland the *rat prostate* is divided anatomically into distinct lobes which are relatively easy to separate from each other. Two ventral and two dorsolateral lobes are usually recognized although some workers define separate dorsal and lateral lobes. (Jesik et al., 1982). It has been suggested that the lateral parts of the dorsolateral lobes possess the closest embryological relationship to the human prostate (Price, 1983). However, the ventral lobes are frequently used as models for the human gland and they are the principal sites for development of spontaneous hyperplasia and prostatic carcinoma in aged rats (Reznik et al., 1981).

The ventral lobes are drained by a series of ducts emptying into four or five main ducts which open into the urethra. In the dorsolateral lobes, groups of two to four acini each drain through a duct directly into the urethra (Jesik et al., 1982). The ease with which lobes of the rat prostate gland can be separated from each other has permitted the clear demonstration of biochemical differences between lobes. Ventral lobes have been shown to contain larger amounts of prostatein and spermine than other lobes (Gerhardt et al., 1983). As in the human gland, the rat prostate also elaborates acid phosphatase.

Other male accessory sex gland structures in the rat include the seminal vesicles, coagulating glands, vas deferens and their associated ampullary glands. Seminal vesicles can be recognized by intense eosinophilic staining of their secretions. Coagulating glands are histologically similar but their secretion is much less eosinophilic and it often appears cracked in conventional preparations (Jesik et al., 1982). The ampullary glands associated with the vas deferens, located on the dorsal surface of the urethra, are lined by columnar epithelium and are also recognized by intensely eosinophilic staining secretions.

The *canine prostate* is a homogeneous structure, not divided into lobes, composed predominantly of epithelial components with relatively little fibromuscular stroma (Habenicht et al., 1987). Histologically, fibrous band-like septa can be recognized. Acid phosphatase is an important hormone-dependent secretion of the canine prostate, although the major secretory component with enzymatic activity in the canine prostate is arginine esterase (Chapdelaine et al., 1984).

Despite the relative homogeneity of the dog prostate gland, regional differences in the response of the prostatic epithelium to hormonal influences are reported. Peri-urethral glands tend to undergo atrophy or squamous metaplasia more readily following androgen withdrawal or oestrogen challenge than subcapsular zones. Subcapsular zones appear to require lower levels of androgen to maintain their secretory function and this may be related to regional differences in vascular perfusion or metabolite patterns (Aumüller et al., 1987). Immunocytochemical study has also shown that there are regional differences in the localization of oestrogen receptors in the canine prostate and these may also account for regional differences in hormonal responsiveness (Schulze and Barrack, 1987).

Surprisingly, the anatomy of the prostate gland of most non-human primates differs considerably from that of the human gland (Habenicht et al., 1987). The gland in most monkeys is divided into a lobular, cranial portion and a compact caudal zone. The cranial lobe shows histological resemblance to the central zone of the human prostate whereas the caudal lobe corresponds more with that of the peripheral zone in man. Unlike the dog, there is an important stromal component. Habenicht and colleagues (1987) have demonstrated that the prostate gland of the cynomolgus monkey possesses the greatest morphological similarity to the human gland. It is not sharply divided into cranial and caudal lobes but possesses a more integral structure, which unlike glands in other non-human primates, completely envelopes the urethra. The cranial and caudal lobes are considered to be homologous to the central and peripheral zones of the human prostate respectively. (Habenicht and EL Etreby, 1988). As in the human gland, it has been shown that both the stromal and glandular components respond to hormonal stimulation, especially the caudal or periurethral zone (Habenicht and El Etreby, 1988).

Paired seminal vesicles of cynomolgus monkeys consist of individual highly convoluted glands containing rounded acini with a simple columnar epithelium. Efferent ducts possess large lumens with papillary infoldings (Habenicht et al., 1987).

Cytochemical and immunocytochemical examination

Cytochemical or immunocytochemical demonstration of acid phosphatase has been shown to be a good indicator of the functional integrity of prostatic secretory cells, particularly as acid phosphatase is a major secretory component which is androgen-dependent in man and laboratory animals. It has been shown that there is a close immunological cross-reactivity of antibody against acid phosphatase from the rat ventral prostate, the canine and human prostate (Terracio et al., 1982; Aumüller et al., 1987).

Other cellular components which can be helpful in the characterization of prostatic changes are cytokeratins, which can be used as markers for prostatic basal cells lying along the base of the glandular epithelium. It has been shown using immunocytochemical analysis of the normal canine prostate that cytokeratins are synthesized in basal rather than glandular cells of the epithelium (Merk et al., 1986). Keratin synthesis appears to be a property of proximal

587

entodermal cells which serve as an embryonic primordium for the developing prostate. It is probable that androgens exert an inhibitory effect on keratin protein synthesis during normal differentiation and maintenance of normal glandular function. As castration or administration of oestrogens is accompanied by loss of the androgen sensitive phenotype and an increase in tonofilaments and cytokeratins, immunocytochemical demonstration of cytokeratins can be a useful indicator of hormone-induced changes (Aumüller et al., 1987). Antibodies to vimentin have also proved of use in the demonstration of hormone induced changes in stromal cells of the prostate.

As in other epithelia, cytochemistry using labelled lectins also has a place in the study of the prostatic epithelium. Surface carbohydrate constituents have been shown to alter in atrophic, metaplastic, hyperplastic, and neoplastic states in the dog prostate gland (Orgad et al., 1984).

It should not be forgotten that endocrine cells are also normal constituents of the prostate gland. Both argentaffin and argyrophilic cells can be found and serotonin activity has been demonstrated in argyrophil cells (Fetissof et al., 1983).

Atrophy

The prostate gland and seminal vesicles of rodents, dogs and primates frequently show a reduction in weight in high dose toxicity studies and this may be associated with histological evidence of atrophy. Whilst these changes can be the manifestation of a direct cytotoxic effect on prostatic glandular cells, they are more commonly the indirect result of disturbances of the pituitary-gonadal axis which is important in the maintenance of accessory sex organ function. These effects can be a result of a primary effect on the hypothalamus or mediated by an effect on testicular steroid production. However, prostatic weight loss and atrophy also occur in high dose toxicity experiments in association with stress and weight loss. These effects, although largely mediated through the pituitary-gonadal axis, do not reflect a specific drug effect on male accessory tissue.

The morphological changes which follow reduction in testosterone levels have been well studied in laboratory animals following castration. Indeed, the rapid weight loss and involution which occurs in the ventral prostate of the rat in the weeks following castration has been used as a model in the study of basic cellular processes involved in tissue involution.

Kerr and Searle (1973) showed that the rapid weight loss which occurs in the ventral prostate of the rat over a period of three weeks after castration is associated with extensive loss of epithelial cells as a result of enhanced cell death, a process known as *apoptosis* [1]. Histologically, there is a progressive decrease in the size of acini, clearly visible from day three onwards. The epithelial cells lose their normal columnar appearance to become cuboidal. Apoptotic bodies, located

---

See footnote next page.

sparsely in epithelial cells in about 5% of normal rat prostatic acini, increase dramatically in castrated rats. Apoptotic bodies are characterized by nuclear and cytoplasmic condensation of epithelial cells with exhuberent budding which gives rise to small, membrane-bound, compact cellular fragments. These apoptotic bodies are mainly Feulgan-positive, compatable with a high content of de-oxyribonucleic acid (Kerr and Searle, 1973). These bodies appear to be either extruded into the lumens of acini or ingested by adjacent cells, notably macro-phages, where they are ultimately degraded by lysosomal enzymes. Light micro-scopic morphometric study of castration effects in the rat prostate has shown that there is a reduction in both epithelial height and cell number in all lobes but changes are most marked in the ventral lobe (Kiplesund et al., 1988).

Epithelial changes in the prostate gland which follow castration appear to be a direct result of androgen withdrawal for they can be completely reversed by concomitant administration of testosterone (Evans and Chandler, 1987).

Investigations from a number of laboratories have also described changes in non-epithelial cells of the prostate of the rat following castration. There is histological evidence of a progressive increase in density of stromal connective tissue following castration. Labelling experiments with tritiated thymidine in the rat ventral prostate after castration have shown that fibroblasts, smooth muscle, and endothelial cells are also reduced in numbers and show a lower labelling index (English et al., 1985).

Studies in mice have shown that the tips and branches of ducts in distal regions near the prostate capsule are lost more readily after castration than more

---

[1] *Apoptosis.* There is increasing evidence that apoptosis is a general cellular phenomenon which plays an opposite but complementary role to mitosis in the homeostasis of cell populations in healthy tissues (Wyllie, 1987). In order to distinguish this form of physiological cell death from other forms of death, the term, apoptosis, derived from the Greek for 'falling of leaves from trees in autumn' has been coined.

Apoptosis has been well-documented in a number of mammalian organs especially those which are endocrine dependent such as adrenal cortex, prostate gland, ovary, endometrium, mammary tissue but also liver, gastro-intestinal tract, thymus, and lymph nodes (Wyllie, 1987).

The key features of this form of cell death are contraction of cell volume, condensation of nuclear chromatin and cellular fragmentation. Cytoplasmic organelles are reasonably well-preserved and exclude substances such as trypan blue. Cells undergoing apoptosis do not provoke an inflammatory reaction but are rapidly phagocytosed by adjacent cells, notably monocytes. Estimates of the half-time that apoptotic cells remain visible under the light microscope are under nine hours (Wyllie et al., 1980; Ijiri and Potten, 1983).

How apoptotic cells are recognized by adjacent cells and monocytes is uncertain. It has been suggested that certain sugar residues such as N-acetyl glucosamine and its dimer N,N'-diacetyl chitobiose which are exposed on the surface of apoptotic cells are recognized by endogeneous lectin-like molecules on monocytes (Duvall et al., 1985).

Although apoptosis can be considered primarily an adaptive process, it may also result from injurious stimuli such as virus infection, ionizing radiation and administration of toxins (Wyllie, 1987). Hence, the borderline between a physiological and pathological increase in apoptosis is not sharp. Evaluation of the phenomenen in toxicity studies requires a thorough evaluation of all salient data including consideration of the dose-response relationship.

proximal segments close to the urethra (Sugimura et al., 1986b). This suggests that distal ducts are particularly androgen-dependent in rodents.

In the castrated dog, acini also atrophy and epithelial cells show a reduced immunocytochemical reaction for secretory acid phosphatase (Aumüller et al., 1987). The loss of acid phosphatase secretion is, therefore, a useful indicator of reduction in secretory function of prostatic epithelium. The glandular atrophy is also accompanied by loss of the androgen-dependent secretory phenotype and an increase in cytokeratins in the epithelium occurs which can be demonstrated by immunocytochemical methods. Aumüller and colleagues (1987) also showed changes in stromal cells in castrated dogs by showing a reduction in immunocytochemical staining for the intermediate filaments of vimentin type.

In castrated cymomolgus monkeys, acini of the caudate lobe (peripheral zone) become more atrophic than those in the cranial lobe or periurethral glands (Habenicht and El Etreby, 1988).

Drugs with anti-androgenic activity, whether mediated directly or through the hypothalamus, can produce similar morphological changes in the male accessory sex glands. A recent example of this phenomenon is provided by an active synthetic analogue of gonadotrophin releasing hormone which produces a decrease in prostatic weight in a number of species, including man. It is believed that this agent produces paradoxical suppression of testosterone production as a result of an inhibition of gonadotrophin release after an initial phase of increased gonadotrophin secretion (Labrie et al., 1978; Blask and Leadem, 1987).

Flutamide, a non-steroidal anti-androgen also produces a decrease in secretory activity and loss of weight of the prostate gland and seminal vesicles when administered to rats, probably also because it deprives these glands of their normal testosterone stimulation (Chapin and Williams, 1989). Under these circumstances, the accessory male sex organs show atrophic changes more readily than the testis. This is presumably because intratesticular androgen concentations are sufficiently high to compete successfully with flutamide given in high doses.

Another example is provided by the histamine H2 blocker cimetidine, which consistently produced decreases in the weight of the prostate gland and seminal vesicles in dogs and rats when it was administered for periods of three or more months (Brimblecombe et al., 1985; Walker et al., 1987). Cimetidine has been shown to possess weak anti-androgenic activity unrelated to H2-receptors which when calculated on a molar basis proved to be over 500 times weaker than cyproterone acetate and over 10 times less than that of spironolactone (Sivelle et al., 1982).

Several benzodiazepines have also been reported to decrease prostatic weight when administered to laboratory animals at high doses, presumably through interference with the hypothalamic-pituitary-gonadal axis (Black et al., 1987).

Despite the variable species and strain-related sensitivity of the testicular germinal epithelium to different oestrogen preparations (see below), administration of oestrogen alone to intact laboratory animals has been shown to consistently decrease the weight and produce atrophy of the male accessory sex organs, particularly the prostate, seminal vesicles, and epididymis (Meistrich et al., 1977; Schardein, 1980a). This effect appears also to be mediated by interference with the production or action of androgens for it has been shown in intact mice that concomitant administration of testosterone can prevent oestrogen-induced changes in the secondary sex glands (Meistrich et al., 1977). Whether these changes are the result of a direct effect of oestrogen on Leydig cells to reduce testosterone production, whether oestrogen acts directly on the secondary sex organs or whether it produces these changes by its inhibitory effects on LH production in the pituitary is not clear.

Weight loss of the prostatic gland and histological evidence of atrophy has also been traditionally ascribed to body weight loss and general stress effects which may be manifest in high dose groups of repeated dose toxicity studies. In view of the complexity of interactions between stress and pharmacological activity and the possibility that test compounds express additional and unexpected specific effects at high doses, attributing prostatic atrophy to inanition and stress, requires careful analysis of all the salient findings.

The effects of stress on the prostate gland have been studied in detail in the rat by Gatenbeck (1986). In these studies, rats were subjected to standardized stress-inducing procedures which included alternating periods of starvation, cold (4°C) or restriction of movements. Rats subjected to these procedures for 10 days showed decreased prostatic weight relative to body weight, accompanied by histological evidence of reduced secretory activity of the glandular epithelium. Acini appeared closer together, separated by condensed stroma containing focal aggregates of lymphocytes, plasma cells and macrophages. Some acini also contained cell debris and inflammatory exudate.

Using a radioactive microsphere technique, Gatenbeck (1986) showed that these histological changes were accompanied by a reduction in blood flow to the prostate gland. In addition, lower plasma testosterone and higher plasma catecholamine levels were found compared with control rats.

It was suggested by Gatenbeck (1986) that these changes were mediated either directly or indirectly by a stress-related decrease in prostatic blood flow. As prostatic blood flow is testosterone dependent, stress stimuli may mediate changes in prostatic blood flow through an effect on the hypothalamic-pituitary gonadal axis with subsequent reduction in testosterone secretion. However, these effects could also mediated through catecholamine-induced increase in vascular resistance (Gatenbeck, 1986).

Dietary alterations have also been shown clearly to produce prostatic changes in rats. Both four- and 18-month-old Long-Evans rats fed a protein-free diet for 20 days developed relatively little change in testicular weight but the weights of the prostate gland and seminal vesicles showed significant reductions in association with reduced testosterone levels (Esashi et al., 1982). Other studies have shown similar reductions in the weights of prostate glands and seminal vesicles of rats following food restriction (Howland, 1975).

Squamous metaplasia

The characteristic response of the prostate epithelium to oestrogen administration both in man and laboratory animals is squamous metaplasia. A variety of in vivo and in vitro studies have shown that squamous metaplasia can be also induced in the rodent prostate by vitamin A deficiency, administration of 3-methylcholanthrene, cyclic adenine nucleotide and prostaglandins E1 and E2 and that these effects can be reversed by retinoid administration (Lasnitzki, 1976; Schaefer et al., 1982). In vitro findings in the mouse ventral prostate have suggested that cyclic adenine nucleotide augmented by prostaglandins E1 and E2 may mediate the process of squamous metaplasia (Schaefer et al., 1982). Squamous metaplasia has also been reported in the human biopsy material in association with prostatic infarction (Mostofi and Price, 1973a).

Squamous metaplasia is characterized histologically by focal or diffuse replacement of the glandular epithelial cells by multilayered cells showing squamous differentiation. Prostastic epithelium showing squamous metaplasia stains well with antikeratin antibodies which may aid recognition of early metaplastic change (Aumüller et al., 1987).

Hyperplasia: dog

The development of prostatic hyperplasia is a common finding in both man and dog with advancing age and for this reason the dog has been widely used as an experimental model for benign prostatic hyperplasia of man.

Glandular prostatic hyperplasia develops spontaneously in beagles and has been found in over 10% of animals between one and two years of age and in 50% of those between four and five years (Berry et al., 1986). The weight of the beagle dog prostate also increases in parallel with these age-related histological changes, the calculated increase being 4.3 gm per year over the first four years of life (Berry et al., 1986). In view of the fact that these changes can occur in quite young beagle dogs, they may be seen in chronic toxicity studies using this species.

Histologically, the hyperplasia of the prostate seen in dogs involves primarily the glandular cells, unlike the human disease which is a variable mixture of proliferating glandular and stromal elements. Appearances range from proliferating and densely packed glands and ducts surrounded by little or no stroma to more complex patterns in which there is a combination of glandular proliferation and papillomatosis with glandular atrophy, cyst formation and mild stromal hyperplasia.

Wilson (1980, 1987) has suggested that the development of hyperplasia in the canine prostate is accelerated by oestrogen which enhances the level of androgen receptors in the gland. This in turn permits androgen-mediated growth in the face of declining androgen function with advancing age. It has been shown using immunocytochemical study that oestrogen receptors develop variably in sub-populations of prostatic epithelial cells in hyperplastic glands of dogs (Schulze and Barrack, 1987). This is presumably a result of induction by oestrogen, consistent with the increase in the oestrogen:androgen ratio which occurs in the dog with advancing age.

Of importance in toxicology is the fact that the development of prostatic hyperplasia in the dog is dependent on the action of sex hormones, for it does not develop in dogs castrated before puberty and its development can be modulated by changes in sex hormone levels.

Focal hyperplasia: rat

Focal prostatic glandular hyperplasia has been well described in association with the development of adenomas and carcinomas in the prostate gland in aged rats of the Lobund Wistar and AC strains (Pollard, 1973; Ward et al., 1980). Careful examination of the prostate gland of more commonly employed strains has shown that this form of hyperplasia is more common in rats than previously believed.

Detailed histological examination of the prostate glands from two year-old Fischer 344 rats from 12 carcinogenicity bioassays conducted by the NCI and NTP showed that 10–20% of rat prostates contained focal proliferative glandular lesions (Resnik et al., 1981). These foci were not macroscopically visible but were observed microscopically localized almost exclusively in the lateral regions of the ventral prostate. These lesions were characterized by papillomatous microglandular or cribriform formations three to five cells thick located in one or more acini. The proliferating cells show rounded or oval hyperchromatic nuclei.

Neoplasia

Prostatic carcinoma is one of the most common cancers of aged men but there are relatively few laboratory animals which frequently develop prostatic cancer spontaneously. Prostatic adenomas and adeno-carcinomas have been described in several strains of rats, including ACI, Wistar and Fischer 344 rats and they probably occur generally in rats more commonly then previously thought (Pollard, 1973; Ward et al., 1980; Reznik et al., 1981). There is no clear consensus of opinion regarding the separation of hyperplasia, adenoma and carcinoma in the rat prostate and the usual general principles are applicable.

Spontaneous rat neoplasms show glandular differentiation and appear to develop mainly in the ventral lobe of the prostate. Histologically, carcinomas are composed of solid sheets or cribriform arrangements of cells which compress and infiltrate adjacent tissues as well as spread along prostatic ducts and into the urethra (Fig. 110). Metastases form relatively uncommonly from this form of carcinoma (Ward et al., 1980; Reznik et al., 1981).

Squamous carcinomas of the prostate gland have been induced in rats following administration of the nitrosamine, N-nitrosobis(2-oxopropyl)amine at a dose of 10 mg per kg body weight per week (Pour, 1981). Histologically, all the

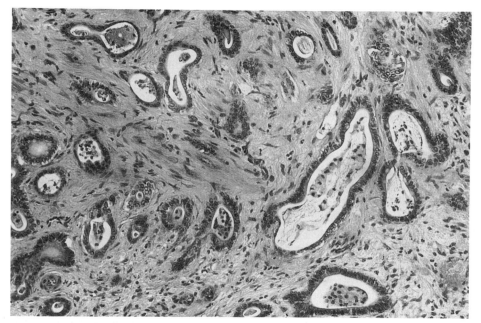

Fig. 110. Prostate gland from a two-year-old Sprague-Dawley rat diffusely infiltrated by a moderately well-differentiated adenocarcinoma. (HE, ×200.)

induced carcinomas were of keratinizing squamous type with focal anaplasia, mostly developing in the suburethral region of the dorsal prostate.

EPIDIDYMIS

Spontaneous or drug-induced lesions of the epididymis are not commonly reported but this may be partly due to the limited sampling which is common practice in toxicity studies (Cardy, 1987).

The epididymis is anatomically and functionally more complex than is apparent in randomly sampled and routinely fixed tissue sections. It has been well studied in the rat where it can be divided into three major regions. The *caput epididymidis* is joined to the superior lateral aspect of the testis by the efferent ductules. The *corpus epididymidis* forms a narrow neck joining the capus to the caudal segment of the epididymis, the *cauda epididymidis*. The epididymus is attached to the testis by a delicate mesentery (White, 1978). Furthermore, the rat epididymis has been subdivided into six histological regions, distinguished by differences in tubular diameter, type and height of columnar epithelium, appearances of basal cells and number of lymphocytes (Reid and Cleland, 1957; Brandes, 1974; White, 1978).

Morphometric analysis of the rat epididymis has shown that tubule diameter increases and tubular wall height and wall density decreases from the caput to the tail (Miller and Killian, 1987). The tubule wall is composed of about 90% of columnar epithelial cells with about 50% lymphocytes and 5% of basal cells. It is probable that the relatively small tubular lumen, the large wall volume and plentiful columnar epithelial cells in the caput region provide the necessary basis for maximal biochemical interaction between columnar epithelial and maturing sperm. In contrast, the large lumen and small tubular wall volume of the caudal region is more suited for storage of spermatozoa (Miller and Killian, 1987).

Histochemical studies have revealed distinct regional variations in enzyme activity in the different regions (Martan, 1969; Weiss, 1983). Both the stereociliated cells (principle or chief cells) and the non-stereociliated cells show an unusually complex pattern of histochemical reactions in different regions and in different species.

Inflammation and sperm granulomas

The epididymis is liable to develop a granulomatous inflammatory process (sperm granuloma) when there is rupture of tubules and ducts with release of mature spermatozoa into the interstitium. This follows trauma to the epididymis or surgical procedures such as vasectomy. Sperm granulomas which form at the site of extravation are composed of a mass of spermatozoa, some of which undergo degradation, surrounded by epithelioid macrophages, granulation tissue, lymphocytes and plasma cells (McDonald and Scothorne, 1987). In experimental animals, vasectomy may also be accompanied by development of sperm granulomas as well as the presence of antisperm antibodies and increased number of lymphocytes in the epididymis (Flickinger, 1985; McDonald and Scothorne, 1987; Miller and Killian, 1987).

Sperm granulomas have also been reported following administration of therapeutic agents in toxicity studies where they may indicate disturbance of the autonomic nervous system (see also Nervous System, Chapter XIII).

Adrenergic antagonists especially guanethidine derivatives and other vasodilating antihypertensive agents have been reported to produce sperm granulomas in the epididymis of rodents (Bhathal et al., 1974; Heywood and James, 1978). Granulomas induced by guanethidine in the rat were shown to bulge from the posteriomedial aspect of the caudal segment of the epididymis. Histological examination showed granulomas composed of a central mass of spermatozoa surrounded by radially arranged epithelioid macrophages and multinucleated giant cells enveloped in an outer layer of vascular connective tissue, lymphocytes, plasma cells and occasional polymorphonuclear cells (Bhathal et al., 1973). The granulomas were associated with microdiverticular and fistulae of the vas deferens at the origin of its straight portion. It was suggested that granulomas resulted as a result of leakage of spermatozoa following rupture of the vas deferens at this site. It was postulated that guanethidine induced loss of contractile ability in the part of the epididymis responsible for emission of semen whilst sparing more proximal parts of the epididymis responsible for movement of spermatozoa along seminiferous tubules. Rupture occurred as a result of spermatozoa continuing to pass from intact seminiferous tubules into the functionally disrupted zone (Bhathal et al., 1973).

Sperm granulomas were also described in the epididymis of rats treated with the salicylanilide antihelmintic, closantel (Van Cauteren et al., 1985). Affected rats developed swelling of the epididymis which histologically was characterized by the presence of sperm granulomas with round cell infiltration, oedema and fibrosis. This phenomenon was not observed in other animal test species and its cause remains uncertain.

Miscellaneous findings

Careful examination of the epididymis from 85 aged Fischer 344 rats revealed a spontaneous segmental degeneration of the epithelial cells characterized by cytoplasmic vacuolation, frequently with accumulation of PAS positive material, epithelial cell necrosis and accumulation of cell debris in the duct lumen (Cardy, 1987). The lesion was localized to a zone comprising the distal part of the caput and the proximal isthmus. The lesion is also found in other strains but its cause is unknown. Testicular atrophy may also be reflected by the lack of mature spermatozoa in the lumen of the epididymis (see below).

TESTIS

Problems relating to fixation of the testis in toxicology studies have been discussed at some length by Lamb and Chapin (1985). Although no fixation is ideal, formalin is undoubtably the least satisfactory when it is followed by routine embedding in paraffin wax. Formalin fixation can produce good results however, when it is followed by embedding in methacylate or epoxy resin (Chapin et al., 1984). For routine needs, immersion fixation in Bouin's, Zenker's or Helly's fluid is usually the most satisfactory, followed by embedding in paraffin wax and staining with haematoxylin and eosin or haematoxylin and PAS.

Later phases of spermatogenesis in laboratory animals can be assessed by analysis of semen and this provides a useful point of comparison with human studies in which the principal method of assessment of drugs on the testis is also analysis of ejaculated semen (Drife, 1987). Semen samples can be obtained from dogs and rabbits by methods using an artificial vagina and from the epididymis of rodents at autopsy or by micropuncture techniques (Puget, 1972; Wyrobek and Bruce, 1975; Wyker and Howard, 1977; Heywood and James, 1978; Taradach, 1986). Assessment of sperm counts and sperm morphology in suspensions or smears can be helpful in assessment of germ cell damage, particularly if examination takes place at appropriately timed intervals following treatment with xenobiotics (Wyrobek and Bruce, 1975). Sperm motility is another method in the evaluation of the function of mature spermatozoa (Taradach, 1986).

In man and laboratory animals, the testes are ovoid paired organs surrounded by a smooth fibrous capsule which is continuous with fibrous septa which divide the testes into a number of compartments or lobules. A posterior thickened portion of the capsule is called the mediastinum which contains blood vessels, lymphatics and the intratesticular part of the *rete testis* from which efferent ductules connect with the *epididymus*.

The lobule of the testis contains several *seminiferous tubules*. Each tubule is a closed loop structure provided with inter-communications but devoid of blind loops or branches. Each arm of the seminiferous tubule opens into the rete testis. The seminiferous tubules contain two important elements, germ cells in varying stages of differentiation and Sertoli cells.

Sertoli cells comprise about 10 or 15% of the total population of tubular cells and they are located towards the base of the tubules. They are characterized by irregular nuclei with vesicular chromatin pattern, prominant nucleoli and eosinophilic granular cytoplasm which contains lipid vacuoles and lipofuscin granules. Ultrastructural study demonstrates the presence of a few oval mitochondria, vesicular and tubular profiles of smooth endoplasmic reticulum, some free ribosomes, lipid droplets, primary and secondary lysosomes. Junctional complexes exist between adjacent Sertoli cells (Rhodin, 1974).

Sertoli cells have several important functions relating to spermatogenesis. One of these is the phagocytosis of residual bodies of spermatids and degenerating sperm cells. Sertoli cells also secrete lactate and to a lesser extent pyruvate and are well-endowed with the appropriate enzymes notably lactate dehydrogenase which catalyzes the interconversion of lactate and pyruvate in the glycolytic pathway (Santiemma et al., 1987). Lactate and pyruvate are important energy substrates for spermatocytes and spermatids and they are more effective than glucose in promoting RNA and protein synthesis by these cells (Jutte et al., 1981; Mita and Hall, 1982).

Another important feature of Sertoli cells is their formation of a meshwork around developing germ cells. The tight junctional complexes between Sertoli cells divide the tubule into basal and inner or adluminal compartments (Dym and Fawcett, 1970). The basal compartment contains spermatogonia and preleptotene spermatocytes whereas the adluminal part contains the remaining primary spermatocytes and more developed forms. A transient third chamber is formed by adjacent Sertoli cells as germ cells move from the basal to the adluminal compartment (Trainer, 1987). This barrier, composed of tight junctional complexes between adjacent Sertoli cells, appears to form the most important part of the blood-testis barrier, preventing direct access of blood borne substances into the adluminal compartment, except by passing through the metabolically active Sertoli cell cytoplasm. Studies with the electron-opaque intercellular tracer, lathanum, have shown that although the myoid cells around seminiferous tubules form a permeability barrier, tight junctions between Sertoli cells are a second and more effective barrier to the penetration of substances through the germinal epithelium (Dym and Fawcett, 1970). All these factors lead to a permeability barrier comparable to that which retards penetration of chemicals to the brain and permeability constants for the two are nearly identical (Dixon and Lee, 1980).

Sertoli cells are believed to be the source of inhibins, non-steroidal inhibitors of FSH (Steinberger and Steinberger, 1976). Inhibins are proteins consisting of two subunits linked by disulphide bridges which are secreted from testicular Sertoli cells or granulosa cells of the ovary in response to FSH from the pituitary, in a reciprocal feedback relationship (Ying, 1987).

Sertoli cells develop cyclical morphological changes. They show alterations in cell volume, nuclear shape, lipid vacuole content, activity of acid phosphatases and thiamine pyrophosphatase as well as changes in volume density of endo-plasmic reticulum at various stages of the cycle of the seminiferous epithelium (Parvinen, 1982).

Germ cells form the predominant cell population of the seminiferous tubules and comprise *spermatogonia, spermatocytes* and *spermatids*. Although there are species differences, spermatogenesis, the process by which spermatogonial stem-cells produce highly differentiated haploid spermatozoa, can be divided into three similar distinct phases in man and laboratory animals. The first phase consists of the formation of spermatocytes as a result of mitotic division of spermatogonia. The second phase is production of spermatids as a consequence of meiotic divisions of spermatocytes. The final phase is the differentiation of spermatozoa from spermatids (Clermont, 1972).

Spermatogonia are situated along the basement membrane. Two forms are recognized, type A which on division gives rise to type B. Spermatogonia are recognized by rounded nuclei, fairly dense chromatin patterns, marginated nucleoli and sparse cytoplasm. After division, type B spermatogonia become primary spermatocytes.

The early forms of primary spermatocytes (proleptotene form) are situated within the basal compartment, side by side with spermatogonia. The various stages of spermatocyte development are recognized by the changes in the filamentous patterns within their round nuclei (Clermont, 1972).

After a relatively long period of gametogenesis, the first meiotic division takes place to give secondary spermatocytes. These haploid cells have short half lives and rapidly undergo second meiotic division to form haploid spermatids. Off-spring of secondary spermatocytes are connected to each other by cytoplasmic bridges and separation occurs late in the spermatid phase.

The term spermatid is usually reserved for all post-meiotic germ cells which have not left the seminiferous tubules (Clermont, 1963), although some authors use the term spermatozoan for the most mature spermatid in the seminiferous tubules. Spermatids are recognized by their dense, round, oval or elongated nuclei, and the presence of an acrosome. The acrosome is composed of muco-polysaccharide which is secreted and accumulated in the Golgi zone and subse-quently forms a cap on one nuclear pole and covers half of the sphere. This eventually becomes the front part of the mature spermatozoan, but it can be recognized in histological sections by its bright staining with the PAS technique. The glycoprotein constituents of the acrosome form the basis for its staining

TABLE 1   *Duration of cycle of seminiferous epithelium and spermatogenesis (from Clermont, 1972)*

Species	Duration in Days	
	Cycle	Approximate duration for spermatogenesis
Rat	12.0	40.0
Mouse	8.6	35.0
Hamster (Mesocricetus auratus)	8.7	35.0
Rabbit	10.9	51.8
Monkey (Macaca mulatta)	10.5	70.0
(Macaca fascicularis)	9.3	37.2
Man	16.0	64.0

patterns with labelled-lectins. In the rat, the acrosome granule and cap phase acrosome stain well with peanut (PNA), Ricinus Communis A1 (RCA 1), Concanavalin (Con A) and wheat germ (WGA) lectins. Following subsequent maturation, these lectin affinities disappear and the mature acrosome is stained by soy bean (SBA), Ulex europaeus 1 (UEA 1) and Dolichos biflorus (DBA) lectins (Arya and Vanha-Perttula, 1984, 1985) (see Table 1, Digestive System, Chapter VII). Lectin probes have also proved useful in the study of the human sperm acrosome (Mortimer et al., 1987).

The transformation of mature spermatids into spermatozoa (termed spermiogenesis) takes place mainly during passage through the epididymus generally in the corpus or proximal cauda, for when spermatozoa leave the confines of the testis they have a poor capacity to fertilize. Maturation is characterized by modification of the structure of nuclear chromatin and tail organelles, loss of spermatid cytoplasmic remnants and an increased capacity for sustained motility (Hinrichsen and Blaquier, 1980).

Although the description of the cellular associations in the seminiferous epithelium have been based on optimally fixed, paraffin embedded, PAS stained sections, these associations have also been clearly defined in semithin sections cut from plastic resin-embedded tissues. These methods usually employ glutaraldehyde as the primary fixative, post fixation in osmium tetroxide and staining of the plastic resin embedded sections with toluidine blue or methylene blue-azure II-basic fuchsin (Russell and Frank, 1978; Ulvik et al., 1982).

For every species each step of spermatogenesis has a constant duration. Furthermore, many spermatogonial stem cells enter spermatogenesis simultaneously and consequently large groups of germ cells evolve synchronously throughout spermatogenesis. As a result of this precise timing, histological examination reveals a limited number of germ cell associations of fixed composition within seminiferous tubules. Spermatids at a particular point in development are always associated with spermatocytes at another precise stage in development. These cell associations follow each other in a certain order at precise time intervals at any given locus in the seminiferous epithelium. This complete series of successive cellular associations appearing at any particular site is considered to represent a *cycle of the seminiferous epithelium* (Clermont, 1972).

The number of stages composing the cycle are species-dependent, and they have been characterized for the rat by Leblond and Clermont (1952), for the mouse by Oakberg (1956) and for man by Clermont (1963). In man, only small areas with a particular association can be identified whereas in the rat these associations occupy longer sections of tubules (Skakkebaek, 1976). Furthermore, in the rat and other mammals, these cell associations are not located at random along the tubules but in a particular order referred to as the wave of the seminiferous epithelium (Perey et al., 1961). This wave is not a prominant feature of the human seminiferous epithelium (Clermont, 1972).

The most precisely defined species differences relate to the timing of the cycle of the seminiferous epithelium. Although reported duration of the cycles determined by labelled tracer studies varies somewhat with technique, there are striking differences between species. These differences have been compared in the classical review by Clermont (1972) (see Table 1). Knowledge of kinetics of these cell associations is important in the analysis of the influence of xenobiotics on mitosis, meiosis and cell-differentiation during spermatogenesis.

A variety of methods have been used for the quantitative or semiquantitative assessment of testicular germ cells in histological sections. Measurement of cross sectional area of seminiferous tubules provide a useful guide in the context of toxicity studies in which fixation procedures and subsequently shrinkage artefact are similar between controls and treated groups.

A method for both human and animal studies involves establishing the germ cell: Sertoli cell ratio in an appropriate number of tubule cross sections (Rowley and Heller, 1971; Skakkebaek and Heller, 1973). This method is based on the concept that Sertoli cells, unlike germ cells are a stable population in adults and are relatively resistant to adverse effects of drugs, chemicals, hormones and ionizing radiation (Skakkebaek, 1976).

Another method involves counting the number of spermatids per tubule cross section. This has been shown to correlate well with seminal fluid sperm counts in man (Sibler and Rodriquez-Rigau, 1981).

A rapid method is a score count in which each tubular section is given a score from one to ten according to the presence or absence of the main cell types arranged in order of maturity (Johnsen, 1970). In man this score count appears to correlate well with sperm count.

Leydig cells (interstitial cells), responsible for the production of testosterone, are located singly or in clusters in the interstitium. These cells possess single rounded vesicular nuclei, one or two nucleoli and a slightly foamy cytoplasm, containing lipid droplets and frequently lipochrome pigment. Ultrastructurally, the cytoplasm shows variable numbers of lipid droplets, abundant vesicular and tubular profiles of smooth endoplasmic reticulum, a fairly prominant Golgi zone and a few mitochondria. In man, characteristic crystalloids (Reinke crystalloids) of protein nature are also in the cell cytoplasm although similar structures are not usually found in Leydig cells of laboratory animals.

The lipid droplets are composed largely of esterified cholesterol, derived from both circulating lipoproteins and from local synthesis, which provides a reservoir of substrate for testosterone biosynthesis. Cholesterol ester is hydrolysed and cholesterol moves to the mitochondria where side chain cleavage to pregnenolone, the rate-limiting step in testosterone biosynthesis, takes place. Pregnenolone is subsequently converted in the endoplasmic reticulum to testosterone and released from the cell (Griffin and Wilson, 1985).

The principle pituitary hormones which control testicular function are luteinizing hormone (LH) and follicle-stimulating hormone (FSH), see Endocrine System, Chapter XII for discussion.

Luteinizing hormone acts through specific receptors on the surface of Leydig cells. Binding of these receptors stimulates membrane-bound adenylate cyclase to catalyze the formation of cyclic AMP. Release of cyclic AMP into the cytoplasm is followed by its binding to the regulatory subunit of a protein kinase with consequent activation of the catalytic subunit of the enzyme. This eventually stimulates the rate-limiting step in testosterone biosynthesis, the conversion of cholesterol to pregnenolone. This in turn enhances production of testosterone. The epithelium of the seminiferous tubule is the main site of action of FSH with binding to the Sertoli cell initiating a similar train of events to luteinizing hormone. There is activation of a cyclic AMP-dependent protein kinase and stimulation of rates of RNA and protein synthesis (Griffin and Wilson, 1985).

Testosterone production by Leydig cells changes with time during the lifespan of many species and these changes may be expressed by alterations in Leydig cell morphology and number, particularly during sexual maturation. It has been shown in the rat that Leydig cell number per testis increases in parallel with testicular weight following birth, accompanied by increases in the surface area of smooth endoplasmic reticulum and inner mitochondrial membrane and decreases in cytoplasmic lipid (Zirkin and Ewing, 1987).

The vascular supply of the testis takes place via the highly coiled, low pressure testicular artery system, which plays an important part in heat exchange. Studies using corrosion casts and scanning electron microscopy have demonstrated two types of capillary in the rat testis. The intertubular capillaries form a dense network with a polyhedral shape and the peritubular capillaries arranged in a ladder-like manner. By contrast in the human testis, the intertubular capillaries form only a loose network and the peritubular capillaries do not show the rope-ladder appearance found in the rat testis (Takayama and Tomoyashi, 1981).

There are a number of other species differences in the organization of the Leydig cells and drainage of the mammalian testis. Fawcett and colleagues (1973) defined three major categories of interstitial tissue organization in the mammalian testis. The first category are those species including rat, mouse, and guinea pig which have relatively small Leydig cell volume (1–5% of testicular volume), minimal interstitial connective tissue but an extensive peritubular lymphatic system. The second category are those species in which clusters of Leydig cells are widely scattered in loose connective tissue drained by prominant lymphatics located centrally in the interspaces. This group comprises a number of species including non-human primates and man. The third category includes a number of non-laboratory animals notably the domestic pig in which the interstitium is almost completely filled with closely packed Leydig cells and associated with sparse lymphatics and little connective tissue.

Interstitial tissue of the testis also contains a number of other cell types notably fibroblasts and macrophages. Macrophages have been described in the interstitial tissues of the normal testes in a variety of different species including man. In rats, testicular interstitial macrophages represent about 20% of cell profiles in histological sections (Miller, 1982). In the rat, they are often observed adjacent to Leydig cells where they are typically rounded, with indented nuclei and cytoplasm more lightly stained than Leydig cells. Ultrastructural study shows they contain mitochondria, dispersed profiles of rough endoplasmic reticulum, a well-developed Golgi complex and numerous lysosomes. Long filopodia and lamellopodia extend from the macrophage into the lymphatic space and there are some unique short cellular processes which extend from apposed Leydig cells into invaginations in the macrophage (Miller et al., 1983). This close anatomical relationship of macrophages with Leydig cells suggests that macrophages posses an important role in testicular function.

In the normal human testis, immunocytochemical study with the monoclonal antibody, LeuM3, believed to specifically bind monocytes and macrophages, showed numerous macrophages around the seminiferous tubules (El-Demiry et al., 1987). It is important to emphasize that lymphocytes were not detected in the interstitial tissues of the normal human testis except for T suppressor/cytotoxic (Leu 2a-positive) lymphocytes in the lining epithelium of the rete testes and within the stromal connective tissue of the rete.

Drugs may effect the testis by a variety of different mechanisms. These have been recently reviewed by Drife (1987). Endocrine control mechanisms can be affected centrally by psychotropic drugs or by negative feedback from circulating sex hormones. Androgen synthesis may be directly inhibited by drugs such as spironolactone or ketoconazole. Heavy metals, particularly cadmium, can damage the blood-testis barrier with subsequent adverse effects on spermatogenesis. Cytotoxic agents directly effect germ cells. Anti-androgens such as cyproterone influence sperm maturation through effects on Sertoli cells or the epididymus. Although some of these different mechanisms are associated with characteristic patterns of testicular pathology, this may not always be evident in routine toxicity studies in view of the limited end-response of the testes to insult. The initial primary damage to one cell population may be obscured by secondary damage to other cells in the testis. Very severe changes may also confound the elucidation of the primary lesion. Since spermatogenesis is an ongoing process, it may be difficult to determine the precise period at which disruption occurred, particularly in repeated-dose experiments.

In addition, adverse effects on fertility may be produced by drug-induced impairement of vas deferans contractility, modification of ejaculation, and decreased sperm motility (Drife, 1987).

Testicular weight

Weighing the testes is a useful adjunct to the macroscopic and microscopic observation, although it provides relatively little detailed information compared with that gained from histological examination of spermatogenesis following good fixation procedures. The size of the testis can also be a useful monitoring tool during the in-life phase of toxicity studies. Heywood and James (1978) showed that the measurement of the dog testis through the scrotal sac using calipers with calculation of cross sectional area using the formula p × length × width/4 was shown to correlate well with the rate of development of the testis in beagle dogs.

Testicular weight remains fairly constant in sexually mature laboratory animals and in human adults. Its weight is relatively unaffected compared with organs such as liver and kidney by underfeeding and low protein diets (Esachi et al., 1982; Pickering and Pickering, 1984). In sexually immature animals, testicular weight is more closely linked to body weight and care is needed in the interpretation of testicular weight group differences in toxicity studies employing younger animals during their growth phase.

This has been clearly demonstrated in a study by James and colleagues (1979) in which testicular size, semen analysis, and histological appearances of testicular biopsies were examined at successive monthly intervals in maturing beagle dogs. A linear correlation between testicular size and body weight was demonstrated in beagles up to about 30 weeks of age, an age at which sexual maturity was reached. Thereafter, testicular weight remained independent of body weight.

In rodents, testicular weight also varies with increasing age, although this depends on species, strain, dietary and housing conditions. In a detailed study of aging dd-mice, it was shown that testicular weight decreased with advancing age after about six months of age (Takano and Abe, 1987). In a study with CD-1 mice housed in different cage densities for 18 months, mice housed most in a cage showed slightly decreased mean body weights as well as lower testicular weights than miced housed singly (Chvédoff et al., 1980).

By contrast, male Fischer rats showed increasing testicular weights with advancing age, probably because of increased numbers of testicular tumours in this strain (Yu et al., 1985). Dietary restriction over the lifetime of rats, however, reduces testicular weight only minimally compared with organs such as the heart, kidney, and liver (Pickering and Pickering, 1984; Yu et al., 1985). Drug-induced effects on the seminiferous epithelium, or hormonal control mechanisms may also lead to reduced testicular weight, usually in association with histological evidence of cell loss (see below).

Inflammation (orchitis) and necrosis

Inflammation and necrosis are relatively uncommon findings in the testicular parenchyma. Adverse effects on the testis usually lead to atrophy of testicular tubules and interstitial fibrosis without inflammation. However, inflammation and necrosis can result from disruption of the blood supply damage to or the blood-testis barrier though which the normally sequestered spermatozoal antigens are exposed to immune attack. Thus, when an inflammatory process is found in the testis care should be exercised in the search for vascular pathology, especially the various forms of spontaneous arteritis found in the beagle dog and rodent (see Cardiovascular System, Chapter III). Cadmium represents the typical example of an agent which can acutely damage the vascular endothelium of the testis. This increases vascular permeability, decreases blood flow toproduce hamorrhagic necrosis and oedema in the testis of laboratory animals (Parizek, 1957; Gunn et al., 1963; Singal et al., 1985).

The classical example of experimental orchitis is provided by autoimmune orchitis in which testicular extracts and Freund's adjuvent are injected with laboratory animals, principally rats and guinea pigs (Tung, 1987). This inflammatory process is believed to be related to the fact that the later stages of germ cells do not develop until sexual maturity is reached and, therefore, their auto-antigens are absent during the development of the immune system. In the normal animal these antigens are tightly sequestered behind adluminal junctions of Sertoli cells in an environment almost completely devoid of lymphocytes. Injection of these antigens with Freund's adjuvent, therefore, can precipitate severe autoimmune damage.

Histologically, this condition is characterized in rats by a focal, frequently perivascular infiltration of the testicular parenchyma by polymorphonuclear and mononuclear inflammatory cells (Nykänen, 1980). Leydig cells show reactive changes and subsequently thickening of the peritubular basement membrane and increased deposition of interstitial collagen occurs. The inflammatory and repair process remains essentially peritubular but tubules are characterized by exfoliation and reduction in height of the germinal epithelium, Sertoli cells become vacuolated and develop numerous cytoplasmic dense bodies and lipid droplets. The epididymis is also frequently involved.

Electron microscopic study using the tracer, lanthanum, shows focal defects in the Sertoli-Sertoli cell junctions suggesting that disruption of the blood-testes barrier is important in the pathogenesis of this condition.

Autoimmune orchitis can also develop spontaneously in the beagle dog where it often occurs in association with autoimmune thyroiditis (Fritz et al., 1976). This form of orchitis is characterized by the presence of focal or diffuse lymphocytic infiltration principally in the interstitium but also involving seminiferous tubular epithelium and the epididymis. The lymphoid infiltrate sometimes contains germinal centres or is admixed with plasma cells, histiocytes and occasional multinucleated giant cells. Variable degrees of degeneration and atrophy of seminiferous tubules are described in association with the inflammatory change. The incidence of both orchitis and thyroiditis in the colony described by Fritz and colleagues (1976) increased with increasing degree of relatedness to certain sibling progenitors, suggesting a hereditary component in its aetiology.

604

Orchitis has been described in mice after neonatal thymectomy (Tung et al., 1987). This process is highly strain dependent and occurs following thymectomy three but not seven days after birth. It is characterized histologically by a focal inflammation with infiltration of lymphocytes and macrophages into seminiferous tubules. Although granular deposits of IgG and C3 are found in affected mice, the sequence of changes suggests that the process is primarily mediated by T-cells. Tung and colleagues (1987) suggested that the development of autoimmune orchitis in certain species and strains may be related to interactions between the hypothalamic-pituitary gonadal-axis and thymic function.

Autoimmune orchitis is also reported in contralateral testes of rats with one ischaemic testis (Harrison et al., 1981). Immunofluorescent studies using the serum of affected rats showed fluorescence of all spermatogenic cells but generally this was brighter in the more mature forms. Leydig cells also showed a reaction with serum. Again, this experiment suggested that spermato-genic damage resulted from an autoimmune response to normally sequestered antigens which were released by the ischaemic insult to the contralateral testis (Harrison et al., 1981).

The question of auto-antigen presentation has also been extensively studied following vasectomy both in man and experimental animals. After vasectomy spermatozoa may escape from the ductus deferens and excite a granulomatous reaction as well as a systemic immune response (Flickinger, 1985; McDonald and Scothorne, 1987; Herr et al., 1987). Histological study of the rat testis after vasectomy has shown depletion of germ cells in the tubules associated with an increase in lymphocytes, particularly in the epididymis (Miller and Killian, 1987). A form of autoimmune orchitis and epididymitis has also been reported in vasectomized rabbits, guinea pigs and non-human primates (Tung, 1987).

Testicular atrophy

Disease processes, age-related degenerative changes, disruption of hormonal control mechanisms, stress, and drug-induced damage to different components of the testis are usually expressed morphologically in a relatively limited way by varying degrees of focal or diffuse atrophy of the seminiferous epithelium. The wide variety of drugs which have the potential to adversely affect spermatogenesis and produce atrophy have been reviewed by Neumann (1984). Drugs may affect the testis directly because of their chemical reactivity or indirectly through an alteration in physiological control mechanisms which maintain reproductive homeostasis.

The least severe changes in the germinal epithelium are commonly described as *maturation arrest*. This is characterized histologically by partial or complete loss of mature spermatids from the adluminal compartment of the seminiferous tubules (Figs. 111 and 112). As the degree of atrophy increases, there is progressive loss of cells undergoing active spermatogenesis so that eventually hypoplasia of all maturing germ cells is apparent. Loss of germ cells can be accompanied by other cytological features such as vacuolation of the germ cell layer and the

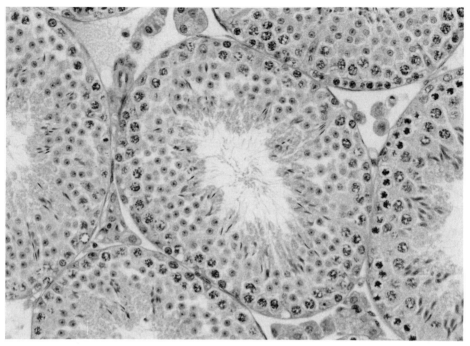

Fig. 111. Testis from a young, untreated CD-1 mouse showing abundant, maturing germ cells. (HE, ×550.)

presence of multinucleated giant cells. The final stages of atrophy are attained when there is total loss of all germ cells including spermatogonia, leaving only the more resistant Sertoli cells (*'Sertoli-only' picture*). Accompanying germ cell loss, the seminiferous tubules become progressively shrunken, develop thickened fibrous walls and eventually reach a totally sclerotic end-stage in which only residual interstitial cells remain.

In the histological assessment of testicular atrophy in routine toxicity studies, it is necessary to search for any additional morphological features which may provide clues to the pathogenesis of the atrophy. It is important to look for morphological alterations in Sertoli cells, blood vessels, Leydig cells, interstitial macrophages, lymphocytes, and connective tissue components. Furthermore, the presence of changes in the epididymus, prostate and other hormone-sensitive organs are also helpful in the overall assessment. It must of course not be forgotten that mature spermatozoa are found in the epididymis and should also be assessed in tissue sections.

Grading of atrophy provides an important component of the assessment and a number of different semi-quantitative scoring schemes have been employed. The distinction between focal and diffuse testicular atrophy is also a source of difficulty for this is often a matter of definition by individual pathologists. This

606

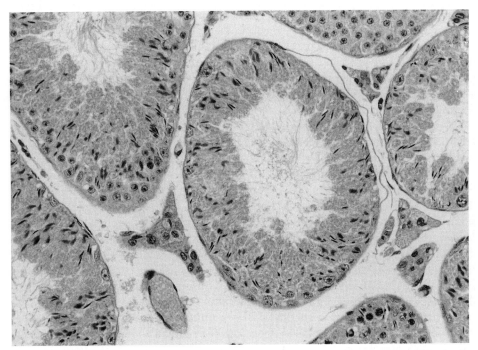

Fig. 112. Testis from a CD-1 mouse treated for two weeks with an antimitotic drug. There is clear loss of germ cells with retention of a few residual spermatids and preservation of Sertoli cells. (HE, ×550.)

is compounded in the problem of bias in sampling of focal atrophic lesions which frequently develop spontaneously in laboratory animals.

Whereas there are a number of different mechanisms for the development of testicular atrophy in toxicity studies, the end result is frequently indistinguishable in histological sections in longer-term studies. However, it is important to distinguish agents which produce their effects directly on germ cells to give rise to morphological abnormalities in spermatogonia, spermatids, or spermatozoa for such agents are frequently considered potential mutagens (Singh et al., 1987). To do this it may be necessary to conduct experiments which are specifically designed to assess the effect of treatment on different stages of the seminiferous epithelium.

This is well illustrated by studies which are designed to assess the effects of cancer chemotherapeutic drugs on the germinal epithelium. Single-dose experiments followed by histological evaluation at intervals which are appropriately timed to coincide with the kinetics of the germinal epithelium of the test species, allow analysis of the particular cell types affected by treatment. Using this approach, single-dose experiments in mice have been able to provide quantitative values and dose-response curves for the killing of specific spermatogenic cells and critically compare the effects of different types of anticancer drugs (Lu and Meistrich, 1979; Meistrich et al., 1982; Wahed et al., 1987).

Differentiated spermatogonia are the most sensitive cells to many anticancer drugs and this is probably related to their short mitotic cycle involving DNA synthesis and cell division. Sensitivity of cells at other stages of the cycle varies with class of anticancer drug, probably as a result of the changes in cell metabolism occurring with maturation (Lu and Meistrich, 1979). However, problems exist in the extrapolation of the results of animal studies performed with cytotoxic anticancer agents to man because of species-specific and age-related differences in the sensitivity of the testis to these agents.

The comparative study of several different anticancer agents by Meistrich and colleagues (1982) showed that the cytotoxic effects of single doses given to mice did not correlate well with their liability to produce prolonged azospermia in man. The reasons for this lack of correlation was unclear, although evaluation of human clinical data is usually complicated by the widespread use of combination chemotherapy (Meistrich et al., 1982).

It is useful to consider species differences in cycling time when comparing results of treatment with anticancer drugs in different species. Understanding of drug disposition is also important, especially the degree to which xenobiotics penetrate into the compartments of the seminiferous tubules. Cyclophosphamide, an alkylating antineoplastic drug, has been shown to impair spermatogenesis in both mice (Lu and Meistrich, 1979) and man (Fairly et al., 1979) but the Syrian hamster seems much more resistant to its testicular effects (Singh et al., 1987). This difference has been ascribed to the inability of this agent to penetrate into the seminiferous tubules in the hamster. The greater sensitivity of young rats to the testicular effects of N-methyltetrazolethiol cephalosporins has been attributed to the greater degree of penetration of these agents into the seminiferous tubules of younger rats compared with older animals (Comereski et al., 1987).

The site of biotransformation of direct acting compounds may also modulate the extent of testicular toxicity. Whereas highly reactive intermediates produced in the liver are unlikely to reach the germinal epithelium in sufficient quantities to produce cell damage, less reactive metabolites may reach the testis to be metabolised to toxic forms by the testis itself. The testis contains sufficient cytochrome P450, mixed function epoxide hydrases, aryl hydrocarbon hydrolases and transferases capable of producing toxic metabolites in close proximity to germ cells (Dixon and Lee, 1980).

Drugs of other therapeutic classes which act indirectly by altering physiological control mechanisms may produce their effects on germinal epithelium following longer periods of treatment. It may be helpful to examine the effects of these drugs in a sequential way in longer term, repeated-dose experiments. An example is the widely used antihypertensive drug methyldopa, which has been shown to produce testicular abnormalities in rats only after several weeks of administration (Dunnick et al., 1986, Chapin and Williams, 1989). Dose-related changes were characterized by decreased numbers of late stage spermatids and germ cells in the testes associated with decreased sperm counts, sperm motility and lower plasma testosterone levels. It was argued that lowered circulating testosterone levels and adverse effects of drug on body weight gain were responsible for the testicular changes (Dunnick et al., 1986). Other antihypertensive drugs, anxiolytics, antipsychotic agents and neuroleptics may also affect the testis in similar way by interference with gonadotrophin secretion (Neumann, 1984). Sex steroids, steroidal antiandrogens and LHRH analogues also produce testicular atrophy when administered for long periods.

Study of the rat testis following administration of clomiphene citrate, a steroidal antiantrogen, cyproterone acetate, oestradiol-17-β, medrogestone or medroxyprogesterone for seven or eight days showed these different agents produced similar morphological changes, notably an increase in degenerating pachytene spermatocytes and late spermatids (Stage VII). As these agents disrupt the hormonal pathways which stimulate the testis at different levels, it was suggested that this pattern of seminiferous cell change is a useful indicator of agents suspected of interfering with hormonal control mechanisms (Russell et al., 1981).

The non-steroidal antiandrogen, flutamide, has also been shown to influence spermatogenesis when administered to rats for long periods although older animals are more resistant to its effects (Viguier-Martinez et al., 1983a,b). This agent is believed to be devoid of progestational or oestrogenic activity but capable of inhibiting androgen activity at several different steps including uptake into tissues, binding to androgen receptors and translocation to the nucleus (Chapin and Williams, 1989). When flutamide was administered to rats seminiferous tubules contained reduced numbers of leptotene spermatocytes and round spermatatids (Viguier-Martinez et al., 1983a,b).

However, the usual histological changes in longer term treatment of rats with agents which disrupt hormonal status is more advanced testicular atrophy. Studies in which rats were treated with oral contraceptives, their oestrogenic or progestogenic components or the synthetic analogue of gonadotrophic releasing hormone (LHRH analogue), buserelin, for two years developed advanced testicular atrophy (Schardein et al., 1970; Schardein 1980a,b; Donaubauer et al., 1987). Treatment of adult male Sprague-Dawley rats with LHRH or potent LHRH analogues for four weeks or more led to total loss of germ cells and a 'Sertoli only' appearance which was associated with reduction in testicular LH and prolactin receptors and decreased plasma testosterone levels (Labrie et al., 1978).

Studies of the testes in man treated for long periods with oestrogens have also demonstrated advanced testicular atrophy or 'Sertoli only' appearances and thickening of the tubular basement membrane. However, light and electron microscopic study of testes showing advanced atrophy has suggested that certain characteristic features remain in Sertoli cells notably the presence of greater numbers of cytoplasmic osmiophilic lipid droplets compared with controls as well as cytoplasmic crystalloid structures and blebs on the nuclear membranes (Lu and Steinberger, 1978). It was suggested that these particular features were characteristic of the suppressed plasma and testicular testosterone levels, undetectable levels of gonadotrophins and elevated plasma and testicular levels of oestrogens which occur following exogenous oestrogen administration (see Fatty Change, below).

Whereas many of these agents which disrupt testosterone and gonadotrophin activity also produce testicular atrophy or reduction in sperm production and fertilizing ability in humans, there are reported species and strain differences in sensitivity to these effects of hormone administration. For instance, doses of 10 μg of oestrodiol benzoate per day inhibits spermatogenesis and produces Leydig cell atrophy in the rat testis but not B6C3F1 mice (Meistrich et al., 1977). Furthermore, the effect of oestrogens on the mouse testis also appears highly strain-dependent (Shimkin et al., 1962; Meistrich et al., 1977). It also should be remembered that agents which only indirectly affect testicular tissue may also require metabolic biotransformation prior to their action and this can also vary between species.

Some agents affect testicular function and produce testicular atrophy neither by interfering with hormonal control mechanisms nor causing primary germ cell damage. Single dose experiments with a novel antispermatogenic agent, AF 1312/TS, in rats showed that primary damage to Sertoli cells was able to produce focal tubular atrophy which involved cells at all stages of the cycle of the seminiferous epithelium (de Martino et al., 1975).

Testicular damage has also been associated with diverse cytoskeletal disrupting agents and it has been suggested that this may be the result of damage to the Sertoli cell cytoskeleton (Boekelheide et al., 1989).

Giant cells

Giant cells are observed in seminiferous tubules under a number of circumstances but as they are frequently associated with tubular atrophy they are usually considered to be an expression of germ cell degeneration. They are found in association with age-related focal testicular atrophy, following efferent duct ligation or as a result of administration of xenobiotics.

The mechanism for the formation of these multinucleated giant cells is unclear. It has been suggested that multinucleated giant cells which form following administration of anticancer drugs result from abnormal meiotic division of germ cells subsequent to mutational events such as induction of translocations and unscheduled DNA synthesis (Lu and Meistrich, 1979). Electron microscopic study of giant cell development in mice following efferent duct ligation has suggested that they result from fusion of germ cells as a result of damage to intercellular bridges (Singh and Abe, 1987). It appears that the membrane-bound dense material which is essential for normal maintenance of intercellular bridges is particularly sensitive to certain types of adverse effect (Torgersen et al., 1982; Singh and Abe, 1987).

Vacuolation, fatty change: Sertoli cells

Sertoli cells are resistant to the adverse effects of xenobiotics but under certain circumstances they become altered and this can be manifest by cytoplasmic

610

vacuolation. A number of antispermatogenic agents which produce testicular atrophy following repeated dose administration have been reported to induce Sertoli cell vacuolation immediately after the onset of treatment. It has been suggested that the subsequent germ cell degeneration occurring with these agents is a direct consequence of functional impairment of Sertoli cells.

An example of this phenomenon is provided by phthalate esters. These are widely distributed in the environment and produce testicular atrophy following repeated dosing of laboratory animals. Several hours after the administration of di-n-pentyl phthalate to young rats, Sertoli cells showed fine pale cytoplasmic vacuolation due to vacuolation of smooth endoplasmic reticulum and loss of mitochondrial succinate dehydrogenase activity associated with inward displacement of germinal cells (Creasy et al., 1983). As Sertoli cell changes preceded degeneration of germ cells, it was suggested that the Sertoli cell may represent the primary site of testicular toxicity of these agents. Similar early cytoplasmic vacuolation have been reported after administration of a number of other anti-spermatogenic agents (Flores and Fawcett, 1972; de Martino et al., 1975; Häusler and Hodel, 1979). These reports all support the concept that Sertoli-cell vacuolation commonly represents a non-specific response to injury (Creasy et al., 1983).

In man, prolonged treatment with oestrogens also produces a characteristic vacuolation of Sertoli cells as a result of accumulation of osmiophilic lipid-like bodies associated with advanced testicular atrophy (Lu and Steinberger, 1978).

Phospholipidosis: Sertoli cells

Lamellated or crystalloid lysosomal inclusions are liable to accumulate in the Sertoli cells of the testes in drug-induced forms of phospholipidosis where they show the typical structural and cytochemical features (see Respiratory System, Chapter V). This predilection is presumably because Sertoli cells are normally engaged in removal and digestion of cellular residues and biomembranes shed from maturing spermatids (Lüllmann-Rauch, 1979).

Atrophy: Leydig cells

As with other endocrine cells, reduced functional demand eventually lead to atrophy of the Leydig cell population of the testis. This has been well documented in both man and laboratory animals following chronic administration of oestrogens or other oestrogenic compounds which have a direct inhibitory effect on testosterone production or suppress gonadotrophin production (Meistrich et al., 1977; Russell et al., 1981; Cameron and Pugh, 1976; Venizelos and Paradinas, 1988; Schulze, 1988).

Leydig cell atrophy accompanying atrophy of the seminiferous tubules both in man and laboratory animals is a morphological feature which serves to distinguish oestrogen-induced testicular atrophy from most other causes, in which there is usually a real or apparent increase in the Leydig cell population.

611

Study of the human testis in patients with prostatic cancer or transexual males treated for long periods of time with oestrogens has demonstrated that there is almost complete loss of Leydig cells. The interstitium of affected testes has been shown to contain fibroblast-like cells with lobulated nuclei, well-developed smooth endoplasmic reticulum, lipid droplets and electron dense cytoplasmic inclusions and it has been suggested that these cells represent immature Leydig cells (Schulze, 1988). However considerable interspecies and strain differences in the sensitivity of the Leydig cell to oestrogens is reported. Oestradiol benzoate in doses of 100 μg per day produces Leydig cell atrophy in rats but not B6C3F1 mice (Meistrich et al., 1977).

Chronic treatment with high doses of testosterone (rather than replacement of subnormal secretion) also produces suppression of Leydig cell function. When plasma testosterone levels rise above the normal range both basal levels of LH and FSH and peak responses following LHRH are diminished (Griffin and Wilson, 1985). This inhibition of the hypothalamic-hypophyseal axis eventually leads to Leydig cell atrophy. Ultrastructural morphometric study of the testis in rats treated with testosterone for periods of up to 12 days has shown that Leydig cells have reduced cytoplasmic smooth endoplasmic reticulum, atrophied Golgi apparatus and to a lesser extent a reduction in mitochondrial volume and surface area of cristae (Mazzochi et al., 1982). These morphological changes are compatable with the concept that the smooth endoplasmic reticulum is the subcellular organelle which is most responsive to changes in functional activity of rat Leydig cells.

Leydig cell hyperplasia, interstitial cell hyperplasia

Leydig cell hyperplasia is a sporadic finding in the testes of aging dogs and rodents and has been reported in the testes of aging men. In some strains of rat, notably the Fischer 344, Leydig cell hyperplasia occurs in quite young animals where it appears to represent a stage in the progression toward Leydig cell neoplasms (Goodman et al., 1979). In man, the development of Leydig cell hyperplasia has been associated with a variety of endocrine disorders which increase pituitary activity. A form of Leydig cell hyperplasia occurs in new born infants as a result of the increased levels of chorionic gonadotrophins and oestrogens in maternal and foetal blood (Mostofi and Price, 1973b).

Histologically, Leydig hyperplasia may be diffuse, focal or multifocal in distribution. Although it can be associated with entirely normal seminiferous tubules, it is more commonly associated with atrophic tubules both in rodents and in man (Honore, 1978; Goodman et al., 1979; Takano and Abe, 1987). Generally, the affected Leydig cells are histologically unremarkable, showing no marked changes in size, no undue pleomorphism or mitotic activity.

In the rat, focal hyperplasia may be nodular in nature, sometimes displacing or effacing adjacent seminiferous tubules. These rounded or nodular foci are composed of Leydig cells which are frequently basophilic in staining characteris-

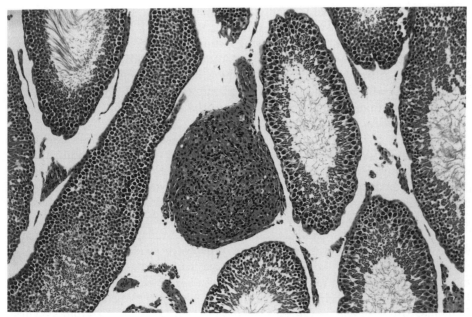

Fig. 113. Testis from an one-year-old Wistar rat showing Leydig cell hyperplasia. This focus, about the size of a seminiferous tubule, was part of a generalised, bilateral process which resulted from prolonged administration of an agent with antiandrogenic properties. (HE, ×300.)

tics and it has been suggested that they represent the earliest stages of the interstitial or Leydig cell tumour in the rat (Ward et al., 1983).

Differentiation of focal hyperplasia from Leydig cell tumour remains therefore somewhat arbitary. Individual foci of hyperplasia are usually considered to be no larger than the diameter of seminiferous tubule and devoid of evidence of compression of adjacent structures (Fig. 113).

In a study of age-related testicular changes in mice, it was demonstrated that the number of Leydig cells increased with advancing age in parallel with the degree and prevalence of seminiferous tubular atrophy (Takano and Abe, 1987). Furthermore, it was shown that at about one year of age Leydig cell accumulation was most marked around foci of atrophied tubules with thickened basement membranes.

Similar spatial associations between atrophied seminiferous tubules and Leydig cell hyperplasia have also been reported in aged rats (Burek, 1978), in old men (Honore, 1978) and in animal testes which have been focally damaged by experimental means (Sato et al., 1981).

The cause of Leydig cell hyperplasia in rodents in advancing age is uncertain, but it appears likely that it results mainly from age-related changes in the hypothalamic-pituitary axis and local control mechanisms. In the rat, it has been shown that aging is accompanied by a reduction in the hypothalamic content of gonadotrophin releasing hormone, a decrease in the capacity of the pituitary to synthesize or release follicle stimulating hormone and luteinizing hormone following injection of gonadotrophin releasing hormone, a lower capacity of the testis to produce testosterone following stimulation with gonadotrophin and a decrease in the number of Leydig cell receptors for luteinizing hormone (Bedrak et al., 1983). Although there may be some inherent decline in steroidogenic capacity of Leydig cells with age, this appears to be relatively small compared with the alterations in function of the hypothalamus and pituitary in the rat (Kaler and Neaves, 1981; Bedrak et al., 1983).

Although it is likely that the age-related increase in Leydig cell population with age is partly a response to declining function of the hypothalamic-pituitary axis, local control mechanisms are important. It has been suggested that the Sertoli cells in atrophied seminiferous tubules elaborate increased amounts of trophic substances which can produce proliferation of Leydig cells around atrophic tubules (Aoki and Fawcett, 1978; Takano and Abe, 1987).

These considerations are important in the assessment of therapeutic agents which give rise to an increase in the prevalence or degree of Leydig cell hyperplasia as well as Leydig cell neoplasia when they are administered to rodents for long periods in chronic toxicity studies or carcinogenicity bioassays. It is not perhaps surprising that drugs which modulate these age-related hypothalamic/pituitary changes or possess an effect on Leydig-cell steroid synthesis can potentiate the development of Leydig cell hyperplasia.

A recent example of this phenomenon occurred in the rat carcinogenicity bioassay performed with the histamine H_2 blocker, cimetidine. Administration of cimetidine for two years produced a mild increase in Leydig cell hyperplasia and greater prevalence of Leydig cell neoplasms in all treated groups compared with controls, associated with reduction in weights of prostate glands and seminal vesicles (Brimblecombe and Leslie, 1984). Cimetidine possesses weak anti-androgenic activity which is not related to its histamine H_2-blocking activity. It has been shown to inhibit the action of testosterone on seminal vesicles and inhibit the binding of tritiated 5α-dihydrotestosterone, an active metabolite of testosterone, to the androgen receptor (Sivelle et al., 1982). It appears probable that this inhibition potentiated the development of an adaptive hyperplasia of Leydig cells. This particlar finding was postulated to have no direct implication for human patients (Brimblecombe et al., 1985) although cimetidine does show a mild antiandrogen effect in less than 1% of patients (Penston and Wormsley, 1986).

A similar increase in prevalence of Leydig cell hyperplasia was also reported in Wistar rats treated daily with high doses of buserelin (HDE 766), a synthetic peptide analogue of gonadotrophin releasing hormone (LHRH), by the subcutaneous route for two years (Donaubauer et al., 1987). Although focal hyperplasia of Leydig cells was noted among control rats in this study, treated animals developed an increase in the prevalence of diffuse Leydig cell hyperplasia. Diffuse hyperplasia was characterized histologically by rows of Leydig cells of variable thickness with increased cytoplasmic lipid between atrophic seminiferous tubules. Increased numbers of Leydig cell neoplasms were also observed in rats treated with buserelin compared with controls, although the distribution among treated groups was not dose-dependent. It was suggested that these findings represented a pharmacodynamic response to buserelin treatment as this drug has been shown to deplete pituitary gonadotrophin and cause loss of gonadal LH and prolactin receptors after long-term administration to rats. It was also argued that these findings had little relevance for the clinical use of buserelin in man as the rat hypothalamic-pituitary Leydig cell axis was unduly sensitive to the effects of this agent.

Flutamide, a non-steroidal antiandrogen indicated for the treatment of prostatic cancer, produced atrophy of the prostate, seminal vesicles and testes after chronic admnistration to rats, associated with Leydig cell hyperplasia and ultimately Leydig cell tumours (Food and Drug Administration, 1980). Mild interstitial cell hyperplasia was also reported in beagle dogs treated for periods of six or twelve months with this agent.

Typically, Leydig cell hyperplasia develops quite slowly during the administration of such agents. Studies in which rats were treated for several weeks with LHRH and synthetic analogues showed that morphological changes in Leydig cells developed only after periods of four weeks (Labrie et al., 1978).

Oestrogen treatment is reported to produce hyperplasia of interstitial cells in some but not all strains of mice. Following long term oestrogen administration, BALB/c mice, slowly developed an increase in Leydig cell number without testicular atrophy whereas C3H mice showed marked loss of testicular weight, tubular atrophy but no increase in the interstitial cells (Shimkin et al., 1962). These observations are of particular interest as the BALB/c strain employed was susceptible to the induction of Leydig cell tumours by oestrogen whereas the C3H strain was resistant to these effects (see below). Shimkin and colleagues (1962) argued that the sequence of changes in BALB/c mice during long-term oestrogen administration were a manifestation of a physiological response which protected spermatogenesis from the adverse effects of oestrogen.

Neoplasia

The classification of testicular neoplasms in laboratory animals is based on that in use in the diagnosis of human testicular tumours. Tumours are grouped into those of *germ cell origin* (seminoma, teratoma), those of *specialized gonadal stroma* (Leydig cell and Sertoli cell tumours, granulosa-theca cell neoplasms) and those arising from *adnexae* and covering membranes and tissues. The testis is also the site of metastatic spread of neoplasms arising in other sites notably lymphomas, leukaemias, and histocytic neoplasms.

As in man, the most important testicular neoplasms which arise spontaneously in animals are seminomas, teratomas, Sertoli cell and Leydig cell tumours. The prevalence of each type varies with species and strain of animal. The interstitial or Leydig cell tumour is undoubtably the testicular tumour type which most commonly occurs in rodent carcinogenicity bioassays and the development of which together with Leydig cell hyperplasia can be influenced by

615

treatment with xenobiotics. Other tumour types are usually only sporadically observed in aged rodents.

The incidence of testicular tumours is higher in the dog then in many other species. They are mostly Sertoli cell tumours or seminomas with a lesser number of Leydig cell tumours being described in most series (Cotchin, 1960; Dow, 1962). However, these neoplasms are uncommonly found among beagles of ages employed in the routine safety studies. Nevertheless, they may be sporadically observed in longer toxicity, particularly, the Sertoli cell tumour which occurs in younger dogs than other tumour types, even in dogs as young as four years of age (Post and Kilborn, 1987).

Testicular neoplasms are very uncommon in non-human primates, although seminomas, Sertoli cell and interstitial cell tumours are occasionally described (Brack, 1988).

Leydig cell tumours: rats

Rats are particularly liable to develop Leydig cell tumours spontaneously with advancing age. They are characteristic of the Fischer 344 strain where they occur in a high proportion of aging males. Although the cause for this high prevalence is not certain, it is probably related to changes in endocrine balance. In the Fischer 344 rat, the development of Leydig cell tumours is associated with age-related decline in plasma testosterone, increases in gonadotrophin levels and decreases in sperm production. Whether these changes are causally related is not entirely clear for the tumours themselves can produce steroid hormones, notably progesterone and these may in turn influence gonadotrophin levels. However, a causal relationship between the development of neoplasia and gonadotrophin levels is suggested by the study of Brown and colleagues (1979) in parabiosed rats. Parabiosis of intact male rats to castrated males or oophorectomized females for about 20 months caused elevated gonadotrophins in the castrate to stimulate the testes in the partner resulting in the development of interstitial tumours.

It has also been shown that the development of Leydig cell tumours in male Fischer rats can be prevented or be delayed beyond a two year observation period by rendering them chronically hyperprolactinaemic either with pituitary implants or treatment with diethylstilboestrol, both of which reduce gonadotrophin levels (Bartke et al., 1985).

Xenobiotics administered to sensitive rats for long periods of time which influence these age-related changes in hormone production have potential to affect the numbers of Leydig cell tumours found at the end of a carcinogenicity bioassay. An example of this phenomenon has been reported in rats following chronic treatment with a novel dihydropyridine calcium channel blocker. The increased prevalence of Leydig cell tumors in treated groups was associated with reduced prolactin levels, decreased testosterone production and an increase in gonadotrophins (Roberts, 1987).

Leydig cell hyperplasia and Leydig cell tumours were also reported in rats following long-term administration of LHRH analogues, buserelin (Donaubauer et al., 1987) and flutamide (Food and Drug Administration, 1988) as well as the histamine H_2 antagonist cimetidine, which at high doses showed an antiandrogenic effect (Brimblecombe and Leslie, 1984).

Microscopically, Leydig cell tumours consist of fairly uniform regular cells with rounded hyperchromatic nuclei and eosinophilic cytoplasm generally similar to normal Leydig cells. The cell cytoplasm may contain vacuoles and spindle cells are sometimes seen. As other neoplasms of the endocrine system, it is frequently difficult to make a clear distinction between benign and malignant neoplasms based solely on cytological criteria. Conventionally, diagnosis of malignancy is based on the degree of anaplasia and mitotic activity and evidence of spread into blood vessels or through the testicular capsule (Mostofi and Bresler, 1976).

Leydig cell tumours: mouse

Both benign and malignant Leydig cell neoplasms develop occasionally in aged mice; Their prevalence can also be increased by administration of agents which alter hormone levels in this species. This is to some extent strain-dependent. BALB/c and A strains appear fairly sensitive to the induction of Leydig cells by oestrogen whereas C3H mice are quite resistant (Shimkin et al., 1962).

In a bioassay performed with tamoxifen in the Alderley Park strain of mice, a high prevalence of Leydig cell tumours were observed in the high dose group and none in the concurrent controls (Tucker et al., 1984). Although the precise mechanism for the tumour development was uncertain, it was subsequently shown that the changes in treated mice were quite similar to those in mice of the same strain treated with oestrogens. It was argued that tamoxifen acted as an oestrogen in mice at the doses utilized in the bioassay and the increase in interstitial tumours was related to this hormonal activity. No testicular tumours were reported in rats treated with tamoxifen, although it should be noted the drug appeared to act as an anti-oestrogen in this species. On this basis the findings in mice were postulated to be of little direct relevance for safety in man where tamoxifen acts primarily as an anti-oestrogen (Tucker et al., 1984).

REFERENCES

AOKI, A. and FAWCETT, D.W. (1978): Is there a local feedback from the seminiferous tubules affecting activity of the Leydig cells? *Biol.Reprod.*, 19, 144–158.

ARYA, M. and VANHA-PERTTULA T. (1984): Distribution of lectin binding in rat testis and epididymis. *Andrologia*, 16, 495–508.

ARYA, M. and VANHA-PERTTULA T. (1985): Lectin staining of rat testis and epididymis: Effect of cytoproterone acetate and testosterone. *Andrologia*, 17, 301–310.

AUMÜLLER, G., SEITZ, J. and BISCHOF, W. (1983): Immunohistochemical study on the initiation of acid phosphatase secretion in the prostate gland. *J.Androl*, 4, 183–191.

AUMÜLLER, G., VEDDER, H., ENDERLE-SCHMITT, U., and SEITZ, J. (1987): Cytochemistry and biochemistry of acid phosphatase. VII: Immunohistochemistry of canine prostatic acid phosphatase. *Prostate*, 11, 1–15.

BARTKE, A., SWEENEY, C.A., JOHNSON, L., CASTRACANE, V.D. and DOHERTY, P.C. (1985): Hyperprolactinemia inhibits development of Leydig cell tumors in aging Fischer rats. *Exp.Aging Res.*, 11, 123–128.

BEDRAK, E., CHAP, Z. and BROWN, R. (1983): Age-related changes in the hypothalamic-pituitary-testicular function of the rat. *Exp.Gerontol.*, 18, 95–104.

BERRY, S.J., STRANDBERG, J.D., SAUNDERS, W.J. and COFFEY, D.S. (1986): Development of canine benign prostatic hyperplasia with age. *Prostate*, 9, 363–373.

BHATHAL, P.S., GERKENS, J.K. and MASHFORD, M.L. (1974): Spermatic granuloma of the epididymis in rats treated with guanethidine. *J.Pathol.*, 112, 19–26.

BLACK, H.E., SZOT, R.J., ARTHAUD, L.E., MASSA, T., MYLECRAINE, L., KLEIN, M., LAKE, R., FABRY, A., KAMINSKA, G.Z., SINHA, D.P. and SCHWARTZ, E. (1987): Preclinical safety evaluation of the benzodiazepine quazepam. *Arzneimittelforschung*, 37, 906–913.

BLASK, D.E. and LEADEM, C.A. (1987): Neuroendocrine aspects of neoplastic growth: A review. *Neuroendocrinol.Lett.*, 9, 63–73.

BOEKELHEIDE, K., NEELY, M.D. and SIOUSSAT, T.M. (1989): The Sertoli cell cytoskeleton: A target for toxicant-induced germ cell lost. *Toxicol.Appl.Pharmacol.*, 101, 373–389.

BRACK, M. (1988): Malignant Leydig cell tumor in a Tupaia belangeri: case report and literature review of male genital tumors in non-human primates. *Lab.Anim.*, 22, 131–134.

BRANDES, D. (1974): Fine structure and cytochemistry of male sex accessory organs. In: D. Brandes (Ed), *Male Accessory Sex Organs*, Chap. 2, pp. 17–113. Academic Press, New York.

BRIMBLECOMBE, R.W. and LESLIE, G.B. (1984): Cimetidine. In: D.R. Laurence, A.E.M. McLean, and M. Weatherall (Eds), *Safety Testing of New Drugs. Laboratory Predictions and Clinical Performances*, Chap. 4, pp. 65–91. Academic Press, London.

BRIMBLECOMBE, R.W., LESLIE, G.B. and WALKER, T.F. (1985): Toxicology of cimetidine. *Hum.Toxicol.*, 4, 13–25.

BROWN, C.E., WARREN, S., CHUTE, R.N., RYAN, K.J. and TODD, R.B. (1979): Hormonally induced tumors of the reproductive system of parabiosed male rats. *Cancer Res.*, 39, 3971–3975.

BUREK, J.D. (1978): Age-associated pathology. In: *Pathology of Aging Rats*, Chap. 4, pp. 29–187. CRC Press, West Palm Beach, Florida.

CAMERON, K.M. and PUGH, R.C.B. (1976): Miscellaneous Lesions. In: R.C.B. Pugh (Ed), *Pathology of the Testis*, Chap. 16, pp. 448–468. Blackwell Scientific, Oxford.

CARDY, R.H. (1987): Segmental degeneration of the epididymis in aged F344 rats. *Vet.Pathol.*, 24, 361–363.

CHAPDELAINE, F., DUBE, J.Y., FRENETTE, G. and TREMBLAY, R.R. (1984): Identification of arginine esterase as the major androgen-dependent protein secreted by dog prostate and preliminary molecular characterization in seminal plasma. *J.Androl.*, 5, 206–210.

CHAPIN, R.E., ROSS, M.D. and LAMB, J.C. (1984): Immersion fixation methods for glycol methacrylate-embedded testes. *Toxicol.Pathol.*, 12, 221–227.

CHAPIN, R.E., and WILLIAMS, J. (1989): Mechanistic approaches in the study oftesticular toxicity: Toxicants that affect the endocrine regulation ofthe testis. *Toxicol.Pathol.*, 17, 446–451.

CHVEDOFF, M., CLARKE, M.R., IRISARRI, E., FACCINI, J.M. and MONRO, A.M. (1980): Effects of housing conditions on food intakes, body weight and spontaneous lesions in mice. A review of the literature and results of an 18-month study. *Food.Cosmet.Toxicol.*, 18, 517–522.

CLERMONT, Y. (1963): The cycle of the seminiferous epithelium in man. *Am.J.Anat.*, 112, 35–45.

CLERMONT, Y. (1972): Kinetics of spermatogenesis in mammals: seminiferous epithelium cycle and spermatogonial renewal. *Physiol.Rev.*, 52, 198–236.

COMERESKI, C.R., BREGMAN, C.L. and BUROKER, R.A. (1987): Testicular toxicity of N-methyltetrazolethiol cephalosporin analogs in the juvenile rat. *Fundam.Appl.Toxicol.*, 8, 280–289.

COTCHIN, E. (1980): Testicular neoplasms in dogs. *J.Comp.Pathol.*, 70, 232–233.

CREASY, D.M., FOSTER, J.R. and FOSTER, P.M.D. (1983): The morphological development of di-n-pentyl phthalate induced testicular atrophy in the rat. *J.Pathol.*, 139, 309–321.

CUNHA, G.R., CHUNG, L.W.K., SHANNON, J.M., TAGUCHI, O. and FUJII, H. (1983): Hormone-induced morphogenesis and growth: Role of mesenchymal-epithelial interactions. *Recent.Prog.Horm.Res.*, 39, 559–598.

DE MARTINO, C., STEFANINI, M., AGRESTINI, A., COCCHIA, D., MORRELLI,M. and SCORZA-BARCELLONA, P. (1975): Antispermatogenic activity of I-p.chlorobenzyl-IH indazol-3-carboxylic acid (AF1312/TS) in rats. III. A light and electron microscopic study after single oral doses. *Exp.Mol.Pathol.*, 23, 321–356.

DIXON, R.L., and LEE, I.P., (1980): Pharmacokinetic and adaption factors involved in testicular toxicity *Fed.Proc.*, 39, 66–72.

DONAUBAUER, H.H., KRAMER, M., KRIEG, K., MEYER, D., VON RECHENBERG, W., SANDOW, J. and SCHÜTZ, E. (1987): Investigations of the carcinogenicity of the LH-RH analogue buserelin (HOE 766) in rats using the subcutaneous route of administration. *Fundam.Appl.Toxicol.*, 9, 738–752.

DOW, C. (1962): Testicular tumors in the dog. *J.Comp.Pathol.*, 72, 247–265.

DRIFE, J.O. (1987): The effects of drugs on sperm. *Drugs*, 33, 610–622.

DUNNICK, J.K., HARRIS, M.W., CHAPIN, R.E., HALL, L.B. and LAMB, I.V.J.C. (1986): Reproductive toxicology of methyldopa in male F344/N rats. *Toxicology*, 41, 305–318.

DUVALL, E., WYLLIE, A.H. and MORRIS, R.G. (1985): Macrophages recognition of cells undergoing programmed cell death (apoptosis). *Immunology*, 56, 351–358.

DYM, M. and FAWCETT, D.W. (1970): The blood-testis barrier in the rat and the physiological compartmentation of the seminiferous epithelium. *Biol.Reprod.*, 3, 308–326.

ECKSTEIN, P. and ZUCKERMAN, S. (1960): Morphology of the reproductive tract. In: A.S. Parkes (Ed), *Marshall's Physiology of Reproduction, Vol. 1*, Part 1, Chap. 2, pp. 43–155. Longmans, London.

EL-DEMIRY, M.I., ELTON, R., HARGREAVE, T.B., JAMES, K., BUSUTTIL, A. and CHISHOLM, G.D. (1987): Immunocompetent cells in human testis in health and disease. *Fert.Steril.*, 48, 470–479.

ENGLISH, H.F., DRAGO, J.R. and SANTEN, R.J. (1985): Cellular response to androgen depletion and repletion in the rat ventral prostate: Auto-radiography and morphometric analysis. *Prostate*, 7, 41–51.

ESASHI, T., SUZUE, R. and LEATHEM, J.H. (1982): Influence of dietary protein depletion and repletion on sex organ weight of male rats in relation to age. *J.Nutr.Sci.Vitaminol.*, 28, 163–172.

EVANS, G.S. and CHANDLER, J.A. (1987): Cell proliferation studies in the rat prostate. II. The effects of castration and androgen-induced regeneration upon basal and secretory cell proliferation. *Prostate*, 11, 339–351.

FAIRLY, K.F., BARRIE, J.U. and JOHNSON, W. (1972): Sterility and testicular atrophy related to cyclophosphamide therapy. *Lancet*, 1, 568–574.

FAWCETT, D.W., NEAVES, W.B. and FLORES, M.N. (1973): Comparative observations on intertubular lymphatics and the organization of the interstitial tissue of the mammalian testis. *Biol.Reprod.*, 9, 500–532.

FETISSOF, F., DUBOIS, M.P., ARBEILLE-BRASSART, B., LANSON, Y., BOIVIN, F. and JOBARD, P. (1983): Endocrine cells in the prostate gland, urothelium and Brenner tumors. *Vichows Arch.[B]*, 42, 53–64.

FLICKINGER, C.J. (1985): The effects of vasectomy on the testis. *N. Engl.J.Med.*, 313, 1283–1285.

FLORES, M. and FAWCETT, D.W. (1972): Ultrastructural effects of the anti-spermatogenic compound WIN-18446 (bis dichloroacetyl diamine). *Anat.Rec.*, 172, 310.

FOOD AND DRUG ADMINISTRATION (1980): Pharmacology and toxicology review of NDA 18-554. (Flutamide) Original summary. December 31, 1980.

FRITZ, T.E., LOMBARD, L.S., TYLER, S.A. and NORRIS, W.P. (1976): Pathology and familial incidence of orchitis and its relationship to thyroiditis in a closed beagle colony. *Exp.Mol.Pathol.*, 24, 142–158.

GATENBECK, L. (1986): Stress stimuli and the prostate gland: an experimental study in the rat. *Scand.J.Urol.Nephrol.*, Suppl 99, 1–39.

GERHARDT, P.G., MEVÅG, B., TVETER, K.J. and PURVIS, K. (1983): A systematic study of biochemical differences between the lobes of the rat prostate. *Int.J.Androl.*, 6, 553–562.

GOODMAN, D.G., WARD, J.M., SQUIRE, R.A., CHU, K.C. and LINHART, M.S. (1979): Neoplastic and non-neoplastic lesions in aging F344 rats. *Toxicol.Appl.Pharmacol.*, 48, 237–248.

GRAYHACK, J.T. (1963): Pituitary factors influencing growth of the prostate. *N.C.I.*, Monogr. 12, 189–199.

GRIFFIN, J.E. and WILSON, J.P. (1985): In: J.D. Wilson and D.W. Foster (Eds), *William's Textbook of Endocrinology*, 7th Edition, Chap. 10, pp. 259–311. Saunders, Philadelphia.

GUNN, S.A., GOULD, T.C. and ANDERSON, W.A.D. (1963): The selective injurious response of testicular and epididymal blood vessels to cadmium and its prevention by zinc. *Am.J.Pathol.*, 42, 685–702.

HABENICHT, U-F., and EL ETREBY, M.F., (1988): The periurethral zone of the prostate of the cynomolgus monkey is the most sensitive prostate part for an estrogenic stimulus. *Prostate*, 13, 305–316.

HABENICHT, U-F., SCHWARZ, K., NEUMANN, F. and EL ETREBY, M.F. (1987): Induction of estrogen-related hyperplastic changes in the prostate of the cynomolgus monkey (Macaca fascicularis) by androstenedione and its antagonization by the aromatase inhibitor 1-methyl-androsta-1,4-diene-3,17dione. *Prostate*, 11, 313–326.

HARRISON, R.G., LEWIS-JONES, D.I., MORENO DE MARVAL, M.J. and CONNOLLY, R.C. (1981): Mechanism of damage to the contralateral testes in rats with an ischaemic testis. *Lancet*, 2, 723–725.

HÄUSLER, A. and HODEL, C. (1979): Ultrastructural alterations induced by two different antispermatogenic agents in seminiferous epithelium of rat testes. *Arch.Toxicol.*, Suppl. 2, 387–392.

HERR, J.C., FLICKINGER, C.J., HOWARDS, S.S., YARBRO, S., SPELL, D.R., CALORAS, D. and GALLIEN, T.N. (1987): The relation between antisperm antibodies and testicular alterations after vasectomy and vasovasotomy in Lewis rats. *Biol.Reprod.*, 37, 1297–1305.

HEYWOOD, R. and JAMES, R.W. (1978): Assessment of testicular toxicity in laboratory animals. *Environ.Health Perspect.*, 24, 73–80.

HINRICHSEN, M.J. and BLAQUIER, J.A. (1980): Evidence supporting the existence of sperm maturation in the human epididymus. *J.Reprod. Fertil.*, 60, 291–294.

HONORE, L.H. (1978): Aging changes in the human testis: A light microscopic study. *Gerontology*, 24, 58–65.

HOWLAND, B., (1975): The influence of feed restriction and subsequent re-feeding on gonadotrophin secretion and serum testosterone levels in male rats. *J.Repro.Fertil.*, 44, 429–436.

IJIRI, K. and POTTEN, C.S. (1983): Response of intestinal cells of differing topographical and hierarchical status to ten cytotoxic drugs and five sources of radiation. *Br.J.Cancer*, 47, 175–185.

JAMES, R.W., CROOK, D. and HEYWOOD, R. (1979): Canine pituitary-testicular function in relation to toxicity testing. *Toxicology*, 13, 237–247.

JESIK, C.J., HOLLAND, J.M. and LEO, C. (1982): An anatomic and histologic study of the rat prostate. *Prostate*, 3, 81–97.

JOHNSEN, S.G. (1970): Testicular biopsy score count: a method for registration of spermatogenesis in human testes: Normal values and results in 335 hypogonadal males. *Hormones*, 1, 2–25.

JUTTE, N.H.P.M., GROOTEGOED, J.A., ROMMERTS, F.F.G., and VAN DER MOLEN, H.J. (1981): Exogenous lactate is essential for metabolic activities in isolated rat spermatocytes and spermatids. *J.Reprod.Fertil.*, 62, 399–405.

KALER, L.W. and NEAVES, W.B. (1981): The steroidogenic capacity of the aging rat testis. *J.Gerontol.*, 36, 398–404.

KERR, J.F.R. and SEARLE, J. (1973): Deletion of cells by apoptosis during castration-induced involution of the rat prostate. *Virchows Arch.*[B]., 13, 87–102.

KIPESUND K.M., HALGUNSET, J., FJÖSNE, H.E., and SUNDE, A., (1988): Light microscopic morphometric analysis of castration effects in the different lobes of the rat prostate. *Prostate*, 13, 221–232.

LABRIE, F., AUCLAIR, C., CUSAN, L., KELLY, P.A., PELLETIER, G. and FERLAND, L. (1978):

Inhibitory effect of LHRH and its agonists on testicular gonadotrophin receptors and spermatogenesis in the rat. *Int.J.Androl.*, Suppl. 2, 303–318.

LAMB, J.C. and CHAPIN, R.E. (1985): Experimental models of male reproductive toxicology. In: J.A. Thomas, K.S. Korach and J.A. McLachlan (Eds) *Endocrine Toxicology*, pp. 85–115. Raven Press, New York.

LASNITZKI, I. (1976): Reversal of methylcholanthrene-induced changes in mouse prostatitis in vitro by retinoic acid and its analogues. *Br.J.Cancer*, 34, 239–248.

LEBLOND, C.P. and CLERMONT, C.P. (1952): Definition of the stages of the cycle of the seminiferous epithelium in the rat. *Ann.NY.Acad.Sci.*, 55, 548–572.

LU, C.C. and MEISTRICH, M.L. (1979): Cytotoxic effects of chemotherapeutic drugs on mouse testis cells. *Cancer Res.*, 39, 3575–3582.

LU, C.C. and STEINBERGER, A. (1978): Effects of estrogen on human seminiferous tubules: Light and electron microscopic study. *Am.J.Anat.*, 153, 11–14.

LÜLLMANN-RAUCH, R. (1979): Drug-induced lysosomal storage disorders. In: J.T. Dingle, P.J. Jacques and I.H. Shaw (Eds), *Lysosomes in Applied Biology and Therapeutics, Vol. 6*, Chap. 3, pp. 49–130. North Holland, Amsterdam.

MARTAN, J. (1969): Epididymal histochemistry and physiology. *Biol.Reprod.*, Suppl. 1, 134–154.

MAZZOCCHI, G., ROBBA, C., REBUFFAT, P., GOTTARDO, G. and NUSSDORFER, G.G. (1982): Effects of a chronic treatment with testosterone on the morphology of the interstitial cells of the rat testis: an ultrastructural stereologic study. *Int.J.Androl.*, 5, 130–136.

MCDONALD, S.W. and SCOTHORNE, R.J. (1987): On the mode of sperm autoantigen presentation to the regional lymph node of the testis after vasectomy in rats. J.Anat., 153, 217–221.

MCNEAL, J.E. (1980): Anatomy of the prostate. *Prostate*, 1, 3–13.

MEISTRICH, M.L., HUGHES, T.J., AMBUS, T. and BRUCE, W.R. (1977): Spermatogenesis in hybrid mice treated with oestrogen and testosterone. *J.Reprod.Fertil.*, 50, 75–81.

MEISTRICH, M.L., FINCH, M., DACUNHA, M.F., HACKER, U. and AU, W.W. (1982): Damaging effects of 14 chemotherapeutic drugs on mouse testis cells. *Cancer Res.*, 42, 122–131.

MERK, F.B., WARHOL, M.J., KWAN, P.W-L., LEAV, I., ALROY, J., OFNER, P. and PINKUS, G.S. (1986): Multiple phenotypes of prostatic glandular cells in castrated dogs after individual or combined treatment with androgen and oestrogen. Morphometric, ultrastructural, and cytochemical distinctions. *Lab.Invest.*, 54, 442–456.

MILLER, S.C. (1982): Localization of plutonium-241 in the testis. An inter-species comparison using light and electron microscopic autoradiography. *Int.J.Radiat.Biol.*, 41, 633–643.

MILLER, S.C., BOWMAN, B.M. and ROWLAND, H.G. (1983): Structure, cyto-chemistry, endocytic activity, and immunoglobulin (Fc) receptors of rat testicular interstitial tissue macrophages. *Am.J.Anat.*, 168, 1–13.

MILLER, R.J. and KILLIAN, G.J. (1987): Morphometric analyses of the epididymis from normal and vasectomized rats. *J.Androl.*, 8, 279–291.

MITA, M. and HALL, P.F. (1982): Metabolism of round spermatids from rats: Lactate as the preferred substrate. *Biol.Reprod.*, 26, 445–455.

MORTIMER, D., CURTIS, E.F. and MILLER, R.G. (1987): Specific labelling by peanut agglutinin of the outer acrosome membrane of the human spermatozoon. *J.Reprod.Fertil.*, 81, 127–135.

MOSTOFI, K.F. and BRESLER, V.M. (1976): Tumours of the testis. In: V.S. Turusov (Ed.), *Pathology of Tumours in Laboratory Animals, Vol. 1, Tumours of the Rat*, Part 2, pp. 135–150. IARC Scientific Publ.No. 6, Lyon.

MOSTOFI, F.K. and PRICE, E.B. (1973)a: Hyperplasia of the prostate. In: *Tumors of the Male Genital System. Atlas of Tumor Pathology*, Second Series Fascicle 8, pp. 182–194. Armed Forces Institute of Pathology, Washington, D.C.

MOSTOFI, F.K. and PRICE, E.B. (1973)b: Tumours of specialized gonadal stroma.In: *Tumors of the Male Genital System, Atlas of Tumour Pathology*, Second series, Fascicle 8, pp. 85–114. Armed Forces Institute of Pathology, Washington, D.C.

NEUMANN, F. (1984): Effects of drugs and chemicals on spermatogenesis. *Arch.Toxicol.*, Suppl 7, 109–117.

NYKÄNEN, M. (1980): Morphology of the rat rete testis in experimental auto-immune orchitis. *Virchows Arch. [B].*, 33, 293–301.

OAKBERG, E.F. (1956): A description of spermiogenesis in the mouse and its use in analysis of the cycle of the seminiferous epithelium and germ cell renewal. *Am.J.Anat.*, 99, 391–413.

ORGAD, U., ALROY, J., UCCI, A. AND MERK, F.B. (1984): Histochemical studies of epithelial cell glycoconjugates in atrophic, metaplastic, hyperplastic, and neoplastic canine prostate. *Lab.Invest.*, 50, 294–302.

PARIZEK, J. (1957): The destructive effect of cadmium ion on testicular tissue and its prevention by zinc. *J.Endocrinol.*, 15, 56–63.

PARVINEN, M. (1982): Regulation of the seminiferous epithelium. *Endocr.Rev.*, 3, 404–417.

PENSTON, J., and WORMSLEY, K.G. (1986): Adverse reactions and interactions with H_2-receptor antagonists. *Med.Toxiol.*, 1, 192–216.

PEREY, B., CLERMONT, Y. and LEBLOND, C.P. (1961): The wave of the seminiferous epithelium in the rat. *Am.J.Anat.*, 108, 47–77.

PICKERING, R.G. and PICKERING, C.E. (1984): The effects of reduced dietary intake upon the body and organ weights, and some clinical chemistry and haematological variates of the young Wistar rat. *Toxicol.Lett.*, 21, 271–277.

POLLARD, M. (1973): Spontaneous prostate adenocarcinomas in aged germ free Wistar rats. *J.N.C.I.*, 51, 1235–1241.

POST, K. and KILBORN, S.H. (1987): Canine Sertoli cell tumor: A medical records search and literature review. *Can.Vet.J.*, 28, 427–431.

POUR, P.M. (1981): A new prostatic cancer model: Systemic induction of prostatic cancer in rats by a nitrosamine. *Cancer Lett.*, 13, 303–308.

PRICE, D. (1963): Comparative aspects of development and structure of the prostate. *N.C.I.*, Monogr. 2, 1–23.

PUGET, A. (1972): Insémination artificielle de la lapine. Aspects technique et résultats. *Rev.Méd.Vét.*, 123, 355–363.

REID, B.L. and CLELAND, K.W. (1957): The structure and function of the epididymis. *Aust.J.Zool.*, 5, 223–254.

REZNIK, G., HAMLIN, M.H., WARD, J.M. and STINSON, S.F. (1981): Prostatic hyperplasia and neoplasia in aging F344 rats. *Prostate*, 2, 261–268.

RHODIN, J.A.G. (1974): Male reproductive system. In: *Histology. A Text and Atlas*, Chap. 33, pp. 675–702. Oxford University Press, New York.

ROBERTS, S. (1987): Presented at PMA Drug Safety Subsection Annual Meeting, October 18–21, 1987, San Antonio, Texas.

ROWLEY, M.J. and HELLER, C.G. (1971): Quantitation of the cells of the seminiferous epithelium of the human testis employing the Sertoli cell as a constant. *Z.Zellforsch.Mikrosk.Anat.*, 115, 461–472.

RUSSELL, L. and FRANK, B. (1978): Characterization of rat spermiogenesis after plastic embedding. *Arch.Androl.*, 1, 5–18.

RUSSELL, L.D., MALONE, J.P. and KARPAS, S.L. (1981): Morphological pattern elicited by agents affecting spermatogenesis by disruption of its hormonal stimulation. *Tissue Cell*, 13, 369–380.

SANTIEMMA, V., SALFI, V., CASASANTA, N. and FABBRINI, A. (1987): Lactate dehydrogenase and malate dehydrogenase of Sertoli cells in rats. *Arch.Androl.*, 19, 59–64.

SATO, K., HIROKAWA, K. and HATAKEYAMA, S. (1981): Experimental allergic orchitis in mice. Histopathological and immunological studies. *Virchows Arch.[A].*, 392, 147–158.

SCHAEFER, F.V., CUSTER, R.P. and SOROF, S. (1982): General process of induction of squamous metaplasia by cyclic adenine nucleotide and prostaglandin in mouse prostate glands. *Cancer Res.*, 42, 3682–3687.

SCHARDEIN, J.L., KAMP, D.H., WOOSLEY, E.T. and JELLEMA, M.M. (1970): Long-term toxicologic and tumorigenesis studies on an oral contraceptive agent in albino rats. *Toxicol.Appl.Pharmacol.*, 16, 10–23.

SCHARDEIN, J.L. (1980)a: Studies of the components of an oral contraceptive agent in albino rats. I. Estrogenic component. *J.Toxicol.Environ.Health*, 6, 885–894.

SCHARDEIN, J.L. (1980)b: Studies of the components of an oral contraceptive agent in albino rats. II. Progestogenic component and comparison of effects of the components and the combined agent. *J.Toxicol.Environ.Health*, 6, 895–906.

SCHULZE, C. (1988): Response of the human testis of long-term estrogen treatment: Morphology of Sertoli cells, Leydig cells and spermatogonial stem cells. *Cell Tissue Res.*, 251, 31–43.

SCHULZE, H. and BARRACK, E.R. (1987): Immunocytochemical localization of estrogen receptors in spontaneous and experimentally induced canine benign prostatic hyperplasia. *Prostate*, 11, 145–162.

SHIMKIN, M.B., SMITH, S.J., SHIMKIN, P.M. and ANDERVONT, H.B. (1962): Some quantitative observations of testicular changes in BALB/c and C3H mice implanted with diethylstilbestrol. *J.N.C.I.*, 28, 1219–1231.

SIBLER, S.J. and RODRIQUEZ-RIGAU, L.J. (1981): Quantitative analysis of testicular biopsy: determination of partial obstruction and prediction of sperm count after surgery for obstruction. *Fertil.Steril.*, 36, 480–485.

SINGAL, R.L., VIJAYVARGIYA, R. and SHUKLA, G.S. (1985): Toxic effects of cadmium and lead on reproductive function. In: J.A. Thomas, K.S. Korach and J.A. McLachlan (Eds), *Endocrine Toxicology*, pp. 149–179. Raven Press, New York.

SINGH, S.K. and ABE, K. (1987): Light and electron microscopic observations of giant cells in the mouse testis after efferent duct ligation. *Arch.Histol.Jpn.*, 50, 579–585.

SINGH, H., HIGHTOWER, L. and JACKSON, S. (1987): Antispermatogenic effects of cyclophosphamide in the Syrian hamster. *J.Toxicol.Environ.Health*, 22, 29–33.

SIVELLE, P.C., UNDERWOOD, A.H. and JELLY, J.A. (1982): The effects of histamine H2-receptor antagonists on androgen actions in vivo and dihydrotestosterone binding to the rat prostate androgen receptor in vitro. *Biochem.Pharmacol.*, 31, 677–684.

SKAKKEBAEK, N.E. (1976): Seminiferous tubules in the adult human testis. In: R.C.B. Pugh (Eds), *Pathology of the Testis*, pp. 38–45. Blackwell, Oxford.

SKAKKEBAEK, N.E. and HELLER, C.G. (1973): Quantification of human seminiferous epithelium. *J.Reprod.Fertil.*, 32, 379–389.

STEINBERGER, A. and STEINBERGER, E. (1976): Secretion of an FSH inhibiting factor by cultured Sertoli cells. *Endocrinology*, 99, 918–921.

SUGIMURA, Y., CUNHA, G.R. and BIGSBY, R.M. (1986)a: Androgenic induction of DNA synthesis in prostatic glands induced in the urothelium of testicular feminized (Tdm/Y) mice. *Prostate*, 9, 217–225.

SUGIMURA, Y., CUNHA, G.R. and DONJACOUR, A.A. (1986)b: Morphological and histological study of castration-induced degeneration and androgen-induced regeneration in the mouse prostate. *Biol.Reprod.*, 34, 973–983.

SUGIMURA, Y., CUNHA, G.R., DONJACOUR, A.A., BIGSBY, R.M. and BRODY, J.R. (1986)c: Whole-mount autoradiography study of DNA synthetic activity during postnatal development and androgen-induced regeneration in the mouse prostate. *Biol.Reprod.*, 34, 985–995.

TAKANO, H. and ABE, K. (1987): Age-related histologic changes in the adult mouse testis. *Arch.Histol.Jpn.*, 50, 533–544.

TAKAYAMA, H. and TOMOYOSHI, T. (1981): Microvascular architecture of rat and mouse testes. *Invest.Urol.*, 18, 341–344.

TARADACH, C. (1986): Evaluation of drug effects on rat and rabbit sperm motility using a modification of Hong's method. *Food.Chem.Toxicol.*, 24, 633.

TERRACIO, L., DOUGLAS, W.H.J., PENNACHIO, D., VENA, R.L. and OFNER, P. (1982): Primary epithelial cell cultures derived from canine prostate: Isolation, culture, and characterization. *Am.J.Anat.*, 164, 311–332.

TORGERSON, M.H., ROVEN, E., STEINER, M., FRICK, J. and ADAM, H. (1982): BCG-induced orchitis: Structural changes during the degeneration of seminiferous tubules of rats and rabbits. *Urol.Res.*, 10, 97–104.

TRAINER, T.D. (1987): Histology of the normal testis. *Am.J.Surg.Pathol.*, 11, 797–809.

TUCKER, M.J., ADAM, H.K. and PATTERSON, J.S. (1984): Tamoxifen. In: D.R. Laurence, A.E.M. McLean and M. Weatherall (Eds), *Safety Testing of New Drugs. Laboratory Predications and Clinical Performance*, Chap. 6, pp. 125–161. Academic Press, London.

TUNG, K. (1987): Immunologic basis of male infertility. *Lab.Invest.*, 57, 1–4.

TUNG, K.S.K., SMITH, S., TEUSCHER, C., COOK, C. and ANDERSON, R.E. (1987): Murine autoimmune oophoritis, epididymo-orchitis and gastritis induced by day 3 thymectomy. Immunopathology. *Am.J.Pathol.*, 126, 293–302.

ULVIK, N.M., DAHL, E. and HARS, R. (1982): Classification of plastic-embedded rat seminiferous epithelium prior to electron microscopy. *Int.J.Androl.*, 5, 27–36.

VAN CAUTEREN, H., VANDENBERGHE, J., HERIN, V., VANPARYS, Ph. and MARSBOOM, R. (1985): Toxicologial properties of closantel. *Drug Chem.Toxicol.*, 8, 101–123.

VENIZELOS, I.D. and PARADINAS, F.J. (1988): Testicular atrophy after oestrogen therapy. *Histopathology*, 12, 451–454.

VIGUIER-MARTNEZ, M.C., HOCHEREAU DE REVIERS, M.T., BARENTON, B. and PERREAU.C. (1983)a: Effect of a non-steroidal antiandrogen, flutamide, on the hypothalamo-pituitary axis, genital tract and testis in growing male rats: Endocinological and histological data. *Acta.Endocinol.*, 102, 299–306.

VIGUIER-MARTNEZ, M.C., HOCHEREAU DE REVIERS, M.T., BARENTON, B. and PERREAU.C. (1983)b: Endocrinological and histological changes induced by flutamide treatment on the hypothalamo-hypophyseal testicular axis of the adult male rat and their incidences on fertility. *Acta.Endocinal.* 104, 246–252.

WAHED, I., BIBBY, M.C. and BAKER, T.G. (1987): Comparative effects of mitozolomide (M&B 39125, NSC 353451) and a series of standard anticancer drugs on mouse testis. *Arch.Toxicol.*, Suppl. 11, 277–280.

WALKER, T.F., WHITEHEAD, S.M., LESLIE, G.B., CREAN, G.P. and ROE, F.J.C. (1987): Safety evaluation of cimetidine: Report at the termination of a seven-year study in dogs. *Hum. Toxicol.*, 6, 159–164.

WARD, J.M., HAMLIN II, M.H., ACKERMAN, L.H., LATTUADA, C.P., LONGFELLOW, D.G. and CAMERON, T.P. (1983): Age-related neoplastic and degenerative lesions in aging male virgin and ex-breeder AC1/seg HapBR rats. *J.Gerontol.*. 38, 538–548.

WARD, J.M., REZNIK, G., STINSON, S.F., LATTUADA, C.P., LONGFELLOW, D.G. and CAMERON, T.P. (1980): Histogenesis and morphology of naturally occurring prostatic carcinoma in the AC1/seg HapBR rat. *Lab.Invest.*, 43, 517–522.

WEISS, L. (1983): *Histology: Cell and Tissue Biology*, 5th Edition, pp. 1038–1043. Elsevier, New York.

WHITE, I.G. (1978): Accessory sex organs and fluids of the male reproductive tract. In: N.J. Alexander (Ed), *Animal Models for Research on Contraception and Fertility*, pp. 105–123. Harper and Row, New York.

WILSON, J.D. (1980): The pathogenesis of benign prostatic hyperplasia. *Am.J.Med.*, 68, 745–756.

WILSON, J.D. (1987): The testis and the prostate. A continuing relationship. *N.Engl.J.Med.*, 317, 628–629.

WYKER, A. and HOWARD, S.S. (1977): Micropuncture studies of the motility of rat testis and epididymis spermatozoa. *Fertil.Steril.*, 28, 108–112.

WYLLIE, A.H. (1987): Apoptosis: Cell death under homeostatic control. *Arch.Toxicol.*, Suppl. 11, 3–10.

WYLLIE, A.H., KERR, J.F.R. and CURRIE, A.R. (1980): Cell death: The significance of apoptosis. *Int.Rev.Cytol.*, 68, 251–306.

WYROBEK, A.J. and BRUCE, W.R. (1975): Chemical inductgion of sperm abnormalities in mice. Proc.Natl.Acad.Sci. USA., 72, 4425–4429.

YING, S-Y (1987): Inhibins and activins: Chemical properties and biological activity. *Proc.Soc.Exp.Biol.Med.*, 186, 253–264.

YU, B.P., MASORO, E.J. and MCMAHAN, C.A. (1985): Nutritional influences on aging of Fischer 344 rats: I. Physical, metabolic, and longevity characteristics. *J.Gerontol.*, 40, 657–670.

ZIRKIN, B.R. and EWING, L.L. (1987): Leydig cell differentiation during maturation of the rat testis: A sterological study of cell number and ultrastructure. *Anat.Rec.*, 219, 157–163.

XI. Female Genital Tract

The potential importance of the effect of xenobiotics on the female reproductive system and the foetus dictates strict regulatory requirements for specific pre-clinical reproductive safety studies which are usually performed in both rodents and rabbits. These studies are conducted with most novel pharmaceutical agents prior to their widespread use among women of childbearing potential.

Reproductive studies are directed primarily towards examination of functional pertubations of reproductive performance and morphological effects on the foetus. Effects of treatment on the morphology of the ovaries, oviducts, uterus, vagina and placenta are usually less well studied in these experiments. Indeed, Maronpot (1987) has suggested that, in general, the characterization and understanding of treatment-induced changes in the female reproductive tract remains lower than for those in many other organs.

This is understandable when it is considered that the female reproductive system is unusual among bodily systems in the number and complexity of its control mechanisms, all of which must operate in order for it to function correctly (Smith, 1983).

Ovarian and reproductive function are intimately linked to hypothalamic and pituitary gland activity. The hypothalamic-pituitary axis serves as the primary control centre for reproductive hormones. Drugs with neuropharmacological activity, notably barbiturates, narcotics and tranquillizers which alter the input of higher brain centres into the hypothalamus can affect gonadotrophin secretion. Such changes disrupt the reproductive system giving rise to infertility, changes in libido and sexual dysfunction (Smith, 1983).

Although drug-induced effects on the reproductive system can be considered to be either mediated directly through action on the peripheral sex organs or indirectly through the hypothalamus, these mechanisms are not sharply separable. For instance, direct damage to the ovaries may in turn lead to loss of feed-back control of the pituitary gland which stimulates the production of more trophic factors, eventually leading to further (tertiary) changes in the sex organs.

Therefore, a constellation of histological findings in the female reproductive system at a particular time point in a toxicity study may represent a combination of primary, secondary and tertiary effects. In addition, treatment-induced changes in reproductive organs also occur in combination with effects in other endocrine organs. This has been the experience in the National Toxicology Program where alterations in reproductive organs induced by a variety of different xenobiotics were commonly found in association with changes in the pituitary gland and adrenal cortex (Maronpot, 1987).

The pathologist should therefore remain aware of these complex inter-relationships and carefully examine endocrine tissues when changes in the reproductive organs are found.

Histopathological evaluation of the female reproductive system is also complicated by the morphological changes which occur during the oestrous or menstrual cycle. Although these cyclic changes are analogous among different laboratory species and man, differences can be sufficient to make interspecies comparison of drug-induced changes in the female reproductive system uncertain. This is particularly true among rodents where the manner in which age-related decline in reproductive function takes place may be quite different between species and strains (Nelson and Felicio, 1985; Felicio et al., 1986).

Age-related cessation of ovulatory function in laboratory animals and in man is proceeded by a transitional phase characterized by increasing variability in ovarian cycling time. This is also highly variable among different strains of both rats and mice (Nelson and Felicio, 1985). These age-related changes in cycling times in rats and mice do not share a common hormonal basis for it has been shown that vaginal cytological profiles and levels of sex steroids and gonadotrophins may be quite different during this period (Nelson and Felicio, 1985; Felicio et al., 1986).

The data suggest that lengthened cycles in aging rats are characterized by an extended preovulatory elevation of oestradiol whereas those of mice are characterized by delayed elevation of oestradiol. The hormonal basis for lengthened cycles may vary within strains and the variation appears age-dependent (Nelson and Felicio, 1985). Although the precise cause of these age-related differences is uncertain, the primary fault frequently appears to be in the hypothalamus. In aging rats the frequent presence of pituitary tumours may be partly responsible for these functional alterations (Meites et al., 1978).

These age-related changes may be modulated by dietary or other environmental factors. For example, housing female rats with males or other females may prolong their cycling lifespan (Nelson and Felicio, 1985). In rats, it has been shown that the integrity of the superior ovarian nerve is necessary for full oestrous responsiveness in cycling rats (Erskine and Weaver, 1988).

General morphology

The oviducts, uterus and vagina are embryonically derived from paired and completely separate Müllerian ducts which become variably fused in a caudocranial manner in higher mammals. The most primitive mammalian arrangement of two separate uteri and cervical canals exists in the rabbit and a number of rodents, including rats and mice.

A slightly more advanced degree of fusion occurs in the guinea pig in which the more caudal cervical segment is fused to form a single lumen so that there are two internal uterine orifices but only a single external os.

In carnivors, the fusion is more complete with two uteri being separated only by a short septal spur. In non-human primates and in man, fusion is generally considered to be complete with formation of a single uterine cavity. In man, only the two oviducts are remaining evidence of development from paired Müllerian structures. These ducts open into the uterine cavity after a long course through the interstitium of the uterine wall. (See review by Eckstein and Zuckerman, 1960a).

Oestrous and menstrual cycles

Four stages of the oestrous cycle are termed *prooestrus, oestrus, metoestrus* and *dioestrus*, separated by a variable period of quiescence, the *anoestrus*.

The first part of the cycle is prooestrus which is characterized by marked change in the reproductive system, but particularly uterine growth and endometrial proliferation. This is followed by the climax of the process, oestrus, at the end of which ovulation usually occurs. If conception results following ovulation, gestation and lactation are followed in some species by a period of anoestrous before the cycle recommences. In some species, particularly rodents, parturition is followed almost immediately by another cycle.

If conception does not occur, which is the usual situation in toxicity studies, oestrus is followed by a short period of metoestrus during which oestrous changes subside. Under some circumstances a longer period referred to as *pseudopregnancy* occurs.

In pseudopregnancy, the changes in the sexual organs are similar to but less marked than those occurring in true pregnancy and is followed either by another oestrous cycle or in some species anoestrus.

In some species, (e.g., rat and mouse) oestrus is succeeded by only a short interval of quiescence, termed dioestrus. This is followed by another prooestrus. This cycle of periods is known as the oestrous and dioestrous cycle. Animals in which oestrus occurs only once in a sexual season are called monoestrous (e.g., dog) whereas those like the rat and mouse in which several cycles occur are referred to as polyoestrous.

Prooestrus and oestrus occur in the follicular phase of the ovarian cycle with ovulation taking place towards the end of oestrus. Metoestrus and dioestrus or pseudopregnancy comprise the luteal phase of the cycle. It should be noted therefore that there are no marked qualitative difference between dioestrus and pseudopregnancy, the latter representing a prolonged dioestrus (Eckstein and Zuckermann, 1960b). These phases therefore correspond to the follicular or proliferative phase and the luteal phase of the menstrual cycle in humans and non-human primates.

Sexual maturity is reached in rats between six and eight weeks of age, although the first oestrus may occur as early as five weeks. In the mouse sexual maturity is reached at about four weeks. In both species the oestrous period occurs every four or five days. The dog, which has a monoestrous cycle, may breed at one year of age although times between cycles are highly variable.

Menstrual cycles in man and rhesus monkeys are classically 28 days although there is some variation in cycle length among Old World monkeys.

VAGINA

Cyclical changes

A key element in the microscopic examination of the vaginal mucosa, is the fact that the morphology of the epithelium shows cyclical changes. Knowledge of these cyclical changes is important in the evaluation of the local irritancy effects of compounds administered vaginally because an inflammatory infiltrate in the mucosa is a normal finding during the oestrous cycle in some species. Furthermore, administration of sex steroids and other agents with hormonal effects may modulate the cyclical changes in the vaginal mucosa.

It was the detailed description of the cyclical changes in the vaginal mucosa by microscopy of both tissue sections and smear preparations in the classical work by Stockard and Papanicolaou (1917) which paved the way for detailed investigation of the oestrous cycle in mammals. From this, developed the study of the cyclical changes in human vaginal smear preparations fixed in alcohol and stained with the polychrome method developed by Papanicolaou (1933), which ultimately gave rise to the development of modern clinical cytology of the genital tract and other organs in disease (Schade, 1960).

Much of the basic literature which relates to the cyclical changes in the vaginal mucosa of laboratory animals and man have been reviewed at length by Eckstein and Zuckerman (1960c).

Well-defined, cyclical changes are observed in the vaginal mucosa of *rats and mice*. Similar, although not identical changes are found in the golden *hamster*.

In dioestus, the vaginal mucosa comprises between three and seven rows of squamous cells, infiltrated by leucocytes. During prooestrus the number of cell layers increases and a granular layer (stratum granulosum) develops. As oestrus approaches, a horny stratum corneum also becomes prominent. During the latter part of oestrus and metaoestrus, the upper layers of the squamous epithelium become desquamated and there is a return of increasing numbers of leucocytes before the cycle is repeated.

In pseudopregnancy and pregnancy the superficial cells of the rodent vaginal mucosa become cuboidal or cylindrical with vacuolation of immediate cell layers. In late pregnacy the superficial cells become mucus-secreting.

These changes may become altered in rats and mice with advancing age as ovarian function declines. As age advances, the vaginal mucosa reflects the lengthening of the oestrous cycles. These vaginal changes differ with strain and species. Generally, increased cornification of the mucosa takes place in rats whereas in mice lengthened cycles are more frequently associated with vaginal leucocytosis (Nelson and Felicio, 1985).

The *rabbit* shows no obvious vaginal cycle in the upper part of the vagina which is lined with a mucus-secreting columnar epithelium. Some cornification is evident during the oestrous cycle in the lowest segment of the vagina which is normally lined by stratified squamous epithelium.

In the *dog*, prominant cyclical changes are evident during the oestrous cycle. Vaginal smear preparations during the oestrous cycle have been well studied in the dog (Schutte, 1967; Fowler et al., 1971). In general terms, as in other species, thickening and cornification of the lining mucosa takes place in prooestrus and oestrus. In anoestrus, the vaginal epithelium comprises two or three layers of low columnar or cuboidal cells. Proliferation occurs in prooestrus which transforms the epithelium into a highly stratified squamous mucosa with a prominant stratum granulosum and stratum corneum. Desquamation and reversion to the columnar pattern occurs in metaoestrus and the epithelium becomes infiltrated by leucocytes.

Cyclical changes in the better studied non-human *primates* such as the rhesus monkey correspond to the general mammalian pattern and are very similar to the changes found in women. There is thickening and cornification of the mucosa in the follicular phase of the cycle with progressive desquamation and vacuolation of cells in the luteal phase followed by leucocytic infiltration and loss of cornified cells in menstruation.

In view of the response of the vaginal epithelium to the hormonal alterations occuring in the oestrous or menstrual cycle, it is not surprising that similar or more marked changes can be induced by exogeneous hormone administration. In women, oestrogen, or oestrogen-dominated oral contraceptives induce cornification of the vaginal epithelium, whereas progesterone limits maturation to intermediate squamous cells (Winkler et al., 1982). Analogous changes occur in laboratory animals.

Inflammation and irritancy potential

The local tolerance or irritancy potential of therapeutic agents intended for vaginal administration is usually evaluated using the vaginal mucosa of laboratory animals. Choice of species is to a large extent dictated by practical considerations and for this reason the rabbit is a commonly used animal, even though the rabbit vaginal mucosa does not histologically resemble that found in man.

Comparison of the vaginal tolerance of spermicidal preparations in rabbits and primates with human clinical experience gained with the same agents, has suggested that the rabbit is a more sensitive species than the non-human primate and that changes induced in the rabbit vagina correspond to clinical findings in man. It was therefore suggested that the rabbit is a reasonably appropriate and practical species to use for this purpose (Eckstein et al., 1969).

Likewise, studies conducted to compare the sensitivities of the vaginal mucosa of rabbit and rat to the non-ionic surfactant, nonoxynol-9 (N-9, p-nonylphenoxypolyethoxyethanol), commonly used in vaginal products, showed greater sensitivity of the rabbit than the rat mucosa (Kaminsky et al., 1985). The high sensitivity of the rabbit vaginal mucosa probably results from the lack of a cornified layer. Therefore, the rabbit is likely to give an exaggerated reaction compared with other laboratory species. Although highly sensitive, the rabbit is an effective model, particularly as comparisons can be more easily made with agents of known vaginal irritancy potential and with products which have an acceptable profile in clinical use.

A comparison of the response of the vaginal mucosa of guinea pigs, beagle dogs and non-human primates (Cebus apella) to intravaginal administration of th antiherpes drug, 2-amino-5-bromo-6-phenyl-4(3H)-pyrimidinone, suggested that the guinea pig vagina was more resistant to that of the other two species (Gray et al., 1984). However, the treatment produced a similar mononuclear infiltration in each species which was generally less severe in keratinized parts of the lining mucosa. Furthermore, macroscopic appearances of the mucosa did not accurately reflect the degree of microscopic changes, underlining the importance of histological assessment for accurate characterization of irritancy potential of drugs on this mucosal surface.

Histological evaluation of irritancy potential is usually conducted by a semi-quantitative analysis, scoring changes such as epithelial exfoliation, haemorrhage, oedema, mucosal necrosis and inflammatory cell infiltrate on a three or four point scale (e.g., minimal, moderate, marked or minimal, slight, moderate, marked). Care needs to be taken with mild inflammatory cell infiltrates for these can be found during the normal oestrous cycle (see above).

CERVIX

The cervix represents the barrier between the uterine cavity and the vagina which is designed to carry out conflicting functions of retaining the conceptus in the uterus and opening at an appropriate time to allow the foetus to be expelled. Its detailed morphology varies between species, notably the degree of fusion of the Müllerian ducts (see above). Fusion is complete in man where a single endocervical canal is present whereas in mice and rats two separate endocervical canals are usually found.

The cervix shows considerable morphological change during pregnancy and labour as well as in advancing age. These changes have been best described in man. Histologically, the upper part of the endocervical canal is covered by columnar mucus-secreting epithelium in continuity with the endometrium. Its vaginal aspect and the lower part of the endocervical canal is covered by stratified squamous mucosa which shows similar cyclical changes to those occuring in the vaginal mucosa. Cyclical changes also occur in the columnar epithelium of the endocervix. In women, these are characterized notably by changes in the quantity and physical characteristics of endocervical mucus.

During the periovulatory period, the cervical mucus is more copious and has been shown to be less acidic and less viscous, a situation which favours penetration of spermatazoa. These differences have been recently demonstrated in the human endocervix by a mucin histochemical procedure which employs sequential saponification, selective periodate oxidation, borohydride reduction followed by PAS and alcian blue staining at pH2.5 (Gilks et al., 1988). This method was developed so that only neutral sugars stain with PAS and acidic ones (O-sulphate esters and carboxyl groups) stain with alcian blue.

The stroma is composed predominantly of dense collageneous tissue mixed with scattered smooth muscle fibres which decrease in number from the upper to lower cervix. In pregnancy and labour in man, there is dissociation and branching of collagen fibres, increases in hyaluronic acid, water and smooth muscle cells (Minamoto et al., 1987).

Epithelial changes: squamous metaplasia

Squamous metaplasia, the process by which mature, non-squamous epithelium is replaced by stratified squamous epithelium is a well described phenomenon in the endocervical canal of both man and laboratory animals. In the human cervix, this process has been shown to develop in stages. Initially, small cuboidal reserve cells develop beneath the columnar epithelium. This is followed by proliferation and differentiation of these cells into immature squamous epithelium. Finally, loss of the overlying columnar cells occurs to leave stratified squamous mucosa (Ferenczy, 1979; Reichart, 1973).

Similar squamous metaplasia occurs in the rat endocervix, after the administration of oestrogenic compounds. Following chronic administration of oestrogens, the squamocolumner junction in the endocervix extends further towards the endometrium (Gitlin, 1954) and may spread to involve the endometrium. Immunocytochemical study of the rat cervical epithelial cells in the presence and absence of oestrogen stimulation has shown that there are alterations in keratin expression during the development of squamous metaplasia (Wright, 1987). Squamous metaplasia appears to develop less readily in the mouse treated with oestrogens.

Adenomatous differentiation, adenosis

Interest in various forms of vaginal and cervical columnar epithelial alterations, especially adenosis, was awakened following reports that these changes were associated with the development of clear cell adenocarcinoma of the cervix and vagina in young women following diethylstilboestol exposure in utero (Robboy et al., 1982). Several animal models have been developed which partly reproduce these changes in women. It appears that the mouse treated prenatally, neonatally or postnatally with synthetic oestrogens is the best rodent model for the study of adenosis and clear cell carcinoma of the cervix and vagina observed in women (Forsberg, 1975; Highman et al., 1977; Ostrander et al., 1985).

Of relevance to routine toxicity testing is the report that long-term administration of diethylstilboestol and 17β-oestradiol to C3H/HeH and C3HeB/Fej mice produced areas of adenosis in the squamous epithelial lining of the cervix and occasionally the vagina (Highman et al., 1977). These alterations were characterized by smooth or papillary surfaces and numerous irregular tubular or glandular downgrowths extending into the adjacent stroma. These downgrowths were lined by variably atypical columnar cells resembling ductal epithelium or endometrial epithelium of secretory type. Most of the lesions were localized around the cervical canal although they also extended over the outer surface of the cervix. Stroma showed oedema and wide separation of fibres and cells by metachromatic mucopolysaccharide. It was of note that similar treatment produced adenosis predominantly in the upper third of the cervix, well above the upper level of the vaginal fornices in C3HeB/FeJ mice. By contrast, lesions were found in the middle and lower thirds of the cervix in C3H/HeJ mice, suggesting that relatively small genetic differences can influence the expression of oestrogen-induced adenosis. These changes were associated with the development of adenocarcinomas of the cervix in some mice of both strains after 52 weeks of treatment with both diethylstilboestrol and 17β-oestradiol, which in some cases appeared to have developed from foci of adenosis.

Long-term administration of combination oral contraceptive steroids to monkeys also produces alterations to the endocervix. These are characterized by dose-related increases in viscid mucous secretion by the endocervical epithelium which is more marked the more potent the progestin component (Valerio, 1989).

UTERUS

Cyclical changes

Cyclical endometrial changes vary between species and alter with advancing age. They are generally characterized histologically by a phase of glandular and stromal proliferation during prooestrus and oestrus whilst follicular maturation occurs. This is followed by a secretory phase during dioestrus, pseudopregnancy or the luteal phase of the menstrual cycle. These changes are relatively marked in the menstrual cycle of non-human primates and in women. Extensive experience with the histopathology of endometrial curettage and biopsy specimens from women has provided an appreciation of the wide range of changes which can occur in the endometrium in normal women as well as in hormonally altered and disease states. By contrast, analogous changes in the uterus of laboratory animals have been less well characterized.

Species differences in the oestrous cycle in laboratory animals with particular reference to older literature have been reviewed in detail by Eckstein and Zuckerman (1960b).

In *rats and mice*, the histological changes in the endometrium during the oestrous cycle are similar. In the *golden hamster* they resemble those in rat and mouse but are considered to be less pronounced.

During dioestrus the rodent uterus is small, poorly vascular with a slit-like lumen lined by columnar cells. In cross-section, the uterine horns are oval with the greatest diameter between the mesometrial and antimesometrial surface. The narrow slit-like lumen is normally oriented in a similar mesometrial-anti-mesometrial plane. In prooestrus the uterine horns enlarge and fill with fluid, Epithelial cells lining the uterine cavity become more cuboidal. These changes reach a maximum during prooestrus, before establishment of oestrus. Oestrus is accompanied by loss of uterine fluid although the uterus itself remains distended. The lining epithelium shows vacuolar degeneration and becomes infiltrated by leucocyte during oestrus but frank epithelial loss and regenerative changes are usually not evident.

In pseudopregnancy, leucocytes disappear and the epithelium and stroma show proliferative changes. Decidual changes may also be seen in the stroma at this stage (see below).

It should be remembered that during aging, the endometrial stroma in mouse, rat and hamster becomes less cellular and accumulates increased amounts of collagen. These changes do not occur uniformly but appear to be most marked in the middle and deep endometrium where they may contribute to age-related decline in uterine function (Wolfe et al., 1942; Craig and Jollie, 1985).

In the *guinea pig*, dioestrus is characterized by glands lined by single layer of ciliated cuboidal or low columnar epithelium showing little or no mitotic or secretory activity. The stroma contains some leucocytes. Prooestrus is accompanied by proliferation of both epithelium and stroma. In oestrus the epithelium becomes columnar and pseudostratified and leucocytes may be found in the stroma beneath the superficial and glandular epithelium.

In the *dog* during anoestrus, the uterus is small and lined by a flattened endometrial epithelium of low columnar or cuboidal type possessing basal nuclei (Figs. 114 and 115). In prooestrus the uterus grows rapidly. It develops mucosal thickening, increased vascularity and accumulation of oedema fluid. Hyperaemia is marked below the surface epithelium and although a few capillaries rupture, collapse of endometrium or development of blood-filled lacunae does not occur. The surface and glandular epithelial cells proliferate and show homogeneous eosinophilic cytoplasm. During oestrus few differences are noted initally but extravasated red blood cells disappear and pigment-containing macrophages appear. The epithelial cells remain proliferative in nature.

In canine pseudopregnancy, there is continued proliferation of uterine glands and surface epithelium and infolding of the mucosa. As the corpus luteum develops, the two layers of endometrium become more evident. There is an inner compact zone containing large number of superficial crypts and a deeper spongy zone containing dilated uterine glands in a scanty stroma. The superficial compact zone becomes transformed into villous processes which project into the uterine cavity. The epithelium overlying the villi becomes composed of large

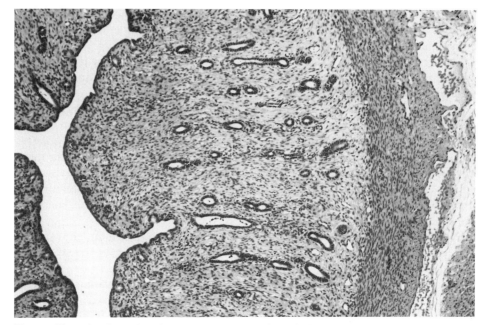

Fig. 114. Normal endometrium from a young untreated beagle dog. (HE, ×150.)

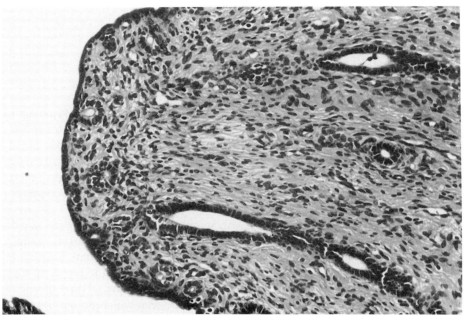

Fig. 115. Higher power view of normal endometrium seen in Figure 114. (HE, ×350.)

vacuolated cells. Regression is characterized by desquamation, liquification and autolysis of the endometrium with little or no overt bleeding.

Cyclical endometrial changes are particularly well characterized in women and they are similar to those described in *non-human primates*, particularly the rhesus monkey. In the early follicular phase of the cycle, the endometrium contains simple, straight glands lined by hyperchromatic cells showing considerable mitotic activity located in loose stroma (*proliferative phase*). In the late follicular phase, proliferation is more marked.

At ovulation, glands develop secretory changes, initially characterized in routine paraffin-embedded sections by subnuclear cytoplasmic vacuolation. Subsequently, these glands then become more coiled and tortuous and show marked secretory activity in the supranuclear cytoplasm. The stroma becomes oedematous and a decidual reaction may develop.

Menstruation is characterized by loss of fluid from the stroma, collapse of capillaries and extravasation of blood in the superficial part of the endometrium.

These cyclical histological alterations are of relevance to the histopathological assessment of treatment-induced endometrial changes in women and laboratory animals for analogous alterations can be induced by appropriate hormone therapy or by drugs which alter endogeneous sex hormone activity (Figs. 116 and 117). It is believed that *oestrogen* stimulates the endometrium by increasing mitotic activity, cell division and the rate of stromal and vascular growth (Winkler et al., 1982). By contrast, *progesterone* is primarily responsible for secretory activity and decidual transformation; it inhibits DNA synthesis, mitotic activity and growth.

A further point here is the potential importance of stroma in the action of steroid hormones on endometrium. The high-affinity steroid receptor proteins appear to reside predominantly on stromal cells and the effect of steroids on endometrial glands may be partly mediated through their action on stromal cells (Cunha et al., 1983).

Decidua, decidual reaction (deciduoma)

A decidual reaction may develop in the endometrial stroma during the luteal phases of the normal oestrous or menstrual cycle and following conception. The term, deciduoma, is frequently used in experimental pathology to define a proliferation of decidual tissue in the non-pregnant animal for the lesion was originally regarded as neoplastic. A decidual reaction or deciduoma is characterized histologically by the presence of large, rounded stromal cells with large round nuclei, prominant nucleoli, abundant eosinophilic cytoplasm, typically containing diastase-fast, PAS-positive granules (Fig. 118). These granules represent membrane-bound cytoplasmic bodies with an electron-dense core sometimes surrounded by small myelin figures (Hart Elcock et al., 1987).

Decidual change can be induced in laboratory rodents and rabbits by various forms of mechanical irritation or trauma, electrical stimulation, instillation of agents such as sesame oil and prostaglandin E_2 (Eckstein and Zuckerman, 1960b; Hart Elcock et al., 1987; Ohta, 1987). However, response to these stimuli appears

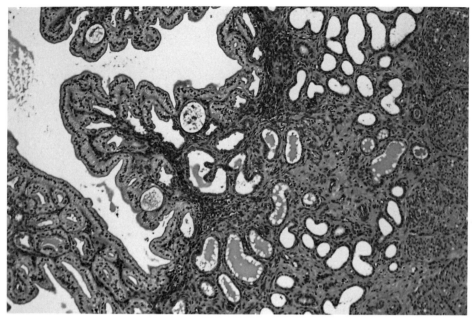

Fig. 116. Endometrium from a beagle dog treated for one month with an aromatase (oestrogen synthetase) inhibitor which produced alteration in circulating sex hormones, presumably reduction of aromatisation of oestrogens and increase in progesterones, accompanied by this secretory endometrial pattern. (HE, ×150.)

to be limited to the late luteal phase of the cycle, suggesting that for induction of decidual change the endometrium must be well-sensitized or primed by progesterone (Eckstein and Zuckerman, 1960b). Studies of deciduogenic activity in rats has suggested that this ability tends to diminish with advancing age although the mechanism for this decline in activity is unclear (Ohta, 1987). Deciduomas may occur spontaneously in rats (Fig. 118) although this is uncommon (Hart Elcock et al., 1987).

Care should be taken to distinguish a florid decidual reaction in rodents from stromal neoplasm showing decidual features.

Decidual changes also develop in women and non-human primates following administration of combination oral contraceptives and at the site of implantation of intra-uterine contraceptive devices (Hughesdon and Symmers, 1978; Wadsworth et al., 1979; Valerio, 1989).

In non-human primates treated for long periods with oral contraceptive drugs, a florid epithelial proliferation termed *epithelial plaque* also develops (Valerio, 1989). This is characterized histologically by the presence of nests of large epithelial cells with atypical nuclei and enlarged nucleoli which grow into the endometrium from the surface epithelium. These growths are believed to be non-neoplastic despite their atypical cytological appearences (Valerio, 1989).

636

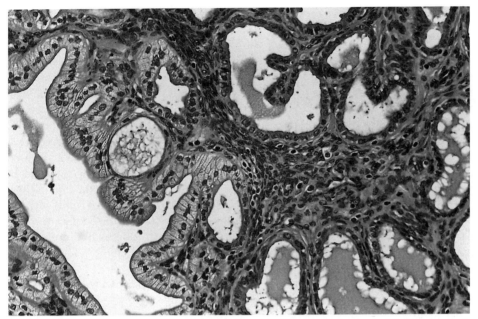

Fig. 117. Higher power view of the endometrium seen in Figure 116 showing epithelial changes in more detail. (HE, ×350.)

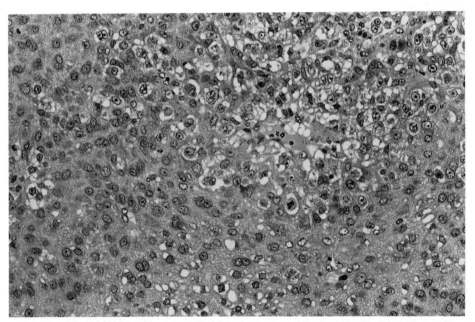

Fig. 118. Endometrium from an untreated Wistar rat showing a marked decidual reaction or "deciduoma". The stroma is composed of large eosinophilic cells containing large rounded nuclei with prominent nucleoli. (HE, ×300.)

Uterine weight and myometrial changes

Although the endometrium shows the most dramatic changes during the oestrous or menstrual cycle, overall uterine size and weight also increases during the oestrous cycle. In rodents, some of these cyclical changes are the result of uterine dilation and accumulation of uterine fluid but the myometrium also increases in thickness. The most dramatic changes in uterine muscle are seen in pregnancy when marked hypertrophy of smooth muscle occurs.

Increases in uterine weight, associated with increased thickness of myometrium or uterine dilation also occur following administration of xenobiotics which mimic these physiological changes. For instance, uterine dilation is reported in rats following treatment with progestins and oestrogens (Schardein, 1980 a,b).

Stilboestrol-treated dogs showed marked increases in uterine weight with an increase in collagen content whereas treatment with the antioestrogen, tamoxifen, produced increases in uterine weight associated with oedema,diminution and fragmentation of collagen (Tucker et al., 1984). These changes resembled the alterations which occur in the oestrous cycle in the dog.

The mouse but not the rat uterus responded by an increase in tone and weight following administration of medroxalol hydrochloride, an antihypertensive agent with predominatly β_1 adrenergic cardiac blocking action with some β_2 and α_1 vasodilatory activity (Gibson et al., 1987). This response was strain dependent. CD-1, CF-1, C3H, DBA/2 and BALB/C strains were quite responsive and C57B2/6 and B6C3F$_1$ strains relatively insensitive.

Adenomyosis

Adenomyosis is characterized by the presence of heterotopic or aberrant endometrial glands and stroma within the myometrium, derived directly from the endometrium. It is distinct from *endometriosis* which is the presence of endometrial tissue outside the uterus, largely confined to man and menstruating non-human primates particularly the rhesus monkey (Schaerdel, 1986; Sternfeld et al., 1988).

Adenomyosis is found in the uterus of man and a number of laboratory animals species notably the mouse. Rats appear more resistant to the development of this change. In man, the diagnosis of adenomyosis is somewhat arbitary with respect to the minimum depth in the myometrium because the normal endometrium can extend fairly deeply into the myometrium. Some authors have used the criterion of one low power microscopic field below the deep endometrial margin, others two low power fields (Hertig and Gore, 1960).

Histologically, islands of adenomyosis in the human uterus are similar to the basal parts of the normal endometrium. Like this zone, they do not usually show the responsiveness to the hormonal changes of the menstrual cycle. Nevertheless, secretory change, cystic or adenomatous hyperplasia and stromal decidual responses are occasionally described in the foci of adenomyosis in man (Hertig and Gore, 1960).

In the narrow uterine horns of laboratory animals such as the mouse, adenomyosis is seen as the extension of fairly unremarkable endometrial glands and stroma into the inner circular or outer longitudinal smooth muscle layers or into connective tissue between the two layers. In mice, glands appear to extend more deeply into smooth muscle on the mesometrial aspect of the uterine horns in the neighbourhood of the larger penetrating blood vessels (Ostrander et al., 1987). Subserosal foci or nodules may also be seen (Mori et al., 1981).

The pathogenesis of adenomyosis is unclear, although hormonal imbalance appears to be a key factor in its development (Güttner, 1980). It has been associated with hyperprolactinaemia in mice (Mori et al., 1981; Huseby and Thurlow, 1982; Nagasawa and Mori, 1982) and in man (Muse et al., 1982), prolonged oestrogen treatment of mice and rabbits (Meissner et al., 1957; Highman et al., 1977; Mori and Nagasawa, 1983) and treatment of mice with progesterone (Lipschütz et al., 1967).

The study of ovariectomized BALB/cCrgl mice treated neonatally with diethylstilboestrol, continuous 17β-oestradiol or progesterone replacement therapy suggested that the hormonal imbalance associated with the development of adenosis was characterized by high levels of circulating *progesterone* (Ostrander et al., 1985).

Atrophy

Loss or suppression of ovarian sex hormone secretion leads to atrophy of the endometrium and uterine myometrium. This can be a spontaneous change in both man and laboratory animals as a result of ovarian aging and loss of function. It can be induced by treatment with agents which damage the ovary or suppress ovarian steroid production for prolonged periods.

An example of this phenomenon is provided by the 10 year toxicity study with norlestrin, an oral contraceptive agent, performed in rhesus monkeys. (Fitzgerald et al., 1982). Treated monkeys showed atrophy of the endometrium which was characterized histologically by reduction in the overall thickness of the endometrium leaving a narrow band of stroma containing a few residual, poorly developed endometrial glands. These appearances were associated with treatment related ovarian atrophy.

Endometrial atrophy, characterized by a reduction in endometrial thickness, loss of endometrial glands and the presence of small endometrial cysts was also reported in dogs treated with the non-progestational androgenic steroid, mibolerone, for periods of up to 9.6 years (Seaman, 1985).

Squamous metaplasia

Squamous metaplasia of the endometrial columnar epithelium is one of the many changes induced in rodents by the administration of oestrogenic compounds although it may also develop spontaneously (Fig. 119). It occurs in mice treated with oestrogens during the prenatal, neonatal or post-natal periods or

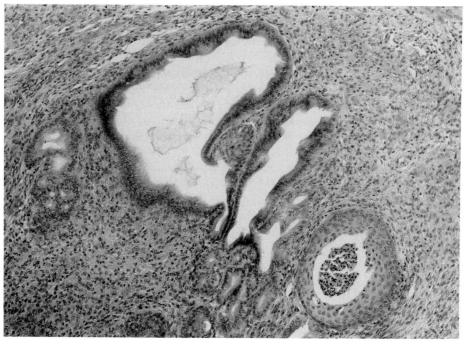

Fig. 119. Endometrium from an untreated 18-month-old CD-1 mouse showing focal squamous metaplasia. (HE, ×200.)

following prolonged oestrogen treatment of mature animals (Loeb et al., 1938; Walker, 1983; Ostrander et al., 1985). Similarly, it occurs in mature rats following exposure to oestrogens 'in-utero' (Rothschild et al., 1988), after prolonged postnatal administration of oestrogens or combination oral contraceptives (Gitlin, 1954; Schardein et al., 1970; Schardein, 1980a,b). Tamoxifen, which tends to act as an oestrogen when given in high doses to rodents also produces squamous metaplasia in the uterus of both rats and mice (Tucker et al., 1984). Histologically, appearances vary but both superficial and glandular epithelium may be affected. Keratinization is not usually prominent although it is associated with cystic hyperplasia and inflammation of the endometrium in oestrogen-treated rodents. It has been suggested that keratinization develops by extension of squamous mucosa from the cervix into the uterine horns. However, it can undoubtably develop by direct metaplasia of columnar endometrial cells, but the mechanisms are complex. As squamous metaplasia has been found in a high proportion of untreated 14-month-old Sprague-Dawley rats and as exposure to oestrogens increases its prevalence, Rothschild and colleagues (1988) have proposed that endometrial squamous metaplasia is an age-related process enhanced

640

by postnatal oestrogenic stimulation or by sensitization of the uterine epithelium by administration of oestrogens at a critical phase of intrauterine development.

Tall columnar epithelium, squamous metaplasia and pyometria are also characteristic of the endometrium in female rats sterilized by a single dose of androgen shortly after birth (Morikawa et al., 1982). It is believed that these morphological changes are also due to a continuous oestrogen effect unopposed by progesterone.

Other studies have shown that continuous oestrogen administration to adult mice produces squamous metaplasia of the endometrium more readily in mice treated with diethylstilboestrol in the neonatal period than in mice untreated in this period (Ostrander et al., 1985). It was shown that diethylstilboestrol treatment in the neonatal period altered the endometrium by inducing the appearance of cuboidal cells beneath the low columnar luminal epithelium, similar to the so-called 'reserve cells' of the human cervix. It appears that these 'reserve' cells are those subsequently induced to undergo proliferation into squamous cells in the presence of excessive oestrogen.

These findings are consistant with those of Wong and colleagues (1982) who showed that, depending on dose of neonatal oestrogen, metaplasia in the endometrium of mice could be ovary (oestrogen) dependent or ovary independent.

The biochemical mechanisms for squamous metaplasia remain uncertain although Schaefer and colleagues (1982) have proposed that its development is mediated by elevated levels of cyclic nucleotides and prostaglandins.

Endometrial hyperplasia

Diffuse or focal (polypoid) hyperplasia of the endometrium is found as a spontaneous change in laboratory animals particularly as age advances. Hyperplasia is associated with age-related decline in sex-hormone levels in which there is often relative oestrogen excess. Oestrogen excess produced by administration of exogenous oestrogens or other xenobiotics with oestrogenic effects also induces endometrial hyperplasia in both laboratory animals and in man. However, there is considerable variation in the reported histological appearances of oestrogen-induced changes in different laboratory animal studies. These differences are partly due to differences in administered compounds, dose and dosage schedule. Other factors are also important. There are differences in responsiveness of the endometrium to oestrogens between different species and strains. Environmental conditions, particularly lighting and diet as well as age of the animal can profoundly affect the reproductive cycle and the final morphological expression of oestrogen-induced changes.

In man, oestrogen therapy or unopposed endogeneous oestrogen excess induces histological changes which can be considered to represent an exaggeration of the normal proliferative phase. Endometrial glands become irregularly dilated or cystic and lined by proliferative, pseudostratifed columnar epithelium containing mitoses but showing little or no secretory activity. These proliferative glands are surrounded by dense, highly cellular stroma. Polyps or polypoid features are also found, presumably a result of the uneveness of responsiveness of the endometrium. Long-term unopposed oestrogen therapy is associated with increasing complexity and atypia of endometrial hyperplasia in women, so it appears that endometrial hyperplasia forms a continuum with frankly invasive endometrial adenocarcinoma (Winkler et al., 1982).

Endometrial hyperplasia induced by oestrogen administration in women is modulated by coadministration of progestins. This has been well-documented in the reports of histological changes induced by combination oral contraceptives. The degree of hyperplasia observed following oral contraceptive administration depends on the dosage of the oestrogenic component, whether administered continuously or cyclically and the time of the cycle at which the tissue biopsy is obtained. In general terms, progestins inhibit the proliferative effects of oestrogens, giving rise to poorly developed stroma which may show a decidual reaction. Long-term administration of oral contraceptives and suppression of ovulation eventually lead to endometrial atrophy (see above).

Likewise, studies in which combination oral contraceptive steroids were administered to non-human primates (mostly rhesus but also cynomolgus monkeys and baboons) have shown similar changes, although the precise appearences vary with dose, type of agent and primate species. Low doses of combination steroids produce mostly proliferative changes whereas mid-doses induce predominatly secretory changes. Endometrial atrophy develops after high dose therapy (Valerio, 1989). Agents with more potent progestational activity are associated with a pleomorphic decidual reaction in the upper endometrium.

Cystic endometrial hyperplasia can be also induced in beagle dogs treated with combination oral contraceptives (Johnson, 1989). Other hormonal modulators may also induce secretory activity (Figs. 116 and 117).

Glandular hyperplasia of the endometrium is a spontaneous finding in a variety of different *mouse strains* as age advances (Reuber et al., 1981). This form of hyperplasia is characterized histologically by an increase in the number of dilated or irregular glands which are lined by hyperchromatic cuboidal or columnar cells with round or oval nuclei and small depots of PAS-positive cytoplasmic mucus. The glands are separated by normal appearing endometrial stroma. The changes are generally diffuse but polypoid glandular growths are also occasionally found (Reuber et al., 1981).

As in the human condition, florid hyperplasia in the mouse may not be easily distinguishable from adenocarcinoma of the endometrium, particularly as endometrial carcinomas also develop spontaneously in mice (Reuber et al., 1981). The distinction can only be made using conventional criteria of cytological atypia, lack of stroma and 'back to back' arranged glands, invasion of the myometrium, serosa and adjacent structures.

Prolonged oestrogen administration also induces hyperplasia and eventually neoplasia of the endometrium in mice. C3H mice tested with diethylstilboestrol or 17β-oestradiol in diet for periods of up to 110 weeks developed elongated irregular or cystic endometrial glands lined by tall, columnar epithelium containing PAS-positive droplets. Hyperplastic glands extended into the myometrium in a form of adenomyosis. The endometrial stroma also showed increased deposition of fine collagen fibres and hyaline material (Highman et al., 1977). In addition, atypical foci were found in the hyperplastic endometrium of some treated mice. These foci were characterized by compactly arranged glands lined by atypical epithelium composed of hyperchromatic cells showing increased mitotic activity (Highman et al., 1977). As in spontaneous changes, the distinction of this form of induced atypical hyperplasia from neoplasia is also difficult, but the same basic principles are applicable.

Cystic and proliferative changes are also found in the endometrium of aging *rats*, in association with the development of endometrial polyps. Likewise, oestrogen administration produces cystic proliferative change in the endometrium, although this is typically associated with dilation of the uterine horns, polymorphonuclear infiltration and secondary changes as a result of an inflammatory process. (Gitlin, 1954; Schardein, 1980a). The altered glandular epithelium is variable in height, being cuboidal, columnar or pseudostratified in nature (Rothschild et al., 1988). Characteristically, squamous metaplasia of the endometrial epithelium is also observed.

Uterine neoplasms

The interest of uterine and cervical neoplasms in safety assessment is due to the oestrogen-sensitive nature of certain tumour types and the fact that oestrogens or xenobiotics which increase the exposure of the female genital tract to endogeneous oestrogens can induce uterine neoplasms in man and experimental animals (IARC, 1979).

It is generally agreed that a broad correlation exists between the tumorigenic effect of oestrogens in laboratory rodents and their carcinogenic activity in the human female genital tract (IARC, 1979; Purchase, 1980). However, the extrapolation of results from individual rodent bioassays in which there are treatment-induced increases in uterine neoplasms to man is made difficult by complex hormonal interactions, particularly in the face of declining activity of an aging rodent reproductive system. In addition, there are clear species and strain differences in the sensitivity and responsiveness of the rodent uterus to sex hormones and other xenobiotics which are reflected by differences in tumour development.

In most laboratory animals, neoplasms of the uterus and cervix are uncommon spontaneous tumours with the notable exception of certain strains of mice (Muñoz et al., 1979). However, a variety of neoplasms occur sporadically in small numbers in rodents and they can be broadly grouped into those of *epithelial* type and non-epithelial or *mesenchymal* tumours.

Epithelial tumours

Epithelial neoplasms of the female tract usually develop in the endometrium, endocervix, exocervix and in the vagina, They may show squamous, glandular or mixed differentiation patterns. Unlike in man, squamous carcinoma of the cervix is uncommon in animals (Cotchin, 1977), although squamous papillomas and squamous carcinomas are occasionally found as spontaneous neoplasms in the lower part of the uterus, the cervix and vagina of laboratory rodents.

Benign glandular neoplasms are found sporadically in the endometrium of laboratory rodents. Although they are usually all considered as *endometrial polyps*, some workers use the term *adenoma*. This underlines the need to carefully characterize the nature of endometrial polyps and define whether they are indeed reactive, hyperplastic or neoplastic in nature. The difficulty of characterizing these polypoid lesions in the rodent endometrium is circumvented by some workers by simply grouping all polyps found in bioassays as benign neoplasms.

Endometrial carcinoma, another important cancer occuring in women is an uncommon spontaneous neoplasm in most laboratory animals except in rabbits and non-human primates. It can be readily induced in rodents by neonatal or long term administration of oestrogens. In the rabbit, endometrial adenocarcinoma is one of the more frequently encountered neoplasms which, as in man, occurs with increased frequency with advancing age and shows varying degrees of differentiation (Baba and Von Haam, 1972; Weisbroth, 1974).

Endometrial polyps

Endometrial polyps are sessile or pedunculated projections of varying proportions of hypertrophied, hyperplastic or neoplastic endometrial glands and stroma. They are found fairly commonly in the uterine cavity of laboratory rodents where they may represent localized areas of hyperplasia, as not all parts of the endometrium are equally responsive to hormonal stimuli (Greaves and Faccini, 1984).

Polyps consisting of projections of highly proliferative epithelium (adenomatous polyps) should be regarded as neoplastic growths in bioassays. It is important to carefully characterize the degree of hyperplasia, cellular atypia and mitotic activity as well as search for any evidence of invasive features in proliferative lesions. It is also helpful to assess the state of adjacent non-polypoid endometrium.

In view of the difficulties in sharply separating the different forms of endometrial polyps occurring in aging rodents, it is common practice to regard them all as neoplasms for statistical analysis.

Endometrial polyps of various types are particularly commonin some strains of rats, presumably a result of altered hormonal status which occur with aging. Burek (1978) described a particularly high prevalence in Wistar-derived (WAG/Rij) rats as they increased in age beyond two years. Adenomatous polyps were reported in increased numbers in Sprague-Dawley rats treated with the progestogenic agent, norethindrone acetate, for two years (Schardein, 1980b).

Adenocarcinoma

Although endometrial and endocervical carcinomas are somewhat variable in cytological features, they are generally characterized in rodents by tall columnar, cuboidal or glandular epithelium arranged in papillary or acinar patterns. The scanty stroma gives rise to a 'back to back' appearance of the acini or papillary structures in well differentiated neoplasms. Varying degrees of cellular stratification, nuclear pleomorphism and mitotic activity are seen. Some neoplasms show poor glandular differentiation.

The neoplasms characteristically infiltrate the myometrium but may show widespread invasion of adjacent extra-uterine tissues. Care needs to be exercised in distinguishing true invasion of the myometrium by adenocarcinoma from the well-ordered infiltration of non-neoplastic endometrium of adenomyosis, particularly liable to occur in the mouse (see above). Cytological criteria are clearly important in this particular respect. Adenosquamous or frankly squamous differentiation is also occasionally reported.

Adenocarcinoma induced by sex steroids and other hormonal manipulation

Administration of oestrogen to adult women has been causally linked to the development of endometrial carcinoma whilst intrauterine exposure to diethylstiboestrol appears to predispose to the development of clear cell adenocarcinomas of the cervix and vagina in girls and young women (IARC, 1979; Robboy et al., 1982). Although administration of oestrogens for long periods to laboratory rodents increases the incidence of neoplasms in a number of organs, the picture with respect to endometrial and cervical cancer is much more confused and different studies with oestrogenic preparations report variable histopathological findings in the uterus.

For instance, in a study in which Sprague-Dawley rats were administered the oral contraceptive agent, norlestrin (98% norethin-drone acetate plus 2% ethylnylestradiol), for two years at doses of 10 and 100 times the human doses, high dose animals developed increased numbers of adenomatous endometrial polyps but no evidence of an excess of endometrial or cervical adenocarcinoma (Schardein et al., 1970). At this high dose, norlestrin presumably possessed predominately oestrogenic effects. Endometrial polyps have also been reported in aged rhesus monkeys following combination steroid therapy (Crossen and Suntzeff, 1950) although only endometrial atrophy followed treatment of rhesus monkeys with the contraceptive norlestrin for 10 years (Fitzgerald et al., 1982).

Administration of diethylstilboestrol or 17β-oestradiol to female C3H mice for long periods is associated with the development of endometrial and endocervical adenocarcinoma (Highman et al., 1977). Therefore, the mouse may represent a more appropriate model for human oestrogen-related uterine neoplasia. However, the sensitivity of mice to the tumorigenic effects of oestrogen varies between strain and among mice of the same inbred strain (Highman et al., 1977; Greenman and Delongchamp, 1986).

Despite the similarity in response of the endometrium to oestrogens by both mouse and man, uterine tumour types may not be histologically comparable. This is best demonstrated by tumours which develop after intrauterine exposure to oestrogens. Intrauterine exposure of the human female foetus predisposes to the development of a highly characteristic, clear cell adenocarcinoma of the cervix and vagina. This neoplasm is composed of solid sheets of clear, glycogen-laden cells or tubules and cystic structures lined by cells witha striking 'hobnail' appearance of prominant protruding nuclei (Robboy et al., 1982). Despite considerable attempts to reproduce this neoplasm in laboratory rodents using intrauterine implants and longer term administration of oestrogens, neoplasms with these precise histological appearances do not develop. (Robboy et al., 1982; Ostlander et al., 1985; Rothschild et al., 1988).

It is also important to note that hormonal derangement of other types also induce adenocarcinoma of the uterus. It was shown that atypical endometrial hyperplasia and adenocarcinoma, some showing squamous metaplasia could be induced in female Spague-Dawley rats sterilized by a single injection of testosterone proprionate two days after birth (Morikawa et al., 1982). The uterine carcinomas were observed only after a fairly long period of about two years. It was suggested they resulted from androgen-induced castration which caused both prolonged oestrogenic stimulation unopposed by progesterone and uterine dysfunction (Morikawa et al., 1982). This illustrates how persistance of both hormonal imbalance and a dysfunctional uterus can lead to endometrial carcinoma.

Mesenchymal neoplasms

The principle mesenchymal tumours found in the uterus and cervix of laboratory rodents are those which resemble endometrial stroma (*stromal sarcoma*) or smooth muscle (*leiomyoma, leiomyosarcoma*). Other mesenchymal tumour types sporadically reported in rats and mice include round cell sarcomas, cystic sarcomas, neurilemmomas, vascular neoplasms, reticulum cell sarcoma type A, as well as mesenchymal neoplasms which contain osteoblastic or chondroblastic differentiation patterns (Stewart et al., 1974; Burek, 1978; Muñoz et al., 1979; Sass, 1981). (See Integumentory System, Chapter I).

The distinction between these tumour types is not always clear cut in view of the variety of appearences which can be seen. Furthermore, mixed patterns of differentiation also occur. As with mesenchymal neoplasms at other sites, histogenesis and terminology of some of these neoplasms remain disputed and variable diagnosis may be used by different authors for essentially identical neoplasms.

Of importance in drug safety evaluation is the fact that the development of stromal and smooth muscle neoplasms of the uterus appears to be hormone-sensitive. This is perhaps not unexpected in view of the hormone-responsive nature of the normal endometrial stroma and myometrium.

Stromal sarcomas

These sarcomas are highly cellular neoplasms resembling normal endometrial stroma which arise mainly in the endometrium. They ultimately replace the endometrium, infiltrate local structures and metastasize widely in the peritoneal cavity. They are well-described in both rats and mice where they develop spontaneously in small numbers with advancing age. They are also induced by local application of genotoxic carcinogens (Baba and von Haam, 1976; Reuber et al., 1981). Analogous stromal sarcomas are also very occasionally observed in the human uterus (Norris and Taylor, 1966).

Histologically, these neoplasms are variable in appearance. They contain cells which range from fairly uniform spindle cells arranged in bundles, showing eosinophilic cytoplasm and moderately pleomorphic nuclei to solid sheets of anaplastic rounded cells with scantly basophilic cytoplasm and hyperchromatic nuclei exhibiting brisk mitotic activity. Large tumours replace the endometrium, infiltrate the myometrium and eventually penetrate the peritoneum to invade other abdominal structures (Reuber et al., 1981; Muñoz et al., 1979).

The weight of the evidence from rat and mouse studies indicates thatthe stromal neoplasms are malignant in biological behaviour. Study of similar human tumours has suggested that biological behaviour correlates with the degree of mitotic activity and the nature of the tumour margins. Benign stromal nodules possess relatively low mitotic activity and expansile, non-infiltrating margins whereas true stromal sarcomas have high mitotic activity and infiltrating margins (Norris and Taylor, 1966).

The histogenesis of stromal sarcomas is somewhat disputed, perhaps in view of their poor differentiation, a degree of overlap with other tumour types and the mixed cellular patterns which can be found, particularly in the mouse (Sass, 1981). Their broad morphological resemblance to normal endometrial stroma in both animals and man favours an endometrial stromal cell derivation. Fine structural examination of human stromal sarcomas has also shown the tumour cells are similar in size and configuration to stromal cells in early proliferative phase endometrium (Komorowski et al., 1970). A primitive stromal cell origin for this and other sarcomas developing in the endometrium is also consistent with the general stem cell concept for the histogenesis of soft tissue tumours at other sites.

The experimental evidence suggests that in certain strains of mice at least, the incidence of uterine stromal sarcomas can be increased by hormonal treatment. For example, sarcomas of the endometrial stroma were observed in BALB/c mice treated with high doses of progesterone for a period of 18 months (Lipschütz et al., 1967). Treatment of C57 black mice with testosterone for their lifespan induced uterine neoplasms with decidual appearances (Van Nie et al., 1961).

Leiomyoma, leiomyosarcoma

Neoplasms composed of spindle cells showing smooth muscle differentiation develop spontaneously in the myometrium of aged laboratory rats, mice and

647

hamsters (Pour et al., 1976; Burek, 1978; Goodman et al., 1980; Kroes et al., 1981; Reuber et al., 1981). Like leiomyomas of the subcutaneous tissues, *leiomyomas* of the uterus are composed of interlacing bundles of uniform spindle cells, typically containing elongated but blunt-ended nuclei and cytoplasmic myofibrils.

A variable degree of interstitial collagen is present ('leiomyofibromas') and larger tumours become hyalinized or develop focal necrosis or mineralization. Leiomyomas are characteristically well-circumscribed and frequently surrounded by a rim of condensed or compressed myometrium. Large tumours distort the myometrium, protrude into the endometrial cavity or extend into the cervix or vagina.

Any substantial degree of nuclear pleomorphism and mitotic activity in smooth muscle tumours is usually considered evidence of malignancy and diagnostic of *leiomyosarcoma*. Leiomyosarcomas invade surrounding tissues and in rodents occasionally produce distant metastases (Reuber et al., 1981).

Although rats treated for long periods with β2-adrenergic receptor agonists develop leiomyomas in the mesovarium (see ovary), uterine leiomyomas were found in increased numbers in CD-1 mice treated for 18 months with medroxalol hydrochloride, an antihypertensive agent with β1-adrenergic cardiac blocking activity with additional β2- and α1-vasodilating (agonist) properties (Sells and Gibson, 1987). In contrast to studies with other agents possessing β2-agonist activity, leiomyomas of the mesovarium did not develop when medroxalol was administered to rats for two years. (Sells and Gibson, 1987).

These treatment-induced uterine neoplasms possessed histological features typical of benign leiomyomas and were located in the myometrium or occasionally in the broad ligament. The neoplasms were also associated with the development of focal hypertrophy and hyperplasia of the myometrium.

Although the precise mechanism for this tumour induction by medroxalol remains unclear, it seems closely related to its pharmacological activity. The compound is devoid of any mutagenic activity and tumour development in mice was prevented by concomitant administration of the β-blocker propranalol (Gibson et al., 1987). Lack of leiomyoma development in treated rats, even though adequate plasma levels and exposure of uterine tissue were achieved, was probably a result of the different sensitivity of rat uterine muscle to the pharmacological effects of medroxalol. Studies in which the force of spontaneous contraction of uterine muscle was examined showed that uterine strips taken from untreated mice showed greater relaxation in response to the β2-agonist effects of medroxalol than rat uterine muscle (Gibson et al., 1987). In addition, spontaneous contraction of uterine muscle strips from mice was completely abolished by pretreatment of the animals with medroxalol for three weeks but only partially in uterine strips from rats given similar treatment. Furthermore mice, unlike rats exhibited increased uterine weight and muscle tone following continuous treatment with medroxalol.

On the basis of these data it was argued that as β2-receptors are believed to predominate in the uterine muscle of non-pregnant mice and rats and that the non-pregnant human uterus shows little or no relaxant response to β2-agonists, it was unlikely that uterine leiomyomas would develop in man in response to treatment with medroxalol (Gibson et al., 1987). This is yet another example of tumour induction by a non-mutagen which may not represent a hazard for man.

Oophorectomized GRS/AFib mice also developed transplantable uterine spindle sarcomas after treatment with oestrogen and progesterone (Briand et al., 1981). These neoplasms were composed of spindle cells with moderately pleomorphic oval or rounded nuclei exhibiting a low level of mitoses. Their appearences were not entirely typical of smooth muscle tumours, for although electron microscopy showed the presence of numerous cytoplasmic myofilaments, there were no focal densities and basal lamina and pinocytotic vesicles were not seen. Both progesterone and oestrogen receptors were also demonstrated on tumour cells using a dextran coated charcoal method (Briand et al., 1981).

Smooth muscle tumours are reported to develop in the female reproductive tract of other species in response to administration of oestrogens. Leiomyomas and leiomyosarcomas were reported in the uterus and vagina of beagle dogs treated for seven years with predominantly oestrogenic oral contraceptive agents (Johnson, 1989). In guinea pigs, a similar oestrogenic effect is so marked that leiomyomas develop in the uterus, spleen, pancreas and kidneys. (Lipschütz and Varglas, 1941). The neoplasms regress on withdrawal of oestrogen. In view of the oestrogen dependancy of these neoplasms, it has been suggested that leiomyomas should be regarded as endocrine-dependent neoplasms although the precise role of oestrogens in their development still remains unclear (Hughesdon and Symmers, 1978).

OVARY

Morphology

The gross anatomy of the ovary is similar between mammalian species although its size, shape, precise location and the form of its peritoneal coverings are variable. It may be located in any position between the caudal pole of the kidney to deep within the pelvis. In addition, the ovary is subject to a wide range of variation in position within a given species, particularly man and dog, after pregnancy has taken place. An ovarian bursa, a sac-like structure formed from the mesosalpinx, is present in most, but not all species. It completely envelopes the ovary in rodents and it is partially absent in man and the anthropoid apes. Interspecies differences in gross morphology have been reviewed in detail by Mossman and Duke (1973a).

In man, the ovary is a uniform structure about three centimeters in maximum diameter enclosed in a fold of peritoneum, the mesovarium. This fold attaches one side of the ovary to the broad ligament. Through the fold, blood vessels, lymphatics and nerves pass to penetrate the ovary at its hilum. In man, as in other mammals, ovarian vessels anastomose at the base of the mesovarium, a feature which allows blood to reach the ovary from either ovarian or uterine vessels to assure good nutrition (Mossman and Duke, 1970b).

The structure of the ovary among non-human primates is variable but in rhesus monkeys and anthropoid primates it is similar to that in man (Eckstein and Zuckerman, 1960a).

In dogs, the ovary is smaller than in man, usually about 1.0 to 1.5 cm in length. It is generally smooth in appearance prior to the onset of oestrous cycle but subsequently it becomes roughened and nodular. The ovaries are embedded in fatty tissue and enclosed in a peritoneal bursa which possesses a slit like opening (Eckstein and Zuckerman, 1960a).

In rats and mice the shape and size of the ovary is dependent on the number and degree of development of Graafian follicles and corpora lutea. Indeed, the slight changes in ovarian weight which occur in rodents during the oestrous cycle are probably related to the development and regression of corpora lutea (van der Schoot et al., 1987). As a result, the ovaries in the rat and mouse appear as grape-like masses of follicles embedded in fatty connective tissue attached to highly convoluted oviducts.

Each ovary in rodents is surrounded by a bursa of the complete type. In rat and mouse, the bursa communicates with the peritoneal cavity through a slit-like opening on the anti-mesometrial side of the bursa at the level of the tip of the uterine horm (Eckstein and Zuckerman, 1960a). This is in contrast to the bursa around the ovary of the hamster which experimental data suggests possesses no communication with the peritoneal cavity (Eckstein and Zuckerman, 1960a).

In this context, it is important to note that direct communication exists between the external environment and the ovary and in most cases also the peritoneal cavity. It appears from studies of the ovary in both women and rats that substances such as talc placed in the vagina or uterine cavity are able to migrate in a retrograde manner to become embedded in the ovary (Henderson et al., 1971, 1986).

Histologically, the ovary can be divided into three main regions, an outer cortex, an inner cortex and a central medulla. The boundary between cortex and medulla is indistinct when the ovary is distorted by large follicles and corpora lutea. The cortex contains the ovarian follicles and corpora lutea and the ovarian blood vessels penetrate into the ovarian stroma through the hilum. The surface of the ovary is continuous with the serosa of the mesovarium and comparable to the peritoneal mesothelium. However, it may not be flattened but cuboidal or columnar in type and in some species it may be pseudostratified. This surface layer is sometimes refered to as the *germinal epithelium*, although it is known to be a specialization of peritoneal (coelomic) mesothelium. For this reason the term 'epithelial' should be used with caution in the context of ovarian pathology.

The evolution of follicular morphology during maturation has been particularly well studied in rodents. It is generally believed that these morphological changes in the rodent ovary are similar to those occurring in man and some of the better studied non-human primates such as the rhesus monkey.

Large numbers of the most immature follicles, *primordial follicles* are present in the cortex of adult animals. The primary oocyte which is in the attenuated prophase of meiotic division is closely enveloped by a single layer of spindle cells or follicular cells. The follicular cells possess desmosomal attachments to the oocyte plasma membrane and it is believed that they provide a route for the transfer of nutrients. The oocyte and follicular cells are surrounded by a basal lamina which separates the primordial follicle from the true ovarian stroma.

At the next stage of development, (*primary follicle*) follicular cells become more cuboidal. Successive divisions of the follicular cells gives rise to the multilayered zona granulosa of the *secondary follicle*. The oocyte continues to enlarge and it forms a band of glycoprotein, the zone pellucida, which separates the oocyte from the inner layer of the follicular cells.

As proliferation of the cells of the zona glomerulosa takes place, adjacent stromal cells outside the basal lamina become arranged in concentric layers and their nuclei become less dense. These cells are referred to as the *theca interna*. The *theca externa* represents an outer layer of more fibrous stromal cells which gradually merges with normal ovarian stroma.

The Graafian follicle forms as cleft-like spaces develop among granulosa cells to form a fluid-filled antrum. At this stage, cells of the theca interna become more rounded or epithelioid in nature but the oocyte ceases to expand.

Following the preovulatory surge of luteinizing hormone, the first meiotic division is completed with extrusion of the first polar body and the formation of the *secondary oocyte* possessing a haploid number of chromosomes. At this stage, the follicle ruptures and the secondary oocyte is extruded into the oviduct. Blood vessels from the theca interna penetrate the basal lamina of the residual follicle to form a corpus luteum composed of granulosa theca cells.

A new corpus luteum is formed each menstrual or oestrous cycle and old corpora lutea degenerate to become fibrous or hyaline in nature (*corpus albicans*) and accumulate in the medulla.

The ovarian stroma is composed of connective tissue spindle cells with morphological characteristics of fibroblasts and smooth muscle cells as well as highly specialized interstitial cells of distinct morphological types. Based on a comparative survey of the interstitial cells in a variety of mammalian ovaries, Mossman and Duke (1973b) classified interstitial cells into several distinct morphological types, including foetal, thecal, stromal and hilar.

Ultrastructural examination of granulosa, thecal and stromal cells show typical features of steroid-secreting cells such as many lipid droplets, well-developed smooth endoplasmic reticulum and oval mitochondria with tubular cristae (Yoshinaga-Hirabayashi et al., 1987).

Hilar cells are found in the ovarian hilum of primates including man. They are similar to Leydig cells of the human testes and may even contain Reinke crystalloids. They are scattered in small groups among the non-myelinated nerve fibres of the hilum but their function is uncertain. The hilum also contains plentiful blood vessels, lymphocytes and supporting stroma.

This basic histological pattern of the ovary is subject to many species and strain variations and these have been discussed in detail by Mossman and Duke (1973b). Differences become more marked with advancing age. This is particularly evident among various strains of laboratory mice in which interstitial cells and stroma differ to a marked degree with advancing age (Russfield, 1967).

Histopathological examination of the ovary is compromised by its complex structure and limitations of sampling. A single section of an ovary may not always include all relevant tissue elements and an appreciation of the age, number and size of follicles and corpora lutea may by inexact. Serial or step sections can provide more information but at increased cost.

Ovarian hormone production and control

To understand the relevance of drug-induced morphological changes in the ovary of experimental animals, it is necessary to consider comparative physiology of gonadal hormone production and control. It is important to be aware that much of our understanding of hormonal control of the ovulatory process in women is based on the study of hypophysectomized rats, supported where technically and ethically possible by data obtained from non-human primates and direct observations in man (Ross, 1985). It is generally believed that the cyclical changes in follicular morphology and sex hormone production observed in the menstrual cycle in man and in non-human primates such as the rhesus monkey are similar to those occurring in the oestrous cycle in the rat (Ross, 1985). Non-human primates, notably rhesus monkey have been used widely in the study of reproductive biology because they have menstrual cycles. Although there are undoubtably differences between some primate species and man in steroid-protein interactions, the metabolism and dynamics of oestrogen and androgens appears very similar between man, rhesus and cynomologous monkeys (Bourget et al., 1988).

The pulsatile release of gonadotrophin releasing hormone (LHRH, GnRH) from the hypothalamus is fundamental to the control of both follicular stimulating hormone (FSH) and luteinising hormone. LHRH, a decapeptide, is released by peptidergic neurones situated in the medial basal hypothalamus and terminating in the median eminance, to flow into the hypophyseal portal circulation to reach the pituitary gland. (See Nervous System and Special Sense Organs, Chapter XIII). The secretion of LHRH is regulated by biogenic amines that link gondadotrophin secretion to the remainder of the central nervous system. This is of potential importance in toxicology because gonadotrophin secretion can be influenced by impulses from the brain such as produced by stress, light-dark cycles and other visual stimuli, olfactory signals of pheromones as well as drugs which interfer with hypothalamic aminergic activity (Reichlin, 1985). For example, endogeneous opioids influence gonadotrophin secretion, morphine and analogues inhibit ovulation and opiate antagonists may induce ovulation (Quigley et al., 1980).

The secretion of LRHR is also modulated by feedback mechanisms involving ovarian hormones. The development of the ovarian follicle is largely under the control of FSH and ovulation is brought about by LH.

Oestrogenic hormones have complex effects on the feedback control of FSH and LH. Depending on dose, time course and previous hormone status, oestrogens can inhibit or stimulate the secretion of gonadotrophins. Administration of a constant dose of oestrogen (or a large amount of androgens) suppresses secretion of FSH and LH, whereas castration or administration of antioestrogenic or antiandrogenic drugs have the opposite effect. The negative feedback effects involve both the pituitary and the hypothalamus for they require the presence of an intact hypothalamus and pituitary gland (Reichlin 1985). Negative feedback is also exerted by a peptide hormone, inhibin, which is derived from germinal cells in the ovary (and testis) (Reichlin, 1985).

A further consideration here is that although a single injection of LHRH brings about a prompt release of both LH and FSH, sustained high levels of LHRH suppress LH and FSH and subsequent gonadal function (Dandow, 1983).

A key feature of the reproductive cycle is the fact that positive feedback is also exerted by ovarian hormones. A pulsatile release of oestrogen is able to sensitize the pituitary-gonadotrophin response to LHRH, stimulating the release of LH and FSH in the normal ovarian cycle. In addition, LHRH secretion appears to be stimulated directly by preovulatory release of oestrogen in both the rat and primate (Kalra and Kalra, 1983; Ferin, 1983).

Gonadotrophins probably exert these effects on target cells in the ovary through specific receptors, the number and distribution of which alters during the reproductive cycle, as a result of changes in the hormonal milieu. For instance, prior to the antral stage, membrane receptors for LH are confined to thecal and other interstital cells and FSH receptors are limited to granulosa cells inside the basal lamina of preantral follicles. Subsequently, LH receptors also appear on granulosa cells (Richards, 1978). Oocytes are devoid of receptors for gonadotrophins and it appears that receptors on follicular cells couple hypothalamic action to follicular and oocyte development. Through their receptors, gonadotrophins stimulate synthesis of sex steroids by ovarian tissues. Granulosa cells, the theca and ovarian stroma possess most, if not all of the enzymatic activity necessary for the synthesis of oestrogens, progestogens and androgens from acetate or cholesterol, although the degree of activity is variable between cell types. Some of these differences have been clearly demonstrated by immunocytochemical means in the rat. (Yoshinaga-Hirabayashi et al., 1987). Steroid enzyme activity appears different from that in the placenta which requires cholesterol as a substrate for production of sex steroids (Korach and Qarmby, 1985).

Granulosa cells have the highest FSH-inducible aromatase activity for the production of oestrogens. The stroma, although capable of producing all sex steroids, normally only produces insignificant amounts compared with the follicular cells and theca.

Mechanisms which control secretion from the corpus luteum are not completely understood. LH, which is released in largest amounts in mid-cycle (mid-cycle surge) causes the luteinization of granulosa and theca cells. Simultaneously, aromatization of androgens to oestrogens is reduced and the quantity of progesterone increased. In rodents prolactin is also a potent luteotrophic factor but in women its role remains controversial (Ross, 1985).

In the rat, prolactin has been shown to possess important luteotrophic and luteolytic properties. It is required for progesterone synthesis in early pregnancy and during lactation. It appears to regulate the luteal receptor for LH (Dunaif et al., 1982).

Prolactin may also be responsible for the lysis of mature corpora lutea during the oestrous cycle, pregnancy and lactation because luteolysis can be prevented by specific inhibitors of prolactin release (Wuttke and Meites, 1971). Immunocytochemical study has shown that prolactin receptors are located in most components of the rat ovary including the ovum but are most heavily concentrated in luteal cells (Dunaif et al., 1982). Evidence for direct inhibition of ovarian function in man and animal species has been reviewed by McNeilly and collegues (1982).

With functional decline of the corpus luteum at the end of the luteal phase of the cycle, there is a reduction in the negative feedback of gonadal steroids with subsequent increase in gonadotrophins, mainly FSH. As a result, another cohort of follicles is recruited for the next cycle.

If conception occurs, foetal chorionic gonadotrophin maintains the corpus luteum. Studies with human chorionic gonadotrophin (hCG) have shown that this hormone binds to the same receptor as LH but its secretion is not subject to the same negative feedback by sex steroids (Haney, 1987). As trophoblasts become the primary producer of steroids, regression of the corpus luteum takes place.

Although the general principles of control of ovarian function appear similar among mammalian species, small functional interspecies differences or variations in sensitivity may assume greater importance in the toxicity testing of high doses of compounds with gonadotrophin or steroid-like activity. For instance in the dog, unlike in man, progestogens stimulate synthesis and release of growth hormone which in turn is a factor in the stimulation of mammary growth and tumour development (Johnson, 1989). Progestogens also have variable degrees of oestrogenic activity among different species and this activity is high in rodents. The agent, tamoxifen, acts as an oestrogen in some species and an antioestrogen in others (Tucker et al., 1984). Even different strains of rat have been shown to respond differently to high doses of oestrogen (Wiklund et al., 1981).

It is worth remarking that it has been shown in rats that the integrity of the superior ovarian nerve, one of the main sources of sympathetic innervation of the ovary, also plays a modest role in the control of oestrous behaviour (Erskine and Weaver, 1988). The function of vagal (parasympathetic) fibres innervating the ovary is poorly understood although it has shown that abdominal vagotomy can disrupt the oestrous cycle in rats (Burden et al., 1981).

Inflammation and necrosis

Overt necrosis and inflammation are uncommon findings in the ovaries of laboratory animals. Treatment-induced oocyte destruction appears to occur principally by a process of atresia (see below) rather than through necrosis and inflammation.

Infections reach the ovary from the exterior via the communication which exists through the vagina and uterine cavity. An example of this phenomenon was reported in B6C3F1 mice used in carcinogenicity bioassays in which an unusually high number of mice developed chronic inflammation and abscess formation in and around the ovary (Rao et al., 1987). This infection was shown to have been the result of opportunistic klebsiella organisms. Although the precise cause for the outbreak was unclear, it appeared related to environmental factors. The lesions were more prevalent in gavage studies than when compounds were administered in diet, topically or by inhalation. They were common in laboratories not routinely flushing the cage rack automated watering manifolds. Careful attention to the sanitization of the automatic watering system reduced the prevalence of this disease. (Rao et al., 1987).

An inflammatory, destructive process can be mediated by auto-immune processes. This has been clearly demonstrated in mice thymectomized at three days of age. Following thymectomy, a high proportion of mice developed an inflammatory infiltrate by three months of age. This was composed of lymphocytes, monocytes, macrophages with some plasma cells and neutrophils in and around ovarian follicles at all stages of development (Tsung et al., 1987). After three months of age the inflammatory process subsided leaving atrophic ovaries containing cells with morphological features of luteal cells. The cause and the inciting antigen was uncertain, although a T-lymphocyte mediated immune mechanism was probably involved. This form of destructive process can be associated with subsequent development of ovarian neoplasia (see below).

Paraovarian fibrosis and inflammation in ovarian tissue was also reported in rats treated for long periods with contraceptive steroids (Lumb et al., 1985).

Oocyte or ovarian follicular degeneration

Oocyte loss has been shown to occur in the human ovary following various forms of cancer therapy including administration of alkylating agents, antimetabolites, antibiotics and vinca alkaloids with and without ionizing radiation (Nicosia et al., 1985). Ionizing radiation alone is also capable of producing oocyte loss in humans (Baker, 1971; Baker and Neal, 1977). By the time the human ovary can be examined histologically following cancer therapy, usually at autopsy, there is oocyte loss is marked and accompanied by focal or diffuse cortical fibrosis and varying degrees of ovarian atrophy or hyperplasia.

It appears that damaged oocytes are eliminated primarily through a process of atresia (Nicosia et al., 1985). The effects of ionizing radiation on the ovary have been quite well studied in laboratory animals. These studies are of interest in the consideration of species differences because dosage of radiation can be well controlled and it is not confounded by the species differences in the disposition and metabolism which occur with chemical agents.

Modest doses of γ radiation destroy immature, primordial oocytes sparing more mature follicles in the ovary of the mouse. The LD50 for these oocytes in young (14 day old) mice is estimated to be only six rad and this represents the highest sensitivity of any known mammalian cell (Dobson and Felton, 1983).

Although the precise cause for this high radiosensitivity is uncertain, micro-dosimetric considerations and autoradiographic studies have suggested that the mouse oocyte cell membrane is particularly sensitive to the damaging effects of radiation (Dobson and Felton, 1983).

The rat ovary responds to ionizing radiation in a qualitatively similar manner but it is considered less sensitive than the mouse ovary. By contrast, in the guinea pig, primordial oocytes appear to be less sensitive to the effects of ionizing radiation than maturing oocytes (Oakberg and Clarke, 1964) suggesting that qualitative differences in oocyte sensitivity also exist between species.

In primates, sensitivity is species-dependent. For instance, squirrel monkey germ cells are highly sensitive to ionizing radiation whereas available evidence suggests that in the rhesus monkey, in common with man, fairly high doses of radiation are required to destroy oocytes. (Dobson and Felton, 1985).

Analogous species differences in oocyte sensitivity to anticancer drugs and other genotoxic chemicals such as polycylic aromatic hydrocarbons also exist although the evidence is confounded by species differences in the disposition and metabolism of these compounds. Again, the mouse oocyte appears to be more sensitive to the effects of these agents than the oocyte of the rat or guinea pig.

Comparative studies of over 70 chemicals including antibiotics and anticancer compounds in juvenile (7–21 days of age) mice have shown that the majority of agents which are capable of destroying oocytes are mutagens and/or carcinogens and produce their effects in a dose-related manner (Dobson and Felton, 1983). Although not all mutagenic-carcinogenic agents are capable of inducing oocyte damage in whole animals, it appears from this work that the activites of these agents are broadly related to their known activity as mutagens or carcinogens.

Undoubtably, the disposition of these agents in the body fluids and ovarian tissue are factors in species differences and it has also been shown that the ovary is itself also capable of metabolising administered compounds to active mole-cules. Some of these factors have been studied with the polycyclic aromatic hydrocarbons benzo(a)pyrene, 3-methylcholanthrene and 7,12-dimethylbenz(a) anthracene which require metabolic activation in order to exert their toxic effects on mammalian cells. These agents are all capable of producing oocyte loss and eventually ovarian neoplasia.

It has been shown in mice that unilateral injection of benzo(a)pyrene is capable of destroying oocytes in the injected but not the contralateral ovary, thus suggesting that the ovary is capable of transforming benzo(a)pyrene to its active metabolites (Mattison et al., 1983).

The ovarian enzymes responsible for the metabolism of polycyclic hydro-carbons are believed to be similar to the hepatic microsomal P450 dependent monooxygenases and epoxide hydrases. In several murine systems the activity of ovarian aryl hydrocarbon [benzo(a)pyrene] hydrolase has been shown to be inducible, although the degree of inducibility among different rodent strains and species does not seem to correlate directly with the destructive activity of these agents. (Mattison et al., 1983).

Nevertheless, species and strain differences in the ovarian sensitivity to polycyclic hydrocarbons are striking. For instance, the destruction of oocytes by 3-methylcholanthracene is greater in C57BL/6N mice compared with the DBA/SN strain (Mattison et al., 1983). The mode of destruction of oocytes occurring with these agents is uncertain but it could result from a direct effect on the oocyte or indirectly by damage to the supporting granulosa-theca cell elements.

In the histological assessment of follicular cell loss, a number of other factors need to be considered. As alluded to previously, the degree of sampling and plane of section are important elements underlying an accurate assessment. Quantitative assessment can be important and it has been proposed that measurement of follicular diameter is a helpful way in which to assess follicular maturation, rather than classifying follicles into arbitary groups. (Ataya et al., 1985).

Another factor is length of dosing period. Long periods of dosing with agents which only damage oocytes at a particular stage of development eventually lead to complete oocyte loss. In addition, it has been suggested that the destruction of large, but not small follicles by a short course of treatment with cyclophospha-mide can damage the steroid producing ability of the ovary, thereby reducing the negative feedback to the pituitary gland. This, in turn leads to increased gonadotrophin secretion which enhances recruitment of immature follicles into mature stages where they can be more readily destroyed (Ataya et al., 1985).

These factors suggest that oocyte destruction by xenobiotics is a complex, multistep process, the expression of which is influenced by species and strain sensitivity, systemic and local metabolism and detoxification, dose and dosage schedule. Part of the assessment of oocyte loss clearly requires critical histopathological analysis using well-prepared histological sections from care-fully designed experiments.

Atrophy

Loss of ovarian weight and histological evidence of ovarian atrophy commonly accompanies the cessation of the cyclical ovarian activity which occurs with aging. This is most frequently observed as a spontaneous alteration in long-term studies using rodents. The relative contributions of ovarian and neuroendocrine factors in the age-related loss of cyclicity is uncertain, although hypothalamic-pituitary impairment may be more important than ovarian age in the rat than in the mouse (Felicio et al., 1986). However, experimental conditions, dietary factors, particularly caloric restriction and the administration of xenobiotics which disturb the hypothalamic-pituitary-gonadal axis may influence the expression of age-related ovarian atrophy. Furthermore, atrophy occurs as a direct result of administration of compounds which damage cellular components of the ovary, block or suppress the normal trophic control of the ovary (Mattison et al., 1983; Mattison, 1983). See also under Inflammation and Necrosis.

Typically, ovarian atrophy is characterized by an organ of small size, devoid of well-developed follicles and corpora lutea. Residual ova and corpora albicans may be evident but the ovarian stroma is characteristically condensed showing hyalinization or fibrosis. Depending on species, strain, age, experimental conditions and the nature of the test agent, these basic histological features may be accompanied by increased number of cystic follicles, ceroid and lipid accumulation in interstitial cells, amyloid and focal interstitial hyperplasia.

These accompanying features provide important clues to the pathogenesis of ovarian atrophy occuring in toxicity and carcinogenicity studies. Russfield (1967) has described the highly variable histological appearences of the aging rodent ovary and noted that strain differences are especially marked among mice. Review of ovarian pathology in Fischer 344 rats and B6C3F1 mice used in the National Toxicology Program (NTP) showed that atrophy occurred ten times more commonly in carcinogenicity bioassays performed in mice than those conducted in rats (Montgomery and Alison, 1987).

Morphological features of ovarian atrophy which is primarily the result of feedback suppression of gonadotrophin secretion are well-illustrated in rodents and primates which were administered high doses of oestrogens, progestogens or combinations of these hormones for long periods of time.

For instance, when C3H mice were fed high doses of 17β-oestradiol or diethyl-stilboestrol for 52 weeks, ovaries were reduced in size and showed atrophy characterized by lack of corpora lutea and accumulation of abundant ceroid pigment. (Highman et al., 1977). Safety studies in which rats or non-human primates were administered the oral contraceptive, norlestrin, or its individual oestrogenic or progestagenic components for long periods also showed treatment-related ovarian atrophy.

When Sprague-Dawley rats were given the combination of 98% ethindrone acetate with 2% ethinyloestradiol (norlestrin) at doses which represented 10 or 100 times the human dose for two years, ovarian atrophy was seen more commonly than in untreated controls (Schardein et al., 1970). Histologically, ovaries in treated rats were characterized by lack of follicular development, absence of corpora lutea and uniform atrophic stroma. Subsequent studies with the oestrogenic component in the same strain of rat at similar doses also showed ovarian atrophy, although it was less marked than in the previous study. Morphologically the changes were similar but more marked than in the concurrent untreated controls (Schardein, 1980a). Although administration of the pure progestogenic component to Sprague-Dawley rats at similar doses for an identical period also inhibited ovulation as shown by an absence of corpora lutea, generalized ovarian atrophy was not observed (Schardein 1980b).

Female Wistar rats treated for 50 weeks with high doses of the progestogen-oestrogen combination quingestanol and quinestrol developed similar ovarian atrophy but associated with chronic suppurative ovarian inflammation (Lumb et al., 1985). However, after withdrawal of treatment for a period of 30 weeks there was considerable regression of these changes and the reappearance of follicular activity.

Long term adminstration of the contraceptive agent, norlestrin, at doses which represented 50 times the human dose, given in a cyclic regimen of 21 days dosing followed by seven days without treatment for 10 years to rhesus monkeys also produced ovarian atrophy (Fitzgerald et al., 1982). Histologically, this atrophy was characterized by reduction in follicular development, as shown by lack of normally maturing follicles and an increase or condensation of stromal cells. These features were believed to be the result of an inhibitory effect of these steroids on hypothalamic-pituitary-gonadal function.

There is increasing evidence that ovarian atrophy in women can result from primary damage to the ovarian follicle complex because treatment of cancer patients with highly reactive antineoplastic drugs is associated with premature ovarian failure (Waxman, 1984). This phenomenon has also been described in laboratory animals treated with these and other genotoxic agents.

Both acute and chronic dosing of rats with the anticancer drug, cyclophosphamide, has been shown to result in a loss in ovarian follicles or *follicular atresia* (Shiromizu et al., 1984, Ataya et al., 1985). Another study in which rats were given single parenteral doses of cyclophosphamide 14 days prior to autopsy, produced a dose-related reduction in total ovarian weight which was associated with a reduction in the number and size of antral but not preantral and primordial follicles (Jarrell et al., 1987). As follicular maturation takes about 19 days in the rat it was suggested that the primary ovarian target for cyclophosphamide is the primodial or small preantral follicle. Although the ovarian follicular loss was associated with reduced levels of circulating oestradiol and progesterone, no elevations in circulating gonadotrophins were reported, consistent with a primary effect on ovarian function.

Ovarian atrophy is also reported in rodent carcinogenicity bioassays of other classes of therapeutic agents. Examples include the antibacterial, nitrofurantoin, which produced necrosis of ovarian follicular epithelium followed by atrophy in mice (Maronpot, 1987; Stitzel et al., 1989) and gentian violet which was associated with ovarian atrophy when fed to mice in the diet for two years (Littlefield et al., 1985).

Cystic change, polycytic ovary, follicular and luteal cysts

A syndrome in which an ovulation is associated with polycystic ovaries has been recognized in women for many years and it is the most frequent cause of secondary amenorrhoea in women associated with increased steroid hormone production (Ross, 1985). In this syndrome, ovaries typically contain many atretic follicles and *follicular cysts* associated with thickening of the ovarian capsule and an increase in stroma (Haney, 1987).

It is believed that this syndrome comprises a number of different conditions, all characterised by altered levels of circulating gonadotrophins, especially LH, with hyperandrogenism and chronic unopposed effects of oestrogens on target organs. The morphological changes appear to be a consequence of anovulation in which large number of atretic follicles are produced with subsequent increase in thecal mass and androstendione production. Thus, any derangement which alters gonadotrophin levels and impedes follicular development could theoretically result in this syndrome (Haney, 1987). The morphological expression of this syndrome in the human ovary is of interest in preclinical drug safety evaluation because similar changes occur spontaneously or can be induced in laboratory animals.

Ovarian *follicular cysts*, believed to be derived from secondary follicles which fail to ovulate are common findings in ovaries of untreated, aged rats and mice. Their incidence is strain dependent although they are most common in some strains of mice (Montgomery and Alison, 1987).

Ovaries from such animals, like those reported in man, are characterized by abundant stroma, atypical cystic follicles and few or no corpora lutea. These changes are associated with persistent oestrus and evidence of excessive oestrogen production such as cystic endometrial hyperplasia (Russfield, 1967; Montgomery and Alison, 1987).

In a study in which CD1 female mice were housed one, two, four or eight to a cage for 18 months, the incidence of ovarian cysts (and cystic endometrial hyperplasia) were lowest in the groups housed eight per cage (Chvédoff et al., 1980). Although the cause for this was not clear, other changes occurred which suggested differences in endocrine status between the different groups in this study.

Similar morphological alterations can also be induced by experimental modification of the hypothalamic pituitary-gonadal axis. Administration of testosterone to newborn female rats permanently modifies the feed-back relationship between the hypothalamus, pituitary and ovary so that at maturity, cyclic ovarian function does not occur and persistent oestrus results. Such animals develop polycystic ovaries with increased production of androgens and oestrogens (Barraclough, 1973). Analogous effects are also reported in preclinical safety studies with therapeutic agents which modify cyclical ovarian activity.

An increase in the number of cystic follicles occurred in the safety studies performed with bromocriptine, an ergot compound which stimulates dopamine receptors and inhibits pituitary prolactin secretion (Richardson et al., 1984). When bromocriptine was given to rats mixed in their feed for 53 weeks, increases in the number of cystic follicles and lower numbers of corpora lutea were found. Increased adrenal weights and decreased pituitary weights were also reported in these female rats. The cause of the cystic changes was not clear but they were associated with features of oestrogen dominance, notably in the endometrium. It is probable that bromocriptine mediated its ovarian effects by its pharmacological activity on the hypothalamic-pituitary gonadal axis (Richardson et al., 1984). In addition, small cystic, poorly formed follicles, or cystic corpora lutea (*luteal cysts*) were also observed in dogs treated with bromocriptine for 62 weeks (Richardson et al., 1984).

Tamoxifen, which is widely used as an antioestrogen in the treatment of human mammary cancer, was also shown to reduce the number of corpora lutea and induce the formation of follicular cysts in the ovaries of Alderley Park strain rats treated for three months (Tucker et al., 1984). The changes were shown to be similar to those produced by clomiphene in the same strain of rats and it was suggested that they resulted from an antioestrogenic activity in the rat which resulted in inhibition of positive feedback of oestrogens on the hypothalamic-pituitary axis (Tucker et al., 1984).

Similar cystic ovarian changes associated with an increase in ovarian weight were also described in the marmoset (Callithrix jacchus) treated with tamoxifen for six months. Tamoxifen acts as an antioestrogen in this species. By contrast, cystic ovarian changes were not produced by tamoxifen in the dog. However tamoxifen is primarily an oestrogen in dogs (Tucker et al., 1984).

Another example of cystic ovarian change occurred when rats were treated for two or four weeks with the progesterone antagonist RU486 (van der Schoot et al., 1987). Ovarian changes were characterised by an increase in weight associated with increased numbers of corpora lutea and cysts compared with untreated controls. Some of the cysts became extremely large or showed variable numbers of luteinized cells along their inner walls. In addition, vaginal cyclicity ceased during treatment and uninterrupted vaginal cornification was observed. Pituitary glands were enlarged. It was postulated that these effects were the result of inhibition of the action of progesterone, giving rise to chronic unopposed oestrogenic effects. However, the precise mechanism remains unclear because similar ovarian changes have not been reported in non-human primates and women treated with RU486. It was suggested that the specific effects of RU486 in the rat could have resulted mainly from an action on the pituitary gland by increasing prolactin secretion (van der Schoot et al., 1987).

CGS 18302B, an inhibitor of aromatase, an enzyme important in the conversion of androgens to oestrogens, was also shown to produce cystic ovaries when administered for 13 weeks to beagle dogs (Arthur et al., 1989). An increase in number of corpora lutea was reported in female rats treated with high doses of the non-steroidal anti-androgen, flutamide, for one year (Food and Drug Administration, 1980).

Bursal cysts

In the rodent, cystic dilation of the ovarian bursa should be distinguished from true ovarian or paraovarian cysts. Dilation of the bursa is particularly common in aged mice (Montgomery and Alison, 1987). Irritating agents such as mineral dusts which reach the ovary from the exterior may disrupt drainage of the bursa into the oviducts and cause bursal dilatation or large bursal cysts which can be

661

associated with reactive proliferative changes in the lining epithelium (Hamilton et al., 1984).

Pigmentation

Accumulation of *ceroid* (lipofuscin) pigment is a common age-related change in stromal cells of the rodent ovary, as in a number of other steroid secreting tissues including Leydig cells and adrenal cortex. In the review of ovaries taken from the National Toxicology Program bioassays in Fischer 344 rats and B6C3F1 mice, yellow-brown, periodic-acid-Schiff-positive and acid-fast ceroid pigment was observed in both species but more commonly in mice (Montgomery and Alison, 1987). Ceroid pigment has been reported commonly in other strains of rats such as the SD/JCL strain (Muraoka et al., 1977). Agents which inhibit steroid synthesis such as the imidazol antifungal drugs also potentiate the appearence of lipofuscin in the rodent ovary Other pigments found in the ovary include haemosiderin, presumably as a result of haemorrhage into follicles and corpora lutea. Melanin is reported occasionally in the pigmented B6C3F1 mouse (Montgomery and Alison, 1987).

Fatty change, lipidosis, phospholipidosis

Interstitial, theca and granulosa cells, typical of steroid-producing cells, contain numerous lipid droplets. Inhibition of the synthesis of steroid hormones may allow the accumulation of lipids in the ovarian stromal cell cytoplasm to give rise to histological appearances of fatty change. An example of this phenomenon occured in rats treated with the imidazole antifungal drug, ketoconazol, for six months (Food and Drug Administration, 1981). Both the adrenal cortex and interstitial cells of the ovaries contained increased lipid associated with lipofusion deposition. Imidazol antifungal agents are known to inhibit a variety of P450-mediated reactions including those involved in steroid synthesis. It has been shown that these agents inhibit the rate of 17β-oestradiol production by the ovary in a dose-dependent manner (Latrille et al., 1987).

A number of the extensive list of amphiphilic, cationic drugs capable of inducing *phospholipidosis* in laboratory animals also produce this change in the ovary, particularly in the corpus luteum (Lüllmann-Rauch, 1979).

Miscellaneous degenerative lesions

A variety of degenerative lesions are found in the ovary, sometimes as manifestation of systemic diseases. These changes include mineralization, osseous metaplasia, hyalinization, amyloidosis and alteration in blood vessels, notably arteritis.

Ovarian hyperplasia

Ovarian weight can increase as a result of increase in follicular or luteal mass or stromal hyperplasia. For instance, rats treated with the progesterone antagonist,

RU486, developed increased ovarian weight which was largely the result of increased luteal mass (van der Schoot et al., 1987). A similar phenomenon has also been reported in rats treated with bromocriptine for a short period of time (two or three ovulation cycles), probably as a result of inhibition of the luteolytic action of prolactin in this species (van der Schoot and Uilenbroek, 1983).

Most forms of ovarian hyperplasia observed in preclinical safety studies are forms of stromal and epithelial hyperplasia in the ovaries of aging rats and mice. Various histological types of hyperplasia are observed. These include diffuse focal *adenomatous* proliferation of epithelial-like cells derived from the surface ovarian cells, *tubular or rod-like Sertoli cell* structures or more typical stromal cells with *thecal or granulosa cell* differentiation.

Many of these hyperplasias are commonly associated with age-related loss of ovarian function (Russfield, 1967). However, they also occur when atrophy of the follicular epithelium is induced by treatment with xenobiotics (Maronpot, 1987; Lemon and Gubareva, 1979). When the antibacterial agent, nitrofurantoin, was administered to mice for two years, follicular atrophy was associated with stromal hyperplasia showing tubule-like differentiation (Maronpot, 1987).

Hyperplasia is not limited to rodents. Hyperplasia of the outer cortex and proliferation of the superficial epithelial layer of ovary was reported in dogs treated with tamoxifen for three months (Tucker et al., 1984). Histologically, the findings were characterized by marked and diffuse proliferation of small dark glandular cells in the widened outer cortex of the ovary. The mechanism was uncertain but appeared to be a result of the oestrogenic activity of tamoxifen in the dog, unlike its antioestrogenic activity in man and other species.

Hyperplasia of smooth muscle tissue in the rat mesovarium in association with smooth muscle tumours has also been reported in rats after long term treatment with β-adrenergic drugs (see below).

Neoplasms

A completely satisfactory classification of ovarian neoplasms remains elusive, partly as a result of the wide range and frequently mixed histological patterns which occur both in man and laboratory animals and the uncertain histogenesis of many tumour types. This difficulty is compounded in drug safety evaluation by the need to group neoplasms according to appropriate histogenetic categories, For instance, use of the term 'sertoliform tubular adenoma' may be an accurate descriptive term for an ovarian neoplasm but leaves open the question of whether such tumours should be regarded as epithelial derived from coelomic mesothelium or whether of sex cord-stroma derivation.

It is often more meaningful, as in the case of mesenchymal tumours, to regard ovarian neoplasms as derived from cells which have the multipotential properties of cells of the indifferent gonad which are able to differentiate along several separate pathways. Tumours can be assigned to groups according to their principle differentiation patterns without the assumption that it developed from a mature or differentiated cell of the same type.

On this basis, neoplasms of the ovary fall into two main groups, those showing principally *epithelial differentiation*, analogous to the superficial ovarian 'germinal epithelium' or coelomic mesothelium (see above) and those exhibiting *sexcord-stromal* differentiation patterns. In addition there is a third type in humans, showing evidence of germ cell differentiation.

Whilst tumours of each type have been clearly descibed in both women and laboratory animals, precise differentiation patterns and prevalence of different subtypes are variable between different species and strains.

Tumour induction in the ovary

Although a number of chemical carcinogens, notably polycyclic hydrocarbons are capable of inducing ovarian neoplasia in rodents (Marchant, 1977; Lemon and Gubareva, 1979), administration of non-genotoxic chemicals and a variety of surgical and other experimental procedures are able to induce ovarian neoplasia in rodents. In many of these experimental systems, hyperplasia and neoplasia of ovarian stroma appears to result as a response to destruction of oocytes and granulosa cells with compensatory increase in pituitary gonadotrophin secretion which in turn stimulates the growth of ovarian stromal cells.

Examples of this phenomenon include ovarian vasoligation, thymectomy of mice at three days of age and genetic deletion using inbred strains of mice (Marchant, 1977) as well as the administration of drugs (Stitzel et al., 1989). Although mutational events cannot be entirely excluded, it appears that even ionizing irradiation of the ovaries of rodents acts primarily by destruction of the ovarian follicular apparatus and the disturbance of hypothalamic-pituitary-gonadal autoregulation (Lemon and Gubareva, 1979).

A number of other procedures which disturb pituitary-gonadal function also lead to ovarian neoplasia. These include intrasplenic ovary grafting to castrated rodents, parabiosis with castrated animals and transplantation of gonadotrophic pituitary neoplasms, all of which result in persistently high levels of circulating gonadotrophin levels. Not surprisingly therefore, chronic exposure of rodents to a variety of different hormonal agents which derange the pituitary-gonadal axis also lead to ovarian tumour induction. Many of these different agents appear to act synergistically. For instance, ovarian tumour induction by carcinogens can also be enhanced by hormonal manipulation (Marchant, 1977). It was also concluded that the increased prevalence of benign tubular adenomas reported in the ovaries of female B6C3F1 mice treated for two years with the antibacterial nitrofurantoin was secondary to the prolonged ovarian atrophy induced in this strain by this drug (Stitzel et al., 1989).

Therefore, the rodent ovary represents yet another example of an organ in which excessive stimulation alone appears capable of causing tumorigenesis. The most frequent cell types induced by these experimental procedures as well as those found spontaneously in laboratory rodents are so-called tubular adenomas and granulosa-theca cell tumours. However, the prevalence of a precise tumour type is dependent on the inducing agent as well as genetic factors. For instance,

664

the most frequent tumour type reported in mice after ovarian irradiation is the tubular adenoma although some strains of mice develop granulosa-thecal cell tumours more commonly after a similar regimen (Marchant, 1977).

Epithelial neoplasms of the ovary

Tumours showing epithelial differentiation are some of the commonest neoplasms in adult women where they account for about two thirds of all ovarian tumours and their malignant forms over 85% of all ovarian cancers (Scully, 1977,1978). The histological varieties of epithelial neoplasm found in women however, are not commonly seen in aged rodents. The neoplasms which show pure cystadenomatous differentiation are usually benign and not particularly common neoplasms in rats and most strains of mice (Frith et al., 1981; Carter, 1968; Gregson et al., 1984; Rehm et al., 1984; Alison et al., 1987b). In rats and mice, this tumour is composed of single or multiple cystic or papillary structures covered by cuboidal or low columnar epithelium sometimes with abundant clear cytoplasm but little or no evidence of mucin secretion (Gregson et al., 1984; Alison et al., 1987a). Malignant cystadenomas occasionally occur in the rat and mouse where they may seed widely in the peritoneal cavity (Gregson et al., 1984).

The term *tubular adenoma* or *tubulostromal adenoma* is used to define the adenomatous proliferation found in the aged mouse ovary which appears to be a result of downgrowth of the surface epithelium, sometimes to involve the entire ovary. The affected ovary contains delicate tubules of tumour cells lined by cuboidal epithelium which are separated by nodules or packets of stromal or sex-cord-like cells which sometimes show luteinization (Alison et al., 1987a).

This term is also used for other adenomatous proliferations composed of variants of tubular structures, particularly in the rat but also in the mouse. These other forms of neoplasm are composed of tubular, gland-like structures lined by cuboidal, columnar or solid cellular structures sometimes showing evidence of minimal mucopolysaccharide secretion (Lemon and Gubareva, 1979; Rehm et al., 1984; Gregson et al., 1984). The stromal component is also variable but it may show luteinization or sclerosis.

A complicating factor in both rat and mouse is the presence of Sertoli-cell differentiation in these tubules. the presence of this form of differentiation has given rise to the term *'Sertoliform tubular adenoma'* (Lewis, 1987; Alison et al., 1987a). It is unlikely that this represents an entirely different tumour entity but rather a clear demonstration of the multipotent nature of certain ovarian tumour cells.

A key diagnostic problem as in many other hormone-sensitive tissues is making the distinction between the various forms of glandular hyperplasia found in the ovary and neoplasia. Here too, it is necessary to apply general criteria for evidence of autonomous growth, such as uniform cellular proliferation, expansion and compression of surrounding normal tissues and structures.

Sex-cord: stromal neoplasms

This group of neoplasms comprises those which show differentiation patterns which resemble those tissues which are believed to derive from the sex cords and specialized ovarian stroma of the developing gonad. These include granulosa cells, theca cells, Sertoli cells, Leydig cells, morphologically undifferentiated sex-cord and stromal derivatives (Scully, 1977, 1978). For practical purposes, they can be divided into two main groups, those showing granulosa and thecal differentiation, termed *granulosa-thecal cell tumours* and those showing Sertoli cell differentiation, the so called *Sertoli cell tumours*. As noted above however mixed granulosa and Sertoli cell types are also seen (Knowles, 1983).

These forms of neoplasms are one of the most common forms of ovarian neoplasms in laboratory rodents and in some strains appear to be the most common neoplasms of advancing age (Alison et al., 1987a).

Granulosa cell and thecal cell tumours

Although pure granulosa cell neoplasms occur in both rats and mice, most show various proportions of both granulosa and thecal cell differentiation. However, the granulosa cell component usually predominates. It is generally believed that this group of neoplasms are morphologically identical to tumours of the same name found in women (Lemon and Gubareva, 1979).

The tumours can be unilateral or bilateral growths. Most contain well-differentiated granulosa cells arranged in sheets, cords or pseudofollicles. The cells are regular, small or moderate sized basophilic cells with a high nuclear-cytoplasmic ratio. Mitotic figures are usually only found with difficulty and the sparse cytoplasm often possesses a granular appearance. These cells may occasionally become luteinized, showing enlargement of cell cytoplasm by accumulation of lipids, a polygonal shape, distinct cell boundaries and eccentric location of nuclei (Lemon and Gubareva, 1979).

The thecal component is also variable in histological appearance, composed of spindle cells which are densely packed and frequently arranged bundles and whorls, with variable degrees of interstitial fibrillar ground substance and hyalinization. Mitotic figures are usually sparse in the thecal component.

These tumours infrequently show evidence of invasion or spread outside the confines of the ovary itself but invasion into periovarian tissue and metastatic spread is occasionally reported in rats (Gregson et al., 1984) and mice (Lemon and Gubareva, 1979).

Occasionally, groups of cells are arranged in a tubular manner surrounding eosinophilic, PAS positive material, features of the so called *Call-Exner body*. This feature is not usually prominant in rodent tumours of this type, but they are occasionally seen in well-differentiated granulosa cell tumours of rodents (Frith et al., 1981).

Whilst granulosa cell tumours are generally found in female rodents of advanced age, they occur spontaneously at four to six weeks in SWR/J and

SWR/Bm inbred strains of mice (Beamer et al., 1985). Breeding experiments suggested that this susceptability is familial in nature being transmitted via the fertilized egg rather than through the milk or placenta.

Fibroma

In women, ovarian fibromas are benign neoplasms composed of collagen-forming spindle cells which most frequently develop in middle age and account for about four percent of all ovarian tumours in women (Scully, 1977). Although some ovarian fibromas may arise from the non-specific fibrous stroma, it is believed that the majority are derived from specialized ovarian stromal cells for they show morphological features which overlap with those of the thecoma (Scully, 1977).

Fibromas are only occasionally reported in the ovaries of laboratory animals. However, an unusually high incidence of ovarian fibromas was reported in dogs treated for long periods with the non-progestational androgenic steroid, milbolerone (Seaman, 1985). This tumour was reported in 12 out of 92 dogs treated with mibolerone at pharmacologically efficacious doses for periods of up to nearly ten years whereas none were found in controls and dogs given exaggerated doses for a similar period. These ovarian tumours presented as firm round nodules in the ovarian medulla or hilar zone or larger rounded or multinodular masses which compressed and distorted the cortex. In some dogs multiple and bilateral tumours were found.

Histological examination revealed that the neoplasms were composed of abundant dense fibrous tissue with a relatively sparse population of fibroblast-like cells. The cell cytoplasm was generally scanty and the nuclei appeared small and angular, rounded or elongated with uniform chromatin patterns.

Although some mitotic figures were observed in the neoplastic cells, the tumours remained well-demarcated from the surrounding tissues and showed no evidence of invasion of metastatic spread, although islands of medullary tubules were embedded in the tumour parenchyma. In addition, spindle cells with histological appearances of smooth muscle cells were also described in some of these tumours.

The precise histogenesis of these neoplasms is uncertain and their occurrence in animals treated with pharmacological and not exaggerated doses of mibolerone remains unclear.

Sertoli cell tumours

These neoplasms are characterized by cytological features and growth patterns of Sertoli cells. Well-differentiated forms are characterized by tubules with lumens lined by fairly uniform columnar cells with oval, basally located nuclei and moderate amounts of eosinophilic cytoplasm. The cells contain moderate amounts of lipid and vacuolation of cytoplasm may also be a prominant feature. Leydig cells may be present between the tubules.

These histological appearances may be mixed with other features, including those of granulosa-theca tumours and tubular adenomas (Knowles, 1983). It is important to note that the tubular adenoma described by a number of authors may contain a significant component showing Sertoli cell-differentiation.

Teratomas

Ovarian neoplasms of primary germ cell origin have been sporadically reported in rodents in small numbers over the past years although they are rare in the mouse and even rarer in the rat.

In the studies of over 400 aged Han:NMRI mice with ovarian neoplasm reported by Rehm et al., (1984), only two animals were found with ovarian teratomas. They consisted of keratinizing squamous epithelium, glandular or intestinal mucosa and connective tissue including bone and cartilage. One of the neoplasms developed in conjunction with a granulosa cell tumour.

Whilst a number of large series of rodent ovarian neoplasms have not contained teratomas, the study of Fischer 344 rats and B6C3F1 mice of Alison and collegues (1987a) reported neoplasms showing germ cell differentiation in both species. Teratomas with mature tissue components were observed only in B6C3F1 mice. These neoplasms comprised a wide variety of well-differentiated tissues including skin, hair, sebaceous glands, melanocytes, skeletal muscle, cartilage and bone. Malignant components were essentially immature nervous tissue commonly showing neural rosette formation. Other forms of germ cell neoplasms reported in this study were seven choriocarcinomas and thirteen ovarian yolk sac carcinomas in the B6C3F1 mice and a single neoplasm of each type in the Fischer 344 rats.

Choriocarcinomas are dark, haemorrhagic cystic lesions composed of rounded cytotrophoblastic cells with centrally located, hyperchromatic or vesicular nuclei between 5 and 10 μm diameter and syncytiotrophoblast composed of large irregular cells with abundant granular cytoplasm with single giant bizarre nuclei or multiple more rounded nuclear forms. Immunocytochemical study of choriocarcinomas in B6C3F1 mice has demonstrated a positive granular staining of syncytiotrophoblast cytoplasm using antiserum to human chorionic gonadotrophin (Alison et al., 1987b).

Miscellaneous neoplasms

A variety of other neoplasms are reported in the ovaries of laboratory rodents. These include lesions of the ovarian surface which are similar to classical mesotheliomas and soft tissue tumours including fibrosarcomas, angiomas, angiosarcomas and metastatic neoplasms. The so called 'cystic sarcoma' (see Integumentory System, Chapter I) also occurs in the ovary of the rat. Caution needs to be exercised in the diagnosis of spindle cell ovarian neoplasm of mesenchymal type for these may be similar to tumours showing marked thecal cell differentiation. A special form of soft tissue neoplasm is the mesovarial leiomyoma.

Mesovarial leiomyomas

Prolonged treatment of rats with several different sympathomimetic drugs has been reported to result in the development of benign smooth muscle neoplasms in mesovarial tissues. These agents have included the β-antagonists, soterenol hydrochloride (Nelson and Kelly, 1971,) mesuprine hydrochloride (Nelson et al., 1972), zinterol and reproterol (Jack et al., 1983), mabuterol (Amemiya et al., 1984) as well as salbutamol and terbutaline sulphate (Gopinath and Gibson, 1987).

Leiomyomas were reported to occur after about one year of treatment with these agents and were described as circumscribed, fusiform, oval or spherical dense, white, nodules or irregular masses in the mesovarium extending into the hilar region of the ovary. They are reported more frequently on the right than the left side (Nelson and Kelley, 1971; Gopinath and Gibson, 1987). Histologically, these neoplasms were typical of leiomyomas found elsewhere in rodents, (see Integumentary System Chapter I) being composed of interlacing bundles and whorls of smooth muscle cells with abundant eosinophilic cytoplasm, oval and elongated nuclei with blunt ends exhibiting little or no mitotic activity. These neoplasms showed sharply defined margins, unlike the associated smooth muscle hyperplastic lesions found in the mesovarium of some treated rats. Hyperplastic areas were characterized by irregular, ill-circumscribed increases in smooth muscle cells, showing no compression or distortion of adjacent tissues.

Gopinath and Gibson (1987) showed that these leiomyomas neither progressed nor regressed following a 44-week post-dose recovery period, subsequent to 80 weeks of treatment with salbutamol. Furthermore, lesions were prevented by concurrent administration of the β-blocker, propranolol.

Rarely, identical neoplasms are found in the mesovarium of untreated rats. Gopinath and Gibson (1987) found four cases in 7748 ovaries from aged, Sprague-Dawley rats.

The pathogenesis of sympathomimetic-induced leiomyomas in the rat is unclear. Certain sympathomimetic agents do not induce these tumours. This property appears limited to those which possess β2-agonist activity. It has therefore been suggested that the tumour development may relate to the presence of specific β2-adrenoceptors in mesovarial smooth muscle cells and that it is the prolonged and intense activation of these particular receptors by β2-agonists which mediate smooth muscle relaxation and which, in turn induces smooth muscle proliferation (Apperley et al., 1978; Gopinath and Gibson, 1987). The tumours do not appear to occur in the mouse following identical treatment nor in man treated with this class of drug (Poynter et al., 1979).

REFERENCES

ALISON, R.H., MORGAN, K.T., HASEMAN, J.K. and BOORMAN, G.A. (1987)a: Morphology and classification of ovarian neoplasms in F344 rats and (C57BL/6XC3H)F$_1$ mice. *J.N.C.I.*, 78, 1229–1243.

ALISON, R.H., LEWIS, D.J. and MONTGOMERY, C.A. (1987)b: Ovarian choriocarcinoma in the mouse. *Vet.Pathol.*, 24, 226–230.

AMEMIYA K., KUDOH, M., SUZUKI, H., SAGA, K. and HOSAKA, K. (1984): Toxicity of mabuterol. *Arzneimittelforschung*, 34, 1680–1684.

APPERLEY, G.H., BRITTAIN R.T., COLEMAN, R.A., KENNEDY, I. and LEVY, G.P. (1978): Characterization of the β-adrenoceptors in the mesovarium of the rat. *Br.J.Pharmacol.*, 63, 345–398.

ARTHUR, A.T., McCORMICK, G.G., RICHIG, J.W., PISACRETA, D.J., SULLIVAN, D.J., IVERSON, W.O. and TRAINER, V.M. (1989): Toxicology evaluation of an aromatase inhibitor, CGS 18320B, in dogs. *Toxicologist*, 9, 253.

ATAYA, K.M., MCKANNA, J.A., WEINTRAUB, A.M., CLARK, M.R. and LEMAIRE, W.J. (1985): A luteinizing hormone-releasing hormone agonist for the prevention of chemotherapy-induced ovarian follicular loss in rats. *Cancer Res.*, 45, 3651–3656.

BABA, N. and VON HAAM, E. (1972): Animal model: Spontaneous carcinoma in aged rabbits. *Am.J.Pathol.*, 68, 653–653.

BAKER, T.G. (1971): Radiosensitivity of mammalian oocytes with particular reference to the human female. *Am.J.Obstet Gynecol.*, 110, 746–761.

BAKER, T.G. and NEAL, P. (1977): Actions of ionizing radiations on the mammalian ovary. In: P.L. Zuckerman and B.J. Weir (Eds): *The Ovary*, Vol. 3, pp. 1–58. Academic Press, New York.

BARRACLOUGH, C.A. (1973): Steroid regulation of reproductive neuroendocrine processes. In: R.O. Greep, E.B. Astwood (Eds). *Handbook of Physiology, Section 7, Endocrinology*. Vol. 2. Part 1. pp. 29–56. American Physiological Society Washington D.C.

BEAMER W.G., HOOPE, P.C. and WHITTEN W.K. (1985). Spontaneous malignant granulosa cell tumours in ovaries of young SWR mice. *Cancer Res.*, 45, 5575–5581.

BOURGET, C., FEMINO, A., FRANZ, C. and LONGCOPE, C. (1988): Estrogen and androgen dynamics in the cynomologous monkey. *Endocrinology*, 122, 202–206.

BRIAND.P., HOU-JENSEN, K., THORPE, S.M. and ROSE, C. (1981): Hormone-dependent uterine sarcomas in GR mice. *Eur.J.Cancer*, 17, 635 –641.

BURDEN, H.W., LAWRENCE, I.E., LOUIS T.M. and HODSON, C.A. (1981): Effects of abdominal vagotomy on the estrous cycle of the rat and induction of pseudopregnancy. *Neuroendocrinology*, 33, 218–222.

BUREK, J.D. (1978): Age-related pathology.In: *Pathology of Aging Rats*. Chap. 4, pp. 29–168. CRC Press West Palm Beach, Florida.

CARTER, R.L. (1968) Pathology of ovarian neoplasms in rats and mice. *Eur.J.Cancer*, 3, 537–543.

CHVEDOFF, M., CLARKE M.R., IRISARRI.E., FACCINI,J.M. and MONRO, A.M. (1980): Effects of housing conditions on food intake, body weight and spontaneous lesions in mice. A review of the literature and results of an 18-month study. *Food Cosmet.Toxicol.*, 18, 517–522.

COTCHIN, E. (1977): Spontaneous tumours of the uterus and ovaries in animals. In: E. Cotchin and J. Marchant (Eds). *Animal Tumors of the Female Reproductive Tract. Spontaneous and Experimental*, Chap. 2, pp. 26–65. Springer Verlag, New York.

CRAIG, S.S and JOLLIE, W.P. (1985): Age changes in density of endometrial stromal cells of the rat. *Exp.Gerontol*, 20, 93–97.

CROSSEN, R.J. and SUNTZEFF, V. (1950): Endometrial polyps and hyperplasia produced in an aged monkey with estrogen plus progesterone. *Arch.Pathol.*, 50, 721–726.

CUNHA, G.R., CHUNG.L.W.K., SHANNON, J.M., TAGUCHI, O. and FUJII, H. (1983): Hormone-induced morphogenesis and growth: Role of mesenchymal epithelial interactions. *Recent Prog.Horm.Res.*, 39, 559–598.

DOBSON, R.L. and FELTON, J.S. (1983): Female germ cell loss from radiation and chemical exposures. *Am.J.Ind.Med.*, 4, 175–190.

DUNAIF, A.E., ZIMMERMAN, E.A., FRIESEN, H.G. and FRANTZ, A.G. (1982): Intracellular localization of prolactin receptor and prolactin in the rat ovary by immunocytochemistry. *Endocrinology*, 110, 1465–1471.

ECKSTEIN, P. and ZUCKERMAN, S. (1960)a: Morphology of the reproductive tract. IN: A.S. Parkes (Ed.). *Marshall's Physiology of Reproduction*. Vol. 1, Part 1, Chap. 2, pp. 43–155. Longmans, London.

ECKSTEIN, P. and ZUCKERMAN, S. (1960)b: The oestrous cycle in the mammalia. In: A.S. Parkes (Ed.). *Marshall's Physiology of Reproduction*. Vol. 1, Part 1, Chap 4, pp. 226–396. Longmans, London.

ECKSTEIN, P. and ZUCKERMAN, S. (1960)c. Changes in the accessory reproductive organs of the non-pregnant female. In: A.S. Parkes (Ed.). *Marshall's Physiology of Reproduction*. Vol. 1, Part 1, Chap. 6. pp. 543–654. Longmans, London.

ECKSTEIN, P., JACKSON, M.C.N., MILLMAN, N. and SOBRERO, A.J. (1969): Comparison of vaginal tolerance tests of spermicidal preparations in rabbits and monkeys. *J.Reprod.Fertil.*, 20, 85–93.

ERSKINE, M.S. and WEAVER, C.E. (1988): The role of ovarian sympathetic innervation in the control of estrous responsiveness in the rat. *Horm.Behav.*, 22, 1–11.

FELICIO, L.S., NELSON, J.F. and FINCH, C.E. (1986): Prolongation and cessation of estrous cycles in aging C57BL/6J mice are differentially regulated events. *Biol.Reprod.*, 34, 849–858.

FERENCZY, A. (1979): Anatomy and histology of the cervix. In: A. Blaustein (Ed.). *Pathology of the Female Genital Tract*. pp. 102 –123. Springer-Verlag, New York.

FERIN, M. (1983): Neuroendocrine control of ovarian function in the primate. *Reprod.Fertil.*, 63, 369–381.

FITZGERALD, J., DE LA IGLESIA, F. and GOLDENTHAL, E.I. (1982): Ten-year oral toxicity study with norlestrin in rhesus monkeys. *J.Toxicol.Environ.Health.*, 10, 879–896.

FOOD AND DRUG ADMINISTRATION (1980): Pharmacology and Toxicology Review of Flutamide *NDA*, 18–554. Washington D.C.

FOOD AND DRUG ADMINISTRATION (1981): Ketoconazole. Summary Basis of Approval. *NDA*, 18–533. Washington D.C.

FORSBERG, J.G. (1975): Late effects in the vaginal and cervical epithelia after injections of diethylstilbestrol into neonatal mice. *Am.J.Obstet.Gynecol.*, 121, 101–104.

FOWLER, E.H., FELDMAN, M.K. and LOEB, W.F. (1971): Comparison of histologic features of ovarian and uterine tissues with vaginal smears of the bitch. *Am.J.Vet.Res.*, 32, 327–334.

FRITH, C.H., ZUNA, R.E. and MORGAN, K. (1981): A morphological classification and incidence of spontaneous ovarian neoplasms in three strains of mice. *J.N.C.I.*, 67, 693–702.

GIBSON, J.P., SELLS, D.M., CHENG, H.C. and YUH, L. (1987): Induction of uterine leiomyomas in mice by medroxalol and prevention by propranolol. *Toxicol.Pathol.*, 15, 468–473.

GILKS, C.B., REID, P.E., CLEMENT, P.B. and OWEN, D.A. (1988): Simple procedure for assessing relative quantities of neutral and acidic sugars in mucin glycoproteins: its use in assessing cyclical changes in cervical mucins. *J.Clin.Pathol.*, 41, 1021–1024.

GITLIN, G. (1954): On the mode of development of stratified squamous epithelium in the rat's uterus following prolonged estrogen administration. *Anat.Rec.*, 120, 637–655.

GOODMAN, D.G., WARD, J.M., SQUIRE, R.A., PAXTON, M.B. REICHARDT, W.D., CHU, K.C. AND LINHART, M.S. (1980): Neoplastic and non-neoplastic lesions in aging Osborne. Mendel rats. *Toxicol.Appl.Pharmacol.*, 55, 443–447.

GOPINATH, C. and GIBSON, W.A. (1987): Mesovarian leiomyomas in the rat. *Environ.Health Perspect.*, 73, 107–113.

GRAY, J.E., WEAVER, R.N., LOHRBERG, S.M. and LARSEN, E.R. (1984): Comparative responses of vaginal mucosa to chronic pyrimidinone-induced irritation. *Toxicol.Pathol.*, 12, 228–234

GREAVES, P. and FACCINI, J.M. (1984): Female genital tract. In: *Rat Histopathology. A Glossary for use in Toxicity and Carcinogenicity Studies*. Chap. 9, pp. 171–186. Elsevier, Amsterdam.

GREENMAN, D.L. and DELONGCHAMP, R.R. (1986): Interactive responses to diethylstilboestrol in C3H mice. *Food Chem.Toxicol.*, 24, 931–934.

GREGSON, R.L., LEWIS, D.J. and ABBOTT, D.P. (1984): Spontaneous ovarian neoplasms of the laboratory rat. *Vet.Pathol.*, 21,292–299.

GUTTNER, J (1980): Adenomyosis in mice. *Z.Versuchstierkd.*, 22, 249–251.

HAMILTON, T.C., FOX, H., BUCKLEY C.H., HENDERSON, W.J. and GRIFFITHS, K. (1984): Effects of talc on the rat ovary. *Br.J.Exp.Pathol.*, 65, 101–106.

HANEY, A.F. (1987): Endocrine and anatomical correlations in human ovarian pathology. *Environ.Health Perspect.*, 73, 5–14.

HART ELCOCK, L., STUART, B.P., MUELLER, R.E. and HOSS, H.E. (1987): Deciduoma, uterus rat. In: T.C. Jones, U. Mohr and R.D. Hunt (Eds), *Genital System*, pp. 140–146. Springer-Verlag, Berlin.

HENDERSON W.J., HAMILTON, T.C., BAYLIS, M.S., PIERREPOINT, C.G and GRIFFITHS, K. (1986): The demonstration of the migration of talc from the vagina and posterior uterus to the ovary in the rat. *Environ.Res.*, 40, 247–250.

HENDERSON, W.J., JOSLIN, C.A.F., TURNBULL, A.C. and GRIFFITHS, K. (1971): Talc and carcinoma of the ovary and cervix. *J.Obstet. Gynaecol.Brit.Commonw.*, 78, 266–272.

HERTIG, A.T. and GORE, H. (1960): Endomyometrium. In: *Tumors of the Female Sex Organs. Part 2. Tumors of the Vulva, Vagina and Uterus*, pp. 177–261. Armed Forces Institute of Pathology, Washington D.C.

HIGHMAN, B., NORVELL, M.J. and SHELLENBERGER, T.E. (1977): Pathological changes in female C3H mice continuously fed diets containing diethylstilbestrol or 17β-estradiol. *J.Environ.Pathol.*, 1, 1–30.

HUGHESDON, P.E. and SYMMERS, W. St C. (1978): Gynaecological pathology. In: *Systemic Pathology*, W. StC. Symmers, (Ed.), 2nd Ed., Vol 4, Chap. 27, pp. 1599–1758. Churchill Livingstone, Edinburgh.

HUSEBY, R.A. and THURLOW, S. (1982): Effects of prenatal exposure of mice to 'low dose' diethylstilbestrol and the development of adenomyosis associated with evidence of hypoprolactinemia. *Am.J.Obstet.Gynecol.*, 144, 939–949.

IARC. (1979): Sex hormones. *Monogr.Eval.Carcinog.Risk Chem.Hum.*, Vol. 21, pp. 131–134. International Agency for Research on Cancer, Lyon.

JACK, D., POYNTER, D. and SPURLING, N.W. (1983): Beta adrenoceptor stimulants and mesovarian leiomyomas in the rat. *Toxicology*, 27, 315–320.

JARRELL, J., YOUNG LAI, E.V., BARR, R., MCMAHON, A., BELBECK, L. and O'CONNEL.G. (1987): Ovarian toxicity of cyclophosphamide alone and in combination with ovarian irradiation in the rat. *Cancer Res.*, 47, 2340–2343.

JOHNSON, A.N. (1989): Comparative aspects of contraceptive steroids. Effects observed in beagle dogs. *Toxicol.Pathol.*, 17, 389–395.

KALRA, S.P. and KALRA, P.S. (1983): Neural regulation of luteinizing hormone secretion in the rat. *Endocr.Rev.*, 4, 311–351.

KAMINSKY, M., SZIVOS, M.M. and BROWN, K.R. (1985): Comparison of the sensitivity of the vaginal mucous membranes of the albino rabbit and laboratory rat to nonoxynol-9. *Food Chem. Toxicol.*, 23, 705–708.

KNOWLES, J.F. (1983): Cancer of rat ovaries: Sertoli cell or granulosa-theca cell tumours? *Br.J. Cancer*, 48, 301–305.

KOMOROWSKI, R.A., GARANCIS, J.C and CLOWRY, L.J. (1970): Fine structure of endometrial stromal sarcoma. *Cancer*, 26,1042–1047.

KORACH, K.S. and QUARMBY, V.E. (1985): Morphological, physiological, and biochemical aspects of female reproduction. In: R.L. Dixon (ed.), *Reproductive Toxicology*, pp. 47–68. Raven Press, New York.

KROES, R., GARBIS-BERKVENS, J.M., de VRIES, T. and van NESSELROOY, J.H.J. (1981): Histopathological profile of a Wistar rat stock including a survey of the literature. *J.Gerontol.*, 36, 259–279.

LATRILLE, F., CHARUEL, C., MONRO, A.M., STADLER, J. and SUTTER, B, Ch, J. (1987): Imidazole antifungal agents reduce production of 17β-oestradiol by rat ovaries in vitro. *Biochem.Pharmacol.*, 36, 1863–1866.

672

LEMON, P.G. and GUBAREVA, A.V. (1979): Tumours of the ovary. In: V.S. Turusov (Ed.): *Pathology of tumours of laboratory animals. Vol. 2, Tumors of the mouse*, pp. 385–410. IARC Scientific Publ. 23, Lyon.

LEWIS, D.J. (1987): Ovarian neoplasia in the Sprague Dawley rat. *Environ.Health.Perspect.*, 73, 77–90.

LIPSCHÜTZ, A., IGLESIAS, R., PANASEVICH, V.I. and SALINAS, S. (1967). Pathological changes induced in the uterus of mice with the prolonged administration of progesterone and 19-nor-contraceptives. *Br.J.Cancer,*

LIPSCHÜTZ, A. and VARGLAS, L., Jr.(1941) Structure and origin of uterine and extragenital fibroids induced experimentally in the guinea pig by prolonged administration of estrogens. *Cancer Res.*, 1, 236–249.

LITTLEFIELD, N.A., BLACKWELL, B.N., HEWITT, C.C. and GAYLOR, D.W. (1985): Chronic toxicity and carcinogenicity studies of gentian violet in mice. *Fundam.Appl.Toxicol.*, 5, 902–912.

LOEB, L., SUNTZEFF, V. and BURNS, E.L. (1938): Growth processes induced by estrogenic hormones in the uterus of the mouse. *Am.J.Cancer*, 34, 413–427.

LÜLLMANN-RAUCH, R., (1979): Drug related lysosomal storage disorders. In: J.T.Dingle, P.J. Jacques and I.H. Shaw (Eds), *Lysosomes in Applied Biology and Therapeutics*, Chap. 3, pp. 49–130. North Holland, Amsterdam.

LUMB, G., MITCHELL, L and DE LA IGLESIA, F.A. (1985) Regression of pathologic changes induced by the long-term administration of contraceptive steroids to rodents. *Toxicol.Pathol.*, pp. 13, 283–295.

MARONPOT, R.R. (1987): Ovarian toxicity and carcinogenicity in eight recent National Toxicology Program studies. *Environ.Health Perspect.*, 73, 125–130.

MARCHANT, J. (1977): Animal models for tumours of the ovary and uterus. In: E. Cotchin and J. Marchant (Eds), *Animal Tumours of the Female Reproductive tract: Spontaneous and Experimental*, Chap. 1, pp. 1–25. Springer-Verlag, New York.

MATTISON, D.R. (1983): The mechanisms of action of reproductive toxins. *Am.J.Ind.Med.*, 4, 65–79.

MATTISON, D.R., SHIROMIZU, K. and NIGHTINGALE, M.S. (1983): Oocyte destruction by polycyclic aromatic hydrocarbons. *Am.J.Ind.Med.*, 4, 191–202.

MCNEILLY, A.S., GLASIER, A., JONASSEN, J. and HOWIE, P.W. (1982): Evidence for direct inhibition of ovarian function by prolactin. *J.Reprod.Fertility*, 65, 559–569.

MEISSNER, W.A., SOMMERS, S.C. and SHERMAN, G. (1957): Endometrial hyperplasia, endometrial carcinoma and endometriosis produced experimentally by estrogen. *Cancer*, 10, 500–509.

MEITES, J., HUANG, H.H. and SIMPKINS, J.W. (1978): Recent studies on neuroendocrine control of reproductive senescence in rats. In: E.L. Schneider (Ed.). *The Aging Reproductive System*. Aging, Vol. 4, pp. 213–135. Raven Press, New York.

MINAMOTO, T, ARAI, K., HIRAKAWA, S. and NAGAI, Y. (1987): Immunohistochemical studies on collagen types in the uterine cervix in pregnant and non-pregnant states. *Am.J.Obstet. Gynecol.*, 156, 138–144.

MONTGOMERY, C.A. and ALISON, R.H. (1987): Non-neoplastic lesions of the ovary in Fischer 344 rats and B6C3F1 mice. *Environ.Health Perspect.*, 73, 53–75.

MORI, T. and NAGASAWA, H. (1983): Mechanisms of development of prolactin-induced adenomyosis in mice. *Acta.Anat.*, 116, 46–54.

MORI, T., NAGASAWA, H. and TAKAHASHI, S. (1981). The induction of adenomyosis in mice by intrauterine pituitary isografts. *Life Sci.*, 29, 1277–1282.

MORIKAWA, S., SEKIYA, S., NAITOH, M., IWASAWA.H., TAKEDA, B. and TAKAMIZAWA, H. (1982): Spontaneous occurence of atypical hyperplasia and adenocarcinoma of the uterus in androgen-sterilized SD rats. *J.N.C.I.*,69, 95–101.

MOSSMAN, H.W. and DUKE, K.L. (1973a): Gross anatomy of the mammalian ovary. In: *Comparative Morphology of the Mammalian Ovary*, Chap. 1, pp.3–33. University of Wisconsin Press, Madison.

MOSSMAN.H.W. and DUKE, K.L. (1973b). Comparative morphology of specific ovarian tissues and

673

structures.In: *Comparative Morphology of the Mammalian Ovary*, Chap. 6, pp. 117–233. University of Wisconsin Press, Madison.

MUNOZ, N., DUNN, T.B. and TURUSOV, V.S. (1979): Tumours of the vagina and uterus. In: V.S. Turusov (Ed.), *Pathology of Tumours in Laboratory Animals*. Vol. 2, Tumours of the Mouse, pp. 359–383. IRAC Scientific Publ. No. 23, Lyon.

MURAOKA, Y., ITOH, M., MAEDA, Y. and HAYASHI, Y. (1977): Histological change of various organs in aged SD-JCL rats. *Jikken Dobutsu Exp.Anim.* 26, 1–12.

MUSE, K., WILSON, E.A. and JAWAD, M.J. (1982): Prolactin hyperstimulation in response to thyrotropin-releasing hormone in patients with endometriosis. *Fertil.Steril.*, 38, 419–422.

NAGASAWA, H. and MORI, T. (1982): Stimulation of mammary tumorigenesis and suppression of uterine adenomyosis by temporary inhibition of pituitary prolactin secretion during youth in mice. *Proc.Soc.Exp.Biol.Med.*, 171, 164–167.

NELSON, J.F. and FELICIO, L.S. (1985): Reproductive aging in the female: An etiological perspective. *Rev.Biol.Res.Aging*, 2, 251–314.

NELSON, L.W. and KELLY, W.A. (1971): Mesovarial leiomyomas in rats in a chronic toxicity study of soterenol hydrochloride. *Vet.Pathol.*, 8, 452–457.

NELSON, L.W., KELLY, W.A. and WEIKEL, J.H. (1972): Mesovarial leiomyomas in rats in a chronic toxicity study of mesuprine hydrochloride. *Toxicol.Appl.Pharmacol.*, 23, 731–737.

NICOSIA, S.V., MATUS-RIDLEY, M. and MEADOWS, A.T. (1985). Gonadal effects of cancer therapy in girls. *Cancer*, 55, 2364–2372.

NORRIS, H.J. and TAYLOR, H.B. (1966). Mesenchymal tumours of the uterus. A clinical and pathological study of 53 endometrial stromal tumours. *Cancer*, 19, 755–766.

OAKBERG, E.F. and CLARKE, E. (1964). Species comparison of radiation response of the gonads. In: W.D. Carlson, and F.X. Gassner (Eds): *Effects of Ionizing Radiation on the Reproductive System*, pp. 11–24. Pergamon Press, Oxford.

OHTA, Y. (1987): Age-related decline in deciduogenic ability of the rat uterus. *Biol.Reprod.*, 37, 779–785.

OSTRANDER, P.L., MILLS, K.T. and BERN, H.A. (1985). Long-term responses of the mouse uterus to neonatal diethylstilbestrol treatment and to later sex hormone exposure. *J.N.C.I.*, 74, 121–135.

PAPANICOLAOU, G.N. (1933). Sexual cycle in human female as revealed by vaginal smears. *Arr.J.Anat.(Suppl)* 52, 519–637.

PLAPINGER, L. and BERN, H.A. (1979): Adenosis-like lesions and other cervicovaginal abnormalities in mice treated perinatally with estrogen. *J.N.C.I.*, 63, 507–518.

POUR, P., MOHR, P., ALTHOFF, J., CARDESA, A. and KMOCH, N. (1976): Spontaneous tumours of common diseases in two colonies of Syrian hamsters. III Urogenital system and endocrine glands. *J.N.C.I.*, 56, 949–961.

POYNTER, D., HARRIS, D.M. and JACK, D. (1978): Salbutamol, lack of evidence of tumour induction in man. *Br.Med.J.*, 6104, 46–47.

PURCHASE, I.F.H. (1980): Inter-species comparisons of carcinogenicity. *Br.J.Cancer*, 41, 454–468.

QUIGLEY, M.E., SHEEHAN, K.L., CASPER, R.F. and YEN, S.S.C. (1980): Evidence for an increased opioid inhibition of luteinizing hormone secretion in hyperprolactinemic patients with pituitary microadenoma. *J.Clin.Endocrinol.Metab.*, 50, 427–430.

RAO, G.N., HICKMAN, R.L., SEILKOP, S.K. and BOORMAN (1987): Utero-ovarian infection in aged B6C3FI mice. *Lab.Anim.Sci.*, 37, 153–158.

REHM, S., DIERKSEN, D. and DEERBERG, F. (1984): Spontaneous ovarian tumours in Han:NMRI mice: Histologic classification, incidence, and influence of food restriction. *J.N.C.I.*, 72, 1383–1395.

REICHART, R.M. (1973): Cervical intraepithelial neoplasia. In: S.C. Sommers (Ed), *Pathol.Annu.*, pp. 301–328. Prentice Hall, New York.

REICHLIN, S. (1985): Neuroendocrinology. In: J.D. Wilson and D.W. Foster (Eds): *William's Textbook of Endocrinology*, 7th Ed., Chap. 17, pp. 492–567. Saunders, Philadelphia.

REUBER, M.D., VLAHAKIS, G. and HESTON, W.E. (1981): Spontaneous hyperplastic and neoplastic lesions of the uterus in mice. *J.Gerontol.*, 36, 663–673.

674

RICHARDS, J.S. (1978): Hormonal control of follicular growth and maturation in mammals: In R.E. Jones (Ed.), *The Vertebrate Ovary*, pp. 331–360. Plenum Press, New York.

RICHARDSON, B.P., TURKALJ, I. and FLÜCKIGER, E. (1984): Bromocriptine. In: D.R. Laurence, A.E.M. McLean and M. Weatherall (Eds): *Safety Testing of New Drugs Laboratory Predictions and Clinical Performance*, Chap. 3, pp. 19–63. Academic Press, London.

ROBBOY, S.J., WELCH, W.R. and PRAT, J. (1982): Intrauterine exposure to diethylstilbestrol. In: R.H. Riddell (Ed.), *Pathology of Drug-Induced and Toxic Diseases*. Appendix to Chap. 13, pp. 325–340, Churchill Livingstone, New York.

ROSS, G.T. (1985): Disorders of the ovary and female reproductive tract. In: J.D Wilson and D.W. Foster (Eds): *William's Textbook of Endocrinology*, 7th Ed. Chap. 9, pp. 206–258, Saunders, Philadelphia.

ROTHSCHILD, T.C., CALHOON, R.E. and BOYLAN, E.S. (1988): Effects of diethylstilbestrol exposure in utero on the genital tracts of female ACI rats. *Exp.Mol.Toxicol.*, 48, 59–76.

RUSSFIELD, A..B. (1967): Pathology of the endocrine glands ovary and testis of rats and mice. In: E. Cotchin and F.J.C. Roe (Eds), *Pathology of Laboratory Rats and Mice*, Chap. 14, pp. 391–466. Blackwell Scientific, Oxford.

SANDOW, J. (1983): The regulation of LHRH action at the pituitary and gonadal receptor level: a review. *Psychoendocrinology*, 8, 277–297.

SASS, B. (1981): Mixed mesenchymal tumours of the mouse uterus. *Lab. Anim.*, 15, 365–369.

SCHADE, R.O.K. (1960): History of cytology. In: *Gastric Cytology. Principles, Methods and Results*, Chap. 2, pp. 4–5. Arnold, London.

SCHAEFER, F.V., CUSTER, R.P. and SOROF, S. (1982): General process of induction of squamous metaplasia by cyclic adenine nucleotide and prostaglandins: Mouse prostate glands. *Cancer Res.*, 42, 3682–3687.

SCHAERDEL, A.D. (1986): Pelvic endometriosis associated with infarctions of the colon in a rhesus monkey. *Lab.Anim.Sci.*, 36, 533–536.

SCHARDEIN, J.L. (1980a): Studies of the components of an oral contraceptive agent in albino rats. 1. Estrogenic component. *J.Toxicol.Environ.Health*, 6, 885–894.

SCHARDEIN, J.L. (1980b): Studies of the components of an oral contraceptive agent in albino rats. 11. Progestogenic component and comparison of effects of the components and the combined agent. *J.Toxicol.Environ.Health*, 6, 895–906.

SCHARDEIN, J.L., KAUMP, D.H., WOOSLEY, E.T. and JELLEMA, M.M. (1970): Long term toxicologic and tumorigenesis studies on an oral contraceptive agent in albino rats. *Toxicol.Appl. Pharmacol.*, 16, 10–23.

SCHUTTE, A.P. (1967): Canine vaginal cytology. I. Technique and Cytological Morphology. *J.Small Anim.Pract.*, 8, 301–306.

SCULLY, R.E. (1977): Ovarian tumors. A review. *Am.J.Pathol.*, 87, 686–720.

SCULLY, R.E. (1978): Common 'epithelial tumors'. In: Tumors of the ovary and maldeveloped gonads. *Atlas of Tumor Pathology*, Second Series, Fascicle, 16, pp. 53–54. Armed Forces Institute of Pathology, Washington, D.C.

SEAMAN, W.J. (1985): Canine ovarian fibroma associated with prolonged exposure to mibolerone. *Toxicol.Pathol.*, 13, 177 –180.

SELLS, D.M. and GIBSON, J.P. (1987): Carcinogenicity studies with medroxal hydrochloride in rats and mice. *Toxicol.Pathol.*, 15, 457–467.

SHIROMIZU, K., TORGEIRSSON, S.S. and MATTISON, D. (1984): The effect of cyclophosphamide on oocyte and follicle number in Sprague-Dawley rats, C57BL/CN and DBA/2N mice. *Pediatr. Pharmacol.*,(New York) 4, 213–221.

SMITH, C.G. (1983): Reproductive toxicity: Hypothalamic-pituitary mechanisms. *Am.J.Ind.Med.*, 4, 107–112.

SNELL, K. (1965): Spontaneous lesions of the rat. In: W.E. Ribelin and J.R. McCoy (Eds), *The Pathology of Laboratory Animals*, pp. 241–300. Charles C Thomas, Springfield. Ill.

STERNFELD, M.D., WEST, N.B. and BRENNER, R.M. (1988): Immunocytochemistry of the estrogen receptor in spontaneous endometriosis in rhesus macaques. *Fert.Steril.*, 49, 342–348.

STEWART, H.L., DERINGER, M.K., DUNN, T.B. and SNELL, K.C. (1974): Malignant schwannomas of nerve roots, uterus and epididymis in mice. *J.N.C.I.*, 53, 1749–1758.

STITZEL, K.A., McCONNELL, R.F. and DIERCKMAN, T.A. (1989) Effects of nitro-furantoin on the primary and secondary reproductive organs of female B6C3F mice. *Toxicol.Pathol.*, 17, 774–781.

STOCKARD, C.R. and PAPANICOLAOU, G.N. (1917): The existence of a typical estrous cycle in the guinea pig: with a study of its histological and physiological changes. *Am.J.Anat.*, 22, 225–283.

TSUNG, K.S., SMITH, S., TEUSCHER, C., COOK, C. and ANDERSON, R.E. (1987): Murine autoimmune oophoritis, epididymoorchitis, and gastritis induced by day 3 thymectomy. Immunopathology. *Am.J. Pathol.*, 126, 293–302.

TUCKER, M.J., ADAM, H.K. and PATTERSON, J.S. (1984): Tamoxifen. In: D.R. Laurence, A.E.M. McLean and M. Weatherall (Eds), *Safety Testing of New Drugs. Laboratory Predictions and Clinical Performance*, Chap. 6, pp. 125–161. Academic Press, London.

VALERIO, M.G., (1989) Comparative aspects of contraceptive steroids: Effects observed in the monkey. *Toxicol.Pathol.*, 17, 401–410.

VAN NIE, R., BENEDETTI, E.L. and MUHLBOCK, O. (1961): A carcinogenic action of testosterone, provoking uterine tumours in mice. *Nature*, 192, 1303.

VAN DER SCHOOT, P., BAKKER, G.H. and KLIJN, J.G.M. (1987): Effects of the progesterone antagonist RU 486 on ovarian activity in the rat. *Endocrinology*, 121, 1375–1382.

VAN DER SCHOOT, P., and UILENBROEK, J. Th. J (1983): Reduction of 5 day cycle length of female rats by treatment with bromocriptine. *J.Endocrinol*, 97, 83–89.

WALKER, B.E. (1983): Uterine tumours in old female mice exposed prenatally to diethylstilbestrol. *J.N.C.I.*, 70, 477–484.

WADSWORTH, P.F., HEYWOOD, R., ALLEN, R.M., (1979). Treatment of rhesus monkeys (Macaca mulatta) with intrauterine devices loaded with levonorgestrel. *Contraception*, 21, 177–184.

WAXMAN, J. (1983): Chemotherapy and the adult gonad: A review. *J.R.Soc.Med.*, 76, 144–148.

WEISBROTH, S.H. (1974): Neoplastic diseases. In: S.H. Weisbroth, R.E. Flatt and A.L. Kraus (Eds): *The Biology of the Laboratory Rabbit*, Chap. 14, pp. 331–375. Academic Press, New York.

WIKLUND, J., WERTZ, N. and GORSKI, J. (1981): A comparison of estrogen effects on uterine and pituitary growth and prolactin synthesis in F344 and Holtzman rats. *Endocrinology*, 109, 1700–1707.

WINKLER, B., NORRIS, H.J. and FENOGLIO, C.M. (1982): The female genital tract. In: R.H. Riddell (Ed.). *Pathology of Drug-induced and Toxic Diseases*, Chap. 13, pp. 297–234. Churchill Livingstone, New York.

WOLFE, J.M., BURACK, E., LANSING, W. and WRIGHT, A.W. (1942): Th effects of advancing age on the connective tissue of the uterus, cervix and vagina of the rat. *Am.J.Anat.*, 70, 135–165.

WONG, L.M., BERN, H.A., JONES, L.A. and MILLS, K.T. (1982): Effect of later treatment with estrogen on reproductive tract lesions in neonatally estrogenized mice. *Cancer Lett.*, 17, 115–123.

WRIGHT, T.C. (1987): Characterization of keratins from rat cervical epithelial cells in vivo and vitro. *Cancer Res.*, 47, 6678–6685.

WUTTKE, W. and MEITES, J. (1971): Luteolytic role of prolactin during the estrous cycle of the rat. *Proc.Soc.Exp.Biol.Med.*, 137, 988–991.

YOSHINAGA-HIRABAYASHI, T., ISHIMURA, K., FUJITA, H., INANO, H., ISHII-OHBA, H. and TAMAOKI, B. (1987): Immunocytochemical localization of 17β-hydroxysteroid dehydrogenase (17β-HSH), and its relation to the ultrastructure of steroidogenic cells in immature and mature rat ovaries. *Arch.Histol,Jpn.*, 50, 545–556.

XII. Endocrine Glands

The capacity of the mammalian organism to function as an integrated unit is made possible by two principle control mechanisms, that of the nervous system and that of the endocrine system. Although the endocrine system has been traditionally regarded as a system of glands capable of releasing chemical mediators which act on targets distant from the site of production, this distinction has become less sharp over recent years. It has become evident that there are intimate links between the nervous and endocrine systems at the level of the hypothalamus and pituitary gland which serves to coordinate the two systems into one control unit. The nervous system also releases chemical substances which not only act as local mediators but also as circulating hormones. Conversely, hormones released by cells in endocrine glands have local effects in the cells in which they are synthesized.

It is particularly important to consider the immense complexity of these inter-relationships in the histopathological assessment of safety studies. Although endocrine organs are usually resistant to direct toxic effects of xenobiotics, they are extremely sensitive to stimulation or inhibition by a variety of trophic or anti-trophic substances and by end-organ feedback. Not only may changes in endocrine organs occur following administration of hormones, hormone modulators, trophic factors and their synthetic analogues but also when high doses of other pharmaceutical agents are administered for long periods with subsequent derangement of endocrine homeostasis. The interpretation of findings in high dose studies is made more difficult by the complex interaction of age, strain, seasonal and circadian periodicity in pituitary, thyroid, parathyroid, gonadal and adrenal hormones, even in laboratory animals raised and maintained in constant laboratory conditions (Wong et al., 1983a,b).

Furthermore, several lines of evidence indicate that the secretory function of endocrine tissue is closely related to proliferation of endocrine cells (Pawlikowski, 1982). This concords with the general observations that a common response to prolonged and excessive glandular stimulation is endocrine hyperplasia and eventually neoplasia. This can lead to major problems in the interpretation of glandular changes in high dose toxicity studies.

677

Interpretation of proliferative changes in glandular tissue in toxicity studies is also clouded by the fact that laboratory animals, particularly rodents, develop hyperplasia and neoplasia of endocrine tissues spontaneously with advancing age, possibly in part as a result of artificial environments and abnormal physiological status. The distinction between hyperplasia, benign and malignant neoplasia on morphological grounds is a further problem which bedevils the interpretation of drug induced changes in endocrine tissue.

Faced with apparent treatment-related changes in endocrine organs, the pathologist needs to fully characterize the changes with particular regard to the cell type involved for this may give important clues to pathogenesis. Critical evaluation of endocrine sensitive tissues such as mammary glands and reproductive organs also provides important information about the nature of changes in endocrine organs.

A powerful tool in the characterization of specific endocrine and neuroendocrine cells and their products is immunocytochemistry (Hökfelt et al., 1980). Immunocytochemical study using antisera to hormones and other antigens in endocrine-sensitive tissue now has an important place in the characterization of the effects of drugs on the endocrine system (El Etreby, 1981). Furthermore, in-situ DNA and RNA hybridization histochemistry with probes complementary to nuclei acid sequences for hormones or polypeptide sequences is another powerful technique for localizing endogeneous products and mRNA coding for specific proteins in individual endocrine cells and studying the changes produced by xenobiotics (Gee et al., 1983; Lloyd and Landefeld, 1986; Chronwall et al., 1987).

Despite the relative frequency with which endocrine pathology is observed in preclinical safety studies, endocrine changes are less commonly observed in subsequent clinical studies in man. In the pilot study by Fletcher (1978) which compared findings in animal safety tests, filed at the Committee on Safety of Medicines (CSM) in England with adverse effects reported in subsequent clinical studies, only about one in ten drugs with hormonal effects in animals showed hormonal effects in man.

Hormones fall into two main groups. The majority are polypeptides of various sizes or aminoacid derivatives. The remainder are steroids derived from cholesterol, either with an intact steroid nucleus or those such as vitamin D and its metabolites with a broken B ring. They are synthesized in a similar way to other cell products by processes and pathways common to many cells. A hormone may not only have multiple actions but a single function can also be controlled by many hormones. This allows fine tuning of control and provides a fail-safe function when one hormone in a series is deficient (Wilson and Foster, 1985).

PITUITARY GLAND

The pituitary gland or hypophysis is composed of an *anterior lobe* or adenohypophysis, embryonically derived from the hypophyseal recess or Rathke's pouch (oropharangeal ectoderm) and a *posterior lobe* or neurohypophysis developing from diencephalic neuroectoderm. The anterior lobe comprises an anterior portion or *pars distalis*, and intermediate lobe or *pars intermedia*, and the *pars infundibularis* or pars tuberalis which represents a dorsal projection or sleeve of cells situated around or along the infundibular stalk. The *median eminance* of the tuber cinereum, the *infundibular stalk* and the *infundibular processes* together make up the neurohypophysis or posterior lobe.

Anterior lobe (adenohypophysis)

The pars distalis is composed of loose cords of variably sized rounded or polygonal cells intimately associated with a rich sinusoidal network. For many years the cells of the pars distalis have been subdivided on the basis of their tinctorial characteristics when stained by alum haematoxylin and eosin or other acidic and basic dyes. The PAS technique is also important for the staining of cytoplasmic granules which contain glycoprotein hormones. However, it is now clear that these light microscopic staining characteristics do not accurately relate to the precise functional subtypes of pituitary cells, particularly when several species need to be considered as in drug-safety evaluation, or in altered physiological or pathological states. Nevertheless, these staining characteristics provide a useful baseline for routine analysis of pituitary cells prior to more detailed structural analysis using the electron microscope or immunocytochemical techniques. Lectin histochemistry provides an additional method for the identification of some cell types by localization of glycosylated prohormones, hormones or other glycoconjugates in rat, dog and human pituitary glands (Komuro and Shioda, 1981; Nakagawa et al., 1986).

In man, *acidophils* or *alpha cells* are typically medium sized, oval or rounded cells with eosinophilic cytoplasm when seen in haematoxylin and eosin stained sections, with cytoplasmic granules usually large enough to be seen by light microscopy. They have been subdivided on the basis of orange G or azocarmine staining, the ultrastructural characteristics of their granules or immunocytochemistry into somatotropes and mammotropes (Rhodin, 1974; Bloom and Fawcett, 1975).

Basophils or beta cells stain relatively poorly with haematoxylin and eosin but their granules stain with the PAS technique, presumably as a result of the presence of glycoprotein hormones. They are subdivided on the basis of special techniques into thyrotrophs and gonadotrophs.

Chromophobes chacteristically stain poorly with all the usual stains including PAS. The typical secretory cell with these staining characteristics is the corticotroph, which secretes adenocorticotrophic hormone or corticotrophin. In addition to chromophobes with secretory properties, the pars distalis contains chromophobes of other types notably the folliculostellate or follicular cells.

The relative proportions of the different cell populations in the pars distalis described by different authors varies with the techniques employed. Light microscopy and the classical histological techniques fail to accurately distinguish all cell populations. Ultrastructural criteria alone have also been shown to be inadequate for the identification of many anterior pituitary cells, particularly cells which are relatively undifferentiated (Hemming et al., 1983). For this reason, the most sophisticated method of cell identification and quantitation of cells in the pars distalis is that of immunocytochemistry employing antisera to the various specific hormones.

Many antisera to pituitary hormones are widely and commercially available and can be employed in different species, including animals used in preclinical safety studies and man. Potential difficulties as a result of common aminoacid sequences in different hormones, differences between the same hormone in different species and the presence of two or more hormones in the same cell can be avoided by use of appropriate fixation and high dilutions of primary antisera in combination with critical absorption techniques using appropriate homologous and heterologous pituitary antigens.

Although somewhat different percentages are recorded between studies, appropriately-controlled immunocytochemical study has revealed that prolactin-containing cells (mammotrophs) are the most abundant in the rat anterior pituitary followed by somatotrophs or growth-hormone containing cells (Dada et al., 1984). Cells which immunostain for prolactin represent 30–50% of the total cell population, although their volume density is much less.

Cells which immunostain for growth hormone represent up to about 20% of the total cell population of the pars distalis in the rat and other types between 2 and 6% (see review by Dada et al., 1984).

In man, percentages of somatotrophs comprise about 50% of anterior pituitary cells whereas prolactin containing cells and corticotrophs each represent about 15–20% of the total, gonadotrophs 10% and thyrotrophs 5% (McNicol, 1987).

Corticotrophs (adrenocorticotrophin, ACTH containing cells)

All corticotropin-related peptides are derived by proteolytic cleavage from a common translational product, pro-opiomelanocortin, a glycoprotein with a molecular weight of 31,000 daltons. The pro-opiomelanotropinergic system consists of corticotrophs, endocrine cells of the intermediate lobe and neurons projecting from the arcuate nucleus of the hypothalamus (O'Donohue and Dorsa, 1982). The pituitary corticotrophs cleave pro-opiomelanocortin into two main secretory products, adrenocorticotrophic hormone (ACTH) and a 91 aminoacid carboxyterminal fragment β-lipotropin (β-LPH). Secondary cleavage of β-LPH to β-endorphin and γ-lipotropin also occurs in the corticotrophs. The ACTH molecule contains the 13 aminoacid sequence of α-melanotropin (α-MSH), although this molecule is formed principally in the intermediate lobe and the neuronal system rather than in corticotrophs (see below). The aminoacid sequence of α-MSH appears to be the same in all mammals studied (O'Donohue and Dorsa, 1982). A second MSH molecule is β-MSH, with an 18 aminoacid sequence common to β-LPH, although this molecule shows considerable interspecies variation.

The secretory products of corticotrophs are, therefore, ACTH, β-lipotropin, and to a lesser extent β-endorphin. The control of secretion is mediated by corticotrophin releasing factor (CRF), a peptide with 41 aminoacid residues released from the hypothalamus as well as through feedback inhibition by the adrenal gland.

Corticotrophs are generally chromophobic when stained with conventional histochemical techniques. However, in a detailed comparative study of pituitary cells which were immunoreactive to anti-porcine ACTH antiserum, Yoshimura and colleagues (1982a) demonstrated considerable interspecies differences in the staining characteristics of corticotrophs with iron haematoxylin and PAS stains, demonstrating the need for caution in the use of classical histochemical techniques among different species.

It is generally considered that corticotrophs in the rat are stellate in shape, with a well-developed Golgi zone, sparse endoplasmic reticulum and a characteristic row of secretory granules approximately 200 nm diameter arranged along the cell membrane. However, the rat cells which are immune-reactive for ACTH may show a variety of different ultrastructural appearances (Yoshimura and Nogami, 1981).

Somatotrophs (growth hormone, GH-producing cells)

Somatotrophs are typically acidophilic cells which stain preferentially with orange G and which elaborate somatotrophin (STH, growth hormone, GH). Growth hormone is important in the control of growth of chondroblasts in the epiphyseal cartilage of long bones. At ultrastructural level, somatotrophs typically possess numerous dense spherical cytoplasmic granules, which in the rat have a diameter of between 350 to 400 nm, and a well-developed rough endoplasmic reticulum and Golgi zone (Rhodin, 1974).

Growth hormone is a single chain peptide with 191 aminoacids which has aminoacid sequences in common with prolactin and placental chronionic gonadotrophin (Daughaday, 1985). It is important to note that humans do not respond to growth hormone from non-primate species due to the different binding specificity of their growth hormone receptors.

Growth hormone secretion is under the control of two hypothalamic peptides, a 44 aminoacid peptide, growth hormone releasing hormone (GRH or somatocrinin) and somatostatin. Somatostatin, which inhibits growth hormone secretion, exists as a 14 or 28 aminoacid peptide.

Some of the effects of growth hormone are mediated indirectly by inducing the formation of somatomedins or insulin-like growth factors structurally similar to proinsulin.

Mammotrophs (lactotrophs, prolactin cells)

These cells secrete prolactin (PRL) which acts on mammary tissue primarily for initiation and maintenance of lactation. Human prolactin is a single chain peptide with 16% of its aminoacid sequence comparable to that of growth hormone.

Prolactin secretion is regulated by dopamine which reaches the anterior pituitary in the portal venous blood to suppress secretion. Negative feedback by prolactin on its own secretion also occurs (Daughaday, 1985). Prolactin-secreting cells are typically acidophilic and widely distributed in the anterior pituitary.

In the rat, prolactin staining-cells are concentrated along the medial border of the anterior adjacent to the intermediate lobe (Phelps, 1986). Quantitative immunocytochemical study has shown that the average percentages and distribution of prolactin cells in rats is similar between both sexes and among Long-Evans, Sprague-Dawley, and Fischer 344 strains (Phelps, 1986).

Prolactin cells are usually small and rounded, but may possess cytoplasmic processes (Dada et al., 1984; Phelps, 1986). Ultrastructural examination of rat mammotrophs reveals sparse, electron dense elipsoid granules measuring between 600 and 900 nm diameter (Rhodin, 1974; Cinti et al., 1985).

In the mouse it is more difficult to distinguish prolactin producing acidophils from somatotrophs on the basis of light microscopic examination and conventional tinctoral characteristics. There is also incomplete cross reactivity between mouse prolactin antigen with anti-rat prolactin antiserum and anti-mouse prolactin antisera need to be used for accurate identification of mouse prolactin-containing cells. (Harigaya et al., 1983).

Gonadotrophs

Gonadotrophs are large rounded basophils with PAS-positive granules resulting from the presence of two glycoprotein hormones, follicule stimulating hormone (FSH) and luteinizing hormone (LH). Gonadotroph granules stain with the labelled-lectin *Limulus polyphemus*, a sialic acid-specific lectin, probably as a result of the abundant sialic acid residues in FSH (Komuro and Shioda, 1981). Ultrastructural study of rat gonadotrophs demonstrates the presence of numerous secretory granules of highly variable size varying from 100 to 300 nm diameter.

FSH and LH as well as human chorionic gonadotrophin are structurally similar glycoproteins composed of two glycopeptide chains linked by hydrogen bonding. The α-chains have a common sequence of 96 residues. The β-chain is unique to each hormone and confers receptor binding specificity. FSHβ and LHβ contain 115 aminoacids and in CGβ 147 aminoacids. Complex carbohydrate side chains are attached to the a subunits. The β chain of FSH and LH have two complex side chains, αLCG five chains. Terminal sialic acid groups are frequently present on the carbohydrate of hCGβ and to a lesser extent FSHβ and probably serve to decrease the metabolic clearance of these hormones compared with thyroid stimulating hormone which possesses a terminal sulphate group. Because of higher sialic acid content, hepatic clearance of FSH is less than LH and its plasma half-life longer. The sequences in common between human chorionic gonadotrophin, FSH and LH provide the basis for the use of some antisera human to chorionic gonadotrophin to be employed in the immunohistochemical stains of gonadotrophins in animals (El Etreby et al., 1980; Komuro and Shioda, 1981).

FSH stimulates gametogenesis in both sexes. In males, it acts on Sertoli cells to enchance spermatogenesis and increases receptors of LH on Leydig cells. In females, FSH acts on granulosa cells, stimulating oestrogen synthesis and follicular development. LH acts on Leydig cells to stimulate testosterone production and the surge in LH secretion is important in follicular rupture and luteinization although not the maintenance of the corpus luteum (see Testis and Ovary, Chapters × and XI).

Regulation of gonadotrophs is under the control of gonadotrophin releasing hormone (LHRH). In males, FSH acts on Sertoli cells to stimulate the secretion of a peptide, inhibin, which in turn inhibits secretion of FSH by gonadotrophs. Inhibition is also found in the ovary but its precise role here has not been confirmed. Female sex steroids, however, can exert a positive feedback on the secretion of FSH and LH in females by a direct effect on gonadotrophs (see review by Daughaday, 1985).

Thyrotrophs

Thyrotrophs secrete thyrotrophic hormone (TSH), which is a glycoprotein structurally similar to FSH and LH, possessing a common α-chain and a distinct β-chain composed of 110 aminoacids, both with attached complex carbohydrate side chains. TSH binds specific receptors on the thyroid cell plasma membrane, as well as those on some other cells such as adipocytes. Its secretion is regulated both by the tripeptide hypothalamic releasing hormone TRH and circulating levels of thyroid hormone.

Thyrotrophs are fairly large polyhedral cells with large nuclei. Cytoplasmic granulesare PAS-positive, moderately electron dense and among the smallest in the anterior pituitary of most species ranging from 100 to 160 nm diameter (Dacheux, 1982; Yoshimura et al., 1982b). The rough endoplasmic reticulum of thyrotrophs is characterized by flattened or slightly dilated cisternae. It should be noted however, that the morphology of thyrotrophs is not entirely static but capable of modification in response to maturation or functional changes (Yoshimura et al., 1982b).

Folliculostellate (follicular) cells

In addition to chromophobes with secretory characteristics, the pars distalis contains another chromophobe devoid of granules which is known as a *folliculostellate* or *follicular cell* (Girod and Lhéritier, 1986). These cells have been documented in man, monkey, dog, mouse, rat, guinea pig, hamster, as well as a variety of other non-laboratory animal species (Girod et al., 1975, 1985; Ishikawa et al., 1983; Girod and Lhéritier, 1986). Common features are their stellate shape and long expanding cytoplasmic processes and lack of cytoplasmic secretory granules. Ultrastructural study shows that adjacent processes interdigitate and form narrow pseudolumens between cells which are lined by microvilli and occasional cilia. The agranular cytoplasm contains a juxtanuclear Golgi, sparse rough endoplasmic reticulum and a few mitochondria (Girod and Lhéritier, 1986). The cells have been shown to contain immune-reactive S100 protein and use of antisera to S100 is a useful light microscopic method for their delineation (Ishikawa et al., 1983; Girod et al., 1985). Their function remains uncertain.

Intermediate lobe

The intermediate lobe is not a distinctive structure in adult man but it is prominant in the human foetus, in non-human primates, dogs and rodents. In the rat, it is composed of 10–15 layers of closely packed cells or melanotrophs which are divided into lobules by fine strands of connective tissue. The main cells are rounded or polyhedral with ovoid smooth nuclei. Small cytoplasmic granules, just visible under the light microscope, stain with PAS and aldehyde fuchsin. These cells or melanotrophs are not entirely homogeneous for darker and lighter staining cells are present throughout the intermediate lobe. A minor subpopulation of non-melanotroph cells with small indented nuclei is also present (Chronwall et al., 1987).

The intermediate lobe of the pituitary gland is part of the pro-opiomelanocortin system and is the major source of α-MSH and β-endophin in the rat (Vaudry et al., 1978). ACTH is also present in the intermediate lobe but possibly as an intermediate product in α-MSH synthesis from the precursor pro-opiomelanocortin (O'Donohue and Dorsa, 1982). The effects of the hormones α-MSH and β-endophin are not well understood. α-MSH has effects on pigmentation and a variety of non-pigmentary effects of uncertain significance (see review by O'Donohue and Dorsa, 1982).

The hormonal secretion of the pars intermedia is complex but appears to be controlled by both inhibitory dopaminergic and stimulatory β-adrenergic receptors (Cote et al., 1982). The dopaminergic terminals which emanate from neurons in the rostral arcuate nucleus of the basomedial hypothalamus terminate directly on intermediate lobe melanotrophs.

Neurohypophysis

The neurohypophysis contains an intrinsic population of cells, the pituicytes and the terminal parts of the axons of secretory neurons, the bodies of which are located in the supraoptic and paraventricular nuclei in the hypothalamus. The fibres from these cells converge upon the median eminence, run down the infundibular stem into the infundibular process where they end, intimately related to the capillary vasculature. Spherical nodules of variable size known as Herring bodies are also present in the fibres and represent secretory material.

Loss of anterior pituitary cell mass occurs under circumstances of reduced demand and this loss may be associated with reduced pituitary weight. Diffuse atrophy of a pituitary cell population also occurs in association with hyperplasia of other cell types (see below) or focally around the margins of an expanding pituitary neoplasm.

Although in rats, aging is undoubtably associated with reduction in the hypothalamic content of releasing hormones and the capacity of the pituitary to synthesize or release FSH, LH and TSH (Bedrak et al., 1983; Chen, 1984), these differences may be partly due to differences in pituitary tumour incidence and their space-occupying effects (Chen, 1984). A decline in volume density of prolactin-containing cells has also been reported in very aged BN/Bikij and WAG/Rij rats when animals with pituitary tumours were excluded from the analysis (Van Putten et al., 1988).

Loss of pituitary cells has been shown to occur with advancing age in man. Quantitative immunocytochemical study has shown that these age-related changes are mainly due to a decline both in the number and size of growth hormone-producing cells, the greatest decline occurring at about the age of 40 (Sun et al., 1984).

Viruses also affect pituitary function without morphological evidence of cell damage. The non-cytopathic lymphocytic choriomeningitis virus which displays a tropism for the murine anterior pituitary gland replicates in somatotrophs resulting in diminished synthesis of growth hormone without evidence of cell necrosis or inflammation (Oldstone et al., 1982).

Reduction of pituitary cells can also occur following pharmacological suppression. Gonadotrophs decrease in number in beagle dogs treated with oestrogens for long periods, although this cell loss is accompanied by concomitant hyperplasia of prolactin-containing cells (El Etreby et al., 1977).

When rats are exposed to low barometric pressure (e.g. 380 mg Hg) for 28 days, the number of thyrotrophs decrease to about 30% of controls, unassociated with significant cytological changes or hypertrophy (Gosney, 1986). Similar changes probably occur in man under hypoxic conditions, although the mechanisms for the changes remain unclear. The mechanisms are undoubtably complex and may be the result of a direct effect of hypoxia on the pituitary gland or on the hypothalamus, perhaps by interference with thyrotrophin release (Gosney, 1986).

Atrophy of the pituitary gland, characterized by generalized loss of cell cytoplasm and undue prominance of vasculature associated with atrophy and tumour development in other endocrine organs has been reported in rats treated with the carcinogens N,N'-2,7-fluorenylene-bisacetamide or N-2-fluorenylacetamide (Morris et al., 1961).

Atrophy of the pars intermedia

Physiological alterations which result in increased activity of the hypothalamus such as water deprivation or lactation may result in involution of the pars intermedia (Russfield, 1975). Treatment of rats with bromocriptine, a dopamine receptor agonist decreases the cell number and thickness of the pars intermedia in association with reduction in synthesis of pro-opiomelanocortin-derived peptides and mRNA (Chronwall et al., 1987).

The thickness of the intermediate lobe in untreated male Sprague-Dawley rats was shown to be $13.2 + 1.0$ cell layers $(n = 6)$ whereas treatment with bromocriptine as a pellet implant for 12 days reduced the thickness of the pars intermedia to $8.4 + 0.6$ cell layers $(n = 8)$ (Chronwall et al., 1987).

Hypertrophy and hyperplasia

In common with other glandular tissues hypertrophy and hyperplasia of the adenohypophysis is liable to result from prolonged or excessive stimulation of its cellular population. Such a response may be physiological in nature as exemplified by the changes occurring in lactation. Other stimuli can be considered excessive or pathological and the pituitary gland may respond in an exaggerated way, although often with features in common with physiological responses.

Although weighing the pituitary gland is a time honoured method for the detection of hypertrophy and hyperplasia, the heterogeneous nature of the pituitary cell population dictates the need for careful microscopic and morphometric analysis with immunostained preparations for the accurate characterization of the degree and nature of hypertrophy and hyperplasia, which often occur in combination. In most long-term rodent studies however, assessment of the pituitary gland is performed using haematoxylin and eosin-stained preparations. In common with other endocrine organs, the diagnosis of proliferative change is somewhat arbitary. Most workers recognise *diffuse and focal hyperplasia*. The term *adenoma* is reserved for growths showing compression of the surrounding parenchyma. Others also recognise *foci of cellular alternation* or *focal cellular hypertrophy* where foci of cells show more abundant cytoplasm without evidence of an increase in cell number.

Diffuse hyperplasia

Diffuse hyperplasia is characterized by a symmetrical enlargement of the anterior pituitary cell gland. However, diffuse hyperplasia affects one or more of the pituitary populations and altered cells are characteristically interspersed with unaffected or even atrophic cells of other types.

Hypertrophy and hyperplasia of the pituitary gland have been particularly well studied in the rat but similar changes appear to occur in other species including man. Of particular interest is the fact that hypertrophy and diffuse hyperplasia occurs spontaneously in aging rats and in response to lactation,

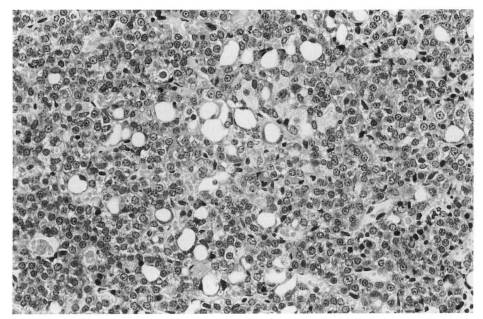

Fig. 120. Anterior pituitary gland from a male Wistar rat treated with a high dose of an antiandrogenic agent. This has produced a catration effect in the pituitary gland characterised by the presence of vacuolated 'castration' cells. (HE ×250.)

surgical resection of endocrine tissue, administration of sex hormones, oral contraceptives, trophic factors and other agents which induce prolonged changes to the endocrine system (Furth et al., 1973). Many of these changes have been better characterized over recent years with the use of immunocytochemistry, electron microscopy and in situ hybridization techniques. The following represents an account of some of these changes.

The effects of gonadectomy on the pituitary gland have been widely investigated since Addison first described alterations in pituitary basophils in castrated male rats. In both male and female castrated rats, gonadotrophs respond by increasing in both size and volume and they become vacuolated at approximately two months after surgery (Figs. 120 and 121). Ultrastructural and immunocytochemical study shows that affected gonadotrophs contain decreased numbers of secretory granules and dilated or vacuolated rough endoplasmic reticulum, both containing follicular stimulatory hormone and luteotrophic hormone (Tixier-Vidal et al., 1975). Some of the dilated residues of rough endoplasmic reticulum fuse to form the large vacuoles typical of the signet ring appearance of 'castration cells'.

Morphometric study of immunostained sections of rat pituitaries showed that females develop a higher percentage of FSH cells following gonadectomy than males and that morphological changes were maximal at three months following surgery (Ibrahim et al., 1986). The morphological features correlated with the

687

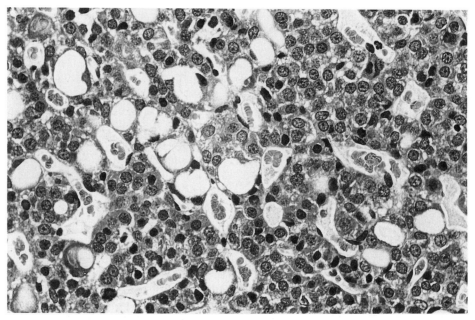

Fig. 121. Same case as in Figure 120 but at a higher magnification. (HE ×400.)

levels of circulating FSH and LH. It is probable that such changes resulting from gonadectomy are the result of both cell division and differentation of monohormonal gonadotrophs as well as more primitive stem cells (Ibrahim et al., 1986).

Typical castration cells, characterised by the presence of large swollen cells with 'signet ring' appearances (Figs. 120 and 121) and containing PAS-positive granules were reported in the pituitary glands of male rats treated for periods of three months or more with flutamide, a non-steroidal antiandrogen (Food and Drug Administration 1980). This drug produced a form of medical castration with testicular and prostate atrophy (see Male Genital Tract, Chapter X).

Biochemical and morphological studies have shown that normal lactation in mammals including man is associated with a physiological hyperplasia of prolactin cells (Sun et al., 1984; Cinti et al., 1985). Morphometric studies of the lactating rat pituitary gland using ultrastructural techniques has shown that prolactin cells show an increase in the amount of cytoplasm which contains prominant Golgi apparatus and abundant rough endoplasmic reticulum, often arranged in concentric rows or whorles termed 'Nebenkern' (Cinti et al., 1985). Furthermore, there is an increase in the total number and secretory activity of folliculostellate cells during lactation (Cinti et al., 1985).

A similar, but exaggerated prolactin cell hyperplasia can be induced by administration of oestrogenic hormones and oral contraceptive agents. Morphological and immunohistochemical study of the pituitary gland of rats treated with diethylstilboestrol or oestradiol for periods of up to 16 weeks has shown enlarged congested glands containing large pituitary cells with large nuclei, prominant nucleoli, numerous mitotic figures and eosinophilic cytoplasm which immunostains for prolactin (Lloyd, 1983; Lloyd and Mailloux, 1987; Niwa et al., 1987). Immunostaining for other pituitary hormones has also shown that normal cells of other types are diffusely scattered among the hyperplastic, prolactin-containing cells.

The increase in pituitary weight and degree of prolactin cell hyperplasia appears time-dependent and serum prolactin levels in rats treated with oestrogen increase in parallel with pituitary hyperplasia (Lyle et al., 1984). However, even after 16 weeks treatment with oestrogens, discrete foci of hyperplasia or nodular changes are not seen.

These changes also parallel the diffuse rather than focal increase in prolactin messenger RNA which can be detected by in situ hybridization histochemistry in rat pituitary glands following increasing duration of oestrogen treatment (Lloyd and Landefeld, 1986).

Florid patterns of diffuse hyperplasias are induced by much longer periods of treatment with high doses of oestrogenic agents, although these changes may be reversible. Female rats given the progestational agent, quingestanol acetate and the oestrogen, quinestrol, in a 2:1 ratio in doses of either 30 mg/kg once weekly or 1.2 mg/kg/day for 50 weeks developed extremely large pituitary glands. The daily treatment schedule resulted in average pituitary weights of 87 mg + 20 mg and the weekly treatment 128 + 29 mg per 100 g body weight (compared with control mean of 5 mg (n = 10)). Histologically, the enlarged glands were characterized by cystic change, telangiectasia, congestion and haemorrhage, chromophobe hyperplasia associated with some atypical cells with large irregular profiles and hyperchromatic nuclei or small cells with dense staining nuclei (Lumb et al., 1985). The pituitary changes were sufficient to produce evidence of displacement of the brain and raised intracranial pressure with resultant early death in some animals. The findings may have been classified as adenomas by some pathologists. However, the particular interest of these findings is that withdrawal from treatment after 50 weeks of treatment was sufficient to reduce pituitary weights by 50% with re-establishment of basophil and acidophil populations, reversal of the vascular changes and disappearance of clinical signs within a period of 30 weeks.

Although some atypical cells remained and one or two nodular pituitary glands were found after the 30 week period of withdrawal from treatment, the results suggested that even most of the florid changes represented chromophobe hyperplasia in which cells were capable of regranulation and reversion to more mature cells following cessation of treatment. These results also highlighted the potential difficulties in making a clear distinction between neoplasia and hyperplasia under these circumstances (see below).

It is also worth noting that different rat strains are variable in their sensitivity to the effects of oestrogens. In a comparative study in which female ACI and Sprague-Dawley rats were administered a similar dose of diethylstilboestrol for periods up to 214, days the ACI rats showed greater increases in pituitary weights and prolactin cell hyperplasia than Sprague-Dawley rats after similar periods of time (Stone et al., 1979; Holtzman et al., 1979). These changes were associated with higher plasma prolactin levels in ACI rats than in the Sprague-Dawley strain.

In another study, Fischer 344 rats showed a far greater increase in pituitary weight than Holtzman rats when treated with similar doses of diethylstiboestrol for periods of twelve weeks (Wiklund et al., 1981).

Administration of high doses of buserelin, a synthetic peptide analogue of the natural gonadotrophin releasing hormone (LHRH) to rats for up to 24 months also produced increased pituitary weights and focal or diffuse hyperplasia of the anterior pituitary associated with reduced weights of the testes and uteri and decreased serum testosterone levels in males and reduced serum progesterone levels in females (Donaubauer et al., 1987).

Thyroidectomy or administration of goitrogens such as thiouracil or propylthiouracil to rats also increase the weight of the pituitary gland and produces an increase in thyrotropin-containing cells. (Purves and Griesbach, 1956; Lloyd and Mailloux 1987). It was shown by Lloyd and Mailloux (1987) that treatment of Fischer 344 rats for six weeks with propylthiouracil produced increases in pituitary and thyroid gland weights, as well as an increase in the percentage of pituitary cells containing immune-reactive TSH prolactin. The positive TSH cells, although more numerous, stained less intensely than cells in control pituitary glands.

Aminoglutethimide, an agent which inhibits several cytochrome P450 mediated hydroxylation steps in steroid synthesis in the adrenal cortex provides another good example of a drug which can induce diffuse pituitary hyperplasia (Dexter et al., 1967; Cash et al., 1967). Aminoglutethimide, previously used as an anticonvulsant (Hughes and Burley, 1970) is currently used in the treatment of certain hormone-sensitive human cancers.

Administration of aminoglutethimide to rats produces hyperplasia of ACTH containing cells. The cells are characterized by increased but variable size with variation in shape and immunostaining intensity with antiserum to ACTH (Zak et al., 1985). These hyperplastic cells were characterized ultrastructurally by irregular, stellate cell margins with long narrow processes, abundant rough endoplasmic reticulum, conspicuous Golgi apparatus and increased number and size of secretory granules. Nuclei contained prominant nucleoli (Zak et al., 1985). Gonadotrophs and thyrotrophs also showed some evidence of hyperplasia, features compatable with the fact that aminoglutethamide also interferes with conversion of androgens to oestrogens and with thyroid synthesis (Pittman and Brown, 1966; Graves and Salhanick, 1979).

Changes in the adrenal cortex and thyroid are reported both in laboratory animals and in humans treated with aminoglutethimide (Hughes and Barley, 1970; see below). It is probable that the stimulation of corticotrophs, gonadotrophs and thyrotrophs is another example of reduced hormone production in target glands leading to lack of feedback suppression with enhancement of the release of the various hypothalamic releasing hormones (Zak et al., 1985).

690

Diffuse hyperplasia of the anterior pituitary gland occurs spontaneously with advancing age in many breeds of dog including the beagle. Immunocytochemical study shows that the changes in advancing age comprise diffuse hyperplasia and hypertrophy of growth hormone-containing cells. The changes are most marked in the dorsal region of the pars distalis of female dogs with proliferative changes or neoplasia in the mammary glands (El Etreby et al., 1980). In some cases, the growth hormone cells appear to infiltrate or encroach into the pars intermedia. A diffuse, increase in prolactin cells is also observed in the pars distalis of older breeding females.

Diffuse hyperplasia and hypertrophy of anterior pituitary cells is also seen in beagle dogs following long-term treatment with sex steroids. An immuno-cytochemical and morphometric study of the pars distalis of female beagles treated with an oestrogen (1.28 mg/kg body weight/week of 17β-oestradiol) by the intramuscular route for 52 weeks showed progressive hyperplasia and hyper-trophy of prolactin-containing cells (El Etreby et al., 1977). These cells were prominant in the ventrocentral area of the pars distalis and showed paler immunostaining using antistera to ovine prolactin than in controls, suggesting subnormal hormone content. Histologically, these cells were large with uniformly spherical or ovoid hyperchromatic nuclei, prominant nucleoli and increased mitotic activity. Cell cytoplasm contained abundant Golgi zones and showed basophilia compatable with abundant rough endoplasmic reticulum. By contrast, gonadotrophs (LH-FSH staining cells) were atrophic, although other cell types appeared unaffected.

Administration of progestagens to dogs produces somewhat different changes. El Etreby and Fath El Bab (1977) showed that treatment of ovariectomized beagles with high doses of a synthetic progestagon (cyproterone acetate) for four weeks produced hyperplasia and hypertrophy of growth hormone producing cells, leaving prolactin-containing cells generally unchanged. It appears that growth hormone plays a major role as a mediator of progestogen induced changes in the beagle dog (El Etreby and Fath El Bab, 1977).

Diffuse hyperplasia of the intermediate lobe

Following transsection of the pituitary stalk or hypothalamic lesions which destroy the supraoptic and paraventricular nuclei, the intermediate lobe of the rat and other species may show hypertrophy and hyperplasia (Russfield, 1975). Hypertrophy and hyperplasia can also result from interference with dopaminergic-control mechanisms by administration of xenobiotics. Chronic treatment of rats with haloperidol, a dopamine receptor antagonist stimulates the secretion of α-MSH and β-endorphin and accelerates the synthesis of pro-opiomelanocortin, associated with an increase in the number of cell layers in the intermediate lobe. The thickened gland contains many dark melanotrophes which do not appear increased in size but contain increase mRNA for pro-opiomelanocortin than controls shown by in situ hybridization (Chronwall et al., 1987).

Hyperplasia of the intermediate lobe is also observed spontaneously in Syrian hamsters with advancing age (Pour et al., 1976).

Focal hyperplasia

Groups or foci of pituitary cells which show altered tinctorial properties and evidence of proliferation without compression of surrounding normal gland or tissues are usually considered *focal hyperplasias*.

If consideration given to the recent classification of pituitary adenomas in which adenomas are characterised by a clearly demonstrable pseudocapsule, *nodular focal hyperplasia* can also be defined. In the rat, these nodular lesions are characterized by islands of hypertrophic cells showing mitoses with cellular and nuclear pleomorphism but not sharply separated from the surrounding tissue by any form of pseudocapsule or condensed reticulin (McComb et al., 1984). In view of the apparent reversibility of some nodular lesions in the rat pituitary gland, it may be appropriate to make this distinction in safety assessment of compounds producing pituitary changes in the rat, although the generally accepted approach is to regard all expansile lesions as neoplastic.

In the dog, focal hyperplasia is also distinguished from diffuse hyperplasia. Focal hyperplasia, in common with pituitary tumours occurs more frequently in untreated, aged female dogs. Focal lesions are particularly common in the ventrocentral and cranial parts of the pars distalis but they are also found in the pars intermedia. The foci are microscopic in size and not sharply demarcated. Cells are variable in size and in tinctorial characteristics. They may contain PAS positive granules but in common with pituitary adenomas (see below) they characteristically stain immunocytochemically with anti-ACTH antisera (El Etreby et al., 1980).

In view of the common aminoacid sequences of ACTH, β-MSH, β-endorphin and β-lipotropin, this immunoreactivity may not represent ACTH but another of these related peptides.

Pituitary neoplasia

Most neoplasms of the anterior pituitary in both man and laboratory animals are considered adenomas. An adenoma of the adenohypophysis can be defined operationally as a homogeneous proliferation of pituitary cells which shows clear histological evidence of compression or displacement of surrounding normal tissues. It is compression which is usually taken as evidence of autonomous behavior. This is characterized by compression of the surrounding tissue to form a pseudocapsule of narrow cords of cells separated by alternating bands of connective tissue, condensed reticulin and capillaries, often best demonstrated by silver staining for reticulin (McComb et al., 1984).

This definition has been applied to both experimental and human pituitary adenomas and has the merit of sharply defining the threshold for the diagnosis of adenoma. It has to be kept in mind, however, that any distinction between adenoma and hyperplasia remains arbitrary. Indeed, as McNichol (1987) has remarked, one of the questions of endocrine pathology is whether adenomas of the pituitary are actually neoplastic because this requires establishment of clonality, which has not yet been achieved.

The distinction between adenoma and carcinoma of the pituitary gland is usually based on histological evidence of the absence or presence of local infiltration or invasion of adjacent structures, notably into brain tissue or bone. This distinction is also arbitary because the benign and malignant biological nature of pituitary tumours is not sharply separable on histological grounds. Carcinomas can simply be considered as more aggressive varients of the same tumour type. Recent experience with pituitary adenomas in man confirms the view that histological appearances do not conform with biological behavior. Although about 10% of pituitary neoplasms found in man possess histological features of local tissue invasion, neoplasms showing unequivocal malignant behavior as evident by dissemination in the cerebral spinal fluid or metastatic spread outside the cranium are extremely rare. However, when they occur they can be quite devoid of cytological expression of malignancy (Scheithauer et al., 1985). Recent guidelines of the National Toxicology Program (NTP) for combining neoplasms for evaluation of rodent carcinogenicity studies have suggested that it is appropriate to group pituitary adenomas and carcinomas for statistical assessment (McConnell et al., 1986).

Pituitary neoplasia: rat

Pituitary adenomas are generally common spontaneous neoplasms in rats although in a few strains their prevalence is low (McComb et al., 1984). Their incidence increases with advancing age and they begin to make an appearance in significant numbers in predisposed strains after about one year of age (Barsoum et al., 1985). In most, but not all strains, female rats are more commonly affected. The reported incidences often vary between laboratories using the same strain of rat and their prevalance may vary with time in the same laboratory using the same strain under identical experimental conditions (Tarone et al., 1981; personal observations).

The reason for predisposition of laboratory rats to the development of pituitary adenomas with advancing age is uncertain. Since the majority of these tumours are composed of prolactin cells, it has been suggested that decreased hypothalamic content of dopamine observed in older rats may be an important factor as dopamine is the main inhibitory factor for prolactin (Prysor-Jones et al., 1983). The higher incidence of pituitary adenomas in females suggests that ostrogens are involved, either by a direct effect on pituitary cells or inhibition of dopamine (Prysor-Jones et al., 1983).

Dietary factors have clearly been shown to influence the incidence of pituitary adenomas in rats. Ad libitum fed Wistar rats were shown to develop significantly more pituitary tumors at two years compared with their counter parts fed the same diet but restricted in quantity by 20% (Tucker, 1979). Wistar rats fed a low protein diet ad libitum developed fewer pituitary adenomas than their counterparts fed a more protein rich diet (Berry, 1986). It is possible that the decreases in prevalence of pituitary adenomas sometimes observed in treated groups in rat carcinogenicity bioassays are also related to the lower body weights and decreased food intake occurring in these groups. Breeding also delays the appearance of pituitary adenomas in female rats (Pickering and Pickering, 1984).

Most pituitary adenomas have, in the past, been considered chromophobe adenomas based on their appearances in haematoxylin and eosin-stained sections. However, their histological appearances are quite variable. They can be highly vascular or haemorrhagic neoplasms with tumour cells arranged in narrow trabeculae or thick cords. They may show solid or nodular growth patterns. Fibrosis and pigmentation is also sometimes prominent. The tumour cells possess variable cytological appearances, ranging from small cells with granular cytoplasm to large highly pleomorphic cells with abundant eosinophilic cytoplasm. Despite these variable histological and cytological features, the largest proportion of spontaneous rat pituitary adenomas contain immunoreactive prolactin (Kovacs et al., 1977; Berkvens et al., 1980; McComb et al., 1984; Barsoum et al., 1985; Berry, 1986; Nagatani et al., 1987). Other adenoma types containing immunoreactive leuteinizing hormone and follicular stimulating hormone (McComb et al., 1985), thyroid stimulating hormone, adrenocorticotrophin, growth hormone and combinations of these hormones (McComb et al., 1984) are observed in smaller numbers in untreated, aged rats. Some adenomas remain totally unreactive to antisera to all the usual pituitary hormones.

A small number of spontaneous pituitary adenomas also develop from cells of the intermediate lobe in the rat, although they are relatively uncommon (Russfield, 1975). Adenomas of the intermediate lobe usually shows immune reactivity to anti-ACTH antiserum (McComb et al., 1984).

Adenomas of the rat adenohypophysis have been reported to follow gonadectomy, long-term administration of oestrogens, gonadotrophin release factor (LHRH) analogues, thyroid ablation, iodine deficiency, administration of goitrogens and various forms of direct pituitary ionizing radiation (Furth et al., 1973; Russfield, 1975; Physicians Desk Reference, 1987). Many of these reports predate the use of immunocytochemistry of pituitary hormones and they do not always describe the pathological changes in sufficient details to make the distinction between hyperplasia and neoplasia based on current criteria.

Although the long-term effects of oestrogens and progestagens on the rat pituitary gland have been extensively studied, the study by Lumb and co-workers (1985) highlights some of the difficulties in the interpretation of pituitary changes induced by these hormones. In this study, massively enlarged pituitary glands, sufficient to cause severe signs of compression of the central nervous system regressed upon withdrawal of treatment raising the possibility that pituitary glands showing quite massive growth may not all contain autonomous neoplastic lesions.

Similar findings were also reported by Treip (1983) who compared the pituitary glands of Wistar rats implanted oestradiol pellets subcutaneously for 230 days with those from which were observed for 110 days after removal of implants at 120 days. Large haemorrhagic pituitary neoplasms were reported in rats implanted for 230 days. Pituitary glands in rats from which implants were removed showed pituitary glands of normal dimensions with only residual disturbance of simusoidal and reticulin pattern, evidence of old haemorrhage and presence of iron pigment.

Treip (1983) postulated that as oestradiol-induced pituitary tumours are totally hormone dependent, they cannot be autonomous neoplasms. However, it was recognised that complete autonomy may not have been achieved in a period of 220 days or that even in regressed pituitary glands potentially neoplastic cells are still present and would eventually become manifest as overt neoplasms with time. (Treip, 1983).

Strain differences may be also important in pituitary tumour induction. In studies in which both female Sprague-Dawley and ACI rats were administered diethylstilboestrol for periods of up to 214 days under identical conditions, prolactin adenomas were described in the pituitary glands of ACI rats, but only focal hyperplasias in Sprague-Dawley rats (Holtzman et al., 1979). These differences were attributed to the different degree to which prolactin cells can be stimulated to grow and produce hormone in the two strains (Stone et al., 1979).

Pituitary neoplasia: mice

In mice, spontaneous pituitary neoplasms are uncommon but they are occasionally observed in advancing age among the strains usually employed in carcinogenicity bioassays. However, these spontaneous neoplasms have been generally less well characterized by immunocytochemistry than those found in rat or man. In the NZY strain however, breeding females commonly develop pituitary chromophobe adenomas as well as mammary carcinomas (Bielschowosky et al., 1956).

As in rats, adenomas of the mouse pituitary can be induced by long-term administration of oestrogens, gonadectomy, various forms of thyroid deficiency, particularly administration of radioactive I^{131} and direct irradiation (Russfield, 1975).

Pituitary neoplasia: hamsters

As in mice, pituitary adenomas are occasionally observed in aged hamsters, and morphologically resemble those in other species (Pour et al., 1976; Bernfeld et al., 1986). However, they have not been well-characterized with immunocytochemical techniques.

Pituitary neoplasia: dog

Pituitary adenomas occur spontaneously in dogs of different breeds including aged beagles (Attia et al., 1980; El Etreby et al., 1980). These expansive nodular lesions are composed of cells with variable cytological appearances. They can be arranged in sheets, trabeculae or in acinar structures. They become large and infiltrate the pars nervosa. They may occur both in the pars distalis and intermedia and can be immunoreactive to antisera to ACTH or MSH related peptides (Attia et al., 1980; El Etreby et al., 1980). Although animals with these pituitary neoplasms often also develop adenomas or nodules of the adrenal cortex, the levels of circulating ACTH are usually low, although cortisol levels have been show to be slightly elevated in affected dogs (El Etreby et al., 1980).

Pituitary neoplasia: man

The most widely used classification of pituitary adenomas occurring in man has been based on their tinctorial properties. They have usually been divided into basophil, acidophil and chromophobe groups. More recently a functional classification of human pituitary adenomas has been proposed based on immuno-cytochemical, ultrastructural, biochemical, and clinical features (Kovacs and Horvath, 1986).

In man the prevalence of pituitary adenomas has generally been considered about 5–10% of all intracranial neoplasms although they may be found more frequently if searched for at autopsy or if modern imaging and biochemical techniques are employed (McNicol, 1987). The most common variety now reported in man is the prolactin cell adenoma (or prolactinoma) followed by the somatroph adenoma (Kovacs and Horvath, 1986).

Treatment of women with oestrogen-containing oral contraceptives is associated with the development of hyperprolactinaemia and amenorrhea and occasionally pituitary adenomas, although the relationship between adenoma development and contraceptive treatment is unclear (Schlechte et al., 1980; Chang et al., 1977; Coulam et al., 1979).

ADRENAL GLAND

Although severe or life-threatening drug-induced lesions in the adrenal gland are uncommon, a literature review by Ribelin (1984) showed that of all reported changes induced by xenobiotics in endocrine glands in laboratory animals, those in the adrenal gland were the most frequently reported. The relatively well characterized structure-function relationships and the limited number of morphological responses to stimulation or injury are helpful in the histological evaluation of drug-induced effects on the pituitary-adrenal axis. The adrenal gland is divided into cortex and medulla. The adrenal cortex is characterized by three layers, the zona glomerulosa, zona fasciculata, and zona reticularis, although there are certain species differences in the organization of these zones.

In man, the zona glomerulosa is not a continuous layer but forms rounded clusters of cells beneath the capsule. This is unlike laboratory species in which the glomerulosa forms a fairly uniform and continuous layer. The zona glomerulosa in the dog is particularly distinct, being characterised by cords and nest of elongated cells, quite different from the more rounded glomerulosa cells in rodents, non-human primates and man. The zona fasciculata constitutes the bulk of cortex in man and laboratory species. The zona reticularis is prominant in man but it is not clearly distinguishable in some rodents, particularly in the mouse where the columns of cells of the fasciculata appear to extend to the medulla (Firth, 1983).

An important feature of the adrenal gland in mammals is the lack of a significant direct arterial blood supply to the deep cortex which depends primarily on blood which has already perfused the outer layers and contains secreted steroids (Neville and O'Hare, 1982). Most blood entering the cortex in the head of the gland ultimately empties into the medulla and this creates a form of corticomedullary portal system. The total blood flow through the adrenal is high in most large mammals. In man it is second only to the flow rate in the thyroid gland (Neville and O'Hare, 1982). In contrast to the arterial blood supply, a single major adrenal vein drains the adrenal gland.

The mouse adrenal cortex is characterized by several unusual features, notably the prominant X-zone, brown degeneration and subcapsular cell proliferation. The review of the mouse adrenal gland by Dunn (1970) still remains one of the key references for most of the older literature. Nussdorfer (1986) provides a more recent review of the anatomy of the adrenal cortex of mammalian species.

X-zone

A characteristic feature in the adrenal gland of mice and some other rodent species is the presence of a fourth cortical layer the so called X-zone, situated immediately adjacent to the medulla. The X-zone appears to be analogous to the foetal cortex of other species and its size, pattern of evolution and degeneration varies with strain, sex and reproductive status (Dunn, 1970). For instance, among strains of white mice, it is thicker in Swiss mice than in C57 or CBA strains (Deacon et al., 1986).

The X-zone is composed of cortical cells which have a denser, more basophilic cytoplasm than cells of the fasciculata. In most strains, the X-zone is not present at birth but makes its appearance by about 10 days. In males, the X-layer subsequently broadens but disappears rapidly as sexual maturity is reached by about 5 weeks (Firth, 1983). The cells become pyknotic leaving a zone of ceroid pigment or 'brown degeneration'. In the female mouse the initial evolution of the X-zone is similar to that in males but it continues to increase in size to reach a maximum at about 9 weeks. However, by this stage lipid vacuoles are visible and they increase in number as the X-zone slowly degenerates over many months. Should pregnancy intervene, rapid involution of the X-zone occurs.

Gonadectomy of prepubertal male and female mice prevents the early involution of the X-zone which widens considerably and degenerates only about five months later. Hypophysectomy causes both the zona fasciculata and X-zone (but not the zona glomerulosa) to degenerate. Deacon and her colleagues (1986) have

697

shown that the morphological expression of the X-zone in Swiss mice depends mainly on luteinizing hormone (LH) and not ACTH, for its involution in the mouse can be prevented by administration of equine LH. It is relatively unaffected by other pituitary hormones. Presumably, gonadectomy of males prevents degeneration of the X-zone by removal of testicular androgens with resultant unopposed secretion of LH. Its rapid disappearance in pregnancy could be due to the presence of ovarian androgens or androgens of other sources (Deacon et al., 1986).

Unlike rat and mouse, the adrenal weight of the Syrian hamster is greater in males than females and this sex difference appears primarily a result of a zona reticularis which is three times thicker in males than in females (Ohtaki, 1979). This adrenal dimorphism may relate to other sex-related characteristics such as seasonal enlargement of the adrenals in males and the sex differences in primary immune response among hamsters (Blazkovec and Orsini, 1976).

The adrenal cortex is capable of secreting all known active steroid hormones comprising progestogens, corticosteroids, mineralocorticoids, androgens and oestrogens. The precursor, cholesterol, is available from both diet or following biosynthetic processes in a number of cells including those of the adrenal cortex. The preferred substrate is, however, plasma cholesterol in the form of low density lipoprotein cholesterol, although high density lipoprotein can act as substrate in some species, including the rat. Cells in the adrenal cortex possess low density lipoprotein receptors which are capable of complexing and internalizing low density lipoproteins for hydrolysis by lysosomes and release of cholesterol (Gwynne and Strauss, 1982).

Hydroxyl groups are placed at all the key positions in the molecule by a series of substrate-specific cytochrome enzymes which requires the presence of NADPH and molecular oxygen (Bondy, 1985). Under normal circumstances the rate limiting step in steroid biosynthesis is the conversion of cholesterol to 20α-hydroxycholesterol, a step which is accelerated by ACTH and is presumably the step also regulated by angiotensin (Temple and Liddle, 1970). The order in which hydroxyl groups are added appears generally unimportant although 17α-hydroxylation apparently does not readily occur after a hydroxyl group has been added to the 21-position. As a result, the relative amounts of cortisol (with a 17α-hydroxy group) and corticosterone (without a 17α group) depends in part on relative rates of 17- and 21-hydroxylation. For this reason, various species may have different abilities to produce cortisol and corticosterone. For example, man, dog and guinea pigs produce predominantly cortisol; in rabbits and rats the major product is corticosterone (Bondy, 1985). However, these ratios are dynamic, for stimulation with ACTH may alter the usual proportions by its stimulation of the production of cortisol rather than corticosterone (Ganjam et al., 1972).

Control of corticosteroid secretion is primarily under the control of ACTH (see Pituitary Gland). ACTH acts on a cell surface receptor and activates cholesterol side-chain cleavage by a cyclic AMP-dependent mechanism which is incompletely understood. However, it may involve increased binding of cholesterol substrate to a cytochrome P450 on the inner mitochondrial membrane which catalyses side-chain cleavage or conversion of cholesterol to pregnenolone (Alfano et al., 1983). There is also some evidence that pro-γ-melanotropin is involved in controlling cholesterol metabolism following stress (Alfano et al., 1983).

Aldosterone formation occurs almost exclusively in the zona glomerulosa and is regulated principally by the renin-angiotensin system. Renin synthesized by the juxtaglomerular apparatus (see Kidney, Chapter IX) acts on angiotensinogen found in the α-2 globulin fraction of the blood to form a decapeptide angiotensin I, the rate limiting step. Angiotensin II, an octapeptide, is formed by the action of a converting enzyme in the circulation on angiotensin I. Finally, the less active angiotensin III is formed by loss of an aminoterminal aspartic acid. Angiotensin II acts mainly to stimulate aldosterone biosynthesis in the zona glomerulosa and to increase peripheral arterial resistance with resultant blood pressure increase. Stimulation does not require activation of the cyclic AMP system but it does require calcium (Elliott et al., 1982). The enzymes involved in aldosterone synthesis appear to be located both in the mitochondria and the smooth endoplasmic reticulum (Tamaoki, 1973; Nussdorfer, 1980).

In addition to the renin-angiotensin system, plasma concentration of sodium and potassium, ACTH, α-MSH and analogues are involved in the control of zona glomerulosa function although undoubtably the interrelationships are complex (Nussdorfer, 1980; Vinson et al., 1984). The finding that pharmacological doses of prolactin influence the function of the zona glomerulosa in rats, raises the possibility that prolactin is also involved in physiological regulation of the zona glomerulosa and is a factor in the development of adrenal changes seen in aged rats. For a complete review of the functional morphology of the zona glomerulosa see Nussdorfer (1980, 1986).

Adrenal cortex

Accessory adrenocortical tissue

A normal variation is the presence of accessory adrenocortical tissue, or rests in laboratory animal species and in man. These are nodules of essentially normal cortex which may be separate from, or attached to, the adrenal gland. They should be distinguished from extruded hyperplasic nodules or neoplasms of cortical cells.

There are considerable species differences in the prevalence of these accessory nodules. In mice, they are particularly common. Hummel (1958) showed that C57L, BALB/c and C58 mouse strains had the highest prevalence (about 60% of animals) and C3H mice a lower prevalence of about 40%. They appear to be more common in mice on the left rather than the right side of the abdomen in a ratio of 4:1.

Inflammation, haemorrhage and necrosis

Although inflammation in the adrenal parenchyma is not frequently found in the adrenal cortex, vascular dilatation, haemorrhage and necrosis are more common changes in man and laboratory animals. Dilated sinusoids, congestion and haemorrhage are often located in the deep cortex, perhaps related to the unique portal vasculature of this zone (Neville and O'Hare, 1982). Blood flow can be enhanced by stress, administration of ACTH and other hormones and therefore, changes in endocrine status may contribute to the development of congestion and haemorrhage. Individual cell cytolysis and focal necrosis may also accompany haemorrhage and congestion.

The cause of hemorrhage and necrosis is not always clear. In man it has been associated with stress, sepsis, burns, myocardial infarction, congestive cardiac failure, acute tubular necrosis hypothermia, hypoxia, vascular thrombosis and treatment with anticoagulants (Neville and O'Hare, 1982).

A number of xenobiotics have the potential to cause necrosis and haemorrhagic infarction in the adrenal cortex of man and laboratory animal species. Examples include acrylonitrile, thioguanine, thioacetamide, 7,12-dimethyl benz(a)anthracene (DMBA), and hexadimethrine bromide (Strauss, 1982). The fat soluble drug O,P'DDD (2,2-bis(2-chlorophenyl-4-chlorophenyl)-1,1-dichloroethane is of particular interest in this context for it has been used to treat unresectable metastatic adrenocortical carcinomas in man (Hutter and Kayhoe, 1966). This agent is highly cytotoxic to adrenal cortical cells, inducing degenerative changes in the adrenal mitochondria and subsequent cellular disruption, primarily in the zona fasciculata and reticularis but largely sparing the glomerulosa (Kaminsky et al., 1962). The dog appears particularly sensitive to the necrotizing effects of this agent, whereas the rat and guinea pig are resistant, with the human adrenal being of intermediate susceptibility (Temple and Liddle, 1970).

Fatty change, lipidosis

Accumulation of lipid is a common phenomenon in the adrenal cortex and occurs under a variety of different conditions. The normal, unstressed cortex contains plentiful lipid droplets, usually about 0.5 μm diameter. It is well established that lipid droplets contain esterified cholesterol (Nussdorfer, 1980). Lipid droplets become larger or more prominent in some species as age advances and in response to other physiological changes. Increased lipid deposition also occurs in the cell cytoplasm of the zona glomerulosa, fasciculata or reticularis following treatment with drugs and other xenobiotics. A number of chemicals which produce fatty change have been reviewed by Yarrington (1983) and Ribelin (1984).

A chemical substance can increase lipid deposition in the adrenal cortex as part of a general cytotoxic phenomenon. It also occurs as a pharmacologically-mediated inhibition of a steroid synthesis pathway which leads to accumulation of cholesterol and steroid precursors. The distinction between these cellular processes by light microscopic examination may not be possible, although the presence of additional histological features may be helpful. For instance, chronic inhibition of steroid synthesis may also lead to adrenocortical hyperplasia by a negative feedback stimulating ACTH production. This may not only produce an accumulation of lipid but also light and electron microscopic evidence of an adaptive hypertrophy and hyperplasia of cells and subcellular organelles. This constellation of changes has been termed *lipid or lipoid hyperplasia* (see below).

A directly cytotoxic phenomenon leads typically to lipid accumulation accompanied by degeneration of cytoplasmic organelles, cell death and atrophy of the cortex. An example of the latter phenomenon is provided by the agent α-(1,4-di-oxido-3-methylquinoxalin-2-yl)-N-methylnitrone. When administered to rats and dogs this agent produces marked vacuolar change in the cortex associated with ultrastructural evidence of lipid accumulation, disruption of smooth endoplasmic reticulum, mitochondrial damage and a prominent phagosomal changes (Yarrington, 1983). This response is eventually followed by cell death, accumulation of cholesterol and lipid droplets in macrophages, and nodular hyperplasia following longer periods of treatment.

It should also be mentioned that accumulation of lipid described above should be distinguished from part of the more generalized phenomenon of phospholipidosis which also can affect steroid producing tissue.

In summary, therefore, it is important to carefully characterize the changes associated with accumulation of lipid material in the adrenal cortex and particularly whether it is associated with hyperplasia, atrophy, or cell damage. This characterization is frequently not attempted in many reports of adrenal changes induced by xenobiotics, although the distinction between simple lipid accumulation and more complex pathologies is not always clear-cut in conventional haematoxylin and eosin stained sections.

Fatty change: imidazole antifungal drugs

The imidazole antimycotic drugs, ketoconazole and clotrimazole, produced lipidosis in the adrenal cortex in toxicity studies performed in both rats and dogs (Tettenborn, 1974; Food and Drug Administration, 1981: Tachibana et al., 1987). Ketoconazole produced increased lipid droplets in the cytoplasm of cells in the zona fasciculata and reticularis in rats, in association with hyperplasia and accumulation of macrophages, ceroid pigment, and eventually some fibrosis. Clotrimazole produced increased lipid vacuolation in the zona reticularis in the subacute and chronic toxicity studies performed in rats, as well as in the zona fasiculata in dogs in parallel toxicity studies (Tettenborn, 1974). As both clotrimazole and ketoconazole have been shown to inhibit a number of cyto-chrome P450-dependent steroidogenic enzyme activities in both the adrenal gland and in other tissues (Mason et al., 1985; Houston et al., 1988; Pont et al., 1982), accumulation of lipid precursors is not perhaps a surprising phenomenon in animals treated with high doses of this class of drug. The finding has relevance to man insofar as this property of inhibition of steroid synthesis has been shown to be of therapeutic benefit in the treatment of hormone-dependent diseases (Allen et al., 1983).

Myeloid bodies, myelinosomes, phospholipidosis

Myeloid bodies may accumulate in the adrenal cortex of laboratory animals as part of a generalized drug-induced phospholipidosis (see also Respiratory System, Chapter V). Histologically, the cortex is characterized by the presence of small dense cytoplasmic inclusions of variable size which are particularly prominent in semithin, plastic embedded sections stained with toluidine-blue (Lüllmann-Rauch, 1979). They are not so easily discernible from other forms of lipid vacuolation in routine paraffin wax exbedded, haematoxylin and eosin stained sections, especially as the normal unstressed cortex is replete with lipid (Fig. 122). Ultrastructural examination shows that these bodies are composed of lamellated or crystalloid, membrane-bound lysosomal inclusions although their precise fine structural features vary with drug and animal species.

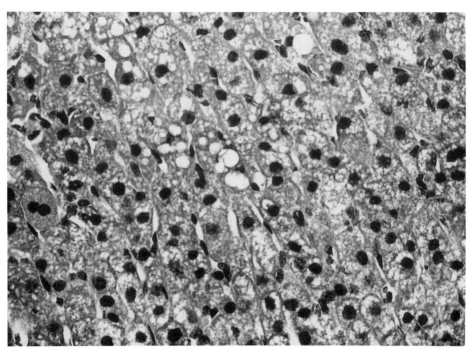

Fig. 122. Adrenal cortex of a Wistar rat treated with an amphiphilic, cationic drug for several weeks. The non-specific, vacuolation of these cortical cells proved to be the result of the accumulation of myelinosomes. (HE, ×400.)

Cytoplasmic bodies, spironolactone or S bodies

Spironolactone bodies are distinct entities found in the adrenal cortex. They are spherical, eosinophilic, lamellar cytoplasmic bodies originally described in cells of the zona glomerulosa in patients treated with the anti-mineralcorticoid compound spironolactone (Janigan, 1963). Spironolactone, a steroid molecule, is known to antagonize the electrolyte effects of aldosterone in target cells at the level of the renal tubules, but it is also capable of inhibition of aldosterone biosynthesis (Corvol et al., 1981).

The spironolactone bodies are found predominantly in the subcapsular layers of the zona glomerulosa and vary from 2 to 25 μm in diameter. The margin of each body is separated from the surrounding cytoplasm by a dense halo. Ultrastructural study shows that they are composed of dense whorls of laminated membranes (Kovacs et al., 1973; Strauss, 1982). Histochemical study demonstrates that the bodies are composed of phospholipids as shown by positive staining with sudan black B, luxol fast blue and acid haematin (Janigan, 1963). Enzyme cytochemical investigation shows that most of these bodies have high activity of 3β-hydroxysteroid dehydrogenase but low activities of glucose-6-phosphate dehydrogenase, succinate dehydrogenase. This suggests that they are composed principally of membranes of smooth endoplasmic reticulum (Aiba et al., 1981). Furthermore, the bodies generally show a paucity of activity of acid phosphatase, non-specific esterase, and other lysosomal enzymes, unlike findings in generalized phospholipidosis. This lack of relationship to lysosomes may be an explanation for the persistence of these bodies after cessation of treatment with spironolactone (Aiba et al., 1981).

These structures have no clear significance for man in terms of safety of spironolactone. It is of note that they are less easily induced in laboratory animals, although similar structures have been noted at ultrastructural level in rats treated with spironolactone (Fisher and Horvat, 1971).

Similar cytoplasmic bodies may represent potentially useful diagnostic clues in the histological diagnosis of cortical neoplasms secreting aldosterone.

Brown atrophy, brown degeneration, lipofuscin or ceroid deposition

A striking feature of the mouse adrenal 'gland is its predisposition to the accumulation of ceroid pigment, particularly in the degenerating X-zone at the corticomedullary interface which may extend to involve the medulla. Histologically, this pigment takes the form of bulky, brown, cell-like masses of finely vacuolated material forming at the inner layer of the cortex. The pigment shows the usual staining characteristics of ceroid being fuchsinophilic, acid fast and negative with Perl's stain for iron. In some strains, especially BALB/c mice, it is a particularly common finding (Dunn, 1970). Its appearance can be potentiated by the administration of oestrogens (Schardein et al., 1967; Dunn, 1970; Highman et al., 1977).

Ceroid pigment is also seen in the rat adrenal gland (Greaves and Faccini, 1984). Lipofuscin was reported in the adrenal glands of rats in the chronic toxicity studies performed with the imidazol antifungal agent, ketoconazole (Food and Drug Administration, 1981; Tachibana et al., 1987). This pigment was observed in association with the accumulation of fat in the zona fasciculata and reticularis. Electron microscopic examination showed that the pigment was localized in lysosomes.

In the aged hamster, dense aggregates of ceroid pigment may also accumulate at the corticomedullary border. Ultrastructural study of the adrenal gland of the hamster has shown that pigment accumulates in cells of the inner zone of the reticularis in macrophages (Nickerson, 1979). Oestrogens are also able to potentiate the appearance of this pigment in the adrenal glands of hamsters (Koneff et al., 1946).

Atrophy of the adrenal cortex: zona glomerulosa

Substances with inhibitory effects on the renin-angiotensin system, or other systems influencing zona glomerulosa function, may produce a reduction in the thickness of this layer and reduce zona glomerulosa cell size.

Morphometric study of the adrenal cortex from rats treated with the inhibitor of angiotensin-converting enzyme, captopril, has shown that there is a significant decrease in the volume of glomerulosa cells, associated with smaller nuclear and mitochondrial volumes and reduced surface areas of mitochondrial cristae and membranes of endoplasmic reticulum (Mazzocchi et al., 1984). These effects were completely abolished by concomitant administration of angiotensin II. When ACTH secretion is suppressed, salt loading, potassium depletion, administration of the mineralocorticoid hormones, aldosterone and deoxycorticosterone as well as β-adrenergic blocker timolol are also able to produce reduction in the thickness of the zona glomerulosa (Mazzocchi et al., 1982; Nussdorfer et al., 1982).

A sulphated mucopolysaccharide, N-formyl-chitosan polysulphuric acid (RO1–8307), was also shown to reduce the width of the zona gloumerulosa when administered to rats for up to four weeks, an effect probably related to its ability to inhibit aldosterone secretion (Abbott et al., 1966).

Prolonged infusion of rats with atrial natiuretic factor (ANF) induced atrophy of the zona glomerulosa and lowering of plasma concentration of aldosterone with changes in plasma renin activity (Mazzocchi et al., 1987a). Morphometric analysis of the adrenal cortex of rats treated with ANF revealed a decrease in the volume of zona glomerulosa cells and their nuclei, a decrease in mitochondrial volume and surface area per cell of mitochondria cristae and smooth endoplasmic reticulum profiles and a concomitent increase in the volume of the lipid droplet compartment. The findings were interpreted to indicate an inhibitory effect of ANF on the steroidogenic capacity of the rat renal zona glomerulosa (Mazzocchi et al., 1987a).

Atrophy of the adrenal cortex: zona fasciculata and reticularis

Excess corticosteroids, whether exogeneous or endogeneous in origin from a steroid-producing neoplasm, lead to loss of adrenal weight and atrophy of the adrenal cortex with relative sparing of the zona glomerulosa.

In a study of the adrenals in dogs treated with 25 mg of hydrocortisone acetate for one year, Bloodworth (1975) demonstrated reduction in thickness of the fascicularis and reticularis with ultrastructural evidence of an increase in extracellular space between individual cells and cell cords, due to an increase in loose collagen. The cells of the fasciculata showed reduction in cytoplasmic lipid, the mitochondria developed plate-like cristae and abundant matrix and there were only modest quantities of smooth endoplasmic reticulum and ribosomes. About 20% of cells in the inner cortex showed cellular degeneration and the accumulation of rounded vacuolated cell debris, membraneous material and pigment. The glomerulosa remained relatively unaltered, although an increase in lipid in this layer was reported (Bloodworth, 1975).

In rats, hydrocortisone or dexamethazone administration produces a similar reduction in the thickness of the cortex, associated with reduction in nuclear size and increased lipid in the zona glomerulosa and fasciculata (Malendowicz, 1973; McNicol et al., 1988). Enzyme cytochemical studies in rats treated with hydrocortisone shows decreased activity of succinate dehydrogenase, NADH2 tetrazolium reductase, ATPase, acid phosphatase and non-specific esterase, although increases in 5'-nucleotidase and alkaline phosphatase are reported (Malendowicz, 1973).

Long-standing atrophy is also characterized histologically by thickening of the fibrous tissue of the capsule of the adrenal gland (Fig. 123). Fibrosis usually does not occur within the gland parenchyma itself. Atrophy of the adrenal cortex may be associated with diffuse fatty change following administration of hydrocortisone and other xenobiotics (Malendowicz, 1973; Yarrington, 1983).

There is evidence that certain hypocholesterolaemic drugs can also decrease the number of lipid droplets in the cells of the zona fasciculata in laboratory animals (Magalhaes et al., 1987). See also below.

Subcapsular proliferation: mouse (subcapsular cell hyperplasia, spindle cell hyperplasia, type A cell hyperplasia)

Spindle or fusiform cell proliferation beneath the adrenal capsule is a common finding in mice as they advance in age, although degree of change varies considerably between different strains. This can appear as a fairly uniform thickening of the capsule, develop as localized, wedged-shaped proliferation beneath the capsule or become an extensive mass replacing much of the cortex. Microscopically, the cells are oval or fusiform with scanty basophilic cytoplasm and little or no mitotic activity (A cells). These cells may be admixed with larger, rounded or polygonal cells with abundant clear or eosinophilic cytoplasm (B

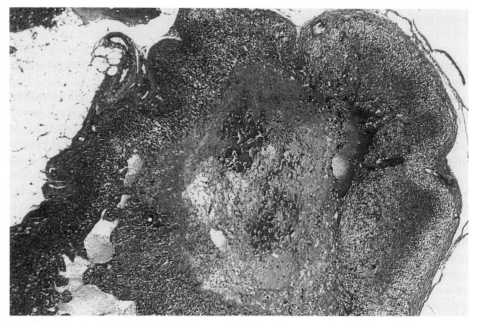

Fig. 123. Adrenal cortical atrophy in a 22-month-old Long-Evans rat that had a cortical adenoma in the contralateral gland. The cortex shows the typical reduction in thickness and the fibrous thickening of the capsule. (HE, ×50.)

cells). In advanced cases it may be difficult to make the distinction between a non- neoplastic proliferative condition and neoplasia.

The mouse is particularly predisposed to the development of this proliferative lesion although its pathogenesis remains uncertain. Similar morphological changes without symptoms have been observed in older men and women, and these may become large enough to be seen by naked eye at autopsy (Carney, 1987). The nature of the spindle cell proliferation in man is also unknown although it has been suggested it may represent metaplasia of adrenal cells into a tissue resembling ovarian stroma (Carney, 1987).

The prevalence of this striking change in the mouse adrenal can be influenced by the effect of housing conditions. In the study by Chvédoff and colleagues (1980) in which Swiss mice were housed for 18 months at densities of one, two, four, and eight in cages 27 × 21 × 14 cm, the prevalence of adrenal subcapsular proliferation showed a parabolic distribution. The lesions were less frequently seen in mice housed one or eight to a cage than in mice housed in groups of two or four. The reason for this pattern remains unexplained, although it was suggested that adrenal activity related to stress of isolation or crowding, may have been an explanation for the parabolic distribution in this study, less stress being present in groups housed two or four to a cage. Gonadectomy also enhances the development of this change in both male and female mice (Dunn, 1970).

Hypertrophy and diffuse hyperplasia of the adrenal cortex: zona fasciculata and reticularis

The adrenal cortex responds to prolonged stress or ACTH administration by an increase in weight associated with higher circulatory levels of adrenal corticoids (Bates et al, 1964; Bloodworth, 1975). It is well recognized that ACTH is a major controlling factor in corticosteroid hormone biosynthesis during stress. An increase in circulating ACTH levels precedes increases in the corticosteroid hormones during stress and this is a result of a coordinated action of both ACTH and pro-γ-melanotropin on cholesterol metabolism (Alfano et al., 1983).

Whether increased adrenal weight is induced by stress or administration of ACTH, its analogues, or other stimulatory agents, it is necessary to consider the concept of metabolic zonation which occurs in the adrenal cortex in order to interprete the histological changes.

The normal resting adrenal gland of healthy, unstressed animals, the adrenal gland in people dying suddenly or surgically excised glands are replete with lipid and the cells of the fasciculata show a foamy, clear cell appearance (clear cells) (Fig. 124).

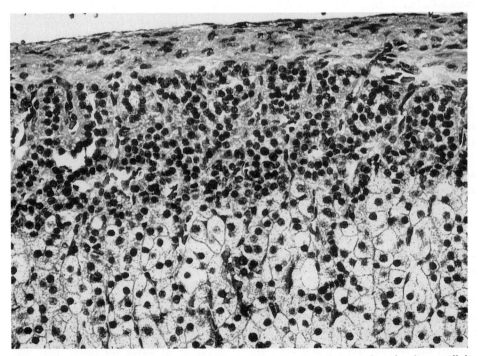

Fig. 124. Normal adrenal cortex from a healthy, unstressed cynomolgus monkey showing a well-defined zona glomerulosa and clear lipid-laden cytoplasm of the cells of the zona fasciculata. (HE, ×250.)

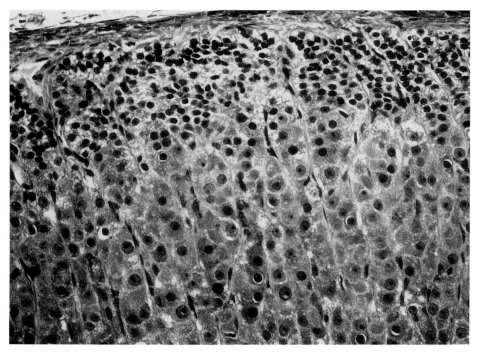

Fig. 125. Adrenal cortex from a cynomolgus monkey which was killed after a period of spontaneous, intercurrent disease. Here, lipid-depleted cells with eosinophilic cytoplasm, typical of an active or 'stressed' adrenal cortex are seen. (HE, ×250.)

In most human autopsy specimens in which death is preceded by more prolonged illness or in animals with diseases, adrenal glands are heavier than in the unstressed state. Similar changes follow ACTH administration. Histologically, the cortical cells show features of increased activity and are referred to as *lipid depleted* or *compact cells*. These cells possess a compact, or dense eosinophilic cytoplasm with reduction in cytoplasmic lipid and large vesicular nuclei with prominent nucleoli (Fig. 125). These changes are reflected at ultrastructural level by a reduction in the number of lipid vacuoles, increased numbers and size of mitochondria, often with vesicular cristae, and prominent endoplasmic reticulum (Symington, 1969; Merry, 1975; Bloodworth, 1975; Neville and O'Hare, 1982).

The shift from clear to compact cells commences at the junction of the fascicular and reticularis. The change progresses outwards towards the capsule when the stress or ACTH stimulus is prolonged until the entire fasciculata is composed of compact cells. Study of the adrenal cortex in rats treated with ACTH for several days has shown that the nuclei of the zona fasciculata and reticularis are larger than controls and those in the fasciculata usually contain one to two nucleoli. In addition, cytochemical study shows increased cytoplasmic activity of acid phosphatase and non-specific esterases, particularly in the zona fasciculata where granules of activity are located in the Golgi area and adjacent to the cell membrane (Malendowicz, 1973). Similar morphological and enzyme cytochemical changes were found in rats treated with metopirone, a specific inhibitor of 11β-hydroxylase presumably as a result a compensatory increase in ACTH secretion.

Following cessation of stress or withdrawal of ACTH administration, a 'reversion reaction' or repletion of lipid occurs. This also occurs from inwards-outwards until all the fasciculata cells have reverted to a clear lipid repleted pattern. It is important to note that the depletion-repletion sequence may not always be entirely regular. When marked stimulation occurs, individual cells may actually undergo degeneration or necrosis (Bloodworth, 1975). Zones of lipid-replete cells may also be seen as islands among lipid depleted cells. This latter effect may be important in the development of focal hyperplasia.

Diffuse hyperplasia of the adrenal cortex has been described in the diabetic mouse mutant C57BL/KsJ db/db associated with other endocrine derangements, including increases in endogeneous catecholamines and adrenal medullary hyperplasia (Carson et al., 1982). Rats treated with high doses of the direct acting vasodilator pinacidil for four to eight weeks also developed diffuse adrenocortical hyperplasia (Arrigoni-Martelli and Finucane, 1985).

Agents with effects on cholesterol synthesis may also produce adrenal cortical hypertrophy or hyperplasia. A seven day infusion of rats with the competitive inhibitor of hydroxymethylglutaryl coenzyme A (HMG-CoA) reductase, lovastatin (mevinolin), produced an increase in the volume of the zona fascicula, associated with increases in the volumes of nuclear, mitochondrial and peroxisomal compartments and decreases in lipid droplets (Rebuffat et al., 1987). Prolonged administration of the hypocholesterolaemic agent 4-aminopyrazolopyridine to rats was also shown to produce an increase in the volume of the zona fasciculata associated with hypertrophy of the smooth endoplasmic reticulum, peroxisomal proliferation and lipid droplet depletion (Mazzocchi et al., 1987b).

Lipid or lipoid hyperplasia

Compounds which inhibit enzymes in the synthetic pathway of corticosteroids induce adrenocortical hyperplasia by a negative feedback mechanism which stimulates ACTH secretion. This hyperplastic process can be accompanied by an accumulation of cholesterol and steroid precursors in the cytoplasm of adrenocortical cells giving rise to a clear cell or foamy appearance, sometimes with cholesterol cleft formation. This constellation of changes has been termed *lipid or lipoid hyperplasia* (Zak, 1983a). Examples of compounds inducing this change include amphenone, aniline and its analogue, aminoglutethimide (Schwarz and Suchowsky, 1963; Kovacs et al., 1971; Malendowicz, 1973).

Aminoglutethimide, an amino derivative of the hypnotic glutethimide, is of particular interest in this context for its effects on the adrenal have been well-characterized and represent a typical form of lipid or lipoid hyperplasia.

Its effects on the endocrine system were first described in man following its introduction as an anticonvulsant in the USA in 1960 (Hughes and Burley, 1970). Although this drug is no longer employed as an anticonvulsant, its endocrine 'side-effects' have found therapeutic use in the treatment of hormone-dependent cancers. Aminoglutethimide inhibits several P450-mediated hydroxylation steps in adrenal cortical biosynthesis, especially cholesterol side chain cleavage (enzymatic conversion of cholesterol to pregnenolone) by suppressing 20α-hydroxylation of the cholesterol side chain (Zak, 1983a). In man, it produces clinical and serum electrolyte manifestations of adrenal cortical insufficiency. Morphological studies of adrenals from patients treated with aminoglutethimide have shown increased gland size, increased thickness of the zona fasciculata associated with increased numbers of cells containing cytoplasmic lipid, but a decrease in thickness of the zona glomerulosa (Camacho et al., 1966; Givens et al., 1968).

Studies in rats and dogs have shown similar morphological changes. A thickened zona glomerulosa is characterized by increased number of cells with pale staining vacuolated cytoplasm containing excess lipid. Some cells may contain small, needle-shaped or rhombic crystals, believed to be cholesterol or cholesterol esters which may evoke cytolysis and be accompanied by foci of inflammation (Marek et al., 1970; Marek and Motlik, 1978; Zak et al., 1985). Histochemical study shows an increase in acid phosphatase activity associated with increased numbers of macrophages (Motlik et al., 1978).

Following continued treatment, necrotic foci became replaced by fibrous tissue and adrenocortical zonation becomes obliterated (Starka and Motlik, 1971; Marek and Motlik, 1975). Ultrastructural study shows increases in cytoplasmic lipid droplets, mitochondrial swelling, and striking intra-mitochondria membrane cavities of up to 6 μm diameter (Marek and Motlik, 1978).

These morphological features are compatible with the concept that by blocking steroid synthesis, aminoglutethimide increases storage of non-utilized natural steroid precursors. Under such conditions there is also a negative feedback mechanism which results in increased ACTH secretion leading to diffuse adrenocorticohyperplasia (Goldman, 1970).

These alterations, following administration of aminoglutethimide, resemble those reported in the rat following subcutaneous administration of aniline which probably also inhibits an early phase of steroidogenesis (Kovacs et al., 1971). The findings are also characterized by adrenal enlargement, accumulation of cytoplasmic lipid droplets and cholesterol crystals, associated with mitochondrial degeneration, proliferation of the smooth endoplasmic reticulum, dilatation of the Golgi and an increase in lysosomes, most pronounced in inner cortical zones.

These changes are different to those produced by metyrapone, an inhibitor of steroid synthesis at the 11β-hydroxylase step. This agent produced an ACTH-like (compact cell) hyperplasia without lipid accumulation in rats (see above). This hyperplasia is associated with increased enzymatic activity of succinate dehydrogenase and NADH2 tetrazolium reductase in contrast to the changes produced by aminoglutethimide (Malendowicz, 1973).

Cyanoketone (WIN 24540), an agent that inhibits microsomal 3β-hydroxysteroid dehydrogenase, therefore blocking the conversion of pregnenolone to progesterone in adrenocortical cells, also induces hypertrophy of the zona fasciculata when administered for several days to rats. Robba and collegues (1987) showed that the hypertrophy induced by cyanoketone was associated with an increase in total mitochondrial volume and smooth endoplasmic reticulum as well as an increase in the volume of lipid droplets and total cholesterol in cells of the zona fasciculata.

Hypertrophy and diffuse hyperplasia of the adrenal cortex: glomerulosa

Compounds, with effects on the regulatory renin-angiotensin system may cause cell enlargement and widening of the zona glomerulosa. Administration of renin or angiotensin II or III not only increases aldosterone secretion but also the thickness of the zona glomerulosa (Bondy, 1985). Angiotensin II is believed to be a potent stimulator of zona glomerulosa growth (Nussdorfer, 1986). Other factors which indirectly stimulate the renin-angiotensin system or affect control mechanisms may also cause thickening of the zona glomerulosa. These include salt depletion, potassium loading, ischaemia, renovascular hypertension and administration of ACTH (Nussdorfer, 1986). Administration of ACTH affects primarily the zona fasciculata but it has been shown in rats that in the absence of other adrenoglomerulotrophic factors, ACTH also stimulates the growth of the zona glomerulosa. ACTH was shown to increase volume of zona glomerulosa cells, nuclei, mitochondria, lipid, surface areas of mitochondrial cristae and smooth endoplasmic reticulum in rats treated with a β-adrenergic blocker and salt loading which suppressed other control mechanisms (Nussdorfer et al., 1982).

Chronic, but not acute, prolactin treatment of rats has also been shown to produce an increase in the volume of the zona glomerulosa, associated with an increase in total cell volume, nuclear volume, mitochondrial volume, lipid droplet volume, increase in surface mitochondrial cristae smooth endoplasmic reticulum (Mazzocchi et al., 1986). This raises the possibility that prolactin is involved in the physiological control of zona glomerulosa and may explain some of the sodium and water retention in hyperprolactinaemia.

Nimodopine, a calcium channel antagonist of dihydropyridine type, produced thickening of the zona glomerulosa associated with increased adrenal weight when administered to rats in high doses for two years, although no nodules or neoplasms were associated with this change (Scriabine et al., 1985). Similar morphological changes were observed in the zona glomerulosa of rats treated with nitrendipine, another calcium channel blocker of similar class (Hoffmann, 1984). The biological significance of this change is uncertain, although another calcium channel blocker has been shown to inhibit secretion of aldosterone by angiotensin II (McAllister et al., 1983) possibly mediated by changes in transmembrane calcium ion flux (Millar and Struthers, 1984).

Focal hyperplasia, foci of cellular alteration, nodular hyperplasia, hyperplastic nodules

Focal alterations and nodules are seen commonly in the adrenal cortex of rats, mice, hamsters, dogs, rabbits, non-human primates, and man with advancing age (Dunn, 1970; Pour et al., 1976; Anderson and Capen, 1978; Appleby and Sohrabi-Haghdorst, 1980).

Their classification has been the source of some dispute, largely as a result of the difficulty in making a clear distinction on histopathological criteria between more florid nodular hyperplasia and adenoma. However, there are a number of reasons why a conservative approach should be adopted in the evaluation of these nodular lesions and the criteria for diagnosis of an adenoma be applied as strictly as in other endocrine organs.

Nodular lesions of the human adrenal cortex, extremely common in advanced age, were long considered to be 'non-functioning' adenomas (Neville, 1978). It is now clear that many of these nodules represent focal hyperplasia. The study by Dobbie (1969) in which a random collection of adrenals obtained from 50 adult human necropsies were subject to detailed three-dimensional study, showed that nodular hyperplasia was a well-defined morphological entity. The lesions were multifocal and bilateral, and situated in any part of the cortex. The smallest or early lesions consisted of small foci or nodules of clear cells. Larger lesions were of varying dimensions, and composed of clear and compact cells with irregular organization of capillaries, some of which developed angiomatous formations or haemorrhage.

A significant correlation was found between the presence of nodules, general cardiovascular disease and pathology of adrenal capsular blood vessels. It was suggested that the focal nodular hyperplasia represents a localized response to loss of cortical cells (segmental atrophy) as a result of focal ischaemia (Dobbie, 1969).

Wexler (1964) has also shown a correlation between the presence of adrenocortical nodules and accelerated vascular disease in male and female rats subjected to repeated breeding sequences. He suggested not only that nodules were a response to adrenocortical hyperactivity induced by repeated breeding, but also that the vascular changes were potentiated by hyperadrenocorticism, analogous to the accelerated vascular and other degenerative changes found in Cushing's syndrome in man.

This association between repeated breeding and adrenocortical nodular hyperplasia concords with the observation by Strauss (1982) that intermittent stimulation by ACTH leads to a picture of nodular hyperplasia, whereas prolonged continuous ACTH administration or stress leads to a diffuse proliferation and lipid depletion of the cortex.

The development of focal hyperplasia of the cortex can be induced or accelerated experimentally by other factors which cause adrenocortical hyper-activity. Castration is one of the most effective methods of inducing focal hyperplasia, particularly in mice (Dunn, 1970). The relationship between gonadectomy and adrenal nodules in mice is, however, highly strain dependent, some strains being highly resistant to nodule development, others quite sensitive (Strickland et al., 1980). It has been proposed that gonadectomy brings about an imbalance in the pituitary-adrenal-gonadal axis leading to increased adrenocorticotrophic activity in the pituitary with production of cortical hyperplasia.

Chemical agents which cause cellular damage or atrophy of the adrenal cortex such as α-(1,4-dioxido-3-methylquinoxalin-2-yl)-N-methyl-nitrone, or dimethyl-benzanthracene also produce a nodular regenerative hyperplasia. The accompanying histological features of fatty change, fibrosis calcification or atrophy help in distinguishing this form of change from neoplasia (Yarrington, 1983; Ribelin, 1984).

Another factor which may increase the appearance of focal adrenocortical hyperplasia is thymectomy of mice at birth (Zak, 1983b). The incidence of adrenocortical nodules can also be influenced by diet. Nodules were found to be more common in hamsters fed various high protein, high fat diets than low protein and fat diets (Birt and Pour, 1985).

Despite certain interspecies differences in morphology, focal hyperplasia of the adrenal cortex is broadly similar between these species including man. Small focal lesions, sometimes termed *foci of cellular alteration* or *focal hypertrophy*, are aggregates of a few cells which differ cytologically from the surrounding normal gland. Nuclei in these foci may be larger and the cytoplasm be clear, finely or coarsely vacuolated, eosinophilic, granular or show other cytoplasmic staining characteristics. Foci arising in the zona glomerulosa in certain strains of rat may be the result of different stimuli to those which influence the appearance of foci in the zona reticularis (Greaves and Rabemampianina, 1982).

As these lesions enlarge and become more nodular, they displace or compress normal surrounding gland and may be termed nodular hyperplasia. They may show a variety of cytoplasmic alterations and nuclei may be larger and more pleomorphic than normal cells. Frequently, a single lesion may be multinodular with one or more different cytological appearances. The large hyperplastic foci may show fatty change or other degenerative alterations and there may be congestion and haemorrhage. By contrast, as in other endocrine glands, neoplasms tend to be solitary, with a much more monomorphic proliferating cell population (see below).

Adrenal medulla

Although the boundary between the cortex and medulla is reasonably demarcated, islands of normal cortical cells may be located deep within the medulla. The close anatomical relationship of the medulla with the cortex poses certain problems in the assessment of the medulla. The medulla cannot be satisfactorily enucleated from the gland. Furthermore, the total weight of the adrenal gland is a poor indicator of medullary weight because the medulla comprises only about 10 to 20% of total adrenal volume in man and laboratory animals (Neville, 1969; Landsberg and Young, 1985). Particular care needs to be

713

taken in the morphometric assessment of the medulla because single measurements of single cross-sections may not be representative of the entire gland. This is especially true of the human medulla which occupies only the head and body of the gland (Neville, 1969). Accurate morphometric assessment of the rat adrenal medulla also requires multiple sections even though the medulla extends throughout the gland in this species (Boelsterli et al., 1984).

The principle cells of the adrenal medulla are the so-called pheochromocytes or chromaffin cells. The term chromaffin is derived from their characteristic darkening on exposure to aqueous solutions of potassium dichromate as a result of oxidation and polymerization of catecholamines (chromaffin reaction). The chromaffin cells are arranged in nests, cords, clumps or alveoli around a rich vascular network of capillaries and sinusoids. Also present are neurones and Schwann cell-like glial cells, the latter staining with immunocytochemical techniques for S-100 protein (Tischler and DeLellis, 1988a). The blood supply is derived both from medullary arteries and a venous portal system draining from the cortex and containing high concentrations of adrenocorticosteroids. The cells are ovoid or polygonal with rounded, frequently eccentric nuclei and finely granular or vacuoled cytoplasm. Following fixation in glutaraldehyde, two types of cytoplasmic granules are apparent in the rat medulla. Cells which contain noradrenaline possess fine brown cytoplasm, whereas adrenaline-containing cells are more eosinophilic in character (Tischler et al., 1985). The chromaffin reaction is less reliable for the detection of catecholamines in tissue sections than fluorescence methods involving use of formaldehyde vapour or glycoxylic acid treatment (Tischler and DeLellis, 1988a). Immunocytochemical methods are generally less well developed for use in the medulla.

Ultrastructural examination of chromaffin cells shows large Golgi zones, small mitochondria, small parallel stacks of rough endoplasmic reticulum and numerous free ribosomes and glycogen particles. The cytoplasm contains numerous chromaffin granules which are characterized ultra-structurally as electron dense, membrane-bound vesicles 0.1 to 0.2 μm diameter. Cells which contain adrenaline are characterised by moderately dense granules whereas noradrenaline containing cells possess granules with an extremely electron-dense core. This differential staining reaction is more marked in the rat than in the human medulla. It is believed to result from the insolublization of noradrenaline but not adrenaline by reaction with glutaraldehyde which is in turn responsible for increased osmiophilic and electron density of noradrenaline-containing granules. (Tischler and DeLellis, 1988a).

The granules have been shown to contain about 20% catecholamines, 35% protein, 20% lipid, and 15% ATP by dry weight (Landsberg and Young, 1985). In addition to catecholamines, there are also small quantities of the opioid peptides met- and leu-encephalin in the adrenal medullary cytoplasmic granules in several species including man (Yoshimasa et al., 1982; North and Egan, 1983; Stern et al., 1981). Other proteins include chromogranins, a family of acidic proteins and dopamine β-hydroxylase (Perlman and Chalfie, 1977). In contrast to catecholamines which are synthesized in the cytosol and taken up into granules, neuro-

714

peptides are synthesised in the rough endoplasmic reticulum and assembled into granules in the Golgi (Tischler and DeLellis, 1988a).

In human adults over 80% of catecholamine stored in the adrenal medulla is adrenalin (Coupland, 1972) although noradrenaline is the principle form in the first-year of life (Neville, 1969). Noradrenaline-containing cells comprise about 10% of the area in the medulla of Long-Evans rats (Tischler et al., 1985). It is probable that the enzyme, phenethanolamine-N-methyl transferase, required for the formation of adrenaline is only acquired after birth and its activity seems to be controlled by adult adrenal cortical hormones perfusing the medulla via the portal system (Neville, 1969). The older literature indicates that a similar decrease in the noradrenaline:adrenaline ratio also occurs with age in cats, dogs, rabbits, and guinea pigs, whereas in rats the ratio changes little (see review by Neville, 1969).

Synthesis of catecholamines takes place principally in the cytosol starting from tyrosine derived from diet or synthesis in the liver. The hydroxylation of tyrosine to L-dopa by the enzyme tyrosine hydroxylase which requires molecular oxygen and a reduced pteridine cofactor, appears to be the rate-limiting step. The aromatic-L-amino acid decarboxylase and dopamine-β-hydroxylase catalyse formation of dopamine and noradrenaline, respectively.

Formation of adrenaline takes place in some cells by the action of the enzyme phenylethanolamine-N-methyltransferase (Landsberg and Young, 1985). Although the biosynthesis takes place principally in the cytosol, catecholamines are stored in the granules which first appear in the Golgi and accumulate in the peripheral parts of the cell cytoplasm.

The regulation of synthesis and release is undoubtably complex but the physiological stimulus for release is acetylcholine originating from the rich network preganglionic sympathetic nerve endings which synapse on chromaffin cells. In common with other endocrine organs, the most common spontaneous or drug-induced lesions of the adrenal medulla are various forms of hyperplasia and neoplasia (pheochromocytoma).

Hyperplasia

Both focal and diffuse adrenal medullary hyperplasia occur in aged laboratory rodents but hyperplasia is particularly common in certain strains of rat where its development can be enhanced by administration of agents which alter hormonal status (Boelsterli and Zbinden, 1985). By contrast, hyperplasia is less commonly reported in the adrenal medulla of man (Tischler et al., 1985). In rodents, the principle diagnostic difficulty is that hyperplasia forms a continuous histological spectrum with undoubted neoplastic growth (pheochromocytoma) of the medulla and unfortunately there are no generally accepted criteria for the separation of hyperplasia from neoplasia in rodents (Strandberg, 1983). This difficulty has given rise to regulatory controversy about the safety of xenobiotics which produce medullary hyperplasias in the rat.

Although Hollander and Snell (1976) resolved this difficulty by dispensing with the concept of hyperplasia and grouped all proliferative lesions of the rat adrenal medulla as pheochromocytomas, this also creates difficulties. The term pheochromocytoma is widely used by pathologists to denote medullary neoplasms in man associated with a particular constellation of clinicopathological findings and it is unreasonable to group small clusters of asymptomatic basophilic cells with such major lesions.

Roe and Bär (1985) used a five point grading system for hyperplasia on a fine-point scale, recognizing that the distinction between their category of severe hyperplasia (grade 5) and benign neoplasia is uncertain. They justified this approach on the basis that the main objective in toxicologic pathology is to distinguish between appearances in control and treated animals and absolute diagnoses are not always necessary. This method undoubtably has the merit of avoiding placing lesions in inappropriate and misleading categories.

Provided a conservative approach is adopted, it is reasonable, as in other endocrine organs, to make the distinction between hyperplasia and neoplasia. This can aid in the comparison between species and help extrapolate results in animals to man. It is nevertheless important that the pathologist adopts precise and consistent criteria for the diagnosis of focal and diffuse hyperplasia and pheochromocytoma, particularly individual studies. Comparison between studies can be aided by adoption of a standard system of nomenclature such as that being developed by the Society of Toxicologic Pathologists.

Diffuse hyperplasia

This cellular process involves most or all of the adrenal medulla and is characterized by an expansion of the medullary volume be increased numbers of chromaffin cells without the formation of nodules. It is often associated with cell hypertrophy. The cells show tinctorial changes, but the expansion takes place diffusely without nodularity or compression of the surrounding adrenal cortex. As in other endocrine organs, morphometric analysis may be necessary to characterise the degree of hyperplasia and the commonly associated cellular hypertrophy (Boelsterli and Zbinden, 1985).

Diffuse hyperplasia may occur spontaneously in rats with advancing age and under conditions in which there has been chronic stimulation of medullary cells. Tischler and his colleagues (1985) have characterized the diffuse hyperplasia occurring in the aging Long-Evans rat. In rats younger than one year of age the medulla was shown to comprise about 8% of the volume of the adrenal gland whereas in older animals the medulla occupied twice this volume. Histologically, the cells in older animals showed slightly more pleomorphic nuclei and were arranged in thicker cords and surrounded by coarser reticulin fibres. The proportions of cell types however remain similar in all groups (Tischler et al., 1985).

Another example of diffuse medullary hyperplasia has also been described in rats exposed to hypobaric hypoxia for 28 days. Hyperplasia was characterized histologically by a distinct clustering of pheochromocytes which showed little or no cellular or nuclear pleomorphism. A characteristic feature was the compression of sinusoids by the hyperplastic cells, and stretching of endothelial cells over the cell clusters in contrast to the widely dilated sinusoids of control rats (Gosney, 1985). These changes were associated with adrenal cortical hyperplasia and increased ACTH levels. The findings were consistent with the concept that medullary hyperplasia occurs as a response to increased requirements for catecholamines in a hypoxic environment (Gosney, 1985). It is not known whether such changes occur in man under similar circumstances.

Diffuse hyperplasia of the adrenal medulla has also been recognized in diabetic mice. In the C57BL/KsJ db/db strain, there is an increase in medullary catecholamine content and increased activity of tyrosine hydroxylase, dopamine-β-hydroxylase and phenylethanolamine-N-methyltransferase. Morphometric analysis showed that the medulla was increased in size by about 30% compared with non-diabetic controls but accompanied by a lower cell density indicating medullary hypertrophy as well as hyperplasia were responsible for the size increase (Carson et al., 1982).

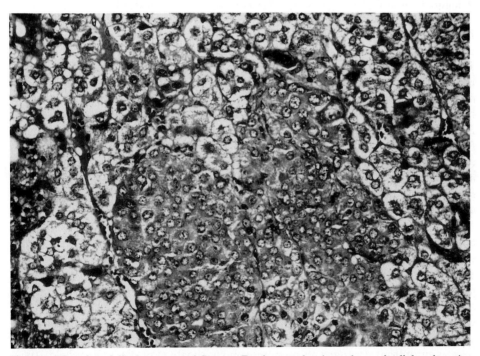

Fig. 126. Adrenal medulla from an aged Sprague-Dawley rat showing a focus of cellular alteration. (HE, ×250.)

Focal hyperplasia

Focal hyperplasia is recognized by the presence of localized aggregates of medullary cells, cytologically distinct from normal cells (Fig. 126). In rodents, cells in these foci usually possess scanty basophilic cytoplasm and enlarged nuclei. Although foci may be multinodular in character (*nodular hyperplasia*) they can be separated from neoplastic growths by the lack of marked compression or disruption of the surrounding tissues, lack of capsule or pseudocapsule and absence of other evidence of autonomous expansile growth. In rats these foci appear to be generally chromaffin negative (Gillman et al., 1953; Bosland and Baer, 1984). Some authors employ the term *basophilic focus* to denote minor foci of tinctoral attentions without other cytological changes.

Neoplasia

The most common neoplasms of the adrenal medulla observed in rodent carcinogenicity bioassays are *pheochromocytomas* and *ganglioneuromas*, both believed to derive from cells of neural crest origin. *Ganglioneuromas*, found occasionally in the adrenal medulla of rats are highly characteristic, being composed of large or small ganglion cells and variable numbers of stromal cells of spindle cell type (Reznik et al., 1980). Although *neuroblastomas*, tumours of immature neuroblasts, are well recognized tumours in the human adrenal medulla in infancy and childhood, they are only occasionally recognised in rodents. When tumours with the distinctive rosette-like clusters of small rounded or ovoid cells are found in rats they do not show other characteristic clinicopathological features of neuroblastomas in man, notably their early age of onset and biological behavior (Hollander and Snell, 1976; Reznik and Ward, 1983).

A *pheochromocytoma* is a tumour of neoplastic pheochromocytes or chromaffin cells. As noted above, pheochromocytomas may be difficult to distinguish from more florid nodular or focal hyperplasia. As with other endocrine tumours it is appropriate to adopt fairly conservative criteria, applicable to both human and rodent neoplasms to aid in interspecies comparisons. Evidence of autonomous growth is provided by compression, displacement, or disruption of the surrounding cortex and soft tissues.

In rats, pheochromocytomas are often found in a background of diffuse adrenomedullary hyperplasia (Tischler et al., 1985). The tumours are highly vascular and consequently haemorrhage, thrombosis and necrosis may be seen. Tumour cell populations are variable. They may be cytologically similar to normal pheochromocytes and be arranged in characteristic cords and nests. The cells exhibit variable degrees of pleomorphism and nuclei appear hyperchromatic with variable mitotic activity. Bizarre multinucleated giant cells may be occasionally present. Other neoplasms are composed of small basophilic cells with scanty cytoplasm arranged in monomorphous sheets (Fig. 127) (Russfield, 1967; Hollander and Snell, 1976; Burek, 1978; Majeed and Harling, 1986).

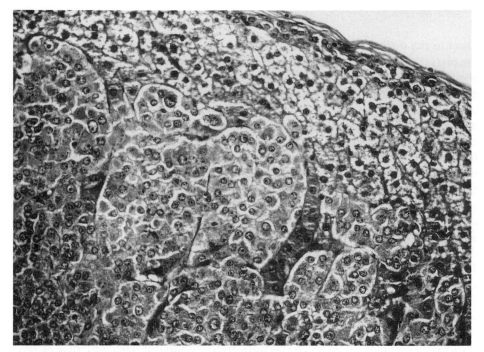

Fig. 127. Edge of a large proliferating pheochromocytoma found in the adrenal medulla of a two-year-old, Sprague-Dawley rat. (HE, ×250.)

In rodents, infiltration of tumour cells into the cortex, spread into capsular or pericapsular connective tissue or blood vessels is usually regarded as evidence of malignant behavior. A cautious application of these criteria is merited for clinicopathological study of human pheochromocytomas shows that benign and malignant pheochromocytomas may have identical appearances. The histological features of penetration of tumour cells outside the adrenal capsule or into vessels and the existance of nuclear and cellular pleomorphism has been associated with a benign clinical behavior (Neville, 1969).

The only absolute criterion for the histological diagnosis of a malignant pheochromocytoma in man remains therefore, the presence of metastatic tumour in organs where chromaffin tissue is not normally found. There is no reason to suppose, based on the few metastasing pheochromocytomas that have been described in rodents, that experimental malignant pheochromocytomas are biologically, fundamentally different from human pheochromocytomas.

In carcinogenicity bioassays performed in the golden hamster, pheochromocytomas are some of the commonest tumours observed (Chvédoff et al., 1984). In mice, they are generally less common spontaneous lesions.

Despite the difficulties in making the distinction between focal hyperplasia and neoplasia on purely histological grounds, it is important to note that the certain strains of rat are particularly liable to develop focal hyperplasia and neoplasia of the adrenal medulla both spontaneously with advancing age and following administration of xenobiotics. In a bioassay conducted to compare the pathology occurring in two different rat strains kept under identical conditions, pheochromocytomas developed in 12% of Long-Evans males but none occurred in females or in male or female Sprague-Dawley rats (Greaves and Rabe-mampianina, 1982). It is generally recognised that male rats are more susceptible to the development of pheochromocytomas than females (Cheng, 1980). Reported incidents of spontaneous proliferative lesions among males of different rat strains vary from 86% to 0% (Tischler and DeLellis, 1988b). Dietary factors may also be important for proliferative lesions of the adrenal medulla appear to develop more commonly in rats fed a high carbohydrate diet (Roe and Bär, 1985).

In a detailed investigation by Tischler and his colleagues (1985), it was shown that the nodular lesions occurring in the adrenal medulla of the Long-Evans rat with advancing age occurred mainly in the juxtacortical region. Cells in the foci and nodules were slightly smaller than normal pheochromocytes but with higher nuclear to cytoplasmic ratio. Cells were hyperchromatic with rounded or oval nuclei showing a greater degree of pleomorphism and mitotic activity than surrounding cells (Fig. 127). Unlike findings in diffuse hyperplasia where the reticulin network is preserved, these focal lesions were shown to progressively displace reticulin fibres. The lesions were bilateral in at least 25% of older rats and often multicentric in single glands and it was suggested that medium sized and large nodular growths were probably neoplastic (Tischler and DeLellis, 1988b).

At ultrastructural level, cells in foci and nodules were characterized by smaller and more homogenous secretory granules than in cells in non-nodular zones but with electron density similar to that observed in normal noradrenaline-containing cells. Biochemical analysis showed that the proliferating cells contained predominantly noradrenaline but with immuno-reactive neurotensin and neuro-peptide.

Focal hyperplasia and pheochromocytoma are also more liable to develop in rats compared with other species following treatment with xenobiotics (Ribelin, 1984). Focal proliferative lesions of the adrenal medulla, including those di-agnosed as pheochromocytoma have been described in the rat following ionizing radiation (Warren et al., 1966), administration of nicotine (Eränkö, 1955; Boels-terli et al., 1984), growth hormone (Moon et al., 1950), a synthetic derivative of retinol (Kurokawa et al., 1985), blocadren, a β-adrenergic blocker, zomepirac, an analgesic (Mosher and Kircher, 1988), reserpine (National Cancer Institute, 1979; Diener, 1988) and a variety of other agents including neuroleptic drugs, lactose and polyols such as sorbitol, mannitol, xylitol and lactitol (Roe and Bär, 1985; Bär, 1988).

Most of the agents which produce hyperplasia and neoplasia, are not genotoxic agents and the mechanisms involved remain unclear. Boelsterli and Zbinden (1985) have suggested that long-term administration of xylitol and other polyols to rats in high doses inhibit catecholamine synthesis. This results in compensatory medullary hypertrophy, hyperplasia and eventually neoplasia.

Roe and Bär (1985) have suggested that the stimulatory effects of the polyols on the rat adrenal medulla are mediated by altered calcium homeostasis. Lactoses and certain polyols are relatively poorly absorbed from the gastrointestinal tract and their presence in the lower ileum is likely to facilitate the absorption of calcium, which may in turn influence adrenal medullary activity. Zomepirac sodium, another agent producing medullary proliferation, may also alter calcium homeostasis because it binds tightly to calcium (Mosher and Kircher, 1988).

Although synthetic retinol acetate has been shown to possess some activity in the Ames test employing certain strains of Salmonella, retinols have been widely used as drugs and food additives and have been shown to possess an inhibitory effect on tumour development in many different systems (Sporn and Roberts, 1983; Moon et al., 1983; Boutwell, 1983). However, when retinol acetate was administered to F344/DuCrj rats, hyperplasia of the medulla and increase numbers of pheochromocytomas were reported (Kurokawa et al., 1985). Similar findings have been reported with other synthetic retinoids (Kamm, 1982).

Although the mechanisms involved in the development of proliferative lesions in the rat medulla following treatment with these agents remains unclear, the sensitivity of the rat medulla, the ubiquitous nature of some of the precipitating agents such as lactose and the lack of direct human counterpart of many of these rat proliferative lesions suggest that these lesions possess little relevance to human safety when found in preclinical toxicity studies.

THYROID GLAND

The thyroid gland is unique among endocrine organs by virtue of the large store and slow overall rate of turnover of hormone, features which probably provide prolonged protection against depletion of circulating hormone levels should synthesis cease (Ingbar, 1985).

The unit of thyroid structure is the follicle, a closed sac of variable size lined by epithelium and containing colloid. Follicles are grouped into lobules each supplied by a terminal branch of an extremely profuse blood supply. Estimates of blood flow to the thyroid parenchyma indicate that it exceeds blood flow to the kidney.

Follicular cells vary in size within the same gland, within the same lobule between different species and between different strains of rodents (Russfield, 1967). A comparative study of dogs in London and Munich showed that thyroids from dogs in Munich contained less colloid and showed taller follicular epithelium than in dogs in London, presumably as a result of differences in iodine intake (Zarrin and Hänichen, 1974). The height of follicular epithelium is a measure of glandular activity, active cells being tall columar cells, whereas inactive cells appear flattened.

Electron microscopy indicates the presence of an uninterrupted basement membrane around follicular cells. Although adjacent follicular cells are separated by a space of fairly constant width, the intercellular spaces are sealed towards the follicular lumen by extensive zonulae occludentes which are quite impervious. Experimental studies have shown that tritiated-inulin with a molecular weight of about 5000 does not pass into follicular colloid (Chow et al., 1965; Chow and Woodbury, 1965, 1970). On the apical surface of acinar cells there is a brush border composed of short, irregular microvilli which project into the colloid. Microvilli are usually about 0.2 μm in height but increase in length in hyperthyroid states.

In resting acinar cells, the nucleus is spherical, relatively poor in chromatin and centrally situated. In more active cells it becomes located near the cell base. Mitochondria and lipid droplets are fairly few in number but lysosomes are quite abundant. Large numbers of free ribosomes and a conspicuous rough endoplasmic reticulum generally distended by amorphous material of low electron density are characteristic electron microscopic features. The Golgi is also a prominent structure situated in a supranuclear or paranuclear position and associated with many small and medium sized vesicles and secretory granules (colloid droplets). The upper part of the cytoplasm is replete with small, moderately electron dense granules or apical vesicles.

The colloid, the principle product of the follicular cells contains mostly thyroglobulin, a glycoprotein composed of 10% carbohydrate, which represents the storage form of thyroid hormones. Its carbohydrate components are composed principally of glucosamine, mannose, fucose, galactose and sialic acid moeities and it possesses a molecular weight of about 660,000. In haematoxylin and eosin stained sections colloid shows variable staining intensity and is reactive with the PAS stain.

Synthesis of the peptide portion of thyroglobulin occurs in the rough endoplasmic reticulum and glycosylation takes place in the Golgi. The protein then moves to the apex of the cell where iodination of tyrosyl residues in the thyroglobulin molecule takes place to give hormonally inactive iodotyrosines. This is followed by coupling of iodotyrosines to give hormonally active iodothyronines, L-tyroxine (T4) and 3,5,3'-L-triiodothyronine (T3). Much of the iodination takes place in the newly synthesized thyroglobulin just before or just as it is extruded into the colloid by exocytosis. The coupling reaction appears to be mediated by endogenous peroxidase activity in the follicular cell of rats and mice. This activity is located in the rough endoplasmic reticulum, subapical vesicles, periluminal colloid and the trans aspect of the Golgi apparatus, the organelles associated with synthesis of thyroglobulin (Sawano and Fujita, 1981). By contrast, granules of absorptive nature are peroxidase negative.

T3 and T4 enter the blood stream after liberation from thyroglobulin by proteolytic cleavage. This takes place in the follicular cell following endocytosis of thyroglobulin to yield colloid droplets which fuse with lysosomes containing active proteases (Doniach, 1967).

The major regulator of thyroid function is pituitary thyrotropin (TSH), the elaboration of which is regulated by a classical type of feedback control by the thyroid gland. Thyrotrophin releasing hormone TRH, a modified tripeptide synthesized by peptidergic neurons in supraoptic and para-ventricular neurones of the hypothalamus, serves to stimulate release and synthesis of TSH after it is transported via the hypophyseal portal system to the pituitary gland (Ingbar, 1985). Although, TRH and thyroid hormones are major regulators of TSH secretion, somatostatin, levodopa, and dopamine may decrease the response of the thyroid to TRH.

The thyroid gland is innervated by both adrenergic and cholinergic fibres which arise from the cervical ganglia and the vagus nerve, respectively. Afferent fibres pass through the laryngeal nerves to regulate the vasomotor system, blood flow, and rate of delivery of TSH, iodide, and other metabolic substrates. In addition, the adrenergic system may influence thyroid function through a direct effect because adrenergic amines influence iodine and intermediary metabolism of the thyroid (Ingbar, 1985).

C-cells (clear cells, parafollicular cells, interfollicular cells, calcitonin-producing cells)

These cells have received particular attention over the last decade. Although their presence was noted in animals for many years, they were only recognized in the human thyroid more recently, probably because they are not numerous and they are unevenly distributed with non-specific histological appearances.

C-cells usually demonstrate light coloured granular cytoplasm in haemotoxylin and eosin stained sections. They are distributed around the follicles, often within the confines of the follicular basal lamina. They can be demonstrated at light microscopic level by argyophil staining methods (eg. Grimelius) or by immunocytochemical staining for calcitonin. Ultrastructural examination shows that they contain abundant electron-dense membrane bound cytoplasmic granules, which in man may be 280 nm in diameter (Type I) or 130 nm dimeter (Type II) (DeLellis et al., 1978). In rats, two classes of granules have also been demonstrated, Type I with a mean diameter of 190 nm, and Type II with an approximate mean diameter of 125 nm (DeLellis et al., 1979). Although mitochondria and Golgi zones are prominent in C-cells, granular endoplasmic reticulum is relatively sparse.

Immunocytochemical study with anti-calcitonin antiserum is the best method for studying the distribution of C-cells within the gland. In man, C-cells appear relatively restricted in distribution being concentrated at the junction of the upper and middle thirds of the lateral lobes along a central axis (DeLellis et al.,

1978). In the rat the C-cells are more widely distributed but with highest concentrations occurring in central regions (DeLellis et al., 1979). C-cells occupy the central parts of the thyroid gland in the Syrian hamster (DeLellis et al., 1987).

In addition to calcitonin, C-cells may elaborate other regulatory substances notably neurotensin (Zeytinoglu et al., 1983).

Inflammation, thyroiditis

Focal aggregates of acute inflammatory cells or mononuclear cells are observed in the thyroid gland of laboratory rodents, dogs and primates but are usually of little biological significance. However, the thyroid gland in both man and laboratory animals is a well recognised site for an intense chronic inflammatory process (chronic thyroiditis) often the result of, or associated with an autoimmune process. Chronic thyroiditis occurs naturally in man, laboratory beagles and certain strains of rat, especially the Buffalo and the BioBreeding/Worcester strains. Lymphocytic thyroiditis can also be induced experimentally in many species by the administration of thyroid extract with complete Freund's adjuvant. This clearly demonstrates that the thyroid gland can be a target of autoimmune attack and animals injected with thyroid extract have been used as models for the elucidation of the mechanisms involved in the human thyroiditis.

Two main forms of thyroiditis are observed in man, a subacute form (de Quervain's subacute thyroiditis) and a chronic thyroiditis (Hashimoto's thyroiditis). The former is less common, frequently seasonal and follows an upper respiratory tract infection or other viral illness such as mumps, influenza, Coxsackie, ECHO or adenovirus infection (Ingbar, 1985). It is a primary destructive condition of follicular epithelium only transiently associated with an autoimmune reaction. Subacute thyroiditis characterised histologically by a patchy or focal infiltration by mononuclear cells, loss of colloid, fragmentation of basement membrane and characteristic granulomas possessing a core of colloid and multinucleated giant cells (giant cell thyroiditis).

Hashimoto's thyroiditis is a more common disease and is believed to be a primary autoimmune disease. It not only shows a familial and female sex predisposition but an association with certain human leukocyte common antigen (HLA) haptotypes. This disease also occurs in subjects with other antimmune diseases and there are circulating anti-thyroid antibodies. Histologically, this condition is characterized by a gland which is diffusely infiltrated by lymphocytes, plasma cells and macrophages associated with active germinal centres. In most cases there is loss of colloid, degeneration of epithelial cells and fragmentation of basement membrane. Some epithelial cells become enlarged, show abundant eosinophilic cytoplasm, characteristics of the so-called Askanazy cells typical of this condition (Meissner and Warren, 1969).

Immunocytochemical analysis of the thyroid glands in Hashimoto's disease have shown that areas of greatest damage are associated with the presence of activated T4 lymphocytes (helper T lymphocytes) often distributed in close

724

relationship to germinal centres of B cell type. Activated T cells of cytotoxic/suppressor types are also found but are scattered throughout the gland often in intimate contact with the thyroid epithelium. Granular immune complexes of IgG type and complement are deposited along the follicular basement membrane mainly in zones spared from major destruction (Aichinger et al., 1985). Increased numbers of dendritic cells are also observed (Kabel et al., 1988). Whilst these findings clearly support the concept that Hashimoto's thyroiditis is mediated by an immune response, they are probably the result of a highly complex avalanche of changes with one immune response initiating a number of others (Rose, 1985).

Among animals employed in toxicology, the beagle dog appears most predisposed to develop a spontaneous chronic thyroiditis similar to that of Hashimoto's disease (Tucker, 1962; Schaffner, 1988). Other dog breeds are also affected (Gosselin et al., 1981; Conaway et al., 1985). Although the aetiology of the spontaneous lymphocytic thyroiditis in dogs is poorly understood, the presence of circulating auto-antibodies and the histological resemblance to Hashimoto's disease in man are highly suggestive of an auto-immune mechanism in this species. Its prevalence in some beagle dog colonies appears to be familiar in nature (Musser and Graham, 1968).

Histologically, this form of spontaneous thyroiditis in the beagle dog is characterized by a multifocal or diffuse infiltration of the interstitium and follicles by lymphocytes, plasma cells and macrophages accompanied by prominent germinal centres. There is loss of colloid, destruction of follicular cells some of which become enlarged with eosinophilic cytoplasm (Tucker, 1962; Fritz et al., 1970). Giant cells may be seen.

Although thyroiditis induced in laboratory animals by injection of thyroid extract and Freund's adjuvant produces thyroid auto-antibodies and thyroiditis with histological features similar to Hashimoto's thyroiditis, studies in dogs have shown that histological appearances do not entirely mimic the spontaneously occurring disease. For instance, injection of dogs with thyroid extract and Freund's adjuvant produced a spectrum of histological changes in the thyroid including an intense granulomatous reaction not usually seen in Hashimoto's thyroiditis in man or chronic spontaneous thyroiditis in the dog.

An example of immune modulation provoking thyroiditis in the beagle dog is provided by the anti-arthritic organic gold compound auranofin. Dogs treated for seven years with auranofin at 30 times the human dose developed hypothyroidism due to chronic lymphocytic thyroiditis in association with other manifistations of an immune disorder including autoimmune haemolytic anaemia and thrombocytopenia (Bloom et al., 1987).

The Buffalo and BioBreeding/Worcester (BB/W) rat strains develop lymphocytic thyroiditis spontaneously with advancing age (Silverman and Rose, 1974; Yanagisawa et al., 1986). Administration of methylcholanthrene, a carcinogenic and immunosuppressive agent, to the thyroiditis sensitive Buffalo rat can increase the incidence of thyroiditis. When this treatment is combined with neonatal thymectomy, all Buffalo rats develop the disease (Silverman and Rose,

1974). Likewise, immunisation of rats with rat thyroid extract and Bordetella pertussis vaccine without complete Freund's adjuvent results in thyroiditis in Buffalo but not Lewis rats (Silverman and Rose, 1975).

Although most rat strains only rarely develop chronic thyroiditis spontaneously, lymphocytic thyroiditis develops in normally resistant rat strains following whole body radiation and thymectomy, suggesting that immunosuppression may lead to development of an autoimmune thyroiditis in conventional rat strains (Penhale et al., 1973). Furthermore, drug-induced immunosuppression has also been reported to induce lymphocytic thyroiditis in Wistar rats, a strain which does not frequently develop thyroiditis spontaneously.

When Wistar rats were given the immunosuppressive compound, frentizole [1-(6-methoxy-2-benzothiazolyl)-3-phenyl urea] for one year they developed chronic thyroiditis when dosing was initiated in immature animals (Kitchen et al., 1979). This condition was characterised histologically by an infiltration of the thyroid by numerous lymphocytes, mixed with plasma cells and macrophages, loss of colloid, follicular cell degeneration and hyperplasia. The changes were more common in males than in females and they were slowly reversible following cessation of treatment. This thyroiditis was probably immune-mediated in view of the presence of circulating antithyroglobulin antibodies and fine granular deposits of IgG and complement in the follicular basement membrane. It was postulated that frentizole acted by depleting suppressor T lymphocytes more than the helper cells, permitting antithyroid antibody formation and development of thyroiditis (Kitchen et al., 1979).

Despite the frentizole-induced changes occurring in the Wistar rat, beagle dogs, rhesus monkeys and ICR mice did not develop these changes in similar studies (Kitchen et al., 1979). Although drug dispositional characteristics may be important in such species differences, it has been suggested on the basis of experiments transferring antithyroid antiserum between different strains of mice and chickens, that the thyroid gland of different strains and species varies in susceptibility to auto-immune damage (Rose, 1985).

Amiodarone, an iodine-containing antiarrhymic drug, is of interest for although its therapeutic use in man is associated with hyperthyroidism and thyroiditis, an autoimmune mechanism may not be involved. This condition is characterised histologically by focal destructive alteration to thyroid acini with macrophage infiltration and fibrosis similar to de Quervain's thyroiditis except for absence of granulomatous changes. The destructive process takes place however in a background of inactive follicles (Physician's Desk Reference, 1987; Lancet, 1987; Brennan et al., 1987; Smyrk et al., 1987). Although an immune mechanism may be important in some cases, the study by Smyrk and collegues (1987) suggested that amiodarone therapy leads to thyroid follicular disruption and release of iodothyronines,with increased levels of thyroid hormones producing thyrotoxicosis, TSH suppression and consequent loss of activity in residual thyroid follicles.

Atrophy

Although atrophy of the thyroid gland follows chronic inflammatory damage, it may also occur as trophic atrophy secondary to diminished secretion of thyroid stimulatory hormone or as a primary degenerative condition of follicular cells. Trophic atrophy is typically characterised histologically by thyroid follicles lined by low cuboidal or flattened epithelium showing little or no evidence of endocytosis and filled by homogenous colloid.

An example of a primary degenerative condition was reported in rats treated for 15 days with gossypol, a compound found in the cotton plant which possesses antifertility properties in male subjects.

Thyroid changes in gossypol treated rats were characterised by the presence of light-staining colloid distending follicles, associated with a dose-dependent focal atrophy and degeneration of follicular cells without associated inflammation (Rikihisa and Lin, 1989). Degenerate follicles appeared distorted and lined by degenerating and pyknotic epithelial cells, some of which were exfoliating into the follicular lumen. Affected rats also showed a dose-related reduction in free thyroxine, triiodothyronine and reverse triiodothyronine, the non-calorigenic and biologically inactive cogener of T3 (Rikihisa and Lin, 1989).

Pigmentation

Coal black pigmentation of the thyroid gland was initially reported in rats, mice, dogs and non-human primates given minocycline, a semi-synthetic tetracycline derivative for periods longer than one month (Benitz et al., 1967). Subsequently, Attwood and Dennett (1976) reported similar discolouration in the thyroid gland in man on long-term treatment with minocycline. These initial findings have been confirmed by a number of other reports in which black discolouration of the thyroid gland in man is associated with minocycline therapy (Saul et al., 1983; Reid, 1983; Gordon et al., 1984; Medeiros et al., 1984; Landas et al., 1986). Unlike tetracycline, minocycline is particularly well distributed to the thyroid (Kelly and Kanegis, 1967).

In all species treated with minocycline, including man, inspection of the cut surface of the thyroid shows striking black discolouration. Histological examination reveals finely granular dark brown pigment in the apical cytoplasm of the follicular epithelium. The pigment is not usually observed in other cells of the thyroid gland although it may occasionally be exfoliated into the colloid or be seen in macrophage-like cells in the interfollicular connective tissue (Reid, 1983; Tajima et al., 1985; Kurosumi and Fujita, 1986).

The pigment posssess histochemical characteristics of melanin pigment. It shows a positive reaction with the Masson-Fontana technique and is bleached by potassium permanganate (Reid, 1983; Tajima et al., 1985). The Perls reaction for iron and the oil-red-O stain are usually negative, although in some human cases the pigment appears to be mixed with lipofusin (Gordon et al., 1984). In all species, ultrastructural study demonstrates that deposition of pigment is primarily lysosomal in nature, characterised by rounded or large irregular eosinophilic bodies associated with lipid or colloid vacuoles. The pigment has also been demonstrated in the cysternae of the rough endoplasmic reticulum in rats given minocycline for over one month (Tajima et al., 1985).

The cause of the pigmentation and its effect on thyroid function is uncertain. Attwood and Dennett (1976) suggested that the pigment was a breakdown product of minocycline which resembled melanin. Subsequent experimental evidence appears to generally support the concept that the pigment is an oxidation product of minocycline with thyroid peroxidases being responsible for the conversion.

Minocycline is easily oxidized to black substances in vitro by the addition of 3% hydrogen peroxide (Reid, 1983). Thin layer chromatography shows that material from the thyroids of minocycline-treated rats possesses identical characteristics to minocycline when mixed with hydrogen peroxide in vitro (Tajima et al., 1985). These authors also showed that at high doses, minocycline also impairs function of the thyroid gland in rats. The total amount of T4 released from the thyroid stimulated by TSH was less than in controls and there was an increased monoiodothyrosine fraction compared with diiodotyrosine (Tajima et al., 1965).

In the original report by Benitz and colleagues (1967) hyperplastic changes in the thyroid and thyroidectomy cells in the pituitary gland were reported, also suggesting minocycline-induced functional changes. This does not appear to occur in humans at therapeutic doses (Saul et al., 1983). Clinical evidence suggests that discolouration of the thyroid associated with minocycline at therapeutic doses in patients is not associated with any adverse functional effects (Gordon et al., 1984). Minocycline has also been associated with pigmentation and discolouration of skin and bone in man (Fenske et al., 1980; McGrae and Zelickson, 1980; White and Besanceney, 1983; Cale et al., 1988; see Integumentary System, Chapter I).

Brown discolouration of the thyroid gland as a result of the accumulation of a lipofucsin pigment has been reported in rats treated with clozapine, a dibenzoazepine antipsychotic drug (Sayers and Amsler, 1977). Although it appears that clozapine is able to promote cellular lipid oxidation in the rat, it was argued that lack of thyroid pigment in mice or dogs given high doses of clozapine and the absence of any detectable functional thyroid changes in man, indicated that the finding of thyroid pigment in the rat did not represent evidence of a hazard to man (Sayers and Amsler, 1977).

Pigments may accumulate spontaneously in the thyroid glands of aging rodents notably iron in the follicular epithelium and colloid as well as lipofuscin (Ward and Reznik-Schüller, 1980).

Hypertrophy and hyperplasia

As in other endocrine organs, increased functional demand is reflected by thyroid enlargement due to cellular hypertrophy and hyperplasia. Hyperplasia may be diffuse or focal in character. Decades of study of surgically excised enlarged human thyroids (goitres) have suggested that continuous or repeated stimulation as a response to a deficiency of thyroid hormone, produces diffuse hyperplasia which eventually develops into a focal or nodular hyperplasia commonly termed adenomatous goitre (Meissner and Warren, 1969).

The term adenomatous goitre is itself a reflection of the difficulty which has been experienced in the differentiation of these focal hyperplastic lesions from true neoplasia in man. A similar difficulty is apparent in the separation of hyperplastic lesions from neoplasia in the thyroid of experimental animals. Many of the focal lesions or nodular growths which would be designated nodular hyperplasia in man are frequently diagnosed as adenomas or cystadenomas in rodents. However, a recent study in the Fischer 344 rat in which the biological properties of focal and nodular proliferative lesions induced in the thyroid by treatment with the antithyroid drug methimazole (1-methyl-2-thiomidazole) were evaluated following withdrawal of treatment, underlines the need for conservative diagnostic criteria in the diagnosis of experimental thyroid nodules. Nodular lesions showing pedunculated or papillary infolding of acinar cells, protrusion of glandular tissue into tissue planes in the thyroid capsule or into thin-walled vascular spaces were found to be completely reversible following cessation of treatment with methimazole compatable with the concept that many of these nodules are not autonomous neoplasms (Todd, 1986).

Such data suggest that biological behavior of nodular thyroid lesions is more comparable between man and laboratory than sometimes believed and it appears quite justified to use the more conservative diagnostic criteria developed for human thyroid lesions in the field of experimental pathology. Whatever classification is adopted, it is important that consistent and clear criteria are chosen to categorise all proliferative lesions in the thyroid glands in individual carcinogenicity bioassays.

Diffuse hyperplasia which accompanies increased thyroid activity in both man and laboratory animals is characterized by a uniform increase in glandular size. Histologically, hyperplastic glands contain irregularly shaped follicles with narrowed lumens and loss of colloid (Figs. 128 and 129). The follicular epithelium becomes infolded, convoluted, stratified or even papillary in structure. The follicular cells appear more columnar than normal with abundant finely vacuolated eosinophilic cytoplasm and enlarged, rounded basally located nuclei. A characteristic change in colloid reported both in primary hyperthyroidism in man and sometimes in thyroid hyperplasia in the rat is the presence of spherical clear vacuoles in the colloid immediately overlying the epithelium (Meissner and Warren, 1969; Heath and Littlefield, 1984). A typical feature in the hyperactive thyroid in rats is an increase in the basophilic staining of colloid in haematoxylin and eosin stained sections. This basophilic substance also may stain with Von Kossa's reaction (Price et al., 1988).

Electron microscopy shows prominent rough endoplasmic reticulum commonly with dilated cisternae, enlarged Golgi, increased numbers of intracytoplasmic droplets, increased numbers of and lengthened surface microvilli and

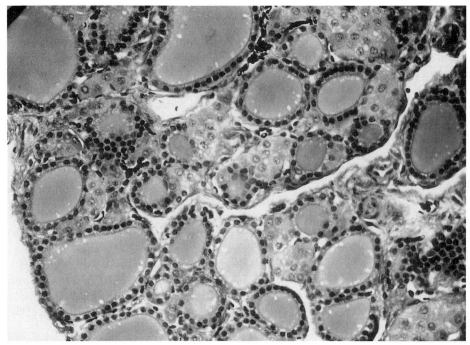

Fig. 128. Normal thyroid from a young untreated beagle dog. (HE, ×250.)

highly developed pseudopodia at the apical surface. Glands may demonstrate histological evidence of increased vascularity.

Focal or nodular hyperplasia both in man and experimental animals is characterised by heterogeneous foci and nodules often within a diffusely hyperplastic thyroid gland. Nodular proliferative zones may either be sharply demarcated or poorly circumscribed but they show neither marked tissue compression nor true capsule formation. They demonstrate mixed or variegated cytological appearances. Follicles may be distended with colloid and lined by inactive flattened cells or be composed of closely packed cellular zones. As in diffuse hyperplasia, a characteristic histological feature is focal papillary infolding of the lining acinar cells. Retrogressive changes including haemorrhage, necrosis, fibrosis, pigment accumulation and the presence of cholesterol clefts may also be found in longstanding hyperplasia both in man and rats.

In summary, hyperplastic nodules can be distinguished from the true adenomas by their lack of marked tissue compression or true capsule, variable structure, their multiplicity or the presence of similar growth patterns in adjacent non-nodular gland.

A wide variety of different agents including therapeutic compounds which have the capacity to inhibit synthesis of thyroid hormones are capable of inducing thyroid hyperplasia and sometimes ultimately neoplasia (see below) following prolonged treatment. These effects occur when the treatment reduces

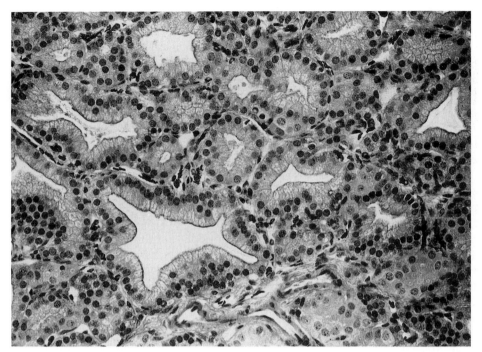

Fig. 129. Thyroid hyperplasia in a beagle dog. There is depletion of colloid, considerable enlargement of the follicular epithelial cells and infolding of the epithelium. (HE, ×250.)

thyroid hormones to subnormal levels and the resultant increase in circulating TSH stimulates enlargement of the thyroid gland. Agents include excess iodine, iodine deficiency, antithyroid thionamides, sulphonylureas, sulphonamides, substituted phenols such resorcinol, and diverse drugs including phenylbutazone, iodopyrine (iodine and antipyrine), ethionamide, 6-mercaptopurine, lithium as well as some plant constituents such as those found in Brassica (Ingbar, 1985). Compounds which affect hepatic clearance of thyroid hormones can also increase thyroid gland activity and produce thyroid hyperplasia.

Excess iodine intake inhibits uptake of iodine by follicular cell blocks peroxidation of iodine, interfers with conversion of diiodotyrosine and monoiodotyrosine, and blocks the release of T3 and T4 which leads to increased secretion of TSH (Nagataki, 1974). Deficiency of iodine results in diminished synthesis of thyroxine, subsequent TSH elevation and thyroid hyperplasia in experimental animals (Axelrod and Leblond, 1955; Denef et al., 1981; Ohshima and Ward, 1986). Iodine containing therapeutic agents such as amiodarone also cause both hypo and hyperthyroidism as well as morphological alterations in the thyroid gland in man (Physician's Desk Reference, 1987; Brennen et al., 1987).

As a class, thionamide compounds are some of the most potent inhibitors of thyroid hormones and they are capable of inducing hyperplasia of the thyroid gland in experimental animals (Todd, 1986). These compounds contain a thiocarbamide group which is responsible for the antithyroid activity (Cooper, 1984). Agents of this class include thiouracil, 6-propylthiouracil and a more potent thioureylene, methimazole (1-methylmercaptoimidazole or Tapazole). Amino-heterocyclic compounds such as para-aminosalicyclic acid, an antituberculous compound, although less potent than thionamides are also capable of producing thyroid hyperplasia. Similarly, sulphonamides are able to induce thyroid hyper-plasia in laboratory animals (Heath and Littlefield, 1984; Takayama et al., 1986). An important feature of the thyroid hyperplasias induced by antithyroid drugs is their reversability following withdrawal of treatment, even after prolonged periods of administration (Todd, 1986).

Another characteristic of thyroid hyperplasia induced by prolonged adminis-tration of antithyroid compounds is the dissociation between function and proliferative activity of the thyroid follicular cells. The hyperplasia of the thyroid gland following treatment of rats with the antithyroid agent aminotria-zole was shown to diminish after one to two months despite continued treatment and continued absence of circulating thyroid hormone (Wynford-Thomas et al., 1982). Although the reason for this dissociation was not clear, it was shown that the levels of circulating TSH and its biological activity remained high and that the decrease in mitotic activity was not a result of decreased TSH activity. It appears that other control mechanisms of thyroid proliferation exist, probably in the follicular cell itself either at a receptor or post-receptor site (Wynford-Thomas et al., 1982).

A key problem in the safety evaluation of such compounds is assessment of probable risk for thyroid changes in therapeutic use in man, based on findings in the thyroid in laboratory species. Although disposition of the test drug in tissues among different species is important for assessment, species differences in the sensitivity of thyroid tissues to these effects of drugs is also reported. For instance, Takayama and colleagues (1986) showed that monkeys were less sensi-tive to the antithyroid effects of propylthiouracil and sulphamonomethoxine than rats at similar dose levels. These agents lowered T3 and T4, decreased incorporation of ^{131}I into thyroid precursors, produced elevation of circulating TSH, increased thyroid weight and diffuse follicular hyperplasia in rats but not primates after five weeks of treatment. Although drug disposition and metabo-lism differences between species were not entirely excluded, in vitro studies suggested that the concentrations of these agents required to inhibit thyroid peroxidase activity were lower in rats than monkeys suggesting tissue sensitivity was an important factor in these species differences.

Other compounds which cause persistent hyperactivity and hyperplasia of the thyroid gland are those which influence the clearance of thyroid hormones. A close metabolic relationship exists between the liver and thyroid gland as hepatic microsomal enzymes play an important part in thyroid hormone deiodinisation and biliary excretion (Anderson and Kappas, 1982; McClain, 1989). Phenobarbi-tone is capable of accelerating thyroxine (T4) turnover and increasing thyroid mass in rats, probably by induction of hepatic thyroxine glucuronyltransferase with subsequent increase in biliary excretion of thyroxine glucuronide (Oppenheimer et al., 1968; McClain, 1989). Treatment of rats for three months or longer with hypolipidaemic drugs clofibrate and fenofibrate or the plasticiser di-(2-ethylhexyl) phthalate was also shown to induce mild hyperplasia of the thyroid gland. This hyperplasia was characterised by reduction in size of follicles which were lined by more cuboidal cells than in untreated controls (Price et al., 1988). The colloid appeared retracted and showed increased basophilic staining in haemotoxylin and eosin stained sections. Follicular cells contained larger and increased numbers of lyosomes, enlarged Golgi apparatus and dilated rough endoplasmic reticulum.

Thyroid hyperplasia was also reported in rats treated with SC 37211, a novel imidazole antimicrobial agent, probably as a result of an increase in hepatic T4 conjugation by the enzyme uridine diphosphate glucoronosyltransferase (Comer et al., 1985). Similarly, thyroid hyperplasia induced in rats by the histamine H_2 antagonist SK and F 93479, may have occurred through a similar mechanism because there was an increase in T4 clearance in treated animals (Brown et al., 1987; Atterwill and Brown, 1988).

It is important to note that there is not always a clear relationship between the degree of hepatic enzyme induction and thyroid hypertrophy or hyperplasia. Female rats treated with simvastatin, a novel competitive inhibitor of HMG CoA reductase for five weeks, developed an approximately 35% increase in serum TSH compared with controls with slightly lower serum thyroxine levels associated with thyroid hypertrophy and liver weight increases (Smith et al., 1989). As simvastatin did not markedly alter hepatic microsomal enzyme activity apart from the induction of HMG CoA reductase, it was suggested that the thyroid changes may have been simply related to the increase in functional liver cell mass and consequent increased capacity for thyroxine clearance.

These instances provide evidence for the existance of a thyroid-liver axis, although in many cases the actual biochemical mechanism linking changes in the two organs remains unclear (Price et al., 1988). Some hepatic enzyme inducers have also been associated with the development of thyroid neoplasia when administered to rats for long periods in carcinogenicity bioassays (McClain, 1989) (see below).

Neoplasia

Distinguishing between focal (nodular) hyperplasia and adenoma and between adenoma and carcinoma of the follicular epithelium on histological grounds remains a problem both in human diagnostic pathology and in preclinical toxicology. The biological behavior of human thyroid neoplasms based on cytological criteria remains unpredictable, even for neoplasms which show morphological features of malignancy. However, as noted above, there are good grounds for the application of similar morphological criteria in the diagnosis of both human and experimental thyroid neoplasms. However, in studies where thyroid neoplasms are found, it is also necessary to critically assess the degree and

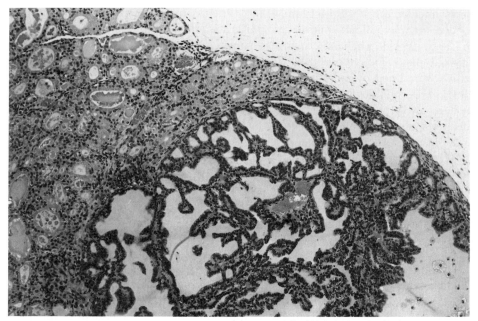

Fig. 130. Thyroid gland, Wistar rat, showing a discrete nodule which is just beginning to compress surrounding parenchyma. It is composed of well-differentiated thyroid epithelium which forms follicles and is thrown into folds and small papillae but shows little or no mitotic activity. This would be generally diagnosed as a thyroid adenoma in toxicological pathology although the biological nature of this type of lesion remains unclear. (HE, ×100.)

prevalence of any associated thyroid glandular hyperplasia as well as looking for evidence of other hormonal derangements and hepatic enlargement.

An *adenoma* is typically a solitary well-encapsulated nodule or mass with a fairly uniform microscopic structure, different in appearance from the surrounding gland. Evidence of autonomous growth is demonstrated by the presence of marked displacement and compression of adjacent gland (Figs. 130 and 131).

Carcinomas of the follicular epithelium have similar growth patterns but are distinguished by the presence of invasion, and not simply cytological atypia. Indeed evidence from both man and experimental animals suggests that the histological features of invasion should be clear-cut and not simply be based on the presence of a few cells entrapped or protruding into the fibrous tissue capsule (Todd, 1986).

Cytological features of adenomas or carcinomas of follicular epithelium in man and laboratory animals are variable but broadly speaking they can be grouped into papillary, acinar and solid subtypes. A particular, if somewhat academic difficulty relates to the diagnosis of papillary neoplasms of the thyroid. In human diagnostic pathology, the papillary adenoma remains a rare tumour and there is a tendancy to denote all thyroid neoplasms with papillary features as carcinomas even in the absence of histological features of invasion. In

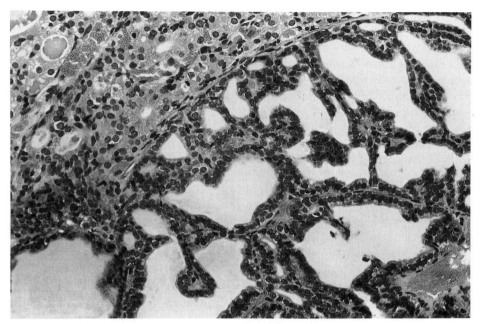

Fig. 131. Higher power view of the nodule seen in Figure 130. (HE, ×250.)

laboratory rodents it is more usual to diagnose thyroid neoplasms with papillary features as adenomas if there is no histological evidence of tissue invasion.

Immunocytochemistry contributes relatively little to the diagnosis of follicular and papillary neoplasms of the thyroid gland, although immunocytochemical study for the presence of calcitonin is useful in the distinction between solid neoplasms of follicular origin from those of C-cell type (see below).

More recently, it has been shown that the nature or degree of rats oncogene expression may reflect the biological nature of human thyroid neoplasms as well as the type of inducing agent in rodent thyroid tumour model systems (Lemoine et al., 1988, 1989).

A few compounds which are powerful genotoxic carcinogens induce thyroid tumours in rodents after short periods of time as part of their spectrum of carcinogenic activity. However, the majority of xenobiotics and experimental procedures which produce thyroid neoplasia in rodents do so only after long periods of time during which there is thyroid hyperplasia as a result of inhibition of synthesis of thyroid hormones or an increase in their degradation and removal (Hill et al., 1989). Examples include low iodine diets, subtotal thyroidectomy, administration of natural goitrogens such as cabbage and rape seed, a number of pesticides and industrial chemicals as well as antithyroid drugs and therapeutic agents which at high doses increase the hepatic clearance of thyroid hormones (Comer et al., 1985; Atterwill and Brown, 1988; Paynter et al., 1988; Hill et al., 1989).

It is generally accepted that thyroid neoplasia is also associated with exposure to ionizing radiation in man and laboratory animals. In man, most of these radiation-associated neoplasias are believed to be papillary carcinomas. In laboratory animals administration of radioactive iodine will induce thyroid neoplasms of follicular cell origin (Doniach, 1957; de Ruiter et al., 1976). This is another example of radiation-induced neoplasia of endocrine tissue and it has been suggested that ionizing radiation acts primarily as an initiator for thyroid neoplasia (Furth, 1963; Wynford-Thomas et al., 1983). However, radiation may also promote the development of thyroid cancer by producing functional impairment of the thyroid gland and subsequent stimulation of prolonged TSH secretion.

Ohshima and Ward (1986) compared the development of thyroid hyperplasia and neoplasia following low iodine diet and the administration of the genotoxic carcinogen, N-nitrosomethylurea. Follicular adenomas and carcinomas were reported after iodine deficient diet alone after 18 months although they were few in number and composed of well differentiated cuboidal epithelium. The incidence of carcinomas was much higher and occurred earlier following N-nitrosomethylurea but their prevalence was potentiated further by iodine deficient diet. These findings suggested that iodine deficiency can act as a promotor for thyroid carcinogens with the increase in TSH acting as a chemical mediator (Ohshima and Ward, 1986). Zbinden (1988) has also recently shown how methimazole, a potent inhibitor of thyroid hormone synthesis, and phenobarbital which stimulates hepatic catabolism of thyroxine, also potentate the development of thyroid hyperplasia and neoplasia induced in rats by N-bis(2-hydroxypropyl) nitrosamine.

The question of species differences in the extrapolation of results in laboratory animals to man is illustrated by the safety evaluation of aminotriazole (amitrole), an antithyroid compound used as a herbicide. This compound, which inhibits thyroid peroxidase, produced increased numbers of thyroid (and pituitary) neoplasms in carcinogenicity bioassays performed in rats but not mice or golden hamsters (Steinhoff et al., 1983). These results correlated with the degree of effect on thyroid function induced by amitrole in these species. These effects were greater in the rat than either in the mouse or hamster. Furthermore, low doses with little or no effect on thyroid function of rats, were also devoid of tumorigenic action. As amitrole is free of mutagenic activity, it was argued that a threshold dose exists for this type of tumorigenic effect below which there is neither disturbance of hormonal balance nor tumour induction (Steinhoff et al., 1983).

Another example of species differences is provided by a novel histamine H_2 antagonist, SK and F 93479. Rats treated with high doses of this drug developed colloid depletion, follicular hyperplasia and eventually follicular adenomas and adenocarcinomas after two years, whereas the thyroid gland of mice and dogs remained eventually unaffected by treatment (Atterwill and Brown, 1988). Special thyroid function studies suggested that SK and F 93479 produced these effects in rats indirectly by increasing thyroxine clearence lowering circulating

736

thyroxine levels and elevating plasma TSH, possibly by affecting receptor interactions occurring at the energy-dependent, high affinity thyroxine uptake sites in the liver (Brown et al., 1987, Poole et al., 1989).

On the basis of comparisons of thyroid follicular cell tumour development in laboratory animals following derangement of thyroid and pituitary homeostasis and epidemiological data relating to thyroid neoplasia development in human populations, it has been suggested that humans are less sensitive than commonly used animal models to the tumour-inducing effects of long-term derangement of thyroid status (Hill et al., 1989). Furthermore, Paynter and colleagues (1988) have also suggested that a threshold for pituitary-thyroid hormonal imbalance exists, below which the risk of neoplasia development in the thyroid is small.

C-Cell hyperplasia and neoplasia

C-cell hyperplasia is characterized by an increase in number and size of the parafollicular cells, either as a focal aggregations or diffusely throughout the gland. In man, C-cell hyperplasia is relatively uncommon but it has been well characterized because it occurs with increased frequency in some families where it is associated with the development of medullary carcinoma and multiple endocrine neoplasia. Hypertrophy and hyperplasia of C-cells also occurs commonly with hypercalcaemia in association with hyper-parathyroidism and toxic goitre.

C-cell hyperplasia and medullary carcinoma is also found in a wide variety of domestic and laboratory animals. It has been well characterised in bulls (Capen and Black, 1974), dogs, cats (Leav et al., 1976) as well as in laboratory rats (DeLellis et al., 1979), mice (Van Zwieten et al., 1983), and hamsters (DeLellis et al., 1987). The sequence of C-cell hyperplasia and medullary carcinoma in the susceptible Long-Evans strain in rat has been shown by DeLellis and colleagues (1979) to be identical to the changes observed in familial medullary hyperplasia in man. Although the stimulus for the initial C-cell proliferation in the rat and in man remains unknown, the results of the immunocytochemical and electron microscopic study by DeLellis and co-workers in rats showed that there is a prolonged phase of diffuse and nodular hyperplasia of C-cells which is accompanied by elevation in serum calcitonin. This precedes the development of medullary carcinoma which in the Long-Evans rat makes its appearance at about one year of age but becomes frequent after about two years.

In the normal rat, proportions of C-cells to follicular cells, colloid and stroma increases progressively with increasing age. In young Long-Evans rats, C-cells form about 4% of thyroid substance when measured morphometrically but at 9–12 months of age they form 7% and nearly 20% in older animals (DeLellis et al., 1979). The distribution of C-cells also extends from a predominantly central one to a more peripheral and even subcapsular localisation.

An interesting point here is that although radioactive iodine(^{131}I) induces follicular cell neoplasia, it has the opposite effect on C-cells. C-cells and C-cell neoplasia were shown to be reduced in aged Long-Evans rats given radioactive iodine compared with the untreated controls (Ott et al., 1987).

With advancing age focal aggregates of C-cells become more prominant. These foci may progress to nodular hyperplasia with distortion, compression and even obliteration of adjoining thyroid follicles. In contrast to the uniformly dense immunocytochemical staining for calcitonin of normal and diffusely hyperplastic C-cells, nodular proliferations show more variable and often weaker staining patterns. They appear frequently more sparsely granulated cells on electron microscopic examination and contain predominantly Type II secretory granules (DeLellis et al., 1979). Despite nodular appearances, DeLellis and colleagues have also shown that there is no evidence of stromal invasion nor disruption of the basement-membrane: a point of distinction from medullary carcinoma.

There are difficulties in the terminology of these lesions. Undoubtably nodular aggregates showing displacement of surrounding gland but no invasion are considered as adenomas by some pathologists. Circumscribed proliferative lesions not showing invasion are being diagnosed as adenomas in the National Toxicology Program carcinogenesis bioassay testing programme (Goodman et al., 1979; 1980). Whether these lesions are autonomous neoplastic growths remains conjecture. In any case, it is appropriate to make the distinction between diffuse, focal, focal nodular hyperplasia (or adenoma) and carcinoma in the diagnosis of C-cell changes in preclinical studies.

Although some Syrian hamsters and certain strains of mice develop medullary carcinomas in an appreciable frequency they appear unassociated with any degree of C-cell hyperplasia unlike the rat (Van Zwieten et al., 1983; Wolfe et al., 1980). Morphometric analysis of the thyroid gland of young dogs has shown that the C-cells become more numerous when the dogs are fed a diet with high calcium content (Goedegebuure and Hazewinkel, 1986).

Medullary carcinoma

A diagnosis of medullary carcinoma is made when nodules or cords of C-cells develop stromal or vascular invasion. In the rat these tumours may be multicentric but in all rodents they show a range of differentiation patterns. Well-differentiated tumours are composed of polyhedral cells with rounded or oval nuclei with moderately granular chromatin inconspicous nucleoli, and low mitotic activity. Tumour cells may be considerably more pleomorphic with enlarged hyperchromatic nuclei and prominent nucleoli. Poorly differentiated medullary carcinomas may exhibit a spindle cell appearance. Stroma is usually fairly scanty although Congo red staining reveals the presence of focal deposits of amyloid in rodent medullary carcinomas.

The most useful diagnostic method for the diagnosis of medullary carcinoma as well as for evaluation of the degree of spread of tumour cells within thyroid tissue is immunocytochemical staining for calcitonin, although poorly differentiated tumours may only show sparse immunoreactivity for calcitonin (DeLellis et al., 1979; 1987). Both human and rat medullary carcinoma cells have been shown to produce other regulatory peptides, particularly the tridecapeptide neurotensin which is found normally in the central nervous system and intestinal tract (Zeytinoglu et al., 1983).

As noted above, medullary carcinoma in the rat is preceded by the development of diffuse and nodular C-cell hyperplasia similar to medullary thyroid carcinoma of familial type in man (DeLellis et al., 1979). By contrast, medullary carcinomas reported in mice and Syrian hamsters appear unassociated with extensive C-cell hyperplasia and therefore resemble sporadic form of human medullary carcinoma (Wolfe et al., 1980; Van Zwieten et al., 1983; DeLellis et al., 1987).

PARATHYROID GLAND

The parathyroid glands are usually examined histologically in conjunction with the thyroid glands. However, their somewhat inconsistent location in the neck and the variability in the plane of sectioning frequently mean that parathyroid glands are not uniformly transected in standard histological sections. Although examination of more than one parathyroid gland in an individual animal may be important in the distinction between hyperplasia and neoplasia, locating every parathyroid gland in routine toxicity studies is usually not necessary for appropriate evaluation of parathyroid function, for this is also reflected in the resorptive surfaces in bone tissue (see Musculoskeletal System, Chapter IV).

In most animal species and in man the parathyroid glands are arranged in two pairs in the anterior part of the neck around the thyroid glands (Capen, 1983). In man, one pair which arises embryonically from the third branchial pouch is situated inferiorly at the anterior or posterior surface of the thyroid gland. The second pair derived from the fourth pouch are located near the upper poles of the thyroid. Their distribution is variable but they are usually located along the lines of descent from pharangeal pouches in embryonic life (Castleman and Roth, 1978). In the dog, the parathyroids are also located in close proximity to the thyroid gland. An external pair derived from the third pharangeal pouch, each measuring between 2 and 5 mm in length, is situated at the upper pole of the thyroid and a smaller pair originating from the fourth pouch is found on the medial surface of the thyroid gland (Capen, 1983).

Rats, mice and hamsters possess only a single pair of parathyroid glands, developing from the third pharangeal pouch and frequently embedded within thyroid tissue on the lateral surface of the superior pole. In all species ectopic parathyroid tissue may be found in the anterior part of the neck and in the thymus gland.

The cells of the parathyroid gland are termed chief cells. Although cytological interspecies variability in chief cell populations are evident, some of these differences are probably a reflection of activity. Inactive chief cells appear rounded or cuboidal with relatively large nuclei and pale-staining cytoplasm. Ultrastructural examination shows relatively electron-luscent cytoplasm with relatively poorly developed organelles including a small Golgi, small mitrochondria, few secretory granules and aggregations of glycogen, neutral lipid and lipofuscin. Active cells have frequently darker staining cytoplasm with increased electron density of cytoplasmic matrix, numerous secretory granules, but paucity of glycogen and lipid (Capen, 1983).

Multinucleated giant cells are reported in parathyroid glands of rats and dogs particularly in hyperactive states (Oksanen, 1980; Capen, 1983). The significance of these cells is uncertain although the cytoplasm of the cells do not contain numerous secretory granules and show degenerative changes.

Oxyphil cells are prominent in the parathyroid glands of adult man and in some animal species, including the hamster but not the rat or mouse. In man the cytoplasm of oxyphil cells are packed with bizarre mitochondria and show high oxidative and hydrolytic enzyme activity (Harcourt-Webster and Truman, 1969). Their significance is uncertain but they do not appear to be involved in active synthesis of parathyroid hormone (PTH).

The cells of the parathyroid are concerned with the elaboration of active parathyroid hormone (PTH), a polypeptide of 84 amino-acids and related peptide precursors, pre-proparathyroid and proparathyroid hormone. Parathyroid hormone is primarily involved in the regulation of blood calcium levels. It exerts its effect by direct action on target cells in the bone and kidney. It acts on bone by increasing activity of osteoclasts and osteoblasts to increase the flow of calcium from the bone to increase blood calcium. If increases in parathyroid hormone are sustained, the active osteoclast population in bone is increased by activation of further progenitor cells. A long-term increase in parathyroid hormone also increases the numbers of osteoblasts in bone with increased bone formation as well as bone resorption. Parathyroid hormone also exerts a direct effect on the proximal renal tubule to block tubular resorption of phosphate with resultant phosphaturia and increased urinary secretion of potassium, bicarbonate, sodium and aminoacids (Capen, 1983). Control of parathyroid secretion is primarily based on the concentration of circulating calcium and to some extent also magnesium ions (Arnaud, 1978).

Although the most common diagnostic difficulties in the parathyroid gland relate to hyperplasia and neoplasia, cells of the parathyroid gland show atrophic changes when suppressed by high calcium diet or high vitamin levels. Using histological criteria such as number of nuclei and mitoses, nuclear/cytoplasmic ratio of chief cells, the presence of cord-like or acinar configuration and palisading of cells, Goedegebuure and Hazewinkel (1986) showed decreased evidence of activity in dogs fed a high calcium diet.

Analagous to the thyroid gland, injection of parathyroid gland extract and Freund's adjuvent may provoke lymphocytic parathyroiditis, degeneration and atrophy (Lupelescu et al., 1968).

Hyperplasia and neoplasia

The diagnosis of neoplasia in the parathyroid gland is subject to similar criteria and the same difficulties as in other endocrine organs.

In man and laboratory animals, hyperplasia may be diffuse, focal or nodular in character. In man, hyperplasia can be recognized by the hypercellular appearances of the glandular parenchyma with chief cells arranged in solid sheets, cords and follicles with loss of stromal fat cells. These changes may be initially multifocal but eventually extend to involve the entire gland. A variable cytological appearance of chief cells with clear, basophilic or eosinophilic cytoplasm may be evident in the parathyroid gland of rat, mouse and hamster (Pour 1983; Pour et al., 1983). In rodents, however, the normal gland is largely devoid of stromal fat rendering the presence or absence of stromal fat of no help in the assessment of hyperplasia. A morphometric study of Long-Evans rats has shown that young adults have a mean maximal area when sectioned longitudinally of 0.3 sq mm. Older rats aged between 9 and 12 months of age showed mild hyperplasia associated with a slight increase in chief cell size, thickened cell cords and a mean glandular area of about 0.6 sq mm. Animals with C-cell hyperplasia or medullary carcinoma of the thyroid gland showed an even greater mean sectional area of about 1.0 sq mm (DeLellis et al., 1979).

Parathyroid hyperplasia appears to be more common among hamsters than in rats or mice. It is often associated with histological evidence of advanced renal disease particularly amyloidosis, nephrocalcinosis and advanced glomerulosclerosis, presumably as a result of calcium loss. It also occurs following low calcium intake and following administration of calcium lowering agents such as calcium ion chelating compounds (Strauss, 1982).

Adenomas are typically sharply demarcated from any residual gland remaining. Any adjacent parathyroid tissue is displaced or compressed and a capsule is inconstantly found. Helpful diagnostic features are found in the contralateral gland in rodents, which show relatively normal or atrophic changes, such as loss of cytoplasm, reduction in cytoplasmic organelles and secretory granules and increased lipid and lipofuscin.

Parathyroid adenomas only occasionally develop spontaneously in aged rodents, although they can be induced. The administration of radio-active iodine is of interest in this context because treatment of neonatal rats with radioactive iodine not only induces neoplasia in the thyroid gland but also in the parathyroid. The close proximity of the parathyroid to the radio-iodine stored in the thyroid gland presumably creates conditions in which the parathyroid gland receives ionizing radiation in a dose sufficient to induce neoplasia. Wynford-Thomas and colleagues (1983) demonstrated that the development of parathyroid adenomas induced by radiation was potentiated by low vitamin D diet. They suggested that radiation acts as an initiator in this situation with the low vitamin diet acting as a promotor through its effects on the parathyroid gland activity.

REFERENCES

ABBOTT, E.C., MONKHOUSE, F.C., STEINER, J.W. and LAIDLAW, J.C. (1966): Effects of sulfated mucopolysaccharide (RO1–8307) on the zona glomerulosa of the rat adrenal gland. *Endocrinology*, 78, 651–654.

AIBA, M., SUZUKI, H., KAGEYAMA, K., MURAI, M., TAZAKI, H., ABE, O. and SARUTA, T. (1981): Spironolactone bodies in aldosteronomas and in the attached adrenals. Enzyme histochemical study of 19 cases of primary aldosteronism and a case of aldesteronism due to diffuse hyperplasia of the zona glomerulosa. *Am.J.Pathol.*, 103, 404–410.

AICHINGER, G., FILL, H. and WICK, G. (1985): In situ immune complexes, lymphocyte subpopulations, and HLA-DR-posit epithelial cells in Hashimoto thyroiditis. *Lab.Invest.*, 52, 132–140.

ALFANO, J., PEDERSON, R.C., KRAMER, R.E. and BROWNIE, A.C. (1983): Cholesterol metabolism in the rat adrenal cortex: acute temporal changes following stress. *Can.J.Biochem.Cell Biol.*, 61, 708–713.

ALLEN, J.M., KERLE, D.J., WARE, H., DOBLE, A., WILLIAMS, G. and BLOOM, S.R. (1983): Combined treatment with ketoconazole and luteinizing hormone releasing hormone analogue: a novel approach to resistant progressive prostate cancer. *Br.Med.J.*, 287, 1766.

ANDERSON, K.E. and KAPPAS, A. (1982): Hormones and liver function. In: L. Schiff and E.R. Schiff (Eds), *Diseases of the Liver*, pp. 167–235, 5th Edn., J.B. Lippencott, Philadelphia.

ANDERSON, M.P. and CAPEN, C.C. (1978): The endocrine system. In: K. Benirschke, F.M. Garner and T.C. Jones (Eds), *Pathology of Laboratory Animals, Vol. 1*, Chap. 6, pp. 423–508. Springer-Verlag, New York.

APPLEBY, E.C. and SOHRABI-HAGHDOOST, I. (1980): Cortical hyperplasia of the adrenal gland in the dog. *Res.Vet.Sci.*, 29, 190–197.

ARNAUD, C.D. (1978): Calcium homeostasis: regulatory elements and their integration. *Fed.Proc.*, 37, 2557–2560.

ARRIGONI-MARTELLI, E. and FINUCANE, J. (1985): Pinacidil. In: A. Scriabine (Ed.), *New Drugs Annual: Cardiovascular Drugs, Vol. 3*, pp. 133–151. Raven Press, New York.

ATTERWILL, C.K. and BROWN, C.G. (1988): Mechanistic studies on the thyroid toxicity induced by certain drugs. *Arch.Toxicol.*, Suppl.12, 71–79.

ATTIA, M.A. (1980): Cytological study on pituitary adenomas in senile untreated Beagle bitches. *Arch.Toxicol.*, 46, 287–293.

ATTWOOD, H.D. and DENNETT, X. (1976): A black thyroid and minocycline treatment. *Br.Med.J.*, 2, 1109–1110.

AXELROD, A.A. and LEBLOND, C.P. (1955): Induction of thyroid tumors in rats by a low iodine diet. *Cancer*, 8, 339–367.

BÄR, A. (1988): Sugars and adrenomedullary proliferative lesions: The effects of lactose and various polyalcohols. *J.Am.Coll.Toxicol.* 7, 71–81.

BARSOUM, N.J., MOORE, J.D., GOUGH, A.W., STURGESS, J.M. and DE LA IGLESIA, F.A. (1985): Morphofunctional investigations on spontaneous pituitary tumors in Wistar rats. *Toxicol.Pathol.*, 13, 200–208.

BATES, R.W., MILKOVIC, S. and GARRISON, M.M. (1964): Effects of prolactin, growth hormone and ACTH, alone and in combination, upon organ weights and adrenal function in normal rats. *Endocrinology*, 74, 714–723.

BEDRAK, E., CHAP, Z. and BROWN, R. (1983): Age-related changes in the hypothalamic-pituitary-testicular function of the rat. *Exp.Gerontol.*, 18, 95–104.

BENITZ, K.F., ROBERTS, G.K.S. and YUSA, A. (1967): Morphologic effects of minocycline in laboratory animals. *Toxicol.Appl.Pharmacol.*, 11, 150–170.

BERKVENS, J.M., VAN NESSELROOY, J.H.J. and KROES, R. (1980): Spontaneous tumours in the pituitary gland of old Wistar rats. A morphological and immunocytochemical study. *J.Pathol.*, 13, 179–191.

BERNFELD, P., HOMBURGER, F., ADAMS, R.A., SOTO, E. and VAN DONGEN, C.G. (1986): Base-line data in a carcinogen susceptible first generation hybrid strain of Syrian golden hamsters: FID Alexander. *J.N.C.I.*, 77, 165–171.

BERRY, P.H. (1986): Effects of diet or reproductive status on the histo-logy of spontaneous pituitary tumors in female Wistar rats. *Vet.Pathol.*, 23, 606–618.

BIELSCHOWSKY, M., BIELSCHOWSKY, F. and LINDSAY, D. (1956): A new strain of mice with a high incidence of mammary cancers and enlargement of the pituitary. *Br.J.Cancer*, 10, 688–699.

BIRT, D.F. and POUR, P.M. (1985): Interaction of dietary fat and protein in spontaneous diseases of Syrian golden hamsters. *J.N.C.I.*, 75, 127–133.

BLAZKOVEC, A.A. and ORSINI, M.W. (1976): Ontogenetic aspects of sexual dimorphism and the primary immune response to sheep erythrocytes in hamsters from pre-puberty through senescence. *Int.Arch.Allergy Appl.Immunol.*, 50, 55–67.

BLOODWORTH, Jr. J.M.B. (1975): The adrenal. In: S.C. Sommers (Ed.), *Endocrine Pathology Decennial 1966–1975*, pp. 391–411. Appleton-Century-Crofts, New York.

BLOOM, J.C., THIEM, P.A., MORGAN, D.G. (1987): The role of conventional pathology and toxicology in evaluating the immunotoxic potential of xenobiotics. *Toxicol.Pathol.* 15, 283–293.

BLOOM, W. and FAWCETT, D.W. (1975): Hypophysis (Pituitary gland). In: *A Textbook of Histology, 10th Edition*, Chap. 18, pp. 503–523. Saunders, Philadelphia.

BOELSTERLI, U.A., CRUZ-ORIVE, L.-M. and ZBINDEN, G. (1984): Morphometric and biochemical analysis of adrenal medullary hyperplasia induced by nicotine in rats. *Arch.Toxicol.*, 56, 113–116.

BOELSTERLI, U.A. and ZBINDEN, G. (1985): Early biochemical and morphological changes of the rat adrenal medulla induced by xylitol. *Arch.Toxicol.*, 57, 25–30.

BONDY, P.K. (1985): Disorders of the renal cortex. In: J.D. Wilson and D.W. Foster (Eds), *William's Textbook of Endocrinology, 7th Edition*, Chap. 22, pp. 816–890. Saunders, Philadelphia.

BOORMAN, G.A. and DELELLIS, R.A. (1983): C-cell hyperplasia, thyroid rat. In: T.C. Jones, U. Mohr and R.D. Hunt (Eds), *Endocrine System*, pp. 192–197. Springer-Verlag, Berlin.

BOSLAND, M.C. and BAER, A. (1984): Some functional characteristics of adrenal medullary tumors in aged male Wistar rats. *Vet.Pathol.*, 21, 129–140.

BOUTWELL, R.K. (1983): The role of retinoids as protective agents in experimental carcinogenesis. In: D.C. McBrien and T.F. Slater (Eds), *Protective Agents in Cancer*, pp. 279–297. Academic Press, London.

BRENNAN, M.D., VAN HEERDEN, J.A. and CARNEY, J.A. (1987): Amiodarone-associated thyrotoxicosis(AAT): Experience with surgical management. *Surgery*, 102, 1062–1067.

BROWN, C.G., HARLAND, R.F., MAJOR, I.R. and ATTERWILL, C.K. (1987): Effects of toxic doses of a novel histamine (H_2) antagonist on the rat thyroid gland. *Food.Chem.Toxicol.* 25, 787–794.

BUREK, J.D. (1978): Age-associated pathology. In: *Pathology of Aging Rats*, Chap. 4, pp. 29–168. CRC Press, West Palm Beach, Florida.

CALE, A.E., FREEDMAN, P.D. and LUMERMAN, H. (1988): Pigmentation of the jawbones and teeth secondary to minocycline hydrochloride therapy. *J.Periodontol.* 59, 112–114.

CAMACHO, A.M., BROUGH, A.J., CASH, R. and WILROY, R.S. (1966): Adrenal toxicity associated with the administration of an anticonvulsant drug. *J.Pediatr.*, 68, 852–853.

CAPEN, C.C. (1983): Structural and biochemical aspects of parathyroid function in animals. In: T.C. Jones, U. Mohr and R.D. Hunt (Eds), *Endocrine System*, pp. 217–247. Springer-Verlag, Berlin.

CAPEN, C.C. and BLACK, H.E. (1974): Animal model of human disease. Medullary thyroid carcinoma, multiple endocrine neoplasia, Sipple's syndrome. Animal model: ultimobronchial thyroid neoplasm in the bull. *Am.J.Pathol.*, 74, 377–380.

CARNEY, J.A. (1987): Unusual tumefactive spindle-cell lesions in the adrenal glands. *Hum.Pathol.*, 18, 980–985.

CARSON, K.A., HANKER, J.S. and KIRSHNER, N. (1982): The adrenal medulla of the diabetic mouse (C57BL/KsJ, db/db): Biochemical and morphological changes. *Comp.Biochem.Physiol.*, 72A, 279–285.

CASH, R., BROUGH, A.J., COHEN, N.N.P. and SATOH, P.S. (1967): Amino-glutethimide (Elipten-Ciba) as an inhibitor of adrenal steroido-genesis. Mechanism of action and therapeutic trial. *J.Clin. Endocrinol.Metab.*, 27, 1239–1248.

CASTLEMAN, B. and ROTH, S.I. (1978): Tumors of the parathyroid glands. In: *Atlas of Tumor Pathology, Second Series*, Fascicle 14, pp. 3–51. AFIP, Washington, DC.

CHANG, R.J., KEYE, W.R.Jr., YOUNG, J.R., WILSON, C.B. and JAFFE, R.B. (1977): Detection, evaluation, and treatment of pituitary micro-adenomas in patients with galactorrhea and amenorrhea. *Am.J.Obstet. Gynecol.*, 128, 356–363.

CHEN, H.J. (1984): Age and sex difference in serum and pituitary thyrotropin concentration in the rat: Influence by pituitary adenoma. *Exp.Gerontol.*, 19, 1–6.

CHENG, L. (1980): Pheochromocytoma in rats: Incidence, etiology, morphology and functional activity. *J.Environ.Pathol.Toxicol.*, 4, 219–228.

CHOW, S.Y., JEE, W.S., TAYLOR, G.N. and WOODBURY, D.M. (1965): Radioauto-graphic studies of inulin, sulfate and chloride in rat and guinea pig thyroid glands. *Endocrinology*, 77, 818–824.

CHOW, S.Y. and WOODBURY, D.M. (1965): Studies on the stromal, luminal and cellular compartments of the thyroid. *Endocrinology*, 77, 825–840.

CHOW, S.Y. and WOODBURY, D.M. (1970): Kinetics of distribution of radio-active perchlorate in rat and guinea pig thyroid glands. *J.Endocrinol.*, 47, 207–218.

CHRONWALL, B.M., MILLINGTON, W.R., GRIFFIN, S.T., UNNERSTALL, J.R. and O'DONOHUE, T.L. (1987): Histological evaluation of the dopaminergic regulation of proopiomelanocortin gene expression in the intermediate lobe of the rat pituitary, involving in situ hybridization and [3H] thymidine uptake measurement. *Endocrinology*, 120, 1201–1211.

CHVEDOFF, M., CLARKE, M.R., IRISARRI, E., FACCINI, J.M. and MONRO, A.M. (1980): Effects of housing conditions on food intake, body weight and spontaneous lesions in mice. A review of the literature and results of an 18-month study. *Food.Cosmet.Toxicol.*, 18, 517–522.

CHVEDOFF, M., FACCINI, J.M., GREGORY, M.H., HULL, R.M., MONRO, A.M., PERRAUD, J., QUINTON, R.M. and REINERT, H.H. (1984): The toxicology of the schistosomicidal agent oxamnaquine. *Drug Dev.Res.*, 4, 229–235.

CINTI, S., SBARBATI, A., MARELLI, M. and OSCULATI, F. (1985): An ultra-structural morphometric analysis of the adenohypophysis of lactating rats. *Anat.Rec.*, 212, 381–390.

COMER, C.P., CHENGELIS, C.P., LEVIN, S. and KOTSONIS, F.M. (1985): Changes in thyroidal function and liver UDP glucuronyltransferase activity in rats following administration of a novel imidazole (SC-37211). *Toxicol.Appl.Pharmacol.*, 80, 427–436.

CONAWAY, D.H., PADGETT, G.A., BUNTON, T.E., NACHREINER, R. and HAUPTMAN, J. (1985): Clinical and histological features of primary progressive, familial thyroiditis in a colony of borzoi dogs. *Vet.Pathol.*, 22, 439–446.

COOPER, D.S. (1984): Antithyroid drugs. *N.Eng.J.Med.*, 311, 1353–1362.

CORVOL, P., CLAIRE, M., OBLIN, M.E., GEERING, K. and ROSSIER, B. (1981): Mechanism of the antimineralocorticoid effects of spirolactones. *Kidney Int.*, 20, 1–6.

COTE, T.E., ESKAY, R.L., FREY, E.A., GREWE, C.W., MUNEMURA, M., STOOF, J.C., TSURUTA, K. and KEBABIAN, J.W. (1982): Biochemical and physiological studies of the beta-adrenoceptor and the D-2 dopamine receptor in the intermediate lobe of the rat pituitary gland: A review. *Neuroendocrinology*, 35, 217–224

COULAM, C.B., ANNEGERS, J.F., ABBOUD, C.F., LAWS, E.R.Jr. and KURLAND, L.T. (1979): Pituitary adenoma and oral contraceptives: A case-control study. *Fertil.Steril.*, 31, 25–28.

COUPLAND, R.E. (1972): The chromaffin system. In: H. Blaschko and E. Muscholl (Eds), *Catecholamines, Handbook of Experimental Pharmacology*, Vol. 33, pp. 16–39. Springer-Verlag, Berlin.

DACHEUX, F. (1982): Ultrastructural localization of thyrotropin (TSH) in the porcine anterior pituitary. *Cell Tissue Res.*, 222, 299–311.

DADA, M.O., CAMPBELL, G.T. and BLAKE, C.A. (1984): Pars distalis cell quantification in normal adult male and female rats. *J.Endocrinol.*, 101, 87–94.

DAUGHADAY, W.H. (1985): The anterior pituitary. In: J.D. Wilson and D.W. Foster (Eds), *Williams Textbook of Endocrinology*, Chap. 18, pp. 568–613. Saunders, Philadelphia.

DEACON, C.F., MOSLEY, W. and JONES, I.C. (1986): The X-zone of the mouse adrenal cortex of the Swiss albino strain. *Gen.Comp.Endocrinol.*, 61, 87–99.

DELELLIS, R.A., MAY, L., TASHJIAN, A.H. and WOLFE, H.J. (1978): C-cell granule heterogeneity in man. An ultrastructural immunocytochemical study. *Lab.Invest.*, 38, 263–269.

DELELLIS, R.A., NUNNEMACHER, G., BITMAN, W.R., GAGEL, R.F., JASHJIAN, A.H., BLOUNT, M. and WOLFE, H.J. (1979): C-cell hyperplasia and medullary thyroid carcinoma in the rat. An immunohistochemical and ultrastructural analysis. *Lab.Invest.*, 40, 140–154.

744

DELELLIS, R.A. and WOLFE, H.J. (1987): New techniques in gene product analysis. *Arch.Pathol.Lab.Med.*, 111, 620–627.

DELELLIS, R.A., WOLFE, H.J. and MOHR, U. (1987): Medullary thyroid carcinoma in the Syrian golden hamster: An immunocytochemical study. *Exp.Pathol.*, 31, 11–16.

DENEF, J.-F., HOUMONT, S., CORNETTE, C. and BECKERS, C. (1981): Correlated functional and morphometric study of thyroid hyperplasia induced by iodine deficiency. *Endocrinology*, 108, 2352–2358.

de RUITER, J., HOLLANDER, C.F., BOORMAN, G.A., HENNEMANN, G., DOCTER, R. and VAN PUTTEN, L.M. (1976): Comparison of carcinogenicity of 131I and 125I in thyroid gland of the rat. In: *Biological and Environmental Effects of Low-Level Radiation*, Vol. 2, pp. 21–33. International Atomic Energy Agency, Vienna.

DEXTER, R.N., FISHMAN, L.M., NEY, R.L. and LIDDLE, G.W. (1967): Inhibition of adrenal corticosteroid synthesis by aminoglutethimide. Studies of the mechanism of action. *J.Clin.Endocrinol.Metab.*, 27, 473–480.

DIENER, R.M. (1988): Case history. Pheochromocytomas and reserpine: Review of carcinogenicity bioassay. *J.Am.Coll.Toxicol.*, 7, 95–105.

DOBBIE, J.W. (1969): Adrenocortical nodular hyperplasia: The aging adrenal. *J.Pathol.*, 99, 1–18.

DONAUBAUER, H.H., KRAMER, M., KRIEG, K., MAYER, D., VONRECHENBERG, W., SANDOW, J. and SCHüTZ, E. (1987): Investigations of the carcinogenicity of the LH-RH analog buserelin (HOE 766) in rats using the subcutaneous route of administration. *Fundam.Appl.Toxicol.*, 9, 738–752.

DONIACH, I. (1957): Comparison of the carcinogenic effect of X-irradiation with radioactive iodine on rat's thyroid. *Br.J.Cancer*, 11, 67–76.

DONIACH, I. (1967): The structure of the thyroid gland. *J.Clin.Pathol.*, 20, 309–317.

DUNN, T.B. (1970): Normal and pathologic anatomy of the adrenal gland of the adrenal gland of the mouse, including neoplasms. *J.N.C.I.*, 44, 1323–1389.

EL ETREBY, M.F. (1981): Practical applications of immunocytochemistry to the pharmacology and toxicology of the endocrine system. *Histochem.J.*, 13, 821–837.

EL ETREBY, M.F. and FATH EL BAB, M.R. (1977): Effect of cyproterone acetate on cells of the pars distalis of the adenohypophysis in the beagle bitch. *Cell Tissue Res.*, 183, 177–189.

EL ETREBY, M.F., SCHILK, B., SOULIOTI, G., TÜSHAUS, U., WIEMANN, H. and GÜNZEL, P. (1977): Effect of 17β-estradiol on cells of the pars distalis of the adenohypophysis in the beagle bitch: An immunocyto chemical and morphometric study. *Endokrinologie*, 69, 202–216.

EL ETREBY, M.F., MÜLLER-PEDDINGHAUS, R., BHARGAVA, A.S. and TRAUTWEIN, G. (1980): Functional morphology of spontaneous hyperplastic and neoplastic lesions in the canine pituitary gland. *Vet.Pathol.*, 17, 109–122.

ELLIOTT, M.E., ALEXANDER, R.C. and GOODFRIEND, T.L. (1982): Aspects of angiotensin action in the adrenal. Key roles for calcium and phosphatidyl inositol. *Hypertension*, 4, 52–58.

ERÄNKÖ, O. (1955): Nodular hyperplasia and increase of noradrenaline content in the adrenal medulla of nicotine-treated rats. *Acta.Pathol. Microbiol. (Scand.)*, 36, 210–218.

FENSKE, N.A., MILLNS, J.L. and GREER, K.E. (1980): Minocycline-induced pigmentation at sites of cutaneous inflammation. *J.A.M.A.*, 244, 1103–1106.

FIRTH, C.H. (1983): Histology, adrenal gland, mouse. In: T.C. Jones, U. Mohr and R.D. Hunt (Eds) *Endocrine System*, pp. 8–12. Springer-Verlag, Berlin.

FIRTH, C.H. and HEATH, J.E. (1983): Adenoma, thyroid, mouse. In: T.C. Jones, U. Mohr and R.D. Hunt (Eds) *Endocrine System*, pp. 184–187. Springer-Verlag, Berlin.

FISHER, E.R. and HORVAT, B. (1971): Experimental production of so-called spironolactone bodies. *Arch.Pathol.*, 91, 471–478.

FLETCHER, A.P. (1978): Drug safety testing and subsequent clinical experience. *J.R.Soc.Med.*, 71, 693–696.

FOOD AND DRUG ADMINISTRATION (1980): Flutamide. Pharmacology and toxicology review of NDA 18–554. Original summary. December 31, 1980.

FOOD AND DRUG ADMINISTRATION (1981): Ketoconazole Summary Basis of Approval NDA 18–533, Food and Drug Administration, Washington.

FRITZ, T.E., ZEMAN, R.C. and ZELLE, M.A. (1970): Pathology and familial incidence of thyroiditis in a closed beagle colony. *Exp.Mol.Pathol.*, 12, 14–30.

FURTH, J. (1963): Influence of host factors on the growth of neoplastic cell. *Cancer Res.*, 23, 21–34.

FURTH, J., UEDA, G. and CLIFTON, K.H. (1973): The pathophysiology of pituitaries and their tumors: Methodological advances. In: H.Busch (Eds), *Methods in Cancer Research*, Vol 10, pp. 201–277. *Academic Press*, New York.

GANJAM, V.K., CAMPBELL, A.L. and MURPHY, B.E.P. (1972): Changing patterns of circulating corticosteroids in rabbits following prolonged treatment with ACTH. *Endocrinology*, 91, 607–611.

GEE, C.E., CHEN, C.-L.C., ROBERTS, J.L., THOMPSON, R. and WATSON, S.J. (1983): Identification of pro-opiomelanocortin neurons in rat hypothalamus by *in situ* cDNA-mRNA hybridization. *Nature*, 306, 374–376.

GILLMAN, J., GILBERT, C. and SPENCE, I. (1953): Pheochromocytoma in the rat. Pathogenesis and collateral reactions and its relation to comparable tumors in man. *Cancer*, 6, 494–511.

GIROD, C. and LHÉRITIER, M. (1986): Ultrastructural observations on folliculo-stellate cells in the pars distalis of the pituitary gland in three rodent species. *Arch.Histol.Jpn.*, 49, 1–12.

GIROD, C., LHÉRITIER, M. and GUICHARD, Y. (1975): Description des cellules folliculo-stellaires dans l'adenohypophyse du singe Macacus irus. *Cr.Acad.Sc.Paris*, 280, 2481–2483.

GIROD, C., TROUILLAS, J. and DUBOIS, M.P. (1985): Immunocytochemical localization of S-100 protein in stellate cells (folliculo-stellate) of the anterior lobe of the normal human pituitary. *Cell Tissue Res.*, 241, 505–511.

GIVENS, J.R., COLEMAN, S. and BRITT, L. (1968): Anatomical changes is produced in the human adrenal cortex by aminoglutethimide. *Clin.Res.*, 16, 441.

GOEDEGEBUURE, S.A. and HAZEWINKEL, H.A.W. (1986): Morphological findings in young dogs chronically fed a diet containing excess calcium. *Vet.Pathol.*, 23, 594–605.

GOLDMAN, A.S. (1970): Production of congenital lipoid adrenal hyperplasia in rats and inhibition of cholesterol side-chain cleavage. *Endocrinology*, 86, 1245–1251.

GOODMAN, D.G., WARD, J.M., SQUIRE, R.A., CHU, K.C. and LINHART, M.S. (1979): Neoplastic and non-neoplastic lesions in aging F344 rats. *Toxicol. Appl.Pharmacol.*, 48, 237–248.

GOODMAN, D.G., WARD, J.M., SQUIRE, R.A., PAXTON, M.B., REICHARDT, W.D., CHU, K.C. and LINHART, M.S. (1980): Neoplastic and non-neoplastic lesions in aging Osborne-Mendel rats. *Toxicol.Appl.Pharmacol.*, 55, 433–447.

GORDON, G., SPARANO, B.M., KRAMER, A.W., KELLY, R.G. and IATROPOULOS, M.J. (1984): Thyroid gland pigmentation and minocycline therapy. *Am.J.Pathol.*, 117, 98–109.

GOSNEY, J.R. (1985): Adrenal corticomedullary hyperplasia in hypobaric hypoxia. *J.Pathol.*, 146, 59–64.

GOSNEY, J.A. (1986): Morphological changes in the pituitary and thyroid of the rat in hypobaric hypoxia. *J.Endocrinol.*, 109, 119–124.

GOSSELIN, S.J., CAPEN, C.C. and MARTIN, S.L. (1981): Histologic and ultra-structural evaluation of thyroid lesions associated with hypothyroidism in dogs. *Vet.Pathol.*, 18, 299–309.

GRAVES, P.E. and SALHANICK, H.A. (1979): Seroselective inhibition of aromatase by enantiomers of aminoglutethimide. *Endocrinology*, 105, 52–57.

GREAVES, P. and FACCINI, J.M. (1984): Endocrine glands. In: *Rat Histopathology. A glossary for use in toxicity and carcinogenicity studies*. Chap. 10, pp. 187–210. Elsevier, Amsterdam.

GREAVES, P. and RABEMAMPIANINA, Y. (1982): Choice of rat strain: A comparison of the general pathology and the tumour incidence in 2-year old Sprague-Dawley and Long-Evans rats. *Arch.Toxicol.*, Suppl. 5, 298–303.

GWYNNE, J.T. and STRAUSS, J.F. III (1982): The role of lipoproteins in steroidogenesis and cholesterol metabolism in steroidogenic glands. *Endocr.Rev.*, 3, 299–329.

HAINES, D.M. and HAINES, W.J. (1985): Experimental thyroid auto-immunity in the dog. *Vet.Immunol.Immunopathol.*, 9, 221–238.

HARCOURT-WEBSTER, J.N. and TRUMAN, R.F. (1969): Histochemical study of oxidative and hydrolytic enzymes in the abnormal human parathyroid. *J.Pathol.*, 97, 687–693.

HARIGAYA, T., KOHMOTO, K. and HOSHINO, K (1983): Immunohistochemical identification of prolactin-producing cells in the mouse adenohypophysis. *Acta-histochem.Cytochem.*, 16, 51–58.

746

HEATH, J.E. and LITTLEFIELD, N.A. (1984): Morphological effects of subchronic oral sulpha-methazine administration on Fischer 344 and B6C3F1 mice. *Toxicol.Pathol.*, 12, 3–9.

HEATH, J.E. and FRITH, C.H. (1983): Carcinoma, thyroid, mouse. In: T.C. Jones, U. Mohr, and R.D. Hunt (Eds), *Endocrine System*, pp. 188–191. Springer-Verlag, Berlin.

HEMMING, F.J., BEGEOT, M., DUBOIS, M.P. and DUBOIS, M.P. (1983): Ultra-structural identification of corticotrophes of the fetal rat. *Cell Tissue Res.*, 234, 427–437.

HIGHMAN, B., NORVELL, M.J. and SCHELLENBERGER, T.E. (1977): Pathological changes in female C3H mice continuously fed diets containing diethyl-stibestrol or 17β-estradiol. *J.Environ.Pathol.Toxicol.*, 1, 1–30.

HILL, R.N., ERDREICH, L.S., PAYNTER, O.E., ROBERTS, P.A., ROSENTHAL, S.L. and WILKINSON, C.F. (1989): Thyroid follicular cell carcinogenesis. *Fundam.Appl.Toxicol.*, 12, 629–697.

HÖKFELT, T., JOHANSSON, O., LJUNGDAHL, A., LUNDBERG, J.M. and SCHULTZBERG, M. (1980): Peptidergic neurones. *Nature*, 284, 515–520.

HOFFMANN, K. (1984): Toxicological studies with nitrendipine. In: A. Scriabine, S. Vanov and K. Deck (Eds), *Nitrendipine*, Chap. 3, pp. 25–32. Urban and Schwarzenberg, Baltimore.

HOLLANDER, C.F. and SNELL, K.C. (1976): Tumours of the adrenal gland. In: V.S. Turusov (Ed.), *Pathology of Tumours in Laboratory Animals, Vol. 1*, Tumours of the Rat, Part 2, pp. 273–293. IARC Scientific Publ. No. 6, Lyon.

HOLTZMAN, S., STONE, J.P. and SHELLABARGER, C.J. (1979): Influence of diethylstibestrol treatment on prolactin cells of female ACI and Sprague-Dawley rats. *Cancer Res.*, 39, 779–784.

HOUSTON, J.B., HUMPHREY, M.J., MATTHEW, D.E. and TARBIT, M.H. (1988): Comparison of two azole antifungal drugs, ketoconazole and fluconazole, as modifiers of rat hepatic mono-oxygenase activity. *Biochem. Pharmacol.*, 37, 401–408.

HUGHES, S.W.M. and BURLEY, D.M. (1970): Aminoglutethimide: A 'side-effect' turned to therapeutic advantage. *Postgrad.Med.J.*, 46, 409–416.

HUMMEL, K.P. (1958): Accessory adrenal cortical nodules in the mouse. *Anat.Rec.*, 132, 281–296.

HUTTER, A.M. and KAYHOE, D.E. (1966): Adrenal cortical carcinoma. Results of treatment with o,p'DDD in 138 patients. *Am.J.Med.*, 41, 581–592.

IBRAHIM, S.N., MOUSSA, S.M. and CHILDS, G.V. (1986): Morphometric studies of rat anterior pituitary cells after gonadectomy: Correlation of changes in gonadotrophs with the serum levels of gonadotropins. *Endocrinology*, 119, 629–637.

INGBAR, S.H. (1985): The thyroid gland. In: J.D. Wilson and D.W. Foster (Eds), *William's Textbook of Endocrinology*, Chap. 21, pp. 682–815. Saunders, Philadelphia.

ISHIKAWA, H., NOGAMI, H. and SHIRASAWA, N. (1983): Novel clonal strains from adult rat anterior pituitary producing S-100 protein. *Nature*, 303, 711–713.

JANIGAN, D.T. (1963): Cytoplasmic bodies in the adrenal cortex of patients treated with spirolac-tone. *Lancet*, 1, 850–852.

KABEL, P.J., VOORBIJ, H.A.M., DE HAAN, M., VAN DER GAAG, R.D. and DREXHAGE, H.A. (1988): Intrathyroid dendritic cells. *J.Clin.Endcrinol.Metab.*, 66, 199–207.

KAMINSKY, N., LUSE, S. and HARTCROFT, P. (1962): Ultrastructure of adrenal cortex of the dog during treatment with DDD. *J.N.C.I.*, 29, 127–159.

KAMM, J.J. (1982): Toxicology, carcinogenicity, and teratogenicity of some orally administered retinoids. *J.Am.Acad.Dermatol.*, 6, 652–659.

KELLY, R.G. and KANEGIS, L.A. (1967): Metabolism and tissue distribution of radio-isotopically labelled minocycline. *Toxicol.Appl.Pharmacol.*, 11, 171–183.

KITCHEN, D.N., TODD, G.C., MEYERS, D.B. and PAGET, C. (1979): Rat lympho cytic thyroidi-tis associated with ingestion of an immunosuppressive compound. *Vet.Pathol.*, 16, 722–729.

KOMURO, M. and SHIODA, T. (1981): Localization of sialic acid-containing hormones in GTH cells and ACTH cells of the rat anterior pituitary. *Cell Tissue Res.*, 220, 519–528.

KONEFF, A.A., SIMPSON, M.E. and EVANS, H.M. (1946): Effects of chronic administration of diethylstibestrol on the pituitary and other endocrine organs of hamsters. *Anat.Rec.*, 94, 169–195.

KOVACS, K. and HORVATH, E. (1986): Tumors of the pituitary gland. In: W.H. Hartmann and

L.H. Sobin (Eds), *Atlas of Tumor Pathology*, Fascicle 21, 2nd Series. Armed Forces Institute of Pathology, Washington.

KOVACS, K., BLASCHECK, J.A., YEGHIAYAN, E., HATAKEYAMA, S. and GARDELL, C. (1971): Adrenocortical lipid hyperplasia induced in rats by aniline. A histologic and electron microscopic study. *Am.J.Pathol.*, 62, 17–34.

KOVACS, K., HORVATH, E. and SINGER, W. (1973): Fine structure and morphogenesis of spironolactone bodies in the zona glomerulosa of the human adrenal cortex. *J.Clin.Pathol.*, 26, 949–957.

KOVACS, K., HORVATH, E., ILSE, R.G., EZRIN, C. and ILSE, D. (1977): Spontaneous pituitary adenomas in aging rats: A light microscopic, immunocytological, and fine structure study. *Beitr.Pathol.*, 161, 1–16.

KUROSUMI, M. and FUJITA, H. (1986): Fine structural aspects on the fate of rat black thyroids induced by minocycline. *Vichows Arch.[B]*, 51, 207–213.

KUROKAWA, Y., HAYASHI, Y., MAEKAWA, A., TAKAHASHI, M. and KUKUBO, T. (1985): High incidences of pheochromocytomas after long-term administration of retinol acetate to F344/Du Crj rats. *J.N.C.I.*, 74, 715–723.

LANCET (1987): Amiodarone and the thyroid: The Janus response. *Lancet ii*, 24–25.

LANDAS, S.K., SCHELPER, R.L., TIO, F.O., TURNER, J.W., MOORE, K.C. and BENNETT-GRAY J (1986): Black thyroid syndrome: Exaggeration of a normal process? *Am.J.Pathol.*, 85, 411–418.

LANDSBERG, L. and YOUNG, J.B. (1985): Catecholamines and the adrenal medulla. In J.P. Wilson, D.W. Foster (Eds),*William's Textbook of Endocrinology*, 7th Edition, chap. 3 pp. 891–965. Saunders, Philadelphia.

LEAV, I., SCHILLER, A.L., RIJNBERK, A., LEGG, M.A., and DER KINDEREN, P.J. (1976): Adenomas and carcinomas of the canine and feline thyroid. *Am.J.Pathol.* 83, 61–122.

LEMOINE, N.R., MAYALL, E.S., WILLIAMS, E.D., THURSTON, V. and WYNFORD-THOMAS, D. (1988): Agent-specific ras oncogene activation in rat thyroid tumours. *Oncogene*, 3, 541–544.

LEMOINE, N.R., MAYALL, E.S., WYLLIE, F.S., WILLIAMS, E.D., GOYNS, M., STRINGER, B. and WYNFORD-THOMAS, D. (1989): High frequency of ras oncogene activation in all stages of human thyroid tumorigenesis. *Oncogene*, 4, 159–164.

LLOYD, R.V. (1983): Estrogen induced hyperplasia and neoplasia in the rat anterior pituitary gland. *Am.J.Pathol.*, 113, 198–206.

LLOYD, R.V. and LANDEFELD, T.D. (1986): Detection of prolactin messenger RNA in rat anterior pituitary in situ hybridization. *Am.J.Pathol.*, 125, 35–44.

LLOYD, R.V. and MAILLOUX, J. (1987): Effects of diethylstibestrol and propylthiouracil on the rat pituitary. An immunohistochemical study. *J.N.C.I.*, 79, 865–873.

LÜLLMANN-RAUCH, R. (1979): Drug-induced lysosomal storage disorders. In: J.T. Dingle, P.J. Jacques and I.H. Shaw (Eds), *Lysosomes in Applied Biology and Therapeutics*, vol. 6, chap. 3, pp. 49–130. North Holland Amsterdam.

LUMB, G., MITCHELL, L. and DE LA IGLESIA, F.A. (1985). Regression of pathological changes induced by long-term administration of contraceptive steroids to rodents. *Toxicol.Pathol.*, 13, 283–295.

LUPELESCU, A., POTORAC, E., POP, A., HEITMANEK, C., MERCUJIEV, E., CHISIU, N., OPRISAN, R. and NEACSU, C. (1968): Experimental investigations on immunology of the parathyroid gland. *Immunology*, 14, 475–482.

LYLE, S.F., WRIGHT, K. and COUINS, D.C. (1984): Comparative effects of tamoxifen and bromocriptine on prolactin and pituitary weight in estradiol-treated male rats. *Cancer*, 53, 1473–1477.

MAGALHAES, M.M., MAGALHAES, M., GOMES, M.L., HIPOLITO-REIS, C. and SERRA, T.A.M. (1987): A correlated morphological and biochemical study on rat adrenal steroidogenesis. *Eur.J.Cell Biol.*, 43, 247–253.

MAJEED, S.K. and HARLING, S.M. (1986): Malignant pheochromocytoma with widespread metastases in the rat. *J.Comp.Pathol.*, 96, 575–580.

748

MALENDOWICZ, L.K. (1973): Comparative studies on the effects of amino-glutethimide, metopirone, ACTH and hydrocortisone on the adrenal cortex of adult male rats. II. Histological and histochemical studies. *Endokrinologie*, 61, 75–93.

MAREK, J. and MOTLIK, K. (1975): Ultrastructural changes of the adrenal cortex in Cushing's syndrome treated with aminoglutethimide (Elipten Ciba). *Virchows Arch. [B]*, 18, 145–156.

MAREK, J. and MOTLIK, K. (1978): Ultrastructure of acute adenocortical damage due to aminoglutethimide (Elipten Ciba) in rats. *Virchows Arch. [B]*, 27, 173–188.

MAREK, J., THOENES, W. and MOTLIK, K. (1970): Lipoide transformation der mitchondrien in Nebennierenrindenzellen nach aminoglutathimid (Elipten Ciba). *Virchows Arch. [B]*, 6, 116–131.

MASON, J.I., MURRY, B.A., OLCOTT, M. and SHEETS, J.J. (1985): Imidazole antimycotics: Inhibitors of steroid aromatase. *Biochem.Pharmacol.*, 34, 1087–1092.

MAZZOCCHI, G. and NUSSDORFER, G.G. (1984): Long-term effects of captopril on the morphology of normal rat adrenal zona glomerulosa. *Exp.Clin. Endocrinol.*, 84, 148–152.

MAZZOCCHI, G., REBUFFAT, P. and NUSSDORFER, G.G. (1987)a: Atrial natriuretic factor (ANF) inhibits the growth and the secretory activity of rat adrenal zona glomerulosa in vivo. *J.Steroid.Biochem.*, 28, 6430646.

MAZZOCCHI, G., ROBBA, C., MENEGHELLI, V. and NUSSDORFEDR, G.G. (1987)b: Effects of ACTH and aminoglutethimide administration on the morphological and functional responses of rat adrenal zona fasciculata to a prolonged treatment with 4-aminopyrazolo-pyrimidine. *J.Anat.*, 154, 55–61.

MAZZOCCHI, G., ROBBA, C., REBUFFAT, P. and NUSSDORFER, G.G. (1982): Effects of sodium repletion and timolol maleate administration on the zona glomerulosa of the rat adrenal cortex: An electron microscopic morpho metric study. *Endokrinologie*, 79, 81–88.

MAZZOCCHI, G., ROBBA, C., REBUFFAT, P. and NUSSDORFER, G.G. (1986): Effects of prolactin administration on the zona glomerulosa of the rat adrenal cortex: Stereology and plasma hormone concentration. *Acta.Endocrinol*, 111, 101–105.

McALLISTER, R.G. Jr., HAMANN, S.R. and PIASCIK, M.T. (1983): Aspects of the clinical pharmacology of verapamil, a calcium- entry antagonist. *Biopharm.Drug Dispos.*, 4, 203–211.

McCLAIN, R.M. (1989): The significance of hepatic microsomal enzyme induction and altered thyroid function in rats. Implications for thyroid gland neoplasia. *Toxicol.Pathol.*, 17, 294–306.

McCOMB, D.J., KOVACS, K., BERI, J. and ZAK, F. (1984): Pituitary adenomas in old Sprague-Dawley rats: A histologic, ultrastructural, and immuno cytochemical study. *J.N.C.I.*, 73, 1143–1166.

McCOMB, D.J., KOVACS, K., BERI, J., ZAK, F., MILLIGAN, J.V. and SHIN, S.H. (1985): Pituitary gonadotroph adenomas in old Sprague-Dawley rats. *J.Submicrosc.Cytol.*, 17, 517–530.

McCONNELL, E.E., SOLLEVELD, H.A., SWENBERG, J.A. and BOORMAN, G.A. (1986): Guidelines for combining neoplasms for evaluation of rodent carcino-genesis studies. *J.N.C.I.*, 76, 283–289.

McGRAE, J.D. and ZELICKSON, A.S. (1980): Skin pigmentation secondary to minocycline therapy. *Arch.Dermatol.*, 116, 1262–1265.

McNICOL, A.M. (1987): Pituitary adenomas. *Histopathology*, 11, 995–1011.

McNICOL, A.M., KUBBA, M.A. and STEWART, C.J.R. (1988): The morphological effects of dexamethasone on the pituitary-adrenal axis of the rat: a quantitative study. *J.Pathol.*, 154, 181–186.

MEDEIROS, L.J., FEDERMAN, M., SILVERMAN, M.L. and BALOGH, K. (1984): Black thyroid associated with minocycline therapy. *Arch.Pathol.Lab Med.*, 108, 268–269.

MEISSNER, W.A. and WARREN, S. (1969): Tumors of the thyroid gland. In: *Atlas of Tumor Pathology, Second Series, Fascicle 4*, pp. 30–52. AFIP, Washington, DC.

MERRY, B.J. (1975): Mitochondrial structures in the rat adrenal cortex. *J.Anat.*, 119, 611–618.

MILLAR, J.A. and STRUTHERS, A.D. (1984): Calcium antagonists and hormone release. *Clin.Sci.*, 66, 249–255.

MOON, R.C., McCORMICK, D.L. and MEHTA, R.G. (1983): Inhibition of carcinogenesis by letinoids. *Cancer Res.*, 43, 2469s–2475s.

749

MOON, H.D., SIMPSON, M.E., LI, C.H. and EVANS, H.M. (1950): Neoplasms in rats treated with pituitary growth hormone. II. Adrenal glands. *Cancer Res.*, 10, 364–370.

MORRIS, H.P., WAGNER, B.P., RAY, F.E., SNELL, K.C. and STEWART, H.L. (1961): Comparative study of cancer and other lesions of rats fed N,N-'2,7,-fluorenylene-bisacetamide or N-2-fluorencylacetamide. NCI Monogr 5, 1–53.

MOSHER, A.H. and KIRCHER, C.H. (1985): Proliferative lesions of the adrenal medulla in rats treated with zomepirac sodium. *J.Am.Coll.Toxicol.* 7, 83–91.

MOTLIK, K., MAREK, J. and STARKA, L. (1978): The influence of aminoglutethimide (Elipten Ciba) on the morphology and function of rat female adrenal cortex in a short-term experiment. *Acta.Univ.Carol.*[Med], (Praha), 24, 131–150.

MUSSER, E. and GRAHAM, W.R. (1968): Familial occurrence of thyroiditis in purebred beagles. *Lab.Anim.Care*, 18, 58–68.

NAGATAKI, S. (1974): Effects of excess quantities of iodine. In: R.O. Greep, E.B. Astwood, M.A. Greer, D.H. Solomon and S.R. Geiger (Eds), *Handbook of Physiology Section 7, Vol. 3*, pp. 329–344. American Physiological Society, Washington, DC.

NAGATANI, M., MIURA, K., TSUCHITANI, M. and NARAMA, I. (1987): Relationship between cellular morphology and immunocytological findings of spontaneous pituitary tumors in the aged rat. *J.Comp.Pathol.*, 97, 11–20.

NAKAGAWA, F., SCHULTE, B.A., SENS, M.A., KOCHIBE, N. and SPICER, S.S. (1986): Lectin cytochemistry of cell types in human and canine pituitary. *Histochemistry*, 85, 57–66.

NATIONAL CANCER INSTITUTE (1979): Bioassay of reserpine for possible carcinogenicity. *Nat.Tech.Inform.Service Publication*, PB 80/217920.

NEVILLE, A.M. (1969): The adrenal medulla. In: T. Symington (Ed.), *Functional Pathology of the Human Adrenal Gland*, Part II, pp. 219–324. Livingstone, Edinburgh.

NEVILLE, A.M. (1978): The nodular adrenal. *Invest. Cell Pathol.*, 1, 99–111.

NEVILLE, A.M. and O'HARE, M.J. (1982): Structure of the adult adrenal cortex. In: *The Human Adrenal Cortex. Pathology and Biology: An Integrated Approach*, Chap. 4, pp. 16–34. Springer-Verlag, Berlin.

NICKERSON, P.A. (1979): Adrenal cortex in retired breeder Mongolian gerbils (Meriones unguiculatus) and golden hamsters (Mesocricetus auratus). Ultrastructural alterations in the zona reticularis. *Am.J.Pathol.*, 95, 347–358.

NIWA, J., MINASE, T., HASHI, K. and MORI, M. (1987): Immunohistochemical, electron microscopic and morphometric studies of estrogen-induced rat prolactinomas after bromocriptine treatment. *Virchows Arch.[B]*, 53, 89–96.

NORTH, R.A. and EGAN, T.M. (1983): Actions and distributions of opioid peptides in peripheral tissues. *Br.Med.Bull.*, 39, 71–75.

NUSSDORFER, G.G. (1980): Cytophysiology of the adrenal zona glomerulosa. *Int.Rev.Cytol.*, 64, 307–369.

NUSSDORFER, G.G. (1986): Cytophysiology of the adrenal cortex. *Int.Rev.Cytol.*, 98, 1–405.

NUSSDORFER, G.G., NERI, G., BELLONI, A.S., MAZZOCCHI, G., REBUFFAT, P. and ROBBA, C. (1982): Effects of ACTH on the zona glomerulosa of sodium-loaded timolol maleate-treated rats: stereology and plasma hormone concentrations. *Acta.Endocrinol.*, 99, 256–262.

O'DONOHUE, T.L. and DORSA, D.M. (1982): The opiomelanotropinergic neuronal and endocrine systems. *Peptides*, 3, 353–395.

OHSHIMA, M. and WARD, J.M. (1986): Dietary iodine deficiency as a tumor promoter and carcinogen in male F344/NCr rats. *Cancer Res.*, 46, 877–883.

OHTAKI, S. (1979): Conspicuous sex difference in zona reticularis of the adrenal cortex of Syrian hamsters. *Lab.Anim. Sci.*, 29, 765–769.

OKSANEN, A. (1980): The ultrastructure of the multi-nucleated cells in canine parathyroid glands. *J.Comp.Pathol.*, 90, 293–301.

OLDSTONE, M.B.A., SINHA, Y.N., BLOUNT, P., TISHON, A., RODRIGUEZ, M., VON WEDEL, R. and LAMPERT, P.W. (1982): Virus-induced alterations in homeostasis: Alterations in differentiated functions of infected cells in vivo. *Science*, 218, 1125–1127.

OPPENHEIMER, J.W., BERNSTEIN, G. and BURKS, M.Z. (1968): Increased thyroxine turnover after stimulation of hepatocellular binding of thyroxine by phenobarbital. *J.Clin.Invest.*, 47, 1399–1406.

OTT, R.A., HOFFMANN,C., OSLAPAS, R., NAYYAR, R. and PALOYAN, E. (1987): Radioiodine sensitivity of parafollicular C cells in aged Long-Evans rats. *Surgery*, 102, 1043–1048.

PAWLIKOWSKI, M. (1982): The link between secretion and mitoses in the endocrine glands. *Life Sci.*, 30, 315–320.

PAYNTER, O.E., BURIN, G.J., JAEGER, R.B. and GREGORIO, C.A. (1988): Goitrogens and thyroid follicular cell neoplasia: Evidence for a threshold process. *Regul.Toxicol.Pharmacol.*, 8, 102–119.

PENHALE, W.J., FARMER, A., McKENNA, R.P. and IRVINE, W.J. (1973): Spontaneous thyroiditis in thymectomized and irradiated Wistar rats. *Clin.Exp.Immunol.*, 15, 225–236.

PERLMAN, R.L. and CHALFIE, M. (1977): Catecholamine release from the adrenal medulla. *Clin.Endocrinol.Metab.*, 6, 551–576.

PHELPS, C.J. (1986): Immunocytochemical analysis of prolactin cells in the adult rat adenohypophysis: Distribution and quantitation relative to sex and strain. *Am.J.Anat.*, 176, 233–242.

PHYSICIAN'S DESK REFERENCE (1987): Cordarone, (amiodarone). 41st Edition, pp. 2157–2159. Medical Economics Co., Oradell, N.J.

PHYSICIAN'S DESK REFERENCE (1987): Lupron (Leuprolide acetate). 41st Edition, pp. 2007–2008. Medical Economics Co., Oradell, N.J.

PICKERING, C.E. and PICKERING, R.G. (1984): The effect of repeated reproduction on the incidence of pituitary tumours in Wistar rats. *Lab.Anim.*, 18, 371–378.

PITTMAN, J.A. and BROWN, R.W. (1966): Antithyroid and antiadrenocorticoid activity of aminoglutethimide. *J.Clin.Endocrinol.Metab.*, 26, 1014–1016.

PONT, A., WILLIAMS, P.L., LOOSE, D.L., FELDMAN, R., REITZ, E., BOCHRA, C. and STEVENS, D.A. (1982): Ketoconzole blocks adrenal steroid synthesis. *Ann.Intern.Med.*, 97, 370–372.

POOLE, A., JONES, R.B., PRITCHARD, D., CATTO, L. and LEONARD, T. (1989): In vitro accummulation of thyroid hormones by cultured rat hepatocytes and the biliary excretion of iodothyronines in rats treated with a novel histamine H_2-receptor antagonist. *Toxicology*, 59, 23–26.

POUR, P., MOHR, U., ALTHOFF, J., CARDESA, A. and KMOCH, N. (1976): Spontaneous tumors and common diseases in two colonies of Syrian hamsters. III Urogenital system and endocrine glands. *J.N.C.I.*, 56, 949–961.

POUR, P.M. (1983): Hyperplasia, parathyroid, hamster. In: T.C. Jones, U. Mohr and R.D. Hunt (Eds), *Endocrine System*, pp. 265–268. Springer-Verlag, Berlin.

POUR, P.M., WILSON, J.T. and SALMASI, S. (1983): Hyperplasia, parathyroid rat. In: T.C. Jones, U. Mohr and R.D. Hunt (Eds), *Endocrine System*, pp. 268–274. Springer-Verlag, Berlin.

PRICE, S.C., CHESCOE, D., GRASSO, P., WRIGHT, M. and HINTON, R.H. (1988): Alterations in the thyroids of rats treated for long periods with di-(2-ethylhexyl) phthalate or with hypolipidaemic agents. *Toxicol.Lett.* 40, 37–46.

PRYSOR-JONES, R.A., SILVERLIGHT, J.J. and JENKINS, J.S. (1983): Hypothalamic dopamine and catechol oestrogens in rats with spontaneous pituitary tumours. *J.Endocrinol.*, 96, 347–352.

PURVES, H.D. and GRIESBACH, W.E. (1956): Changes in the basophil cells of the rat pituitary after thyroidectomy. *J.Endocrinol.*, 13, 365–375.

REBUFFAT, P., MAZZOCCHI, G. and NUSSDORFER, G.G. (1987): Effect of long-term inhibition of hydroxy-methylglutaryl coenzyme A reductase by mevinolin on the zona fasciculata of the rat adrenal cortex. A combined morphometric and biochemical study. *Virchows Arch.*[B], 54, 67–72.

REID, J.D. (1983): The black thyroid associated with minocycline therapy. A local manifestation of a drug-induced lysosomal/substrate disorder. *Am.J.Clin.Pathol.*, 79, 738–746.

REZNIK, G. and WARD, J.M. (1983): Ganglioneuroma, adrenal rat. In: T.C. Jones, U. Mohr and R.D. Hunt (Eds), *Endocrine System*, pp. 30–34. Springer-Verlag, Berlin.

REZNIK, G., WARD, J.M. and REZNIK-SCHÜLLER, H. (1980): Ganglioneuromas in the adrenal medulla of F344 rats. *Vet.Pathol.*, 17, 614–621.

RHODIN, J.A.G. (1974): Hypophysis. In: *Histology, A Text and Atlas*, Chap. 20, pp. 428–439. Oxford University Press, New York.

RIBELIN, W.E. (1984): The effects of drugs and chemicals upon the structure of the adrenal gland. *Fundam.Appl.Toxicol.*, 4, 105–119.

RIKIHISA, Y. and LIN, Y.C. (1989): Effect of gossypol on the thyroid in young rats. *J.Comp.Pathol.*, 100, 411–417.

ROBBA, C., MAZZOCCHI, G., GOTTARDO, G., MENEGHELLI, V. and NUSSDORFER, G.G. (1987): Effects of prolonged treatement with cyanoketone on the zona fasciculata of rat adrenal cortex. A combined morphometric and biochemical study. *Cell Tissue Res.* 250, 599–605.

ROE, F.J.C. and BÄR, A. (1985): Enzootic and epizootic adrenal medullary proliferative disease of rats: Influence of dietary factors which affect calcium absorption. *Hum.Toxicol.*, 4, 27–52.

ROSE, N.R. (1985): The thyroid gland as source and target of auto-immunity. *Lab.Invest.*, 52, 117–119.

RUSSFIELD, A.B. (1967): Pathology of the endocrine glands, ovary and testis of rats and mice. In: E. Cotchin, F.J.C. Roe (Eds), *Pathology of Laboratory Rats and Mice*, Chap. 14, pp. 391–467. Blackwell, Oxford.

RUSSFIELD, A.B. (1975): Pituitary tumors. In: S.C. Sommers (Ed.), *Endocrine Pathology Decennial 1966–1975*, pp. 41–79. Appleton-Century Crofts, New York.

SAUL, S.H., DEKKER, A., LEE, R.E. and BREITFELD, V. (1983): The black thyroid: Its relation to minocycline use in man. *Arch.Pathol.Lab Med.*, 107, 173–177.

SAWANO, F. and FUJITA, H. (1981): Some findings on the cytochemistry of the thyroid follicle epithelial cell in rats and mice. *Arch.Histol.Jpn.*, 44, 439–452.

SAYERS, A.C. and AMSLER, H.A. (1977): Clozapine. In: M.E. Goldberg (Ed.), *Pharmacological and Biochemical Properties of Drug Substances, Vol. 1*, pp.1–31. American Pharmaceutical Association, Academy of Pharmaceutical Science.

SCHAFFNER, J-C. (1988): Lymphocytic thyroiditis in beagle dogs. *Arch.Toxicol.* Suppl.12, 110–113.

SCHARDEIN, J.L., PATTON, G.R. and LUCAS, J.A. (1967): The microscopy of 'brown degeneration' in the adrenal gland of the mouse. *Anat.Rec.*, 159, 291–309.

SCHEITHAUER, B.W., RANDALL, R.V., LAWS, E.R., KOVAKS, K.T., HORVATH, E. and WHITAKER, M.D. (1985): Prolactin cell carcinoma of the pituitary. Clinicopathologic, immunohistochemical and ultrastructural study of a case with cranial and extracranial metastases. *Cancer*, 55, 598–604.

SCHLECHTE, J., SHERMAN, B., HALMI, N., VAN GILDER, J., CHAPLER, F., DOLAN, K., GRANNER, D., DUELLO, T. and HARRIS, C. (1980): Prolactin-secreting pituitary tumours in amenorrheic women: A comprehensive study. *Endocr.Rev.* 1, 295–308.

SCHWARZ, W. and SUCHOWSKY, G.K. (1963): Die Wirkung von Mefopiron und Amphenon B auf die Nebennierenninde der Ratte. *Virchows Arch.[A].*, 334, 270–278.

SCRIABINE, A., BATTYE, R., HOFFMEISTER, F., KAZDA, S., TOWART, R., GARTHOFF, B., SCHLÜTER, G., RÄMSCH, K-D and SCHERLING, D. (1985): Nimodipine. In: A. Scriabine (Ed.), *New Drugs Annual: Cardiovascular Drugs*, Vol. 3, pp. 197–218. Raven Press, New York.

SILVERMAN, D.A. and ROSE, N.R. (1974): Neonatal thymectomy increases incidence of spontaneous and methylcholanthrene-enhanced thyroiditis in rats. *Science*, 184, 162–163.

SILVERMAN, D.A. and ROSE, N.R. (1975): Spontaneous and methylcholanthrene-enhanced thyroiditis in BUF rats. II Induction of experimental autoimmune thyroiditis without complete Freund's adjuvent. *J.Immunol.*, 114, 148–150.

SMITH, P.F., GROSSMAN, S.J., GORDON, L.R., MACDONALD, J.S. and GERSON, R.J. (1989): Studies on the mechanism of simvastatin induced thyroid hypertrophy in the rat. *Toxicologist*, 9, 196.

SMYRK, T.C., GOELLNER, J.R., BRENNAN, M.D., CARNEY, J.A. (1987): Pathology of the thyroid in amiodarone-associated thyrotoxicosis. *Am.J.Surg.Pathol.*, 11, 197–204.

SPORN, M.B. and ROBERTS, A.B. (1983): Role of retinoids in differentiation and carcinogenesis. *Cancer Res.*, 43, 3034–3040.

STARKA, L. and MOTLIK, K. (1971): The influence of injected amino-glutethimide on the morphology of rat adrenal cortex and adrenal metabolism of progesterone. *Endocrinologie*, 58, 75–86.

STEINHOFF, D., WEBER, H., MOHR, U. and BOEHME, K. (1983): Evaluation of amitrole (aminotriazole) for potential carcinogenicity in orally dosed rats, mice and golden hamsters. *Toxicol.Appl.Pharmacol.*, 69, 161–169.

STERN, A.S., JONES, R.N., SHIVELY, J.E. et al., (1981): Two adrenal opioid polypeptides: proposed intermediates in the processing of proencephalin. *Proc.Natl.Acad.Sci.* USA. 78, 1962–1966.

STONE, J.P., HOLTZMAN, S. and SHELLABARGER, C.J. (1979): Neoplastic responses and correlated plasma prolactin levels in diethylstibestrol-treated ACI and Sprague-Dawley rats. *Cancer Res.*,39, 773–778.

STRANDBERG, J.D. (1983): Hyperplasia, adrenal medulla, rat. In: T.C. Jones, U. Mohr and R.D. Hunt (Eds), *Endocrine System*, pp. 18–22. Springer-Verlag, Berlin.

STRAUSS, F.H. (1982): The endocrine system. In: R.H. Riddell (Ed.), *Pathology of drug-induced and endocrine diseases*, Chap. 20, pp. 631–648. Churchill Livingston, New York.

STRICKLAND, J.E., SAVIOLAKIS, G.A., WEISLOW, O.S., ALLEN, P.T., HELLMAN, A. and FOWLER, A.K. (1980): Spontaneous adrenal tumors in the aged, ovariectomized NIH Swiss mouse enhanced retrovirus expression. *Cancer Res.*, 40, 3570–3575.

SUN, Y-K, XI, Y-P, FENOGLIO, C.M., PUSHPARAJ, N., O'TOOLE, K.M., KLEDIZIK, G.S., NETTE, E.G. and KING, D.W. (1984): The effect of age on the number of pituitary cells immunoreactive to growth hormone and prolactin. *Hum.Pathol.*, 15, 169–180.

SYMINGTON, T.S. (1969): The adrenal cortex. In: T.S. Symington (Ed), *The Functional Pathology of the Human Adrenal Gland*, Part II, pp. 3–216, Livingstone, Edinburgh.

TACHIBANA, M., NOGUCHI, Y. and MONRO, A.M. (1987): Toxicology of fluconazole in experimental animals. In: R.A. Fromtling (Ed.) *Recent Trends in the Discovery, Development and Evaluation of Antifungal Drugs*, pp. 93–102. J.R. Prous Science.

TAJIMA, K., MIYAGAWA, J-I, NAKAJIMA, H., SHIMIZU, M., KATAYAMA, S., MASHITA, K. and TARUI, S. (1985): Morphological and biochemical studies on minocycline-induced black thyroid in rats. *Toxicol.Appl.Pharmacol.*, 81, 393–400.

TAKAYAMA, S., AIHARA, K., ONODERA, T. and AKIMOTO, T. (1986): Antithyroid effects of propylthiouracil and sulfamonomethoxine in rats and monkeys. *Toxicol.Appl.Pharmacol.*, 82, 191–199.

TAMAOKI, B.I. (1973): Steroidogenesis and cell structure. Biochemical pursuit of sites of steroid synthesis. *J.Steroid Biochem.*, 4, 89–118.

TARONE, R.E., CHU, K.C. and WARD, J.M. (1981): Variability in the rates of some naturally occurring tumors in fischer 344 rats and CC57BL/6N × C3H/HeN)F1 (B6C3F1) mice. *J.N.C.I.*, 66, 1175–1181.

TEMPLE, T.E. and LIDDLE, G.W. (1970): Inhibitors of adrenal steroid biosynthesis. *Ann.Rev. Pharmacol.*, 10, 199–218.

TETTENBORN, D. (1974): Toxicity of clotrimazole. *Postgrad. Med.J.*, Suppl. 50, 17–20.

THIELE, J. and REALE, E. (1976): Freeze-fracture study of the junctional complexes of human and rabbit thyroid follicles. *Cell Tissue Res.*, 168, 133–140.

TISCHLER, A.S., DELELLIS, R.A., PERLMAN, R.L., ALLEN, J.M., COSTOPOULOS, D., LEE, Y.C., NUNNEMACHER, G., WOLFE, H.J. and BLOOM, S.R. (1985): Spontaneous proliferative lesions of the adrenal medulla in aging Long-Evans rats. Comparison to PC12 cells, small granule-containing cells, and human adrenal medullary hyperplasia. *Lab.Invest.*, 53, 486–498.

TISCHLER, A.S. and DELELLIS, R.A. (1988)a: The rat adrenal medulla. I. The normal adrenal. *J.Am.Coll.Toxicol.*, 7, 1–19.

TISCHLER, A.S. and DELELLIS, R.A. (1988)b: The rat adrenal medulla. II. Proliferative lesions. *J.Am.Coll.Toxicol.*, 7, 23–41.

TIXIER-VIDAL, A., TOUGARD, C., KERDELHUE, B. and JUTISZ, M. (1975): Light and electron microscopic studies on immunocytochemical localization of gonadotrophic hormones in the rat pituitary gland with antisera against ovine FSH, LH, LHβ, and LHa. *Ann.NY.Acad.Sci.*, 254, 433–461.

TODD, G.C. (1986): Induction and reversibility of thyroid proliferative changes in rats given an antithyroid compound. *Vet.Pathol.*, 23, 110–117.

TREIP, C.S. (1983): The regression of oestradiol-induced pituitary tumours in the rat. *J.Pathol.* 141, 29–40.

TUCKER, W.E. (1962): Thyroiditis in a group of laboratory dogs. *Am.J.Clin. Pathol.*, 38, 70–74.

TUCKER, M.J. (1979): The effect of long-term food restriction on tumours in rodents. *Int.J.Cancer*, 23, 803–807.

VAN PUTTEN, L.J.A., VAN ZWIETEN, M.J., MATTHEIJ, J.A.M. and VAN KEMENADE, J.A.M. (1988): Studies on prolactin-secretory cells in aging rats of different strains. I. Alterations in pituitary histology and serum prolactin levels as related to aging. *Mech.Ageing.Dev.*, 42, 75–90.

VAN ZWEITEN, M.J., FRITH, C.H., NOOTEBOOM, A.L., WOLFE, H.J. and DELELLIS, R.A. (1983): Medullary thyroid carcinoma in female BALB/c mice. A report of 3 cases with ultra-structural immunohistochemical and transplantation data. *Am.J.Pathol.*, 110, 219–229.

VAUDRY, H., TONON, M.C., DELARUE, R., VAILLANT, R. and KRAICER, J. (1978): Biological and radioimmunological evidence for melanocyte stimulating hormones (MSH) of extrapituitary origin in the rat brain. *Neuroendocrinology*, 27, 9–24.

VINSON, G.P., WHITEHOUSE, B.J., BATEMAN, A., HRUBY, V.J., SAWYER, T.K. and DARMAN, P.S. (1984): α-MSH analogues and adrenal zona glomerulosa function. *Life Sci.*, 35, 603–610.

WARD, J.M. and REZNIK-SCHÜLLER, H. (1980): Morphological and histochemical characteristics of pigments in aging F344 rats. *Vet.Pathol.*, 17, 678–685.

WARREN, S., GROZDEV, L., GATES, O. and CHUTE, R.N. (1966): Radiation-induced adrenal medullary tumors in the rat. *Arch.Pathol.*, 82, 115–118.

WEXLER, B.C. (1964): Correlation of adrenocortical histopathology with arteriosclerosis in breeder rats. *Acta. Endocrinol.*, 46, 613–631.

WHITE, S.W. and BESANCENEY, C. (1983): Systemic pigmentation from tetra-cycline and minocycline therapy. *Arch.Dermatol.*, 119, 1–2.

WIKLUND, J., WERTZ, N. and GORSKI, J. (1981): A comparison of oestrogen effects on uterine and pituitary growth and prolactin synthesis in F334 and Holtzman rats. *Endocrinology*, 109, 1700–1707.

WILSON, J.D. and FOSTER, D.W. (1985): Hormones and hormone action. In: *Williams Textbook of Endocrinology*, 7th Edition, Section 1, pp. 1–8. W.B. Saunders, Philadelphia.

WOLFE, H.J., DELELLIS, R.A., JACKSON, C.E., GREENWALD, K.A., BLOCK, M.A. and TASHJIAN, A.H. (1980): Immunocytochemical distinction of hereditary from sporadic medullary carcinoma. *Lab.Invest.*, 42, 111.

WONG, C.C., DÖHLER, K-D., ATKINSON, M.J., GEERLINGS, H., HESCH, R-D. and VON ZUR MÜHLEN, A. (1983)a: Circannual variations in serum concentrations of pituitary, thyroid, parathyroid, gonadal and adrenal hormones in male laboratory rats. *J.Endocrinol.*, 97, 179–185.

WONG, C.C., DÖHLER, K-D., GERRLINGS, H. and VON ZUR MÜHLEN, A. (1983)b: Influence of age, strain, and season on circadian periodicitiy of pituitary, gonadal and adrenal hormones in the serum of male laboratory animals. *Horm.Res.*, 17, 202–215.

WYNFORD-THOMAS, D., STRINGER, B.J.M. and WILLIAMS, E.D. (1982): Dissociation of growth and function in the rat thyroid during prolonged goitrogen administration. *Acta.Endocrinol.*, 101, 210–216.

WYNFORD-THOMAS, V., WYNFORD-THOMAS, D. and WILLIAMS, E.D. (1983): Experi mental induction of parathyroid adenomas in the rat. *J.N.C.I.*, 70, 127–134.

YANAGISAWA, M., HARA, Y., SATOH, K., TANIKAWA, T., SAKATSUME, Y., KATAYAMA, S., KAWAZU, S., ISHII, J. and KOMEDA, K. (1986): Spontaneous autoimmune thyroiditis in Bio Breeding/Worcester (BB/W) rats. *Endocrinol.Jpn.*, 33, 851–861.

YARRINGTON, J.T. (1983): Chemically induced adrenal lesions. In: T.C. Jones, U. Mohr and R.D. Hunt (Eds), *Endocrine System, Monograph on Pathology of Laboratory Animals*, pp. 69–75. Springer-Verlag, Berlin.

YOSHIMURA, F. and NOGAMI, H. (1981): Fine structural criteria for identifying rat corticotrophs. *Cell Tissue Res.*, 219, 221–228.

YOSHIMURA, F., NOGAMI, H. and YASHIRO, T. (1982)a: Comparative-immunohistochemical study of the mammalian pituitary corticotrophs. *Okajimas Folia.Anat.Jpn.*, 56, 709–728.

YOSHIMURA, F., NOGAMI, H. and YASHIRO, T. (1982)b: Fine structural criteria for pituitary thyrotrophs in immature and mature rats. *Anat. Rec.*, 204, 255–263.

YOSHIMASA, T., NAKAO, K., OHTSUKI, H. et al., (1982): Methionine-enkephalin and leucine-enkephalin in human sympathoadrenal system and pheochromocytoma. *J.Clin.Invest.*, 69, 643–650.

ZAK, F. (1983)a: Lipid hyperplasia, adrenal cortex rat. In: T.C. Jones, U. Mohr and R.D. Hunt (Eds), *Endocrine System*, pp. 80–84. Springer-Verlag, Berlin.

ZAK, F. (1983)b: Nodular cortical hyperplasia, adrenal thymectomized mouse. In: T.C. Jones, U. Mohr and R.D. Hunts (Eds), *Endocrine System*, pp. 75–80. Springer-Verlag, Berlin.

ZAK, M., KOVAKS, K., McCOMB, D.J. and HEITZ, P.U. (1985): Amino-glutethimide-stimulated corticotrophs. An immunocytologic, ultrastructural and immunoelectron microscopic study of the rat adenohypophysis. *Virchows Arch.[B].*, 49, 93–106.

ZARRIN, K. and HÄNICHEN, T. (1974): Comparative histopathological study of the canine thyroid gland in London and Munich. *J.Small Anim.Pract.*, 15, 329–342.

ZBINDEN, G. (1988): Hyperplastic and neoplastic responses of the thyroid gland in toxicological studies. *Arch. Toxicol.*, Suppl. 12, 98–106.

ZEYTINOGLU, F.N., GAGEL, R.F., DELELLIS, R.A., WOLFE, H.J., TASHJIAN, A.H., HAMMER, R.A. and LEEMAN, S.E. (1983): Clonal strains of rat medullary thyroid carcinoma cells that produce neurotensin and calcitonin. Functional and morphological studies. *Lab.Invest.*, 49, 453–459.

ZEYTINOGLU, F.N., GAGEL, R.F., DELELLIS, R.A., WOLFE, H.J., TASHJIAN, A.H., HAMMER, R.A. and LEEMAN, S.E. (1983): Clonal strains of rat medullary thyroid carcinoma cells that produce neurotensin and calcitonin. Functional and morphological studies. *Lab.Invest.*, 49, 453–459.

XIII. Nervous System and Special Sense Organs

The complexity of neurotoxicological assessment has been lucidly described by Mailman (1987) who has suggested that the number of potential molecular and biochemical targets for the neurotoxic effects of xenobiotics is so large that there is little likelihood that a single test or test battery will effectively screen all neurotoxicants. To a certain extent, this is reflected in the histopathological assessment of the nervous system, particularly if insufficient attention is given to fixation, tissue sampling, sectioning and staining procedures. For this reason, it is important to employ a comprehensive approach to neuropathological assessment. The pathologist needs to consider structure-activity relationships, pharmacological activity and disposition of the test compound, notably its degree of penetration through the blood-brain or blood-nerve barrier. He or she should also attempt to relate these data to clinical observations in the in-life phase of toxicity studies. Following these considerations, he is far better placed to appropriately focus his histopathological examination with the judicious application of special fixation, embedding and staining methods to the appropriate parts of the nervous system.

It should not be forgotten that the nervous system interacts in a complex way with other body systems and that neurotoxic effects may be manifest by alterations in other organs. For instance, damage to the trigeminal ganglion may be associated with corneal ulceration. Spermatic granulomas in the epididymis may follow drug-induced effects on the non-adrenergic neurones supplying the vas deferens (see Male Reproductive System, Chapter X).

Conversely, drug-induced changes in peripheral organs, experimental or environmental factors may produce secondary effects in the nervous system, frequently mediated through the hypothalamus. Damage to the testis or adrenal glands can alter the hypothalmamic-hypophyseal axis with subsequent repercussions on animal behaviour (Bondy, 1985). Neuroendocrine and immune systems have also been shown to be involved in bidirectional communication. Cells of the immune system both produce biologically active peptides and possess receptors for hormones (Weigent and Blalock, 1987). Although our understanding of these multisystem interactions is far from complete, there is clearly considerable capacity for multisystem interaction in the whole animal following administration of high doses of potent therapeutic agents.

Clinical and behavioural assessment

An important part of toxicological assessment of the central and peripheral nervous system is good clinical observation during the in-life phase of safety studies. Whilst laboratory animal housing conditions are not always conducive to critical neurological assessment, well-trained and experienced veterinary and technical staff can frequently achieve a high degree of expertise in the detection of changes in animal comportment, posture, gait, coordination, muscle tone and behavioural patterns in the daily routine. Added to this are alterations in feeding patterns, loss of appetite, emesis, vomiting and other more general changes which may be effects of alterations in the functioning of the autonomic nervous system.

Alder and collegues (1986) have shown how a systematized approach to general clinical observation using a check list approach for recording of general behavioural and physical signs in the conventionally housed rat can provide a considerable degree of sensitivity in the detection of changes induced by psychotherapeutic drugs. The key to this approach is possessing systems whereby such voluminous data can be effectively recorded, organised and analysed in a coherent manner.

Naturally, the nature of the housing and husbandry conditions are of particular importance in the critical assessment of neurological or behavioural changes. For instance, careful observation of beagle dogs in large runs clearly has greater potential for detection of change than when animals are housed in cages where natural movement is restricted.

The place of special neurobehavioural tests in routine toxicological assessment of potential therapeutic agents is less clear. Whereas these tests may represent more precise probes of animal behaviour, they do not represent completely validated methods for the prediction of specific effects in man. For this reason, they may provide little additional predictive information that cannot be obtained by careful, general clinical assessment of treated animals followed by detailed histopathological study in the context of the pharmacological and dispositional data of the test drug. Nevertheless, these special studies, sometimes referred to as second tier tests, may have a place in the characterization of effects initially detected in more conventional studies (Reiter, 1987). Indeed, they have to a certain extent become embodied in some regulatory guidelines, particularly those referring to environmental or industrial chemicals for which little other pharmacological or dispositional data may exist.

Histopathological assessment

It is generally believed that neurotoxic effects are characterized by morphological changes in the nervous system and that pharmacodynamic effects are not

757

manifest by pathological alterations in nervous tissue. Whereas this is a useful concept, the borderline between pharmacological and toxicological effects is not sharp, particularly when potent pharmacological agents are administered at high doses. A further difficulty relates to the detail and quality of the neuropathological examination.

This difficulty is accentuated by the concept that neuropathology is considered to be a separate branch of pathology requiring a more detailed understanding of the anatomy and physiology of the nervous system and knowledge of special histological techniques than usually possessed by general histopathologists.

Regulatory concerns about the quality of neuropathological assessment in the context of toxicity studies is highlighted by the very detailed guidelines published by the Environmental Protection Agency (1985) concerning fixation, sampling, dehydration, embedding, sectioning, staining and assessment of brain, spinal cord, ganglia and nerves in experimental neurotoxicity studies.

In routine toxicity studies, most laboratories employ immersion fixation of the brain, spinal cord and nerves in conventional fixatives followed by paraffin wax embedding and preparation of haematoxylin and eosin stained sections.

This appears to be acceptable as a screening procedure provided its limitations are recognized and special techniques are employed in appropriate situations. Artefacts produced by immersion fixation of rodents brains in toxicity studies have been reviewed by Garman (1990).

Krinke (1988) has made the valid point that the only credible approach for establishing a no-effect dose level when there are pathological changes in the central nervous system is histopathological examination following optimum perfusion fixation of the brain. Likewise, Spencer and collegues (1980) have demonstrated the superiority of special fixation techniques, resin embedding and semithin sections in the characterization of neurological lesions in experimental toxicity studies, especially in the study of the temporal development of cellular changes and location of the primary site of cell damage.

Whether conventional or special histological techniques are employed, the extent and nature of the sampling and sectioning of a complex organ such as the brain and spinal cord is of paramount importance. It should be sufficiently extensive to include grey and white matter from the cerebrum, cerebellum, brain stem, spinal cord, spinal ganglia and peripheral nerves, paying particular attention to those areas which may be preferentially affected by xenobiotics. Key areas include the basal ganglia, substantia nigra, dentate nucleus, Purkinji cells and optic tracts. Despite the relative impermeability of the blood-brain barrier to many molecules, it is also important to consider those regions located principally around the third and fourth venticles which are supplied by blood vessels with fenestrated endothelium allowing a more rapid and extensive exchange of plasma filtrate. These regions are frequently those which contain hormone-producing cells or hormone receptors or have other functions requiring more direct contact with circulating substances. They include the neurohypophysis, median eminence, pineal, area postrema, organum vasculosum of the lamina terminalis, subfornical and subcommisural organs as well as the choroid plexus (Jacobs, 1980). The choroid plexus is of special interest to general pathologists as it is frequently a target for systemic disorders including those of autoimmune type and those produced by xenobiotics and it can be a pathway by which toxic substances reach the brain substance (Levine, 1987).

Producing histological sections consistently from precise parts of the brain represents a difficult task, particularly from the small rodent brain. For this reason a metal template or matrix for slicing blocks can be helpful in producing consistent sections. Standard sections produced in this way can be important in the assessment of specific brain structures, particularly when use is made a stereotoxic atlas for the brain anatomy of animal species (reviewed by Palkovits, 1983).

Reference sections or photographs of sections obtained from a group of male and female control animals can also be useful for the general pathologist when assessing brain sections in toxicity studies (Krueger, 1971).

Immunohistochemical, cytochemical and ultrastructural techniques

The complexity and heterogeneity of the nervous system lends itself well to immunohistochemical study. Immunocytochemical localisation of neurotransmitters, receptor proteins in combination with anterograde tracing with the labelled lectin, Phaseolus vulgaris (PHA), represent powerful techniques in the demonstration of connections, transmitters and receptors in neuroanatomy (reviewed by Luiten et al., 1988). These methods possess potential in the characterization of the effects of xenobiotics on the nervous system. Some of this potential has been demonstrated in the immunohistochemical characterization of the effects of glutamate on releasing hormones in the hypothalamus and median eminence of the rat brain.

Monosodium glutamate has been shown to selectively destroy neurons of the arcuate nucleus in the hypothalamus (see below). The arcuate nucleus is the main source of growth hormone releasing factor (GRF) in the both the rat, non-human, primates and man. The neurone bodies in the arcuate nucleus can be demonstrated immunocytochemically using antisera to GRF, although in both rats and non-human primates, pretreatment with colchicine may be necessary to increase peptide content in cell bodies (Bloch et al., 1983, 1984) to improve their immunostaining. However, immunocytochemical staining of GRF is able to demonstrate the presence of GRF-immunoreactive nerve fibres which project to the median eminence to end in contact with portal vessels without colchicine pretreatment. In rats tested with monosodium glutamate, Bloch and collegues (1984) were able to demonstrate loss of GRF immune reactive fibres in the median eminence whilst the distribution of axons containing corticotrophin-releasing factor and luteinizing hormone-releasing factor was identical to those in untreated controls (Fig. 132).

Bloch (1985) has also demonstrated how in-situ hybridization methodology

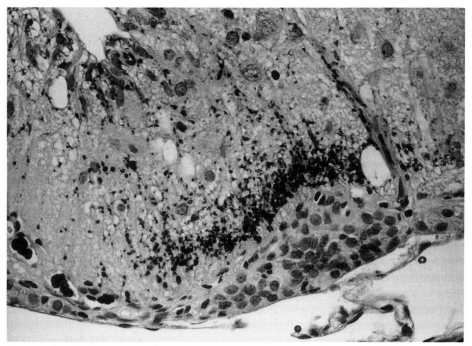

Fig. 132. Section of median eminence from a normal Wistar rat stained immunocytochemically for gonadotrophin releasing hormone (LHRH). (Formalin fixed, immunoperoxidase, ×400.)

detecting messenger RNA can be used to identify and localize cell populations producing neuropeptides in brain tissue sections fixed in formalin.

The widely distributed cytochromes P450 are also present in the brain where they are involved in both the metabolism of endogenous steroids and xenobiotics. They have also been demonstrated in sections in both neurones and glial cells of the rat brain using immunocytochemical staining (Köhler et al., 1988). Of particular interest is the demonstration of induction of cytochrome P-450 in the mouse brain following phenytoin administration (Volk et al., 1988). Specific cytochrome P450 enzymes involved in steroid synthesis have also been demonstrated immunocytochemically in rat brain as well as in adrenal cortex (Le Goascogue et al., 1987).

Another important antigen in the central nervous system is glial *fibrillary acidic protein* (GFA). This protein possesses a molecular weight of about 48,000 daltons and was originally isolated by aqueous extraction from old, fibril-rich plaques from human brain tissue altered by multiple sclerosis. The protein was subsequently purified by ammonium sulphate and isoelectric precipitation and polyacrylamide gel electrophoresis. Immunocytochemistry using antisera to GFA can detect glial cells in paraffin wax embedded brain sections and represents a powerful staining method for the study of normal and pathologically altered glial cells in the pathology of human tissues (Rubinstein, 1982). This protein has been

760

shown to be similarly distributed in adult rat brain (Ludwin et al., 1978) and in rat peripheral nervous tissue (Nada and Kawana, 1988).

The *S100 protein* in glial cells and Schwann cells in the nervous tissue of man and laboratory animals and although not specific for these cells, may be helpful in tumour diagnosis (Kahn et al., 1983; Van Eldik et al., 1986; Gough et al., 1986).

An isoenzyme of *enolase*, (2-phospho-D-glycerate hydrolase), an enzyme which catalyzes the interconversion of 2-phosphoglycerate and phosphoenolpyruvate in the glycolytic pathway, is found in large quantities in neurones (Schmechel, 1985). Although the neurone specific γ-subunit has been demonstrated in non-neural cells, its high level of expression in normal neurons has enabled its use as a neurone-specific marker.

Monoclonal antibodies against macrophage determinants can delineate microglial and other macrophage populations in the brain (Jordan and Thomas, 1988). Likewise, antisera against B and T lymphocytes as well as labelled lectins can also be used in the study of the immune system in the nervous system.

Indeed, the potential of immunocytochemical techniques in the study of neurotoxicity is so great in routinely fixed materials, that it is more logical to develop these techniques than spend undue effort in developing some of the more capricious classical neuropathological staining techniques.

Quantitive enzyme cytochemistry, although less widely used, also has potential for the study of enzymatic alterations in the structurally heterogenous tissue of the nervous system (Kugler, 1988).

As in the study of the toxicity of these organs, electronmicroscopy has an undoubted place in neurotoxicological assessment. It can permit visualization of fine structural changes as well as be combined with cytochemical or immunocytochemical techniques for a more functional analysis of drug-induced changes (Jones, 1988).

Blood-brain barrier

The presence of the blood-brain barrier is an important feature in the disposition of xenobiotics. Paul Ehrlich originally demonstrated over a 100 years ago that intravenously injected dyes failed to enter the brain substance even though other organs were stained. Many subsequent studies with tracers of various molecular weights have confirmed this finding. This barrier appears to be the result of the special characteristics of most endothelial cells lining cerebral vasculature, particularly their very tight cell junctions and paucity of micropinocytic vesicles and possibly their relative lack of contractile protein and inability to produce mechanical stress at tight junctions (Jacobs, 1980).

The blood-brain barrier is impermeable to most tracers such as horseradish peroxidase (molecular weight 40,000, diameter 5–6 nm), cytochrome C (molecular weight 12,000), and microperoxidase (molecular weight 2,000, diameter 2 nm). Ionic lanthanum with a hydrated diameter of 0.92 nm does not penetrate the usual capillaries in the CNS, although it does penetrate those of the choroid plexus (Bouldin and Krigman 1975). Despite this relative impermeability, it is clear that the capillary wall interface is important in the transfer of essential substances such as glucose, oxygen and essential aminoacids. Indeed, the blood brain-barrier is far more complex than the simple restriction of tracers of defined molecular weights suggest. Lipid soluble substances penetrate more freely through the lipoprotein membranes. Electrical charge may also be important.

Special transport systems are also found. These transport systems are localized on both the brain and blood side of the blood-brain barrier. Some are carrier-mediated transport systems for a number of nutrients as well as thyroid hormones. Receptor-mediated systems appear particularly important in peptide transport, notably insulin and transferrin. Although steroid hormones and free fatty acids are highly lipid soluble and are transported through the barrier by lipid mediated transport, it has been shown that these substances can be transported even when bound to proteins, a phenomenon termed plasma protein-mediated transport (See review by Pardridge, 1988).

It is important to note that the permeability of the blood-brain barrier may be altered by pathological states such as hypertension, irradiation, adminstration of hypertonic solutions and a number of xenobiotics such as those which inhibit cerebral metabolic processes (Jacobs, 1988). Clearly, any agent which has the capability to disrupt the cerebral endothelial cells has potential to affect the blood-brain barrier.

The existence of a blood-nerve barrier should also be noted because of the peripheral nerves are also protected by relatively impervious layers, the perineurium, epineurium and the intrafascicular connective tissue or endoneurium. Like blood vessels of the brain, the vasculature of the epineurium and perineurium is relatively impermeable, although perhaps the channels are somewhat larger than those in the brain.

Certain zones of the blood-nerve barrier are more permeable to some tracers, particularly dorsal root and autonomic ganglia. Fenestrated blood vessels appear to be more prominent in these zones (Jacobs, 1980).

One of these zones deserving particular mention is the area postrema, a spongiform vascular body protruding into the lumen of the fourth ventricle. This is the site of a separate chemoreceptor emetic trigger zone, sensitive to agents such as apomorphine, morphine, cardiac glycosides, nicotine and L-dopa. It may be a particular target in cancer chemotherapy-induced emesis in man (Edwards, 1988). In view of the relative permability of this zone to xenobiotics, it may also be involved in the central triggering of emesis in high-dose preclinical toxicity studies.

Recent studies with the anticancer agent, cisplatin have shown that drug-induced release of serotonin from damaged enterochromaffin cells in the intestine may be important in the induction of nausea by cytotoxic drugs. It has been shown that nausea induced by cisplatin can be prevented by administration of a selective antagonist of serotonin S3 receptors (Cubeddu et al., 1990). These receptors are located in sympathetic and parasympathetic and fibres in the enteric nervous system and their activation appears capable of triggering the vomiting centre via the vagus. Similar serotonin S3 receptors are also found in high concentrations in the area postrema-nucleus tractus solitarii region suggesting that serotonin can also mediate nausea and vomiting via a central action (Cubeddu et al., 1990).

Immune systems

Immune responses in the central nervous system are modified by its unique cellular and functional organization and the presence of the blood-brain barrier. Although the leucocytes in the cerebrospinal fluid (CSF), are derived from blood-forming tissues, they are present in different proportions to those in the peripheral circulation. The number of polymorphonuclear cells in the CSF is low compared with the peripheral blood and lymphocytes are largely of T-cell type.

The diversity of circulating and resident monocyte-macrophage cells is reflected in the central nervous system (reviewed by Jordan and Thomas, 1988). Microglial cells are the largest population of resident cells in the cortex and grey matter which are believed to be derived from monocyte precursors. Several different forms have been described, some of which bear macrophage surface markers such as Mac-1 and glycoproteins with sugar residues bound by specific lectins (Mikaye, 1984). Other intrinsic macrophages have been described in the meninges, the ventricular surface of the ependyma and in the choroid plexus. As in other tissues, blood-derived macrophages may leave the circulation and migrate to the surrounding brain when damaged occurs (Jordon and Thomas, 1988).

Immune responses in the central nervous system have been divided into two main types. There are those which can be considered a normal response to foreign antigen ending in its elimination and those which result in pathological changes, frequently involving auto-immune phenomena.

The normal response was characterized in a series of studies of experimental encephalitis in mice infected with the Sinbis virus conducted by Griffin and collegues (1987). They showed that the early response to virus replication was characterized by perivascular accumulation of mononuclear cells and increased members of mononuclear cells in the CSF. Immunocytochemistry showed that at this stage, the perivascular cuffs comprised only T-cells. As the specific immune response to virus developed, monocytes and B lymphocytes increased in number. In addition, Lyt-1 positive (helper/inducer) cells increased although the percentage of Lyt-2 (cytotoxic/suppressor) cells remained stable. Thus, it was postulated by Griffin and colleagues (1987) that T helper/inducer cells were the first to arrive at the site of virus replication in the CNS and were subsequently responsible for the production of lymphokines and chemotaxic factors needed to recruit B cells and monocytes. Although perivascular cuffing and increased numbers of CSF cells occurred at about the same time after infection, the number of cells in the CSF reached a peak at about four to five days whereas the maximum parenchymal response occurred later, between about six and ten days.

Some of the effector cells were shown also to be natural killer cells (Griffin and Hess, 1986). A similar range of changes has been reported in some forms of encephalitis occurring in man (Johnson et al., 1985, 1986).

This basic response which leads to elimination of virus could be distinguished from other forms of experimental encephalitis such as lymphocytic choriomeningitis or experimental allergic encephalitis in which myelin basic protein is the disease-inducing component. In these forms of demyelinating conditions, T lymphocytes and macrophages appear to be important cellular effector cells (Sobel et al., 1984). Lyt-1 cells appear to mediate acute allergic encephalitis in the mouse (Hauser, 1984).

Careful histological assessment and scoring of such cellular reaction to viral antigen, neuronal degeneration and loss as well as the non-specific response to cell damage, is an important component of neurovirulence testing of live poliomyelitis vaccines in cynomolgus monkeys (Boulger, 1973; Chino et al., 1984).

Species and sex differences

In the study by Fletcher (1978) in which the toxicity profiles of 45 novel therapeutic agents were compared with adverse findings in subsequent clinical studies, a reasonable degree of correlation of effects on the nervous system was recorded. However, effects such as ataxia and convulsions seen in high-dose acute experiments correlated poorly with subsequent effects in man.

Krinke (1988) has pointed out how certain anatomical and metabolic features of the rat brain have the potential to influence the predictability of neurotoxic effects for man. The rat cerebral hemispheres are devoid of gyri such that the high susceptability of the sulci of the human brain to ischaemia and hypoxia cannot be observed in studies using the rat. It has been agreed that relative insensitivity of the rat brain to methylphenyltetrahydropyridine (MPTD), a metabolite of which has a high affinity for neuromelanin, is a result of the paucity of neuromelanin in the rat substantia nigra compared with man and non-human primates (D'Amato et al., 1986).

Sex differences also occur in some brain regions both in hypothalamic and preoptic areas as well as in the cerebral cortex (Gorski et al., 1987; Diamond, 1987). In this respect the rat brain has been the most critically assessed. It has been shown that there is a different pattern of brain development between male and female Long Evans rats. In the adult male rat the right cortex is thicker than the left and in the female, the cortex is thicker on the left (Diamond, 1987). These differences appear to relate to the greater number of neurones and glia per unit area in the right cortex in male rats and in the left cortex in females. Furthermore, the hippocampal-dentate complex is thicker on the right in males and on the left in females. It has also been shown that these differences can be modulated by manipulation of sex hormones by gonadectomy, although different zones of the rat cortex are not all equally responsive to hormone levels (Diamond, 1987). Analogous differences have been reported in man but they are less well characterized.

Classification of neurotoxic lesions

Although as other organs, the nervous system is subject to malformations, inflammory, dystrophic and neoplastic disease. Toxic substances tend to produce their primary effects in one cell type. For this reason, Schaumberg and Spencer (1979) suggested that a useful way to classify neurotoxic lesions was according to the principle cellular target site, i.e. *nerve body, axon, myelin sheath, glial cell* or associated cellular structures such as *blood vessels, meninges* and *choroid plexus*. Whilst this classification undoubtably provides a logical basis for the development of concepts about mechanisms involved in particular toxicities, it should be underlined that in order to classify lesions in this way, detailed and exhaustive neuropathological study may be required. The frequent presence of secondary and tertiary changes in other cell populations can make simple descriptive terminology most appropriate, at least before more detailed investigations can be undertaken.

BRAIN

Lesions of nerve body, neuronopathies

Damaged neurones show a variety of different appearances. They may be vacuolated, swollen or shrunken or dark staining degenerate cells with indistinct Nissl substance. Related glial cells typically show reactive cytoplasmic changes and proliferate around damaged neuronal cell bodies to give rise to so called 'satellosis'. Immunocytochemical staining for glial fibrillary acidic protein is a particularly useful method for demonstrating reactive glial changes. It is important to search for evidence of reactive glial alterations for they confirm that the changes occurred during life and are not simply a result of fixation artefact or agonal factors.

Neuronal loss may occur in discrete and quite focal regions of the brain. Morphometric analysis following perfusion fixation represents a powerful tool for precisely defining the nature and distribution of neuronal cell loss in experimental toxicity studies performed with neurotoxic agents (Robertson et al., 1987).

Although a number of industrial and environmental chemicals have been shown to directly destroy neurones in the central nervous system, novel therapeutic agents which possess this property at potentially therapeutic levels are unlikely to be developed for clinical use. A striking example of this phenomenon was reported in preliminary toxicity studies performed in rhesus monkeys with a tetrahydropyridine, a cerebral dopamine agonist intended for use as a anti-pschychotic drug (Barsoum et al., 1986).

Monkeys tested for periods of up to 29 days developed clinical evidence of akinesia, rigidity, tremors and abnormal posture. Pathological examination showed a variable pattern of diffuse cortical atrophy which was most marked in occipital and parietal lobes. Histological examination of these zones showed diffuse neuronal damage or loss involving cerebral cortex as well as substantia nigra and corpus striatum. Damaged neurones showed a variety of cytological changes including swelling, cytoplasmic vacuolation, coarse eosinophilic vacuolation, loss of Nissl substance, cell shrinkage and pyknosis.

It was suggested by Barsoum and colleagues (1986) that the findings in these primates were similar to the Parkinson-like syndrome reported in man and non-human primates after administation of an illicit narcotic which contained 1-methyl-4-phenyl-1,2,3,6-tetrahydropyridine or MPTP (Davis et al., 1979; Langston and Ballard, 1983, Burns et al., 1983).

Whilst the neuronal damage induced by MPTP and other similar agents is dramatic, neuronal cell loss has been reported in laboratory animals treated with drugs active in the central nervous system and which are widely used in man. However, the significance of some of these findings for human safety still remain quite unclear.

Particularly important in the consideration of drug-induced neuronal damage is the concept of excitotoxic mechanisms proposed by Olney (1980). Based on structure-activity relationships using glutamate, aspartate and a variety of structurally similar aminoacids, Olney (1980) proposed that these and similar agents possess the potential to produce neuronal damage through their ability to cause excitation and depolarization of the nerve cell by a common species of receptor located on dendrosomal membranes. It was argued that when such agents are present in excessive concentrations in the vicinity of neuronal membranes, they induce a continuous state of depolarisation and sustained increase in plasma membrane permeability. Ultimately energy-dependent homeostatic mechanisms in the cell are overwhelmed and cell damage and death occurs (Olney, 1980). Specific groups of neurones may be preferentially involved by virtue of receptor specificity, cell sensitivity or the variable degree of penetration through the blood-brain barrier.

This concept has considerable potential importance in drug safety assessment because glutamate is a major natural excitatory transmitter in many pathways in the central nervous system and its receptors are only beginning to be more clearly characterized (Strange, 1988). Therefore, agents with glutamate-like properties or xenobiotics causing excitation of other receptor classes may have the potential to cause adverse effects in brain tissue if excessive concentrations at receptor sites are achieved.

In this context therefore, the pathological changes following administration of glutamate and similar compounds are of general interest in safety assessment. Neuronal cell damage resulting from systemically administered glutamate appears to be primarily related to the disposition of the administered compounds. Damage occurs in neurones exposed to high concentrations of the compound, notably the retina and the arcuate nucleus, the latter probably as a result of the nature of the blood brain barrier at this site. Although many studies with glutamate have been performed with young or neonatal animals, adults also develop brain damage although higher doses are usually necessary.

Early lesions are seen less than one hour after systemic administration of glutamate. In most species, there is early swelling of dendrosomes, followed by degenerative changes in the cell body. Typically, affected neurons show dense pyknotic nuclei within clear or empty cytoplasm. Axons from neurones not damaged directly by glutamate are typically unaffected, even though they may be located close to the primary site of damage, a process which has been termed an axon-sparing cytopathological reaction (Olney, 1980).

As noted previously, immunocytochemical staining of the arcuate nucleus and median eminence of rats treated with monosodium glutamate has shown quite specific loss of cells and axons containing growth hormone-relasing factor (GRF). Indeed, a considerable range of neuroendocrine changes occur following damage to the arcuate nucleus by glutamate and similar compounds. These may be shown by obesity, stunting and reproductive failure (Olney, 1980).

Clinical use of anticonvulsants and neuroleptic drugs is associated with a variety of adverse clinical signs related to the nervous system but whether these agents are the cause of structural damage to neurones or are directly responsible for neuronal loss in man is the cause of some dispute.

In man, anticonvulsant therapy may produce mental impairement, cerebellar and brain stem dysfunction including ataxia, dysarthria, nystagmus and increase in seizure frequency (Beghi et al., 1986). In animals treated with the widely used anticonvulsant drug, phenytoin, a reduction in the number of Purkinje cells in the cerebellum has been reported (Alcala et al., 1978). Likewise, degeneration of Purkinje cells has also been reported in epileptics treated with phenytoin (Ghatak et al., 1976). However, in rats treated with phenytoin, careful quantitative analysis of Purkinje cells following perfusion fixation showed a reduction in Purkinje cells only at acutely toxic doses at which severe ataxia and tremor were evident and profound decreases in firing rate of Purkinje cells were recorded by electrophysiological means. (Puro and Woodward, 1973).

Chronic treatment with gradually increasing doses to reach a high dose without overt cerebellar signs produced no microscopic evidence of cerebellar injury (Puro and Woodward, 1973). These finding suggested that damage to the Purkinje cells were a non-specific, high dose effect only. In an analogous way, cerebellar degeneration in epileptics can be correlated with the number of repeated seizures and it has been suggested that the loss of Punkinje cells results not from phenytoin therapy itself but from hypoxia or other form of damage due to seizures (Dam, 1982). This hypothesis is fully consistent with the concept that abnormal nerve cell firing leads to excessive metabolic demand which cannot be supported by the normal compensatory increases in blood flow so that neuronal cell damage occurs (Salcman et al., 1978).

A similar situation applies to other classes of therapeutic agents, especially the major tranquillizers such as phenothiazines, thioxanthenes and butyrophenones. Although these drugs have been of major benefit in the treatment of psychiatric disease, their clinical use is associated with a number of side effects in the nervous system. Several clinical forms of these adverse effects are described, notably drug-induced Parkinsonism, akathisia, acute dystonic reactions and a more serious chronic tardive dyskinesia (Marsden and Jenner, 1980). Although each of these syndromes may possess a different pathogenesis, they all appear to involve disturbance of the central dopaminergic system.

Some of the clinical side effects can be reproduced in laboratory animals and these experimental models have been used in the study of mechanisms responsible the side effects in man (Marsden and Jenner, 1980). Although some animal studies have suggested that neuronal cell loss can occur in the corpus striatum as a result of long-term treatment with these agents (Pakkenberg et al., 1973, Nielson and Lyon, 1978), post-mortem studies of the brain in patients have produced no clear evidence of a direct drug-induced neuronal cell loss which could not be explained by the disease progression or normal aging (Jellinger, 1977).

This debate about possible structural damage induced by these widely used and clinically important drugs for which there is a large amount of experience, underlines the potential difficulties faced in the risk assessment when nervous system effects are produced in animals by entirely novel drugs for which no human data exists.

Peripheral neurones

Some agents selectively damage nerve cells situated outside the blood brain barrier, presumably because of the relative permeability of blood vessels around the ganglia. For instance, doxorubicin can produce alterations in the dorsal root and Gasserian ganglia and sympathetic neurones when given in high doses to laboratory animals, although not apparently in man (Cho, 1977; Cho et al., 1980). Treatment produces an initial pallor of the nuclei, loss of chromatin and eventually loss of Nissl substance, increased numbers of neurofilaments, cytoplasmic vacuolation and finally neuronal cell loss with Wallerian degeneration of sensory neurones in the spinal dorsal roots, posterior columns and peripheral nerves. The reason for the interspecies differences is unclear.

Phospholipidosis

Cationic amphiphilic drugs, notably chloroquine, tricyclic antidepressants, chlorphentermine and tamoxifen may produce the accumulation of phospholipids or polar lipids in the lysosomes of neural cells within the cerebrum, cerebellum, spinal cord, dorsal root ganglia, neurosecretory cells of the hypothalamus and retinal ganglion cells (Lüllmann et al., 1975; Lüllmann-Rauch, 1979; Lüllman and Lüllmann-Rauch, 1981). Morphologically, these inclusions are similar to those occurring in phospholipidosis in other organs. They are characterized by the presence of numerous crystalloid or lamellar inclusions in the cytoplasma of the cell bodies (perikarya) of the neurones. Chloroquine, unlike most other agents producing phospholipidosis, induces only lamellated forms. As in other cell types, these inclusions are difficult to visualize in routine haematoxylin and eosin stained sections but can be seen under the light microscope in semi-thin, toluidine blue-stained sections and at ultrastructural level.

An additional feature of nerve cells affected by phospholipidosis, is the accumulation of polymorphic, dense autophagic inclusions in axons and axon terminals (Lüllman-Rauch, 1979). This accumulation of autophagic vacuoles can be massive, particularly in neurosecretory cells where the membrane-limited inclusions contain recognizable structures including mitochondria and neurosecretory granules. However, the lamellated or crystalloid structures observed in the neural cell bodies are usually absent from these axonal inclusions. Lüllmann-Rauch (1979) has suggested that the large number of autophagic vacuoles in axons may be the result of the reduction in supply of functional lysosomal hydrolytic enzymes to the axon as a result of the phospholipidosis in the nerve cell bodies. The function implications of these changes in the neurons has not been well studied, although some of these drugs are reported to cause neurological changes associated with demyelinisation in man. However, the relationship between phospholipidosis and neuropathy remains uncertain (Lüllmann-Rauch, 1979).

Vacuolation

Vacuoles appear in histological sections of neural tissue for a number of quite different reasons and it is important that when they are found within the context of toxicity studies that they are adequately characterized. Although vacuolation can affect neuronal cell bodies and glial cells, vacuoles typically occur in white matter of the brain and myelinated peripheral nerves as a result of alterations to myelin. However, it should be noted that conventionally prepared paraffin embedded sections of brain from most laboratory animal species including rodents, dogs and non-human primates, may show numerous moderately-sized round vacuoles in white matter which may contain amorphous eosinophilic or basophilic material (Garman, 1990). These changes are probably artefacts but their precise mode of development is unclear. Their presence may be disconcerting in the histological assessment of the brains from animals treated with drugs with activity on the nervous system for although they are typically found in untreated control animals, individual variation in numbers of vacuoles and group differences may be quite marked for no clear reason.

Vacuolar encephalopathy, vacuolar degeneration of aged rats and mice

Vacuolation of the cerebral white matter without any cellular reaction is a notable spontaneous change in aged rats although its precise cause is unknown. It has been suggested that prevalence of vacuoles can be increased in a quite non-specific ways by chronic administration of a variety of different xenobiotics (Gopinath et al., 1987)

Increasing numbers of vacuoles may be also seen in the major fibre tracts of the brains of mice with advancing age. In B6C3F1 hybrids, vacuoles were found most commonly in the corpus callosum, tapetum, hippocampal fimbria and fornix, optic tract, optic nerve and the cingulum (Sheldon, 1990). Their onset can be delayed by food restriction.

Drug-induced vacuolation: myelin

A number of quite unrelated therapeutic agents have been reported to produce vacuolation of the white matter or peripheral nerve sheaths in laboratory animals. Among these are drugs in widespread clinical use, some of which have been associated with neurological side effects in man. The variable distribution and time course of development of these vacuoles, interspecies and dosage differences make the risk assessment for man a complex issue. This is illustrated by a number of examples.

Vacuolation of the white matter and peripheral nerves have been reported in several species of laboratory animals following systemic administration of high doses of hexachlorophene, an agent used as an antimicrobial in soaps, cosmetics and therapeutic products. Its effects have been best studied in the rat which shows increase in brain weight associated with diffuse vacuolation of the cerebral white matter and peripheral nerves when high blood levels of hexachlorophene are achieved by oral, parenteral or topical administration (Towfighi et al., 1974; Towfighi 1980). Semi-thin sections and ultrastructural study have shown that these vacuoles are the results of intramyelinic oedema which produces separation of the intraperiod lines of myelin lamellae. Although these changes appear to be largely reversible, high exposure to hexachlorophene may result axonal degeneration in cerebral white matter and optic nerves. Similar changes are evident in peripheral nerves and nerve roots. The mechanism is obscure but it is of note that similar findings have been reported in both children and adults when high tissue levels of hexachlorophene are achieved (Towfighi, 1980).

More recently, focal, reversible vacuolation of white matter was reported in Sprague-Dawley and pigmented Lister-Hooded rats treated for 90 days with high dose of vigabatrin (γ-vinyl GABA), an enzyme-activated, irreversible inhibitor of GABA transaminase (Butler et al., 1987). This agent is indicated for the treatment of epilepsy not well controlled by other drugs.

Treated rats showed reduced body weight gain and some animals developed convulsions towards the end of the study. Simple vacuoles associated with local oedema were described in the white matter of the cerebellum, particularly near the roof nuclei but also in the cerebellar folia, pons, thalamic tract, internal capsule, optic tracts and white matter of the hippocampus. Myelin stains showed no evidence of demyelination but ultrastructural study revealed separation of the outer laminae of the myelin sheath along the interperiod line. These changes were associated with disorganization of the outer nuclear layer of the retina of Sprague-Dawley but not Lister-Hood rats.

Heywood and colleagues (1978) showed acute focal vacuolation of the medulla oblongata in rhesus monkeys treated with a novel antifertility agent, 1-amino-3-

chloro-2-propanol. Clinically, animals developed mild periods of incoordination and loss of balance but histological examination showed vacuolation with oedema, moderate glial proliferation the presence of myelin-laden macrophages and early nerve fibre degeneration in focal zones in the medulla.

Another drug which produces vacuolation of the white matter in laboratory animals is the antituberculous drug isoniazid (Cavanagh, 1967; Blakemore et al., 1972; Blakemore 1980). This agent appears to produce a primary effect on the axon in man. Nevertheless, the findings in animals treated with isoniazid serve to illustrate the interspecies differences in susceptability which can occur in nervous system toxicity.

The major pathway for the metabolism of isoniazid in man is by acetylation, the main enzyme being N-acetyltransferase present in the soluble fraction of hepatocytes. Slow acetylators of isoniazid tend to develop a peripheral neuropathy which can be ameliorated or prevented by administration of pyridoxine. Convulsions, visual disturbances, muscle twitching, dizzyness, ataxia euphoria and stupor are also occasionally reported in man. Principle pathological alterations reported in clinically affected patients are largely limited to a Wallerian-type degeneration of both myelinated and unmyelinated peripheral motor nerves associated with a denervation type atrophy of skeletal muscle.

The rat is relatively insensitive to the toxicity of isoniazid but high doses produce a dose-dependent peripheral neuropathy similar to that reported in man. This is an axonal degeneration most marked in the distal segment of both motor and sensory nerves although motor nerves are most affected. Regenerative changes are also observed if treatment continues. Histologically, changes in nerves are characterized by multifocal periaxonal vacuolation with subsequent axonal degeneration similar to that seen in Wallerian degeneration and chromatolysis of ventral motor neurones (Blakemore, 1980).

The dog is more sensitive to isoniazid and it has been suggested that this is due to a failure to acetylate isoniazid because of an absence of appropriate enzymes in this species. However, in the dog there is extensive vacuolation of white matter and to some extent in grey matter when high acute or modest subchronic doses are administered (Blakemore, 1980). The vacuolation is most marked in the thalamus, mid-brain, medulla and cerebellum with the subcortical and hippocampal white matter being also affected in sub-chronic studies. Vacuoles were shown to be a result of separation of the intraperiod lines of the myelin sheaths associated with changes in oligodendrocytes, notably cellular swelling and nuclear pyknosis. Astroglial hypertrophy also occurs after prolonged dosing. In the dog, the principle cell affected appears to be the oligodendrocyte, although unlike the changes in the rat they appear to be prevented or reversed by pyridoxine or nicotinamide administration. Blakemore (1980) has suggested that the oligodendrocyte changes do not represent a specific cellular toxicity but rather imply a drug-induced requirement for increased oligodendrocyte metabolism. The difference between isoniazid-induced changes in dog and rat are striking but all findings possess certain elements common to findings in man.

Perivascular vacuolation of the cerebral cortex and white matter associated with shrunken, degenerate and acidophilic nerve cell bodies has been shown to occur in rats following carotid artery infusions of hyperosmolar solutions of mannitol or urea (Salahuddin et al., 1988). These authors showed that under these circumstances, extravasation of albumin occurred, suggesting tht hyperosmolar solutions can cause significant opening of the blood-brain barrier with subsequent risk to brain damage from injected solutions.

Demyelination

An example of primary drug-induced demyelinization is that which occurred in dogs following intravenous infusion of the antifungal agent amphotericin B methyl ester for periods of up to 12 weeks (Ellis et al., 1988). Treatment was associated with severe clinical signs after completing the course of amphotericin B but at autopsy the brains showed no macroscopic abnormality. By contrast, histological examination showed widespread loss of myelin, most marked in subcortical cerebral white matter, especially in centrum ovale and frontal lobes as well as in periventricular white matter, corpus callosum, white matter of the cerebellum and brain stem. This was most clearly demonstrated in sections stained for myelin. Although no actual vacuolation of white matter was described by these authors, other cellular changes indicating myelin damage were noted including decrease in the number of oligodendrocytes and the presence of reactive astrocytes with gemistocytic cytoplasm and bulbous cytoplasmic bodies. Sudanophilic debris was seen in the interstitium. Plump, perivascular macrophages laden with sudanophilic lipid scattered in the white matter were prominant.

Phosphotungstic acid haematoxylin (PTAH) and GFAP stains revealed a fine network of glail fibres in affected zones and Bodian's stain showed scattered, swollen or fragmented axons. Some endothelial proliferation was noted in severely affected areas.

Although the mechanism for the development of the demyelination remains unclear, it may be related to the property of amphotericin B and related polyene macrolides to alter cell membranes by interacting with membrane sterols to disrupt myelin membrane permeability (Ellis et al., 1988).

Similar clinicopathological findings have been reported in patients treated with high intravenous doses of amphotericin B methyl ester. Indeed, the similarity of findings in man and animals under analogous regimens underlines the need for careful consideration of the route and period of dosing as well as the levels of tissue exposure to drug in the design of toxicity studies. Shorter term studies with amphotericin B methyl ester showed none of these pathological changes in the nervous system.

Axonal lesions

Primary damage to the distal segments of axons appears to be one of the most common forms of adverse drug reaction involving the nervous system. A large number of different drugs have been reported to cause a pure sensory or mixed sensorimotor neuropathy (Argov and Mastaglia, 1979). These drugs include antimicrobials such as isoniazid, ethambutol, ethionamide, nitrofurantoin and metronidazole, antineoplastic drugs especially vinca alkaloids, cardiovascular agents perhexiline and hydrallazine, hypnotics, psychotropics and anticonvulsants as well as antirheumatic gold salts and indomethacin (Argov and Mastaglia, 1979; Schaumburg and Spencer, 1979). Some authors have found that damage to axons is also more common in routine experimental toxicity testing than other forms of neuronal damage (Gopinath et al., 1987).

Morphologically, silver impregnation techniques such as Bodian's stain show disruption and fragmentation of axons with focal increases in argyrophilia. Axonal degeneration is usually accompanied by secondary demyelination when myelinated axons are involved, characterized by the presence of myelin spheroids and lipid or myelin-laden macrophages.

Of particular interest in drug safety assessment is the distal axonal degeneration limited to the central nervous system of dogs treated with high doses of clioquinol (5-chloro-7-iodo-8-hydroxyquinoline). This agent was originally produced as a topical antiseptic but found widespread use as an oral antiparasitic agent where it was associated with toxic encephalopathy and subacute myelo-optico-neuropathy in Japan. In the latter syndrome, there was degeneration of axons and secondary changes in myelin in the distal gracilis fasciculus and corticospinal tracts (Schaumberg and Spencer, 1980).

The toxicity of clioquinol has been extensively investigated in the dog where toxicological manifestations depend less on actual dose than the degree of absorption and exposure levels achieved. High blood levels can be better achieved in fed rather than fasted animals. Histological changes have been characterized in dogs given high doses of clioquinol for 25 weeks (Schaumburg et al., 1978; Worden et al., 1978). Changes included axonal swelling and degeneration, disruption of myelin with aggregation of myelin-laden macrophages and some astrocyte activation in dorsal ventromedial and lateral columns of the spinal cord and in the optical nerve but not in peripheral nerves, spinal and autonomic ganglia. These pathological changes were associated with evidence of a motor deficit as well as pallor of the optic papilla and sluggish pupillary light reflexes. The pathological changes in these dogs resembled those reported in the man treated with clioquinol, but their precise pathogenesis remains uncertain.

Vascular lesions

Generalized vascular pathology may also involve cerebral vessels, although, as in the case of spontaneous arteritis of the beagle dog, meningeal arteries are those which appear more predisposed to systemic conditions.

Vessels of the choroid plexus are also more predisposed to changes which involve the systemic circulation by virtue of their similarity in structure and function to those in the glomeruli. However, most xenobiotics appear to act on the choroid epithelium rather than its blood vessels and stroma (Levine, 1987).

However, by virtue of the unique structural features of the cerebral blood vessels, they may be involved in disease processes or drug-induced disorders which spare the systemic circulation. A recent example of this phenomenon was reported in beagle dogs treated with high doses of the cholesterol-lowering drug, lovastatin, a competitive inhibitor of the rate limiting enzyme of cholesterol synthesis, 3-hydroxy-3-methylglutaryl coenzyme A (HMG CoA) reductase (Berry et al., 1988).

In these studies, normal beagle dogs were given up to 180 times the human therapeutic dose of lovastatin which reduced serum cholesterol levels to nearly 10% of their pre-test values. However, at this high dose, a variety symptoms of mainly neurological nature occurred suddenly from about 11 days onwards. These signs comprised hypoactivity, ataxia, evidence of dogs walking into objects, recumbancy, vomiting, ptyalism, tremors, tetanic and chronic convulsions.

The brains of affected dogs showed histological evidence of widespread, multifocal perivascular oedema and haemorrhage particularly in grey matter but also to a lesser extent in white matter. There was exudation of homogeneous eosinophilic material and small vessels showed fibroid degeneration and reactive hyperplasia of the endothelium. The changes were widespread in the cerebrum, cerebellum and brain stem but amygdala and frontal cortex were most affected. Large cerebral vessels were spared. These changes were associated with axonal degeneration. Optic nerves showed retrolaminal vacuolation of adjacent fascicles with fusiform axonal swelling close to the retina.

Ultrastructural study demonstrated clear evidence of vascular degeneration which primarily involved endothelial cells. Endothelial cells were characterized by distension of rough endoplasmic reticulum cysternae with fine granular material and electron luscent membrane-bound cytoplasmic vacuoles. The primary nature of the vascular changes was also demonstrated histologically by the presence of extravasated horseradish peroxidase injected during life. Thus, it was suggested that the brain lesions and symptoms were essentially ischaemic in nature.

Although the precise mechanism for endothelial damage was unclear, it only occurred at high doses in dogs and was limited to high multiples of the human dose. It was argued by Berry and colleagues (1980) that as particularly high blood drug levels were achieved in the dog but not other species and that cerebral vascular endothelium has low reductase activity and limited capacity for induction, the special susceptability of small vessels of the central nervous system to lovastatin could be explained.

Inflammation: choroid plexus

Inflammation may develop in the choroid plexus for a variety of reasons, including viral, bacterial a protozoal infections, immune complex diseases and drug-induced disorders (Levine, 1987). Inflammation of the choroid plexus (choroid plexitis) has been reported in rats given cyclophosphamide by the subcutaneous route, a process which was enchanced by concomitant administration of endotoxin (Levine and Sowinski, 1974).

Vacuolation: choroid plexus

As the choroid plexus is a target for a variety of systemic disorders, it is perhaps not surprising that systemic drug-induced changes such as phopholipidosis may also be expressed at this site. This was reported in rats and non-human primates following treatment with disobutamide, a piperidine ring antiarrhythmic compound (Koizumi et al., 1986). This agent produced typical phospholipid-type lamellar inclusions in epithelial cells in an extensive number of organs including smooth muscle, cardiac muscle and macrophages in rat, dog and cynomologous monkeys.

Vacuoles characterised ultrastructurally by lamellated lysomal inclusions were also found in the epithelial cells of the choriod plexus in both rats and monkeys but not dogs. It was shown by Koizumi and colleagues (1986) that these differences in response were due to species differences in the penetration of disobutamide into CSF and its uptake by the choroid plexus, underlining the importance of disposition data in species comparisons.

Several piperazine and piperidine immune modulatory compounds which produced hydropic vacuolation in proximal renal tubules and in cells of the splenic red pulp in rats were also shown to produce a similar vacuolation in the epithelial cells of the choroid plexus (Levine and Sowinski, 1977).

Neoplasia

It is generally accepted that most experimental intracranial and peripheral nerve neoplasms, with few exceptions, fall into the categories defined by the histogenic classification of human neoplasms originally proposed by Bailey and Cushing (1926) and currently defined in the latest WHO classification (Zülch, 1980). However, as all the various subtypes described in man have not been well characterized in laboratory animals and as only conventional histological techniques are usually employed in carcinogenicity bioassays, a relatively simple classification has considerable merit.

The prevalence of brain tumours in rodents used in bioassays is highly variable between different species and strains and between different laboratories using the same strain. The aged rat appears to develop brain tumours more commonly than either the mouse or hamster, with incidences of over 5% reported in some colonies of rats (Sumi et al., 1976). However, as pointed by Koestner (1986) an important and frequently ill-defined variable among different laboratories is the detail of histological sampling.

As many tumours or tumour-like lesions in the brains of rats and mice have been shown to be small, sampling can be a critical element in the incidence of reported spontaneous intracranial neoplasms in these species. Furthermore, sampling bias combined with a general low incidence of these neoplasms, may lead to misleading intergroup differences which may reach statistical significance in a particular bioassay.

Another important biological feature of brain neoplasms in the rat and mouse is their increasing prevalence with advancing age, which parallels the situation in man where the peak incidence of malignant glial tumours occur in the sixth decade (Jones, 1986; Weller, 1986). Lifetime studies in some strains of rats have shown that there is a fairly rapid increase in the prevalence of brain tumours after an age of about 24 months (Solleveld et al., 1986). Therefore, particular care in the interpretation of group differences is needed in studies in which group differences in survival occur.

Another general feature of spontaneous brain neoplasms is their frequently greater prevalence in male rats (Fitzgerald et al., 1974; Gopinath, 1986) and male mice (Fraser, 1986). This corresponds to the slightly greater number of deaths from brain tumours reported in the human male population in England and Wales (Jones, 1986).

In view of the potential for error in the interpretation intergroup differences in the numbers of brain neoplasms in carcinogenicity bioassays as a result of their low incidence, age and sex relationships and sampling bias, Koestner (1986) has proposed that certain criteria should be met before and test substance is designated as neurocarcinogen. There should be a reliable and consistent increase in brain-tumour incidence in treated animals beyond the expected control range. A decrease in the age at which tumours appear or possibly a decline survival should occur. The effect should show a dose-relationship, a shift to less differentiated tumour types should occur and preneoplastic lesions should be evident. Although these criteria are undoubtably stringent, they are helpful guidelines in the critical biological analysis of any statistically signficant intergroup differences in the prevalence of nervous system neoplasms in carcinogenicity bioassays.

The principle tumour groups are those showing neuroectodermal or neurogenic differentiation, those arising from meningeal tissue and their derivatives and tumours developing in a more peripheral location from nerve sheath elements. In addition, there is a group of miscellaneous neoplasms developing in other structures such as the pineal gland, choroid plexus and the lymphoreticular system. The typical medulloblastoma of childhood is not often reported as a spontaneous neoplasm in laboratory rats and mice.

Neuroectodermal tumours

These are frequently grouped together as *gliomas*, the term used to designate primary tumours of the central nervous system which show astrocytic, oligodendroglial and/or ependymal differentiation. Spontaneous rodent glial neoplasms have been best studied in the rat where they occur quite commonly and where they are morphologically similar to those induced in animals by neurocarcinogens such as nitrosoethylurea and other alkylating agents (Mennel and Zülch, 1976).

776

Reviews of spontaneously occurring neuroectodermal tumours in a number of mouse strains have nevertheless indicated that a similar range of these neoplasms also occur in this species (Morgan et al., 1984; Fraser, 1986).

In some rat strains, neuroectodermal neoplasms form the most common subtype of neoplasm in the cranial cavity (Gopinath, 1986). There is a tendancy for them to be located in the cerebral hemispheres, although their diffuse spread may at times render their localization somewhat arbitary. Macroscopically, they appear as swollen areas in the brain or cord of variable colour and texture which may appear relatively well-demarked to the naked eye. A surprising feature noted by a number of authors is a relative lack of apparent clinical abnormalities in many cases (Gopinath, 1986) although as in human cases symptomology and prognosis is highly dependent on tumour location (Weller, 1986). Indeed although rare, when gliomas occur in the spinal cord of rats severe posterior paralysis is reported (Adams and Crowley, 1987).

Although macroscopic appearances and low-power light microscopy may suggest that these neoplasms are well circumscribed, frequently tumour cells infiltrate into the surrounding brain parenchyma. Tumour cells show a variable degree of maturity. Well-differentiated astrocytomas are characteristically composed of elongated or angular cells with eosinophilic cytoplasm, indistinct cell margins and oval hyperchromatic nuclei containing inconspicuous nucleoli. Oligodendrogliomas are composed of cells with clear cytoplasm, distinct cell borders and smaller dense-staining nuclei.

Frequently tumours are not well-differentiated. Many are composed of proliferating pleomorphic cells with scattered bizarre giant cells and zonal necrosis, often surrounded by a pseudopallisade of radially arranged tumour cells. Mixed astrocytic and oligodendrocytic elements also occur quite frequently in some reported series (Krinke et al., 1985). Haemorrhage and iron pigment deposition may occur and vascular or endothelial proliferation may be a prominent feature.

Characterization of an *ependymoma* is more contentious, although they are reported in the rat (Mennel and Zülch, 1976; Dagle et al., 1979; Krinke et al., 1985). The recognition of these in man depends on the presence of ependymal elements or rosettes with a well-defined central lumen and the demonstration of cilia or blepharoblasts, the latter representing basal bodies of cilia (Rubinstein, 1972). Those reported in the rat by Krinke and colleagues (1985) and Gopinath (1986) possessed pseudorosette patterns and protruded into venticules but structures diagnostic of ependymal cell differentiation were not demonstrated. Therefore unequivocal evidence of ependymal differentiation has not been confirmed in many reported cases.

A notable feature of rat gliomas described by Krinke and colleagues (1985) was their lack of immunohistochemical staining for glial fibrillary acidic protein (GFAP). The contrasts with the positive staining of neoplastic astrocytes found in human tumours, although the extent of staining is inversely proportional to the anaplastic nature of the neoplasm (Rubinstein, 1982). Thus, the lack of reactivity to antisera to GFAP may be related to their poor differentiation.

In laboratory mice, neuroectodermal neoplasms present similar histological appearances and mixed forms are also found (Morgan et al., 1984). Neoplasms may be poorly differentiated and spread widely through white matter without marked distortion of the brain (Fraser, 1986).

Focal gliosis, microtumours, covert astrocytomas

Extensive histological sectioning of the brain of aging rats and mice shows small lesions composed of increased numbers of glial cells (Solleveld et al., 1986; Fraser, 1986). These lesions are sometimes diagnosed as gliomas, particularly if there is evidence of cellular atypia. However, there is little evidence to indicate whether such lesions progress to become typical gliomas. Indeed, in the study by Fraser (1986), these foci showed a peak incidence in mice at 200 days, suggesting that regression of a proportion of these lesions does occur. Although these lesions should be recorded in carcinogenicity bioassays, the term, *focal gliosis*, appears the most appropriate.

Mesenchymal tumours

Meningiomas develop from cells forming the meninges and their derivatives in the meningeal space. In man, they are characterized by a highly variable range of histological appearances and it has been suggested that this reflects the adaptive potential of the progenitor arachnoid cell itself (Rubinstein, 1972). The variability of histological appearances of meningeal tumours is reflected in experimental tumours, notably in the rat, where they more commonly develop than in the mouse. This has given rise to some controversy concerning the origin of the so called granular cell tumour which develops in the rat cranial cavity. Most of the evidence suggests that this tumour is simply a varient of meningioma arising from a similar progenitor cell to other meningeal neoplasms (Mitsumori et al., 1987a).

In some, but not all series of rat bioassays, the meningioma is the most frequently found primary tumour in the cranial cavity (Burek 1978; Krinke et al., 1985). They are usually found in close association with the surface coverings of the brain where they are sharply delineated and compress adjacent brain structures. They may occasionally spread diffusely over the cerebral surface and infiltrate into the Robin-Virchow spaces.

Histologically in the rat, they present three major appearances. They may contain fibroblastic, epithelioid or granular cell types, although mixed forms occur.

Fibroblastic forms are composed of spindle cells arranged in bundles and sometimes showing whorl formation. Variable amounts of collagen and reticulin are formed and concentric concretions (psammoma bodies) are occasionally described (Burek, 1978). Cellular pleomorphism and mitotic acivity may be sufficiently marked and associated in infiltrative patterns of growth to merit the diagnosis of sarcoma.

Some neoplasms show more typical epitheloid appearance, possessing regular ovoid nuclei and moderately abundant cytoplasm with distinct cell margins.

A particularly common type is composed of polygonal or elongated cells with finely granular, eosinophilic cytoplasm containing PAS-positive, diastaste-resistant granules (*granular cell tumour, granular cell meningioma, granular cell myoblastoma*). Electron microscopic examination reveals the presence of cytoplasmic, membrane-bound, electron dense bodies, intermediate filaments and desmosome like structures between cells (Mitsumori et al., 1987b). Immunocytochemical study has shown the presence of vimentin but an absence of keratin, S-100 and GFAP in these tumours, features all fully consistent with menigeal arachnoid cell differentiation (Mitsumori et al., 1987b).

Although far less common, tumours of meningeal type and occasionally a granular cell tumour with PAS positive intracytoplasmic granules may occur in the mouse (Morgan et al., 1984).

In both rat and mouse, a variety of other mesenchymal neoplasms are reported to develop in the cranial cavitety, notably soft tissue sarcomas showing vascular or fibrobastic differentiation.

Other neoplasms

Malignant reticulosis, believed to represent a neoplastic proliferation of lymphoreticular cells within the central nervous systems, is traditionally diagnosed in domestic animal species and in the laboratory rats (Luginbühl et al., 1968; Dagle et al., 1979; Krinke et al., 1985). In the rat, use of this diagnosis has been contested on the basis that few diagnoses have been confirmed using appropriate cell marker studies (Solleveld et al., 1986). Clearly, these data are not easily obtained as frozen tissue is necessary for adequate demonstration of most of the surface markers of lymphoreticular cells (see Haemopoietic and Lymphatic Systems, Chapter III). Nevertheless, growth characteristics and cytological features suggest that neoplastic proliferation of lymphoreticular cells can occur within the central nervous system.

As generally reported in the rat, malignant reticulosis is characterized histologically by multifocal and frequently perivascular infiltration of a highly cellular, solid growth of tumour cells. Cells appear lymphoid in character or resemble microglia, but the histological picture can be confounded by the presence of reactive glial cells both in and around neoplastic masses. Reticulin is demonstrable particularly in perivascular locations (Dagle et al., 1979; Krinke et al., 1985).

A variety of other primary neoplasms are occasionally found in the cranial cavity of rats and mice, notably pineal tumours, teratomas and lipomas, which are frequently located in the choroid plexus. Schwanomas and ganglioneuromas also develop in cranial nerve roots (see below).

SPINAL CORD, SPINAL NERVE ROOTS, PERIPHERAL NERVES

The pathology of the spinal cord is similar to that of the brain. Changes occurring in peripheral nerves and nerve roots as a result of xenobiotic administration have been for convenience described previously. One spontaneous condition of the peripheral and spinal nerves of common occurrence in the aged rat which can confound the interpretation of long-term toxicity studies deserves separate comment. This condition, termed *spinal radiculoneuropathy* or *degenerative myelopathy*, is a spontaneous degenerative condition of the peripheral nerves found in association with lesions in the spinal cord and spinal nerve roots which is described in several rat strains (Burek et al., 1976; Cotard-Bartley et al., 1981; Krinke et al., 1981).

Histologically, the condition is characterized by focal swelling of myelin sheaths or overt segmental demyelinization accompanied by myelin-laden foamy macrophages. A granulomatous reaction may also be seen. The sciatic and tibial nerves appear to be most commonly affected (Cotard-Bartley et al., 1981) but other nerves involved include lumbar spinal nerve roots, spinal tracts and the corda equina (Burek, 1978). Skeletal muscle inervated by affected nerves may also become atrophic (Fig. 36) (Burek et al., 1976).

The cause of this condition is unknown, although electron microscopic examination suggests that primary damage occurs in the myelin. However, Krinke (1983) has suggested that the damage may develop as a response to primary changes in the distal axon for he showed that distal axonal changes occured before typical changes developed in the myelin sheaths. Although the cause of this degenerative condition is uncertain, it may be exacerbated by treatment with xenobiotics.

Neoplasia

Spontaneous peripheral nerve tumours are reported only sporadically in aging laboratory rats (Gough et al., 1986) mice (Ward et al., 1979) and hamsters (Pour et al., 1979). They can be successfully induced in rats by the administration of ethyl and methyl nitrosourea (Koestner et al., 1972). Accurate light microscopic diagnosis of experimental nerve sheath neoplasms is complicated by their histological similarities to a number of other soft tissue neoplasms and the fact that they may not possess features that are typical of neoplasms of this class found in man. The less well-differentiated spindle cell sarcomas induced in rats by ethyl or methyl nitrosourea do not frequently exhibit light microscopic features of schwannomas found in man, despite the fact that Schwann cell differentiation has been shown using electron microscopic examination during their early development (Koestner et al., 1972).

This difficulty extends to the spontaneous undifferentiated sarcoma of rats with cystic appearances because this neoplasm possesses certain light microscopic characteristics found in Schwann cell tumours induced by nitroureas and contains immune-reactive S100 protein (see Integumentary System, Chapter I).

Typical Schwann cell neoplasms (*schwannoma, neurinoma, neuroma*) which develop in rodents are characterized by interlacing bundles of elongated spindle cells resembling peripheral nerve and show the classical palisading of nuclei (Antoni's B areas). Ultrastructural examination of neoplasms of this type occurring spontaneously in Wistar rats showed that the cells possess a distinct external lamina, interdigitating cytoplasmic processes and intracytoplasmic concentric lamellae, regularly spaced with a periodicity of about 15 nm (Gough et al., 1986). Although S100 is widely distrubuted in rat tissues, these tumours were shown by Gough and colleagues (1986) to express S100.

In view of the difficulty of making the diagnosis of Schwann cell tumour in less well differentiated cases, particularly if electron micrographs of well-preserved tissue is not available, it is often more prudent to use a term such as undifferentiated sarcoma.

Although *paragangliomas* are also uncommon neoplasms in laboratory rodents, they possess fairly well-defined and characteristic histological features and do not usually represent diagnostic problems. They tend to occur in a distribution which parallels the para-axial distribution of the mammalian paraganglionic system. In man, most paragangliomas are found in the head and neck region or the mediastinum, but the retroperitoneum is a more common site in the Fischer 344 rat (Hall et al., 1987). They have been well-characterized in the Fischer 344 rat where they are composed of dense, variably sized nests or 'Zellballen' often outlined by a prominant reticulin pattern (Hall et al., 1987). The tumour cells are of two main types. One population is characterized by abundant granular eosinophilic cytoplasm with indistinct cell margins, containing central round or oval vesicular nuclei. The other population is composed of smaller, elongated cells with eosinophilic cytoplasm and oval hyperchromatic nuclei. Agyrophilic cytoplasmic granules can be demonstrated in most tumours and electron microscopic examination reveals these to be electron dense granules surrounded by a smooth membrane.

Mitotic figures are uncommon but the tumour cells frequently infiltrate blood vessels and produce intravascular or pulmonary tumour emboli.

Another well-defined neoplasm of the peripheral nervous system is the *ganglioneuroma* (see Endocrine System, Chapter XII).

EYE

The concerns about potentially disabling or irreversible adverse effects of drugs on the human eye, places ocular assessment in preclinical toxicity studies in a prominant and sensitive position. In conventional subacute and chronic toxicity studies, the eyes are usually monitored at regular intervals during the dosing period by ophthalmoscopy and slit lamp biomicroscopy. These techniques are sensitive and able to detect quite minor changes in the cornea, lens or retina. Unfortunately, conventional histological processing using immersion fixation and paraffin embedding are quite limited for the detection of minor changes seen by biomicroscopy. Therefore it is important that special morphological techniques using careful fixation, double paraffin wax embedding, semithin plastic embedded sections or electron microscopy are employed to characterize any drug-induced lesions observed during the dosing phase of the study.

It is important to appreciate that the eye is a highly complex organ with diverse physiology and structure. It is served by multiple neural pathways which can be the site of the action of a wide range of undesirable pharmacological effects of drugs both at or above the therapeutic range of blood and tissue concentrations. Some of these effects reported in man, such as diplopia occurring with anticonvulsant therapy (Beghi and Di Mascio, 1986), may be difficult to predict from experimental studies using animals.

Despite the concern that drug-induced eye changes in man are likely to be associated with severe tissue damage and irreversible functional changes, reported eye changes are actually quite variable in nature and severity. For instance, corneal deposits which occur following administration of the anti-arrhymic drug, amiodarone, are reversible following cessation of treatment and usually not associated with visual impairment (D'Amico et al., 1981). By contrast, retinal changes induced by large doses of chloroquine may be irreversible and progressive after cessation of treatment and be associated with visual impairment (Davidson and Rennie, 1986).

Assessment of the relevance of drug-induced changes in the eye of laboratory animals is complicated by species differences in eye structure and physiology. For instance, the rate of aqueous humour formation varies between species. Although blood vessels of the iris and ciliary bodies possess non-fenestrated endothelium, tight zonulae occludens are present in mouse, non-human primate and man, but gap junctions of 4 nm are present between muculae occludens in the rat (Szalay et al., 1975).

The tapetum, a light reflecting structure, is found in the choroid of dogs but not rat, mouse, rabbit, most non-human primates and man. Albino rats and mice commonly used in drug-safety evaluation have eyes which are devoid of melanin, unlike eyes of dogs, non-human primates and man, so that compounds which produce toxicity through their melanin binding properties may not exert their effects in eyes of albino animals.

Technical considerations

Routine histological techniques for light microscopy of the eye leave much to be desired. Usually formalin or formal saline are avoided and metallic fixatives such as Zenker's or Davidson's fluid are employed prior to paraffin wax embedding and preparation of haematoxylin and eosin stained sections. Undoubtably, electron microscopic examination of appropriately selected and fixed samples of altered structures within the eye is a useful adjunct in the characterization of changes observed during ophthalmoscopy or slit lamp biomicroscopy.

Various types of plastic embedding and preparation of reasonably sized, semithin sections form particularly useful methods for high resolution light microscopy of drug-induced changes in the eye. This avoids the highly selective sampling necessary for ultrastructural examination, yet provides far better resolution of cellular changes than can be provided by paraffin embedding.

Conjunctiva

Inflammation of the conjunctiva is seen sporadically in laboratory animals in response to infections, airbourne dusts and pollutants. More severe conjunctivitis is usually observed in association with corneal inflammation or inflammation in other structures of the anterior segment of the eye (see cornea for discussion).

Harderian and lacrymal glands

The harderian gland is a well-developed gland in the orbit of the rat, mouse and hamster, composed of tubuloalveolar endpieces with wide lumens but devoid of an intraglandular duct system. It secretes lipid-containing substances by a merocrine mechanism. In rodents, the secretions contain variable amounts of porphyrin pigment (see review by Sakai, 1981).

The harderian glands exhibit sexual dimorphism. More prominant porphyrin deposits are observed in female rodents. Castration, administration of androgens or oestrogens can moderate the pigment content of the harderian glands in rodents (Saki, 1981; Spike et al., 1985). In rats, dietary pantothenic acid deficiency may also lead to accumulation of porphyrin and eventually hypertrophy of the harderian gland (Eida et al., 1975).

The rodent eye is also equipped with one intraorbital and one extraorbital lacrymal gland composed of serous cells, structurally similar to those found in the parotid gland.

Chromodacryorrhea

This is a condition characterized by an excessive secretion of red secretions from the harderian gland which may be mistaken for blood (Harkness and Rigeway, 1980). Chromodacryorrhea may precipitated by stress, local irritation as well as administration of cholinergic drugs.

Inflammation

Small foci of non-specific chronic inflammation are found sporadically in harderian or lacrymal glands in laboratory animals. More severe inflammatory changes are much less common, although they may be associated with inflammation of salivary glands.

An example of this phenomenon is observed in rats infected with the sialodacryoadenitis virus. Harderian and lacrymal glands are also predisposed to develop acute and chronic inflammation, oedema and necrosis in response to this infection.

Severe inflammation of the lacrymal gland is not commonly reported in mice, although a form of keratoconjunctivitis sicca associated with a lymphocytic infiltrate in lacrymal glands has been reported to occur spontaneously in NZB/NXW F_1 hybrid mice. The inflammatory process was more common in females and found not only in lacrymal glands but also submandibular and parotid tissue. A peak in the lacrymal gland lymphoid infiltrate occurred in mice between about 24 and 29 weeks of age, corresponding to a time of maximum immune responsiveness of this strain (Gilbard et al., 1987).

Xenobiotic-induced inflammation in the rodent lacrymal or harderian glands is less commonly reported than in the dog lacrymal tissue. Localized necrotizing inflammation of the rodent harderian gland has been reported in association with the orbital bleeding technique (McGee and Maronpot, 1979).

In dogs, inflammation and atrophy has been reported in the lacrymal, nictitans and parotid salivory glands following adminsitration of 5-aminosalicylic acid for one year (Joseph et al., 1988). The changes were more common in female dogs and were associated with keratoconjunctivitis (see below). Histological examination of the lacrymal and nictitans glands revealed atrophy of the glandular tissue in association with a lymphoid cell infliltration. Joseph and colleagues (1988) suggested these findings were probably not of relevance to man in view of lack of reports of keratoconjunctivis sicca in man following the clinical use of the prodrug of 5-aminosalicylic acid, salicylic acid, for many years.

Similar changes have been reported in dogs treated with phenazopyridine, although the lacrymal glands not only showed inflammation and atrophy but also accumulation of a brown pigment (Slatter, 1973).

Neoplasia

Primary neoplasms of harderian and lacrymal glands occur spontaneously in aged rats, mice and hamsters (Goodman et al., 1979; Sheldon et al., 1983), although they are more common and best characterized in mice. Most neoplasms are adenomas showing papillary, cystic or acinar differentiation. Adenocarcinomas are reported in mice where they may invade local tissue or metastasize to the lungs (Sheldon et al., 1983).

Cornea

The normal cornea is transparent because the diameter of collagen fibrils and interfibrillar distance is less than half the wave length of light and this minimizes light scattering. Alteration of this arrangement by an inflammatory process, oedema or the deposition of abnormal substances, creates stromal spaces which are wider than half the wave length of light with consequent light scattering and corneal cloudiness or opacity (Grayson, 1979; Spangler et al., 1982).

Lesions of the cornea can be divided into two main groups, those primarily caused by an inflammatory process (*keratitis*) and those which are essentially degenerative in nature or the result of abnormal depositions in the corneal substance (*dystrophies*). However, the division between these two groups is not sharp, for healed inflammatory lesions may give rise to appearance of dystrophy and the deposition of abnormal substances such as calcium in the cornea may be a result of prior inflammatory damage.

During the course of conventional toxicity studies, repeated ophthalmoscopic examination reveals a number of spontaneous alterations in the optical charateritistics of the cornea, particularly among aging rodents. Many of these spontaneous changes are minor or transient focal opacities which are not detectable histologically and presumably represent the effects of trauma, minor infection or the irritent properties of dust and ammonia developing from bedding and food stuff in animal housing.

When corneal changes are produced by treatment, it is important that they are accurately characterized and an attempt made to distinguish lesions which result from a pharmacological disturbance in corneal defence mechanisms from those which are caused by a primary, direct effect on corneal tissue.

Inflammation (keratitis)

Spontaneous inflammation of the cornea and conjunctiva with or without subsequent scarring and opacity varies with the laboratory animal population and the prevalence of causative organisms. The laboratory rat is more liable than either mouse or hamster to develop keratitis spontaneously, principally as a result of infection with the sialodacryoadenitis virus (Taradach and Greaves, 1984). However, the ocular sequelae of this infection are infrequent. In laboratory beagles, keratitis is found only occasionally in most laboratories, probably related to environmental factors of dust and bedding as well as infections, but it may be exacerbated when ocular defence mechanisms are depressed following administration of high doses of active pharmacological agents.

Induced corneal and conjunctive inflammation is primarily associated with topical administration of irritant substances or exposure to irritant vapours. Changes induced are dependent on the severity of the insult and vary from oedema and mild inflammation to severe inflammation, erosion, ulceration with epithelial hyperplasia and keratinization, features typical of inflammation processes in other epithelial surfaces.

Comparison of the ocular irritant effects of propylene glycol monopropyl ether vapour between Sprague Dawley and Fisher 344 rats, Hartley guinea pigs and New Zealand white rabbits showed species and strain differences in corneal sensitivity. Although in all these animals, conjunctivitis and keratitis was induced by the vapour, only the Fischer 344 rat developed irreversible mineralization, vascularization, stromal splitting and fibrosis of the cornea (Klonne et al., 1988).

Although the testing protocol of Draize using direct administration of irritant substances into the eye of rabbits is now less frequently employed, studies using this model have shown that damage to the eye is generally greater following local administration of alkaline substances than acidic chemicals, although concentration and duration of contact with the eye before washing are also important factors (Murphy et al., 1988).

Systemic administration of drugs may also cause corneal inflammation. Drugs or their metabolites may be secreted into lacrymal fluid where they may exert irritant local effects. More frequently, xenobiotics damage defence mechanisms with inflammation, infection and subsequent opacities.

Drug-induced opacities have been reported in the eyes of experimental animals following administration of narcotic analgesics (Fabian et al., 1967; Roerig et al., 1980). Administration of single doses of the long acting narcotic analgesic, 1-α-acetylmethadol, to male Sprague-Dawley rats produced localized opacities in the cornea, mainly in central, nasal or infero-nasal regions between three and five days after dosing (Roerig et al., 1980). Histologically, lesions were variable in severity but generally characterized by thickened corneal epithelium exhibiting loss of cellular polarity, hyalinization of the basement membrane, stromal vascularization, spindle cell proliferation and small numbers of inflammatory cells. In some animals, frank corneal perforation and intense inflammation was also found. Although the precise cause was not clear in this instance, it was suggested that corneal changes resulted from pathophysiological mechanisms involving adverse effects on corneal sensory innervation, blinking or tear formation, rather than a direct chemical effect on the corneal epithelium. Rats rendered tolerant to morphine were partly protected from these corneal effects of 1-α-acetylmethadol (Roerig et al., 1980).

Lacrymal gland dysfunction in which there is a change in the quantity or quality of the tear fluid may give rise to the the changes of *keratoconjunctivitis sicca*. This condition is found in Sjogren's syndrome in man and similar findings have been documented in NZB/NZW F_1 hybrid mice in which a lymphocytic infiltration develops spontaneously in lacrymal tissue and in rabbits with surgically excised lacrymal glands (Beitch 1970; Gilbard et al., 1987). A form of keratoconjunctivitis sicca has been reported in dogs treated with an antispasmodic agent which produced a diminution in lacrymal secretion (Majeed et al., 1983). A similar condition has been reported in dogs following administration of a number of sulphonamides and the non-sulphonamide, 5-aminosalicyclic acid, all associated with a diminution in the aqueous fraction of tear fluid (Joseph et al., 1988).

Histological findings in keratoconjunctivitis, typically include flattening and desquamation of the superficial corneal epithelial cells with ultrastructural evidence of stunting and loss of cell surface microplicae, decreased density of cell cytoplasm in superficial epthelial cells and disruption of anterior cell membranes (Gilbard et al., 1987). There may be an inflammatory overlay with varying degrees of inflammation, vascularization and proliferation of fibroblasts (Majeed et al., 1983).

Ketatoconjunctivitis sicca reported in dogs after treatment with 5-aminosalicylic acid was associated with atrophy in lacrymal, nictitans and parotid salivary glands and lymphoid cell infiltraton, suggestive of a cell mediated immune reaction in these tissues (Joseph et al., 1988).

Neovascularization

Neovascularization of the normally avascular cornea is a complex multifactorial process. In most instances vascularization accompanies an inflammatory process in the cornea and conjunctiva and it is believed that leucocytes and activated macrophages and their chemical products are involved in the mediation of this process (Klintworth and Burger, 1983). Dietary factors are also potentially important. Blood vessels develop in the cornea of laboratory animals fed diets deficient in tryptophan, lysine, riboflavin, vitamin A or trace metals such as zinc (Carter-Dawson et al., 1980; Leure-Dupree, 1986).

Detailed morphological examination of the vascularization process in rats maintained on a zinc deficient diet for up to seven weeks showed the development of thin-walled capillaries lined by non-fenestrated epithelium, accompanied by nerve fibres and primitive Schwann cells devoid of basal lamina (Leure-Dupree, 1986). No inflammatory changes were observed in this model although some inflammation may have been an early event occurring prior to examination of the eyes.

Corneal dystrophy: mineralization, band keratopathy

Mineral deposits form in the cornea particularly along the basement membrane and in the subepithelial stroma in both man and laboratory animals. In man, this condition, known as *calcific band keratopathy* is associated with alterations in calcium metabolism which accompany hyperparathyroidism, hypercalcaemia of malignancy and excessive vitamin D therapy but it also follows localized damage or dessication of the cornea.

Similar mineralization occurs spontaneously in different strains of laboratory rats and mice, including those such as Fischer 344, Sprague Dawley and Wistar rats and CD-1 mice which are commonly employed in toxicity and carcinogenicity studies (Greaves and Taradach, 1984; van Wincle and Balk, 1986, Bellhorn et al., 1988; Losco and Troup, 1988). It is also reported in diabetic mice of the KK strain which have increased serum alkaline phosphatase values (Mittle et al., 1970) and MRL mice possessing features of hyperparathyridism (Hoffman et al., 1983). Furthermore, similar mineral deposits form in rats as a result of the corneal dessication which follows administration of morphine (Fabian et al., 1967) and in rabbits in association with local trauma and vitamin D excess (Fine et al., 1968; Muirhead and Tomazzoli-Gerossa 1984).

The lesions are morphologically similar in both rats and mice although the degree and extent of mineralization and the severity of secondary changes vary with animal strain, age and experimental conditions. The lesions are usually located centrally in the cornea, occupying an elliptical zone corresponding to the palpebral fissue region.

Early histological changes are those of basophilic granularity along the epithelial basement membrane. This increases to become a continuous mineralized plaque extending along the basement membrane and into the superficial stroma.

The PAS stain shows partial thickening of the basement membrane. At this stage, Von Kossa and alizarin red stains are usually weakly positive suggesting the presence of calcium and phosphate (Losco and Troup, 1988). In more advanced lesions, disruption of the basement membrane and overlying epithelium occurs, giving rise to necrosis, inflammation, a foreign body reaction and scarring.

Ultrastructural study of the affected corneas of Fischer 344 rats has shown the presence of extracellular, electron-dense crystals or granules with an opaque core, a luscent periphery and laminated arrays of alternating light and dark rings which energy dispersive x-ray analysis shows to be composed of calcium and phosphorous (Losco and Troup, 1988).

The cause of this condition in rodents is uncertain. However, calcium is present at or near saturation concentrations in corneal stromal tissues and quite small changes in the corneal microenvironment can cause calcium to precipitate (O'Conner, 1972). Therefore, it has been postulated that change in pH or ionic concentrations of tear fluid can be instigating factors (Bellhorn et al., 1988). As the prevalence of corneal opacities, including those produced by mineralization in different colonies of mice, was shown to be related to cage cleaning frequency, van Winkle and Balk (1988) suggested that factors in the cage environment, notably the presence of urease positive bacteria and ambient cage ammonia levels, were important pathogenic factors. Whatever, the precise pathogenesis, it is clear that the prevalence and severity of this condition can be modulated by quite minor changes in calcium balance and corneal homostasis, including those produced by high doses of some therapeutic agents (Kaplun and Barishak, 1976).

Vacuolation, phospholipidosis

Some cationic amphiphilic drugs which are associated with generalized phospholipidosis, produce lipidosis-like alterations in the cornea. This phenomenon has been reported in the cornea of patients treated with drugs such as chloroquine and amiodarone (D'Amico et al., 1981). Unlike some other adverse effects of these drugs, the deposits which form in the human cornea are usually reversible and associated with little or no visual impairment (Davidson and Rennie, 1986). Experimental studies with these agents have shown that the rat cornea may also develop phospholipidosis (Lüllmann and Lüllmann-Rauch, 1981; Drenkhahn et al., 1983). However, Drenkhahn and colleagues (1983) have suggested the reaction of the rat cornea may be less marked in this respect with agents such as chloroquine and quinacrine than the human cornea.

Histologically, the cornea shows clear lipidosis-like alterations in corneal epithelial cells which are characterized in semithin toludine-blue stained sections as irregular, dense-staining cytoplasmic inclusions (Drenkhahn et al., 1983). Ultrastructural examination reveals typical lamellated and crystalline-like inclusions.

Pigmentation

Pigmentation of the cornea can follow haemorrhage in the anterior chamber. Pigmentation is reported in man following long term parenteral therapy with compounds containing gold in which the metal deposits as golden yellow particles in the anterior layers of the cornea (Davidson and Rennie, 1986).

Uveal tract

Although ophthalmological examination of laboratory rats, mice, hamsters and beagle dogs reveals a number of minor developmental anomalies such as persistent pupillary membranes, pupillary strands, ectopic pupil and coloboma, inflammatory, degenerative and neoplastic processes are quite uncommon (Taradach and Greaves, 1984). When uveal inflammation, haemorrhage, fibrosis or attachment of the iris to the lens (synechia) is observed, this usually is the result of trauma or an inflammatory process developing in the anterior chamber of the eye.

Drug-induced morphological changes in the uveal tract of laboratory animals are rarely reported. Perhaps not surprisingly, however agents which produce generalized phospholipidosis, also induce typical cellular changes in the iris. For instance, in dogs but not rats treated with the piperidine antiarrhymic drug, disobutamide, vacuolation typical of phospholipidosis was found in the pigmented epithelial cells of the iris (Koizumi et al., 1986).

Oedema and dilatation of intramuscular spaces of the ciliary body has been reported in the eyes of cynomolgus monkeys following the topical application of prostaglandin F2α probably related to reduced intraocular pressure and increase in uveoscleral outflow (Lütjen-Drecoll and Tamm, 1988).

Lens

The lens in a transparent, biconcave structure composed of modified epithelial cells. It is surrounded by an elastic capsule which is an exaggeration of a PAS-positive basement membrane, devoid of elastic fibres which acts as a sieve for large molecules. The anterior and equatorial surfaces contain a superficial layer of cuboidal cells with their apexes facing the lens substance. At the equator, the cell cytoplasm elongates anteriorly and posteriorly to form long cells or lens fibres. At the periphery of the lens the nuclei are visible and arranged in an arc or lens 'bow'. Lens fibres form throughout life and move towards the centre of the lens where cytoplasmic condensation and nuclear pyknosis occurs. Thus, older fibres accumulate in the centre or *nucleus* of the lens and younger fibres are found in the outer layer or lens *cortex*. Lens sutures forming a 'Y' pattern in the centre of the lens represent junctions of apposed lens fibres (Rhodin, 1974; Martin and Anderson, 1981).

The transparency of the lens is dependent on the solubility of its constituent cellular proteins, unlike the cornea which depends on a precise arrangement of collagen fibrils (Schmidt and Coulter, 1981). In man and laboratory animals at least 50% of the lens is composed of water which contains various proportions of three types of soluble proteins termed crystallines. Insoluble proteins are found mainly in the nucleus of the lens where older lens fibres are found, associated mainly with cell membranes. Lens proteins are in an immunologically privileged site, being protected from humoral and cellular components of the immune system by the lens capsule. However rupture of the capsule may bring about lens-induced autoimmune uveitis.

The integrity of the lens is dependent on the diffusion of nutrients directly from tissue fluids, mainly the aqueous humour. The lens epithelium is the principle site of energy production of the lens which is used for transport of inorganic ions and aminoacids by an active process involving Na^+ and K^+ activated ATPase. The principle source of energy is glucose which undergoes anaerobic glycolysis forming lactic acid which diffuses into the aqueous humour.

The rate of glycolysis is controlled by hexokinase and the rate of entry of glucose into the lens. If glucose concentration increase, the levels of glucose-6-phosphate also rise and this in turn limits the rate of glycolysis and excessive accumulation of lactic acid (Schmidt and Coulter, 1981).

In the face of very high blood glucose levels such as occur in diabetes mellitus, activation of aldose reductase occurs. This provides an alternative route of metabolism giving rise to sorbital.

Disturbance of the metabolic equilibrium of the lens or interaction of xenobiotics with crystalline proteins may lead to adverse changes in the lens fibres resulting *opacity* or *cataract*. Particular care is necessary in the use of the term cataract. Slit lamp investigations have shown that minor lens opacities can occur in essentially normal laboratory animals and reversible opacities can be induced by a variety of non-specific and specific adverse stimuli (Frauenfelder and Burns, 1970).

In the context of drug safety assessment, the term *cataract* is used by some authors to denote a state of permanence and reserved for irreversible opacities present at birth, advanced or unequivocally progressive opacities in adult animals (Taradach and Greaves, 1984). However, other workers define cataracts as *any* lens opacity which can be detected by standard ophthalmoscopy. Hence, it is vital in preclinical safety studies that terminology for lens lesions is clearly defined and the nature of any induced lesions precisely described.

Cataracts have been shown to develop in a number of different ways. They may result from the effects of toxic metabolites of ingested xenobiotics or from accumulation of naturally occurring products such as sorbital and peptides. They may also develop in states of disordered metabolism through dietary deficiences or from direct physical damage to lens fibres by ionizing radiation (Schmidt and Coulter, 1981). Xenobiotics or their metabolites may also interact non-enzymatically with crystallines to give rise to protein aggregates which in turn may cause light scatter (Karim et al., 1988).

Histological appearance

Biomicroscopy shows that a wide range of spontaneous, age-related lens alterations occur in laboratory animals. These may be focal or diffuse opacities or alterations in optical density involving the anterior or posterior cortex or the lens nucleus (Taradach and Greaves, 1984). The histological appearance of spontaneous lens opacities and cataracts have probably been best characterized in the rat. Lens fibres may show tinctoral changes, swelling or ballooning with cytoplasmic granulation. Frank cell degeneration with vacuolation or accumulation of basophilic debris or eosinophilic globules may also be found. Displacement or degeneration of the regularly aligned nuclei in the lens bow may also be a feature of lens damage. The subcapsular epithelial cells may likewise show degenerative alterations, notably nuclei pyknosis, fragmentation, cytoplasmic vacuolation and eosinophilic globule formation (Balazs et al., 1970).

Cataracts and lens opacities are well described in dogs but in most beagle colonies lenticular changes are of a minor nature and are regarded as normal variations (Taradach and Greaves, 1984). In a review of cataracts and opacities induced by a range of unnamed drugs, Heywood (1971) suggested that the development of drug-induced cataract in dogs followed two distinct routes after a latent period of a few days to several months.

One group of cataracts were initiated at the equator by the development of small vacuoles showing an opaque halo which extended in superficial lens fibres, towards the poles along sutural planes. The progression of this type of change to complete cataract could occur in a few days.

The second group of cataracts were initiated at the posterior pole by the development of broad white suture lines with feathery edges which was followed by the development of a triangular opacity around the sutures. This form of lesion appeared to develop slowly over a period of several months (Heywood, 1971).

Histologically, early opacities at the posterior suture lines are characterized by swelling of lens fibres as they abut on the sutures. Progression to complete cataract is evident by cystic degeneration and accumulation of cell debris, including rounded eosinonophilic globules near the suture lines.

The anterior lens epithelium appears to be the primary site of dysfunction in cataracts induced by long term steroid therapy for increased numbers of intercellular clefts have been observed in the lens epithelium of patients with steroid-induced cataracts (Karim et al., 1988). Several mechanism may be responsible for these changes: mechanical forces pulling epithelial cells apart, increased transport of sodium into the basolateral spaces causing osmotic swelling, increased entry of sodium across apical membranes causing increased sodium pump activity, inhibition of the sodium pump causing general swelling, a direct effect of steroids on the lateral membrane surface or an effect on lens epithelial cell growth (Karim et al., 1988).

The development of drug-induced and dose-related lens opacities or cataracts in one or more of the test species in preclinical studies performed on a novel therapeutic agent is cause for concern. It may be particularly difficult to predict likely risk for man and the degree of clinical monitoring necessary to exclude a drug-induced effect in patients treated with a novel drug, especially as cataracts occur spontaneously in aged subjects.

Some of the potential strain and species differences are illustrated by acetaminophen (Tylenol), a widely used analgesic and antipyretic which has been shown to cause cataracts in mice (Shichi et al., 1978). It has been shown that there are considerable species and strain differences in sensitivity to acetaminophen caractogenesis. In studies in mice, it was shown that acetaminophen-induced cataracts developed more readily in C57BL/6 mice than in DBA/2 mice but this effect appeared to be independent of the hepatic biotransformation and hepatic toxicity of acetaminophens in these strains (Lubek et al., 1988).

The cholesterol lowering agent lovastatin, a competitive inhibitor of 3-hydroxy-3-methylglutaryl coenzyme A reductase (HMG CoA reductase), produced lens opacities in dogs but not rats, mice or monkeys treated for long periods of high doses (MacDonald et al., 1988). These opacities occurred in low incidence but in a dose-related distribution. They commenced as an increase in density of suture lines in the posterior region of the lens, followed by an increase in vacuolation near the junction of the sutures. Eventually, they progressed to full cataract. Similar lens changes have been reported with other HMG CoA reductase inhibitors (MacDonald et al., 1988). As the lens findings only occurred in the dog at drug exposures far in excess of those achievable at maximum human dose, it was argued by MacDonald and collegues (1988) that cateracts were unlikely to develop in patients as a result of lovastatin therapy. Although no drug-induced lens changes have been reported in patients using HMG CoA reductase inhibitors, there was clearly a need to monitor for this closely in clinical trials.

Retina

The ophthalmological appearances of the retina and its basic anatomy and physiology in the usual laboratory animals used in toxicology has been well documented (Rubin, 1974; Martin and Anderson, 1981). It is the most complex part of the eye comprising ten anatomical layers which can be recognized in routine histological sections.

The outer layer is the supportive pigmented epithelium or *pars pigmentosa*. The remaining nine layers comprise the sensory epithelium or *pars nervosa* in which photosensory outer and inner segments of rods and cones are separated from the external nuclear layer by an external limiting membrane. This membrane represents densities of zonular adherens which join the inner segments of rods and cones to Müller cells and Müller cells to each other. Müller cells are generally regarded as highly specialized astrocytes developing from neuroectoderm but different structurally from astrocytes in the retina (Lewis et al., 1988).

The external nuclear layer, containing the cells bodies of rods and cones is adjacent to the outer plexiform layer or synapse zone. Here, there are synapses between joining axons of photoreceptors and dendrites of the horizontal and bipolar cells and processes of Müller cells. The inner nuclear layer contains the nuclei of horizontal cells, bipolar cells, Müller cells and amacrine cells. The inner plexiform layer is the synaptic zone between first and second order neurones which is located below a single layer of ganglion cells. The axons of the ganglion cells which converge to also form the optic nerve, form an inner nerve fibre layer on the retina. This is covered by an internal limiting membrane composed of processes of Müller cells (Martin and Anderson, 1981).

Although these different retinal layers are clearly delineated in routinely fixed, paraffin embedded, haematoxylin stained sections, the use of plastic enbedded semithin sections, improves the appreciation of fine detail of the retinal layers at light microscopic level.

Immunocytochemical techniques are also helpful in the delineation of retinal cell populations. Immunocytochemical study of the rat retina has shown that the non-neuronal elements, Müller and astrocytic cells stain with antisera to S100 protein, although Müller cells stain less intensely than astrocytes (Kondo et al., 1984).

Antibodies to cellular retinaldehyde binding protein and glutamine synthetase also label Müller cells but not astrocytes whereas glial fibrillary acidic protein can be found in both glial and Müller cells (Lewis et al., 1988).

A particularly important aspect of retinal anatomy is the blood-retinal barrier, which like its counterpart in the brain, helps to maintain retinal integrity by regulation of fluid and metabolite exchange as well as prevent access of large molecules from the blood stream. The blood-retinal barrier is a function of the endothelial plasma membrane resulting from the presence of tight junctions and a low level of endocytosis coupled with an apparant lack of transendothelial vesicular transport from the blood (Essner, 1987).

A similar barrier exists in the vessels of the optic nerve (Peyman and Apple, 1972) and the iris (Rapoport, 1977) although the latter barrier shows a more variable response to experimental conditions than the other barriers.

The retina is basically a similar in structure in rodents, dogs and primates although there are certain differences which may be of some relevance in toxicology. For instance, the absence of melanin from the retina of albino rat and mouse strains may provide the basis for greater resistance to the harmful effects of compounds which accumulate in melanin containing cells. The hamster retinal pigment epithelium has been shown to possess a melanin pattern different from that found in mice and this could also form the basis for interspecies differences in retinal toxicity (Buyukmihci and Goehring-Harmon, 1982).

Tapetal cells forming the *tapetum lucidum* are a modified part of the underlying choroid which reflects light after it passes through the retinal layers. This aids vision under conditions of low ambient light intensity. It is present in the dog but not man and rodents.

In the dog it is located in the dorsal segment of the ocular fundus. It is composed of angular cells arranged in up to 15 layers at the centre, thining out to a single layer at its periphery near the optic nerve.

Tapetal cells possess round nuclei with prominant nucleoli and slender cytoplasmic rods which are electron-dense following osmium fixation (Martin and Anderson, 1981). Intercellular spaces are wide and contain abundant elastic fibres. It has been suggested that as the tapetum is a species-specific structure not found in man, that drug-induced alterations in the tapetum may have little or no relevance for man (Heywood, 1974).

Retinal toxicity is one of the most important ocular side effects of a number of drugs employed therapeutically in man. Examples include chloroquine, quinine, chlorpromazine and thioridize (Davidson and Rennie, 1986). Unfortunately, the difficulty of obtaining good retinal tissue sections precludes accurate histological characterization of some of these lesions, limiting correlation of findings in man with those induced in laboratory animals. It is therefore particularly important to characterize both the ophthalmoscopic and histological appearances as well as the evolution of retinal alterations found during the course of toxicity studies in the preclinical phase of development of a novel therapeutic agent and define the mechanism or mechanisms involved. Without precise characterization of induced retinal lesions and reasonable case for not expecting damaging retinal effects in man, it is clearly quite difficult to argue for the therapeutic use of a novel drug with such properties. It is also important to carefully exclude drug-induced retinal damage in toxicity studies when a particular drug is shown to bind melanin pigment in autoradiographic studies using pigmented rats.

Retinal atrophy

Atrophy is the most common alteration seen in the retina of laboratory animals, where it may appear spontanously or be induced by xenobiotics. It is usual to classify retinal atrophy in laboratory animals according to pathogenesis because histological characteristics of retinal atrophy are common to most types of atrophy (Bellhorn, 1981).

Classification of retinal atrophy

Senile retinal atrophy
Hereditary retinal atrophy
Nutritional retinopathy
Post inflammatory atrophy
Atrophy following glaucoma
Toxic retinopathy
Phototoxic retinopathy

These categories are not entirely distinct because hereditary factors may interact with age related alterations, ambient light and xenobiotic induced toxicity.

Hereditary retinal atrophy

Rats: Retinal atrophy occurring spontaneously in albino rats is usually considered to be a senile alteration or related to the adverse effects of high ambient light intensity. Hereditary retinal degeneration has been characterized in some rat strains, notably the Roayl College of Surgeons (RCS) strain (Dowling and Sidman, 1962) and the Wag/Rij rat (Lai et al., 1975).

In both albino and pigmented RCS rats, hereditary retinopathy develops in the first few weeks of life, probably as a result of relative inability to phagocytose shed rod outer segment discs. This results in photoreceptor degeneration which can be prevented by pigment epithelial transplantation (Li and Turner, 1988). Histologically, there is a loss of photoreceptor cells, evident by the reduction in the number of nuclei in the outer nuclear layer and the persistence of foci of debris between the pigment epithelium and retinal cells (von Sallman and Grimes, 1972).

In the Wag/Rij there appears to be a primary degeneration of the photoreceptor cell body starting at about one month of age and within a period of one year this lead to total loss of outer retinal cells (Li et al., 1975).

Whilst the early onset of retinal degeneration in these strains is characteristic of a hereditary condition, a genetic predisposition to retinal degeneration in other strains cannot be excluded.

Mice: Hereditary degeneration is a more prevalent condition in laboratory mice. It was reported by Brückner in 1951 in Switzerland and it was shown to be inherited in an autosomal recessive manner. The condition probably corresponds to the so called, rodless retina, described in 1924 in other mice by Keeler. A morphologically similar retinal degeneration has also been noted in routine subacute toxicity studies performed using young CD-1 mice so the pathologist should be alert to this possibility when looking at the eyes of mice (Taradach and Greaves, 1984).

Dogs: Although hereditary retinal degeneration is a well described phenomenon in some dog breeds, it is described only rarely in beagles (Heywood, 1974).

Senile retinal atrophy

Weisse and colleagues (1974) demonstrated loss of cells from both the inner and outer nuclear layers of the peripheral retina in aging albino rats of the Chbb/THOM strain. Similar morphological findings have been documented in aging Fischer 344 (Li et al., 1978, 1979) Sprague-Dawley (Taradach and Greaves, 1984; Lin and Essner, 1987) and Wistar-Furth rats (Lin and Essner, 1988). However, the precise pathogenesis of these changes are uncertain. It is not entirely clear whether some of these changes is genetically programmed or senile in nature. Similar changes may also occur in quite young rats. It has been suggested that these age-related changes in Fisher 344 rats may be linked to the migration of photoreceptor cells into the subretinal space and derangement of the nutritive function of Müller's cells (Li et al., 1979).

Ultrastructural examination of the age-realated retinal changes in Sprague-Dawley rats has shown that early degenerative changes occur in the pigment epithelium, notably in the basal plasma membrane and subsequently in the photoreceptor cells (Lin and Essner, 1987). The degenerative process of the pigment epithelium was shown to allow permeation of injected horseradish peroxidase from the choroid into the retina. On this basis it was argued that these age-related retinal changes may represent a primary defect in the pigment epithelium.

Analagous age-related changes have not been well characterized in mice or hamsters. A senile form of atrophy is reported in aged dogs, but it is seldom seen in the young beagle dog employed in toxicity studies.

Light induced retinal atrophy

The retina of the albino rat is very sensitive to the effects of light. It shows an age-related sensitivity to short periods of exposure to high light intensity and longer term exposure to relative normal levels of artificial lighting even when there are regular periods of light and darkness (Weisse et al., 1974). Studies of the rat retina in animals housed under controlled light conditions have shown that in contrast to age-related retinal atrophy which tends to occur at the periphery of the retina, changes induced by light tends to be more marked in the posterior pole (Noell et al., 1966; Weisse et al., 1974). Histologically, the changes are similar to those found in other forms of atrophy and characterized by a progressive loss of the nuclei from the outer nuclear layer followed by loss of inner retinal layers and proliferation of retinal vessels (Weisse et al., 1974).

Post inflammatory atrophy

Inflammation rarely occurs in the posterior segment of the eye in laboratory animals but may occasionally occur and lead to retinal damage and atrophy. An epidemic of multifocal serous chorioretinitis was described in beagle dogs during toxicity studies characterized histologically by focal retinal detachment, focal accumulation of serous fluid between photoreceptors and focal loss of the outer nuclear layer (Weisse et al., 1981). The disease occurred mainly during the summer months but no transmissible agent was identified.

Very occasionally, focal retinitis, choroiditis and retinal atrophy is observed in association with larva migrans (Rubin and Saunders, 1965). In non-human primates, chorioretinal changes are usually the result of traumatic damage and frequently unilateral, although spontaneous macular degneration is reported (Bellhorn, 1981).

Drug-induced atrophy

Retinal atrophy induced by xenobiotics may morphologically resemble atrophy found spontaneously, particularly among rodents (Bellforn, 1981). However, some drugs induce cytological changes in particular retinal cells or cell layers in association with retinal atrophy and it is important to characterize the nature of such changes when induced by a novel therapeutic agent.

Retina-phospholipidosis, lipidosis

Drugs which are capable of inducing generalized phospholipidosis may produce similar alterations in the cells of the retina. In rats, these agents produce the typical lamellated or crystalloid inclusions in retinal pigment epithelium, neural cells and Müller cells. These can be characterized in semithin toluidine blue-stained sections by the presence of dense closely packed cytoplasmic inclusions (Drenkhahn and Lüllmann-Rauch, 1978; Lüllmann-Rauch, 1979; Lüllmann and Lüllmann- Rauch, 1981). Studies in rats with a number of different cationic amphiphilic drugs have shown that the distribution of these cellular alterations within the retinal cell population varies with the particular drug. For instance, chloroquine and 4, 4' diethyl-aminoethoxyhexestrol were shown to affect mainly neurons and Müller cells whereas triparanol affected pigment epithelium and Müller cells and chlorcyclizine altered both pigment epithelium and sensory retinal cells to a similar extent (Drenkhahn and Lüllmann-Rauch, 1978).

It was suggested that some of the differences between drugs are due to their different affinities for particular polar lipids. The retinal pigment epithelium is particularly at risk because of its normal role in the phagocytosis of large amounts of shed discs of membranous material from the tips of rod outer segments (Lüllmann-Rauch, 1979).

Whereas the use of some of these cationic amphiphilic drugs is associated with the development of retinopathy in man, the role of phospholipidosis in this process is not always clear. In dogs, tapetal cells may also show lipidosis-like vacuolation following treatment with catronic amphiphilic agents (Ruben et al., 1989), although the relevance of this distribution of lipidosis for man is unclear.

Atrophy-tapetum

In beagle dogs, the tapetum lucidum has been reported to show degenerative changes and atrophy following administration of a number of different classes of therapeutic agents including the β-adrenergic blocking agent, SCH 19927 (Schiavo et al., 1984), ethambutol (Cappiello and Layton, 1965), a macrolide antibiotic, rosamicin (Massa et al., 1984), an imidazo quinazoline (Shiavo et al., 1972) and an aromatase inhibitor, CGS 14796C (Schiavo et al., 1988).

Ophthalmoscopic examination of affected eyes typically shows loss of tapetal reflectivity with the development of focal, mottled or diffuse zones of pigmentation similar to that found in non-tapetal zones of the fundus. Histologically, these pigmented areas are represented by degeneration, thinning or total loss of tapetal cells with litle or no alterations in pigment epithelium. Ultrastructural examination of tapetal cells of dogs treated with the aromatase inhibitor, CGS 14796C, showed evidence of cellular degeneration and cytoplasmic autophago-

797

cytic vacuolation (Shiavo et al., 1988). As the tapetum is a non-regenerating structure, the changes are usually irreversible. Drug-induced discolouration of the tapetum can also occur without histological evidence of damage (Massa et al., 1984).

Why the tapetum should be singled out for the damaging effects of xenobiotics is, in most cases, unclear. It has been suggested that some of these agents may affect the tapetum by chelating metals, particularly zinc, which is found in high concentrations in dog tapetal cells (Cappiello and Layton, 1965; Figueroa et al., 1971).

Although it is widely accepted that drug-induced tapetal effects are without toxicological significance for non-tapetal species including man (Schiavo et al., 1988), cautious assessment of all the relevant data about a novel agent in several species remains an essential part of this evelution.

This is illustrated by ethambutol, an effective antituberculous drug. Clinical use of ethambutol, is associated with loss of visual acuity in some patients although the precise mechanism is uncertain. However, ethambutol also produces tapetal changes in the dog probably by virtue of its zinc chelating properties for it has been shown that zinc tissue levels in the dog tapetum lucidum decrease following treatment (Figueroa et al., 1971). It was therefore suggested by Figueroa and colleagues (1971) that although the human eye does not possess a tapetum, the retina and choroid contain relatively high zinc concentration so it is conceivable that ethambutol-induced eye changes in man are also linked to its zinc chelating properties.

EAR

The ear is divided anatomically into three principle regions, the *external ear* comprising the auricle, the external auditary meatus with modified sebaceous glands, the *middle ear* or tympanic cavity and the *inner ear* which contains the sensory structures involved in hearing and equilibrium.

The comparative anatomy of the middle ear cavity in man and rat has been reviewed by Albiin and colleagues (1986). In both species, the tympanic cavity can be divided into an epitympanum or attic space, a mesotympanum and hypotympanum. Air-filled cavities corresponding to the human mastoid cells are not found in the rat. In man and rat, the lining mucosa is formed of tracts with both ciliated and secretory cells, with other areas particularly over the epitympanum, being covered by single squamous or cuboidal epithelium (Albiin et al., 1986). Ciliated and secretory cells become extended over greater areas of the cavity in pathological conditions, notably otitis media.

The function and structure of the cochlea is not readily assessed within the context of conventional toxicity studies. Most of the audiometric techniques are too time consuming or complex for routine application in toxicity studies. The small size and well protected position within the temporal bone make provision of good histological techniques technically demanding and they can only demon-

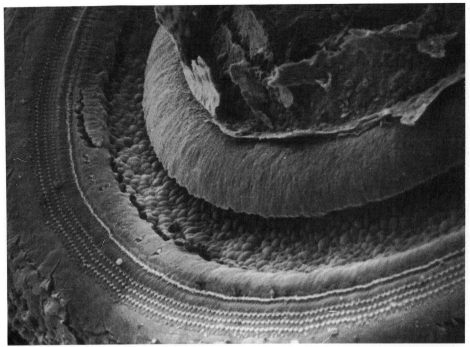

Fig. 133. Scanning electron micrograph of part of the apical turn of the organ of Corti from the rat. Sensory hair cells have been exposed by removal of the Reissner's membrane and the tectorial membrane from the limbus. This and the following figures by courtesy of Dr N.G. Read. (SEM ×450.)

strate small numbers of sensory cells. As the anatomy of the guinea pig ear makes it easier to expose the inner ear structures using standard surface preparation techniques than in other experimental species (Engström 1964), this species is frequently employed in studies of ototoxicity.

Astbury and Read (1982a) have demonstrated how scanning electron microscopy of the critical point dried cochlea of both rats and non-human primates can be employed in routine toxicity studies (Figs. 133 and 134). Using this technique on the cochlea of rats treated with kanamycin, Astbury and Read (1982b) showed the presence of stereotyped morphological damage to the reticular organ of Corti, similar to that reported for kanamycin-induced ototoxicity in the guinea pig. The changes were time and dose related, starting in the outer hair cells at the base and progressing to the apex of the cochlea with subsequent loss of inner hair cells following changes to the cuticular plate (Fig. 135). It was also noted that fairly extensive morphological changes occurred before a shift in the startle response (Preyer reflex) to a range of different auditary frequencies.

In addition, it has been shown that degenerative changes also occur in the vestibular ganglion cells in animals treated with aminoglycosides, although

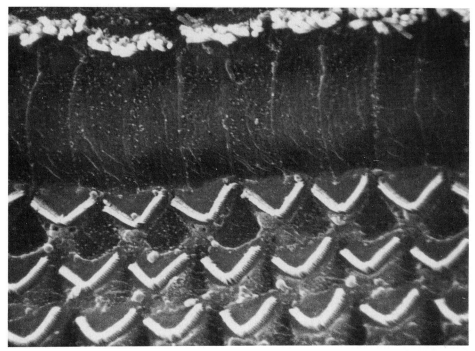

Fig. 134. Higher power view of the reticular lamina of the Organ of Corti from a rat. The single row of inner hair cells is separated from the outer hair cells by the rectangular plates of the inner pillar cells. The outer hair cells are arranged in three precise rows. (SEM ×4400.)

whether such changes are a primary direct effect of drug or retrograde degeneration following damage to sensory epithelium is disputed (Sera et al., 1987).

External ear (pinna)

The external ear is affected by inflammatory and neoplastic conditions similar to those occurring elsewhere in the skin and subcutaneous tissues. The protruding auricle is particularly liable to traumatic damage. In mice it can be used as a convenient site for mechanistic studies of skin irritancy (see Skin and Subcutaneous Tissue, Chapter I). A number of more specific conditions may occasionally be seen in the external ear of rats, notably auricular chondritis and carcinomas of the auditory subaceous glands.

Auricular chondritis in rats

This striking condition of the auricular cartilage occurs spontaneously in several strains of rats (Chiu and Lee, 1983; Prieur et al., 1984), even in rats aged only a few months. It can also be induced by immunization of rats with type II collagen (Cremer et al., 1981; McCune et al., 1982).

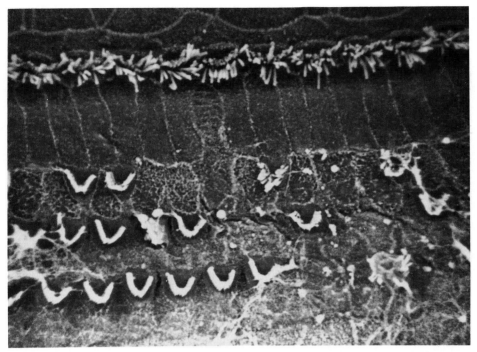

Fig. 135. Similar view to that in figure 134 but taken from a rat in which the organ of Corti was damaged by systemic administration of kanamycin. A number of outer hair cells have been lost and replaced by expanded support cells. (SEM ×2800.)

Clinically, bilateral erythematous nodules are observed on the pinnae. Histologically, the normal cartilage of the pinna is focally disrupted by proliferative granulomatous inflammation composed of a mixture of lymphocytes, plasma cells, neutrophils, macrophages, foreign body giant cells and proliferating fibroblasts. The maturity of the inflammatory infiltrate is variable from area to area. Some zones appear quite quiescent with zones of marked fibrogenesis and prominant vasculature. A further striking feature in less inflammed but disrupted zones is the presence of discrete, irregular nodules of immature cartilage composed of a pale eosinophilic matrix and numerous chondroblasts.

The cause of this condition is not known but is has been suggested that the condition results from an autoimmune reaction to the type II collagen present in cartilage (Prieur et al., 1984).

Carcinoma

Carcinomas of the auditary sebaceous glands develop as localized infiltrating growths located in the vicinity of the external auditory meatus (Pliss, 1973). Histologically, they are composed of infiltrating masses of squamous cells frequently showing considerable keratinization as well as sebaceous features. They infiltrate locally, produce ulceration of the overlying skin, erode bone and produce distant metastases notably in the lung.

REFERENCES

ADAMS, S.W. and CROWLEY, A.M. (1987): Posterior paralysis due to spontaneous oligodendroglioma in the spinal cord of the rat. *Lab.Anim.Sci.*, 37, 345–347.

ALBIIN, N., HELLSTRÖM, S., STENFORS, L-E., and CERNE, A. (1986): Middle ear mucosa in rats and humans. *Ann.Otol.Rhinol. Laryngol.*, 95, Suppl. 126, 2–15.

ALCALA, H., LERTRATANANGKOON, K., STENBACH, W., KELLAWAY, P. and HORNING, M.G. (1978): The Purkinje cell in phenytoin intoxication: Ultrastructural and Golgi studies. *Pharmacologist*, 20, 240.

ALDER, S., CANDRIAN, R., ELSNER, J. and ZBINDEN, G. (1986): Neurobehavioral screening in rats. *Meth.Find Exptl.Clin. Pharmacol.*, 8, 279–289.

ARGOV, Z. and MASTAGLIA, F.L. (1979): Drug-induced peripheral neuropathies. *Br.Med.J.*, 1, 663–666.

ALEU, F.R., KATZMAN, R. and TERRY, R.D. (1963): Fine structure and electrocyte analysis of cerebral oedema induced by alkyltin intoxication. *J.Neuropath.Exp.Neurol.*, 22, 403–413.

ASTBURY, P.J. and READ, N.G. (1982)a: Improved morphological technique for screening potentially ototoxic compounds in laboratory animals. *Br.J.Audiol.*, 16, 131–137.

ASTBURY, P.J. and READ, N.G. (1982)b: Kanamycin induced ototoxicity in the laboratory rat. A comparative morphological and audiometric study. *Arch.Toxicol.*, 50, 267–278.

BAILEY, P. and CUSHING, H. (1926): A classification of the gliomata. In: *A Classification of the Tumors of the Glioma Group on a Histiogenetic Basis with a Correlated Study of Prognosis*, pp. 53–95. Lippincott, Philadelphia.

BALAZS, T., OHTAKE, S. and NOBLE, J.F. (1970): Spontaneous lenticular changes in the rat. *Lab.Anim.Care*, 20, 215–219.

BARSOUM, N.J., GOUGH, A.W., STURGESS, J.M. and de la IGLESIA, F.A. (1986): Parkinson-like syndrome in nonhuman primates receiving a tetrahydropyridine derivative. *Neurotoxicology.*, 7, 119–126.

BEGHI, E., and DIMASCIO, R. (1986): Antiepileptic drug toxicity: definition and mechanism of action. *Ital.J.Neurol.Sci.*, 7, 209–222.

BEGHI, E, DIMASCIO, R. and TOGNONI, G. (1986): Adverse effects of anticonvulsant drugs: a critical review. *Adv.Drug Ac.Pois. Rev.*, 2, 63–86.

BEITCH, I. (1970): The induction of keratinization in the corneal epithelium. A comparison of the 'dry' and vitamin A deficient eyes. *Invest.Ophthalmol.*, 9, 827–843.

BELLHORN, R.W., (1981): Laboratory animal opthalmology. In: K.N. Gelatt (Ed.): *Textbook of Veterinary Ophthalmology*, Chap. 19, pp. 649–671. Lea and Febiger, Philadelphia.

BELLHORN, R.W., KORTE, G.E. and ABRUTYN, D. (1988): Spontaneous corneal degeneration in the rat. *Lab.Anim.Sci.*, 38, 46–50.

BERRY, P.H., MACDONALD, J.S., ALBERTS, A.W., MOLON-NOBLOT, S., CHEN, J.S., LO, C-YL., GREENSPAN, M.D., ALLEN, H., DURAND-CAVAGNA, G., JENSEN, R., BAILLY, Y., DELORT, P. and DUPRAT, P. (1988): Brain and optic system pathology in hypocholesterolemic dogs treated with a competitive inhibitor of 3-hydroxy-3-methylglutaryl coenzyme A reductase. *Am.J.Pathol.*, 132, 427–443.

BLAKEMORE, W.F. (1980): Isoniazid. In: P.S. Spencer, and H.H. Schaumburg, (Eds). *Experimental and Clinical Neurotoxicology*, Chap. 33, pp. 476–489. Williams and Wilkins, Baltimore.

BLAKEMORE, W.F., PALMER, A.C. and NOEL, P.R.B. (1972): Ultrastuctural changes in isoniazid-induced brain oedema in the dog. *J. Neurocytol.*, 1, 263–278.

BLOCH, B. (1985): L'hybridation in situ: Méthodologie et application à; l'analyse des phénomènes d'expression génique dans les glandes endocrines et le système nerveux. *Ann.Endocrinol.*, 46, 253–261.

BLOCH, B., BRAZEAU, P., LING, N., BOHLEN, P., ESCH, F., WEHRENBERG, W.B., BENOIT, R., BLOOM, R. and GUILLEMIN, R. (1983): Immunohistochemical detection of growth hormone-releasing factor in brain. *Nature*, 301, 607–608.

BLOCH, W., LING, N., BENOIT, R., WEHRENBERG, W.B. and GUILLEMIN, R., (1984): Specific depletion of immunoreactive growth hormone-releasing factor by monosodium glutamate in rat median eminence. *Nature*, 307, 272–273.

BONDY, S.C. (1985): Especial considerations for neurotoxicological research. *CRC.Crit.Rev.Toxicol.*, 14, 381–402.

BOULDIN, T.W. and KRIGMAN, M.R. (1975): Differential permeability of cerebal capillaries and choroid plexus to lanthanum ion. *Brain Res.*, 99, 444–448.

BOULGER, L.R. (1973): The neurovirulence test for live poliomyelitis vaccine. *J.Bio.Stand.*, 1, 119–138.

BRÜCKNER, R. (1951): Spaltlampenmikroskopie und Ophthalmoskopie am Auge von Ratte und Maus. *Doc.Ophthalmol.*, 5–6, 452–554.

BUREK, J.D. (1978): Age associated pathology. In: *Pathology of Aging Rats*, Chap. 4, pp. 29–167. CRC Press, West Palm Beach Fl.

BUREK, J.D., VAN DER KOGEL, A.J. and HOLLANDER, C.R. (1976): Degenerative myelopathy in three strains of aging rats. *Vet. Pathol.*, 13, 321–331.

BURNS, R.S., CHIUEH, C.C., MARKEY, S.P., EBERT, M.H., JACOBOWITZ, D.M. and KOPIN, I.J. (1983): A primate model of Parkinsonism: Selective destruction of dopaminergic neurones in the pars compacta of the substantia nigra by N-methyl-4-phenyl-1,2,3,6-tetrahydropyridine. *Proc.Natl.Acad.Sci.*, 80, 4546–4550.

BUTLER, W.H., FORD, G.P. and NEWBERNE, J.W. (1987): A study of the effects of vigabatrin on the central nervous system and retina of Sprague-Dawley and Lister-Hooded rats. *Toxicol.Pathol.*, 15, 143–148.

BUYUKMIHCI, N. and GOEHRING-HARMON, F. (1982): Histology and fine structure of the hamster retinal pigment epithelium. *Acta.Anat.*, 112, 36–46.

CAPPIELLO, V.P. and LAYTON, W.M. (1965): A one year study of ethambutol in dogs: Results of gross and histopathologic examinations. *Toxicol. Appl. Pharmacol.*, 7, 844–849.

CARTER-DAWSON, L., TANKA, M., KUWABARA, T. and BIERI, J.G. (1980): Early corneal changes in vitamin A deficient rats. *Exp.Eye Res.*, 30, 261–268.

CAVANAGH, J.B. (1967): On the pattern of changes in peripheral nerves produced by izoniazid intoxication in rats. *J.Neurol. Neurosurg.Phychiat.*, 30, 26–33.

CHINO, F., KODAMAN, H., HARA, M. and KOMATSU, T. (1984): Evaluation of the neurovirulence test of oral poliovaccines in Japan during the period 1963–1982. *Jpn.J.Med.Sci.Biol.*, 37, 233–240.

CHIU, T, and LEE, K.P. (1983): Auricular chrondropathy in aging rats. *Vet.Pathol.*, 21, 500–504.

CHO, E.S. (1977): Toxic effects of adriamycin on the ganglia of the peripheral nervous system: a neuropathological study. *J. Neuropathol.Exp.Neurol.*, 36, 907–915.

CHO, E.S., SPENCER, P.S. AND JORTNER, B.S. (1980): Doxorubicin. In: P.S.Spencer, and H.H.Schaumburg, (Eds): *Experimental and Clinical Neurotoxicology*, Chap. 30, pp. 430–439. Williams and Wilkins, Baltimore.

COTARD-BARTLEY, M.P., SECCHI, J., GLOMOT, R., and CAVANAGH, J.B. (1981): Spontaneous degenerative lesions of peripheral nerves in aging rats. *Vet.Pathol.*, 18, 110–113.

CREMER, M.A., PITCOCK, J.A., STUART, J.M., KANG, A.H. and TOWNES, A.S. (1981): Auricular chondritis in rats: An experimental model of relapsing polychondritis induced with Type II collagen. *J.Exp. Med.*, 154, 535–540.

CUBEDDU, L.X., HOFFMANN, I.S., FUENMAYOR, N.T. and FINN, A.L. (1990): Efficacy of ondansetron (GR 38032F) and the role of serotonin in cisplatin-induced nausea and vomiting. *N.Engl.J.Med.*, 322, 810–816.

DAGLE, G.E., ZWICKER, G.M. and RENNE, R.A. (1979): Morphology of spontaneous brain tumors in the rat. *Vet.Pathol.*, 16, 318–324.

DAM, M. (1982): Phenytoin toxicity. In: D.M. Woodbury, J.K. Penry, C.E. Peppenger (Eds): *Antiepileptic Drugs*, pp. 247–256. 2nd Edition, Raven Press, New York.

D'AMATO, R.J., LIPMAN, Z.P. and SNYDER, S.H. (1986): Selectivity of the Parkinsonian neurotoxin MPTP: Toxic metabolite MPP$^+$ to neuromelanin. *Science*, 231, 987–989.

D'AMICO, D.J., KENYON, K.R., RUSKIN, J.N. (1981): Amiodarone keratopathy: drug induced lipid storage disease. *Arch. Ophthalmol.*, 99, 257–261.

DAVIDSON, S.I. and RENNIE, I.G. (1986): Ocular toxicity from systemic drug therapy. An overview of clinically important adverse reactions. *Med.Toxicol.*, 1, 217–224.

DAVIS, G.C., WILLIAMS, A.C., MARKEY, S.P., EBERT, M.H., CAINE, E., REICHERT, C.M. and KOPIN, I.J. (1979) Parkinsonism secondary to intravenous injection of meperidine analogues. *Psychiat.Res.*, 1, 249–254.

DIAMOND, M.C. (1987): Sex difference in the rat forebrain. *Brain Res. Reviews*, 12, 235–240.

DOWLING, J.E. and SIDMAN, R.L. (1962): Inherited retinal dystrophy in the rat. *J.Cell Biol.*, 14, 73–109.

DRENKHAHN, D., and LÜLLMANN-RAUCH, R. (1978): Drug-induced retinal lipidosis: Differential susceptibilities of pigment epithelium and neuroretina toward several amphiphilic cationic drugs. *Exp. Mol.Pathol.*, 28, 360–371.

DRENKHAHN, D., JACOBI, B. and LÜLLMANN-RAUCH, R. (1983): Corneal lipidosis in rats treated with amphiphilic cationic drugs. *Arzneimittelforschung*, 33, 827–831.

EDWARDS, C.M. (1988): Chemotherapy induced emesis-mechanisms and treatment: a review. *J.R.Soc.Med.*, 81, 658–662.

EIDA, K., KUBOTA, N., NISHIGAKI, T. and KIKUTANI, M. (1975): Harderian gland. V. Effect of dietary pantothenic acid deficiency on porphyrin biosynthesis in harderian gland of rats. *Chem.Pharm.Bull. (Tokyo)*, 23, 1–4.

ELLIS, W.G., BENCKEN, E., LE COUTEUR, R.A., BARBANO, J.R., WOLFE, B.M. and JENNINGS, M.B. (1988): Neurotoxicity of amphoteracin B methyl ester in dogs. *Toxicol.Pathol.*, 16, 1–9.

ENGSTRÖM, H., ADES, H.W. and HAWKINS, J.E. (1964): Cytoarchitecture of the organ of Corti. *Acta.Oto-Laryngol.Suppl.*, 188, 92–99.

ENVIRONMENTAL PROTECTION AGENCY (1985): Neuropathology. *Fed.Reg.*, 50, 39461–39463.

ESSNER, E. (1987): Role of vesicular transport in breakdown of the blood retinal barrier. *Lab.Invest.*, 56, 457–460.

FABIAN, R., BAND, J. and DROBECK, H. (1967): Induced corneal opacities in the rat. *Br.J.Ophthalmol.*, 51, 124–129.

FIGUEROA, R., WEISS, H., SMITH, J.C., HACKLEY, B.M., McBEAN, L.D., SWASSING, C.R. and HALSTEAD, J.A. (1971): Effect of ethambutol on ocular zinc concentration in dogs. *Am.Rev.Res.Dis.*, 104, 542–594.

FINE, B.A., BERKOW, J.S. and FINE, S. (1968): Corneal calcification. *Science*, 162, 129–130.

FITZGERALD, J.E., SCHARDEIN, J.L. and KURTZ, S.M. (1974): Spontaneous tumours of the nervous system in albino rats. *J.N.C.I.*, 52, 265–273.

FLETCHER, A.P. (1978): Drug safety test and subsequent clinical experience. *J.R.Soc.Med.*, 71, 693–696.

FRASER, H. (1986): Brain tumours in mice, with particular reference to astrocytoma. *Food.Chem.Toxicol.*, 24, 105–111.

FRAUNFELDER, F.T. and BURNS, R.P. (1970): Acute reversible lens opacity: carried by drugs, cold, anoxia asphyxia, stress, death and dehydration. *Exp.Eye Res.*, 10, 19–30.

GARMAN, R.H. (1990): Artefacts in routinely immersion-fixed nervous tissue. *Toxicol.Pathol.*, 18, 149–153.

GHATAK, N.R., SANTOSO, R.A. and McKINNEY, W.M. (1976): Cerebellar degeneration following long-term phenytoin therapy. *Neurology*, 26, 818–820.

GILBARD, J.P., HANNINEN, L.A., ROTHMAN, R.C. and KENYON, K.R. (1987): Lacrymal gland, cornea, and tear film in the NZB/NZWF, hybrid mouse. *Curr.Eye Res.*, 6, 1237–12.

GOODMAN, D.G., WARD, J.M., SQUIRE, R.A., CHU, K.C. and LINHART, M.S. (1979): Neoplastic and non-neoplastic lesions in aging F344 rats. *Toxicol.Appl.Pharmacol.*, 48, 237–248.

GOPINATH, C. (1986): Spontaneous brain tumours in Sprague-Dawley rats. *Food.Chem.Toxicol.*, 24, 113–120.

GOPINATH, C., PRENTICE, D.E. and LEWIS, D,J. (1987): The nervous system. In: *Atlas of Experimental Toxicological Pathology. Current Histopathology Vol 13,* Chap. 9, pp. 137–144. MTP Press, Lancaster.

GORSKI, R.A., GORDON, J.J., SHRYNE, J.E. and SOUTHHAM, A.M. (1978): Evidence for a morphological sex difference within the medial preoptic area of the rat brain. *Brain Res.,* 148, 333–346.

GOUGH, A.W., HANNA, W., BARSOUM, N.J., MOORE, J. and STURGESS, J.M. (1986): Morphologic and immunohistochemical features of two spontaneous peripheral nerve tumours in Wistar rats. *Vet. Pathol.,* 23, 68–73.

GRAYSON, M. (1979): Diseases of the cornea. In: *Diseases of Lipid Metabolism,* pp. 388–395. Mosby, St Louis.

GRIFFIN, D.E. and HESS, J.L. (1986): Cells with natural killer activity in the CSF of normal and athymic nude mice with acute Sindbis virus encephalitis. *J.Immunol.,* 136, 1841–1845.

GRIFFIN, D.E., HESS, J.L. and MOENCH, T.R. (1987): Immune responses in the central nervous system. *Toxicol.Pathol.,* 15, 294–302.

HALL, L.B., YOSHITOMI, K. and BOORMAN, G.A. (1987): Pathologic features of abdominal and thoracic paragangliomas in F344/N rats. *Vet.Pathol.,* 24, 315–322.

HARKNESS, J.E. and RIDGEWAY, M.D.(1980): Chromodacyorrhea in laboratory rats (Rattus norvegicus). Etiological considerations. *Lab.Anim.Sci.,* 30, 841–844.

HAUSER, S.L., WEINER, H.L., BHAN, A.K., SHAPIRO, M.E., CHE, M., ADRICH, W.R. and LETVIN, N.L. (1984): Lyt-1 cells mediate acute murine experimental allergic encephalomyelitis. *J.Immunol.,* 133, 2288–2290.

HEYWOOD, R. (1971): Drug-induced lenticular lesions in the dog. *Br. Vet.J.,* 127, 301–303.

HEYWOOD, R. (1974): An unusual case of retinal atrophy in the beagle dog. *J.Small Anim.Pract.,* 15, 189–191.

HEYWOOD, R. (1974): Drug-induced retinopathies in the beagle dog. *Br. Vet.J.,* 130, 564–569.

HEYWOOD, R., SORTWELL, R.J. and PRENTICE, D.E. (1978): The toxicity of 1-amino-3-chloro-2-propanol hydrochloride (CL 88,236) in the rhesus monkey. *Toxicology,* 9, 219–225.

HOFFMAN, R.W., YANG, J.E., WAGGIE, K.S., DURHAM, J.B., BURGE, J.R. and WALKER, S.E. (1983): Band keratopathy in MRL/l and MRL/n mice. *Arthritis and Rheum.,* 26, 645–652.

HRUBAN, Z. (1984): Pulmonary and generalized lysosomal storage disorders induced by amphiphilic drugs. *Environ.Health Perspect.,* 55, 53–76.

JACOBS, J.M. (1980): Vascular permeability and neural injury. In: P.S. Spencer and H.H. Schaumburg (Eds): *Experimental and Clinical Neurotoxicology,* Chap 8, pp. 102–117. Williams and Wilkins, Baltimore.

JELLINGER, K. (1977): Neuropathologic findings after neuroleptic long-term therapy. In: L. Roizin, H. Shiraki and N. Grcevic (Eds): *Neurotoxicology,* pp. 25–42. Raven Press, New York.

JOHNSON, R.T., BURKE, D.S., ELWELL, M., LEAKE, C.J., NISALAK, A., HOKE, C.H. and LORSOMRUDEE, W. (1985): Japanese encephalitis: Immunocytochemical studies of viral antigen and inflammatory cells in fatal cases. *Ann.Neurol.,* 19, 567–573.

JOHNSON, R.T., INTRALAWAN, P. and PUAPANWATTON, S. (1986): Japanese encephalitis: Identification of inflammatory cells in the cerebospinal fluid. *Ann.Neurol.,* 20, 691–695.

JONES, H.B. (1988): The role of ultrastructural investigations in neurotoxicology. *Toxicology,* 49, 3–15.

JONES, R.D. (1986): Epidemiology of brain tumours in man and their relationship with chemical agents. *Food.Chem.Toxicol.,* 24, 99–103.

JORDAN, F.L. and THOMAS, W.E. (1988): Brain macrophages: questions of origin and interrelationships. *Brain Res.Rev.,* 13, 165–178.

JOSEPH, E.C., BETTON, G.R., BARNETT, K.C. and FACCINI, J.M. (1988): The toxicology and pathology of 5-aminosalicylic acid keratoconjunctivitis sicca in the beagle dog. *Toxicologist,* 8, 131.

KAHN H.J., MARKS, A., THOM, H. and BAUMAL, R. (1983): Role of antibody to S100 protein in diagnostic pathology. *Am.J.Clin.Pathol.,* 79, 341–347.

KAPLUN, A. and BARISHAK, R.Y. (1976): Appearance of keratitis in laboratory mice: influence of azathioprine and meticorten. *Lab. Anim.* 10, 105–109.

KARIM, A.E.A., JACOB, T.J.C. and THOMPSON, G.M. (1988): The human lens epithelium; morphological and ultrastructural changes associated with steroid therapy. *Exp.Eye Res.*, 48,, 215–224.

KEELER, C. (1924): The inheritance of a retinal abnormality in white mice. *Proc.Natl.Acad.Sci.USA*, 10, 329–333.

KLINTWORTH, G.K. and BURGER, P.C. (1983): Neovascularization of the cornea: Current concepts of its pathogenesis. *Int.Ophthalmol. Clin.*, 23, 27–39.

KLONNE, D.R., DODD, D.E., BALLANTYNE, B. and LOSCO, P.E. (1988): Multispecies comparison of corneal lesions produced during a two-week vapor exposure to propylene glycol monopropyl ether. *Toxicologist*, 8, 130.

KOESTNER, A. (1986): The brain-tumour issue in long-term toxicity studies in rats. *Food Chem.Toxicol.*, 24, 139–143.

KOESTNER, A., SWENBERG, J.A. and WECHSLER, W. (1972): Experimental tumors of the nervous system induced by resorptive N-nitrosourea compounds. *Prog.Exp.Tumor Res.*, 17, 9–30.

KÖHLER, C., ERIKSSON, L.G., HANSSON, T., WARNER, M. and AKE-GUSTAFSSON, J.(1988): Immunohistochemical localization of cytochrome P-450 in the rat brain. *Neurosci.Lett.*, 84, 109–114.

KOIZUMI, H., WATANABE, M., NUMATA, H., SAKAI, T. and MORISHITA, H. (1986): Species difference in vacuolation of the choroid plexus induced by the piperidine-ring drug disobutamide in the rat, dog and monkey. *Toxicol.Appl.Pharmacol.*, 84, 125–148.

KONDO, H., TAKAHASHI, H. and TAKAHASHI, Y. (1984): Immunohistochemical study of S-100 protein in the postnatal development of Müller cells and astrocytes in the rat retina. *Cell Tissue Res.*, 238, 503–508.

KRINKE, G. (1983): Spinal radiculoneuropathy in aging rats: Demyelination secondary to neuronal dwindling? *Acta. Neuropathol.(Berl)*, 59, 63–69.

KRINKE, G.J. (1988): Effects of neurotoxins on the nervous system of rats. In: *The Nervous System of Laboratory Animals*. A Histopathology Seminar, International Life Science Institute, Hannover.

KRINKE, G., NAYLOR, D.C., SCHMID, S., FRÖHLICH, E. and SCHNIDER, K. (1985): The incidence of naturally occurring primary brain tumours in the laboratory rat. *J.Comp.Pathol.*, 95, 175–192.

KRINKE, G., SUTER, J. and HESS, R. (1981): Radicular myelinopathology in aging rats. *Vet.Pathol.*, 18, 335–341.

KRUEGER, G. (1971): Mapping of the mouse brain for screening procedures with the light microscope. *Lab.Anim.Sci.*, 21, 91–105.

KUGLER, P. (1988): Quantitative enzyme histochemistry in the brain. *Histochemistry*, 90, 99–107.

LAI, Y-L., JACOBY, R.O. and JONAS, A.M. (1978). Age-related and light-associated retinal changes in Fischer rats. *Invest. Ophthalmol.Vis.Sci.*, 17, 634–638.

LAI, Y-L., JACOBY, R.O., JONAS, A.M. and PAPERMASTER, D.S. (1975): A new form of hereditary retinal degeneration in Wag/Rij rats. *Invest.Ophthalmol*, 14, 62–67.

LAI, Y-L., JACOBY, R.O. and YAO, P.C. (1979): Animal model: peripheral degeneration in rats. *Am.J.Pathol.*, 97, 449–452.

LANGSTON, J.W. and BALLARD, P.A. (1983): Parkinson's disease in a chemist working with 1-methyl-4-phenyl-1,2,3,6-tetrahydropyridine. *N.Engl.J.Med.*, 309, 310.

LE GOASCOGNE, C., ROBEL, R., GOUEZOU, M., SENANES, N., BAULIEU, E-E. and WATERMAN, M. (1987): Neurosteroids: cytochrome P-450 scc in rat brain. *Science*, 237, 1212–1215.

LEURE-DUPREE, A.E. (1986): Vascularization of the rat cornea after prolonged zinc deficiency. *Anat.Rec.*, 216, 27–32.

LEVINE, S. (1987): Choroid plexus: Target for systemic disease and pathway to the brain. *Lab.Invest.*, 56, 231–233.

LEVINE, S. and SOWINSKI, R. (1974): Cyclophosphamide-induced cerebral and visceral lesions in rats: enhancement by endotoxin. *Arch.Pathol.*, 98, 177–182.

806

LEVINE, S. and SOWINSKI, R. (1977): T-lymphocyte depletion and lesions of the choroid plexus and kidney induced by tertiary amines in rats. *Toxicol.Appl.Pharmacol.*, 40, 147–159.

LEWIS, G.P., ERICKSON, P.A., KASKA, D.D. and FISHER, S.K. (1988): An immunocytochemical comparison of Müller cells and astrocytes in the cat retina. *Exp.Eye Res.*, 47, 839–853.

LI, I. and TURNER, J.E. (1988): Inherited retinal degeneration in the RCS rat: Prevention of photoreceptor degeneration by pigment epilthlial cell transplantation. *Exp.Eye Res.*, 47, 911–917.

LIN, W-L., and ESSNER, E. (1987): An electron microscopic study of retinal degeneration in Sprague-Dawley rats. *Lab.Anim.Sci.*, 37, 180–186.

LIN, W-L. and ESSNER, E. (1988): Retinal dystrophy in Wistar-Furth rats. *Exp.Eye Res.*, 46, 1–12.

LOSCO, P.E. and TROUP, C.M. (1988): Corneal dystrophy in Fischer 344 rats. *Lab.Anim.Sci.*, 38, 702–710.

LUBEK, B.M., AVARIA, M., BASU, P.K. and WELLS, P.G. (1988): Pharmacological studies on the in vivo cataractogenicity of acetaminophen in mice and rabbits. *Fundam.Appl.Toxicol.*, 10, 596–606.

LUDWIN, S.K. and ENG, L.F. (1976): The topographical distribution of S-100 and GFA proteins in the adult rat brain: An immunohistochemical study using horseradish peroxidene-labelled antibodies. *J.Comp.Neurol.*, 165, 197–209.

LUGINBÜHL, H., FANKHAUSER, R. and McGRATH, J.T. (1968): Spontaneous neoplasms of the nervous system in animals. *Prog.Neurol.Surg.*, 2, 85–164.

LUITEN, P.G.M., WOUTERLOOD, F.G., MATSUYAMA, T., STROSBERG, A.D., BUWALDA, B. and GAYKEMA, R.P.A. (1988): Immunocytochemical applications in neuroanatomy. Demonstration of connections, transmitters, and receptors. *Histochemistry*, 90, 85–97.

LÜLLMANN-RAUCH, R. (1979): Drug-induced lysosomal disorders. In: J.T. Dingle, P.J. Jaques and I.H. Shaw (Eds): *Lysosomes in Applied Biology and Therapeutics 6*, Chap 6, pp. 49–130. North Holland, Amsterdam.

LÜLLMANN, H. and LÜLLMANN-RAUCH, R. (1981): Tamoxifen-induced generalized lipidosis in rats subchronically treated with high doses. *Toxicol.Appl.Pharmacol.*, 61, 138–146.

LÜLLMANN, H., LÜLLMANN-RAUCH, R. and WASSERMAN, O. (1975): Drug-induced phospholipidoses. *CRC Crit.Rev.Toxicol.*, 4, 185–218.

LÜTJEN-DRECOLL, E. and TAMM, E.(1988): Morphological study of the auterior segment of cynomolgous monkey eyes following treatment with prortaglandin F_2 α. *Exp.Eye Res.*, 47, 761–769.

MACDONALD, J.S., GERSON, R.J., KORNBRUST, D.J., KLOSS, M.W., PRAHALADA, S., BERRY, P.H., ALBERTS, A.W. and BOKELMAN, D.L. (1988): Preclinical evaluation of lovastatin. *Am.J.Cardiol.*, 62, 16J–27J.

MAILMAN, R.B. (1987): Mehanisms of CNS injury in behavioural dysfunction. *Neurotoxicol.Teratol.*, 9, 417–426.

MAJEED, S.K., PRENTICE, D.E. and HEYWOOD, R. (1983): A form of kerato-conjunctivitis sicca in dogs treated with an anti-spasmodic compound. *J.Pathol.*, 140, 133.

MARSDEN, C.D. and JENNER, P. (1980): The pathophysiology of extrapyramidal side-effects of neuroceptic drugs. *Psychol.Med.*, 10, 55–72.

MARTIN, C.L. and ANDERSON, B.G. (1981): Ocular anatomy. In: K.N.Gelatt (Ed.): *Textbook of Veterinary Ophthalmology*, Chap 2, pp. 12–121. Lea and Febiger, Philadelphia.

MASSA, T., DAVIS, G.J., SHIAVO, D.M., SINHA, R.J., BLACK, H.E. and SCHWARTZ, E. (1984): Tapetal changes in beagle dogs. II Ocular changes after intravenous administration of a macrolide antibiotic-rosamicin. *Toxicol.Appl.Pharmacol.*, 72, 195–200.

McCUNE, W.J., SCHILLER, A.C., DYNESIUS-TRENTHAM, R.A, and TRENTHAM, D.E. (1982): Type II collagen-induced auricular chondritis. *Arthritis Rheum.*, 25, 266–273.

McGEE, M.A. and MARONPOT, R.R. (1979): Harderian gland dacryoadenitis in rats resulting from orbital bleeding. *Lab.Anim.Sci.*, 29, 639-641.

MENNEL, H.D. and ZÜLCH, K.J. (1976): Tumours of the central and peripheral nervous system. In: V.S. Turusov (Ed.): *Pathology of Tumours in Laboratory Animals Vol 1. Tumours of the Rat, Part 2*, pp. 295–311. IARC Scientific Publ. No. 6, Lyon.

MIKAYE, T. (1984): Identification of neonatal brain macrophages by lectin histochemistry. *Acta.Histochem.Cytochem.*, 17, 279–282.

MITTLE, R., GALIN, M.A., OPPERMAN, W., CAMERINI-DAVALOS, R.A. and SPIOR, D. (1970): Corneal calcification in spontaneously diabetic mice. *Invest.Ophthalmol.*, 9, 137–145.

MITSUMORI, K., MARONPOT, R.R. and BOORMAN, G.A. (1987)a: Spontaneous tumors of the meninges in rats. *Vet.Pathol.*, 24, 50–58.

MITSUMORI, K., DITTRICH, K.L., STEFANSKI, S., TALLEY, F.A. and MARONPOT, R.R. (1987)b: Immunohistochemical and electron microscopic study of meningeal granular cell tumors in rats. *Vet.Pathol.*, 24, 356–359.

MORGAN, K.T., FRITH, C.H., SWENBERG, J.A., McGRATH, J.T., ZÜLCH, K.J. and CROWDER, D.M. (1984): A morphologic classification of brain tumors found in several strains of mice. *J.N.C.I.*, 72, 151–160.

MUIRHEAD, J.R. and TOMAZZOLI-GEROSA, L. (1984): Animal models of band keratopathy. In: K. Tabbara and R. Cello (Eds): *Animal Models of Ocular Disease*, pp. 221–232. Thomas, Springfield.

MURPHY, J.C., OSTERBERG, R.E., SEABAUGH, V.M. and BIERBOWER, G.W., (1982): Ocular irritancy responses to various pHs of acids and bases without irrigation. *Toxicology*, 23, 281–291.

NADA, O. and KAWANA, T. (1988): Immunohistochemical identification of supportive cell types in the enteric nervous system of the rat colon and rectum. *Cell Tissue Res.*, 251, 523–529.

NIELSON, E.B. and LYON, M. (1978): Evidence for cell loss in corpus striatum after long-term treatment with a neuroleptic drug (flupenthixol) in rats. *Psychopharmacology*, 59, 85–89.

NOELL, W.K., WALKER, V.S., KANG, B.S. and BERMAN, S. (1966): Retinal damage by light in rats. *Invest.Ophthalmol.*, 5, 450–473.

O'CONNER, G.R. (1972): Calcific band keratopathy. *Trans.Am.Ophthalmol.Soc.*, 70, 58–81.

OLNEY, J.W. (1980): Excitotoxic mechanisms of neurotoxicity. In: P.S. Spencer and H.H. Schaumberg (Eds): *Experimental and Clinical Neurotoxicology*, Chap. 19, pp. 272–294. Williams and Wilkins, Baltimore.

PAKKENBERG, H., FOG, R. and NILAKANTAN, B. (1973): The long-term effects of perphenazine enanthate on the rat brain. Some metabolic and anatomical findings. *Psychopharmacolgia(Berl)*, 29, 329–336.

PALKOVITS, M. (1983): Stereotaxic map, cytorachitectonic and neurochemical summary of the hypothalamic nuclei. In: T.C. Jones U. Mohr and R.D. Hunt (Eds): *Endocrine System*, pp. 316–331. Springer-Verlag, Berlin.

PARDRIDGE, W.M. (1988): Recent advances in blood-brain barrier transport. *Ann.Rev.Pharma-col.Toxicol.*, 28, 25–39.

PEYMAN, G.A. and APPLE, D. (1972): Peroxidase diffusion processes in the opticnerve. *Arch.Oph-thalmol.*, 88, 650–654.

PLISS, P.G. (1973): Tumours of the auditory sebaceous glands. In: V.S. Turusov (Ed.): *Pathology of Tumours in Laboratory Animals, Vol. I, Tumours of the Rat, Part 1*, pp. 23–30. IARC Scientific Publ. No. 5, Lyon.

POUR, P., ALTHOFF, J., SALMASI, S.Z., and STEPAN, K. (1979): Spontaneous tumors and common diseases in three types of hamster. *J.N.C.I.*, 63, 797–811.

PRIEUR, D.J., UUNG, D.M. and COUNTS, D.F. (1984): Auricular chrondritis in fawn-hooded rats: A spontaneous disorder resembling that induced by immunization with type II collagen. *Am.J.Pathol.*, 116, 69–76.

PURO, D.G. and WOODWARD, D.J. (1973): Effects of diphenylhydantoin on activity of rat cerebellar Purkinji cells. *Neuropharmacology*, 12, 433–440.

RAPOPORT, S.I. (1977): Osmotic opening of blood-brain and blood-ocular barriers. *Exp.Eye Res.25.Suppl.*, 499–509.

REITER, L.W.(1987): Neurotoxicology in regulation and risk assessment. *Dev.Pharmacol.Ther.*, 10, 354–368.

RHODIN, J.A.G. (1974): Eye. In: *Histology. A Text and Atlas*, Chap. 35, pp. 750–772. Oxford University Press, New York.

ROBERTSON, D.G., GRAY, R.H. and DE LA IGLESIA, F.A. (1987): Quantitative assessment of trimethyltin induced pathology of the hippocampus. *Toxicol.Pathol.*, 15, 7–17.

ROERIG, D.L., HASEGAWA, A.T., HARRIS, G.J., LYNCH, K.L. and WANG, R.I.H. (1980): Occurrence of corneal opacities in rats after acute administration of 1-α-acetylmethadol. *Toxicol.Appl.Pharmacol.*, 56, 155–163.

RUBIN, L.F. (1974): Atlas of Veterinary Ophthalmoscopy. Lea and Febiger, Philadephia.

RUBIN, L.F. and SAUNDERS, L.Z. (1965): Intraocular larva migrans in dogs. *Pathol.Vet.*, 2, 566–573.

RUBINSTEIN, L.J. (1972): Classification and grading. In: *Tumors of the Central Nervous System. Atlas of Tumor Pathology Second Series Fascicle 6*, pp. 7–17. Armed Forces Institute of Pathology, Washington DC.

RUBINSTEIN, L.J. (1982): Diagnostic applicability of GFA protein immunoperoxidase staining. In: *Tumors of the Central Nervous System. Supplement, Fascicle 6, Second Series*, pp. 21–30. ArmedForces Institute of Pathology, Washington DC.

SAKAI, T. (1981): The mammalian harderian gland: Morphology, biochemistry and physiology. *Arch.Histol.Jpn.*, 44, 299–333.

SALAHUDDIN, T.S., JOHANSSON, B.B., KALIMO, H. and OLSSON, Y. (1988): Structural changes in the rat brain after carotid infusions of hyperosmolar solutions. A light microscopic and immunohistochemical study. *Neuropathol.Appl.Neurobiol.*, 14, 467–482.

SALCMAN, M., DEFENDINI, R.L., CORRELL, J. and GILMAN, S. (1978): Neuropathological changes in cerebellar biopsies of epileptic patients. *Ann.Neurol.*, 3, 10–19.

SCHAUMBURG, H.H. and SPENCER, P.S. (1979): Toxic models of certain disorders of the nervous system: a teaching monograph. *Neurotoxicology*, 1, 209–220.

SCHAUMBURG, H.H. and SPENCER, P.S. (1980): Clioquinol. In: P.S. Spencer and H.H. Schaumburg (Eds): *Experimental and Clinical Neurotoxicology*, Chap 27, pp. 395–406. Williams and Wilkins, Baltimore.

SCHAUMBURG, H.H., SPENCER, P.S., KRINKE, G., THOMANN, P. and HESS, R. (1978): The CNS distal axonopathy in dogs intoxicated with clioquinol. *J.Neuropathol.Exp.Neurol.*, 37, 686.

SCHIAVO, D.M. (1972): Retinopathy from administration an imidazo quinazoline to beagles. *Toxicol.Appl.Pharmacol.*, 23, 782–783.

SCHIAVO, D.M., GREEN, J.D., TRAINA, V.M., SPAET, R. and ZAIDI, I. (1988): Tapetal changes in beagle dogs following oral administration of CGS14796C, a potential aromatase inhibitor. *Fundam.Appl.Toxicol.*, 10, 329–334.

SCHIAVO, D.M., SINHA, D.P., BLACK, H., ARTHAUD, L., MASSA, T., MURPHY, B.F., SZOT, R.J. AND SCHWARTZ, E. (1984): Tapetal changes in beagle dogs, 1. Ocular changes after oral administration of a beta-adrenergic blocking agent, SCH 19927. *Toxicol.Appl.Pharmacol.*, 72, 187–194.

SCHMECHEL, D.E. (1985): γ-Subunit of the glycolytic enzyme enolase: Nonspecific or neuron specific? *Lab.Invest.*, 52, 239–242.

SCHMIDT, G.M. AND COULTER, D.B. (1981): Physiology of the eye. In: K.N. Gelatt (Ed.): *Textbook of Veterinary Ophthalmology*, Chap. 44, pp. 129–159. Lea and Febiger, Philadelphia.

SERA, K., HARADA, Y., TAGASHIRA, N., SUZUKI, M., HIRAKAWA, K. and OHYA, T. (1987): Morphological changes in the vestibular epithelia and ganglion induced by ototoxic drug. *Scanning Microscopy*, 1, 1191–1197.

SHELDON, W. (1990): The effects of a calorically restricted diet upon the occurrence of a spontaneous leucodystrophy in old B6C3F1 female mice. IX International Symposium of Society of Toxicologic Pathologists, Ottawa, Canada.

SHELDON, W.G., CURTIS, M., KODELL, R.L. and WEED, L. (1983): Primary harderian gland neoplasms in mice. *J.N.C.I.*, 71, 61–68.

SHICHI, H., GAASTERLAND, E.E., JENSEN, N.M. and NEBERT, D.W. (1978): Ah Locus: Genetic differences in susceptibility to cataracts induced by acetaminophen. *Science*, 200, 539–541.

SOBEL, R.A., BLANCHETTE, B.W., BHAN, A.K. and COLUIN, R.B. (1984): The immunopathology of experimental allergic encephalitis. 1. quantitative analysis of inflammatory cells in situ. *J.Immunol.*, 132, 2392–2401.

SOLLEVELD, H.A., BIGNER, D.D., AVERILL, D.R., BIGNER, S.H., BOORMAN, G.A., BURGER, P.C., GILLESPIE, Y., HUBBARD, G.B., LAERUM, O.C., McCOMB, R.D., Mc-GRATH, J.T., MORGAN, K.T., PETERS, A., RUBINSTEIN, L.J., SCHOENBERG, B.S., SCHOLD, S.C., SWENBERG, J.A., THOMPSON, M.B., VANDEVELDE, M and VINORES, S.A. (1986):Brain tumors in man and animals. Report of a workshop. *Environ.Health Res.*, 68, 155–173.

SPANGLER, W.L., WARING, G.O. and MORRIN, L.A. (1982): Oval lipid corneal opacities in beagles. V. Ultrastucture. *Vet.Pathol.*, 19, 150–159.

SPENCER, P.S., BISCHOFF, M.C. and SCHAUMBURG, H.H. (1980): Neuropathological methods for the detection of neurotoxic disease. In: P.S. Spencer and H.H. Schaumburg (Eds): *Experimental and Clinical Neurotoxicology*, Chap 50, pp. 743–757. Williams and Wilkins, Baltimore.

SPIKE, R.C., JOHNSON, H.S., McGADEY, J., MOORE, M.R., THOMPSON, G.G. and PAYNE, A.P. (1985): Quantitative studies on the effects of hormones on structure and prophyrin biosynthesisin the harderian gland of the female golden hamster. 1. The effects of ovariectomy and androgen administration. *J.Anat.*,142, 59–72.

STERMAN, A.B. and SCHAUMBURG, H.H. (1980): Neurotoxicity of selected drugs. In: P.S. Spencer and H.H. Schaumburg (Eds): *Experimental and Clinical Neurotoxicology*, Chap. 41, pp. 593–612, Williams and Wilkins, Baltimore.

STRANGE, P.G. (1988): The structure and mechanism of neurotransmitter receptors. Implications for the structure and function of the central nervous system. *Biochem.J.*, 249, 309–318.

SUMI, N., STAVROU, D., FROHBERG, H., and JOCHMANN, G. (1976): The incidence of spontaneous tumours of the central nervous system of Wistar rats. *Arch.Toxicol.*, 35, 1–13.

SZALAY, J., NUNZIATA, B. and HENKIND, P. (1975): Permeability of iridalblood vessels. *Exp.Eye Res.*, 21, 531–543.

TARADACH, C. and GREAVES, P. (1984): Spontaneous eye lesions in laboratory animals: Incidence in relation to age. *CRC Critical Rev.Toxicol.*, 12, 121–147.

TOWFIGHI, J. (1980): Hexachlorophene. In: P.S. Spencer, and H.H. Schaumburg (Eds): *Experimental and Clinical Neurotoxicology*, Chap 31, pp. 440–455. Williams and Wilkins, Baltimore.

TOWFIGHI, J., GONATAS, N.K. and McCREE, L. (1974): Hexochlorophene-induced changes in central and peripheral myelinated axons of developing and adult rats. *Lab.Invest.*, 31, 712–721.

VAN ELDIK, L.J., JENSEN, R.A., EHRENFRIED, B.A. and WHETSELL, W.O. (1986): Imunohistochemical localization of S100β in human nervous system tumours using monclonal antibodies with specificity for the S100β polypeptide. *J.Histochem.Cytochem.*, 34, 977–982.

VAN WINKLE, T.J. and BALK, M.W. (1986): Spontaneous corneal opacities in laboratory mice. *Lab.Anim.Sci.*, 36, 248–255.

VOLK, B., AMELIZAD, Z., ANAGNOSTOPOULOS, J., KNOTH, R., and OESCH, F. (1988): First evidence of cytochrome P450 induction in the mouse brain by phenytoin. *Neurosci.Lett.*, 84, 219–224.

VON SALLMAN, L. and GRIMES, P., (1972): Spontaneous retinal degeneration in mature Osborne-Mendel rats. *Arch.Opthalmol.*, 88, 404–411.

WARD, J.M., GOODMAN, D.G., SQUIRE, R.A., CHU, K.C. and LINHART, M.S. (1979): Neoplastic and non-neoplastic lesions in aging (C57BL/6N x C3H/HeN)F, (B6C3F₁) mice. *J.N.C.I.*, 63, 849–854.

WEIGENT, D.A. and BLALOCK, J.E. (1987): Interactions between the neuroendocrine and immune systems: Common hormones and receptors. *Immunol.Rev.*, 100, 79–108.

WEISSE, I., SEITZ, R. and STEGMAN, H. (1981): Eine multifokale seröse Chorioretinitis beim Beagle. *Vet.Pathol.*, 18, 1–12.

WEISSE, I., STÖTZER, H. and SEITZ, R., (1974): Age and light-dependent changes in the rat eye. *Virchows.Arch.[A.]*, 362, 145–156.

WELLER, R.O. (1986): Brain tumours in man. *Food.Chem.Toxicol.*, 24, 91–98.

WORDEN, A.N., HEYWOOD, R., PRENTICE, D.E., CHESTERMAN, H., SKERRETT, K. and THOMANN, P.E. (1978): Clioquinol toxicity in the dog. *Toxicology*, 9, 227–238.

ZÜLCH, K.J. (1980): Principles of the new World Health Organization (WHO) classification of brain tumours. *Neuroradiology*, 19, 59–66.

Subject index

renal osteodystrophy, 153
bone marrow, 77-85
    atrophy, 84
    hyperplasia, 85
    hypocellularity, 84
brain, 765-779
    axonal lesions, 772-773
    demyelination, 772
    gliosis, focal, 778
    neoplasia, 775-779
    neuronopathies, 765-768
    phospholipidosis, 768-769
    vacuolation, 769-772
    vascular lesions, 773-774
bromocriptine, 12-14, 16-17, 68, 257, 424, 513,
    539, 660-661, 663
bronchial associated lymphoid tissue (BALT),
    196-198
bronchus
    see lung
bucetin, 551
bupivicaine, 169
bupropion, 438
buserelin, 609, 614-615, 617, 690
busulphan, 208
BW58C, 532, 538
BW540C, 532, 538
BW134U, 12
BW755C, 306

C-cells, 723-738
    hyperplasia, 737-738
caecum
    see intestine, large
caerulein, 449
caffeine, 6, 291, 348
calcium channel blockers, 232, 237, 281-282,
    616, 711
captopril, 81, 424, 512-514, 543, 704
carcinoid tumour
    stomach (glandular), 321-323
carcinoma
    auditory sebaceous gland, 801-802
    bladder, 560
    liver, 439-441
    mammary gland, 61-64
    pancreas, exocrine, 459-460
    skin, 21-22
cardiomyopathy, hamster, 234-235
carmustine, 208
carotene, 13-14
cartilage, 156-164
    atrophy, 162
    degeneration, 158-162

cataract, 790-792
cephalosporins, 79, 83, 608
cervix, 630-632
    adenosis, 631-632
    metaplasia, squamous, 631
CGS 14796 C, 797-798
CGS 18302 B, 661
chlorcyclizine, 210, 797
chlordiazepoxide (Librium), 53
chloroquine, 12-13, 174-175, 214, 244, 279, 768,
    788
chlorphentermine, 210, 213, 263, 768
chlorpromazine, 13, 443
cholangioma, 436
cholestasis, 442-444
chondrosarcoma, 154
choroid plexus, 774-775
    inflammation, 774-775
    vacuolation, 775
chromodacryorrhea, 783
CI-918, 449
CI-936, 449
CI-959, 232-233
cimetidine, 79, 83, 323-325, 590, 614, 617
cinoxacin, 156
ciprofibrate, 456
ciprofloxacin, 159
cirrhosis, 438-439
cisplatin, 441, 541, 549, 762
CL 115, 574, 299
clavulanic acid, clavulanate, 402
clindamycin, 356
clioquinol, 773
clofibrate, 171-172, 406-408, 733
clonidine, 348
closantel, 596
clotrimazole, 701-702
clozapine, 728
colchicine, 173, 402, 447, 523
colon
    see intestine, large
colitis, 355-363
congestion
    lung, 207
    spleen, 102-103
conjunctiva, 783
contact dermatitis, 7-9
cornea, 784-789
    dystrophy, 787-788
    inflammation, 785-786
    mineralisation, 787-788
    neovascularisation, 787
    phospholipidosis, 788
    pigmentation, 789

813

bone marrow, 85
bronchus, 214-216
C-cell, 737-738
endometrium, 641-643
forestomach, 297-300
gingiva, 281-282
intestine, large, 364-367
intestine, small, 346-349
islets of Langerhans, 468-469
Leydig (interstitial) cell, 612-615
liver, 403-406
lung, 214-216
lymph nodes, 98-100
juxtaglomerular apparatus, 543-544
mammary gland, 53-57
ovary, 662-663
pancreas, exocrine, 451-453
parathyroid gland, 740-741
pituitary gland, 686-692
prostate gland, 592-593
salivary gland, 291-292
skin, 18
spleen, 108
stomach (glandular), 314-320
thymus, 114
thyroid, 728-733
urothelium, kidney, 548-549
urothelium, bladder, 557-560
hyperplastic nodule
adrenal cortex, 712-713
liver, 426-438
pancreas, exocrine, 457-459
hyperpyrexia (hyperthermia), malignant, 172
hypertrophy
adrenal cortex, 707-711
blood vessels, pulmonary, 265-267
blood vessels, systemic, 261-262
heart, 231-233
intestine, small, 346-349
liver, 403-406
renal tubular, 539-540
juxtaglomerular apparatus, 543-544
pancreas, exocrine, 451-452
pituitary gland, 686-692
salivary gland, 291-292
skeletal muscle, 177
stomach (glandular), 314-316
thyroid, 728-733

ibopamine, 513
ibuprofen, 340
ICI 17,363, 345-346
ICI 53,072, 407-408
ICI 125,211 (tiotidine), 321, 324

ICI 153,110, 258, 262, 348
ICI 162,848, 323
ileum
see intestine, small
imidazole antifungals, 404, 406, 424, 602, 662, 701-702, 704
immune complex deposition, 513-515
immunocytochemistry
heart, 230
islet cell neoplasms, 470-471
intestine, small, 327-333
Langerhans cell, 2-3
lung, 196-198
lymphoid cells, 87-95
nasal mucosa, 190
renal, 506-507
mammary gland, 52
mesenchymal neoplasms, 25-26
myocardium, 230
nervous system, 759-761
prostate gland, 587-588
skeletal muscle, 166
skin, 2-3
stomach (glandular), 302-303
immunotoxicology, 85-87
implantation
skeletal muscle, 170
subcutaneous, 11, 34-36, 154
indacrinone (MK-196), 540
indomethacin, 306-307, 339-340, 361
infarction
heart, 233
kidney, 542
infection
intestine, large, 356-359
intestine, small, 334-339
lung, 200-203
skeletal muscle, 170-171
skin, 3-5
infestation
intestine, large, 359-361
intestine, small, 334-339
lung, 201-202
skin, 3-5
inflammation
adrenal cortex, 700
cornea, 785-786
epididymis, 595-596
forestomach, 296-297
heart, 233-241
intestine, large, 355-363
intestine, small, 334-341
islets of Langerhans, 462-468
lacrimal gland, 783-784

intestine, small, 353-354
  mammary gland, 52
mucus depletion
  stomach, 308-309
muzolimine, 527
myeloid bodies, myelinosomes
  adrenal cortex, 702
  kidney, 525
  liver, 419-420
myocarditis, 233-241
myopathy, spheromembranous, 173-174

naevus (benign melanoma), 22
nafenopin, 409
nail loss (onychoptosis), 11-13
nalidixic acid, 159
nasal sinus, 189-192
  inflammation, 191-192
  ulceration, 191-192
nasopharynx, 189-192
necrosis
  adrenal cortex, 700
  bone, 146
  heart, 233-241
  liver, centrilobular, 412-413
  liver, focal, 412
  liver, periportal, 413
  liver, single cell, 413-414
  ovary, 655
  renal papilla, 544-545
  renal tubular, 523-525
  salivary gland, 288-290
  skeletal muscle, 166-170
  skin, 3-13
  testis, 603-605
neomycin, 366
neoplastic nodule, liver, 426-441
nephroblastoma, 551-552
neuroectodermal tumours, 776-778, 780-781
neuronopathies, 765-768
neurotoxicology, 756-765
nicorandil, 245
nicotinamide, 471
nifedipine, 281
nimodopine, 711
nitrendipine, 711
nitrofurantoin, 416, 659, 664, 773
nitrosation
  stomach, 323-325
nitrous oxide, 172
nonoxynol-9, 630
noradrenaline (norepinephrine), 231-232, 236-237, 251, 253
norfloxacin, 159

norlestrin, 53, 70, 639, 645, 658-659
nose, 189-192
nystatin, 523

oedema
  lung, 206-207
  skin, 7
oesophagus, 294-295
  impaction, 294
  irritation studies, 295
  megaoesophagus, 294-295
oestrogens, 13, 53, 67-68, 120, 150, 155-156, 438, 443, 449, 541, 590-593, 609-612, 615-617, 631-632,638-642, 645-646, 649, 658-660, 688-691, 694-695, 703-704, 783
oestrogen-progestogen combinations, 16, 53-56, 64, 68-71, 263, 420, 425-427, 438, 440-441, 443, 467, 562, 636, 638-642, 649, 655, 658-659, 688-689, 696
omeprazole, 79, 314, 321-322
Oppenheimer effect, 34-36
oral cavity, 278-283
orchitis, 603-605
oropharynx, 278-283
osteitis fibrosa, 153
osteodystrophy, 153
osteomalacia, 147-148
osteonecrosis, 146
osteopetrosis, 152-153
osteoporosis, 146-147
osteosarcoma, 153-156
osteosclerosis, 148-152
ouabain, 523
ovary, 649-669
  atrophy, 657-659
  cysts, 659-662
  degeneration, follicular, 655-657
  fatty change, 662
  hyperplasia, 662-663
  inflammation, 655
  lipidosis, 662
  necrosis, 655
  neoplasia, 663-669
  phospholipidosis, 662
  pigmentation, 662
  polycystic, 659-661
oxamniquine, 446
oxazepam, 438
oxfenicine, 232, 240, 244
oxodipine, 282
oxolinic acid, 159
oxyphenbutazone, 291
oxyphenisatin, 416